HISTORICAL COLLECTION

SIGNS AND SYMPTOMS

Applied Pathologic Physiology and
Clinical Interpretation

Contributors

ELISHA ATKINS

DAVID PRESTWICK BARR

RICHARD H. FREYBERG

EDWIN F. GILDEA

ROBERT GOLDSTEIN

HELEN GOODELL

LAWRENCE E. HINKLE

JOHN L. HORNER

H. H. HYLAND

HAROLD JEGHERS

E. CHARLES KUNKLE

WILLIAM M. LANDAU

BERNARD S. LIPMAN

DANIEL S. LUKAS

CYRIL MITCHELL MACBRYDE

EDWARD MASSIE

HERBERT MESCON

ROGER S. MITCHELL

JAMES L. O'LEARY

ROBERT PAINE

STEPHEN ROTHMAN

LEON SCHIFF

HENRY ALFRED SCHROEDER

ARTHUR L. SHAPIRO

JOHN R. SMITH

OTHMAR C. SOLNITZKY

EUGENE ANSON STEAD, JR.

RICHARD W. VILTER

RAY DAVID WILLIAMS

STEWART G. WOLF

HAROLD G. WOLFF

Signs and Symptoms

Applied Pathologic Physiology and Clinical Interpretation

Edited by

CYRIL MITCHELL MacBRYDE, A.B., M.D., F.A.C.P.

ASSOCIATE PROFESSOR OF CLINICAL MEDICINE, WASHINGTON UNIVERSITY
SCHOOL OF MEDICINE; ASSISTANT PHYSICIAN, THE BARNES HOSPITAL;
DIRECTOR, METABOLISM AND ENDOCRINE CLINICS, WASHINGTON UNIVER-
SITY CLINICS, ST. LOUIS, MISSOURI

FOURTH EDITION
WITH 233 FIGURES AND 4 COLOR PLATES

PHILADELPHIA   MONTREAL

J. B. LIPPINCOTT COMPANY

Contributors

Elisha Atkins, A.B., M.D.
Associate Professor of Medicine, Yale University Medical School; Assistant Attending Physician, University Service, Grace-New Haven Community Hospital, New Haven, Conn.; Attending Physician West Haven V. A. Hospital.

David Preswick Barr, A.B., M.D., Sc.D., LL.D.
Emeritus Professor of Medicine, Cornell University Medical College; Consultant Physician, The New York Hospital, New York.

Richard H. Freyberg, M.D.
Clinical Professor of Medicine, Cornell University Medical College; Director, Department of Rheumatic Diseases, Hospital for Special Surgery, New York Hospital–Cornell University Medical College, New York.

Edwin F. Gildea, M.D.
Wallace Renard Professor of Psychiatry, Department of Psychiatry, Washington University School of Medicine; Psychiatrist-in-Chief Emeritus, Barnes, Renard and Affiliated Hospitals, St. Louis.

Robert Goldstein, A.B., M.D.
Associate Professor of Medicine, New York Medical College; Director of the Hematology Section of the Department of Medicine; Associate Attending Physician, Flower and Fifth Avenue Hospitals; Associate Visiting Physician, Metropolitan Hospital.

Helen Goodell, B.S.
Research Fellow, Cornell University Medical College, New York.

Lawrence E. Hinkle, Jr., M.D.
Clinical Associate Professor of Medicine, Cornell University Medical College; Director of the Human Ecology Study Program at New York Hospital–Cornell Medical Center, New York.

John L. Horner, M.D.
Instructor in Medicine, Washington University School of Medicine; Consultant in Gastroenterology, Washington University Clinics; Assistant Physician, Barnes Hospital, St. Louis.

H. H. Hyland, M.D., F.R.C.P. (London), F.R.C.P. (Canada)
Associate Professor of Medicine Emeritus, University of Toronto; Consulting Physician, Toronto General Hospital, Wellesley Hospital, Toronto, and Sunnybrook (D.V.A.) Hospital, Toronto.

Harold Jeghers, M.D.
Professor and Director, Department of Medicine, Seton Hall College of Medicine and Dentistry; Director, Department of Medicine, Jersey City Medical Center, Jersey City, New Jersey; Consultant in Medicine, Boston City Hospital, Boston.

E. Charles Kunkle, M.D.
Professor of Neurology, Duke University School of Medicine; Neurologist and Chief of Neurology Division, Duke University Medical Center, Durham, N. C.

William M. Landau, M.D.
Professor of Neurology, Division of Neurology, Washington University School of Medicine; Assistant Neurologist, Barnes Hospital; Chief of Service, Unit I Neurology, City Hospital, St. Louis; Consultant, Jefferson Barracks Veterans Administration Hospital; Assistant Neurologist and Electroencephalographer, Jewish Hospital, St. Louis.

Bernard S. Lipman, A.B., M.D., F.A.C.P.
Assistant Professor of Clinical Medicine, Emory University Medical School; Director of Heart Station, St. Joseph Hospital; Co-Director of Glenville Giddings Cardiac Clinic, St. Joseph Hospital; Visiting Physician and Consultant Cardiologist, Grady Memorial Hospital; Regional Consultant in Cardiology to the Veterans Administration, Atlanta.

Daniel S. Lukas, A.B., M.D.

Associate Professor of Medicine, Cornell University Medical College; Director, Cardio-Pulmonary Laboratory and Associate Attending Physician, New York Hospital–Cornell Medical Center, New York.

Cyril Mitchell MacBryde, A.B., M.D., F.A.C.P.

Associate Professor of Clinical Medicine, Washington University School of Medicine; Assistant Physician, Barnes Hospital; Director, Metabolism and Endocrine Clinics, Washington University Clinics, St. Louis.

Edward Massie, A.B., M.D., F.A.C.P., F.A.C.C.

Associate Professor of Clinical Medicine, Washington University School of Medicine; Director of Heart Stations, Barnes Hospital and Jewish Hospital, St. Louis; Director, Cardiovascular Clinic, Washington University Clinics; Area Consultant in Cardiology to the Veterans Administration.

Herbert Mescon, M.D.

Professor and Chairman, Department of Dermatology, Evans Memorial Department of Clinical Research, Massachusetts Memorial Hospitals, and Department of Medicine, Boston University School of Medicine, Boston University Medical Center.

Roger S. Mitchell, B.A., M.D.

Head, Division of Pulmonary Disease, University of Colorado School of Medicine; Director, Webb-Waring Institute for Medical Research; Consultant to Veterans Administration Hospital, Denver; Consultant in Pulmonary Disease, Veterans Administration, St. Louis Area; Consultant to Fitzsimons General Hospital, Denver.

James L. O'Leary, M.D.

Professor and Head of Neurology, Division of Neurology, Washington University School of Medicine; Neurologist-in-Chief, Barnes Hospital; Consultant, Cochran and Jefferson Barracks Veterans Administration Hospitals; Head of Neurology, Homer G. Phillips City Hospital, St. Louis.

Robert Paine, M.D.

Assistant Professor of Clinical Medicine, Washington University School of Medicine; Assistant Physician, Barnes Hospital; Chief of Medical Service, St. Luke's Hospital, St. Louis.

* Stephen Rothman, M.D.

Professor Emeritus, Department of Medicine (Dermatology), University of Chicago.

Leon Schiff, Ph.D., M.D.

Professor of Medicine, University of Cincinnati College of Medicine; Director, Gastric Laboratory, Cincinnati General Hospital.

Henry Alfred Schroeder, A.B., M.D., F.A.C.P.

Associate Professor of Physiology, Dartmouth Medical School, Hanover, New Hampshire; Director of Research, Brattleboro Retreat, Brattleboro, Vermont.

Arthur L. Shapiro, M.D.

Clinical Assistant Professor of Dermatology, The Chicago Medical School; Associate in Dermatology, Mount Sinai Hospital; Active Staff, Jackson Park Hospital, Chicago.

John R. Smith, A.B., A.M., M.D.

Associate Professor of Medicine and Chief, Cardiovascular Division, Washington University School of Medicine; Assistant Physician, Barnes Hospital, St. Louis.

Othmar C. Solnitzky, A.M., Ph.D., M.D.

Professor of Anatomy, Department of Anatomy, Georgetown University School of Medicine, Washington, D. C.

Eugene Anson Stead, Jr., B.S., M.D.

Professor of Medicine and Chairman, Department of Medicine, Duke University School of Medicine; Physician-in-Chief, Duke Hospital, Durham, N. C.

Richard W. Vilter, A.B., M.D.

Professor of Medicine and Director, Department of Internal Medicine, University of Cincinnati; Director, Department of Medicine, Cincinnati General Hospital.

* Deceased.

Ray David Williams, M.S., M.D.

Assistant Professor of Clinical Medicine, Washington University School of Medicine; Assistant Physician, Barnes Hospital; Associate Physician, St. Luke's Hospital; Active Staff, Missouri Baptist Hospital, St. Louis.

Stewart G. Wolf, M.D.

Professor and Head, Department of Medicine, University of Oklahoma Medical Center; Head, Psychosomatic and Neuromuscular Section, Oklahoma Medical Research Foundation, Oklahoma City.

*Harold G. Wolff, A.M., M.D.

Anne Parrish Titzell Professor of Medicine (Neurology), Cornell University Medical College; Attending Physician, The New York Hospital, New York.

* Deceased

Preface to the Fourth Edition

This book approaches diagnosis as the physician must when studying patients. It is dedicated to the proposition that the physician with the most complete insight into the processes of illness is best equipped to aid the patient. We are here concerned with *understanding the processes* which result in manifestations of the disabilities and derangements of disease. In each chapter a major sign or symptom is analyzed and the operations and interrelationships of the various factors in its causation (whether in anatomy, pathology, physiology, chemistry or psychology) are considered and wherever possible are clarified and logically related.

The field we are here concerned with is largely that of applied pathologic physiology, but on the one hand we delve back into the "pre-clinical" sciences for basic information and on the other we range forward into medical diagnosis. The chief aim in the treatment of every subject discussed is the development of understanding and insight into the disturbed mechanisms resulting in abnormal clinical evidence. In this book we attempt to synthesize and integrate the available relevant information, from sources often fractionated and scattered, so as to make it meaningful and useful in the explanation of how and why certain signs and symptoms develop.

This volume is of multiple authorship, deriving breadth and strength from the varied talents of 31 contributors, but the 35 chapters are not an assemblage of unrelated monographs. Much effort has been devoted to properly interrelate the various parts of the book and to present in general an integrated approach and a similar logical, systematic treatment of each subject. An outline heads each chapter. Liberal use is made of illustrations, diagrams and tables. The present edition contains about 30 per cent more of such learning and teaching aids than the previous one. Very complete reference lists follow each chapter, specific reference numbers being employed throughout the text, to encourage exploration of original medical literature.

Workers in medical fields today need to be constantly and increasingly aware of two phenomena of our times: one, that in recent years and extending back only two or three decades, there has been dramatic and explosive progress in all the sciences auxiliary to medicine; the other, that as our knowledge widens and deepens it is ever more evident that all the branches of science are interrelated and interdependent. It is to be hoped that with *assimilation* of all the new information becoming available there will come not only multiplication, extension and refinement of our technical skills—but wisdom: new concepts and insights enabling us to make good use of the treasures yielded by the march of science. Fortunately, as understanding develops, seeming complexities and contradictions often dissolve and isolated facts and masses of seemingly unrelated observations frequently are found to form logical patterns—as logical and intelligible in the life sciences as in the physical sciences. As more thorough perceptions evolve concerning biological phenomena, the various sciences are recognized as simply different approaches, differing tools of measurement and study. We have too often been limited in our understanding, being forced into inaccurate or incomplete concepts as we attempt to explain living processes in the terms of the restricted viewpoints within one or more basic methods of investigation. Syntheses among the various scientific disciplines concerned with living things are becoming ever more possible, especially within the past decade, and our compartmentalized thinking is yielding to a realization of the essential unity of the biological sciences.

Recent advances in the basic sciences and in the "preclinical" medical sciences have been widespread and rapid; many new technical aids in the study of disordered physiology have proved valuable. Formation of many fresh and illuminating perceptions has become possible in the years since the previous edition of this book was written. Much of the material has therefore been completely rewritten and all has been thoroughly revised.

In general we feel that the newly available knowledge and the clearer concepts have been made to pervade the volume throughout. A few instances may be cited. In Chapter 1 better understanding of patient-physician interrelationships and fresh psychological approaches are made use of in the study of the technic of interviewing and examining the patient.

In Chapter 2 recent progress in medical genetics is drawn upon to clarify mechanisms concerned in normal and abnormal growth and development. The recent elucidation of the structure and functions of DNA and RNA in heredity and in the transmission of the genetic code is also discussed in this chapter, with the idea that the nucleic acids are now considered the chemical counterparts of the previously entirely conceptual entities called genes. Here also are considered the influences upon the developing embryo and fetus of immunologic processes, hormones, drugs, and radiation—all of these being practical modern problems receiving of necessity much recent worldwide attention.

Vasospasm, resulting in high blood pressure and other vasospastic disorders, is better understood now that more is known of the chemical factors causing it and relieving it (Chapter 12).

Humoral factors resulting from neuronal excitation and associated with pain have received increased attention recently and are discussed in the several chapters dealing with pain (Chapters 3, 4, 6, and 7). Neurohumoral transmitting agents concerned in hyperexcitability and in fatigue states and new understanding of their action through use of drug tranquilizers and energizers are reviewed in Chapter 25.

Several different types of lymphography have proved valuable lately in identifying and localizing disorders of the lymphatic system, as discussed in Chapter 23. Immunologic processes, some of them autoimmune mechanisms, have recently been implicated in many diseases, especially hematologic conditions (Chapter 24).

New concepts concerning states of consciousness are reviewed in Chapter 26. Study of muscle disorders involves recently developed technics and new insights as indicated in Chapter 27.

Dr. Sara M. Jordan, Dr. William G. Lennox, Dr. Richard A. Portis, Dr. Stephen Rothman and Dr. Harold G. Wolff have died since preparation of the last edition and are sorely missed. They all contributed greatly in previous editions and in their teachings elsewhere to promote the approach to medical studies on which this book is based.

Ten new contributors to this new edition bring fresh insight and add much wide-ranging information gleaned from their special fields.

The editor is grateful to his colleague, Dr. Edward H. Reinhard, for critically reviewing certain sections. To Mr. Brooks Stewart (Medical Editor) and to Mr. Stanley A. Gillet (Production Editor, Medical Department) of the Lippincott Company, go special thanks for constructive and efficient cooperation. To my wife, Anita Koehler MacBryde, deep gratitude for devoted assistance during long hours spent in checking proofs and references.

Finally, the editor and all who have contributed to this volume express gratitude to those who have found in this book a work which integrates the preclinical sciences with clinical medicine. We trust that this thoroughly revised and considerably enlarged fourth edition will prove to be increasingly useful to practicing physicians, to teachers and students of medicine, and to all who labor to understand and relieve the diseases of man.

CYRIL MITCHELL MACBRYDE

Preface to the First Edition

How convenient it would be for the physician if the new patient were able to announce: "I have a gastro-intestinal disturbance," or, "My trouble is nephritis." A perusal of the usual textbooks of diagnosis or of medicine would lead one to believe this might be the case, for the chapters consider "infectious diseases," "intoxications," "deficiency diseases," "metabolic diseases," "respiratory diseases" and so on, in rigorous order, as though every sick person carried his presumptive diagnosis labeled on his chest. Where in such textbooks can the doctor seek help when the patient confronts him complaining, for example, of severe epigastric pain, or of headache, or of jaundice?

One must admit that monographic development of the complete picture of a disease is an important means of medical education, but there are serious defects in a system which encourages us to force the ailing person into a compartment, no matter how poorly it may fit him. It is widely recognized by experienced clinicians that a skillfully taken history, with a careful analysis of the chief complaints and of the course of the illness, will more frequently than not indicate the probable diagnosis, even before a physical examination is made or any laboratory tests are performed. A master diagnostician I know says: "Let me take the history and I will accept any good intern's word on the physical findings." In other words, even today the accomplished physician can learn more in the majority of cases from what his patient says, and the way he says it, than from any other avenue of inquiry. If one doubts this, let him remember that pain in one of its thousands of guises is by far the most common presenting symptom. How handicapped we would be if the patient could not tell us that he had pain, or where it was, or its nature, or duration, or radiation!

A useful aid in the interpretation of symptoms consists in grouping them together to form quickly recognizable complexes or syndromes. Every medical student learns that "dermatitis, diarrhea and dementia" means pellagra, and that "tremor, tumor and tachycardia" indicates hyperthyroidism. The veriest medical tyro knows that a chill, a pain in the chest and rusty sputum could hardly signify anything but pneumonia. Little medical rhymes, hallowed by word-of-mouth transmission to successive medical generations, honor *ileus,* "the symptom-complex known throughout the nation, characterized by pain, vomiting, tympanites and obstipation," and epilepsy, "the aura, the cry, the fall, the fits, the tonus, the clonus, the involuntary defecation." Indelibly stamped in many a physician's mind lies *"Charcot's triad"* of INSular (multiple or disseminated) sclerosis: Intention tremor, Nystagmus and Scanning speech. Frequently, however, in the commonly recognized syndromes very little is understood as to the actual origin or mechanism of production of the primary symptoms and signs. Thus these tricks, these aids to memory, lull us into a false complacency, based too often upon very little real knowledge.

The physician today has many technics available to assist him in making accurate diagnoses. He can peer into the recesses of the body: bronchoscopy, gastroscopy, thoracoscopy, peritoneoscopy, cystoscopy; he can study the shadows cast by the body's parts upon the x-ray film: simple x-ray, laminography, kymography, cholecystography, encephalography, gastroenterography, pyelography, bronchography; he can remove blood or lymph or abnormal fluid accumulations for physical and chemical analysis; he can remove bits of tissue from the surfaces or the cavities of the body and study them under the microscope and in the chemical and physiologic laboratory; the action potential, the very currents of life itself, he can record and analyze in the electro-encephalogram and the electrocardiogram. However, without an understanding of the meaning of symptoms, how useless are these refined diagnostic technics! They are but tools which are only as valuable as the mind which directs them. The informed mind will understand the meaning of the specific type of mucosal defect seen through the bronchoscope in relation to the patient's symptom of hemoptysis. The high icterus index observed in the laboratory study of a patient's serum has significance of one type if associated with recurrent attacks of right upper quadrant pain, but of another when found in association with a shrinking liver during pregnancy.

No mechanical measures can take the place of careful consideration of the patient's complaints. No device, be it ever so clever mechanically, electrically or chemically, can serve as a substitute in the art of medicine for the informed mind of the physician. The physician's ability as a diagnostician will determine the nature and the efficacy of the treatment he chooses to employ. His ability to diagnose will depend in only a minor degree upon his ability to use special technical measures. He must know when to use them, which tests to select, and how to interpret the physical findings, as well as the special laboratory tests. The physician's judgment in these matters will depend largely upon his ability to analyze and interpret symptoms.

This book attempts, so far as present knowledge permits, to give the basis for analysis and interpretation of some of the commonest symptoms which bring patients to the physician. Emphasis is placed upon the pathologic physiology of the symptom, while its correlation with other symptoms and with physical and laboratory evidence is considered as important but secondary in the diagnostic method. Our knowledge concerning many of these symptoms is incomplete, but it is rapidly expanding. Although the final word often cannot be said, critical and analytical thinking in the manner followed in these chapters should prove productive for us all: patient, practitioner, professor and student.

CYRIL MITCHELL MACBRYDE

Contents

SIGNS AND SYMPTOMS

Applied Pathologic Physiology and
Clinical Interpretation

1

The Study of Symptoms

CYRIL M. MACBRYDE

Definitions. As broadly and generally employed the word *symptom* is used to name any manifestation of disease. Strictly speaking, symptoms are subjective, apparent only to the affected person. *Signs* are detectable by another person and sometimes by the patient himself. Pain and itching are symptoms; jaundice, swollen joints, cardiac murmurs, etc., are physical signs. Some phenomena, like fever, are both signs and symptoms. In this chapter the word symptom is often used to denote any evidence of disturbed physiology perceived by the patient or the physician.

PATIENT AND PHYSICIAN: THE INTERVIEW

The patient comes to the physician because he has a problem and wants help. The problem may be a simple one requiring only a health survey for school, employment, insurance or for personal information, and the patient may have no complaints. Nevertheless, the physician may disclose in the course of such an examination one or more signs or symptoms of significance.

In this book we are concerned primarily with the study of the patient who presents himself with a disturbing sign or symptom. A sign or a symptom occurring in any person is not an isolated phenomenon: it may have multiple interrelationships including causes, associated phenomena and effects. There may be interrelationships evidencing various types of disturbed physiology, and there is always a subjective, psychological component, sometimes of minor but often of major importance. The responses of the patient to his disorder, his reactions to it and understanding of it are essential and often deeply revealing parts of the history. The young and inexperienced physician is often apt to neglect or to feel scorn for emotional and psychological manifestations unless they constitute well-defined and therefore "interesting" neuroses or psychoses. The physician who fails to utilize opportunities to consider and evaluate subjective aspects of the illness and confines his efforts unduly to objective data is not studying the patient as a whole and may be misled into inaccurate or incomplete conclusions and solutions.

1

To derive the fullest possible potential from the history, the physician must become skilled in eliciting the patient's story. Securing a meaningful history requires an interpersonal relationship, involving give-and-take cooperation between two strangers about one's intimate problems. With the patient distressed and distracted, the physician sometimes inexpert or inexperienced, and time pressing, it is small wonder that many histories are inadequate. Since amassing laboratory data requires much less skill and experience, technical approaches are often overemphasized in the diagnostic work-up.

The technical and the scientific aspects of medicine can be learned largely through reading and study; not so the arts and the skills required in the interpersonal parts of the patient-physician relationship. The clinical ability to secure a good history is an art developed by imitation of accomplished preceptors and by pr ice and experience. One must not confuse the accumulation and the interpretation of technical data (no matter how clever and helpful or even decisive) with the development of true insight into human problems.

The patient's attitude toward the physician should be analyzed as the history is being obtained. It will depend on his background and on elements in the present situation, including responses to the appearance, the attitude, the actions and the words of the physician. Excessive hopes or dependence must be forestalled. Insufficient trust in the doctor or anger or secretiveness may defeat the patient's objective in seeking medical help. The skillful physician guides the patient's attitude into desirable channels.

The physician's attitude toward the patient requires self-study. His emotions will respond to those of the patient and he must be aware of and evaluate his own emotional resonances. The physician must direct his own attitudes, words and actions into a pattern most apt to promote the patient's welfare. Certain ingredients we take for granted in a good physician: medical knowledge and self-confidence based upon competence, emotional self-control in the face of stress, dignity, kindness, graciousness and good manners. The patient usually becomes aware of these quickly even during a first interview.

In addition to these characteristics, other important qualities required of the physician who is skillful in interviewing are: interest, acceptance, warmth and flexibility.

The physician's concern for his patient is conveyed by his actions, rather than by a statement. Confidence and cooperation of the patient are not secured by saying "Trust me. I am trying to help you." It is best not to handicap oneself with such a bald, obvious and superfluous remark, which may give the patient pause and make him distrustful. Proceed with the job at hand; the patient by his own observations will soon know whether you care about him and his problem.

In the art of interviewing there is no substitute for genuine interest not only in the patient's problems but in the patient as a person. In trying to obtain a truly valuable history the physician will do well to keep these points in mind:

1. **Interest** springing from the desire to understand and to help, is evident to the patient; as a rule, the patient responds by answering questions and telling his story so as to assist the doctor as much as possible. Frequently, realization that the doctor really cares about him as a person, not just as "a case" of illness, will remind the patient of aspects of his problem and lead to illumination of facets of the situation of great diagnostic importance.

2. **Acceptance** of the patient is essential. The physician must not reveal moral judgments he may have or his own emotional responses in regard to attitudes or behavior or statements of his patient. This does not necessarily imply approval, but the physician must be tolerant and understanding. The physician must be objective in evaluating the patient's story. In addition, he should convey to the patient his belief that the patient also is trying his best to be objective.

3. **Warmth and Empathy.** No one can ever actually share the experiences of another person, but the effort to do so always brings one person closer to another. The physician who can combine sensitive in-

sight and understanding (without over-sympathizing or sentimentalizing) with a sensible objective approach to the patient's problem will usually win quickly the patient's friendship and confidence.

4. Flexibility. The topics selected and the direction of the inquiry stem naturally (at least in the beginning) from the patient's presenting complaints. As the story is developed, the picture of the present illness will emerge. Then past history, family history and other related subjects will be explored. This is the usual course along which the interviewer gently guides his patient in order to secure a coherent history which may be recorded in some logical order. However, the physician will often find that adherence to a rigid pattern is a handicap and that the apparent wanderings of the patient's talk may be highly revealing. Frequently, what at first seems to be only a bypath will be found to be the main highway.

Sometimes the topics that the patient **avoids** are the most significant ones. If he shies away, changes the subject, becomes irritated, anxious or confused, the interviewer may explore a more neutral area for a while, returning to the sensitive topic more productively later.

Therefore, the expert interviewer must be flexible and prepared to allow the patient to vary the order in which topics are discussed. The interviewer may learn much by allowing the subject to run on freely with his story: he will observe what the patient wants to emphasize and thus may learn what seems to be important to the patient, or what his motives are.

The responses of the physician must be flexible, natural and appropriate. As a rule, the medical interview is serious business, but the physician tries to keep it upon a constructive, optimistic level. He should respond with hopeful reassurance to the depressed patient, but not with excessive cheerfulness. To the patient who is anxious or fearful he should offer some basis for confidence and courage. If the patient is ill at ease, angry or suspicious, the physician may establish more relaxed and friendly cooperative relations by discussing briefly a mutual interest, or by inquiring into the possible causes for the patient's disquieting attitude before continuing the study of his medical problems.

The accomplished physician develops a technic in securing the history, and his technic must vary from patient to patient, and according to circumstances. Knowledge of medicine and an understanding of human beings are limitless fields of endeavor; the physician's skill in obtaining the patient's story and interpreting it will grow in proportion to his progress in these very complex fields.

ANALYZING AND INTERPRETING SYMPTOMS

THE IMPORTANCE OF THE HISTORY

Symptoms are apt to appear some time before striking physical signs of disease are evident and before laboratory tests are useful in detecting disordered physiology. For this reason, and because a careful, detailed, properly analyzed and interpreted history usually leads the physician more directly toward the correct conclusion than any other diagnostic method, one should never neglect to elicit an accurate and sufficiently detailed history.

Persons vary greatly in their abilities to observe and describe their symptoms; intelligence, education and verbal proficiency differ so much that eliciting a lucid and coherent account demands flexibility and adaptability. Routine or mechanical recording of data does not constitute a medical history. The emotional status of the patient colors his story; his background and environment always will condition his responses to stimuli as well as his efforts to describe such responses. Evaluation and perception of the patient as a person proceed simultaneously with the process of learning about his immediate symptoms.

So productive of insight, so apparently simple, so truly complex: "taking the history" involves analysis and interpretation and requires the highest order of medical skill.

"Of all the technical aids which increase the doctor's power of observation, none comes even close in value to the skillful use of spoken words —the words of the doctor and the words of the patient. Throughout all of medicine, use of words is still the main diagnostic technic."[1]

THE PATIENT QUESTIONNAIRE

There is no doubt that a detailed printed history form to be filled in by the patient can be of great assistance under certain circumstances. When time permits and the patient is not acutely ill, and for use in health surveys, etc., such a record of medical history may help to prevent omission of significant data and may save the physician much time.[7]

It might be suggested that such a multipaged questionnaire be presented to the patient *after* the initial history is obtained by the physician if and when the intellectual, physical and emotional status of the subject encourage such a method of assembling information. Such a detailed health record would then be very useful for later more incisive or pertinent inquiry by the physician.

However, when the patient's complaint is urgent or he is emotionally disturbed, as is usually the case in illness, he must of course not be confronted with a routine printed form or by a clerk or physician following any routine method of approach to his problem. The approach must vary appropriately with the problem and with the person affected.

No impersonal inquiry into the patient's complaints, no mechanical system, no tabular compilation with check marks or crosses or pressed buttons or electronic computers can substitute in diagnosis or care of the patient for personal interest and acquaintance by the physician with each individual, unique human being and with his particular problem.

TIME WITH THE PATIENT

The most successful physician in the field of diagnosis is often simply he who devotes sufficient effort and time to discussion of the patient's problems with the patient himself.

Too often the physician fails to take full advantage of the phase of his work which is frequently the most productive: *repeated* conversation with and examination of his patient. The first history and physical examination can usually be substantially and significantly supplemented later, especially after there has been establishment of rapport (a good, friendly cooperative relationship) directed toward solving the patient's problems.

Important points in the history and in the physical examination are frequently elicited only after patient and physician have gotten to know each other and have learned to work together.

In a recent time study of the activities of 2 medical interns on a university service in a teaching hospital[8] it was found that "contrary to some expectation, a very small amount of the intern's time was spent with patients"! The authors very properly regard their teaching program as "similar in philosophy, design and standards of performance to that at any other prominent university teaching hospital in the United States." It is pointed out that no definite conclusions or recommendations can be evolved from this limited pilot study. However, "results of this study stimulate questions concerning postgraduate programs. . . ." Among these questions were: "Do attending physicians sufficiently encourage interns to broaden their experience of patient-doctor contact? When does the doctor in training learn how to relate himself to patients?"[8]

It seems that at present we are going through a prolonged phase of overemphasis in both undergraduate and in postgraduate medical teaching upon mechanical and laboratory assessment of patients. There is danger that physicians will be more concerned with the study of diseases than the study of patients. There is now probably excessive involvement of the doctor-in-training in technical matters, with insufficient emphasis on the learning of clinical skills. Students of medical education have proposed steps which should be heeded to bring about a halt in the decline of clinical tradition.[12]

There should be no conflict (although at present there is much) between the two approaches. Certainly we need all the help that laboratory science can render us in understanding man's diseases, but we must use all our new scientific knowledge plus all available clinical acumen in the service of the patient.

Physicians must have technical skills and make maximum intelligent use of them and of laboratory procedures in the study of the ill person, but not excessive and maldirected use.

One reason that doctors tend to become better technicians but poorer true physicians is that it is much more difficult and takes much more time to deal with the *patient + disease* than with the *disease* only. The true physician devotes sufficient time and applies his best efforts not just to assembling information, not just to recording data, not just to determining what the disease is, but equally to each of these problems: how is this particular person affected? (physically, emotionally, mentally, socially, etc.); also — what relief can be offered? (not just physically, but in *all the ways he is affected* and needs help).

Those who intend to develop superior ability in the art of diagnosis must be prepared to spend many hours learning how to talk with patients and how to obtain not just adequate but highly significant, truly rewarding medical histories.

CONDUCT OF THE INTERVIEW

Satisfactory use of the physician's abilities or of the information available from the patient cannot be made under adverse conditions. A private room should be available. No third person should be present. Neither patient nor physician should feel under pressure to be elsewhere or otherwise employed.

Time and skill are required in obtaining an informative and sufficiently complete history. The physician must not hurry, nor must he seem hurried. All his attention must be devoted to the patient, who must feel that the doctor is interested, sympathetic and eager to help. The interview should be uninterrupted and conducted in privacy and quiet. The purpose is to get the patient to talk, so that the doctor can listen and learn. The doctor says only enough to keep the patient's story going. Each statement of the patient must be considered in relation to the aid it may furnish in understanding his chief complaints or symptoms. The patient may not present the story of his difficulties well, or in logical order: he may use misleading words in describing his symptoms; he may omit important relevant information. All these defects may be corrected if the physician *asks the proper questions* —not merely to fill in spaces on a printed form, but to develop the story. It is best to let the patient tell his story in his own words whenever possible. Many patients will present a coherent and concise description of the development of the presenting symptoms. When, however, the patient wanders, or when important facts are omitted, pointed questions are necessary. Care must be taken that the answer is not implied in the question—that the questions are not leading.

Often patients are confused about anatomic terms: to some, "the stomach" includes the whole abdomen; to others, any discomfort in the back is located in "the kidneys." Descriptions of sensations are often misleading. "Pain" is employed to include almost any kind of discomfort, such as itching, aching, smarting and burning, as well as true pain. "Dizziness" may mean vertigo or faintness. One must not simply put down the patient's words; one must make certain of *what he means.* For example, a patient may complain of pain in his heart, but inquiry may reveal that the discomfort is epigastric—not related to exertion, but relieved by food, thus suggesting not heart disease but peptic ulcer. Sometimes alternating constipation and diarrhea are complained of, but the fact may be omitted that diarrhea never occurs unless a cathartic is taken. The patient may present symptoms of goiter and nervousness, but may not yield the information, until after careful questioning, that the goiter had been present for years and had not increased in size, and that the nervous symptoms came on after recent marital difficulties. Careful cross-questioning is often necessary in the process of analyzing the patient's symptoms. Sometimes the physician will have to pursue a symptom, and often he may have difficulty in getting the patient to decide which one or two of his complaints are the most distressing. For example, he may have to elicit more data about progressive weight loss, unemphasized by the patient, and may devote less attention to the patient's favorite topic of insomnia.

Often the entire analysis of the symptom is not possible on the basis of the patient's story alone, and important information is obtainable from the spouse or another member of the family, or from friends. This is particularly true in relationship to fatigue and to nervous symptoms. For example, the cause of backache and exhaustion in one woman seemed obscure until her husband came in to report that she had stubbornly insisted on painting the fence, a job she said he had been neglecting. Her real difficulty was emotional, not physical; her nervous symptoms were due to domestic problems.

Thus symptoms may be considered as primary, when directly related to the basic cause, or secondary or even tertiary, when more remotely related. In the instance just cited, the backache was not a primary symptom: it did not indicate disease present in the back. It was secondary to an emotional situation. A young man had visual difficulty; various lenses were tried before it was discovered that he had an unequal but bilateral proptosis; the latter was found to be associated with hyperthyroidism. A man had pains in the arms and the legs characteristic of peripheral neuritis; the neuritis was found to be due to thiamine deficiency; the thiamine deficiency seemed to result from alcoholism. One might stop here, but the alcoholism was not the final diagnosis—it was a *symptom* of an underlying severe neurosis. Not until one had traced through the steps in the pathologic physiology from the tertiary symptom neuritis → thiamine deficiency → alcoholism → psychic disorder did one have a true *diagnosis,* the result of "understanding through" or thoroughly.

The physical examination and any necessary laboratory studies can be directed much more intelligently after a careful, complete and exact history is obtained. The hurried physician is apt to hope that the laboratory will give him the diagnosis and may be tempted to skimp on the history to save the time, the effort and the thought it requires. However, sufficient time and effort to get a clear story are usually well repaid, while the hours, the work and the expense devoted to unnecessary laboratory tests are notorious.

The trouble with most histories is, first, that they are too short and, second, that they are taken without pursuing the main points far enough and completely enough. Printed history forms can lead to bad habits and shallowness of inquiry. Perhaps a blank page and an untrammeled interest and curiosity are better. Probably best of all is to take only brief notes while listening to the patient; writing is distracting to patient and physician—the written summary can be put down later. One must not feel that because he has a printed blank to fill out, questions must be asked routinely, always in the same order. The spaces on the blank are useful reminders, but the nature of the patient's trouble and the informed mind of the physician must govern the course of the questioning and the development of the story. Skill must be used in excluding extraneous material, while care is necessary at the same time to obtain as much as possible of the information that will prove helpful.

As a rule, organic disorders cause clearcut symptoms, while emotional or nervous disorders are apt to be presented by the patient as a number of poorly defined, apparently unrelated complaints. That is, they seem to be unrelated until one discovers the nervous trouble responsible for the various symptoms, such as headache, indigestion and insomnia.

Sometimes the patient is too ill or too excited to give or to be bothered with giving a complete history. The most essential facts are then obtained from him as quickly as possible, or from a companion or a relative. Later the complete story may be obtained.

Each Patient Unique

We need a properly balanced, scientific-humanistic, interrelated approach to the study of each patient and his problems. The investigation should include appropriate psychological, physical, laboratory, quantitative and mechanical assessment plus full consideration of the special features which make every single clinical study unique—different in some aspects from every other, although possibly also similar in many ways. The physician must attempt to acquire as much information as possible about the individual affected because in every case there are special peculiarities in the constitution of the subject which personalize his disease and differentiate it from the same disease in other patients. His specific constitution will consist of interrelated psychic and somatic elements.

The clinician will understand that illness is related to the *patient as a whole* and to his *life history* in its entirety, not just to his medical history (past diseases). One should learn about *positive aspects* of the patient's life: aims, ambitions, accomplishments, pleasures, recreations. Knowledge of constructive factors brings insight and provides material for assisting the patient. Often it is of tremendous help to the physician to visit the *patient's home* and to get to know his immediate family. Thus one may be able to integrate his sickness into his life history: to relate it to his home, his job, his parents, spouse, children, his economic and social problems, etc. One can learn much in this broader approach to obtaining a medical history, not only about symptoms of obvious psychological origin but about disorders usually considered as primarily physical.

Many conditions are greatly influenced by various tensions or frustrations, and by the attitudes of others (whether the patient is pitied, loved, feared or respected, etc.). Often one may discover environmental aspects of importance in regard to home or neighborhood or working conditions: light, heat and cold, dust, noise, stairs to climb, etc. Knowledge concerning ability to secure rest, or interest or engagement in hobbies or cultural activities may prove valuable.

PSYCHE AND SOMA

In the study of each sign or symptom, or in the formulation of a complete concept of an illness as it involves the particular person, evaluation of the psychological aspects are necessary as well as thorough consideration of the primarily physical elements. For example, in some cases of vascular hypertension, or of headache, or of peptic ulcer, or of dermatitis, psychological factors may prove most important, while in other cases physical causes and effects may predominate. In each disorder there are various combinations of these elements even though the presenting symptoms or chief complaints may at first seem highly similar as they occur in various persons.

Modern psychosomatic concepts of health and illness have taught us that there is close interrelation, even integration, between psyche and soma. At times more attention must be paid to one aspect than the other, but in man neither aspect should be dealt with alone. Realization of the variety of aspects but the basic unity of each person is the essence of modern medicine's attempt to study each person *individually* and as *a whole,* as a unique, complex but integrated entity.

CHIEF COMPLAINTS AND PRESENT ILLNESS

Information concerning the onset and the course of development of the patient's symptom, its nature, quality, duration, intermittent or cyclic character, etc., helps in analysis of the true nature of the symptom. Such an analysis of one or more chief presenting complaints constitutes the part of the medical history usually recorded under the heading of *present illness.* "The complaints of the patient—fragmentary expressions of the underlying disease— should be used as *leads* . . . [which] can be followed to the actual seat of disease."[2] The present illness should be described by the patient in detail, and where parts are missing, or helpful information is lacking, the physician should get the patient to fill in, round out or dig deeper to obtain as full a story as possible. Symptoms are not always what they seem. Was the black stool accompanied by abdominal pain or preceded by indigestion? Or, perhaps, was it preceded by the taking of bismuth powders? Was the pain in the left chest and the left arm really precipitated by exertion, or only by motion of the left shoulder? Is the shortness of breath caused only by exertion, or does it occur at rest and result from nervous tension and hyperpnea? Is the blood really coughed up in a case of suspected hemoptysis, or does it come from the nose, the pharynx or the mouth? In suspected jaundice, has the patient been taking Atabrine, or could it be carotinemia? Often the fact that back pain is at its worst on rising in the morning suggests that the patient sleeps on an excessively soft mattress and consequently has back strain, while pain increasing during the day suggests postural or arthritic factors related to occupation. Getting all such related details may prevent one from being led astray and may sharply narrow the diagnostic possibilities.

When the symptoms suggest involvement particularly of one organ or system, one should attempt to determine whether or not any of the other possible symptoms associated with disorders of that system or organ have been present. For example, if polyuria has suggested possible diabetes, one should inquire concerning polydipsia, polyphagia, weakness, fatigue, weight loss, etc. Or if costovertebral pain has suggested renal or ureteral disease, one should find out whether there has been pain referred to the genital region, or dysuria, frequency, hematuria, etc.

A typical day or a typical attack should be described. The physician may thus learn much about the time of occurrence, the precipitating factors, correlation with the day's activities, times of recurrence, factors which give relief and other informative phenomena related to the symptom.

In recording the history one should first list the chief complaints in the order of their severity, noting the duration of each.

Often the duration, or time of onset, or some periodicity of attacks or intervals of relief will furnish important clues. "My headaches began about 2 years ago, a few weeks after my mother died." Follow the clue—note that the patient is linking the symptom to psychic trauma. "My asthma came on in the summer, went away while we were in the mountains, but came back on the desert ranch." Possibly due to allergy to ragweed and to horse dander?

"The dermatitis started on a Sunday; it gets better during the week but usually flares up on Sundays." Possibly due to dyes in the ink of Sunday rotogravure or color sections?

One should then take up each complaint in order, following its course throughout the present illness. Even when the physician is unable to get the patient to give an orderly account, the written record should be ordered, consecutive, compact and complete but not verbose.

THE ASSOCIATION OF SYMPTOMS: SYNDROMES

Certain disorders in physiology are characterized by the association of two or more related symptoms or signs. Investigation of either symptom will then lead to a further understanding of the related complaints and of the basic disease. For example, it is useful to know that a convulsion was preceded by carpopedal spasm, for that suggests hypocalcemia, whereas a convulsion preceded by hunger and perspiration suggests hypoglycemia. Likewise, vomiting accompanied by right lower abdominal pain and muscle spasm may indicate appendicitis, while vomiting with headache and failing vision leads one to suspect increased intracranial pressure.

One must be alert to recognize characteristic groupings of certain signs and symptoms (syndromes). Often the anatomical location of the cause may be suggested (e.g.: scalenus anticus s., Horner's s., Ménière's s.) or the organ or tissue or system involved (Banti's s., Cushing's s.) or the etiology (Korsakoff's s., Plummer-Vinson s.), etc.

It is important, however, not merely to learn by rote, for instance, that sore tongue, pallor, digestive disorders and numbness in the extremities suggest pernicious anemia, but to try to understand as thoroughly as possible *how* these symptoms happen to be related and *why* the disease process results in these particular manifestations.

THE PATIENT'S ATTITUDE TOWARD HIS SYMPTOMS

Much can be learned from the manner and the method used by the patient in telling his story. If he is obviously over-sensitive and apprehensive, the interpretation of his complaints must usually differ from that of similar complaints of a calm and unemotional person. If he is exaggerating or minimizing his symptoms, evaluation must be correspondingly adjusted, and motives must be sought. While the physician is taking the history he has an excellent chance to form preliminary impressions of the patient's personality.

Only rarely can a sick person present a relatively objective account of the illness. More often than not, the patient's presentation of his story to the physician is colored by (1) *emotional reaction* or (2) *motivation.* Among frequently encountered emotional states are: *fear,* which sometimes operates to limit information, sometimes leads to excessive emphasis and elaboration; *embarrassment,* usually leading to fragmentary or misleading statements; *anger,* resentment or rebellion at being ill, which often causes the afflicted person to blame others in his family, his employer, his physician, or some element in his environment. Anger is often the expression of guilt feelings; sometimes anger is used as a cover for or defense reaction against anxiety or fear.

Among motives, one must consider first the usual one—the patient tries in his own way (which may be misguided) to assist the physician, because he wants relief. One must consider the patient's self-diagnosis, but beware of accepting it uncritically. For example, beware of the patient who has "just a little cough"—it may be tuberculosis; or "just a little constipation"—it may be rectal carcinoma. Second, consider motives which might lead to overemphasis or malingering: compensation neuroses, etc. Third, remember motives leading to discounting of the importance of symptoms: ambition, religious faith wrongly employed, etc. We should teach our patients that it is admirable not to exaggerate symptoms, but it is foolish to be reticent or to conceal clues. A symptom which may seem minor to the patient could prove important in the development of the diagnostic picture.

EVOLUTION OF SYMPTOMS

Not only must the presenting symptom or symptoms be clearly understood, but they must be followed in their *development* from the onset to the date the history is obtained. Data should be sought indicating any alteration or *change* in the symptom. Has the pain changed its location? Has it changed in severity or nature? Is it now accompanied by any new phenomena? Was it first in the epigastrium and relieved by food or alkali, but now not so relieved? Did the ankle edema at first disappear upon recumbency, but does it now persist all night?

The course, or evolution of each sign or symptom forming the clinical picture of the present illness should be traced so that the significance of alterations may be considered in regard to possible changes in the pathologic physiology.

ELABORATION OF THE HISTORY

Every effort should be made to get a good history at the first interview. Later, further study of the patient's story may prove to be important. Often a useful procedure is repetition or elaboration or further cross-questioning concerning certain points in the history after some information is obtained from the physical examination or the laboratory tests. For example, a patient who has very dry or thickened skin will be questioned further about loss of energy, sensitivity to cold, drowsiness and other symptoms that may be due to hypothyroidism. Or, if leukocytosis is revealed, further evidence of possible infection may be sought. Or, if a cardiac murmur is discovered, inquiry is pursued concerning previous episodes of joint soreness, or febrile illness.

PAST HISTORY

The history of previous illnesses and health problems should be reviewed, and in some instances fully explored, particularly when information of help in understanding the present complaint is elicited. No listing of "measles, mumps, whooping cough and chickenpox in childhood" is sufficient if, in the history of a man with edema, the information is omitted that he had scarlet fever and albuminuria as a child. Inquiry concerning trauma may be pursued particularly if joint pain or back pain is the chief symptom. A careful analysis of the diet and inquiry concerning appetite, diarrhea, vomiting or digestive disorders are indicated when weight loss is prominent. The process of taking the history of past illnesses, as of present disease, should not be pointless and systematic but pointed and varied to draw out the maximum amount of pertinent information.

FAMILY HISTORY

It is not sufficient to ask if there are any known familial diseases. Such a vague and general question is usually answered in the negative. If a patient has symptoms suggesting thyrotoxicosis, one is especially interested in and must inquire specifically about the occurrence of goiter or nervous troubles in the family. Or if migraine is suspected, one inquires particularly about headaches, epilepsy and allergic or nervous disorders. When a growth or developmental problem is being studied, these characteristics of the close relatives are investigated. When an infectious disease, such as tuberculosis, is suspected, one should learn whether or not the patient could have been exposed to a relative suffering from it. If there is a question of allergic disease, inquiry is made concerning hay fever, hives, asthma and other allergic manifestations in the family. In other words, every effort should be made by *specific inquiry* to determine whether or not the family history will yield data helpful in understanding the patient's problems. When an hereditary trait is suspected, a diagram of the pedigree may clarify the nature of the disease.

MARITAL HISTORY

Much may often be learned by inquiry concerning domestic and sexual happiness, the health of the spouse, the number of children, pregnancies and miscarriages, housing conditions, diet, infections within the family and family problems affecting husband, wife or children.

SOCIAL HISTORY

In certain instances, especially of nervous or emotional disorders, the social history is of great importance. It may also bear important relationships to the understanding of obviously organic disease. For example, it is important to know about the excessive use of tobacco by a patient with toxic amblyopia, or about alcoholism in a patient with vitamin deficiencies or jaundice, or about *what caused* the poor food habits when malnutrition or vitamin deficiency is suspected, or about the emotional factors which may precipitate attacks of angina pectoris or peptic ulcer symptoms.

Information is obtained about the patient's education, home and family life, economic status, ambitions and interests, country and climate of residence, business and social life, recreations, sex experiences, habits and all the personal factors that may assist the physician in *understanding him more completely as an individual*. When sympathetically obtained and skillfully developed, such knowledge often is most important in revealing the origin and the nature of the patient's difficulties.

OCCUPATIONAL HISTORY

Certain occupations expose persons to particular hazards, such as muscular or joint strain, nervous tension, animal infections or animal products, dusts, gases, chemicals, heat and abnormal lighting conditions, unhygienic surroundings and the possible presence of infected insects. It often is necessary to know what kind of work the patient does and under what conditions. Not only the physical conditions of the work itself, but relationships with employers and fellow workers may be important in determining, for example, whether irritability, headache, undue fatigue, tremor or increasing inefficiency and inaccuracy may be a result of work problems.

The occupations of children likewise should be studied. School progress and conditions and play habits and environment may be related to the patient's symptoms.

INTERPRETING SYMPTOMS

The history consists largely in an analysis of the presenting symptom or symptoms and of the associated information that may be pertinent. The next step usually employed in the diagnostic method is the physical examination, and thereafter certain laboratory procedures may be utilized. The physician who pursues as far as possible the logical processes of reasoning based upon and initiated by his analysis of the symptoms often finds that he can understand the pathologic physiology leading to the complaints even with no data but the history. Thinking through as far as possible toward a diagnosis and writing down preliminary *diagnostic impressions* at the end of the history are useful clinical exercises. Such a practice enables one to perform the *physical examination* with *discrimination and curiosity*, not as a routine requirement. For example, if symptoms have suggested a blood dyscrasia, particular attention is paid to the skin color, the mouth and the tongue, and to the lymph nodes and the spleen, or, if the patient has had rheumatism, the heart and the tonsils are studied with special care.

When certain diagnostic possibilities are under consideration, the choice of certain *special studies, tests* and *laboratory procedures* is logical. *Purpose, discrimination* and a *guided curiosity* depending upon the problem and the data yielded by the history and physical examination should direct the choice of special tests and laboratory studies. Other irrelevant studies may be omitted, and time, expense and discomfort to the patient may be avoided. Thus, if epigastric distress relieved by food is present, gastroscopy, gastric analysis and x-ray studies of the gastrointestinal tract may promptly yield the diagnosis. Or if pain that may originate in the ureter is present, a urinalysis and an x-ray may at once give positive evidence of a kidney stone.

Interpretation of symptoms leads the clinician to choose valuable laboratory tests but to avoid compilation of useless data. He will secure blood sugar tests in diabetes but not a sugar tolerance test. He will avoid bone marrow puncture or liver biopsy puncture if the hematologic or hepatic diagnostic pictures are already clear. The wise doctor will protect his patient from even slight dangers or small pains or minimal expenses unless possible gains warrant them. He will not order a battery of tests in the hope that his shotgun diagnostic method will accidentally score a bull's-eye.

Studies[3,4] have found that from 30 to 40 per cent of persons consulting internists and diagnosticians have psychoneuroses. These psychoneuroses may cause many of the symptoms discussed in the various chapters in this book: chest pain, backache, headache, malnutrition, obesity, nervousness, fatigue, to name just a few. It is not possible nor is it advisable for the average doctor to refer all such patients to psychiatrists. Often the mechanism of production of the symptom can be elucidated and the patient can be relieved through simple measures by the general physician. Careful history with proper interpretation of symptoms will reveal which patients are to be included in this large group with functional "nervous" symptoms.

Possibly 60 per cent of patients may be expected to have an organic basis for their symptoms. As one diagnostician has sagely pointed out,[4] *clinical-pathologic conferences* offer excellent training in the differential diagnosis of fatal diseases with an anatomic substratum, but there are many organic illnesses which are functional and nonfatal, and the clinician must be interested not only in the diagnosis of anatomic disease but in the personality of victims of disease. Study of differential diagnosis based upon autopsies[5] is recommended highly, but one must keep in mind that fortunately a large percentage of the clinician's practice will have similar symptoms with much less dire implications.

It has been estimated that "about 55 per cent of all internal diseases can be diagnosed from aspect and history alone, an additional 20 per cent by physical examination and another 20 per cent by laboratory tests. The rest of the patients remain undiagnosed, regardless of whether they get well or die."[4]

Since so much depends upon it, the history, with its careful analysis of the patient's symptoms, deserves the physician's utmost attention and effort. Many believe that this is the greatest art in medicine.[6] With Bauer[4] the author feels that taking the history *and interpreting it* certainly constitute the greatest art.

Interpretation may be faulty if based upon inaccurate or incomplete information. Therefore, analysis of the symptom or symptoms must precede interpretation. With a good history the physician, by virtue of his knowledge of the mechanisms of disease, of pathologic physiology and of the causation of signs and symptoms, may arrive at a tentative conclusion concerning the malady present.

In recent years there has been ample demonstration that not only functional "nervous" symptoms may result from emotional or psychic disorders, but that organic disease may be so caused. *Psychosomatic illness* is common, and the more familiar the physician is with the two-way interplay of mental and emotional factors with body physiology and even with body structure, the better he will be able to interpret signs and symptoms.

Usually diagnosis of an illness and removal of its cause is a welcome contribution to the patient's general health. One must realize, however, that in many chronic illnesses the handicap comes to play an essential part in the patient's life—so important sometimes that he may not gracefully part with it. For example, a man who for years had suffered with peptic ulcer was dramatically cured by gastrectomy and for the first time in years was free of pain. Surprisingly, instead of being happy he became depressed and attempted suicide. It became evident that his stomach symptoms had served as a crutch or excuse to spare him from stress or unpleasant situations. His symptoms were gone and so was his protection.[1] Therefore we must consider: what does this symptom mean to this patient?

Symptoms must be interpreted. One must determine not only what the symptom is, but what part it plays in the patient's life—*how it affects him.* Does the nausea interfere with taking regular meals, does it come at night, has it caused weight loss? Does the dyspnea get worse with exercise or recumbency? Has it led to loss of a job?

Study of the *patient's body* through the usual physical examination, supplemented if indicated by special examinations, is next in order, with the *emphasis* of the examination depending upon the results of thorough consideration of the complaints and the history. The laboratory studies that offer hope of giving additional pertinent data may then be selected. The diagnostic study must be guided throughout by consideration of the patient's complaints. Unrelated physical findings or laboratory data of interesting or important nature may be discovered, but one's primary aim should be the detection of the cause of the symptoms. Thus may we progress in the understanding of disease and in the development of means to relieve or cure it.

REFERENCES

1. Bird, B.: Talking With Patients, Philadelphia, Lippincott, 1955.
2. Cabot, R. C.: Differential Diagnosis, Philadelphia, Saunders, 1915.
3. Allan, F. N., and Kaufman, M.: Nervous factors in general practice, J.A.M.A. 138: 1135, 1948.
4. Bauer, Julius: Differential Diagnosis of Internal Diseases, New York, Grune, 1955.
5. Harvey, A. McG., and Bordley, J.: Differential Diagnosis, Philadelphia, Saunders, 1955.
6. Platt, R.: Two essays on the practice of medicine, Lancet 2:305, 1947.
7. Forkner, Claude E.: Record of medical history, Arch. Int. Med. 106:22, 1960.
8. Payson, H. E., Gaenslen, E. C., and Stargardter, F. L.: Time study of an internship on a university medical service, New England J. Med. 264:439, 1961.
9. Wittkower, E. D., and White, K. L.: Bedside manners, British M. J. 1:1432, 1954.
10. Meares, A.: The Medical Interview, Springfield, Ill., Thomas, 1958.
11. Stevenson, I.: Medical History Taking, New York, Hoeber-Harper, 1960.
12. Ruesch, J.: Declining clinical tradition, J.A.M.A. 182:110, 1962.

2

Growth and Sex Development

CYRIL M. MACBRYDE

DEFINITIONS

Growth is accomplished by cell multiplication and results in augmentation of mass or size, without regard to development, function or specialization. Examples of pure growth are (1) the continued multiplication of chicken-heart cells in Alexis Carrel's potentially immortal tissue culture, (2) certain malignant tumors. In the one case there is an experimental situation which lacks the guiding influences which normally would result in the development of a mature, functioning myocardium. In the other the normal controlling influences have been lost or deranged.

Development is the process which leads to differentiation into specialized functional tissues. It normally occurs concurrently with growth.

Maturation may be considered the end result of normal growth and development.

Accurate definition of the terms *growth* and *development* is not merely a matter of semantics. Diagnosis and understanding of growth and development problems involve insight into the part played by each of these processes.

FACTORS INFLUENCING GROWTH AND DEVELOPMENT

Growth and development of the human organism begin with the fertilization of the ovum. The rate and extent of growth and the type and the completeness of development are influenced by many factors, especially these:

INTRINSIC INFLUENCES

1. The inherent properties of the fertilized ovum, which depend upon the characters present in the chromosomes of the sperm and the ovum and upon their man-

13

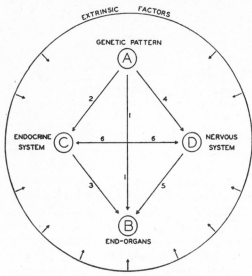

Fig. 1. Pathways through which genetic factors may influence the growth, the development or the "constitutional pattern" of an individual. (Adapted from Bauer, J.: Constitution and Disease, ed. 2, New York, Grune)

ner of combination: the result gives the genetic pattern.

2. Endocrine factors
3. Nervous system factors
4. End-organ factors

EXTRINSIC INFLUENCES

1. Nutritional factors
2. Other factors: mechanical, thermal, ionic (radiation), immunologic, toxic, chemical, infectious

The new cell formed by the union of the male and the female gametes constitutes the first cell of the new human being. In relation to time and the life cycle of the individual the factors influencing its growth and development may be grouped as follows:

1. Genetic influences from parents (hereditary factors)
2. Genetic (mitotic) accidents in early embryonic growth; (mosaicism, etc.)
3. Factors affecting embryo and fetus (maternal, fetal and placental hormones; maternal nutrition, mechanical influences, drugs, toxins, anoxia, infection, immunologic disorders, irradiation)
4. Factors affecting infant and growing child: "environment," including the multi-

plicity of extrinsic factors which are operative during the long post-natal period of human growth and development.

The terms *congenital* and *inherited* are often used loosely and confusingly. It would seem best to separate and define them. *Inherited* should refer to traits transmitted from parents to offspring. *Congenital* should exclude hereditary characters—it implies that the organism is born with the condition, but that the condition is acquired after formation of the zygote (the fertilized ovum). Thus most genetic traits are hereditary, but some are acquired or congenital (genetic (mitotic) accidents, see above). The infant may be born with congenital defects from maternal rubella or with congenital syphilis: these disorders are acquired in utero, they are not inherited.

Genetic Influences. The pattern of genes or "genotype" laid down in the fertilized ovum determines the plan for the future growth, the development and the biologic constitution of the individual. Their influence probably is exerted in the embryo through the formation of chemicals which operate as hormones or catalysts. At a later fetal period certain tissues become specialized into endocrine glands; other tissues become organized into the nervous system, the skeletal system, the circulatory system, the gastrointestinal system, the liver, the muscles, the skin, etc., and certain functions become delegated to these specialized tissues and organs. It seems clear that genetic factors continue throughout life to influence body growth and function, either by direct action on the tissue end-organs or indirectly through the endocrine and the nervous systems.

The relationships discussed above are illustrated in Figure 1.

Hereditary differences in genetic patterns or genetic mutations may account directly for variations in body build, various congenital anomalies of growth, and constitutional differences in the endocrine patterns of individuals. A large part of the direct A → B pathway is concerned with genetic control of enzyme activity. Derangement may sometimes be expressed as hereditary metabolic disease. Genetic factors determine constitutional differences in the nervous system also, and the nervous system influences growth and development both directly and through the endocrine system. These factors of hereditary nature may be considered *intrinsic factors*.

Extrinsic Factors. In addition to these intrinsic factors there are a number of *extrinsic factors* which affect growth, differentiation and development. Among these are: (1) *the supplies* of certain substances such as amino acids, carbohydrates, lipids, minerals, vitamins and oxygen necessary for the building of body tissues, (2) *the ability* of the body to *assimilate* and *transport* these, and (3) the normal activity of numerous *enzymes* concerned in their utilization. Severe malnutrition or disease injurying the tissues or impairing cardiovascular, gastrointestinal, renal or hepatic functions may exert an unfavorable influence upon the growth of the organism as a whole, or upon some part of it. Malnutrition during childhood delays growth, and malnutrition preceding or during adolescence, retards sex development and the adolescent growth spurt.

Extrinsic factors may operate during prenatal as well as during postnatal life, as shown by congenital abnormalities occurring if the mother has rubella during the first trimester of pregnancy, or has severe malnutrition, or is subjected to radiation, or is exposed to certain chemical influences, or ingests certain drugs.

Prenatal extrinsic influences of importance therefore include all these categories: (1) nutritional, (2) mechanical, (3) chemical, (4) hormonal, (5) irradiation, (6) infectious, (7) immunologic, (8) anoxic, (9) prematurity of birth.[30]

Rubella occurring in the first trimester of pregnancy causes a high incidence of abortions and stillbirths and results in abnormalities in about 20 per cent of living offspring. The abnormalities include various combinations of the following disorders particularly (listed in order of decreasing frequency): congenital heart disease, cataracts and microphthalmia, deafness and mental deficiency. The earlier in pregnancy

the rubella occurs, the higher the incidence of abnormal infants: if during the first month, about 50 per cent; during the second month 15 to 20 per cent; during the third month 7 to 10 per cent. Affected viable infants tend to be small and to be retarded in somatic and mental development.

Prenatal syphilis may produce generally retarded growth and many lesions, especially interstitial keratitis, skeletal involvement with "saddle nose" and "sabre shins," Hutchinson teeth, mental deficiency, etc.

Immunologic disorders caused by incompatibility between the maternal blood and that of the infant may seriously interfere with growth and development (erythroblastosis; kernicterus, etc.).

Mechanical factors sometimes acting prenatally include: trauma, ectopia, amniotic bands, abnormal fetal position, oligohydramnios.

Anoxia of the embryo may cause damage resulting from faulty placental function.

Drugs. A tragic syndrome of multiple deformities, especially of the extremities (phocomelia) has resulted from maternal ingestion of a *sedative drug* (thalidomide) in early pregnancy. In a 2-year period hundreds of cases appeared, chiefly in West Germany. It is estimated that 3,500 to 4,000 cases will be reported, although the drug is no longer marketed.[23]

The great need for caution concerning drugs taken by pregnant women cannot be overemphasized.

Radiation.[26] An increasing hazard to growth and development is man-made radiation. Exposure may result from diagnostic or therapeutic roentgen rays or from radioisotopes (medically employed, or from fallout from atomic explosions or contamination from radioactive wastes).

Exposure may affect:

1. The *gonads,* producing genetic changes (mutations) in developing ova or sperm which may be transmissible to offspring.

2. The *embryo* or the *fetus* in utero. Major malformations (including microcephaly in particular) have been described in infants born to pregnant women exposed to radiation in the atomic explosions at Hiroshima and Nagasaki.[11]

Carbohydrate Metabolism
diabetes mellitus
pentosuria
fructosuria
glycogen deposition diseases
galactosemia
hyperbilirubinemia

Amino Acid Metabolism
familial goiter
phenylketonuria
tyrosinosis
alkaptonuria
albinism
primary hyperoxaluria and oxalosis
maple-syrup urine disease

Lipid Metabolism
essential familial hyperlipidemia
infantile amaurotic family idiocy
Niemann-Pick disease
Gaucher's disease

Steroid Metabolism
adrenogenital syndrome

Purine and Pyrimidine Metabolism
gout
xanthinuria
oroticaciduria
beta-aminoisobutyricaciduria

Metal Metabolism
Wilson's disease
hemochromatosis
periodic paralysis
adynamia episodica hereditaria
pseudohypoparathyroidism

Porphyrin Metabolism
porphyrias

Blood and Blood-Forming Tissues
hereditary spherocytosis
drug-induced hemolytic anemia
hereditary methemoglobinemias
hemoglobinopathies and thalassemia
blood-clotting factors

Renal Tubular Transport
familial hypophosphatemia and vitamin D-resistant rickets
Fanconi syndrome
renal glycosuria
renal tubular acidosis
vasopressin-resistant diabetes insipidus
glycinuria
cystinuria
Hartnup disease

Circulating Enzyme or Plasma Protein Deficiency
hypophosphatasia
hereditary hypoproteinemias
acatalasia

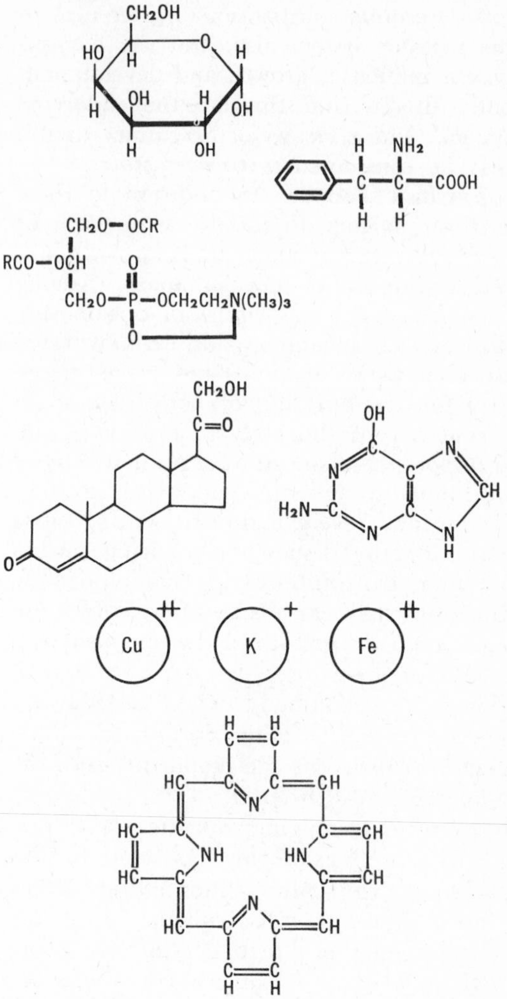

Fig. 2. A working classification of inherited metabolic disorders. (After Stanbury, *et al.*;[20] and Hsia, D. Y.: Pictoclinic 9:3, 1962, the Ames Co.)

Note that of the 10 groups, 7 are based upon the type of metabolic abnormality, and 3 upon the presumed site of action of the hereditary defect.

3. The body generally or certain organs or tissues other than the gonads. These are called *somatic* effects. Absorbed nuclides may localize or be generally distributed. The more harmful radioisotopes tend to localize: plutonium and strontium in bone; cesium in bone; iodine in the thyroid gland.

The isotope strontium[90] emits beta rays and has a 30-year half-life. It therefore offers the greatest biologic hazard, as it is retained in the body and behaves chemically much like calcium. It has caused bone tumors in mice and dogs and possibly leukemia in mice. It is assumed to be harmful to man, but as yet no lesions have been noted.

An important feature of irradiation effects is that they may be long-delayed, appearing many months or many years after exposure. There may be no symptoms or only mild ones occurring soon after the inciting dose, or there may be apparent healing or minor chronic disorders—then very late serious consequences may appear such as skin cancer, thyroid cancer, leukemia, osteogenic sarcoma, chronic nephritis, cataract, osteitis or dermatitis.[26]

Diagnosis of the causes of growth and development problems requires familiarity with all of the above basic concepts.

Types of Genetic Disorders

First one must determine whether or not the condition is primarily genetic. Genetic disorders may be grouped into 4 main types.

Type 1, in which genetic factors *act directly* upon body tissues or end-organs. Examples are seen in: (A) abnormalities such as mongolism, gonadal agenesis (Turner's syndrome), testicular tubular dysgenesis (Klinefelter's syndrome), osteogenesis imperfecta, arachnodachtyly (Marfan's syndrome), achondroplasia, hypertelorism and "primordial dwarfism," (B) various constitutional types of body build, often directly inherited, (C) differences in the size of sex organs such as the penis or the breasts, or in the degree of sensitivity of such organs to hormone stimulation, (D) constitutional tendencies to obesity or leanness, (E) certain diseases in which specific cells of the nervous system degenerate (e.g. Huntington's chorea), (F) red-green color blindness, (G) the antigens which characterize the various blood types, (H) skin, hair and eye pigmentation, and in many other characters.

Type 2, in which genetic factors give rise to constitutional differences in the *endocrine status* of certain individuals or families, certain types of habitus, different times and patterns of puberty, tendency to diabetes, or thyrotoxicosis, etc.

Type 3, in which genetic factors may cause certain abnormalities in the *nervous system*. Anomalies of the hypothalamus, in one or more of its centers, may alter directly the body metabolism or may act indirectly through the pituitary or some other endocrine gland (some cases of sexual precocity, some cases of diabetes insipidus, etc.).

Type 4, in which genetic abnormalities result in the inactivation of a normal enzyme. This mechanism is believed to be that which accounts for most if not all of the inherited metabolic diseases, often designated as inborn errors of metabolism.[9] (See Fig. 2.)

Approach to the Problem

Thus, when confronted by a patient exhibiting a growth or development problem, the physician must consider:

1. Is it genetic or congenital, and unrelated to the endocrine system?

2. Is it perhaps primarily genetic or congenital, but operating secondarily through an endocrine mechanism?

3. Is it perhaps primarily genetic or congenital but operating secondarily through a neural mechanism?

4. Is there merely a constitutional difference in the growth or endocrine pattern of minor significance which may be only a temporary deviation from the average normal pattern of development?

5. Is the condition due to a specific endocrine disorder or neural disorder (pituitary dwarfism, acromegaly, tumor or disease affecting the hypothalamus, etc.).

6. Is the abnormality the result of nutritional factors, systemic disease or other extrinsic influences?

GENETIC ASPECTS

Recent progress in the study of human genetics has been rapid. In 1956 Tijo and Levan showed that the normal number of human chromosomes is 46 rather than 48. New technics in human cytogenetics have been developed so that studies of human chromosome patterns in various conditions have been greatly facilitated. Many recent discoveries are fundamental, permitting new insight into the determination of sex and into the etiology of many disorders and diseases.

CYTOLOGIC TESTS OF SEX

A great impetus to chromosomal investigation arose from the important discovery in 1949 by Barr and his associates of the existence of a distinctive chromocenter, the sex chromatin, in intermitotic nuclei of females and its virtual absence from the nuclei of males. Cells for sex chromatin study may be obtained from simple buccal scrapings, biopsies of tissues, or cell cultures. In nearly all instances the subject's sex, as indicated by the simple and rapid sex chromatin determination, corresponds with the chromosomal sex as revealed by chromosomal analysis, a difficult technical procedure even in skilled hands, and one which also requires experience and judgment in its interpretation. When the sex chromatin does not correspond with the apparent sex of the subject, or when sex anomaly is present either with or without other evidences of developmental aberrations or hereditary or congenital abnormalities, determination of the karyotype may be advisable.

In the normal female there are two X chromosomes, and the cells show the sex chromatin body. In normal males the sex chromosomes are XY, and the sex-chromatin body is absent. The usual or expected number of chromatin bodies is one less than the number of X chromosomes in the cell.

The sex chromatin is about 1 μ in diameter and is typically located against the inner surface of the nuclear membrane.

Three procedures are now available for rapid cytologic sex determination and study of sex anomalies.[2]

1. Oral Smear Method. Over 40 per cent of nuclei in mucosal smears contain the sex chromatin (Fig. 3) if the subject is a chromosomal female. This mass of chromatin is lacking in smears from chromosomal males. The simplicity of this procedure makes it the usual method of choice.

2. Skin Biopsy Method. Nuclei in cells from the spinous layer of the epidermis reveal the characteristic chromatin body in over 50 per cent of cells from females, none in males.

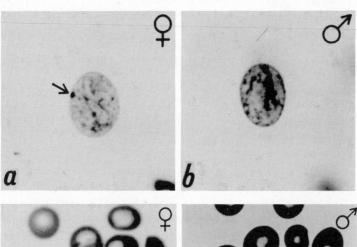

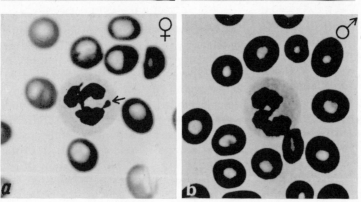

FIG. 3. Nuclei from an oral mucosa smear (1800 ×). (a) Nucleus with sex chromatin, from a female. (b) Without sex chromatin, from a male. (Grumbach and Barr.)

FIG. 4. Two neutrophil white blood cells. (a) With an accessory nuclear lobe ("drumstick"). (b) Without the accessory lobe. (Grumbach and Barr.)

3. Neutrophil Method. In chromosomal females an average of 2 to 3 per cent of neutrophil leukocytes have a small accessory nuclear lobule that presumably contains the sex chromatin. This particular characteristic "drumstick" lobule does not occur in males (Fig. 4).

Chromosomal Analysis

Each somatic cell of all normal human beings characteristically contains 46 chromosomes: 44 autosomes and 2 sex chromosomes. The chromosomal constitution (karyotype) of any person may be determined by study of cells cultured from peripheral blood, bone marrow or other tissues. In unusual cases it is advisable to analyze cells from several different tissues, since in rare cases the chromosomal patterns may differ (mosaicism).

Human chromosomes at the metaphase of mitosis are recognizable as longitudinally doubled rodlike structures, the halves of which are joined only at the centromere. Each chromosome has a mate somewhere

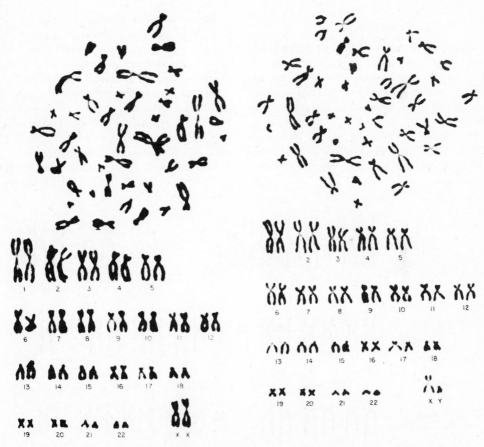

Fig. 5. (*Left*) Appearance of the chromosomes of a dividing human cell at metaphase. Each chromosome is longitudinally doubled, the chromatids (potential daughter chromosomes) being held together at their respective centromeres. (*Bottom*) Karyotype of a normal human female showing twenty-two pairs of autosomes and an XX sex chromosome constitution. This was constructed from the preparation above by sorting and matching homologous pairs of chromosomes.

(*Right*) Chromosomes of a dividing human cell at metaphase; from a male. (*Bottom*) The chromosome constitution of a normal human male containing 22 pairs of autosomes and an XY sex chromosome complex. (Barr, M. L., and Carr, D. H.: Canad. M. A. J., 83:979)

in the nucleus which can be matched with it, the two constituting a homologous pair. Homologous *autosomes* (nonsex chromosomes) from the cells of the same or of different persons do not differ significantly either in relative length or in centromere position. The two members of each pair are identical in appearance except for the sex chromosomes of the male. In the male one first identifies 22 pairs of autosomes; there will then remain the 2 sex chromosomes: one is large, called X, and one small, called Y. In the female the 2 X chromosomes make a matched homologous pair (Fig. 5).

Terminology[18]

Genotype denotes the genetic constitution of an individual organism, regardless of external appearance. Probably no two human beings (excluding, possibly, identical twins) have ever had the same genotype.

Phenotype is the apparent or externally visible type with characteristics that may be independent of the hereditary type (genotype).

Meiosis is a specialized type of cell division resulting in reduction of the number of chromosomes from the somatic (diploid) number to the half (haploid) number in the sperm and ova, fertilization then restoring the somatic number in the zygote.

Nondisjunction is a type of abnormal chromosomal behavior during nuclear division, occurring either in mitosis or meiosis. During anaphase the longitudinally doubled chromosomes or the members of a pair of homologous chromosomes fail to separate. As a result one daughter cell receives both chromosomes, the other neither of the pair.

Mutation is a change in a gene. When a mutant gene is present in a germ cell it may produce hereditary variations. Mutation occurs spontaneously or may result from radiation, chemical alterations, etc.

Mosaicism is the presence of genetically dissimilar cells within various tissues of the same organisms; the body contains 2 or more stem lines of cells with different chromosome numbers or constitution.

Karyotype is the group of characteristics (number, size and form) identifying a par-

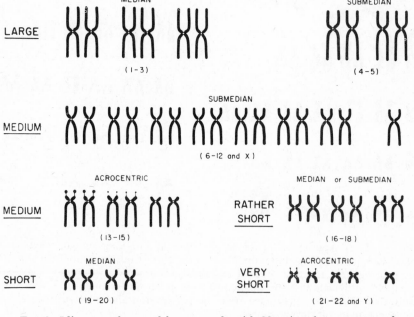

Fig. 6. Idiogram of normal human male with 22 pairs of autosomes and an XY sex chromosome constitution. The chromosomes are arranged in seven groups according to their length and centromere position. The classification is in accordance with an international system of nomenclature adopted in Denver, Colorado. (After Sohval[18])

ticular chromosome constitution. The human karyotype is obtained by sorting and matching the individual mitotic chromosomes of a number of single cells as visualized in drawings or photographic enlargements. The pairs of chromosomes are then systematically arranged according to their lengths and centromere positions. According to the Denver system, the autosome pairs are numbered 1 to 22 in descending order of length (Fig. 6).

KARYOTYPES IN HUMAN DISORDERS

The principal disorders in which human chromosomes have been analyzed may be grouped as follows:

1. A large variety of sexual anomalies
2. Persons (usually mental defectives) with more than 2 X chromosomes
3. Mongolism
4. A heterogeneous assortment of conditions exhibiting multiple congenital anomalies
5. Leukemia.

SEXUAL ANOMALIES[18]

1. Pseudohermaphroditism. Elements of both sexes are present in the genital tract, but the gonads are either testes or ovaries, and accordingly the condition is designated male or female pseudohermaphroditism. Sex chromatin and karyotype correspond to the gonadal sex.

In the special variety of male pseudohermaphroditism known as *testicular feminization* the person is chromatin-negative (indicating genetic maleness) but appears to be a female. Sex chromatin determination should be done in all women with primary amenorrhea, since some may actually be males with this syndrome and removal of the testicular tissue may be advisable (possibility of carcinoma).

2. True Hermaphroditism. In some cases of true hermaphroditism (in whom both ovarian and testicular tissues are present) the sex chromatin may be positive, (in approximately two thirds of 25 cases studied), in others, negative. Of 9 unquestionably true hermaphrodites 7 were chromatin-positive and each of these showed the karyotype of a normal human female (46XX). Two

were chromatin-negative, with male karyotypes (46XY). An intersex patient who "may be" a true hermaphrodite was chromatin-negative and showed a mosaic chromosome constitution (45/46XO/XY). The occurrence of sex mosaicism in true hermaphroditism would not be surprising—rather one might expect it in persons with gonadal tissue of both sexes.

A point of great interest in connection with the karyotypes of some patients with true hermaphroditism is that testicular tissue may be present without the presence of a Y chromosome. This suggests that the normal Y chromosome is not the only important factor in the initiation of male differentiation.

3. Klinefelter's Syndrome. Persons with this disorder constitute the most frequent type of human sex anomaly. They are phenotypically male with anatomic derangement of the testes (sclerosing tubular fibrosis, seminiferous tubular dysgenesis, microorchidism) and functional impairment (sterility and androgen deficiency). Gynecomastia is frequent. About 50 per cent of such patients are chromatin-positive. This suggests the presence of two X chromosomes, and the karyotype in the majority of the chromatin-positive cases is 47XXY. Very few karyotype analyses have been reported in chromatin-negative subjects with Klinefelter's syndrome. One patient had 46XY (normal male type) and another 46/47XY/XXY mosaic. The karyotype usually found in this syndrome, 47XXY, is apparently the result of nondisjunction of the sex chromosomes during gametogenesis of either parent.

4. Turner's Syndrome. Persons with this anomaly are phenotypic females with normal type but undeveloped female genitalia and failure to have normal puberty with development of the usual secondary sex characteristics. The gonads are represented by vestigial fibrous streaks. A number of other congenital anomalies may be present. About 80 per cent of these apparent females are chromatin-negative. The karyotype of the majority of persons with chromatin-negative Turner's syndrome may be said to be neither male nor female (45XO). All humans have one X chromosome; in normal males the second of the sex pair is a Y, in females it is a second X, while in Turner's syndrome it is missing. In several patients with this disorder a 45/46XO/XX mosaic karyotype has been reported.

In Turner's syndrome, as in Klinefelter's syndrome, the clinicopathologic constellation of anomalies is highly variable. Both disorders apparently may result from nondisjunction during gametogenesis of either parent.

5. Mongolism. In this disorder in the majority of instances there is an additional, small acrocentric chromosome, making the modal number 47. The extra chromosome has been identified most often as one of the two smallest autosomes, usually number 21. Several patients have been reported who have the trisomy-21 condition and also have an XXY sex chromosome constitution (48 chromosomes). They clinically have both mongolism and chromatin-positive Klinefelter's syndrome.

Miscellaneous

Karyotype analysis has been carried out in more than 40 congenital abnormalities and hereditary disorders (other than mongolism and sexual anomalies) with apparently normal chromosomal constitution being found in the great majority.[18] As yet no characteristic chromosomal abnormality has been found for example in any of the following conditions: achondroplasia, Albright's syndrome, arachnodactyly (Marfan's syndrome), primordial dwarfism, pituitary dwarfism, Fröhlich's syndrome, Gaucher's disease, Laurence-Moon-Biedl syndrome, muscular dystrophy, neurofibromatosis, osteogenesis imperfecta, phenylketonuria, etc. The genetic defects which no doubt account for such conditions are by present technics ultramicroscopic—not yet visualized.

Multiple Congenital Abnormalities

Chromosomal aberrations have been found in a number of nonmongoloid subjects, usually mentally defective, chiefly infants with a variety of serious anomalies including cardiac, cerebral and renal defects, etc. Two examples of autosomic trisomy syndromes other than mongolism are recorded (D_1 trisomy, with 4 cases reported and 18-trisomy,[24] with 13 cases reported).

The other chromosomal aberrations are various and as yet form no recognizable specific clinical entities or syndromes.

Acquired Chromosomal Anomalies

In most of the disorders so far discussed, the chromosomal derangements are present in the gamete (ovum, or sperm, or both) and the zygote carries the aberration as the first cell of the new organism and later cells show it as the cells multiply and the tissues and organs develop.

When the karyotype is originally normal but abnormalities arise later in life, we are dealing with acquired chromosomal abnormalities.

Two types of acquired anomalies are known:

1. In most cases of chronic myeloid *leukemia* there is deletion of part of 1 of the 2 smallest autosomes (21 or 22).

2. Roentgen ray irradiation of the spine or 100 mc. of radioiodine produces a brief but abundant crop of chromosomal anomalies.

In other forms both of acute and of chronic leukemia chromosomal aberrations in number and form have been reported in bone marrow cells and skin cells. Since mongolism is now recognized as caused by a chromosomal defect, it is of particular interest that mongoloids have a high incidence of leukemia.

Radiation therapy produces changes in chromosomes observed in cultures of blood cells of patients after roentgen ray therapy over the spine.

Radioactive iodine therapy of thyroid carcinoma with ablative doses (100 mc.) has also resulted in chromosome changes in blood cell cultures.

Implications. Various types of cancer and leukemia are known to be caused by radiation. There is no certainty at present that ultramicroscopic genic changes or more massive visible chromosomal aberrations are prerequisites for cancerous growth but present evidence is at least highly suggestive that genic changes may cause malignant growth and that radiation may induce such changes.

MUTATIONS IN GERM CELLS

Mutations may arise in germ cells (ova or sperm) if gonads are exposed to irradiation. Radiation-induced genetic changes in germ cells may become phenotypically apparent in later generations. In these days of increasing radiation exposure this problem is of grave concern.

Other mutagenic agents affecting the germ cells may possibly include temperature changes, viruses, toxins, chemicals and drugs.

SEX DIFFERENTIATION

The distinction in our society between male and female is expected to be absolute, whereas actually there is wide variation in the maleness of males and femaleness of females. Many normal persons have some characteristics usually considered typical of the opposite sex; it is difficult to define the limits of normality, for the range is wide.

The "sex" of any person is the final result of a number of components. The components are usually of one gender and conform to the sex chromosomal pattern established in the zygote at the time of fertilization. As emphasized by Van Wyk,[25] there are nevertheless possible influences operating at every level from the earliest cellular chromosomal components to the levels which include the influences of environment, social pressures and psychological factors.

In studying Table 1 one should remember that each component is developed from bipotential primordia which have the capacity of differentiating in either direction. At each level of sexual organization a widely variable range of development is possible; also the type and the degree of differentiation at each stage will in turn affect development in the successive stages.

DETERMINATION OF SEX

Sex may be considered from two chief viewpoints: (1) phenotypic or apparent sex and (2) genotypic sex, which may or may not be the same.

Human beings may be grouped (as to sex types) thus:

1. Normal females
2. Normal males
3. Essentially neuter states (phenotypic females: Turner's syndrome)
4. Mixed sex (true hermaphroditism)
5. Female pseudohermaphroditism (most often due to fetal adrenocortical hyperplasia, but may result from other androgenic influences)
6. Male pseudohermaphroditism
7. Modified males (partially feminized)
   A. Testicular feminization (phenotypic females, genetic males)
   B. Klinefelter's syndrome (phenotypic males, genetically modified males)
8. Modified females (partially virilized). These genetic females have various degrees of masculinization due to androgen-producing ovarian tissue (Stein-Leventhal syndrome; arrhenoblastoma) or from adrenocortical hyperplasia or tumor, etc. The virilism may be evident at birth, because of fetal hormonal influences, and result in pseudohermaphroditism, or may develop in a previously normal girl or adult woman.

SEX DETERMINANTS

Two types of sex determinants are involved:

1. Genetic, determining the "true" sex.

Normally one of each pair of homologous chromosomes is derived from each parent. In addition to a single set of 22 autosomes, all ova contain one X chromosome. Each sperm contains a single set of 22 autosomes plus either an X or a Y chromosome. Fertilization of any egg by an X sperm results in an XX zygote destined to develop into a female. Fertilization by a Y sperm forms an XY zygote destined to become a male.

2. Hormonal, including

A. The maternal hormonal milieu (important, since man is a placental animal, with a relatively long exposure to influences affecting the developing embryo and fetus *in utero*). Hormones which may affect the offspring include the normal maternal hor-

TABLE 1. NORMAL SEX DIFFERENTIATION: CONSTITUENTS OF SEXUAL CONSTITUTION

COMPONENT	HOW IDENTIFIED	DERIVED FROM	FACTORS DETERMINING DIFFERENTIATION
Chromosomal sex	Direct chromosomal count of cells grown in tissue culture	Parental germ cells	*Normal:* Chromosomal composition of sperm *Abnormal:* Nondisjunction of parental germ cells during meioses; mitotic nondisjunction
Nuclear sex	Buccal smear; Sections of peripheral tissues	Sex chromatin	Requires two X chromosomes to be positive (?)
Gonadal sex	Histologic appearance	Medullary and cortical components of primitive bipotential gonad	Sex-determining genes on X and Y chromosomes; Medullary and cortical inductor substances; Environmental factors in fetus?
Genital ducts	Pelvic exploration	Müllerian ducts Wolffian ducts	Duct-organizing substances of fetal testis

External genitalia	Inspection
	 Urethroscopy
		Genital tubercle
		 Urethral folds
		 Labioscrotal folds
		 Urogenital sinus
			Androgen from:
			   fetal testis
			   fetal adrenal
			   maternal circulation
			   End-organ sensitivity

Hormonal sex	Secondary sex characteristics (excretion of 17-ketosteroids and estrogens not reliable)	Secretory cells of testes, ovaries and adrenals	Differentiation of gonads: Differentiation of biosynthetic enzymes; End-organ sensitivity
Gender role	Social comportment; Mannerisms and dress; Direction of sex drive	Neuter at birth	Assigned sex of rearing; Attitudes of others; Conformity of external appearance

Table 1. Factors determining, identifying, and influencing sex differentiation. (Van Wyk, J. J. *in* Williams: Textbook of Endocrinology, ed. 3, p. 516, Philadelphia, Saunders.)

mones, abnormal maternal hormones or administered hormones.

    B. Hormones from the subject's own gonads.

    C. Hormones from the subject's other tissues (adrenal cortex and other hormone-producing tissues or tumors).

    Gonadal ridges appear in the human embryo at about the 4th week of gestation. Their structure is identical in male and female embryos until the 7th week. The cellular cortex of the indifferent gonad has the potentiality of developing into an ovary, the medulla into a testis.

    Whether the indifferent gonad becomes an ovary or a testis depends upon female-determiners and male-determiners in the genes. If the somatic cells of the gonad are XX, the cortical germ cells proliferate more than the medullary cells, and an ovary results; if XY, the medullary cells take over, resulting in a testis. Further control of sexual development apparently depends largely upon various hormonal influences, but genetic influences upon sex development do not cease entirely once the gonad type is established. Secondary sex characters as well as general somatic characters appear to be subject to genes probably present in both sex chromosomes in either sex as well as in autosomes.

    Since normal females have XX sex chromosomes, and normal males XY, apparently a single Y chromosome is a sufficiently strong sex determinant to overcome the influence of a single X chromosome. Indeed, a single Y overcomes the influence of *two* X chromosomes in the XXY configuration of Klinefelter's syndrome and the phenotype is male and the gonads are male, although the presence of the second X impairs male development.

In Turner's syndrome the subject may be considered (in typical cases with complete gonadal agenesis) as essentially neuter. All humans have at least one X chromosome, but the person with this syndrome has neither the other X chromosome to cause femaleness nor the Y chromosome to cause maleness. The XO state is as a rule accompanied by actual absence of recognizable gonadal tissue. Such persons are phenotypic females with undeveloped breast tissue, infantile uterus and vagina, etc. It seems probable that the subject develops as an apparent female because of the combined effects of the single X chromosome plus the hormonal influence of the maternal milieu (normally strongly feminine).

Testicular tissue may apparently be present (some cases of true hermaphroditism) in the absence of a Y chromosome, but in normal or abnormal persons, whenever a Y chromosome is present, testicular tissue is present. There may also be autosomal male determiners.

A genetic explanation for the female body development in the type of male pseudohermaphroditism called testicular feminization is lacking. The phenotype is female, genotype male, with undescended testes which seem to produce estrogen rather than androgen.

The concept of hormonal determination of sexual traits is not in conflict with genetic sex determination. Hormones are among the chief means by which the genetic constitution of the embryo directs its own development, both sexual and somatic. Later the fetus is subject to its own hormones, to the normally strongly female hormones of the mother, and to any abnormal hormones which may reach it through the mother. The hormonal milieu of the developing organism determines its characteristics, as well as do other influences in its environment (supply of nutrients, infection, etc.), both prenatally and throughout life.

In *female pseudohermaphroditism*[4] we may find, for example:

1. Subjects with associated malformations (apparently primarily genetic disorders, often lethal)

2. Subjects without associated malformations

    A. Fetal androgenic influence (adrenogenital syndrome)

    B. Maternal androgenic influence

        a. Due to treatment during pregnancy with androgens or certain progestational type hormones, especially of the nor-19 group

        b. Functional deviation of steroid metabolism (usually with some virilizing symptoms, probably most often due to hyperadrenocorticism)

        c. Virilizing tumor during pregnancy (arrhenoblastoma; rare).

In *male pseudohermaphroditism* further insight into the processes of sex development is made possible by study of these genotypic males who exhibit failure of the fetal testis to bring about complete male differentiation of the genital ducts and external genitalia. Here the situation differs from that in female pseudohermaphroditism. In the female, deviations toward intersex may be thought of as due to a *positive* androgenic influence. However, in the male, deviation toward the opposite sex (in the absence of the very rare occurrence of estrogen-producing tissues or tumors) is a *negative* condition, depending upon the degree of deficiency of virilizing influences.

Almost a complete spectrum has been described ranging from simulant females to almost normal males. One may visualize this spectrum as beginning with the neuter subject (gonadal agenesis—certain cases of Turner's syndrome). In such subjects with complete absence of virilizing influence the apparent sex is female, for reasons previously discussed. With increasing degrees of androgen supply the inherent human tendency toward femaleness is partially overcome and the apparent sex becomes ambiguous, the genital duct systems may be partly female and partly male and the external genitalia may also exhibit mixed characters: phallus and vagina, etc.

GENETIC DISORDERS WITH NORMAL KARYOTYPES

In this discussion we have been concerned chiefly with the dramatic but relatively gross chromosomal abnormalities which accompany certain clinical disorders. Two points now need emphasis:

1. Morphologic chromosomal abnormalities often occur without any known clinical disorder resulting therefrom

2. The great majority of genetic abnormalities occur as the result of the chemical characteristics present in one or more genes, without detectable structural or morphological chromosomal aberration.

At present we believe that the genes are the basic, ultramicroscopic, intramolecular units of heredity and that they are arranged linearly at definite points (loci) in a chromosome. Apparently genes function by controlling enzymatic action.

Certain abnormal genes produce specific biochemical disorders in human beings. Examples are phenylketonuria and galactosemia, both of which produce severe mental deficiency. In both of these the basic biochemical defect is fairly well understood and attempts at treatment have met with some success. See Figure 2 for a working classification of inherited metabolic diseases.[20]

BIOCHEMICAL GENETIC DISORDERS IN HUMAN HEREDITARY DISEASES

Genes are parts of chromosomes and it should be possible someday to define them in terms of specific molecular structure. It seems highly probable that genes consist of chemical substances called deoxyribonucleic acids (DNA), which are typically found only in chromosomes.[31]

"The ultimate basis of biogenetic traits resides in some 20 thousand pairs of genes. The term gene refers to that subdivision of chromosomes which conveys a unit biochemical message."[33] Recently investigators have, by growing cell lines in tissue cultures and by quantitatively analyzing their enzymatic contents, made a beginning at intercepting the biochemical message conveyed by certain genes in some conditions and at interpreting the message in precise biochemical language.[34,35] In the understanding of human genetics such studies constitute a breakthrough of high significance and great promise.

Skin cells, obtained from patients with galactosemia or acatalasia, maintain in cultures the enzymatic defect characteristic of these diseases, even after the cells have increased their numbrs by many times. The persistence of the enzymatic defects in culture is obviously of far greater importance than simply to furnish another method of demonstrating that a specific enzyme is defective in these metabolic diseases. It means that we now have available human cell lines with particular "markers" (that is, specific biochemical characteristics) which will make it possible to investigate a number of fundamental unsolved problems in the biochemical-genetic aspects of human hereditary metabolic diseases.

Cell cultures with "markers" may prove to be useful in further studies on the nature of the enzymatic defects at a molecular level. It is believed that hereditary diseases associated with enzyme deficiencies are due to alterations in the genetic material (DNA), which via RNA (ribonucleic acid), directs the synthesis of enzyme protein. The defective DNA may result in the formation of a slightly altered enzymatic protein structure which has little or no catalytic activity, or the DNA alteration may be such that no protein analogous to the enzyme is formed. Examples of both these possibilities are found among bacterial mutations.[36] The best example of protein structure variants in man is the family of abnormal hemoglobins.[37]

As yet we know little about the actual structural abnormalities of the enzymes deficient in metabolic diseases except that there is a lack of catalytic activity, and we know even less about the molecular changes in the corresponding genetic material (DNA). Tissue culture cells may be useful in these studies and have several obvious advantages over biopsy or autopsy material.[35]

Insight and understanding of the basic mechanisms of heredity gained from studies such as those discussed should apply not only to rare defects. Biochemical studies in the field of genetics have as yet been concerned primarily with relatively rare abnormalities. The biochemistry and genetics of many common defects is less well understood, largely because most rare defects are caused by practically complete absence of a normal metabolic process, while the more common defects may be correlated not with the absence of a biochemical reaction, but with a quantitative abnormality. Genes, by regulating biochemical processes, determine not only striking disorders but also less striking ones, and above all, much of the variability among normal human beings.[31]

Insight into the biochemistry of genetic variation has already provided tools for overcoming genic deficiencies. For example: infants with galactosemia can be helped by removing galactose (milk) from their diets; mental deficiency of phenylketonuric infants may be prevented by supplying diets low in phenylalanine; diabetes mellitus may be controlled by supplying the deficient pancreatic secretion, insulin; pernicious anemia may be controlled with vitamin B_{12}.

MEDICINE AND EUGENICS

Not only are physicians and other scientists in this field responsible for trying to correct or at least partially to control the *results* of genetic disorders *after* they have occurred, but they are confronted with the challenge of applying the new and rapidly advancing knowledge of genetics in many other ways. Among these responsibilities is the providing of information and advice to individuals and couples about marriage and the production of children, to governments, medical agencies and industry about the control of mutagenic agents, and to society in general about possible ways which may be feasible (but may or may not be desirable) of planning and effecting more direct intervention by man into human evolution.

In recent years factors largely detrimental to a genetically fit human population have rapidly increased. We are confronted by certain progressing elements in our culture, especially: (1) increasing exposure through modern technology to mutagenic agents, ionizing and chemical; and (2) interference with natural selection by current social and medical developments. Technologic and cultural changes are producing effects upon the human population at a speed with which genetic adaptation cannot keep pace.

To prepare physicians for their much wider future role, encompassing responsibilities in relation to human genetics, the horizons of medical education must be greatly broadened. Added to the traditional concern of medicine for the individual must be concern for the whole human species. A prime factor in meeting this role must be ever closer cooperation between physician and geneticist.[33]

METHODS OF STUDYING GROWTH AND DEVELOPMENT

It is of great importance to recognize deviations from normal growth and development as early in life as possible, for early recognition may lead to correction. Even in later childhood, during adolescence or adult life, proper diagnosis may permit great improvement through appropriate therapy.

Assessment of the state of growth and development requires: (1) a knowledge of norms at various ages during the usual period of progressive growth and development; (2) a knowledge of the levels acceptable as adult or mature; (3) an understanding of the limits of the deviations which may be considered as "normal"—that is, due to constitutional variants.

Categories to be specifically evaluated include:

1. Skeletal development and teeth
2. Tissue and organ status: muscles, fat storage, skin and nails, scalp hair, etc.
3. Sexual development
4. Mental development

Data to evaluate growth and development is secured by a complete general medical examination with special emphasis upon certain aspects of all three chief avenues of inquiry: (1) the history, (2) the physical examination and (3) laboratory studies.

History. 1. THE FAMILY HISTORY is analyzed for possible hereditary abnormalities and special family constitutional traits. A diagram (pedigree) showing members of the family with certain characteristics or disorders may be very useful.

Whenever possible the family history should include:

Health record of grandparents and parents

Height and weight of all grandparents

Father's height and weight and age at onset of puberty

Mother's height and weight and age at onset of puberty, menarche and menopause

Siblings' growth and health records

Information about more distant relatives (aunts, uncles, cousins, etc.) and any tendencies toward unusual growth or sex development, obesity, etc.

Data about thyroid disorders, diabetes or other endocrine disorders in the family

Information about water supply and geographic area of residence in relation to endemic goiter.

2. THE PAST HISTORY should include all pertinent information concerning:

A. Prenatal period. Any abnormality during pregnancy such as unusual weight gain, goiter, signs of myxedema, unusual pigmentation, glycosuria; any medication such as thyroid, insulin, sedatives; any infection, such as rubella.

B. Birth. First child?—or number of previous births; duration of labor; type of delivery; condition at birth; birth weight; any evidences of birth injury during neonatal period.

C. Nutrition. Type of feeding during infancy; weight gain record; digestive or nutritional disorders; past and recent appetite, diet and dietary habits.

D. Diseases. Systemic disease, infectious disease, especially if related in time to onset of presenting complaints or abnormalities.

E. Operations. Time of removal of appendix, tonsils or other operation in relation to onset of symptoms.

F. Injuries. Type and time-relationship to symptoms.

G. Chronologic record of growth and development:

All available data about actual *heights* and *weights* at specified ages. Any unusual growth features or changes in rate of growth. Growth in past year.

Weight history. Striking changes in weight and any correlation with dietary habits, physical activities, or sex development.

Osseous development. Time of closure of fontanelles; any data obtained previously by roentgenograms of bones.

Dentition. Time of appearance of first tooth; number of teeth at 1 year, at 2 years, etc. Ages at which certain deciduous teeth were lost and permanent teeth appeared.

Physical and mental performance. Age of holding up head, sitting, standing and walking. First words, first sentences formed at what age? Learning ability: progress and grades in school.

Sexual development. Earliest signs of puberty: sex hair, genitalia, breasts, acne, menses, voice.

3. THE CHIEF COMPLAINTS AND PRESENT ILLNESS are analyzed as to their character and time of onset. For example: did the growth retardation antedate the severe infectious disease? Or, did the sudden acceleration of growth occur at time of appearance of the first pubic hair? Has sluggishness, constipation and dry skin appeared in recent years when growth rate decreased (suggesting thyroid deficiency)? Any headaches, visual disturbances, neurologic signs or polyuria (suggesting an intracranial lesion)?

The Physical Examination. In addition to the usual complete general physical examination (including neurologic and ophthalmologic observations) certain data should be noted when evaluating possible growth and developmental abnormalities.

1. General appearance. The chief characteristics of the patient apparent on inspection should be noted: normal size, dwarfed or tall, obese or thin; pale or plethoric, muscular or asthenic; hairy or beardless; active or sluggish; cool or warm;

TABLE 2. NORMAL MEASUREMENTS IN RELATION TO AGE (FEMALE)*

AGE	HEIGHT	WEIGHT	SPAN	UPPER MEAS.	LOWER MEAS.	RATIO U/L	HEAD	CHEST	ABDO-MEN
Birth	19.9	7.5	19.0	12.6	7.3	1.73	13.6	13.6	13.2
1 Mo.	21.5	9.7	20.5	13.5	8.0	1.69	14.9	14.1	13.6
2 Mos.	22.7	11.2	21.4	14.2	8.5	1.67	15.7	15.3	15.0
3 "	23.7	12.7	22.4	14.8	8.9	1.66	16.3	16.0	15.7
4 "	24.6	14.1	23.3	15.2	9.4	1.62	16.7	16.5	16.2
5 "	25.3	15.5	24.3	15.6	9.7	1.61	17.1	16.8	16.5
6 "	26.0	16.2	24.8	16.0	10.0	1.60	17.3	17.0	16.8
7 "	26.6	16.9	25.3	16.3	10.3	1.58	17.5	17.2	17.0
8 "	27.1	17.6	25.8	16.6	10.5	1.58	17.7	17.4	17.2
9 "	27.6	18.2	26.2	16.8	10.8	1.56	17.8	17.6	17.3
10 "	28.1	18.8	26.7	17.0	11.1	1.53	18.0	17.8	17.4
11 "	28.6	19.5	27.2	17.3	11.3	1.53	18.1	17.9	17.5
12 "	29.0	20.1	27.7	17.5	11.5	1.52	18.2	18.1	17.6
15 "	30.2	21.3	28.7	18.1	12.1	1.50	18.5	18.4	17.9
18 "	31.4	23.2	30.1	18.7	12.7	1.47	18.7	18.7	18.2
21 "	32.4	24.4	31.1	19.2	13.2	1.45	18.9	19.0	18.4
24 "	33.4	25.7	32.1	19.6	13.8	1.42	19.0	19.2	18.6
30 "	35.1	27.7	33.6	20.4	14.7	1.39	19.2	19.6	18.9
36 "	36.7	29.8	35.1	20.9	15.8	1.32	19.4	20.0	19.1
42 "	38.2	31.9	36.6	21.5	16.7	1.29	19.6	20.4	19.3
48 "	39.6	34.0	38.1	22.0	17.6	1.25	19.7	20.7	19.5
54 "	40.9	36.2	39.7	22.4	18.5	1.21	19.9	21.0	19.7
60 "	42.2	37.7	40.7	22.9	19.3	1.19	20.0	21.4	19.9
5½ Yrs.	43.4	40.2	42.3	23.2	20.2	1.15	20.1	21.7	20.0
6 "	44.6	42.0	43.3	23.7	20.9	1.13	20.1	22.0	20.2
6½ "	45.7	44.0	44.4	24.1	21.6	1.12	20.2	22.3	20.4
7 "	46.8	47.2	46.0	24.4	22.4	1.09	20.3	22.7	20.5
7½ "	47.9	49.5	47.1	24.7	23.2	1.06	20.3	23.0	20.7
8 "	48.9	52.0	48.2	25.0	23.9	1.05	20.4	23.4	20.8
8½ "	49.9	54.6	49.3	25.4	24.5	1.04	20.5	23.8	21.0
9 "	50.9	57.4	50.4	25.7	25.2	1.02	20.5	24.2	21.2
9½ "	51.9	60.7	51.5	26.1	25.8	1.01	20.6	24.6	21.5
10 "	53.0	63.6	52.6	26.7	26.3	1.01	20.7	25.0	21.8
10½ "	54.1	67.2	53.7	27.2	26.9	1.01	20.8	25.5	22.1
11 "	55.3	72.4	55.3	27.7	27.6	1.00	20.9	26.1	22.4
11½ "	56.5	76.2	56.3	28.2	28.3	1.00	20.9	26.6	22.8
12 "	57.6	80.6	57.5	28.7	28.9	0.99	21.0	27.1	23.2
12½ "	58.7	85.1	58.5	29.2	29.5	0.99	21.1	27.6	23.6
13 "	59.7	90.0	59.7	29.7	30.0	0.99	21.2	28.1	23.9
13½ "	60.6	95.4	60.8	30.3	30.3	1.00	21.3	28.5	24.2
14 "	61.4	101.4	61.3	30.6	30.8	0.99	21.4	28.9	24.5
14½ "	62.0	104.5	62.4	30.9	31.1	0.99	21.5	29.3	24.7
15 "	62.5	107.7	63.0	31.2	31.3	1.00	21.6	29.6	24.8
15½ "	62.9	110.9	63.6	31.4	31.5	1.00	21.7	29.9	25.0
16 "	63.2	110.9	63.6	31.6	31.6	1.00	21.7	30.1	25.1
16½ "	63.5	114.2	64.2	31.8	31.7	1.00	21.8	30.3	25.2
17 "	63.7	114.2	64.2	31.9	31.8	1.00	21.8	30.5	25.3
17½ "	63.9	117.5	64.8	32.0	31.9	1.00	21.8	30.7	25.4
18 "	64.0	117.5	64.8	32.1	31.9	1.01	21.9	30.8	25.5
18½ "	64.0	117.5	64.8	32.1	31.9	1.01	21.9	30.8	25.5
19 "	64.0	117.5	64.8	32.1	31.9	1.01	21.9	30.9	25.6
19½ "	64.0	117.5	64.8	32.1	31.9	1.01	21.9	30.9	25.6
20 "	64.0	117.5	64.8	32.1	31.9	1.01	21.9	31.0	25.7

* From Williams, R. H.: Textbook of Endocrinology, ed. 2, p. 587, Philadelphia, Saunders.

TABLE 3. NORMAL MEASUREMENTS IN RELATION TO AGE (MALE)*

AGE	HEIGHT	WEIGHT	SPAN	UPPER MEAS.	LOWER MEAS.	RATIO U/L	HEAD	CHEST	ABDOMEN
Birth	20.2	7.4	19.1	12.7	7.5	1.69	13.9	13.8	13.4
1 Mo.	21.9	10.4	21.1	13.7	8.2	1.67	15.2	14.3	13.8
2 Mos.	23.1	12.0	22.0	14.4	8.7	1.65	16.0	15.6	15.2
3 "	24.1	13.6	23.0	15.0	9.1	1.65	16.6	16.4	16.0
4 "	25.0	15.0	24.0	15.5	9.5	1.63	17.0	16.9	16.5
5 "	25.7	15.8	24.4	15.9	9.8	1.62	17.4	17.2	16.8
6 "	26.4	17.3	25.4	16.3	10.1	1.61	17.7	17.5	17.1
7 "	27.1	18.0	25.9	16.6	10.4	1.61	17.9	17.7	17.3
8 "	27.6	18.7	26.4	16.9	10.7	1.58	18.1	17.9	17.5
9 "	28.1	19.4	26.9	17.2	10.9	1.58	18.2	18.0	17.6
10 "	28.6	20.0	27.3	17.4	11.2	1.55	18.4	18.2	17.7
11 "	29.1	20.7	27.8	17.6	11.5	1.53	18.5	18.3	17.8
12 "	29.5	21.4	28.3	17.9	11.6	1.54	18.6	18.5	17.9
15 "	30.7	22.7	29.3	18.5	12.2	1.52	18.9	18.8	18.2
18 "	31.9	24.6	30.8	19.2	12.7	1.51	19.1	19.1	18.5
21 "	32.9	25.9	31.8	19.6	13.3	1.47	19.3	19.4	18.7
24 "	33.9	27.2	32.7	20.0	13.9	1.44	19.4	19.7	18.9
30 "	35.7	29.2	34.2	20.8	14.9	1.40	19.6	20.2	19.2
36 "	37.3	32.0	36.2	21.3	16.0	1.33	19.8	20.6	19.5
42 "	38.8	34.0	37.7	22.0	16.8	1.31	20.0	21.0	19.8
48 "	40.2	35.5	38.8	22.5	17.7	1.27	20.1	21.4	20.0
54 "	41.5	37.7	40.3	22.9	18.6	1.23	20.3	21.7	20.2
60 "	42.7	39.3	41.4	23.4	19.3	1.21	20.4	22.1	20.4
5½ Yrs.	43.9	41.9	42.9	23.7	20.2	1.17	20.4	22.4	20.6
6 "	45.0	43.9	44.0	24.0	21.0	1.14	20.5	22.7	20.9
6½ "	46.1	45.9	45.1	24.3	21.8	1.11	20.5	23.0	21.1
7 "	47.2	48.1	46.2	24.7	22.5	1.10	20.6	23.3	21.3
7½ "	48.2	50.4	47.3	24.9	23.3	1.07	20.7	23.7	21.5
8 "	49.2	52.8	48.6	25.3	23.9	1.06	20.7	24.0	21.8
8½ "	50.2	55.3	49.8	25.7	24.5	1.05	20.8	24.3	22.0
9 "	51.2	58.0	51.0	26.0	25.2	1.03	20.9	24.6	22.3
9½ "	52.2	61.0	52.2	26.4	25.8	1.02	20.9	25.0	22.5
10 "	53.2	64.3	53.4	26.8	26.4	1.02	21.0	25.3	22.8
10½ "	54.2	67.7	54.5	27.1	27.1	1.00	21.0	25.7	23.0
11 "	55.2	71.2	55.6	27.5	27.7	0.99	21.1	26.1	23.3
11½ "	56.2	74.7	56.7	27.9	28.3	0.99	21.2	26.6	23.6
12 "	57.1	78.3	57.9	28.3	28.8	0.98	21.2	27.0	23.9
12½ "	58.0	82.0	59.1	28.7	29.3	0.98	21.3	27.5	24.2
13 "	58.9	85.8	60.2	29.1	29.8	0.98	21.4	28.0	24.6
13½ "	59.8	89.8	61.3	29.5	30.3	0.97	21.5	28.6	25.0
14 "	60.7	92.0	61.9	29.9	30.8	0.97	21.6	29.1	25.4
14½ "	61.6	96.5	63.0	30.3	31.3	0.97	21.7	29.7	25.9
15 "	62.4	101.4	64.1	30.7	31.7	0.97	21.8	30.3	26.4
15½ "	63.2	103.9	64.7	31.1	32.1	0.97	21.9	31.0	26.8
16 "	64.0	109.0	65.8	31.5	32.5	0.07	22.0	31.7	27.2
16½ "	64.7	111.7	66.4	31.9	32.8	0.97	22.1	32.3	27.5
17 "	65.4	117.7	67.5	32.2	33.2	0.97	22.2	32.9	27.8
17½ "	66.0	121.0	68.1	32.5	33.5	0.97	22.3	33.3	28.0
18 "	66.6	124.4	68.6	32.8	33.8	0.97	22.4	33.7	28.2
18½ "	67.1	127.8	69.2	33.2	33.9	0.98	22.4	34.1	28.4
19 "	67.5	131.4	69.8	33.4	34.1	0.98	22.5	34.4	28.5
19½ "	67.8	135.0	70.4	33.6	34.2	0.98	22.5	34.6	28.6
20 "	68.0	135.0	70.4	33.7	34.3	0.98	22.5	34.7	28.7

* From Williams, R. H.: Textbook of Endocrinology, ed. 2, p. 588, Philadelphia, Saunders.

dry or sweating; calm or nervous; intelligent or mentally retarded.

Note also any features suggestive of recognized syndromes such as cretinism, mongolism, etc.

2. Stature and proportions

Height: note deviation from average for age

Ratio between upper and lower measurements and deviation from normal

Type of body build: width of shoulders, depth of chest, width of hips, depth of pelvis; size of abdomen, flat or protuberant; proportions of extremities to trunk

Head and face: size and shape of head, fontanelle; general configuration of face, development of jaw; eyes, spacing, palpebral fissures; nose, width, height of bridge, length; mouth, lips, palate

Neck: length, webbing

Spine: normal or abnormal curves or length

Extremities: proportions of segments; size and shape of hands and feet, length of fingers and toes, development of nails

3. Muscle structure and development

4. Adipose tissue: normal, deficient or excessive; type of distribution

5. Skin: color, pigmentation, striae, temperature, texture, acne

6. Hair: scalp, axillary, pubic and general body hair, beard

7. Teeth: note which deciduous or permanent teeth are present, also size of teeth, spacing, any abnormal arrangement

8. Sex development: size of breasts, amount of pubic and axillary hair, development of genitalia, voice changes

STANDARDS FOR COMPARISON
STATURAL GROWTH

Height and Body Proportions. As suggested by Wilkins, seven simple measurements are sufficient, and complex anthropometric measurements are not necessary: (1) standing height; (2) span (from fingertip to fingertip); (3) lower segment, measured from the top of the symphysis pubis to the floor; (4) upper segment, derived by subtracting lower segment from total height; (5) circumference of head; (6) circumference of chest; (7) circumference of abdomen.

In Tables 2 and 3 are given average normal measurements for females and males from birth to age 20 years as compiled by Wilkins from data of Shelton and Engelbach.

Body proportions normally change as growth progresses. A convenient and clinically useful way to determine whether the length of the trunk and the extremities are normally proportionate is by use of the ratio of the upper measurement to the lower measurement. At birth this is approximately 1.7:1. The legs grow more rapidly than the trunk, so that by 10 or 11 years of age the upper and the lower segments become approximately equal and remain in approximate ratio of 1:1 thereafter.

Deviations from normal $U:L$ ratios may be seen in various conditions and thus be of assistance in diagnosis. Some examples are:

1. Hypothyroidism. There is delay in both growth and maturation of skeletal proportions, so the $U:L$ ratio remains high, revealing relative immaturity of proportions in relation to the patient's age.

2. In some hypogonadal (eunuchoid) persons of both sexes, the limiting influence of gonadal hormones on length of extremities is weak or delayed, permitting unusual growth in length of arms and legs. In such persons the $U:L$ ratio may be considerably less than 1, the lower measurement may exceed the upper by inches, and the span may exceed the height.

3. In achondroplasia, the arms and the legs are short, while the trunk and the head may be normal in size.

4. In conditions which affect the spine, limiting its growth or causing compression or collapse of vertebrae, the spine is shortened and the $U:L$ ratio may be less than normal for the age.

Velocity of Growth. The most rapid rate of growth is accomplished during the early months of fetal life. In general there is a decrease in the velocity of growth from the fourth month of fetal life until full adult size is reached and growth ceases. A study done 200 years ago by de Montbeillard upon his son (Fig. 7) remains one of the best and it, like subsequent longi-

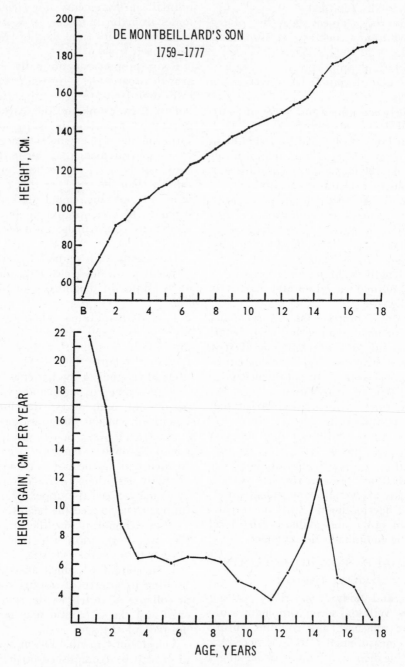

FIG. 7. Growth in height of de Montbeillard's son from birth to 18 years, 1759–1777. *(Top)* distance curve, height attained at each age; *(Bottom)* velocity curve, increments in height from year to year. (Data from Scammon, 1927, Amer. J. phys. Anthrop.) (Tanner, J. M.: Growth at Adolescence, Oxford, Blackwell)

tudinal growth records, shows clearly the decrease in velocity with two interruptions. At 6 to 8 years of age there is a mild "juvenile growth spurt," and at 13 to 15 years of age there is a true reversal when the marked "adolescent growth spurt" appears.

The adolescent spurt occurs in all normal children, but varies greatly in time of onset, intensity and duration. In boys, on the average, it begins at 12½ years of age and is over by 15 years of age. It is responsible for an average gain in height of about 8 in. (range 4 to 12 in.) and an average accompanying gain in weight of about 40 lbs. (range 15 to 65 lbs.). The *peak velocity* averages about 4 in. (10 cm.) per year, which is (it is rather surprising to note) the rate at which the boy was growing at age 2 years.

In girls the adolescent spurt begins about 2 years earlier than in boys, lasts on the average from ages 10½ to 13, and is smaller in magnitude, the peak velocity averaging 3¼ in. (8 cm.) per year. In girls the average gain in height is about 6 inches, in weight about 23 lbs. The sex difference is shown in Figure 8, giving velocity growth curves for girls and boys.

The difference in height between adult men and women is largely the result of the adolescent spurt, since prior to it, boys and girls average practically the same in height.

In gonadal agenesis there is no adolescence and therefore no adolescent growth spurt; the height eventually attained is consequently less than average by 6 or 8 inches, the extent of the normal spurt.

THE GENERAL GROWTH CURVE applies to the skeleton as a whole and also to the muscles and the viscera in the thorax and

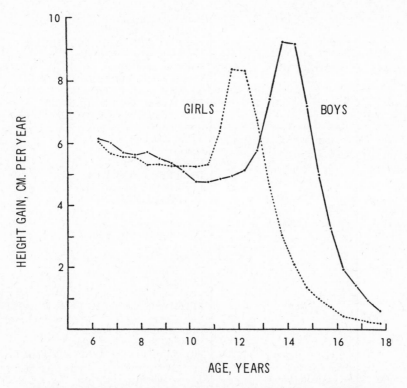

FIG. 8. Adolescent spurt in height growth for girls and boys. The curves are from subjects who have their peak velocities during the modal years 12 to 13 for girls, and 14 to 15 for boys. (Actual mean increments, each plotted at center of its ½-year period. Data from Shuttleworth, 1939, Tables 23 and 32) (Tanner, J. M.: Growth at Adolescence, Oxford, Blackwell)

TABLE 4. NORMAL OSSEOUS DEVELOPMENT (1 TO 5 YEARS*†)

AGE	JOINT	CENTERS PRESENT
At birth	Knee (Lat.)	DISTAL EPIPHYSIS OF FEMUR PROXIMAL EPIPHYSIS OF TIBIA
	Ankle (Lat.)	TALUS, CUBOID CALCANEUS
At 1 year	Wrist (AP)	CAPITATE HAMATE DISTAL EPIPHYSIS OF RADIUS
	Shoulder (AP)	EPIPHYSIS OF HEAD OF HUMERUS
	Hip (AP)	EPIPHYSIS OF HEAD OF FEMUR
	Ankle (Lat.)	Talus, Cuboid Calcaneus EXTERNAL CUNEIFORM DISTAL EPIPHYSIS OF TIBIA
At 2 years	Shoulder (AP)	Epiphysis of Head of Humerus GREAT TUBEROSITY OF HUMERUS
	Elbow (AP)	CAPITELLUM OF HUMERUS
	Ankle (Lat.)	Talus, Cuboid Calcaneus External Cuneiform Distal Epiphysis of Tibia DISTAL EPIPHYSIS OF FIBULA
At 3 years	Wrist (AP)	Capitate, Hamate Distal Epiphysis of Radius TRIQUETRUM (TRIANGULARIS) EPIPHYSES OF PHALANGES EPIPHYSES OF METACARPALS
	Ankle (AP)	Talus, Cuboid Calcaneus External Cuneiform Distal Epiphysis of Tibia EPIPHYSES OF METATARSALS INTERNAL CUNEIFORM
At 4 years	Wrist (AP)	Capitate, Hamate Distal Epiphysis of Radius Triquetrum Epiphyses of Phalanges Epiphyses of Metacarpals LUNATE
	Hip (AP)	EPIPHYSIS OF GREAT TROCHANTER
	Knee (Lat.)	Distal Epiphysis of Femur Proximal Epiphysis of Tibia PROXIMAL EPIPHYSIS OF FIBULA
	Ankle (Lat.)	Talus, Cuboid Calcaneus External Cuneiform Distal Epiphysis of Tibia Distal Epiphysis of Fibula Epiphyses of Metatarsals Internal Cuneiform MIDDLE CUNEIFORM, NAVICULAR

TABLE 4 (*Continued*). NORMAL OSSEOUS DEVELOPMENT (5 TO 15 YEARS)

AGE	JOINT	CENTERS PRESENT†
At 5 years	Wrist (AP)	Capitate, Hamate Distal Epiphysis of Radius Triquetrum Epiphyses of Phalanges Epiphyses of Metacarpals Lunate MULTANGULUM MAJUS (TRAPEZIUM) NAVICULAR (SCAPHOID)
	Elbow (AP)	PROXIMAL EPIPHYSIS OF RADIUS
	Knee	Distal Epiphysis of Femur Distal Epiphysis of Tibia Distal Epiphysis of Fibula PATELLA

AGE		JOINT	APPEARANCE OF	UNION OF
6 years		Wrist (AP)	Multangulum minus (trapezoid); Distal epiphysis of ulna	
		Elbow (AP)	Internal condyle of humerus	
		Shoulder (AP)		Head and greater tuberosity of humerus
7 years		Hip (AP)		Ischium and pubis
8 years		Knee (AP)	Depression for semilunar cartilage	
		Ankle (Lat.)	Epiphysis of calcaneus	
9 years		Elbow (Lat.)	Trochlea of humerus; olecranon (chief center)	
10 years		Wrist (AP)	Pisiform	
		Hip (AP)	Epiphysis of lesser trochanter of femur	
11 years		Elbow (AP)	External condyle of humerus	
		Knee (Lat.)	Tubercle of tibia	
12 years		Elbow (AP)		Trochlea and capitellum of humerus
Boys	Girls			
14 years	13–14 years	Elbow (Lat.)		Olecranon with ulna
		Hip		Primary centers of os coxae at acetabulum
		Ankle (Lat.)		Epiphysis of calcaneus
15 years	14–15 years	Elbow (AP)		Proximal epiphysis of radius
		Hip (AP)		Trochanter and head of femur

TABLE 4 (*Continued*). NORMAL OSSEOUS DEVELOPMENT (15-16 TO 20 YEARS)

AGE		JOINT	APPEARANCE OF	UNION OF
BOYS	GIRLS			
16 years	15 years	Wrist (AP)		Epiphyses of metacarpals and phalanges
		Ankle (AP)		Epiphyses of metatarsals and phalanges
		Shoulder	Coracoid and acromion	
		Hip	Secondary centers of os coxae	
17 years	16 years	Hip	Crest of ilium	
		Shoulder	Angle of scapula	Coracoid
18–19 years	17 years	Wrist (AP)		Distal epiphyses of radius and ulna
		Ankle (AP)		Distal epiphyses of tibia and fibula
		Shoulder (AP)	Sternal end of clavicle	Acromion
19–20 years	18 years	Wrist (AP)		Distal epiphysis of radius Distal epiphysis of ulna
		Shoulder (AP)		Head of humerus Greater tuberosity of humerus
		Knee (AP)		Distal epiphysis of femur Proximal epiphysis of tibia Proximal epiphysis of fibula

* Compiled from Shelton, Stuart and other sources. (From Williams, R. H.: Textbook of Endocrinology, ed. 2, p. 591, Philadelphia, Saunders.)

† Those that have newly appeared are printed in capitals.

the abdomen. However, certain parts of the body have distinctive growth curves which do not follow the general pattern of slow gain to maturity at age 18 or 20 (upper curve, Fig. 7).

Tissues showing different curves are:

1. Central nervous system. The brain, the spinal cord, the eye, the auditory mechanism, etc., grow very rapidly in early life, reaching almost their maximum size within a few years as does the head (but not the face).

2. Lymphoid tissues, including thymus, tonsils, adenoids, etc., normally reach their peak size at puberty, then decline to adult levels.

3. Reproductive tissues (gonads and accessory organs) remain infantile and quiescent until puberty, when growth suddenly begins and continues rapidly through adolescence. The special growth changes accompanying *pregnancy* in the uterus, the vagina, the breasts and elsewhere apparently are due to hormonal effects from pituitary and placenta.

HEAD AND FACE. The head and the face are of particular interest; it is a matter of common observation that the changes of adolescence are mirrored in the face, and that maturation into adult status is reflected by facial changes. Head length, breadth and circumference reach about 96 per cent of adult values at 10 years of age. However, there is an acceleration of slight degree in head length and breadth at adolescence with peak increments of only about 2 mm. a year.

Changes in the face are of greater degree, especially in the mandible. In childhood the mandible lags behind the rest of the face in development; at adolescence the mandible grows the fastest. Between the ages of 12 and 20, only about 6 per cent of mature growth remains to be completed in the cranial base, but about 25 per cent of the ramus height of the mandible is accomplished in this period. The body of the mandible also accelerates in anteroposterior length and in depth from lower incisor teeth to point of chin. The maxilla becomes more prominent also, so altogether, prognathism of upper and lower jaws increases, but the lower more than the upper. At adolescence there is also a distinct acceleration of nose growth, especially in the anteroposterior dimension. There is a definite but subtle change in facial muscle size and subcutaneous tissue distribution in the face with unmistakable maturation in the facial expression. Changes similar to those occurring at normal adolescence are seen with precocious puberty in boys and girls. Failure of facial maturation is seen in *hypogonadism* and maturation occurs when sex hormones are supplied in treatment.

With deficient *growth hormone,* the facial features remain infantile. With excessive growth hormone, the jaw is heavy, the nose and the ears large, the teeth spaced, the lips and the soft tissues of face thickened. These changes may be only of mild degree in gigantism, but become striking in acromegaly.

In the *cretin* the bridge of the nose remains flat, broad and undeveloped as in the newborn, so the eyes seem widely spaced, and the nose is short and retroussé. The cretin may also have thickened rough skin but he *looks young,* at 2 years of age like an infant of 4 or 5 months, or at 6 years of age like a child of 2 years.

In *gonadal agenesis* there is maturation of the features to some degree in spite of the failure of development of other characteristics of adolescence. At adult age the subject has a face that seems half or partially mature, the jaw and chin remain poorly developed and the body appears to be that of a prepubertal female.

In *progeria* the face becomes prematurely senile, with features sunken and drawn and nose thin and beaklike.

In *primordial dwarfism* there is normal facial maturation, just as there is normal sex maturation.

Osseous Development. The stage of osseous development or the "bone age" may be determined by roentgenograms of the epiphyseal centers. There may be considerable scattering of apparent bone age in different centers, therefore it is desirable to obtain roentgenograms of several centers rather than to rely upon the development of a single group of bones, for example, those of hand and wrist. The tables compiled by Shelton (Table 4) permit fairly accurate estimation by roentgenograms of the bone age of any person.

There is a fairly wide range of rate of ossification in normal persons and an absolute norm cannot be given. As emphasized by Shelton and Skeels, the careful tabulations of Todd are useful but must not be taken to mean that minor variations of months in bone development are clinically significant. It is now generally agreed, even by Todd's successors, Greulich and Pyle, that variations of plus or minus one year in the carpal index are within the range of normal.

From birth to 4 years of age the development of the carpal centers is essentially the same for both sexes. From the ages of 4 to 10, girls are about 6 months to a year ahead of boys. During puberty, girls gain still more in osseous development so that at 13 years of age girls are about 2 years ahead of their masculine contemporaries.

Union of the epiphyses and skeletal maturation begins a year or two earlier in girls, and growth in the length of the bones is terminated earlier. Union of the distal epiphysis of the femur, for example, one of the last to close, is complete in the average girl at 18 years of age, but not in the average boy until 20 years of age. This *longer growth period* in males is another factor added to the *greater growth spurt at adolescence* which explains the greater average height of males.

The most severe retardation of carpal maturation and epiphyseal development is seen in cretins and in patients with juve-

TABLE 5. CHRONOLOGY OF DENTITION*

Tooth			First Evidence of Calcification	Crown Completed	Eruption	Root Completed	Root Resorption Begins
	Name	Number					
Deciduous Teeth	Lower central incisors	L. I	5th month in utero	4 mos.	6–8 mos.	1½–2 yrs.	5–6 yrs.
	Upper incisors	U.I & II	5th month in utero	5 mos.	8–10 mos.	1½–2 yrs.	5–6 yrs.
	Lower lateral incisors	L. II	5th month in utero	5 mos.	10–14 mos.	1½–2 yrs.	5–6 yrs.
	Canines (cuspids)	III	6th month in utero	9 mos.	16–20 mos.	2½–3 yrs.	6–7 yrs.
	First molars	IV	5th month in utero	6 mos.	12–16 mos.	2–2½ yrs.	4–5 yrs.
	Second molars	V	6th month in utero	10–12 mos.	20–30 mos.	3 yrs.	4–5 yrs.
Permanent Teeth	Upper Jaw						
	Central incisor	1	3–4 mos.	4–5 yrs.	7–8 yrs.	10 yrs.	
	Lateral incisor	2	1 yr.	4–5 yrs.	8–9 yrs.	11 yrs.	
	Canine (cuspid)	3	4–5 mos.	6–7 yrs.	11–12 yrs.	13–15 yrs.	
	First bicuspid	4	1½–1¾ yrs.	5–6 yrs.	10–11 yrs.	12–13 yrs.	
	Second bicuspid	5	2–2¼ yrs.	6–7 yrs.	10–12 yrs.	12–14 yrs.	
	First molar	6	At birth	2½–3 yrs.	6–7 yrs.	0–10 yrs.	
	Second molar	7	2½–3 yrs.	7–8 yrs.	12–14 yrs.	14–16 yrs.	
	Third molar	8	7–9 yrs.	12–16 yrs.	17–30 yrs.	18–25 yrs.	
	Lower Jaw						
	Central incisor	1	3–4 mos.	4–5 yrs.	6–7 yrs.	9 yrs.	
	Lateral incisor	2	3–4 mos.	4–5 yrs.	7–8 yrs.	10 yrs.	
	Canine (cuspid)	3	4–5 mos.	6–7 yrs.	10–11 yrs.	12–14 yrs.	
	First bicuspid	4	1¾–2 yrs.	5–6 yrs.	10–12 yrs.	12–13 yrs.	
	Second bicuspid	5	2¼–2½ yrs.	6–7 yrs.	11–12 yrs.	13–14 yrs.	
	First molar	6	At birth	2½–3 yrs.	6–7 yrs.	9–10 yrs.	
	Second molar	7	2½–3 yrs.	7–8 yrs.	12–13 yrs.	14–15 yrs.	
	Third molar	8	8–10 yrs.	12–16 yrs.	17–30 yrs.	18–25 yrs.	

*Holt, and McIntosh: Pediatrics, ed. 12, New York, Appleton-Century-Crofts.

nile myxedema, but less marked degrees of retardation of osseous development are observed also in pituitary and nutritional growth deficiencies. Therefore carpal development may be considered a physiologic time clock, but retardation of bone age does not indicate the etiology of such a deficiency.

Osseous abnormalities should be sought in roentgenograms of bones and epiphyses. When *hypothyroidism* exists during the period when the cartilages usually undergo ossification, "stippled epiphyses" may be formed. These changes must be distinguished from those of *osteochondritis deformans,* which is a degenerative process occurring in an epiphysis previously normally formed.

In *chondrodystrophy* the epiphyses may be irregular and show multiple centers of ossification, but usually the metaphyses of the long bones are so misshapen that it is easy to distinguish it from hypothyroid epiphyseal dysgenesis. Occasionally the changes of chondrodystrophy are confined to the epiphyses, and distinction can only be made by failure to respond to thyroid therapy.

Rickets and other nutritional and metabolic disorders may be identified by characteristic bone changes.

DENTAL DEVELOPMENT

The development and growth of the teeth are affected chiefly by the same factors controlling other types of skeletal maturation. Abnormalities in the formation of the tooth buds as revealed by roentgenography are probably more significant than eruption of teeth (which may depend upon the growth of the alveolar process). When complete growth studies are done, both formation of tooth buds and time of eruption of teeth should be noted. Table 5, from Holt and McIntosh, gives the chronology of dentition, which should be correlated with the chronology of skeletal development, sex development, etc.

MENTAL DEVELOPMENT

Mental development can be judged fairly accurately in the average child by obtaining records of performance in school work and comparing with the average for age. In situations requiring more accurate and detailed assessment, evaluation by a trained psychologist or psychiatrist may be indicated, with use of special psychometric tests such as the Wechsler (Adults' and Children's Scales), the Stanford-Binet (children over 2 years) and the Cattell (infants) tests. Results may be expressed as the intelligence quotient (I.Q.), or as the mental age, to compare with height age, bone age and chronological age.

Mental Subnormality may be separated into its two major components, retardation and deficiency. Mental *deficiency* includes conditions in which "the mental capacities themselves are diminished as a result of pathological causes, as opposed to environmental causes which may lead to mental *retardation*." The word retardation implies the influence of possibly removable or reversible conditions. It is important to remember that hereditary, congenital or organic brain disease may result in various degrees of mental functional impairment which may be further retarded by adverse environmental factors; and also that mental deficiency is only one constituent of organic brain disease—that it is frequently associated with other disabilities in the continuum such as cerebral palsy and epilepsy.[11]

In various countries studies have revealed that from 1 to 4 per cent of persons are considered educationally subnormal and a further 6 to 9 per cent are so dull as to require special assistance within the normal school system. Modern medicine with antibiotics and improved care for premature infants plays a major role in increasing the survival rate of those with brain damage. About 40,000 infants weighing 1,500 Gm.

or less at birth are born in the United States every year. Approximately 40 per cent, or 16,000, now survive, and 20 per cent of these survivors are mentally defective.

Hereditary and Congenital Mental Deficiency. The hereditary and congenital disorders which interfere with growth and development often are also associated with mental deficiency.

GENETIC DISORDERS. Two types may be distinguished:

1. Genetically transmitted metabolic errors
2. Chromosomal aberrations.

Although some 300 diseases due to genetically transmitted errors of metabolism have been recognized, only a few of these are associated with mental deficiency and the incidence of any individual syndrome is extremely small. Among these are: phenylketonuria, Hartnup disease, Wilson's disease (hepatolenticular degeneration), galactosemia, idiopathic hypoglycemia, sucrosuria, lipochondrodystrophy, infantile amaurosis, Niemann-Pick disease, the infantile form of Gaucher's disease, and nonendemic goitrous cretinism.

Among chromosomal aberrations with mental deficiency the Klinefelter 47XXY syndrome is frequent. The incidence is about 0.26 per cent among newborn boys. This syndrome accounts for about 0.75 per cent of institutionalized male mental defectives.

The most common chromosomal disorder in mentally defective females is the so-called "superfemale" (preferably "metafemale") or XXX syndrome. It is estimated that the syndrome appears in less than 0.1 per cent of all female births, but accounts for about 0.7 per cent of institutionalized female mental defectives.

In the syndrome of gonadal agenesis (45XO, Turner's syndrome) there is usually no associated mental deficiency.

In mongolism (47 trisomy-21 syndrome) there is severe mental deficiency. The incidence is about 3 per 1,000 births, with a striking relationship to age of the mother. In the maternal age group of 20 to 24 years, the incidence is one mongoloid per 3,500 births; for the maternal age group

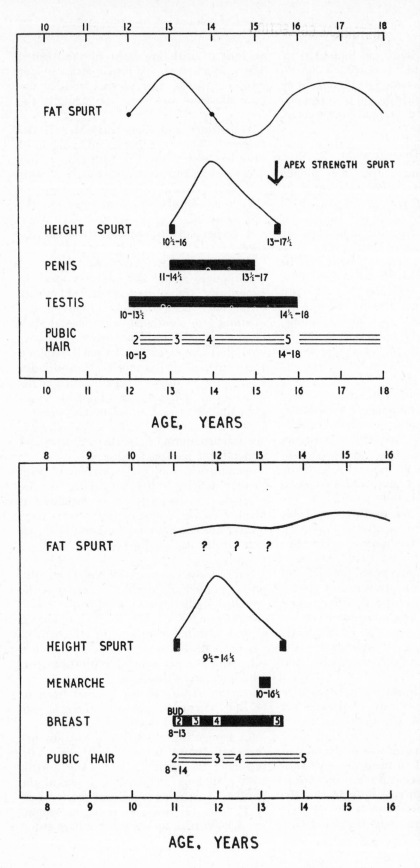

FIG. 9. Diagram of sequence of events in adolescence in boys. An average boy is represented; the range of ages within which each event charted may begin and end is given by the figures placed directly below its start and finish. (Tanner, J. M.: Growth at Adolescence, ed. 2, Oxford, Blackwell)

FIG. 10. Diagram of sequence of events at adolescence in girls. An average girl is represented; the range of ages within which some of the events may occur is given by the figures placed directly below them. (Tanner, J. M.: Growth at Adolescence, Oxford, Blackwell)

of 40 to 44 years, one per 70 births; for the group over 45, one per 38 births. In the 1st year patients with mongolism constitute about 12.5 per cent of the 1.5 per cent of infants who are defective. Mortality in mongolism is extremely high, only about 40 per cent surviving for 5 years. About 40 per cent fail to live 1 month and less than 50 per cent survive the 1st year.

PRENATAL FACTORS. Adverse extrinsic influences which may operate prenatally and which may affect the fetus, causing mental deficiency and possibly other congenital disturbances in growth and development, include:

1. Nutritional disorders
2. Mechanical factors
3. Drugs, chemicals and toxins
4. Hormones
5. Infections (syphilis, rubella, febrile illness, etc.)
6. Immunologic factors
7. Irradiation
8. Anoxia
9. Prematurity of birth.[30]

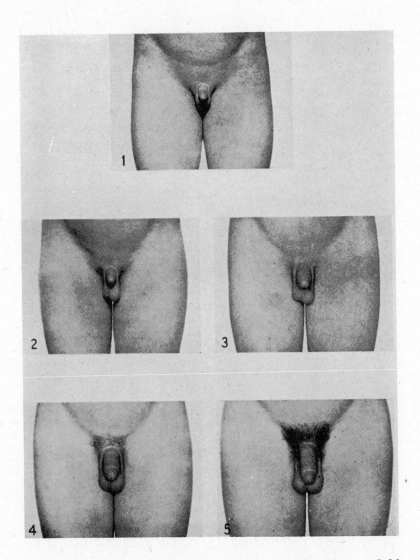

FIG. 11. Standards for genitalia maturity ratings in boys. (Tanner, J. M.: Growth at Adolescence, Oxford, Blackwell)

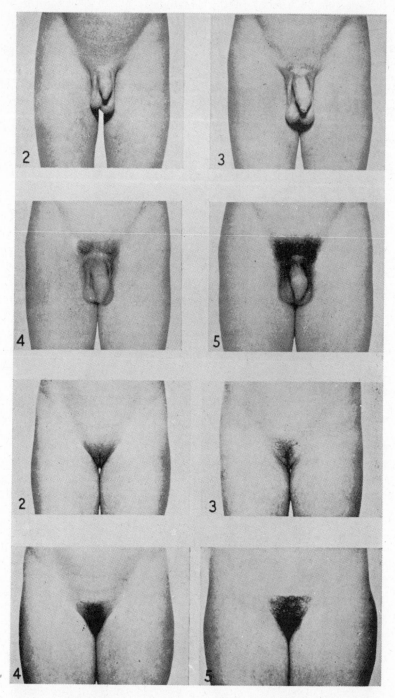

FIG. 12. Standards for pubic hair ratings in boys and girls. (Tanner
J. M.: Growth at Adolescence, Oxford, Blackwell)

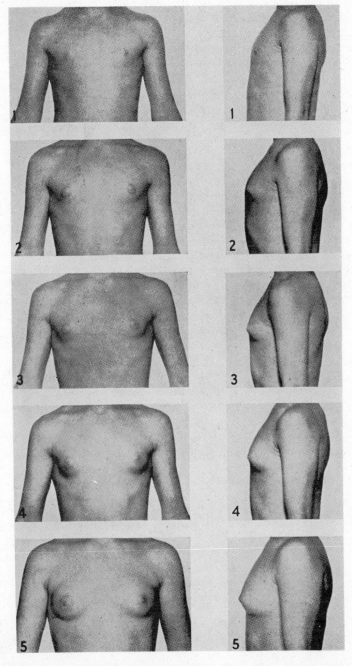

FIG. 13. Standards for breast development ratings during adolescence. (Tanner, J. M.: Growth at Adolescence, Oxford, Blackwell)

SEXUAL DEVELOPMENT

Many studies have shown that there is wide variation in the time when sex development begins. Nevertheless there is a fairly constant pattern, the sequences of which are more regular than the time of onset. The *average normal* time of occurrence and sequence of appearance of sex characteristics as compiled by Seckel is shown in Table 6.

The physician will find it valuable to train himself to observe and record the relative degrees of development of sex organs and secondary sexual characteristics. Fairly accurate quantitative methods are available: one may note pubic hair, development of genitalia or development of breasts on a scale of 1 to 5. (See Figs. 9, 10, 11, 12 and 13.)

When possible one should also make measurements of breasts, penis, testes, etc., which may be compared with norms, and with subsequent measurements of the same person to determine changes (Fig. 14).

In the female, measurements may be made of breasts and areolae; and relative development may be noted of the labia, the clitoris and the vagina; one attempts to palpate uterus and ovaries and judge their size and maturity.

In the male, development of scrotum is noted, testes measured, penis length and circumference measured and prostate is palpated, voice maturity is judged.

In both sexes location and amount of sex hair is noted and presence and amount of seborrhea or acne.

There must be a clear distinction between the *average* age of adolescence and the *normal* age of adolescence. The average beginning of pubertal change in boys is noted at age 10 to 11, but many perfectly normal boys begin at age 9, and some perfectly normal boys do not begin until age 16 or 17. The range of normal is, therefore, seen to be quite wide. For example, Figure 15 shows that stage 4 of pubescence (according to the scale of Fig. 14) is reached

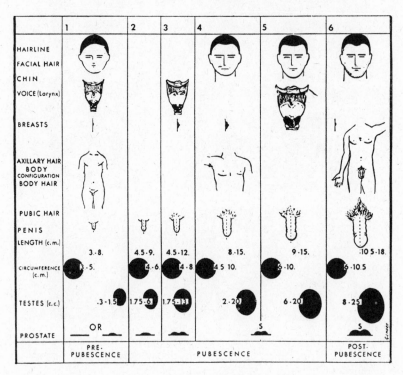

FIG. 14. Stages of sexual development and maturation. (Schonfeld, Wm. A.: Primary and secondary sexual characteristics, Am. J. Dis. Child. 65:535)

TABLE 6. AVERAGE APPROXIMATE AGE AND SEQUENCE OF
APPEARANCE OF SEXUAL CHARACTERISTICS IN BOTH SEXES*

AGE, YEARS	BOYS	GIRLS
9–10		Growth of bony pelvis. Budding of nipples
10–11	First growth of testes and penis	Budding of breasts. Pubic hair
11–12	Prostatic activity	Changes in vaginal epithelium and the smear. Growth of external and internal genitalia
12–13	Pubic hair	Pigmentation of nipples. Mammae filling in
13–14	Rapid growth of testes and penis. Subareolar node of nipples	Axillary hair. Menarche (average 13½ yrs., range 9–17 yrs.). Menstruation may be anovulatory for first few years
14–15	Axillary hair. Down on upper lip. Voice change	Earliest normal pregnancies
15–16	Mature spermatozoa (average 15 yrs., range 11¼–17 yrs.)	Acne. Deepening of voice
16–17	Facial and body hair. Acne	Arrest of skeletal growth
21	Arrest of skeletal growth	

* From Wilkins, L.: The Diagnosis and Treatment of Endocrine Disorders in Childhood and Adolescence, Springfield, Thomas (after Seckel).

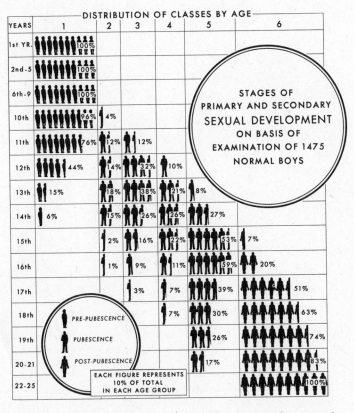

FIG. 15. (Schonfeld, Wm. A.: Primary and secondary sexual characteristics, Am. J. Dis. Child. 65:535)

by 10 per cent of *normal* boys during the 12th year, 21 per cent during the 13th year, 26 per cent during the 14th year, 22 per cent during the 15th year and 11 per cent during the 16th year. There remain 14 per cent of *normal* boys who have not reached this stage by the 16th birthday, but attain it during the next year or two.

Similarly, normal girls may show pubescent changes at 8 years of age, or not until age 17, and menses may begin normally anytime from 9 to 17 years of age, but the average menarche appears at 13½ years of age.

METHODS OF RECORDING STAGES AND CHANGES IN GROWTH AND DEVELOPMENT

Very useful charts have been devised by Burgess (Fig. 16) showing the growth of children, giving the mean height and the percentile deviations from this mean at different ages. For example, a boy 11 years old may be found to be 53 in. tall. By plotting on the chart, we find that average height for age 11 is 55 in. and that only 25 per cent of boys his age are as short as he. Subsequent measurements of height may be plotted on the chart and the influence of treatment may be noted, with any changes in the percentile grouping.

Not only height deviations from normal but the status and progressive changes in the patient's bone age, mental age and other respects may be recorded on a simple chart suggested by Wilkins (Fig. 17). Such a method permits comparison of the rate of statural growth with other types of development. For this purpose one compares height age with bone age and mental age. Sexual age and dental age also could be recorded and followed chronologically, and all the chief elements of growth and development visualized.

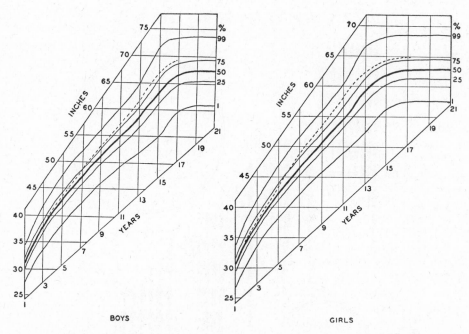

BOYS   GIRLS

Fig. 16. Charts adapted from M. A. Burgess show height of American boys and girls at various ages, the horizontal lines being inches and the vertical lines years. The diagonal curves represent percentile distributions in the population. The 50 percentile curve represents the mean or average. The dotted curves show the way the growth of a particular child may be charted and illustrate the fact that a normal child may frequently pass from one channel to another. (Wilkins, L.: The Diagnosis and Treatment of Endocrine Disorders in Childhood and Adolescence, Springfield, Thomas)

PATHOLOGIC PHYSIOLOGY OF GROWTH DISORDERS

There are many types of disease and some genetic or hereditary conditions which result in small stature.

The various clinical causes of subnormal growth are given in Table 7. Analysis of the various etiologic agents shown in the table reveals that each of them operates through one or more of 4 basic influences which control growth: (1) genetic, (2) central nervous system, (3) nutritional, (4) endocrine.

Nutritional inadequacy may (1) directly retard growth through lack of calories, certain minerals or vitamins, or protein; or (2) indirectly retard growth, since malnutrition may impair hormone function and thus secondarily lead to stunted growth. Malnutrition if prolonged may impair pituitary function. Diets deficient in protein decrease the synthesis of pituitary hormones. Microscopic examination of the pituitary in malnourished persons has revealed atrophy and degenerative lesions. The adrenal glands in malnourished persons are smaller than normal and show evidence of lipid depletion. In malnutrition the excretion of 17-ketosteroids is abnormally low. Starvation results in decreased secretion of gonadotropic hormones and signs of sex failure. Examination of the ovaries of chronically malnourished women has revealed them to be atrophic. The secretion of pituitary thyrotropic hormone, as well as that of the gonadotropic factor, apparently is diminished also by malnutrition, as the thyroid gland becomes atrophied and involuted.

Experimental studies reveal lack of response of animals to growth hormone who lack either calories, protein or certain vitamins. Further discussion of the many important interrelationships between nutrition and growth is given in the excellent reviews by Ralli and Dumm,[14] and by Tanner.[22]

ENDOCRINE INFLUENCES ON GROWTH

Four glands of internal secretion are concerned primarily in the regulation of growth: the pituitary, the thyroid, the gonads and the adrenal cortex.

The growth hormone of the anterior lobe of the pituitary gland is responsible for growth of the skeleton, the muscles and the viscera.

Pituitary gonadotropic hormones initiate and regulate growth and differentiation of the gonads.

The sex hormones (androgen and estrogen) control the growth and the develop-

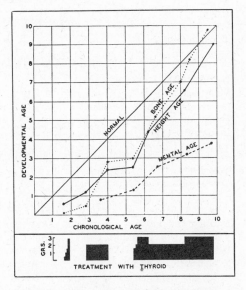

Fig. 17. Chart illustrates method of following and comparing growth and development. Chronologic age is plotted horizontally and developmental age vertically. The patient's "height age" indicates that he has the height of an average child of the same sex of the age specified. Such a chart permits a comparison of the rate of growth with that of osseous and mental development.

The case shown is a cretin whose thyroid medication was omitted during two periods because of failure of the parents to cooperate. The resulting retardation in growth and development are shown. By this method of charting, inadequate treatment sometimes is detected by a lag in growth and development, even when other signs of deficiency are not obvious. (Wilkins, L.: The Diagnosis and Treatment of Endocrine Disorders in Childhood and Adolescence, Springfield, Thomas)

TABLE 7. ETIOLOGIC CLASSIFICATION OF SUBNORMAL GROWTH*

I. GENETICALLY DETERMINED PURE GROWTH DEFICIENCY

A. PRIMORDIAL DWARFISM—PYGMIES   B. NORMAL SMALL-STATURED PERSONS

II. GENETIC DISORDERS WITH GROWTH DEFICIENCY PLUS OTHER SYSTEMIC DEFECTS

A. GONADAL APLASIA   C. MULTIPLE ANOMALIES
B. MONGOLISM

III. GENETIC SKELETAL DISORDERS

A. ACHONDROPLASIA   C. CLEIDOCRANIAL DYSOSTOSIS
B. OSTEOGENESIS IMPERFECTA

IV. INHERITED METABOLIC DISEASES
(See Fig. 2)

V. ACQUIRED SKELETAL DISEASE

A. TUBERCULOSIS   B. JUVENILE OSTEOCHONDRITIS (SCHEUERMANN'S DISEASE)

VI. PRENATAL (INTRAUTERINE) DISORDERS

A. NUTRITIONAL   F. IMMUNOLOGIC
B. MECHANICAL   G. IRRADIATION
C. DRUGS, CHEMICALS, TOXINS   H. ANOXIA
D. HORMONES   I. PREMATURITY
E. INFECTIONS (SYPHILIS, RUBELLA, ETC.)

VII. ANOMALIES OF CARDIOVASCULAR AND RENAL SYSTEMS

A. CONGENITAL HEART DISEASE   C. FIBROCYSTIC PULMONARY DISEASE
B. CONGENITAL POLYCYSTIC KIDNEYS

VIII. NUTRITIONAL DISTURBANCES

A. INADEQUATE FOOD, VITAMIN, AND MINERAL INTAKE
1. Starvation and mixed dietary deficiencies
2. Anorexia nervosa
3. Rickets

B. INADEQUATE ABSORPTION AND UTILIZATION OF ESSENTIAL NUTRIENTS
1. Achylia gastrica
2. Sprue
3. Cystic fibrosis of pancreas
4. Celiac disease
5. Hepatic cirrhosis and other chronic liver disease
6. Diabetes mellitus

C. DEFICIENCIES ASSOCIATED WITH CHRONIC INFECTIONS AND OTHER DISEASES INCREASING CATABOLISM
1. Tuberculosis
2. Intestinal parasites
3. Chronic osteomyelitis
4. Malignancies
5. Malaria
6. Syphilis
7. Bronchial asthma

IX. ENDOCRINE DISEASES

A. DEFICIENCY OF INTERNAL SECRETIONS
1. Anterior pituitary somatotropic deficiency
2. Cretinism and juvenile hypothyroidism
3. Diabetes mellitus (causes defective utilization of nutrients)

B. EXCESSIVE OR PREMATURE SECRETION OF HORMONES PRODUCING PRECOCIOUS EPIPHYSEAL UNION
1. Constitutional and neurogenic pubertas praecox
2. Precocious puberty associated with polyostotic fibrous dysplasia (Albright's syndrome)
3. Macrogenitosomia praecox due to adrenal tumor or hyperplasia (adrenogenital syndrome, Cushing's syndrome)
4. Interstitial cell tumor of testis
5. Granulosa cell or theca cell tumor of ovary

* Adapted from Shelton, E. K., and Skeels, R. F.: Ciba Clinical Symposia 3:184.

ment of the accessory organs of reproduction. Androgens promote protein anabolism and increase retention of the nitrogen, potassium, calcium and phosphorus needed for building protein tissues and bone. Estrogens have similar but generally less potent anabolic activity.

Pituitary thyrotropin is necessary to growth and activity of the thyroid gland.

The thyroid hormone is needed for all growth but specifically and especially for differentiation.

The adrenal cortex secretes, among other hormones, androgenic steroids which promote tissue anabolism. The relatively low biologic potency of the adrenal androgens makes them unimportant in males with normal testicular function. In the female, however, they are important to counteract the catabolic adrenal steroids.

The glucocorticosteroids of the adrenal are antianabolic or catabolic. They divert amino acids from the formation of protoplasm toward the synthesis of carbohydrate and fat. When present in greater than physiologic amounts and unbalanced by anabolic influences they may inhibit growth; such may be the case in Cushing's syndrome or during steroid therapy.

Pituitary Influence

In pituitary dwarfism there is infantilism, with failure of maturation as well as of growth. There is a concomitant inadequacy of all of the anterior pituitary hormones, including the thyrotropic, the gonadotropic and the adrenocorticotropic, not a lack of pure "somatotropin" alone. The pituitary dwarf has a symmetrical, normal body configuration but retains relatively infantile proportions and looks much younger than the actual age, tending to remain apparently the age of onset of the pituitary deficiency. Facial features are delicate, the skeleton gracile, the genitalia infantile. Obesity is absent unless there is associated hypothalamic damage. Intelligence is usually normal unless there is associated brain damage (from tumor, encephalitis, etc.).

In adult life complete pituitary failure results in Simmonds' disease, with signs of thyroid, gonadal and adrenocortical deficiency.

Excessive anterior pituitary activity with overproduction of pituitary growth hormone after epiphyseal closure results in acromegaly; before closure it is responsible for gigantism.

Pituitary somatotropins (growth hormones) are proteins. Those obtained from different animal species vary considerably in structure. The primate growth hormones are composed of only a single unbranched peptide chain, compared to the larger branched peptide chains of the bovine hormone. Simian or human growth hormones produce somatotropic effects in man, nonprimate hormones do not.

The human pituitary gland is quite rich in growth hormone. Assays have not revealed significant differences in the hormone content of glands of children, normal adults and elderly persons. Direct bioassays of human growth hormone in serum have been done for investigative purposes, but are impractical in clinical work. Measurement of a serum factor which promotes sulfate incorporation into chondroitin sulfate in cartilage in vitro has revealed that variations in the level of this factor are dependent upon the amount of growth hormone present. Growth hormone apparently promotes the formation of the component called sulfation factor. Assays by sulfation factor measurement reflect the activity of circulating growth hormone. Results of such assays reveal a range in growing children similar to that found in normal adults, low levels in hypopituitarism, high levels in acromegaly.[5]

Sulfation factor assays of growth hormone activity of human serum are low after hypophysectomy, in pituitary dwarfism and in Sheehan's syndrome.[5,38,39,40]

Almqvist *et al.*[40] found, among normal persons, low sulfation factor levels in early infancy and slightly higher values in children aged 8 to 15 years. No differences were observed between normal adults and aged persons.

After administration of human growth hormone the sera of pituitary dwarfs is found to exhibit higher levels of sulfation factor activity.

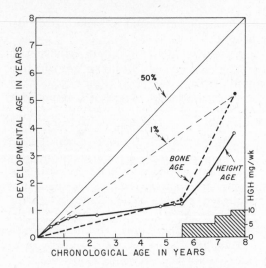

FIG. 18. Developmental chart for a boy with hypopituitary dwarfism. Before growth hormone treatment his height was below the first percentile curve. Note the excellent growth following human growth hormone administration. (From Daughaday and Parker: Pituitary in Disorders of Growth, Disease-a-Month, Chicago, Year Book)

Among short children there is an impressive number of low sulfation levels. However, it is as yet difficult to evaluate the accuracy of sulfation factor activity in the diagnosis of hyposomatotropism in the absence of clearly defined pituitary deficiency.[39]

Nearly all patients with low sulfation levels who were treated with human growth hormone showed good growth response. None of the patients with normal sulfation factor activity showed a good response to treatment with growth hormone.[38,39]

In 8 pituitary dwarfs treated by Daughaday and Parker for periods of 17 to 105 weeks, the growth rates rose to normal or above normal levels in all cases.[38] In 3 patients the annual growth rate was twice normal. In one boy started on treatment with human growth hormone at age 5½ years, growth in height has been at a rate of 4.7 in. per year for 2 years (Fig. 18). This response to human growth hormone is quite remarkable and convincing, revealing that patients previously growing at one fourth the normal rate can be stimu-

lated to grow at twice the normal rate, an acceleration of 800 per cent.

When rapid growth is induced by growth hormone the epiphyseal plates become wider. In pituitary giants and others who continue to grow beyond the usual age of growth cessation, the epiphyses may remain open. The ultimate dimensions of skeletal growth depend upon growth rate and duration of growth. The final length of the long bones is determined by the time of union of the epiphyses. The cause of the fusion and the relative roles of growth and gonadal hormones is incompletely understood. The tempting concept that epiphyseal union may occur when growth hormone secretion might suddenly decelerate at the end of the adolescent growth spurt is confounded by two observations: (1) no such decline in growth hormone secretion has yet been demonstrated; (2) in human hypopituitary dwarfs the epiphyses remain open. One might conclude therefore that gonadal hormones must bring about epiphyseal closure and thus terminate growth. Testosterone accelerates both epiphyseal ossification and fusion, and estrogen has been thought to act similarly. Recent observations have shown that estrogen may inhibit growth without hastening fusion.

Thyroid Influence

Thyroid hormone exerts its most important influence during the early months and years of life, when growth and development are most rapid. It promotes pure growth but is especially necessary for the processes of differentiation. Without the synergistic or the catalytic effect of the thyroid, the anabolic effects of the pituitary and the gonadal secretions are insufficient to produce a normally grown mature person, and the potentialities for normal development lie dormant within the organism. It seems that the thyroid hormone does not of itself produce growth, but when it is given in proper amounts to a thyroid-deficient organism, there is a rapid release of "stored-up" growth potential. This phenomenon is most spectacular when a severe cretin or a patient with childhood myxedema is given thyroid replacement therapy. Probably the pituitary must elaborate growth hormone as the result of such a restoration of normal metabolism because very little growth results from treatment of pituitary dwarfism with desiccated thyroid.

The degree of dwarfing and severity of other symptoms in cretinism or childhood myxedema depend upon (1) the age at onset of the thyroid deficiency, and (2) the degree of thyroid hormone lack. There may be slight or prolonged delay in walking, talking and teething. The infant or child is sleepy, clumsy, constipated. The skin is thick and dry, the tongue large and often protruding. Sexual development is delayed, and body proportions tend to be infantile. Bone age is less than chronologic age. Mentality may be impaired seriously.

Gonadal Hormone Influences

The ultimate dimensions reached by any person depend upon the rate at which growth occurs and the duration of growth. The gonadal hormones are concerned with the adolescent growth spurt and with bringing about the termination of linear growth. At puberty there is apparently not only a sudden increase in pituitary gonadotropic hormone activity but also in pituitary adrenotropic activity. In males there is an increase in testicular androgen, in females an estrogen increase from the ovaries and in both sexes an increase of adrenal androgen secretion. The androgen stimulates increase in height and promotes muscular development, tissue growth and weight gain. Androgens eventually promote epiphyseal closure. Estrogens act similarly but less potently. The sex hormones apparently act in two ways in bringing about cessation of linear growth: (1) directly to cause epiphyseal fusion; (2) indirectly by inhibition of the production of growth hormone by the pituitary.

It has been postulated that the adolescent growth spurt of the female results from the stimulus furnished by androgens from the adrenal cortex. It seems more likely that in both boys and girls the sudden acceleration of growth at adolescence is due to sex stimulus, because when such stimulus is lacking there is no spurt. The sex stimulus to somatic growth may result not only from a sudden rise in the secretion of gonadal hormone, but also from specific release at adolescence of the growth capacity inherent in all normal body cells by virtue of the presence in each cell of a second sex chromosome.

The primary stimulus which initiates adolescence arises in the central nervous system, is transmitted from hypothalamus to pituitary and thence to the endocrine system. In the human sexless, agonadal state, with the 45XO chromosomal aberration, the subject usually attains a height shorter than average by 6 to 8 inches (the growth increment normally occurring during adolescence). Such persons also remain less sturdy in bone and muscle development (less mesomorphic) than average. Two factors may be operative in producing the shorter stature and the lighter bones and muscles in gonadal aplasia (Turner's syndrome): (1) the direct genetic result of the lack of the second sex chromosome in all body cells; (2) lack of gonadal hormone.

Lack of the second sex chromosome is known to result in a number of anomalies other than failure of gonadal development. This important chromosome may carry powerful *growth-promoting genes* in addition to *genes determining sex*. Either the second large X chromosome or the small Y chromosome would seem to be necessary and adequate to support the growth surge during the 3 or 4 year period of normal adolescence. At this point one should recall that lack of sex hormones resulting from prepubertal castration results in reduced mesomorphism but does not limit linear growth. In regard to the genetics of growth it seems highly significant that the 45XO karyotype associated with gonadal aplasia is the only known human chromosomal configuration characterized by monosomy (absence of one of a pair of chromosomes normally present). Presumably absence of one chromosome of any one of the autosomic pairs is lethal.

Apparently loss (or gain) of sex chromosomes is relatively well tolerated. Perhaps this is at least partly because there is a normal variation in the number of the two kinds of sex chromosomes: a normal zygote may have 2 X's or only 1; it may have a

TABLE 8. DIAGNOSIS OF DWARFISM AND SEXUAL RETARDATION IN CHILDHOOD

DISEASE*	DEGREE OF DWARFING	MUSC. DEVEL.	FEATURES	CONGENITAL DEFECTS	SEXUAL DEVEL.	SKELETAL PROPORTIONS	EPIPHYSEAL OSSIFICATION & FUSION	BONE CHANGES	URINARY GONADOTROPINS	URINARY 17-KETOSTEROIDS
Gonadal aplasia	+	Good	Mature	Webbed neck; cubitus valgus; coarctation of aorta; skeletal abnormalities	Infantile	Normal boyish	Slightly retarded	Osteoporosis in older girls	Elevated	Normal or low
Pituitary infantilism	+ to +++	Asthenic	Immature	—	Infantile	Normal	Retarded +++	Osteoporosis	Low	Low
Eunuchoidism	Tall	Fair to poor	Immature but wrinkled	—	Infantile	Long extremities	Retarded ++	Osteoporosis and epiphysitis	Variable Elevated	Low
Hypothyroid	+++	Fair	Puffy	—	Delayed	Infantile	Retarded +++	Epiphysitis	Low	Low
Delayed adolescence	+	Good	Immature	—	Delayed but eventually normal	Normal	Slightly retarded	—	Low for age	Low for age
Primordial dwarfism	+ to +++	Good	Mature	—	Normal	Normal	Normal	—	Normal	Normal
Sexual precocity	Tall child; short adult	Herculean	Precociously mature	—	Precociously advanced	Mature	Prematurely advanced	—	Normal or high	Normal or high

*Other diseases to be considered are:
1. Bone diseases: (a) chondrodystrophy; (b) rickets (all types); (c) osteogenesis imperfecta; (d) disease of the spine; (e) dysostosis multiplex.
2. Nutritional or metabolic disorders: (a) celiac syndrome; (b) chronic renal disease; (c) hepatic insufficiency; (d) nutritional defects; (e) chronic infections.
3. Circulatory and respiratory disorders: (a) congenital malformations of the heart; (b) extensive chronic pulmonary disease.
4. Mongolism
5. Progeria
(From Gordan, G. S., and Lisser, H.: Endocrinology in Clinical Practice, p. 315, Chicago, Year Book Pub.)

single Y or none. It is XX or XY. Whatever the reason, the only form of monosomy yet recognized is sex-chromosome monosomy (single X or so-called XO).

One X is apparently necessary for human survival. No living human being with a YO sex chromosome constitution has as yet been discovered. Also, most cases with extra chromosomes have involved the sex chromosomes.[12]

Although the person with a single sex chromosome may survive, the subject is essentially neuter and has limited somatic growth, probably primarily because of the lack of the second sex chromosome rather than from the lack of gonadal hormones. Another reason for doubting that the lack of sex hormones leads to limitation of linear growth is that when a full complement of sex chromosomes are present and prepubertal castration occurs in either sex, linear growth continues and eunuchoid proportions develop, with long extremities, excessive height and late closure of the epiphyses.

Central Nervous System Influences

The anterior lobe of the pituitary appears to be under the control of the hypothalamus. Damage to the hypothalamus or of the adenohypophysis (from craniopharyngiomata, vascular lesions, etc.) may result in dwarfism. Usually the dwarfism is accompanied by other evidences of hypothalamic-pituitary derangement: hypogonadism or precocious puberty, diabetes insipidus, somnolence, obesity or emaciation, disturbed thermal regulation, etc. Headache and signs of impingement upon the optic nerves (visual field defects) may be present. The term *Fröhlich's syndrome* (which has been much misused) should be restricted to instances of dwarfism with obesity and hypogonadism.

When the hypothalamus has been damaged, the triggering mechanism which activates the pituitary may not be set into operation, and the changes of adolescence, with the usual growth spurt may not appear.

DISTINGUISHING FEATURES IN DEFICIENT GROWTH

Some types of dwarfism are not difficult to identify. Table 8 shows the chief distinguishing features for the types of dwarfism which present diagnostic problems.

Since the etiology of dwarfism is closely interrelated with the causes of sexual retardation, and deficiencies in both spheres are apt to occur together, it may be quite difficult to determine the cause of stunted growth before the late teens. The conditions especially hard to distinguish are (1) delayed adolescence, (2) hypopituitarism, (3) primordial dwarfism and (4) the syndrome of gonadal agenesis.

The majority of *children* with stunted growth are examples of simple *delayed growth and delayed adolescence,* who eventually grow and mature normally without treatment. The bone age and general development remain 1 to 4 years below normal but advance at the normal rate. When osseous development reaches about the 12 year level, sexual development begins and the adolescent growth spurt occurs. In these instances, epiphyseal union is late, so average or near normal height may be attained.

Dwarfs who mature sexually at about the average time (primordial) usually have normal bone age. Sexual development often begins when the bone age reaches 12 or 13 years. If one finds a bone age of 8, one does not expect signs of puberty for several years. If the patient is 12 years old, he is probably therefore not a primordial dwarf. If the bone age is 12 and the dwarfed patient's age is about 12, he is probably a primordial dwarf and one may anticipate signs of sexual maturation soon.

Persons with dwarfism associated with gonadal agenesis are apt to have other genetic defects (webbed neck, coarctation of the aorta, etc.). They are stocky, not gracile like pituitary dwarfs. The bone age is only slightly low in gonadal agenesis but is much retarded in pituitary deficiency. The former tend to have more pubic and more axillary hair and to be taller, reaching 52 to 58 in. The gonadotropin titer is high in gonadal aplasia (after age of expected puberty), and low in pituitary dwarfism.

RELATIVE FREQUENCY OF DIFFERENT TYPES OF SUBNORMAL GROWTH

Among 442 children with subnormal growth Wilkins[29] found almost 50 per cent

TABLE 9. RELATIVE FREQUENCY OF TYPES OF SUBNORMAL GROWTH*

TYPE	CASES	PER CENT
Constitutional delayed growth and adolescence................	130 ⎰	
Cases with retarded bone age but still too young to diagnose....	67 ⎱	44.6
Primordial dwarfism without congenital anomalies	91	20.5
Dwarfism with gonadal aplasia............................	48	10.9
Genetic and congenital dwarfism with somatic anomalies	23	5.2
Hypothyroidism..	53	12.0
Hypopituitary or hypothalamic		
Tumors or cysts....................................	11 ⎰	
Idiopathic..	19 ⎱	6.7
Total...	442	100.0

* From data of Wilkins, L. *in* Williams, R. H.: (Textbook of Endocrinology, ed. 3, Philadelphia., Saunders.)

to have "constitutional delayed growth and adolescence" without genetic defect and without endocrine disorder. These patients are slow in growth but eventually become normal adults without treatment (see Table 9).

The next largest group were primordial dwarfs with no other anomalies, constituting 20.5 per cent of the 442 cases. Over 10 per cent of the patients had gonadal aplasia. A varied group of genetic and congenital dwarfed patients with other somatic anomalies accounted for over 5 per cent of cases.

Although endocrine causes are commonly considered responsible for most cases of subnormal growth, they accounted for only 18.7 per cent of this large series. Two thirds of the endocrine cases were due to hypothyroidism. The remaining one third of the endocrine cases (6.7 per cent of the total series) were children with subnormal growth due to pituitary or hypothalamic disorders.

Excessive Stature. The pathologic physiology of extreme height is less complex than that of dwarfing. There are essentially only three types: (1) constitutional or genetic tall stature (primordial gigantism, normal tall-statured persons); (2) primary hypogonadism; and (3) pituitary gigantism.

The genetic type of tallness occurs in certain families. Just as pygmies illustrate genetic small stature, certain other racial strains such as some African tribes are unusually tall.

When the gonadal secretion is inadequate during the period when normal epiphyseal closure should occur, the limbs may continue to grow in length, so that height becomes excessive and body proportions are abnormal. Such persons with eunuchoidal proportions have a span which exceeds the height and a lower measurement which exceeds the upper.

True pituitary gigantism is rare. Body growth is proportionate and only if growth hormone excess persists beyond epiphyseal closure do the physical evidences of acromegaly appear. The cause, as in acromegaly, is functioning eosinophilic hyperplasia or tumor of the anterior pituitary. The sella turcica is expanded or eroded and there may be impingement upon the optic nerves with visual field defects.

PATHOLOGIC PHYSIOLOGY OF SEX DEVELOPMENTAL DISORDERS

The basic sex structures are formed in the developing fetus because of the genetic pattern. See the discussion earlier in this chapter under Genetic Aspects and Determination of Sex.

The embryonic gonad is bipotential (may develop into either a testis or an ovary). In gonadal agenesis with only a single X chromosome neither gonad develops. Apparently, the embryologic development of a gonad depends upon the presence of 2 sex chromosomes. If 2 X chromosomes are present in the embryonic gonad, the cortex of the primitive gonad becomes dominant and an ovary develops. The ovary produces ovarian hormones and these bring about development of the Müllerian duct system and female differentiation.

If the bipotential embryonic gonad contains cells with a Y chromosome, regardless of the number of X chromosomes, development of the medullary part of the primitive gonad occurs, with differentiation into a testis. The testicular tissue produces androgenic hormone. Both tissue and hormone are necessary to induce embryologic regression of the Müllerian (female) duct system, to induce development of the Wolffian (male) ducts and differentiation of the bipotential embryonic external genitalia into those of a male.

In the newborn infant there may be present for a few days or a week or two some hyperplasia of the breasts in both sexes, and some vaginal changes in the female indicative of estrogen effect from the placenta.

In the male infant there may be some enlargement of the penis and of the testes which subsides soon after birth. In the first 4 to 6 weeks of life Leydig cells are present in the testes. They then disappear, not to reappear until adolescence. These changes may be attributed to maternal chorionic gonadotropin.

Throughout childhood, before any signs of adolescence, small quantities of estrogen and of androgen may be detected in the urine of both sexes, and there is no difference in the amounts found in the two sexes.

There is no *gradual* increase in the secretion of such hormones during the prepuberal years. It is possible that the hormones found in the preadolescent urine are produced by the adrenal cortex.

Suddenly there is an increase in gonadal development and in the secretion of sex hormones. The dramatic phenomenon of adolescence apparently is initiated by the pituitary. The factors which are responsible for the activation of this function of the pituitary are not known. There is some evidence that the triggering stimulus comes from the hypothalamus. So perhaps the *basic event* in adolescence is a maturation of certain centers in the *nervous system*. Certain tumors or diseases of the hypothalamus have been associated with premature or delayed sex development. Certainly there are familial and racial differences in the age of onset of puberty, probably due to hereditary genetic factors.

At puberty there is apparently not only sudden increase in pituitary gonadotropic activity, but also in pituitary adrenocorticotropic activity. There is an increase in the amount of adrenal androgen, indicated in girls by the appearance of sex hair and by increased urinary 17-ketosteroid secretion.

Agonadism

Persons with gonadal aplasia (also called Turner's syndrome and ovarian agenesis) are truly *neuter* human beings if one judges by the fact that neither ovarian nor testicular tissue is present. However, they are apparent females with sexual infantilism and short stature. They do have breast tissue, a uterus, a vagina, etc., capable of responding to stimulus with ovarian hormones. Mentality is usually normal.

In 55 instances of this syndrome, multiple congenital anomalies occurred in a high percentage,[7] including a broad shield-like chest with widely spaced hypoplastic nipples, cubitus valgus, micrognathia, epicanthal folds, high palate, low-set ears, short webbed neck, low hairline in back, numerous pigmented nevi, telangiectases in skin and bowel, hypoplastic nails, idiopathic hypertension, coarctation of the aorta, lymphedema of hands and feet, cutis laxa, keloid formation, strabismus, ptosis, cataracts, deafness, renal anomalies, etc. The condition is genetic in origin, with 45XO karyotype. Estrogen therapy produces breast and vaginal development. Sexual intercourse may be normal; but such patients are of course sterile.

Hypogonadism

Male Hypogonadism. The testes have two roles: one hormonal, the other reproductive. They consist primarily of the seminiferous tubules; the interstitial (Leydig) cells produce androgen. Androgen has growth-promoting and anabolic effects in addition to promoting the development of secondary male sex characteristics. Prominent in fetal testes, Leydig cells disappear shortly after birth and do not reappear until adolescence. The output of 17-ketosteroids is low until the 8th or 9th year and then increases fairly rapidly throughout adolescence. Usually the earliest sign of androgenic effect is increased vascularity of the penis and the scrotum; this is soon followed by pigmentation and thickening of the scrotal skin and growth of the prostate. Next there is growth of the penis, appearance of pubic hair, enlargement of the larynx, deepening of the voice, increased secretion of sebaceous glands and acne. Growth of the beard comes later.

Prepubertal testicular enlargement precedes the appearance of androgenic effects and is due chiefly to proliferation of seminiferous tubules stimulated by pituitary gonadotropins.

Testosterone, principal androgen secreted by the Leydig cells, is not a ketosteroid but is metabolized to 17-ketosteroids and excreted in the urine, accounting for 30 per cent of the 17-ketosteroid excretion in normal males (the other 70 per cent coming from the adrenal cortex). The androgenic effects of testosterone are much more potent under normal conditions than those of the adrenal steroids.

Better understanding of abnormalities of male sex development has been promoted by recent advances, among which are (1) greater knowledge of normal and pathological testicular cytology through biopsies; (2) sex chromatin body studies to establish genetic sex; (3) chromosomal analyses, elucidating many genetic anomalies, and (4) wider use of improved hormonal assays for 17-ketosteroids and 17-hydroxysteroids, pituitary gonadotropins, etc.

1. IN PRIMARY TESTICULAR FAILURE in preadolescent boys, pubertal changes fail to appear and body proportions become eunuchoid. In postadolescence, body proportions having already been established, testicular failure causes osteoporosis; the genitalia become relatively small; pubic, axillary and facial hair become sparse; muscles become flabby (loss of protein anabolic factor) and libido and potentia are diminished. Androgen excretion is low;

gonadotropin excretion is high. Fat deposits increase in mammary and trochanteric regions. In addition to deficiency of androgenic function, the testis may present germinal epithelial failure with little or no production of spermatozoa.

Klinefelter's syndrome is one of the most common examples of hypogonadism and is characterized by a genetically determined defect of the germinal epithelium (karyotype XXY), seminiferous tubule failure, small, firm testes, gynecomastia, eunuchoidism and frequently mental deficiency. The sex chromatin pattern is of positive (female) type because of the two X chromosomes, but genotype and phenotype are male, because of the presence of the Y chromosome.

Testicular biopsy[25] reveals two main features: (1) hyalinization of the seminiferous tubular membranes and (2) clumping of the Leydig cells. The hyalinization of the tubules does not occur prior to puberty, but then proceeds rapidly. There is great variation between cases in degree of Leydig cell function and degree of eunuchoidism; urinary gonadotropin is elevated. There is azoospermia and sterility in 95 per cent of cases.

In some *idiopathic* cases the clinical syndrome and testicular biopsy resemble those of Klinefelter's syndrome but the sex chromatin is negative, and the karyotype normal XY.

Acute orchitis develops in 15 to 25 per cent of males having epidemic parotitis. In young boys there is usually no testicular damage but at puberty or in adults damage to seminiferous tubules and to Leydig cells may result.

Irradiation may cause testicular damage, more often tubular, producing infertility, but Leydig cells may atrophy also, producing varying degrees of androgen deficiency.

2. HYPOGONADOTROPIC HYPOGONADISM (see Fig. 20) produces a clinical picture similar to that of primary testicular eunuchoidism of preadolescent onset. Since it may be due to involvement of the pituitary by tumor, possible indications of such should be sought. When the gonadal failure is secondary to pituitary failure, urinary gonadotropin secretion is low or absent; when

the eunuchoidism is of primary testicular origin, urinary gonadotropins are high.

Hypogonadism may occur with other types of pituitary involvement (dwarfism, acromegaly, gigantism, Cushing's disease, Simmonds' disease, etc.).

Hypothalamic disorders may be characterized by hypogonadism, usually accompanied by other evidence of involvement of the central nervous system (obesity, diabetes insipidus, neurologic signs) and by hypogonadotrophic signs.

Female Hypogonadism. The ovaries, like the testes, serve a dual role, producing germ cells (the ova) and sex hormones (estrogen and progesterone). Estrogen from the ovary and androgen from the adrenal cortex bring about development of the secondary sex characteristics. Usually the onset of puberty is signalled by growth and

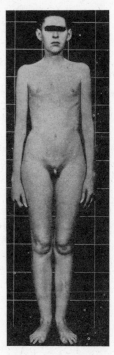

Fig. 20. Hypogonadotropic hypogonadism. Age 25, bone age 17, height 67.7 (average height for male age 25: 65.8-68.0-70.2 in.). The patient's genetic destiny was perhaps to be shorter than his present height. This is an excellent example of the complex interplay between genetic and acquired factors in the processes of growth. Wide-open epiphyses in late adolescence enabled him to grow over a longer period than normal, but his genes (mother, 64.0 in.; father, 66.0 in.) did not permit the development of disproportion between upper and lower body segments typical of eunuchoids.

Figures 19 and 20 from Shelton, E., and Skeels, R.: Growth and Development, Ciba Clinical Symposia 3: No. 6.

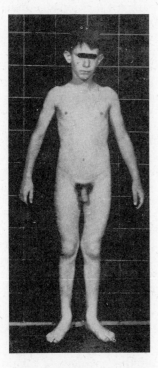

Fig. 19. Pubertas praecox. Age 6, bone age 12, height 56.0; urinary 17-ketosteroids 18.9 mg. per 24 hours; exploration of both adrenals negative for tumor (average height for male, age 6: 43.5-45.0-46.5 in.).

development of the nipples and the areolae. Estrogen is responsible for the development of the nipple and the duct structures of the breasts, the labia minora, the vulva, the vagina, the uterus and the tubes. Vaginal growth is accompanied by formation of rugae and change of the epithelium to the stratified squamous type. Vaginal smear studies permit assessment of estrogenic effect.

Progesterone promotes development of the alveoli of the breasts. Cyclic control through the hypothalamus and pituitary gonadotropins regulates ovulation and secretion of estrogen and progesterone. After normal adolescence such cyclic ovarian activity acts upon the uterus to produce menstruation.

Sexual hair growth on the pubis and in the axillae is due to *androgen*. Androgen is responsible for seborrhea and acne and possibly for development of the labia majora (female analogue of the scrotum). When androgen is present in excess it causes enlargement of the clitoris and other signs of virilization.

1. IN PRIMARY OVARIAN DEFICIENCY a eunuchoid type of body growth occurs; there is amenorrhea and failure to develop secondary sex characters. Postadolescent removal of or damage to the ovaries seems to cause less disturbance than castration in the male. Menstruation ceases, of course, but there may be little breast atrophy or loss of libido. Nervous symptoms and vasomotor instability with hot flashes may be troublesome. Loss of the anabolic effect of estrogen may result in serious osteoporosis. Gonadotropin titers are high.

2. HYPOGONADOTROPIC HYPOGONADISM may occur in the female with eunuchoidal characteristics resembling those occurring from primary preadolescent ovarian deficiency.

PANHYPOPITUITARISM with signs of gonadal failure as a prominent feature may occur as the result of infarction of the anterior pituitary in women suffering from hemorrhage and shock at childbirth. When signs of hypopituitarism are severe, with profound weakness and cachexia, the term Simmonds' disease usually is used. Milder forms, with amenorrhea, loss of pubic and axillary hair, etc., often have been termed Sheehan's syndrome.

HYPERGONADISM

Pubertas Precox. In either sex, precocious activation of the gonads may occur with resultant premature puberty. There is premature development of the secondary sex characteristics and the adolescent spurt in growth comes on early. Because of the premature spurt the child may for a time be tall for his age (Fig. 19), but ultimately stature is less than normal due to early epiphyseal union. The cause for premature puberty is often obscure and the patient may go on to live quite a normal life. Occasionally at necropsy hypothalamic lesions or pineal tumors have been found. In a few instances a functioning neoplasm (possibly amenable to surgical extirpation) has been found in ovary, testis, or adrenal.

In the more common constitutional or neurogenic pubertas precox, excretion of 17-ketosteroids and estrogens is increased to levels corresponding to the physiologic or apparent sex age of the patient, rather than the actual age. In patients with interstitial cell tumors of the testis or with functioning adrenal cortical tumors, androgen secretion is much higher than in normal adult males. Estrogen excretion in females with granulosa cell or theca cell tumors of the ovary is higher than in normal adult females.

COMMON ABNORMAL GROWTH AND SEX PATTERNS

The chief patterns discussed in this chapter may be grouped as follows:

1. Subnormal statural growth
   A. Without sex disorder (genetic; primordial)
   B. With sex deficiency
   C. With precocious development
2. Excessive statural growth
   A. Without sex disorder (acromegaly; gigantism)
   B. With sex deficiency (eunuchoidism)
   C. With precocious sex development (temporary statural spurt)
3. Sexual hypofunction
   A. With normal stature
   B. With deficient stature (delayed adolescence; hypogonadotropism)
   C. With excessive stature (eunuchoidism)
4. Sexual hyperfunction

When *isosexual* (that is, the excessive sex hormone corresponds to the sex of the patient), excessive gonadal hormones usually cause premature statural growth spurt, and later premature epiphyseal union with permanent subnormal dimensions.

When *heterosexual* (excess estrogen in the male or excess androgen in the female), excessive gonadal hormones cause mixed patterns discussed in the section below.

SPECIAL ABNORMAL GROWTH AND SEX PATTERNS

So far in this chapter we have discussed the mechanisms which may result in deficient or excessive growth and in deficient or premature sex development. The chief types of clinical disorders associated with such conditions have been analyzed on the basis of the pathologic physiology involved.

There are a number of other clinical disorders which are not connected so directly to straightforward alterations in growth and sex development, but are closely related to them. Many of these conditions are characterized by the development in a person of one sex of features considered characteristic of the other.

Adiposogenital Dystrophy. In either sex one not infrequently sees obese children with retarded adolescence. The syndrome is more striking in boys because of the apparent feminization: fat padding in breast region and about hips, knock knees, and small genitalia (which often appear even smaller, being buried in fat).

Height may be subnormal, normal, or often above normal. When dwarfing is present and the obesity and hypogonadism are striking, one may find other evidences of pituitary or hypothalamic damage and be able to make a diagnosis of true Fröhlich's syndrome. Usually, however, one finds no evidence of such organic lesions. It seems likely that a functional disorder of the hypothalamic-pituitary mechanism is present. Often there is eventual normal sex maturation, but if delay is sufficient, therapy is indicated.

Gynecomastia. At adolescence the majority of boys have mild temporary pubertal gynecomastia, consisting of a small palpable nodule 2 to 3 cm. in diameter under the areola. Such nodes nearly always disappear within a few months or a year or two. Presumably an estrogenlike hormone causes the breast growth. It may come from the testes or the adrenals. There is usually no lack of testicular hormone. Among 1,855 boys from 10 to 16 years of age, gynecomastia was present in 38.7 per cent, with a peak incidence of 64.6 per cent at age 14 to 14½.[13] In 23 per cent of the gynecomastia cases, it was unilateral (right 15 per cent, left 8 per cent). In most cases the nodules were present only for some months, but among the cases followed, they were persistent for 2 years in 27 per cent and for 3 years in 7.7 per cent.

In adult life gynecomastia may occur as the result of testicular damage or disease. It may also result from testicular tumor, cryptorchidism, cirrhosis of the liver, feminizing tumors of the adrenal, pituitary tumor, starvation and impairment of liver function.

Breast growth has occurred in males being treated with estrogens, testosterone, desoxycorticosterone, chorionic gonadotropin or adrenal cortical hormones.

The mechanisms resulting in gynecomastia are not always clear. In males there is a small anlage of breast tissue which apparently can respond if (1) estrogen is supplied; (2) a steroid hormone similar to estrogen is present in excess (? transformed to estrogen in the body); (3) testicular function is diminished; or (4) conjugation and inactivation of the small amount of estrogen in the blood is not performed normally by the liver.

In cirrhosis or starvation, probably both factors 3 and 4 are operative.

Undescended Testes (Cryptorchidism). In about 30 per cent of male infants born prematurely, one or both testes are undescended. This condition is found in only about 10 per cent of full-term births. The testes frequently descend spontaneously during childhood or adolescence, but about 2 per cent of boys reach puberty with an undescended testis.

DIAGNOSIS is important and depends upon palpation. Physiologic ectopy (migratory testes) depends upon the power of the cremaster muscle to retract the gonad into the canal in the groin. This may be overcome by putting the boy in a warm bath.

The cause of testicular ectopy is often not evident. Presumably chorionic gonadotropin furnished in late fetal life brings about usual normal descent. Two groups of patients may be subject to cryptorchidism:

1. Those with anatomic defects: short gubernaculum, tight internal ring, adhesions, impatent canal, etc.

2. Those with an endocrine disorder; failure to descend is associated with imperfect development of the testis, and other evidence of testicular deficiency either primary, or secondary to pituitary deficiency. Bilateral cryptochidism is seen more often when there is hormonal deficiency.

The warm intra-abdominal temperature interferes with development of tubules and production of spermatozoa and if the condition is bilateral results in sterility. Eventually the cryptorchid gonads may atrophy, and even if initially there was adequate androgenic hormone, androgenic lack may supervene.

Cryptorchidism is frequent in eunuchoid patients—this may signify that failure of descent resulted from poor development of the testes, particularly if both testes are undescended, or if one is cryptorchid and the other descended but atrophic.

Untreated men with bilateral ectopy excrete about one half the normal androgen level.

Therapy with chorionic gonadotropin will cause descent in many cases of cryptorchidism in boys and may prevent serious spermatogenic damage and relieve or prevent androgenic deficiency.

Virilism. Excessive adrenal androgen secretion during fetal life results in pseudohermaphroditism in the female. When such a hormonal abnormality occurs in preadolescent, adolescent or adult life, there is hirsutism, amenorrhea and absence or atrophy of breasts, enlargement of the clitoris, increased muscle mass and development of male rather than female body contours. When the adrenocortical hyperplasia is bilateral, Addison's disease may occur, with signs of salt deficiency.

Heterosexual signs in the prepubertal or adult female may be due to *adrenocortical lesions* (hyperplasia, adenoma, carcinoma) or *ovarian disease* (arrhenoblastoma, Leydig cell tumor, luteoma, polycystic disease, adrenal rests).

The clinical pictures produced by androgenic hormones arising in the various ovarian and adrenocortical regions are so similar that differentiation is often difficult. Attempts are made by perirenal air injection and pyelography to visualize adrenal masses. Hormone assays may be helpful. Very high levels of 17-ketosteroids (40 mg. per day or more) in the urine suggest adrenocortical carcinoma. If cortisone therapy will diminish urinary 17-ketosteroid excretion, the cause is probably bilateral adrenal cortical hyperplasia.

Attempts are made to palpate pelvic masses. Pelvic exploratory operation may be advisable.

Cushing's syndrome may occur, with hirsutism, amenorrhea, obesity, osteoporosis, tendency toward diabetes and poor musculature. The 17-ketosteroid output is elevated moderately; 17-hydroxysteroid output is high—the catabolic steroid effect is preponderant over the anabolic, even though there is evidence of increased androgen secretion.

Hirsutism. Hirsutism without any other signs suggesting masculinization is not uncommon. Brunette women of Mediterranean antecedents are more hirsute than the blonder, Nordic types. Many women can be considered to have genetic hypertrichosis, since similar hair growth will be found to occur among mother, aunts and sisters.

When hirsutism appears during adolescence it is most often essential or idiopathic—that is, not related to an endocrine abnormality. When it appears later in a previously nonhirsute woman, a causative lesion should be sought.

Even when hirsutism is not accompanied by other signs and symptoms, it is advisable to measure 17-ketosteroid excretion on a day midway between menstrual periods. In idiopathic hirsutism values may be normal (5 to 15 mg.) or up to 25 mg.

Hair follicles, when once matured, require very little androgen to maintain growth. Therefore, even when 17-ketosteroid excretion is normal, it is possible that (1) an earlier temporary hyperadrenocorticism may have been present, or (2) the end-organs (the hair follicles) are more sensitive than usual to normal amounts of androgen.

Hermaphroditism. A true hermaphrodite has gonads of both sexes. In some instances there is an ovary on one side and a testis on the other. More often there are ovotestes bilaterally, or one ovotestis and one testis or one ovary. There are various combinations of the sex characteristics seen in such truly *intersex states*.

Usually genetic causes are invoked to account for such intersex combinations. However, it is known that in certain animals gonadal differentiation may be reversed more or less completely by the administration of sex hormones during fetal life. It thus seems possible that nongenetic or hormonal factors may be responsible for the development of ovotestes in the human.

Pseudohermaphroditism. Females with ovaries but male development of some of the accessory organs are called *female pseudohermaphrodites.* This condition is usually due to congenital adrenal hyperplasia. Other possible causes are discussed earlier in this chapter in the section on determination of sex. The 17-ketosteroid excretion is high during the first few months of life (2 mg. per 24 hours or more, compared to the normal of less than 0.5 mg.). Excess androgen activity is manifested by clitoral hypertrophy, rapid somatic growth of masculine type, and early appearance of pubic hair.

Males with testes, but female type development of genitalia are called *male pseudohermaphrodites.* In distinct contrast to the female pseudohermaphrodite, there is no sign of excessive hormone secretion, no acceleration of somatic growth and no precocious sexual development. At puberty the secondary sexual characteristics may follow either a male or a female pattern.

Testicular feminization[19] is a form of male pseudohermaphroditism which includes apparent females with definite signs of spontaneous apparently female gonadal hormone activity at puberty but with male sex chromatin pattern and male gonads. The chromosomal constitution is 46XY. The condition is familial and is transmitted exclusively through the maternal line. The disorder seems to be transmitted either by a sex-linked recessive or by a sex-limited dominant mutant gene. Since the gene defect is not closely linked to either of 2 sex-linked genetic conditions (hemophilia and color blindness), evidence favors the latter hypothesis.

This syndrome should be suspected when breast development occurs but axillary and pubic hair are sparse or absent, the vagina is rudimentary, short and blind, external genitalia are normal female type and there is primary amenorrhea. A chromatin-negative skin biopsy or buccal smear and surgical disclosure of testes and rudimentary or absent internal female organs will confirm the diagnosis. The relatively high incidence of testicular neoplasms in this syndrome indicates prompt surgical castration. In this disorder with its characteristic feminization without virilization (no facial or body hirsutism, no hypertrophy of clitoris or male body contours, etc.), the testes seem to be the source of adequate amounts of estrogen but fail to produce appreciable quantities of androgen. After removal of the testicular tissue, postoperative estrogen levels fall practically to zero. Preoperative 17-ketosteroid levels are normal and remain so after operation (suggesting adrenocortical source of this steroid in these patients). After removal of the testes "menopausal" symptoms may occur, with breast atrophy, loss of estrogen effect upon the vaginal smear and a rise in the urinary gonadotropin titer.

Distinction should be made between the true intersex states (true hermaphroditism) in which gonads of both sexes are present, and pseudohermaphroditism of the various male and female varieties.

LABORATORY TESTS IN GROWTH AND DEVELOPMENT STUDIES

No attempt will be made here to list completely or to describe in detail all of the adjuncts to the history and physical examination which are useful in growth and development studies. We will outline the chief avenues of approach and discuss briefly some of the more pertinent points.

1. Studies of the cellular elements of the blood may reveal anemia or other blood disorders with characteristics suggesting possible causative factors.

2. Urinalysis may disclose diabetes, renal impairment, etc.

3. Blood chemical studies: blood sugar (diabetes, hypoglycemia); urea nitrogen (renal disorders); calcium, phosphorus, phosphatase (bone disease); cholesterol, protein-bound iodine (thyroid disorders); lipids (inherited metabolic diseases), etc.

4. Urinary chemical studies: phenylketonuria; aminoaciduria and renal glycosuria and renal hyperphosphaturia (Fanconi syndrome); etc.

5. Roentgenologic studies: skull (sella turcica, pituitary disorders); bones, for bone age, epiphyseal closure, bone diseases, etc.

6. Hormonal assays.

7. Thyroid up-take of I^{131}.

8. Determination of the basal metabolic rate.

9. Cytogenetics.

Growth Factors. GROWTH HORMONE. A practical clinical method for the measurement of growth hormone in body fluids is greatly needed. Bioassay technics have proved to be laborious, prohibitively expensive and in general not sensitive enough to be of use clinically. A sensitive growth hormone assay would be highly significant in determining whether subnormal growth is due to pituitary deficiency or will have to be otherwise explained. When body size is excessive we could determine whether excess somatotropin is the cause. In acromegaly we could ascertain whether the condition is "burned-out" or still active and whether treatment is indicated.

Recent investigative work has resulted in the development of methods which measure indirectly the growth hormone levels present in human sera under various conditions. In the evaluation of levels of circulating growth hormone two methods have received considerable attention: (1) the measurement of the hormone in sera by sensitive immunoassay techniques; (2) measurement of a serum factor which promotes chondroitin sulfate synthesis. Growth hormone apparently promotes the formation of the sulfation factor, and assays of the amount of this factor have revealed (in both experimental and clinical studies) variations in the levels of growth hormone present. Sulfation factor assays of human sera have shown a "normal" range of somatotropin activity in growing children and in normal adults, low levels in hypopituitarism (after hypophysectomy, in pituitary dwarfism and in Sheehan's syndrome) and high levels in acromegaly.[5,38,39,40]

As yet such studies have necessarily been confined to a few research centers. It is to be hoped that a clinically practical method of measuring circulating somatotropin can soon be made more widely available.

THE SERUM PHOSPHORUS level is elevated in the presence of high amounts of circulating growth hormone. It is relatively high in growing children, in acromegalics, and in postmenopausal or castrated individuals (perhaps due to pituitary hyperactivity). It can be lowered by the administration of gonadal hormones.

THE SERUM ALKALINE PHOSPHATASE apparently is secreted by the osteoblasts, and its level (in the absence of liver disease) is an index of osteoblastic activity and of bone formation.

Gonadotropins. The anterior lobe of the pituitary gland secretes three hormones which exert important effects upon the gonads: (1) follicle-stimulating hormone (FSH); (2) interstitial cell-stimulating hormone (ICSH; luteinizing hormone, LH); (3) lactogenic hormone (prolactin; luteotropic hormone, LTH).

In the female these pituitary hormones are responsible for the growth, the maturation and the expulsion of the ova and for the production of ovarian hormones by the ovary. In the male they stimulate spermatogenesis and the production of androgen.

These protein pituitary hormones cannot as yet be assayed chemically. Bioassays are of clinical value in a number of conditions. Pituitary failure results in a diminution of secretion of the gonadotropins and secondarily leads to lack of development or atrophy of the gonads, with consequent atrophy of the target organs: penis, prostate, seminal vesicles; uterus, vagina, etc. Secretion of the gonadotropic pituitary hormones is controlled by the level of circulating androgen or estrogen. A decrease in the sex steroid causes stimulation of gonadotropin production; an increase causes depressed gonadotropin output.

Gonadotropin appears in the urine of girls at about 11 years of age, usually many months or a year before the first menstruation. In boys gonadotropins appear at about 12 to 13 years of age.

In adult women there is a fluctuating level varying with the menstrual cycle, usually with a peak at midmonth just before ovulation. In pregnancy large amounts of gonadotropin appear in blood and urine (produced by chorionic tissue—basis for pregnancy tests).

In adult men moderate amounts of gonadotropic hormone may be demonstrated regularly in the urine.

EXCESS GONADOTROPINS. Abnormally high gonadotropin may be found in:

1. Functional hyperactivity of the pituitary in response to gonadal failure: agenesis, orchitis or oophoritis (after mumps, etc.), failure of descent of testes after puberty, cystic disease of the ovaries, trauma and castration. In women with the approach of the menopause there is often an increase in gonadotropins. This increased hypophyseal activity may persist for years in some women and is believed to be responsible for "hot flashes" and other menopausal symptoms. In men at the "male climacteric" the increase in gonadotropins is not as consistent or as great as in women.

2. Increased production by chorionic tissue: hydatidiform mole, chorionepithelioma.

3. Certain malignant tumors of the testis.

DECREASED GONADOTROPINS. Diminution in gonadotropin in blood and urine may be found in:

1. Panhypopituitarism; Simmonds' disease, chromophobe pituitary tumors.

2. Hypogonadotropic hypogonadism: specific failure of gonadal stimulation without complete pituitary failure.

3. Estrogen or androgen excess. Endogenous gonadal hormone causes decrease in gonadotropic activity. Hormones used exogenously act similarly. Testosterone is relatively ineffective but estrogen administration will diminish gonadotropin secretion. Use of this fact is made in treating carcinoma of the prostate.

Androgens. About two thirds of the androgenic substances present in the urine of males is secreted by the adrenal cortex, about one third originates in the testes. In adult females there is normally about two thirds as much androgen excreted in the urine as in males, all apparently from the adrenal cortex. True androgenic levels may be determined by bioassay, but chemical determination of the 17-ketosteroids usually is employed. These are believed to be excretory transformation products of testicular and adrenocortical hormones. Since some of the 17-ketosteroids are only weakly androgenic or even biologically inactive, the values obtained are not equivalent to those of bio-assay. In most instances, however, the colorimetric 17-ketosteroid assays and the biologic values are roughly parallel.

Children under 6 years of age usually excrete less than 1 mg. 17-ketosteroid per day; 7 to 12 years, average 3.7 mg.; 12 to 15 years, average 7.5 mg.[21]

Adult men excrete normally 8 to 20 mg. daily. Adult women excrete 5 to 15 mg. daily.

INCREASED 17-KETOSTEROID VALUES are found in adrenocortical carcinoma, adrenocortical hyperplasia, and interstitial cell tumor of the testis. Arrhenoblastoma of the ovary is associated with normal or only moderately increased levels. Boys with pubertas precox have high 17-ketosteroid values.

The highest 17-ketosteroid values have been reported in adrenocortical carcinoma, but there is much overlapping with cases of adrenocortical hyperplasia. The slight increase observed in arrhenoblastoma (despite considerable hirsutism and clitoral hypertrophy) may be explained by secretion of such tumors of androgen which is not excreted as 17-ketosteroids.

DECREASED 17-KETOSTEROID VALUES may be found in primary or secondary hypofunction of the adrenal cortex or interstitial cells of the testes: hypopituitarism, hypogonadism, adrenocortical deficiency, especially; also in hypothyroidism, liver disease, malnutrition, debilitating illness and marked physical fatigue.

THE ACID PHOSPHATASE CONTENT OF THE PROSTATIC FLUID obtained after prostatic massage provides a simply determined index of androgenic activity. Kirk, Eisenstein and MacBryde[10] examined the prostatic exprimate in 71 normal boys between the ages of 11 and 16½ years. There was an increase in the mean acid phosphatase values from 50 units per ml. of prostatic fluid at age 11 to 8,700 units at age 16 to 16½ (Fig. 21). In adult males the average was 14,000 units per ml. In elderly men there is a decrease in the values.

In adolescent boys there was a good correlation between the acid phosphatase values and the clinical signs of sex development. The method has been found to be useful as a simple laboratory means of confirming clinical diagnoses of male hypogonadism. Results of treatment with gonadotropin or testosterone also may be followed by this method. One may determine whether the testicular deficiency is primary or secondary by whether response is obtained (a rise in acid phosphatase titer) to gonadotropin therapy. A failure to secure a rise after adequate treatment indicates primary gonadal deficiency.

Estrogens. Estradiol is apparently the primary estrogen secreted by the ovary. The liver converts estradiol to biologically inactive substances and to estrogens of lower activity (estrone and estriol). Estrogens in the urine are believed to represent about 5 to 10 per cent of those secreted.

Estrogens may be determined by bioassay of serum or of urinary extracts, by chemical (colorimetric or fluorometric) methods, or by cytologic examination of vaginal smears.

The newborn infant is in a state of hyperestrogenism (hormone from maternal circulation) which disappears within 10 days after birth. Small amounts of estrogen are detectable in childhood (probably of adrenal origin) in both males and females. At age 8 to 10 years, girls show

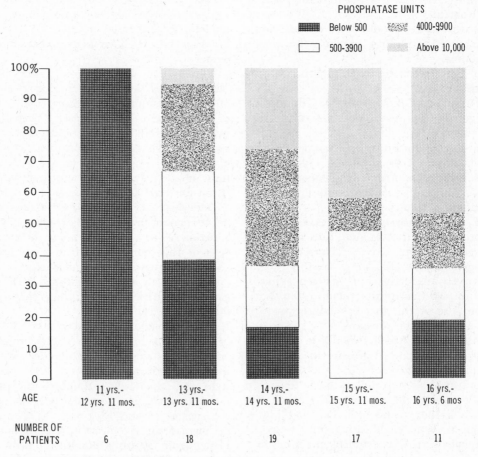

FIG. 21. The acid phosphatase concentration of the prostatic exprimate in 71 normal boys 11 to 16½ years of age. (Kirk, Eisenstein and MacBryde[10])

increases above the level of boys, then the slow increase yields to a sharp rise shortly before the menarche.

In women there is a cyclic pattern of estrogen production, with two peaks each month, one at about the time of ovulation, and the other at the height of corpus luteum activity (21st to 24th day), then a drop in the immediately premenstrual phase.

As the menopause approaches, the cyclic fluctuations become shallower. The estrogen secretion decreases at first rapidly, then more slowly during the postmenopausal years.

In pregnancy estrogen titers reach very high levels; the increased estrogen comes from the corpus luteum during the first two months, thereafter chiefly from the placenta.

In the urine of normal adult men there is found about one-half the estrogen present in the urine of normal adult women.

EXCESS ESTROGEN. In precocious puberty in girls the estrogen titer is high for the age. Granulosa cell tumors, thecomas, and luteomas usually are accompanied by moderate increase of estrogen in blood and urine. In tumor or hyperplasia of the adrenal cortex there may be very high estrogen titers.

Functional ovarian disorders may occur with persistent high plateau of estrogen production and alternate amenorrhea and bleeding from a hyperplastic endometrium (metropathia hemorrhagica).

In hepatic functional impairment there may be no increase in estrogen production but various degrees of failure in estrogen degradation and excretion, therefore a higher level of circulating estrogen results. Persons with such disorders (cirrhosis, hepatitis) may manifest signs of hyperestrogenism: menstrual disorders in the female; gynecomastia and testicular atrophy in the male.

ESTROGEN DEFIENCY may during the reproductive period in women result from either primary or secondary ovarian failure: hypopituitarism, hypogonadism. The distinction must be made by gonadotropin assays: such titers are low if the pituitary is at fault, high if there is primary ovarian failure.

Estrogen excretion is diminished in the male castrate; apparently, therefore, a portion of the estrogen in normal male urine is of testicular origin.

Cytogenetics. The simplest way to determine genetic sex is usually by search of buccal smears for the characteristic chromatin body present in females and absent in males. Another rapid method involves the recognition of the accessory lobules ("drumsticks") of neutrophil leukocytes in females. True chromosomal sex can only be determined by expert and experienced analysis of cells of peripheral blood, bone marrow or other tissues grown in tissue culture. In nearly all instances the subject's sex by the rapid method will correspond with results of the chromosomal method.

For clarity in distinguishing the two methods, both of which are aimed at determining *genetic sex* and the second of which may give much additional information, it is suggested that results of the first method be designated as *nuclear sex positive* (female) or *negative* (male), and the results of the second as *chromosomal sex*.

For further discussion of the technics, results and significance of recent studies in the fast-moving field of cytogenetics, see earlier sections of this chapter on Genetic Aspects and on Determination of Sex, and consult the references.

REFERENCES

1. Bauer, J.: Constitution and Disease: Applied Constitutional Pathology, ed. 2, New York, Grune, 1945.
2. Barr, M. L., *in* Montagu, M. F. A., ed.: Genetic Mechanisms in Human Disease, p. 118, Springfield, Ill., Thomas, 1961.
3. Cantarow, A., and Trumper, M.: Clinical Biochemistry, Philadelphia, Saunders, 1962.
4. Carpentier, P. J., and Potter, E. L., *in* Montagu, M. F. A., ed.: Genetic Mechanisms in Human Disease, pp. 166-202, Springfield, Ill., Thomas, 1961.
5. Daughaday, W. H.: Somatotropin, *in* Williams, R. H., ed., Textbook of Endocrinology, ed. 3, pp. 30-38, Philadelphia, Saunders, 1962.

6. Gordan, G. S., and Lisser, H., eds.: Endocrinology in Clinical Practice, Chicago, Year Book Pub., 1953.

7. Haddad, H. M., and Wilkins, L.: Congenital anomalies associated with gonadal aplasia: review of 55 cases, Pediatrics 23:885-902, 1959.

8. Holt, L. E., McIntosh, R., and Barnett, H. L.: Pediatrics, ed. 13, New York, Appleton, 1962.

9. Hsia, D.: Inborn Errors of Metabolism, Chicago, Year Book Pub., 1959.

10. Kirk, J. E., Eisenstein, A., and MacBryde, C. M.: The acid phosphatase concentration of the prostatic exprimate during normal puberty, J. Clin. Endocrinol. 12:338-345, 1952.

11. Knobloch, H., and Pasamanick, B.: Mental subnormality, New England J. Med. 266: 1045-1051; 1092-1097, 1962.

12. Lennox, B.: Chromosomes for beginners, in Montagu, M. F. A., ed.: Genetic Mechanisms in Human Disease, pp. 553-569, Springfield, Ill., Thomas, 1961.

13. Nydick, M., Bustos, J., Dale, J. H., Jr., and Rawson, R. W.: Gynecomastia in adolescent boys, J.A.M.A. 178:449-454, 1961.

14. Dumm, M. E., and Ralli, E. P.: Hormonal control of metabolism, in Wohl, M. G., and Goodhart, R. S., eds.: Modern Nutrition in Health and Disease, ed. 2, Philadelphia, Lea & Febiger, 1960.

15. Schonfeld, W. A.: Primary and secondary sexual characteristics in males from birth through maturity, Am. J. Dis. Child. 65:535, 1943.

16. Shelton, E. K., and Skeels, R. F.: Growth and development, Ciba Clinical Symposia 3:183-215, 1951.

17. Shuttleworth, F. K.: The Sexual Maturation and Physical Growth of Girls, Age Six to Nineteen, Monograph, Soc. Res. Child Development, Vol. II, No. 5, 1937.

18. Sohval, A. R.: Recent progress in human chromosome analysis and its relation to the sex chromatin, Am. J. Med. 31:397-441, 1961.

19. Southren, A. L., and Saito, A.: The syndrome of testicular feminization, Ann. Int. Med. 55:925-931, 1961.

20. Stanbury, J. B., Wyngaarden, J. B., and Frederickson, D. S.: The Metabolic Basis of Inherited Disease, New York, McGraw-Hill, 1960.

21. Talbot, N. B., Sobel, E. H., McArthur, J. W., and Crawford, J. D.: Functional Endocrinology from Birth through Adolescence, Cambridge, Harvard, 1952.

22. Tanner, J. M.: Growth at Adolescence, ed. 2, Springfield, Ill., Thomas, 1962.

23. Taussig, H.: A study of the German outbreak of phocomelia, J.A.M.A. 180:1106-1114, 1962.

24. Uchida, I. A., et al.: 18-trisomy syndrome, New England J. Med. 266:1198-1201, 1962.

25. Van Wyk, J. J.: Disorders in sex differentiation, in Williams, R. H., ed.: Textbook of Endocrinology, ed. 3, pp. 515-558, Philadelphia, Saunders, 1962.

26. Warren, S.: Radiation protection, New England J. Med. 264:705-711, 1961.

27. Watson, E. H., and Lowrey, G. H.: Growth and Development of Children, ed. 4, Chicago, Year Book Pub., 1962.

28. Wilkins, L.: The Diagnosis and Treatment of Endocrine Disorders in Childhood and Adolescence, ed. 2, Springfield, Ill., Thomas, 1957.

29. ————. Influence of endocrine glands upon growth and development, in Williams, R. H., ed.: Textbook of Endocrinology, ed. 3, Philadelphia, Saunders, 1962.

30. Montagu, M. F. A.: Prenatal Influences, Springfield, Ill., Thomas, 1962.

31. Stern, C.: Principles of Human Genetics, ed. 2, San Francisco, Freeman, 1960.

32. Clarke, C. A.: Genetics for the Clinician, Springfield, Ill., Thomas, 1962.

33. Neel, J. V.: A Geneticist Looks at Modern Medicine, The Harvey Lectures, Series 56, p. 127, Academic Press, New York, 1960-61.

34. Krooth, R. S., and Weinberg, A. N.: Studies on cell lines developed from the tissues of patients with galactosemia, J. Exp. Med. 113:1155, 1961.

35. Bunim, J., Krooth, R., Weinberg, A., Howell, R., La Du, B., and Seegmiller, J.: Biochemical abnormalities in hereditary diseases, Ann. Int. Med. 57:472-497, 1962.

36. Suskind, S. R.: Gene function and enzyme formation, in McElroy, W. D., and Glass, B., eds.: The Chemical Basis of Heredity, p. 123, Baltimore, Johns Hopkins Press, 1957.

37. Ingram, V. M.: Hemoglobin and Its Abnormalities, Springfield, Ill., Thomas, 1961.

38. Daughaday, W. H., and Parker, M. L.: The Pituitary in Disorders of Growth, in Disease-a-Month, Chicago, Year Book, 1962.

39. ————: Sulfation factor measurement as an aid in the recognition of pituitary dwarfism, J. Clin. Endocrinol. and Metab. 23:638-650, 1963.

40. Almqvist, S., et al.: Sulfation factor activity of human serum, Acta endocrinol. 35:381, 1960; 36:31, 566, 577, 1961.

3

Pain

CYRIL M. MACBRYDE

DEFINITION

Pain is a disagreeable sensation produced by the action of stimuli of harmful nature. Physicians and philosophers have studied pain for centuries, and many conflicting views have arisen concerning it. A popular view until fairly recently was that pain was simply a feeling state, an emotional reaction like that of pleasure. However, it is now clear that pain is a specific sensation, not only perceived as such, but provided with a special and separate mechanism for detection of the noxious stimuli and for transmission of the pain impulses.

The pain perception may be, and usually is, accompanied by a feeling or emotional state as well as by other reactions of physical nature, so that the entire pain experience is apt to be complex in nature.

DUAL ASPECTS OF PAIN

The pain sensation itself must be differentiated as completely as possible from *the reactions* which usually accompany it. It is of value to the physician to understand the location and the intensity of the pain, as well as its other attributes, such as its quality, time of occurrence, etc. However, since pain is entirely subjective,

the physician is dependent upon what the patient tells him and upon his interpretation of the patient's reactions to the pain. Whenever the subject is able to be relatively objective in describing his discomfort, dissociating his reactions from his actual sensations, the task of discovering the origin of the pain is usually much easier. Thus, the person who is able to tell how he at first had epigastric distress, then nausea and vomiting, and that the pain finally settled in the right lower side of the abdomen, is much more apt to have appendicitis promptly diagnosed than the person who is weeping and excited and states that "my whole stomach hurts." The physician should assist the patient in discriminating between *pain* and *reaction*.

The *total manifestations* of the complex pain experience are, however, of interest and value to the physician, for he must strive to understand not only the physical origin of the pain but also physical, emotional and psychological reactions to the distressing experience.

When pain originates from a peripheral stimulus, travels the usual pathways and is perceived normally, it may be thought of as "direct" and its interpretation is not difficult. However, there is tremendous variation among human beings in their physical, emotional and psychological responses to equivalent stimuli, so that even in a relatively simple pain situation there are many modifying influences. In less simple instances, as in referred pain and the pain of causalgia and of phantom limb, the apparent source of the pain as perceived by the patient may be widely misleading. The ultimate perception of pain depends more upon the interpretation in the cerebral cortex than upon the characteristics of the original stimulus.

Psychogenic Pain. Pain not only comes to the brain or ego but may emanate from it. There are two fundamental types of psychogenic pain: (1) *conversion* pain of hysteria and (2) *functional pain* originating from an emotional disorder, causing muscle tension or vasodilation, etc., and the latter effects then setting up pain responses (e.g.: tension backache, tension headache, gastrointestinal pain).

ANATOMY AND PHYSIOLOGY OF PAIN

End-Organs. Cutaneous pain is aroused by stimulation of certain structures in the skin. These are special groups of the finer myelinated and unmyelinated nerve fibers bearing free endings. Pain is carried chiefly by myelinated nerve fibers, 3 to 6 μ in diameter. These fibers have a characteristically short refractory period and chronaxia and convey impulses at a rate of 15 (or less) to 30 meters per second. Pain also results from the stimulation of certain unmyelinated fiber groups such as the smaller, finer class C fibers of Gasser, which conduct more slowly (less than 2 meters per second). The peripheral endings of pain fibers arborize in the tissues and are lacking in recognizable specialized anatomic end structures. These nerve fibers and endings are arranged in a plexiform, interlocking pattern. It has long been known that pain can be elicited only by stimulating certain spots on the skin: any adequate stimulus to these spots produces pain; a less than adequate stimulus does not cause the sensation of touch or any other sensation. Until recently it has been accepted that nerve endings in such a "pain spot" were

specific for pain, but newer studies indicate that such fibers may carry impulses for touch, as well as pain.

The receptor endings are distributed richly on the body surface, but there are relatively few in deep somatic structures and viscera, none in the parenchyma of the central nervous system and the lungs, which are insensitive to pain.

About 1890 it was discovered that the skin is not everywhere uniformly sensitive to all aspects of a stimulating object. Some spots give rise to sensations of warmth but not of cold or pain; others respond only to a cold stimulus and with a sensation of coldness; still others respond only with sensations of pressure or pain. Cutaneous sensibility is punctiform or pointlike in its distribution. Touch is divided into several separate senses: pressure or touch, warmth and cold.

The separation of pain as a separate modality of sensation was more difficult because pain sensations can be aroused from virtually every spot stimulated. However, the criterion for *an adequate stimulus* for pain or any other special sense is not whether a stimulus can be perceived, but whether it is the form of energy to which the receptor is *most* sensitive. The best quantitative illustration is that the warmth end-organs of the skin are nearly 2,000 times as sensitive to radiant heat as are the intermingled pain-sensitive nerve endings.[35]

Several kinds of energy are adequate to elicit pain: mechanical, electrical, extremes of heat and cold, and a wide variety of chemical stimuli. Therefore, the pain-ending is not specialized to react to a single form of energy but reacts to extreme degrees of several kinds of stimulation. Increasing degrees of heat first stimulate warmth receptors, then at about 44.9° C, commence to stimulate pain endings. At about 44° to 45° C, irreversible damage to the skin occurs (demonstrable histologically), and accompanying release of chemical substances such as histamine is expected.

A chemical action as the ultimate pain stimulus might explain certain pathologic pain responses (such as itch and hyperalgesia) which may persist long after the noxious agent is removed. Very light stimulation to the same fine free nerve-endings which subserve pain can initiate tickle or itch sensations. Low concentrations of histamine cause itch, high concentrations cause pain.

Sensory Unit. Recent studies indicate the existence of a "sensory unit," consisting of many nerve endings, all branches of a single fiber, connected with a single cell in the dorsal root ganglion. Apparently the area of skin or cornea supplied by such a single unit is about one centimeter in diameter. It seems that many pain fibers supply overlapping sensory units to a given area, but there is no connection between the endings of the fibers of different units.

Nerves Conducting Pain Impulses. The myelinated and unmyelinated nerve fibers have different speeds of conduction, the greatest conduction velocity being in the myelinated fibers, the slowest in the unmyelinated. The nerve fibers are gathered together into peripheral nerves, each supplying a certain cutaneous area. The nerves become rearranged into nerve plexuses and finally enter the spinal canal to form dorsal ganglia. The fibers are reformed into the posterior root which enters the cord as a number of rootlets in the line of the posterior lateral sulcus and these in entering break up into medial and lateral filaments.

All the pain fibers enter the spinal cord through the dorsal root ganglia. There are two varieties of pain, superficial pain and deep pain, and the routes of their conduction by the sensory fibers differ considerably. Stimuli from the surface of the body originate impulses that are usually carried in the somatic nerves and thus enter the spinal cord more or less directly through the dorsal roots. Superficial pain impulses therefore follow a relatively simple pathway as compared with the deep pain impulses that may be conducted to the central nervous system by a variety of routes. Some of the deep pain impulses are carried by pain fibers attached to blood vessels at first, later joining autonomic nerves. Some deep pain fibers are associated with autonomic nerves from the beginning; others join with somatic nerves.

Fibers which conduct pain impulses may travel directly to the posterior root ganglia in somatic nerves or indirectly in sympathetic trunks and through sympathetic ganglia to the posterior root ganglia via the white rami communicantes.

The Spinal Pathway. The lateral filaments carry the pain fibers, both myelinated and unmyelinated. They enter Lissauer's tract, ascend for a short distance, then end in the gray matter of the posterior horn. Here new neurones arise and cross through the anterior commissure of the spinal cord, then reform in the lateral spinothalamic tract, where they ascend to the lateral nucleus of the optic thalamus.

In the spinal cord the spinothalamic tracts convey the nerve fibers that transmit the pain impulses. When these tracts are interrupted, pain only is absent from the areas concerned, touch and temperature sensations being retained.

Pain Perception. In the thalamus arise new neurones which ascend to the sensory portion of the cerebral cortex. In the simplest conduction of the pain impulse, three neurones take part: spinal ganglionic, spinothalamic, and thalamocortical. See the illustrations of pain pathways in Chapter 7 and in Chapter 10. The cerebral cortex ultimately receives the pain impulses, and is necessary for localization and evaluation of intensity. The thalamus is important in the integration of pain. There is awareness of pain at the thalamic level, but the cortex is required for distinction of point of origin, quality and degree.

Increasing the intensity of the stimulus results in perception of increasing degrees of pain intensity.[17]

The spreading of a noxious stimulus over a larger area does not increase the *intensity* of the resulting pain. However, the dimensions "extension" and "duration" are of great significance in the over-all *reaction* of a person to pain.

A useful scale for evaluating pain has been devised, which may be employed to evaluate pain from clinical conditions by matching it with experimentally induced pain.[17] The experimental pain is induced by thermal radiation (for pricking pain) or by pressure (for aching pain). There are 21 just noticeable differences (jnd's) between the threshold and the "ceiling pain." The term "dol" is used to signify an arbitrary unit equivalent to the sum of 2 jnd's. There is surprising uniformity in the evaluation of pain on the "dol" scale by normal subjects.

Pain perception is describable by most persons according to four categories:

1. *Quality:* burning, pricking, aching, or various combinations of these qualities.

2. *Intensity:* expressed in "dols" ranges from zero to $10\frac{1}{2}$ for pricking or aching pain. The scale for burning pain, the third quality, has not been defined.

3. *Extension:* means localization in the body, and also the "size and shape" of the pain: at a point, along a line or in three dimensions.

4. *Duration:* includes all temporal aspects of the pain: cramping, lightning, throbbing, pulsating, etc., time of onset, duration.

The Stimulus. Evidence at present available indicates that tissue tension or chemical irritants (or both) furnish the adequate stimulus to initiate the nerve impulse of pain. When pain results instead of other sensations, such as pressure, heat or cold, etc., tissue damage is either present or imminent.

The threshold of pain lies just at the threshold of tissue damage: if the noxious stimulus is maintained for sufficiently long, tissue destruction results. Pain is an indication of the *rate* of tissue damage rather than the amount or the seriousness of the damage. Thus extensive wounds may be painless, whereas slight wounds may be extremely painful, due to a progressive increase in tissue damage. Pain is a warning that tissue damage is *in progress,* rather than an indication of potential or existing tissue injury.

Whether all pain depends upon a single *ultimate stimulus* is not yet clear. One theory is that an adequate noxious stimulus results in partial denaturing of the cellular proteins of the endings of the nerve fibrils; such a change being caused by thermal, mechanical, chemical or electrical energy.[18] The pain fiber is depolarized and impulses are transmitted along it which are interpreted by higher centers as pain.

Armstrong *et al.*[40] have extracted pain-producing substances from blister fluid and inflammatory exudates. Blister fluid and other inflammatory exudates and plasma become powerful pain-producing agents when brought into contact with glass. Two substances or types of substances are thus formed:

1. A protein (globulin) which probably acts like a proteolytic enzyme; this can produce pain by direct action on nerve endings, or perhaps by acting on a substrate in plasma to form a second substance.

2. A polypeptide resembling "bradykinin" or "kallidin" (which are formed from plasma in other ways). The name "plasma kinin" is used to describe these polypeptides.[40,42]

Both the active protein and the polypeptide are very unstable in plasma or exudates.

Wolff *et al.*[36] have identified a polypeptide called "neurokinin" obtained from painful headache sites. In addition to the neurokinin, headache fluid was found to contain a proteolytic enzyme capable of forming neurokinin, presumably by cleavage of a plasma globulin. Neurokinin was produced at nerve endings by antidromal neuronal excitation. Apparently an intact nerve mechanism is essential to its production. Neurokinin is a powerful vasodilator. Injected intradermally, neurokinin plus the protease produce pain and erythema, lower pain threshold and increase capillary permeability.

Studies so far indicate that plasma kinin and neurokinin are both polypeptides and have similar properties but are not identical. Thus it seems that the polypeptide released at the site of headache pain may not be the same as that in blister fluid and inflammatory exudates.

Serum apparently produces pain because of the serotonin it contains. Serum brought into contact with glass produces the same active pain-producing agents as does plasma.

The pain-producing plasma globulin has been shown to initiate blood clotting and to increase capillary permeability.

Thus plasma when activated by contact with a foreign surface has produced all the essential elements of inflammation: dolor, rubor, calor and tumor. Similar changes apparently result from humoral substances obtained from the site of headache pain. It may be that damage to tissue cells initiates changes in the surrounding blood or tissue fluids which lead to these sensory and vascular phenomena.

Injury to tissues might release or cause to be formed several pain-producing agents: the active plasma globulin, one or more polypeptides, histamine from mast cells, and 5-hydroxytryptamine (serotonin) from disintegrating platelets. If present in high enough concentration these substances could cause pain by direct stimulation of nerve endings;[40,41] in lower concentrations they might sensitize nerve endings and thus produce *primary hyperalgesia* (which is the most characteristic sensory feature of inflammation).[42]

It must be emphasized that the above series of reactions constitutes a working hypothesis. As yet we have no proof that we may thus explain the chemical component of pain, or that the usual common stimulus which initiates the pain impulse is chemical.

Certain observations are interesting in this connection. *Nettle stings* contain pain-producing concentrations of acetylcholine, histamine and serotonin. *Wasp venom* contains high concentrations of histamine and serotonin and also a pain-producing polypeptide resembling that found in plasma.

Present evidence suggests that the pain of injury or inflammation is due to histamine, serotonin and the plasma pain-producing substances, acting individually or in concert.[42] These may constitute Lewis' "pain-producing metabolites."[2]

Intensity of the stimulus and intensity of pain perceived are correlated. That the correlation is close and can be graded according to a scale of pain units or dols is maintained by some authorities[14,17,18] and denied by others.[19,20,43]

In general, the threshold for pain stimuli is higher than for touch, pressure and temperature; accordingly various kinds and degrees of these other sensations may be appreciated without necessarily provoking painful sensation. Usually any stimulus twice as intense as the minimal stimulus giving pain will damage tissue.

PSYCHOLOGY OF PAIN

There are always two aspects of pain—the perception and the reaction. While the nature and the severity of the noxious stimulus may be the same, the reactions to the same pain (that is, the *suffering*) differ widely among persons and in the same person at different times. Some of the reactions are physical; some are psychological. In the following chapters, therefore, the psychological reactions to pain in the various parts of the body necessarily receive consideration. No matter what the site of origin of the pain, certain factors tend to influence the psychological responses, among which are:

Integrity of Nervous System. The integrity of the end-organs, the conductive pathways and the perceptive centers. Obviously any diminution in sensation caused by nerve lesions reduces all reactive responses.

State of Consciousness. Consciousness is not an "all or none" entity. There are numerous stages, ranging from neurologic coma up through deep sleep, light sleep, reverie, increasingly alert states to the peak condition of unallayed alertness in which the greatest variety of cortical and subcortical connections are possible. The meaning of a sensory stimulus such as pain depends upon one's position *at the time* in the spectrum of consciousness. Past and present experience has a symbolic meaning which can distort, exaggerate, minimize, magnify or caricature a sensation.[28,29,38]

Total Pain Load. When pain impulses are reaching the perceptive centers along many pathways, responses are greater than if there is a single pain. When pain is intense, greater reactions are as a rule to be expected than when of lesser degrees.

Training. Persons who because of race, education or previous environment have been taught that pain is to be accepted without show of emotion are less apt to exhibit weeping, crying out, flight or fight reactions, etc., to pain. Others in whose family or school training such reactions have been condoned may show violent emotional reactions, considering it proper so to respond, either consciously or unconsciously.

Previous Experience. Conditioning through previous experience with pain has a profound effect upon response to it. The reactions may be either increased or decreased, depending upon the person and the previous pain circumstances. Extremely severe pain may at first be borne rather stoically by a relatively stable person. Repetition of the experience may engender such fear that anticipation alone may cause profound emotional and physical reactions with vomiting, or syncope, etc. Less stable personalities may respond similarly to even mild or moderately disagreeable stimuli.

On the contrary, again depending upon the personality make-up of the subject, repetition of painful experiences may develop either fortitude or resignation, with progressive decrease in the psychologic responses, sometimes to the point where practically no reaction is evident.

Knowledge and understanding of the origin and the significance of the pain greatly influence the subject's responses. Uncertainty or fear of dire import exaggerates responses. Thus, a woman with a breast nodule in fear of cancer often suffers pain until it is discovered to be a benign lesion, whereupon all discomfort disappears. Children often react violently to minor hurts until they understand that they will be of little consequence or of short duration.

Attention and distraction exert profound effects in modifying reaction to pain. The soldier who sustains serious injury but is unaware of it until out of the heat of combat, the athlete who is unconscious of his painful lesion until the excitement of the game is over, are examples of this. Likewise, the response to pain may be increased by attention, as exemplified by the patient with every faculty focused on the insertion of a venipuncture needle.

Fatigue may change the reaction to pain in various ways. Weariness and exhaustion may be so great that attention wanders from the injury. Or, in the opposite direction, fatigue may sometimes so vitiate the powers of resistance and self-control that even minor discomfort precipitates profound psychologic responses, such as crying out, weeping, attempts at flight or withdrawal.

Anxiety, Tension and Fear. The severity of suffering from a given painful stimulus depends largely upon emotional factors. The emotional state at the time will depend largely upon the *significance* of the pain to the patient. Measures to relieve anxiety may *dissociate* the pain from responses to it: the pain is still perceived but suffering is reduced or abolished.[29] Such results have been obtained with ataractic drugs, electroshock therapy, prefrontal lobotomy and psychotherapy. The patient may state that the pain is still there but he just does not care. Mounting anxiety tends to greatly increase suffering.

Pain associated with pleasurable emotion may cease to be recognized as pain: as when associated with sexual or religious ecstasy, or the return of sensation to a paralyzed analgetic limb. Women who experience "childbirth without fear" may be relatively indifferent to the pains of parturition.[30]

Suggestion is commonly supposed to alter at least the reaction to pain, if not its threshold. However, in at least one study,[21] neither normal nor psychoneurotic patients responded to suggestion with any significant change in threshold or reaction.

Religious or hysterical mental states may cause considerable dissociation of pain perception from reaction to pain. When under such influences, subjects may undergo unbelievably severe trauma without exhibiting evidence of experiencing pain.

SIGNIFICANCE OF PAIN TO THE AFFECTED PERSON

When pain is transitory or not severe one is apt soon to forget it. If, however, the pain experience is severe or recurrent or prolonged, the personality of the subject is affected. The possible ways that suffering may produce different psychological patterns in various types of personalities cannot be discussed fully here. However, we may mention certain common patterns:

1. The affected person may become resigned, patient, but with a brave "carry-on" attitude.

2. He may become resigned, but de-

pressed with resultant withdrawal, "give-up" or suicidal tendencies.

3. He may become stoic, indifferent to his own pain and sometimes to that of others.

4. He may become vindictive, revengeful, want to strike back; cruelty to self and others may become manifestations: masochism, sadism.

5. He may become fearful, apprehensive, anxious, irritable.

6. He may become tolerant, philosophical, kind, sympathetic with other sufferers.

Various combinations of these different types of effects may result in various persons. The pattern of response may become fixed in some subjects but in others may vary from time to time, or there may be progression from one type of pattern to another as the pain experience is repeated, or extended or modified.

Given a fairly severe or repeated painful stimulus of a standard intensity, one may observe in the *same subject* various physical and emotional reactions at different times, depending upon

1. State of consciousness: alert, drowsy, etc.

2. Whether rested or fatigued

3. Whether apprehensive, calm, etc.

4. Whether distracted from or concentrating upon the pain or its causes.

Among *various persons* subjected to such a painful stimulus of standard intensity, physical and emotional responses will depend upon all of the above variable factors applying to all subjects, plus differences between subjects dependent upon:

1. Past experience with pain in general

2. Significance of the particular type of pain to the affected person as an individusual: "Is this just a test?" or "Does this mean I have a cancer?"

3. What is expected: the pressures on the individual at least to try to conform to the standards of his society, especially of his own group. In some groups wailing and writhing is expected or condoned; in others even minimal reactions are regarded as contemptible.

It must be remembered that the responses or reactions mentioned above may be partly conscious and voluntary, partly subconscious or autonomic. The same pain might result in precipitate flight in one subject, in stoical immobility in another, and in shock and loss of consciousness in still another.

The physician studying the patient suffering from pain is concerned with:

1. *Discovering the cause* of the pain, so that if possible, it may be eliminated

2. *Observing the reactions* of the subject to the pain: these (physical, emotional and psychological) may help greatly in understanding of the patient as a person; various responses to pain may in themselves require further major study and treatment

3. *Evaluating the impact or significance* of the pain experience upon the subject as a whole person: including not only his pain perceptions and reactions but his psychological make-up, his philosophy, etc.

THE PHYSICIAN AS INTERPRETER

Here we must remind ourselves that the physician himself cannot be a completely objective observer. He, like the patient, is a human being with his own individual constellation of hereditary and environmental influences. His education in the sciences, in psychology and sociology, should be of great help to him, but if his own personal experience of suffering with pain is scant, so may his understanding of it in another person be limited. A person who has known little or no true pain will be handicapped in evaluating pain in another.

On the basis of his medical training, supplemented by all the education and the experience that he has gained in actually working with suffering patients, the physician must interpret (from the history, the physical examination and all special adjunctive tests) what the pain means *medically* as concerns the patient's body and also, *often even more significant,* what it means in regard to his total personality.

Thus in some persons a migraine attack or an ulcer pain or precordial distress may be a personal temporary inconvenience, whereas in others pains of apparently similar character and severity may become dominant influences not only in the patient's own life but also that of his family, business associates, etc.

The physician frequently finds the solution of pain problems simple, especially if the cause of the pain is transitory. However, when the pain is severe or recurrent or chronic, interpretation of the pain experience in all its aspects may be quite complex.[38]

PHYSICAL RESPONSES TO PAIN

Pain of some types excites not only the conscious but the unconscious automatic defense reactions, largely through stimulation of the sympathetic nervous system and an outpouring of adrenalin: the blood is withdrawn from the skin, the brain and the gastrointestinal tract and forced into the muscles, the blood pressure rises, the pulse rates increases, the pupils dilate, etc. This type of reaction is particularly characteristic of the response to superficial pain; that is, pain originating on the body surface.

Deep pain, especially if severe, is more apt to cause a sudden failure of the defense reactions — weakness, prostration, bradycardia, a fall in blood pressure, often nausea and vomiting, sweating and pallor, and sometimes syncope. Man and other animals subjected to such pain usually seek quiet, rest, inactivity and withdrawal, rather than activity and flight or combat.

Continued pain has been demonstrated to have deleterious action upon vital organs, such as the heart[6] and the kidneys.[5] Pain may initiate physical reactive patterns, usually recognizable as protective in nature, for example: elevation of arterial blood pressure, cardiac arrhythmias, cardiospasm, disturbances of gastric and colonic function,[12] occlusion of nasal passages with cr without lacrimation, etc.[14] If such reactions are long continued or frequently repeated, functional disorders may result, and eventually tissue damage may result from the responses to pain.

Frequently the physical attitude will indicate pain and sometimes suggest its location—grasping the painful head, crouching or pressing upon the cramping abdomen, etc. The facial expression of true pain— the pinched features, the pallor, the clammy skin, the dilated pupils, the knotted brow—cannot be imitated by the malingerer: these, with the intermittent involuntary cry or groan and the characteristic writhing or bodily contortions, present an unmistakable picture of suffering.

PAIN THRESHOLD

Pain, unlike other sensations, may be provoked by a variety of stimuli. Both superficial and deep pain can be provoked by mechanical, thermal, electrical or chemical stimuli. Superficial pain may be evoked by pricking, by heat or by chemical agents; deep pain may be caused by pressure, by stretching, by electrical stimulation (such as faradic current) or by chemical means.

The threshold of pain is not far removed in intensity from the trauma causing actual tissue damage. When pain is felt, danger to the tissues is usually imminent. As a rule, any intensity of stimulus of double (or greater) the minimal pain stimulus destroys tissue.

Hardy[18] and his co-workers believe that the pain threshold and the threshold for tissue damage are one and the same. He states "pain results from noxious stimulation which indicates the beginning of damage to the pain-fiber ending."

By choosing a stimulus of controlled and measured intensity one may determine the *lowest perceptible intensity of pain;* this is the pain threshold.

Wolff[1] and his co-workers[17,18] found that the threshold for pain in man was remarkably uniform. The stimulus which just provoked pain (the minimal or threshold stimulus) varied within only 5 per cent in each subject. In a group of 200 subjects of both sexes, from 10 to 80 years of age, the threshold stimulus varied within only 15 per cent. In all the tests the stimulus used was radiant heat applied to the skin.

In these studies, no effect upon the threshold was apparent from the emotional state, or after enforced wakefulness. However, if because of defects in concentration or attention, or due to fatigue, lethargy, suggestibility or prejudice, the subject was unable to focus on the test, the pain threshold varied widely and unpredictably.

Other investigators have found that the "normal" experimental pain threshold is neither constant from man to man, nor is it constant in a given person from time to time.[20] Beecher states that the threshold varies widely because it is not a true perception, and experience and value judgments (conditioning) enter unavoidably into its determination.[43]

When an intensely painful stimulus is applied to one body area, there is simultaneous elevation of the threshold of pain in other body areas (phenomenon of extinction[26]). This may result in partial or total failure to perceive pain arising from one source at a time when simultaneous noxious stimuli of equal or greater intensity (or significance to the person) are in operation and are causing pain from another source.

Perception of pain can be altered by lesions of the central nervous system which elevate the pain threshold.

HYPERALGESIA

The threshold for pain may be lowered by traumatic deformation, denudement, inflammation or injury of tissues near the nerve endings subserving pain.

Hyperalgesia is the term used to describe the state in which ordinarily non-noxious stimuli become capable of producing pain or in which noxious stimuli induce pain of greater intensity than they normally do. Two broad types of hyperalgesia may be distinguished:[14] (1) that due to a lowered pain threshold; (2) that due to other mechanisms and occurring with a normal pain threshold.

The peculiar hyperalgesia of *peripheral neuropathy* is of type 1: there is a differential effect upon the two types of cutaneous pain—the "burning" pain threshold may be greatly lowered, while the "pricking" pain threshold is elevated.[7]

An important part of the mechanism responsible for primary or Type 1 hyperalgesia is the local release of a chemical substance which lowers pain threshold. There may be several such substances such as neurokinin,[36,40,41,42] plasma kinin, histamine, serotonin, etc. See the discussion earlier in this chapter under The Stimulus.

Local tissue changes such as those of hyperemia and inflammation result in type 1 hyperalgesia of skin and mucous membranes both on the surface and lining the viscera. When the stomach is engorged, normal forceful contractions may be painful. Sunburn may lower the pain threshold of the skin by as much as 50 per cent.

Type 2 or secondary hyperalgesia is discussed below in the section Deep Pain, because it is often associated with referred pain from noxious stimuli to deep structures, and is of diagnostic importance. However, it is important to note that cutaneous hyperalgesia may be associated with either deep or superficial injury. Secondary hyperalgesia occurs in undamaged tissues the innervation of which is in the same or adjacent segments to that of the site of the injury (Figs. 76, 77 and 78, pp. 238, 239 and 240).

ANESTHESIA AND ANALGESIA

Local anesthetization can raise or obliterate the threshold. When analgesics are given to the subject, the pain threshold is raised. Pain itself was found to be a powerful antagonist of analgesics such as morphine.

Analgesics such as alcohol and morphine seem to have a much greater effect upon the reaction to pain or the emotional or the alarm response to it than upon the perception of pain. That is, the pain is felt in the same intensity or but little diminished, but the subject loses the anxiety and the other reactions that usually accompany the perception of pain.[22]

Wolff[1] found that the threshold for the emotional alarm reaction varied widely from subject to subject and in the same subject from time to time. It was usually below the pain threshold but sometimes above it. The alarm reaction could be elicited by painful or nonpainful stimuli, when the latter had become symbols of painful or dangerous experience.

SUPERFICIAL PAIN

Two types of cutaneous pain have been described by a number of investigators. Bigelow, Harrison and Wolff[1] believe their studies show that there are two qualities of cutaneous perception, while Lewis[2] and Gasser[3] emphasize a difference in speed. One type of pain is abrupt in onset and has a *pricking* quality that terminates quickly, while the other has a slower onset and has a *burning* quality. The types of discomfort and their relative speed may be observed by pressing a pin into the skin. The first pain is bright, sharp and quick; it terminates, and, from persistence of the original stimulus, the slow, burning pain is shortly felt. According to Gasser,[3] the first pain is carried mainly by the larger myelinated fibers conducting at a rate between 10 and 90 meters per second, while the second pain is carried mainly by small fibers called C fibers at a rate between 0.6 and 2 meters per second.

According to Wolff,[1] there is a real difference in quality, as well as time difference, between the quicker, or pricking, and the slower, burning types of cutaneous pain. He feels that the latter type of pain is similar to that experienced on the glans penis and on some mucous membranes, and regards it as truly an intermediate between superficial and deep pain.

That the two types of cutaneous pain can to some extent be dissociated is shown by observations in which nerves subjected to asphyxia exhibit a rise in threshold to pricking pain, but a fall to burning pain. It seems likely that in peripheral neuritis, or in pain due to pressure on nerve roots, etc., true hyperalgesia of this type does exist.

Superficial pain, sometimes called direct pain, is localized accurately to the point of disturbance. It may be associated with hyperalgesia, paresthesia, analgesia, tickling or itching.

DEEP PAIN

Pain which does not arise from surface structures, but from deeper structures such as the periosteum, the muscles and the viscera, has certain characteristics as to quality, localization and associated phenomena that distinguish it from superficial pain.

Quality. Deep pain feels deep—has a duller, aching nature as compared with the bright, sharp sensation of surface pain. This quality is essentially the same no

matter in what tissue or organ the sensation arises, although there are certain characteristic additional features of pain from particular sites that will be described later.

Duration. Surface pain is apt to be of shorter duration; deep pain tends to persist for a considerable period of time. It may have variations in intensity and be described as throbbing or cramping, boring or crushing, or often as aching, or if less intense, as hurting or soreness.

Localization. Deep pain is more diffuse, usually seems to originate in a wider area, and the site of origin of the pain is less accurately perceived.

Deep pain is apt to feel as if it were 3-dimensional and occupied space; superficial pain is more apt to be felt as a point or line or surface.

The accuracy of sensory localization (a function of the cerebral cortex) depends largely upon the relative abundance of sense organs present in the various regions and upon the frequency with which the whole sensory circuit is employed. For example, surface localization is highly accurate on the hands, the lips and the tongue, since these structures are employed to a great extent in identifying objects and are richly supplied with sensory nerve endings. On the back, localization is relatively crude because of the smaller number of sense organs and because of the lack of cortical training in recognition of the various back areas. A similar generalization may be made in regard to the deeper structures: those more frequently stimulated by contacts giving rise to sensory impulses are fairly well localized (muscles, periosteum of bones lying near the surface, etc.).

Hyperalgesia occurring at the site of the original noxious stimulus has been called primary, while that occurring at a distance is called secondary. Secondary hyperalgesia is promptly abolished when the original noxious stimulation ceases. Noxious stimulation of an area of referred pain is often productive of more discomfort than similar stimulation of an uninvolved region. The actual threshold of the area for cutaneous pain, however, is not altered.[8]

The association of superficial hyperalgesia with deep pain and the effects of anesthetization of the skin in modifying deep pain have caused much recent study and controversy.[16] Referred pain may occur with or without associated hyperalgesia; also with or without pain and tenderness induced by secondary muscle spasm. Skin or muscle procainization in the area of referred pain may modify greatly pain from visceral or other deep noxious stimulation, but the pain cannot be eliminated until the primary afferent impulses are terminated, or chemically or surgically blocked at their source.[24,25]

Muscle Contraction and Tenderness. Segmental hypersensitivity also must explain the muscle contraction occurring so often in association with deep pain, and the accompanying tenderness. The muscle spasm may sometimes be so pronounced and intense that the muscles become the dominant source of the pain.

Segmental spread of pain is observed frequently; that is, the pain may not remain confined to the original segment, but the false localization may spread into one or more neighboring spinal cord and skin segments. This is particularly apt to occur with very intense or prolonged deep pain. In coronary occlusion, for example, the pain often spreads from the skin areas supplied by the first four or five thoracic segments to the areas supplied by the lower, then the upper, cervical segments.

The spread of pain is a central, not a peripheral, effect. The spread is not dependent upon afferent impulses from the tissues into which spread occurs.[8]

Autonomic responses to deep pain include most frequently pallor and sweating; often there is nausea, vomiting, sometimes bradycardia, a fall in blood pressure, faintness, syncope, even death in shock.

VISCERAL PAIN

The viscera, when healthy, give no sensation, but when diseased or subjected to traction or tension, they may give rise to severe pain. The reason that inflammation or edema or vascular engorgement makes a previously insensitive organ highly sensitive is not known. Wolf and Wolff[4] showed that the normal healthy gastric mucosa gave no pain in response to stimuli intense enough to cause pain in other sites, but that when the mucosa was inflamed, congested or edematous, the same stimuli resulted in painful sensations. True visceral pain, therefore, does exist. The sensation coming from a viscus is usually rather poorly localized because of the relative paucity of nerve endings and because of the relative lack of use of the sensory pathway and consequent lack of cortical training in identifying the organ or part of the organ affected. It is generally agreed that the parietal peritoneum, in response to certain types of noxious stimulation, may give rise to pain. In the severe cramping type of pain associated with vigorous contractions of part of the gastrointestinal tract, where does the pain arise? Lewis,[2] reviewing the available evidence, concluded that contractions of the muscle of the gut did not give rise to painful sensations, and that traction on mesenteric attachments must explain it. Wolf and Wolff,[4] however, present quite convincing evidence that the muscularis, the serosa and the visceral peritoneum may give rise to pain when under abnormal tensions.

Localization of Visceral Pain: Referred Pain. Visceral pain may at first be felt as within the body in the approximate location of the viscus, but soon, and more intensely, the pain is apt to be falsely localized and referred to a surface area of the body. The sensation from the viscus is referred to the site of peripheral distribution of the afferent nerves from certain skin areas, the particular site depending upon the spinal cord segment receiving the afferent fibers from the viscus. The nerves of cutaneous sensation have a definite segmental distribution (see Fig. 76, p. 238), and, therefore, visceral pain is quite regularly falsely localized or referred to certain segmental surface areas, the area indicating more or less accurately the possible viscus involved. The site in which the pain is falsely localized depends not only upon the particular spinal cord segment and corresponding skin segment, but upon the part of the segment most accustomed to feel pain. The cerebral cortex is here again apparently involved on the basis of previous training, experience or conditioning. The exact mechanism of how the pain sensation is changed from an interior to an apparently exterior phenomenon is not too well understood. One theory is that it is simply a fault of cortical function; the site of surface localization is mistakenly chosen simply because of the relatively higher number of nerve endings and because of the fact that pain from the segment usually comes from the surface. Another theory is that afferent impulses from the viscus, on entering the spinal cord, lower the threshold to impulses from the skin, so that the normal stimuli acting upon the surface may thus cause pain. The latter theory seems an adequate explanation for the associated phenomena of hyperesthesia and hyperalgesia frequently found in the corresponding skin area, but not for the falsely localized pain itself.

White, Sweet and others[23,24,34] have shown that surgeons can eliminate pain in visceral disease by cutting viscerosensory fibers within the peripheral sympathetic trunks, the posterior spinal roots, or the anterolateral quadrant of the spinal cord with the larger mass of sensory afferent fibers from the surface of the body. Interrupting the *cutaneous* inflow alone from the segment concerned will not stop pain of visceral origin.

Deep Somatic Pain

Pain of segmental distribution associated with segmental tenderness of the skin is in a large percentage of instances due to somatic rather than to visceral disease. Irritation of the trunks, the ganglia or the roots of the spinal sensory nerves may give rise to pain that simulates that of visceral disease. For example, the injection of hypertonic saline solution into an interspinous ligament results in referral of the pain to the peripheral distribution of the corresponding segmental nerve, with accompanying tenderness and muscular rigidity.[2] If the first lumbar interspinous ligament is injected, loin or scrotal pain

similar to that caused by ureteral stone may occur; injection of the eighth cervical interspinous ligament causes pain like that of angina pectoris. The same type of pain, the same false localization and the same reflex effects may in some instances be produced from deep somatic structures and from certain viscera. (Often, however, referred somatic pain does not follow a simple segmental pattern.[9]) Intercostal neuralgia may simulate intrathoracic visceral disease, and abdominal-wall neuralgia may simulate intra-abdominal visceral disease. Among the commoner conditions that cause deep somatic pain are spinal deformities, arthritis of the spine, spinal cord tumors, tumors involving the vertebrae and ruptured intervertebral disks.

Segmental neuralgia from such lesions usually is associated with significant segmental tenderness, whereas the referred pain arising from visceral disease is not. Paravertebral nerve block may be very successful in relieving pain of segmental somatic origin[25] but does not relieve the pain of visceral disease.[14,34]

Usually *hyperalgesia* is described in the area of referred pain from deep somatic stimuli. However, Feinstein[27] has found *hypoalgesia* as more characteristic. He also found (from studies based on paravertebral muscle injections of neck and back) that areas of referred pain were roughly segmental, with much overlapping and many differences in location from the conventional dermatomes.

Three Kinds of Deep Pain

To summarize, three varieties of deep pain may be recognized: (1) *True visceral and deep somatic pain.* This type of pain is felt *in situ*, at the point of noxious stimulation. It may or may not be associated with referred pain. (2) *Referred pain.* This falsely projected pain is felt at a site other than and often some distance from the site of the stimulus; it is felt in an area supplied by the same or adjacent neural segments. (3) *Pain from secondary skeletal muscle contraction.* There may be central spread of excitation within the spinal cord, with resultant effector activity including muscle contraction which may itself then act as a source of painful stimuli.

Clinical Variations. In some instances, the severity of the Type 1 *in situ* pain may be the most intense and one or more of the varieties of referred pain may be present in lesser degree.

In other instances the referred pain may predominate, and there may be little or no pain felt *in situ*. Under such circumstances, local procainization at the site of referred pain may relieve pain and muscle spasm sufficiently to give complete or almost complete relief, at least temporarily.

When the cause of the deep pain is temporary, and the original noxious stimulus is gone, procainization may seem to have removed the cause of the pain. However, when the original cause persists, the referred pain phenomena recur with or without the true deep *in situ* pain. To terminate such pain, elimination of the noxious stimulus is necessary by removing the cause or blocking it at its source.

CENTRAL PAIN

Central pain is pain perceived by the subject, but for which no peripheral cause exists. Central pain occasionally is caused by organic lesions of the sensory gray matter and sensory tracts of the central nervous system, but most instances of central pain are due to persistence of perception after the peripheral stimulus has ceased.

Central pain occurs in causalgia (after injury to peripheral nerve trunks) and in cases of phantom limb. Another example is that occurring in herpes, long after the herpetic lesion has healed and even after dorsal rhizotomy.

Patients suffering from certain lesions of the thalamus or of the spinothalamic tracts complain of constant or frequently recurring pain, usually not localized, sometimes indicated as occurring in one lateral half of the body or in an entire extremity. Apparently some inhibitory control is removed, so that stimuli of normal intensity are interpreted as causing pain.[11]

CLINICAL MANIFESTATIONS OF PAIN

Since pain is subjective, but offers, if properly understood, a valuable key to the patient's disease, the patient's complaint and his reactions to his discomfort deserve careful analysis and interpretation. The physician should have the patient describe his pain as accurately as possible as to its nature and exact location, pointing to the spot. Often, for example, a pain described as "in the stomach" may actually by pointing be found to be in the lower abdomen, or one "in the leg" will really be in the buttock or the thigh. Time of occurrence, spread, severity, constancy or recurrent or intermittent nature should be elicited. Associated phenomena should be observed or their character ascertained from the history.

Under certain conditions the perception of pain may be facilitated or inhibited. It is important to study not only the pain itself but the patient who has the pain, for the same stimulus produces varying results in various individuals and even in the same individual if conditions are altered.

Let us consider somewhat more fully the significance of pain facilitation and inhibition, the means of judging the severity of pain, and the implications of certain qualities and time characteristics.

FACILITATED PAIN

The sense-perceptive centers in the brain after repeated stimulation become hypersensitive. It is probably for this reason that the chronic rheumatic through exacerbations of the pain is able to predict changes in the weather. The habitual pain pathway responds like a sensitive barometer to changes in the atmospheric pressure and the temperature.

The patient who has had a chronic cholecystitis and still has the typical gallbladder pain after the gallbladder has been removed is a trying and familiar problem to many a physician. Slight structural changes at or near the original site of the production of pain seem to cause stimuli to flow easily along the old smooth wellworn channels. Or in more physiologic language, resistance at the synapses is reduced in a frequently used pathway.

The cortical threshold may be lowered generally as well as locally. In certain illnesses, such as pneumonia and malaria, marked general hyperalgesia occurs. Neurasthenics may actually be so hypersensitive to pain that pricking the finger for a blood count may cause real anguish and leave a tender spot for days. In hysteria only one arm or one skin area may be hypersensitive.

INHIBITED PAIN

Age, Training. Certain individuals are less sensitive to pain than the average, while certain others are more sensitive than the average. The marked differences in apparent sensitivity to pain are chiefly in the response or reaction to pain, since carefully measured true *pain thresholds are remarkably uniform.* Emotional attitudes toward pain can greatly alter perception of the stimulus. Studies have shown that in any one individual sensitivity is learned by the infant, increases to adult life, then gradually diminishes. Blows small infants receive are often apparently felt much less than they would be by an adult. The learning process in regard to pain involves the *emotional, reactive* components rather than the physical components. Education and protection usually cause increased sensitivity. Habituation and exposure to a rigorous environment usually diminish pain perception. Individuals can by will power and training greatly control their pain perception. Persons of asthenic body type are usually more sensitive than persons of sthenic habitus.

Race. Persons of certain races, such as Jews and Latins, are as a rule more sensitive to pain. The Anglo-Saxon or the Nordic type of person is apt to be relatively less sensitive (i.e., less reactive).

The factors mentioned tend to be characteristic of the individual. However, temporary alterations occur. These may result in lessened acuity of the pain sense, as in anger, fear or excitement. Hysteric analgesia is an example of pain inhibition.

PAIN SEVERITY

The severity of the pain experience involves both the *intensity* of the purely sensory phenomenon and the *reactions:* physical, emotional and psychological.

Both the sensation and the reactions to it are important to the physician in guiding diagnosis and therapy.

The physician's estimate of the severity of pain must depend upon several factors:

General impression as to the patient's general sensitivity: age, race, training, emotional state, truthfulness, relative objectivity in describing his symptoms, etc.

Face. Pallor, brow furrowed, lips drawn, teeth clenched, eyes fixed, pupils dilated —hippocratic facies.

Body position. Examples:

Peritonitis: Horizontal, quiet, hands lightly on abdomen or lying at sides.

Colic: Rolled up, pressing on painful point, kneeling on bed.

Joint or limb: Holding limb in protected position.

Muscle rigidity. Involuntary muscle spasm: broken bone, peritonitis.

Activity. Usually ceases with severe pain. Exception: Colic, often accompanied by rocking, kneeling, etc.

Blood pressure and pulse rate. Increase usually; if pain is very severe, blood pressure may fall (shock).

Associated signs. Vomiting, fever, sweating, jaundice, leukocytosis, etc.

Emotional Reactions. Fear, excitement, anger, depression, weeping and other emotional states reflect as a rule the *significance* of the pain to the subject. Anxiety increases the patient's estimate of the intensity of the pain and his emotional responses to it.

The patient's description of the severity of his pain must not be accepted without interpretation based on the above factors. The patient may consciously or unconsciously exaggerate or minimize his symptoms. If he consciously exaggerates he is called a malingerer.

QUALITY OF PAIN

Patients differ in their ability to describe symptoms accurately, and they often differ in the words used to describe the quality of sensations. They usually refer them to something similar previously experienced. Characteristic descriptive terms are:

In aneurysmal erosion: boring, pounding

In bones: deep, aching, boring

In muscles: sore, aching

In colic: twisting, griping, cramping, recurs in waves

In angina: compression, constriction, comes on with exertion, great weight, agonizing, impending death

In pleuritis: stabbing, knifelike, with each breath

In peptic ulcer: burning, sharp, associated with hunger, relieved by food or alkali, occurs at night

In tabes: lightning-like, shooting, stabbing

In neuritis: burning, stinging

In neuralgia: sharp, cutting, paroxysmal, intermittent

In causalgia: burning, peculiar stinging (paresthesiae)[10]

In burns, blisters, superficial skin lesions: burning, smarting, stinging, hot.

TIME OF OCCURRENCE OF PAIN

Duration. It is highly unlikely that an extremely intense pain *can* be felt over a long period of time, for pain of great intensity usually means that the nerve endings themselves are being destroyed, and when they are destroyed, the pain is apt to diminish or cease.[18] An exception, when severe pain is experienced over long periods, is causalgia, when the nerve trunk itself is damaged.

The descriptive terms used to describe various *qualities* of pain involve *time* as a dimension: sticking, pricking, flashing, shooting, stabbing are adjectives implying *momentary* sensations of various severity. Burning, throbbing, boring, cramping, griping, twisting, pressing, crushing, aching imply discomfort of *longer duration* or recurrent in point of time. Soreness and tenderness or hurting mean pain or discomfort provoked by touch or pressure upon or motion of a part.

Pain from organic disease is seldom constant. When a patient says he has the same pain constantly, the diagnosis is usually psychoneurosis. At least, great care must be shown in accepting such a statement. Organic pain varies because the nerve centers tire periodically, and thus give respite, and because organic etiologic factors usually vary from time to time.

Periodic or Seasonal. Peptic ulcer pain seems to recur often in spring and in fall. Such seasonal variations may be due to change in diet. Ulcer pain tends to recur at intervals of weeks or months and to occur daily for several weeks. Gallbladder pain tends to occur in severe attacks lasting only a few minutes or hours, or perhaps a day or more, with relative freedom for weeks or months.

Time of Day. Certain pains are made worse by mental or physical activity. They usually, therefore, occur during the day. Examples are:

1. Neurasthenic pain
2. Locomotor pain: rheumatism, flat foot, sciatica
3. Eye pain
4. Gastrointestinal pain
5. Morning sinus pain: no chance to drain at night, congested in the morning.

Night Pain. Night pain is usually characteristic of organic disease, especially if it awakens the patient.

Some types of psychogenic pain may be more frequent at night, especially when the patient is freed of the distractions of the day, becomes anxious and fearful and suffers from insomnia.

Night is largely devoted to autonomic nerve control, and thus is the time of vagus and parasympathetic activity. Therefore, ulcer pain and colics characteristically come at night. The pain of rheumatic affections and of tuberculous and other joint disease may be chiefly nocturnal, for then the protective muscle contraction of the day is often relaxed and involuntary movement occurs.

ADVERSE PHYSICAL EFFECTS OF PAIN

Pain may, through its widespread reactions influencing the nervous system and the circulation, cause profound disturbance in the function of vital organs. Shock from pain may be so profound that death results. Pain may cause a significant decrease in the blood supply to the kidney, with failure of kidney function and a fall in urine output. The relative ischemia may be of no serious consequence to previously unimpaired kidneys, but when the kidneys were diseased, such a transient decrease in renal circulation has caused death.[5] Physiologic responses to pain may adversely affect heart function, as indicated by the electrocardiograph.[6] If the heart were previously normal, such changes might not be significant, but if it were already damaged, such an additional insult might be serious in its consequences.

Peripheral nerve damage may cause profound deleterious tissue changes in the area of distribution of the nerve.[33]

ADVERSE PSYCHOLOGICAL EFFECTS OF PAIN

There are two general types of reaction which are apt to occur in response to pain, either (1) mobilization for resistance or flight with anger or fear as dominant emotions, or (2) immobilization or withdrawal often with feelings of weakness, sickness and fear. The first or hyperdynamic type of response is associated with sensations of excitement, and autonomic responses of tachycardia, elevated blood pressure and increased capacity for muscular effort. The second or hypodynamic type of response is associated with muscular weakness, faintness, nausea, low blood pressure and bradycardia.

Resistance or flight or withdrawal may be protective and thus not adverse to the organism's welfare.

Repeated or prolonged pain is apt to cause fear, depression, insomnia, anorexia, irritability and nervous tension. Interrupting the pain or abolishing it may have profound salutary effects upon the patient's morale and emotional balance.

FUNCTION OF PAIN

Pain is often looked upon as a great enemy of mankind. Philosophers have debated whether man would be happier in a world free of pain; some have considered pain simply as a necessary contrast so that pleasure can be appreciated.

From the standpoint of a highly developed organism such as man, the sensation of pain acts primarily as an important alarm signal which usually sets into operation a *protective mechanism*. It is possible for persons congenitally without the pain sense, or in whom pain pathways have been surgically interrupted, to make certain compensatory adjustments to environment.[13,15] Stimuli of harmful nature may become associated with injury or the danger of injury so that the alarm and the defense reactions may be called into play without the occurrence of the perception of pain.[31] However, such persons are handicapped, and are less perfectly equipped to withstand the hazards of the environment. Repeated traumatic incidents may be endured unconsciously when pain is absent, with resultant severe tissue damage, as in the deep perforating ulcers of the feet in tabes dorsalis. Man has learned that certain stimuli warn of the imminence of pain or tissue damage and defense reactions are more often than not initiated without pain actually being experienced. Pain is not the only warning of the danger of injury, but it is a very important one. Moreover, it is the final warning, for shortly beyond the normal pain threshold lies the threshold of tissue destruction.

Pain is therefore not man's enemy, but his ally. Pain alerts the subject; it is an aid in a world full of possible injurious influences. Pain is still more significantly the ally of the physician, for it acts as an indicator to him of disease in the patient. It brings the patient to him before the lesion is far advanced, often in the stage when the disease process may be halted, when healing may be brought about. Pain acts not only as the notifier of the presence of disease but as an indicator of its location. Thus, adequate analysis and interpretation of the symptom pain, probably more often than of any other symptom, are instrumental in leading to correct diagnosis.

SUMMARY

Each pain experience may be thought of as consisting of three parts:

1. Reception of the pain stimulus and conduction of the pain impulse by nerves.

2. Perception of pain in higher centers (thalamus, cerebral cortex).

3. The reactions to pain: (a) physical, (b) emotional, (c) psychological.

Pain is a sensation, a subjective phenomenon, which does not exist until it is registered in consciousness. Pain always appears in a certain *context* that determines the significance of the subjective experience. The context varies greatly between subjects, and in the same subject may differ from time to time.

In quality pains can be grouped into three basic types: (1) bright, pricking; (2) burning; (3) deep, aching.

Pain normally operates as an alerting or alarm signal; it warns of the imminence of danger, the presence of peripheral damage or of central distress. The perception of pain usually is part of a protective mechanism which sets into operation defensive or withdrawal reactions valuable in preserving the integrity of the organism.

Occasionally, pain may serve no useful purpose and be damaging to the subject not only psychologically but physically. In such instances pain itself can be a disease and its elimination may be necessary to preserve health or life.

Study of pain as reported to him by patients and of the many phenomena associated with pain as observed in patients is particularly rewarding to the physician. Understanding of pain in its varied aspects constitutes a primary approach to a large proportion of man's diseases and disabilities.

This chapter is concerned with certain basic and general considerations of pain; subsequent chapters analyze a number of special types and locations of pain.

REFERENCES

1. Wolff, H. G.: Some Observations on Pain, Harvey Lectures 1943-1944, Series 39:39-95.
2. Lewis, T.: Pain, New York, Macmillan, 1942.
3. Gasser, H.: Pain-producing impulses in peripheral nerves, Proc. A. Research Nerv. Ment. Dis. 23:46, 1943.
4. Wolf, S., and Wolff, H. G.: Human Gastric Function, an Experimental Study of a Man and His Stomach, New York, Oxford, 1943 and 1947.
5. Wolf, G.: The effect of pain on renal function, Proc. A. Research Nerv. Ment. Dis. 23:358, 1943.
6. Gold, H., Kwit, N., and Modell, W.: The effect of extracardiac pain on the heart, Proc. A. Research Nerv. Ment. Dis. 23:345, 1943.
7. Bigelow, N., Harrison, I., Goodell, H., and Wolff, H. G.: Studies on pain, J. Clin. Investigation 23:503, 1945.
8. Wolff, H. G., and Hardy, J. D.: The nature of pain, Physiol. Rev. 27:167, 1947.
9. Travell, J., and Bigelow, N.: Referred somatic pain does not follow a simple segmental pattern, Federation Proc. 5:106, 1946.
10. Livingston, W. K.: Pain Mechanisms; A Physiologic Interpretation of Causalgia and Related States, New York, Macmillan, 1943.
11. Kendall, D.: Some observations on central pain, Brain 62:253, 1939.
12. Almy, T. P., and Tulin, M.: Alterations in colonic function in man under stress. Experimental production of changes simulating irritable colon, Gastroenterology 8:616, 1947.
13. Kunkle, E. C., and Chapman, W. P.: Insensitivity to pain in man, Proc. A. Research Nerv. Ment. Dis. 23:100, 1943.
14. Wolff, H. G., and Wolf, S.: Pain, ed. 2, Springfield, Ill., Thomas, 1958.
15. McMurray, G. A.: Experimental study of a case of insensitivity to pain, Arch. Neurol. Psychiat. 64:650, 1950.
16. Hardy, J. D., Wolff, H. G., and Goodell, H.: Experimental evidence on the nature of cutaneous hyperalgesia, J. Clin. Investigation 29:115-140, 1950.
17. ———: Pain Sensations and Reactions, Baltimore, Williams & Wilkins, 1952.
18. Hardy, J. D.: The nature of pain, J. Chron. Dis. 4:22-51, 1956.
19. Haugen, F. P.: Current concepts of the pain process, J. Chron. Dis. 4:4-10, 1956.
20. Beecher, H. K.: Limiting factors in experimental pain, J. Chron. Dis. 4:11-21, 1956.
21. Chapman, W., Finesinger, J. and Chesley, G.: The effect of direct suggestion on pain sensitivity, J. Nerv. Ment. Dis. 118:19-26, 1953.
22. Kornetsky, C.: The effects of anxiety and morphine on the anticipation and perception of painful radiant thermal stimuli, J. Compar. Physiol. Psychol. 47:130-132, 1954.
23. White, J. C.: Conduction of pain in man; observations on its afferent pathways within spinal cord and visceral nerves, A.M.A. Arch. Neurol. Psychiat. 71:1-23, 1954.
24. White, J. C., and Sweet, W. H.: Pain; Its Mechanisms and Neurosurgical Control, Springfield, Ill., Thomas, 1955.

25. Judovich, B., and Bates, W.: Pain Syndromes: Treatment by Paravertebral Nerve Block, Philadelphia, Davis, 1950.

26. Berlin, L., *et al.*: Studies of pain; the relation of pain threshold and pain intensity to the phenomenon of extinction, Trans. Am. Neurol. A. 229-231, 1953.

27. Feinstein, B., *et al.*: Experiments on pain referred from deep somatic tissues, J. Bone Joint Surg. 36A:981-997, 1954.

28. Schiller, F.: Consciousness reconsidered, A.M.A. Arch. Neurol. Psychiat. 67:199-227, 1952.

29. Rome, H. P.: The problem of pain, Proc. Staff. Meet. Mayo Clin. 31:221-226, 1956.

30. Read, G. D.: Childbirth Without Fear, New York, Harper, 1944.

31. Kipnis, D. M., *et al.*: Experimental studies on insensitivity to pain, Trans. Am. Neurol. A. 105-110, 1954.

32. Yonge, K. A.: Pain: direct, referred and displaced, Canad. M.A.J. 71:430-438, 1954.

33. Bilisoly, F. N.: Vasodilatation, lowered pain threshold and increased tissue vulnerability, A.M.A. Arch. Int. Med. 94:759-773, 1954.

34. Sweet, W. H.: *in* Handbook of Physiology, Section I: Neurophysiology, Chap. 12, Vols. 1 and 2, Baltimore, Williams & Wilkins, 1959-60.

35. Ruch, T. C., and Fulton, J. F.: Medical Physiology and Biophysics, p. 300f., 350f., Philadelphia, Saunders, 1960.

36. Chapman, L. F., Ramos, A., Goodell, H., Silverman, G., and Wolff, H. G.: A humoral agent implicated in vascular headache of the migraine type, Arch. Neurol. 3:223-229, 1960; Trans. Am. Neurol. Assn. 85:42-45, 200-202, 1960.

37. Wolstenholme, G., and O'Connor, M., eds.: Pain and itch: nervous mechanisms *in* Ciba Foundation Study Group No. 1, Boston, Little-Brown, 1959.

38. Buytendijk, F.: Pain, Its Modes and Functions, Chicago, Univ. Chicago Press, 1962.

39. Keele, K. D.: Anatomies of Pain, Springfield, Ill., Thomas, 1957.

40. Armstrong, D., Jepson, J. B., Keele, C. A., and Stewart, J. W.: Plasma pain-producing substance, J. Physiol. 135:350, 1957.

41. Armstrong, D., *et al.*: Chemical excitants of cutaneous pain, J. Physiol. 120:326, 1953.

42. Wright, S.: Applied Physiology, ed. 10, (revised by Keele, C. A., and Neil, E.), London, Oxford, 1961.

43. Beecher, H. K.: The measurement of pain, Pharmacol. Rev. 9:59-209, 1957; Pathology and experiment in advancing study of subjective responses, with emphasis on pain *in* Beecher, H. K. ed.: Disease and the Advancement of Basic Science, Cambridge, Harvard, 1960.

4

Headache*

HAROLD G. WOLFF

(May 26, 1898—February 21, 1962)

PATHOPHYSIOLOGY
OF HEADACHE

Headaches fall into two major categories as regards their origin: (1) those that arise mainly as a result of stimulation of intracranial structures, and (2) those that occur on stimulation of tissues which lie on the outside of and adjacent to the skull.

PAIN-SENSITIVE STRUCTURES OF THE HEAD

The pain sensitivity of the tissues covering the cranium, the cranium itself and most of the intracranial structures has been

*Revised by Helen Goodell, Lawrence E. Hinkle, Jr., and E. Charles Kunkle.

ascertained from a series of patients during surgical procedures on the head by using a variety of stimuli. Some of the "pain pathways" and the mechanisms of headache are defined.

1. Of the tissues covering the cranium, all are more or less sensitive to pain, the arteries being especially so.

2. Of the intracranial structures, the great venous sinuses and their venous tributories from the surface of the brain, parts of the dura at the base, the dural arteries and the cerebral arteries at the base of the brain, the 5th, the 9th and the 10th cranial nerves and the upper 3 cervical nerves are sensitive to pain.

3. The cranium (including the diploic and the emissary veins), the parenchyma of the brain, most of the dura, most of the pia-arachnoid, the ependymal lining of the ventricles and the choroid plexuses are not sensitive to pain.

Stimulation of the pain-sensitive intracranial structures on or above the superior surface of the tentorium cerebelli resulted in pain in various regions in front of a line drawn vertically from the ears across the top of the head. The pathways for this pain are contained in the 5th cranial nerve.

Stimulation of the pain-sensitive intracranial structures on or below the inferior surface of the tentorium cerebelli resulted in pain in various regions behind the line just described. The pathways for this pain are contained chiefly in the 9th and the 10th cranial nerves and the upper 3 cervical nerves.

Intracranial diseases commonly cause headache through more than one mechanism and by involvement of more than one pain-sensitive structure. From the data available, 6 basic mechanisms of headache from intracranial sources have been formulated: headache may result from (1) traction on the veins that pass to the venous sinuses from the surface of the brain and displacement of the great venous sinuses; (2) traction on the middle meningeal ar-

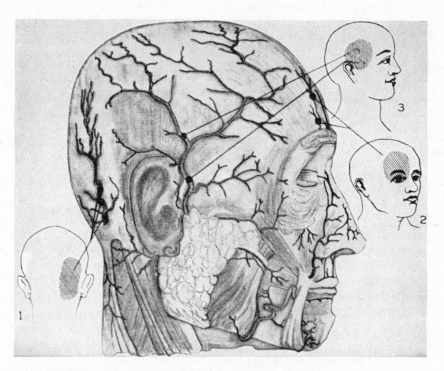

Fig. 22. The arteries of the scalp. Solid circles indicate the points of stimulation causing pain. The diagrams show the areas of pain following the stimulation of (1) the occipital arteries, (2) the supraorbital and frontal arteries and (3) the superficial temporal artery. (Ray and Wolff: Arch. Surg. 41:817)

teries; (3) traction on the large arteries at the base of the brain and their main branches; (4) distension and dilatation of intracranial arteries; (5) inflammation in or about any of the pain-sensitive structures of the head; and (6) direct pressure or traction by tumors on cranial and cervical nerves containing many pain-afferent fibers from the head.

Traction, displacement and inflammation of pain-sensitive venous structures, arteries, cranial and upper cervical nerves are chiefly responsible for headache arising from intracranial structures.

Headache from intracranial disease is usually referred pain. Local tenderness of the scalp may serve as an index to the structures responsible when a lesion produces direct irritation of pain-sensitive structures. However, disease of remotely separated pain-sensitive structures may cause pain and hyperalgesia in identical areas. Sepsis or fever of any origin may be associated with headache, but this is not referred pain. Pain referred to the head from disease of tissue elsewhere than the head does not occur, with the rare exception of pain in the jaw or the neck with angina pectoris. In paraplegics, headache may be associated with excessive distention of the urinary bladder or the rectum. Such headache results from dilatation of cranial vessels, secondary to a rise in systemic arterial pressure.

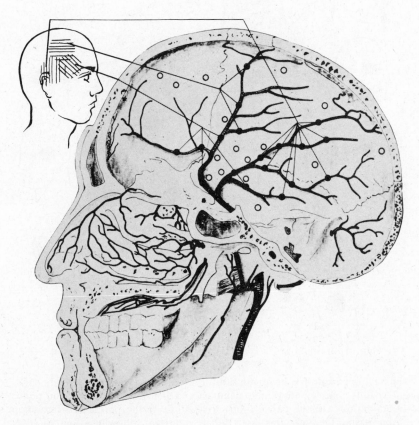

Fig. 23. Middle meningeal artery. Open circles indicate the point of stimulation of the dura without pain. Solid circles indicate the point of stimulation causing pain. The diagram shows three overlapping areas of pain in the parietotemporal region resulting from stimulation of different portions of the artery and its branches.

Mechanism of Headache Associated with Changes in Intracranial Pressure

The headache so frequently associated with abnormally high or low cerebrospinal fluid pressure has long been the subject of contradictory speculations. In a study of headache associated with changes in intracranial pressure, headache was regularly induced in normal erect human subjects by the free drainage of approximately 20 ml. of cerebrospinal fluid (about 10% of the total CSF volume), the estimated vertex pressure falling to between minus 220 and minus 290 mm. from a normal of approximately minus 130 mm.

The headache which often follows lumbar puncture has predictable and unique features, all of which indicate its similarity

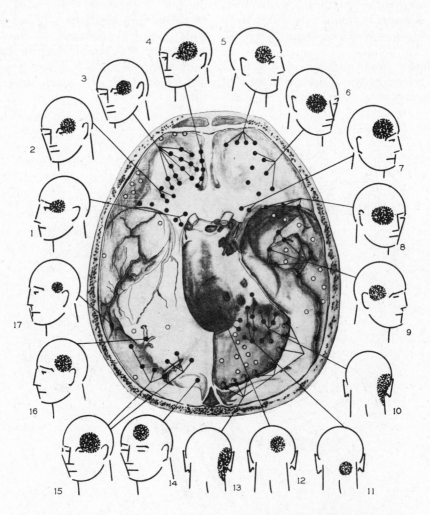

Fig. 24. The dural floor of the skull, the tentorium cerebelli and the adjacent venous sinuses and venous tributaries. Open circles indicate the points of stimulation without pain. Solid circles indicate the points of stimulation causing pain. The diagrams show the areas of pain following stimulation of: (1–8) the dura of the floor of the anterior fossa, (9–17) the middle meningeal artery, (10–12) the dura of the floor of the posterior fossa, (13) the inferior wall of the transverse sinus, (14) the superior wall of the torcular Herophili, (15) the superior wall of the transverse sinus and upper surface of the tentorium cerebelli and (16) the inferior cerebral veins. (Ray and Wolff: Arch. Surg. 41:825)

to the drainage headache. It may appear a few hours to several days after lumbar puncture, lasting a variable period of days or, rarely, weeks. The pain is a dull, deep ache and may be throbbing. It is usually bifrontal and often also suboccipital. In the latter position it may be associated with moderate stiffness of the neck. Like drainage headache, postpuncture headache was shown to be associated with a decrease in cerebrospinal fluid volume as evidenced by a fall in cerebrospinal fluid pressure. It was completely eliminated by the intrathecal injection of an amount of saline equal to that of spinal fluid removed. Its intensity was reduced by change from the erect to the horizontal position or by head flexion or extension. Its intensity was increased by bilateral jugular compression and by shaking the head (lowered "jolt threshold").

Therefore, the usual variety of postpuncture headache is similar in type and mechanism to the headache induced by drainage of cerebrospinal fluid. Its behavior suggests that it is caused chiefly by dilatation and traction upon pain-sensitive intracranial venous structures. It is probably secondary to the loss of cerebrospinal fluid removed for analysis, plus the prolonged leakage of fluid through the dural hole in the lumbar sac produced by the operator's needle. Prevention is facilitated by the use of a small bore lumbar puncture needle.

The headache so often associated with increased intracranial pressure has generally been assumed, but never proved, to be related to the increased pressure. Yet elevation of intracranial pressure in normal human subjects to abnormally high levels failed to cause headache. Headache homolateral to the lesion in a patient with a brain tumor was induced by lowering the intracranial pressure, but could not be induced by elevation of the pressure to a high level of 550 mm. That increased intracranial pressure is not the dominant factor in headache associated with brain tumor is suggested by an analysis of 72 patients in whom headache occurred almost as commonly (82%) in 23 patients without increased intracranial pressure as it did (94%) in 49 patients with increased pressure.

Hence, increased intracranial pressure is neither a prime nor an essential factor in the headache that may be associated with it.

From these data it is concluded that the headache associated with either decreased or increased intracranial pressure results from traction upon or displacement of pain-sensitive intracranial structures and is independent of generalized intracranial pressure changes per se.

BRAIN-TUMOR HEADACHE

The Quality and the Intensity of Brain-Tumor Headache. The headache associated with brain tumor is of a deep, aching, steady, dull nature. It is not rhythmic and seldom throbs. It is usually intermittent, but in one tenth of the patients it is continuous. The headache is sometimes severe, but rarely is it as intense as that of migraine or of the headache associated with rupture of cerebral aneurysm, meningitis or certain febrile illnesses or of that induced by certain drugs. It is usually diminished in intensity by acetylsalicylic acid, or cold packs applied to the scalp, both indications of its moderate intensity. It rarely interferes with sleep. It may be aggravated by coughing, or straining at stool, and sometimes it is worse in the erect than in the recumbent position. It is commonly aggravated also by the onset of a minor infection. If there is any variation in intensity during the 24-hour cycle, it is worse in the early morning.

Even when the tumor directly compresses or extensively stretches cranial nerves containing pain afferents, the pain is not equal in intensity to that of tic douloureux and indeed is often mild or absent.

One rare form of very intense headache may be encountered in patients in the terminal phase of brain tumor. This headache is generalized, paroxysmal and agonizing and it may precede stupor or death. The pain may last for 30 seconds to half an hour and may disappear suddenly.

Unless the pain is severe, nausea with tumor headache is slight. Vomiting occurs with displacement or compression of the medulla and is sometimes projectile (perhaps because it is unexpected when unaccompanied by nausea). The headache when occipital or suboccipital is sometimes associated with "stiffness" or aching of the muscles of the neck and tilting of the head toward the side of the tumor. The possibility of brain tumor should be appraised, (1) whenever severe and/or persistent headache begins in a patient who upon careful questioning reveals that he has not had headache previously; and (2) whenever a change occurs in the site, the quality, the intensity and the temporal features of the head pain in those with a long history of headaches.

The Mechanism of Brain-Tumor Headache. Brain-tumor headache is produced by traction upon and displacement of intracranial pain-sensitive structures, chiefly the large arteries, veins and venous sinuses and certain cranial nerves. There are two types of traction which operate singly or in combination: local traction by the tumor upon adjacent structures; and distant traction by extensive displacement of the brain, either directly by the tumor, or indirectly by ventricular obstruction (internal hydrocephalus). Brain tumor may in addition press directly upon cranial nerves.

Headache as an aid in the localization of brain tumor is limited in its value by two facts: the headache may be remote from the site of its production and the site of production of headache may be remote from the tumor.

In spite of these limitations, when it is interpreted in terms of known principles of intracranial pain production and pain reference, the headache of brain tumor may significantly aid in the diagnosis and the localization of the lesion. The following generalizations are useful:

1. Although the headache of brain tumor is often referred from a distant intracranial source, it approximately overlies the tumor in about one third of all patients.

2. Brain-tumor headache in the absence of papilledema is of great localizing value. In about two thirds of such patients the headache immediately overlies or is near the tumor; in all, when unilateral, it is on the same side as the tumor.

3. Headache is almost always present with posterior fossa tumor but may be absent with any of the common types of supratentorial tumor.

4. Headache is usually the first symptom of posterior fossa tumor and is almost always over the back of the head, except in cerebello-pontile angle tumors.

5. The headache of cerebello-pontile angle tumors is frequently and sometimes solely postauricular on the side of the tumor.

6. Headache is the first symptom of one third of supratentorial tumors and is rarely in the back of the head unless associated with papilledema.

7. When headache associated with brain tumor is both frontal and occipital it indicates extensive displacement of the brain and has little localizing value.

8. Brain-tumor headache is usually intermittent, but when it is continuous its value in localization is greatly enhanced. The history of the site and the distribution of headache, whether it was initially and predictably on the left or the right, frontal or occipital, may indicate the site of a lesion. In some instances intracranial tumor is manifested by induced frontotemporal headache following sudden head rotation or jolting. If the induced headache is unilateral the lesion is usually on the side of the head pain.

EXPERIMENTAL EVIDENCE ON
INTRACRANIAL VASCULAR MECHANISMS
OF HEADACHE

The association of headache following intravenous histamine injection with increase in the amplitude of the intracranial arterial pulsations has been demonstrated photographically. Simultaneous records of systemic arterial blood pressure, cerebrospinal fluid pressure, temporal artery pulsations and intracranial pulsations were made (Fig. 25). Such experimentally induced headaches were abolished by increasing the intracranial pressure, thereby giving extramural support to the cerebral arteries at the base of the brain. The demonstrated correlation is further evidence that headache can arise from dilatation and stretching of the pain-sensitive pial and dural arteries and their surrounding tissues.

PRESSOR HEADACHE

Rapid and extreme increase in intravascular pressure in the arteries within the head will induce headache in most persons. Thus, on bladder distention in paraplegics with lesions about T-6 a systemic pressor response is evoked which is associated with severe headache. This is abolished by increasing the intracranial pressure, demonstrating its intracranial origin. This phenomenon has been attributed by Whitteridge (1947) to a pressor reflex undamped by the usual compensatory alterations in peripheral resistance. It is most marked when the cord lesion is high thoracic or cervical.

Coincident with the pressor response, facial flushing and a moderate to intense anterior headache are noted. The reaction subsides spontaneously after a few minutes. Preliminary studies by Thompson and Witham (1948) have shown that the pressor response and headache can be blocked by prior administration of a tetra-ethyl ammonium salt. Especially relevant is the observation by Schumacher and Guthrie (1949) that the headache can be eliminated by the artificial elevation of intracranial cerebrospinal fluid pressure by the intrathecal injection of saline. Therefore, it is probable that this variety of headache stems from distended intracranial arteries.

The massaging of a pheochromocytoma with subsequent sudden paroxysmal hypertension is associated with severe headache. Likewise, too rapid infusion of norepinephrine with sudden and extreme rise in systemic arterial blood pressure will cause headache.

No headache resulted from experimental bladder and large bowel distention in intact humans. It is inferred that in normal persons with constipation or with urinary retention, the mechanism of any associated headache is not directly related to the viscus distention or to large bowel contraction.

Headache does not depend upon the integrity of sensation from the superficial tissues. The extracranial and the dural arteries play a minor role in contributing to the pain of headache experimentally in-

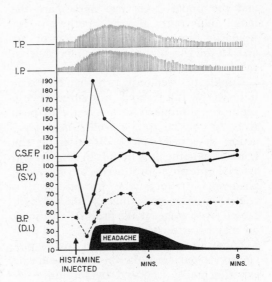

FIG. 25. Diagrammatic representation of the course of events during headache produced by histamine in subject G. The headache was most severe with rising blood pressure, and it should be noted that at this time the cerebrospinal fluid pressure is returning to its resting level from the high point reached after the injection of histamine. Increase in amplitude and rate of the temporal pulse (T.P.) and of the intracranial pulsation (I.P.) are indicated in the upper two shaded areas. The line C.S.F.P. indicates the cerebrospinal fluid pressure in millimeters of Ringer's solution. Systolic blood pressure is indicated by the heavy black line at B.P.S.Y., and the diastolic blood pressure is indicated by the broken line at DI.

duced by histamine. Cerebral arteries, principally the large arteries of the base of the brain, including the internal carotid, the vertebral and the basilar arteries and the proximal segments of their main branches, are chiefly responsible for the quality and the intensity of such headache. Although there may be other less important afferent pathways for the conduction of impulses interpreted as headache following injection of histamine, (1) the 5th cranial nerve on each side is the principal afferent pathway for headache resulting from dilatation of the supratentorial cerebral arteries and felt in the fronto-temporo-parietal region of the head, and (2) the 9th and the 10th cranial and the upper 3 cervical nerves are the most important afferent pathways for headache resulting from dilatation of the arteries of the posterior fossa and felt in the occipital region of the head.

Kunkle has demonstrated that headache induced by intravenous histamine is also promptly eliminated by exposure to positive "G" of 3.0 to 3.6 (centrifugal force acting in a head-to-foot direction on the human centrifuge). The fall in intracranial arterial pressure produced by increased positive G reduces the pressure within cranial arteries and thus eliminates pain caused by average blood pressure thrusting on relaxed arterial walls.

These findings lend support to the previously stated formulation that headache experimentally produced by histamine results from the stretch of the walls of the intracranial vessels during the period in which they are hypotonic and unable adequately to absorb the shock of the systemic arterial pressure, as it returns to normal levels soon after the drug injection. (See Fig. 25.)

Headache Associated with Fever

Observations of the amplitude of pulsations of the cranial arteries during headache associated with experimentally induced fever showed that the spontaneous increase and decrease of intensity of the headache paralleled the change in amplitude of pulsations in these arteries.

The observation was made, moreover, that increasing the cerebrospinal fluid pressure in the subarachnoid space reduced the intensity of fever headache (Pickering). From fragmentary data it is likely that the headaches associated with acute infections, sepsis, bacteremia, nitrites, anoxia, hunger, hypoglycemia, caffeine-withdrawal, "hangover" and postconvulsive state are similarly due primarily to the distention of intracranial arteries.

Headache Resulting from Traction Upon Intracranial Structures

Head Jolting. In many normal subjects sudden and vigorous head movement will elicit a fleeting headache in the frontal or temporal area on one or both sides.

For test purposes, a brisk rotary head movement to one side and back to the midposition is carried out actively by the instructed subject. The maximum force of such a jolt can be recorded by means of a miniature accelerometer gripped between the teeth. In this way it is possible to measure in approximate terms the threshold force for induced jolt headache.

Kunkle has shown that the threshold to jolt headaches as here defined is usually very low in association with diffuse inflammation of intracranial meningeal and vascular structures, as in meningitis, and may be moderately low with distortion of intracranial anchoring vessels, as with brain tumor. Such evidence strongly suggests that jolt headache results from traction by the brain as it shifts in position within the skull case, exerted chiefly upon the major arteries which anchor the brain at its base. With inflammation or sustained displacement of intracranial veins, particularly those tributory to the superior sagittal sinus, the pain from head jolting may arise in part from venous traction. The jolt threshold is greatly lowered during states in which intracranial arteries are known to be dilated, as after the injection of histamine. On the other hand, the threshold is not lowered in normal subjects during procedures which induce distention of intracranial veins, as with straining or bilateral jugular compression.

For these reasons the rotary jolt maneuver is doubly useful: it produces an instructive experimental headache, and may be an aid in the detection of intracranial sources in clinical headaches (Fig. 26).

Other Features of Traction Headache. When headaches arise from sustained displacement of any or several of the structures anchoring the brain, the pain may be aggravated by coughing or straining, measures which produce sudden fluctuations in intracranial arterial, venous and cerebrospinal fluid pressures. The intensity of the headache is not reduced by compression of surface arteries of the head or by the administration of vasoconstrictor drugs.

The Headache Associated with Meningitis. The headache of meningitis is primarily related to the lowered pain threshold of inflamed tissues and structures within or adjacent to the coverings of the brain. Though generalized, the inflammatory changes are usually most marked in the basal dura and the pia and the adjacent blood vessels and nerves at the base of the brain. Under these circumstances even slight jolting of the head and the usually painless arterial dilatation and distention during each cardiac systole become painful—thus the characteristic throbbing headache.

Special Mechanical Stresses in Relation to Vascular Headache. When the human subject is turned to the inverted position the adaptive response includes an increase in vasoconstrictor tone in the head, in which both the internal and external carotid branches share. Headache associated with arterial dilatation has in some instances been eliminated completely during this postural adaptation.

A vasomotor reaction of opposite type may occur following an abrupt fall in cranial arterial pressure. This is seen most dramatically in man in a unique circumstance: during the phase of release from exposure to centrifugal force in the head-to-seat direction—increased positive G

(Kunkle *et al.*, 1948). Presumably, in an attempt to maintain cranial circulation during such mechanical stress, there is a decrease in constrictor tone in head vessels, for, as the centrifugal force subsides and cranial arterial pressure rises to normal, flushing of the face is briefly observed. At this point in some subjects a transient headache develops. This symptom can conveniently be termed rebound vascular headache; whether the pain is principally intracranial or extracranial in origin has not been determined. A comparable reaction may explain the occasional occurrence of a trivial and fleeting headache in some individuals a few seconds after suddenly standing up from a recumbent position.

MIGRAINE HEADACHE

Incidence. It has been said that migraine headache is the commonest complaint of civilized people, though few reliable data exist concerning its frequency. Grimes found that "of 15,000 individuals examined in general practice with reference to migraine, 1,200 or 8 per cent were afflicted." There are all gradients of migraine complaint from the most severe and disabling illness to trifling symptoms, and it is safe

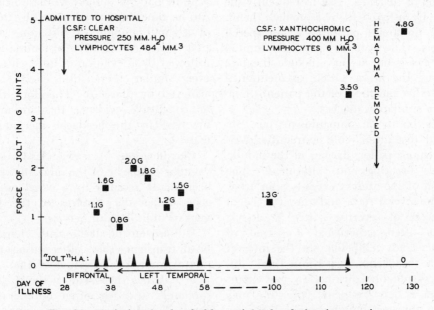

FIG. 26. Variation in threshold to "jolt" headache—in a patient with left temporoparietal subdural hematoma.

to say that less than half the migraine victims ever consult a physician. It is a difficult syndrome to investigate because it usually disappears under conditions of intensive laboratory study. Therefore, development of knowledge of the pathogenesis of migraine headache has been slow.

Hereditary Aspects. In the family pedigrees of 119 patients with the migraine type of vascular headache there were found to be 343 relatives with migraine, distributed in as many as 5 generations. Migraine occurred in the children of families having relatives with migraine with the following frequencies: 69.2 per cent when both parents had migraine; 44.2 per cent when one parent had migraine; and 28.6 per cent when neither parent had migraine. Applying genetic concepts to these data, the hereditary character of migraine became highly significant; it appears that inheritance of the migraine headache trait is through a recessive gene with a penetrance of approximately 70 per cent.

Definition. The outstanding feature of the migraine syndrome is periodic headache, usually unilateral in onset, but which may become generalized. The headaches are associated with irritability and nausea, and often with photophobia, vomiting, constipation or diarrhea. Not infrequently the attacks are ushered in by scotomata, hemianopia, unilateral paresthesia and speech disorders. The pain is commonly limited to the head, but it may include the face and even the neck. Often, as mentioned above, other members of the patient's family have similar headaches.

Other bodily accompaniments are abdominal distention, cold extremities, vertigo, tremors, pallor, dryness of the mouth, excessive sweating and "chilliness." The duration of the attacks extends from a few hours to several days and they can be of any degree of severity. After an attack, patients often experience a period of buoyancy and well-being. In the interval between headaches, gastrointestinal disturbances, notably constipation, may occur. Diarrhea is less frequent. Migraine may begin at any age, though commonly during adolescence. No age, social, intellectual or economic group is immune. There are many variants of the migraine attack and some phase of the syndrome other than headache may become the presenting complaint.

One variety has features special enough to justify separate description. It is unilateral, of high intensity, brief, burning and boring in character, and many attacks occur in quick succession, sometimes several in a 24-hour period, for several days or weeks, followed by remissions lasting months or years; hence the name, *cluster headache.* The pain involves the region of the eye, the temple, the neck and often one side of the face, and may spread into the teeth and extend into the shoulder on the involved side. Associated manifestations are profuse watering and congestion of the conjunctiva, rhinorrhea and nasal obstruction, increased perspiration, redness of the skin, and swelling of the temporal vessels. Kunkle, in a study of 90 patients, pointed to the unique tempo of the recurrence of cluster headaches as its most striking feature, although in a few patients the attacks occur sporadically instead of in groups. The thesis that endogenous histamine may be responsible for cluster type headache is based on the facts (1) that unilateral headache in patients subject to these headaches can be experimentally induced by injection of a small amount of histamine and (2) that "desensitization" to histamine is often followed by alleviation of headaches. However, similar therapeutic effects can be achieved by placebos. Therefore, there is no conclusive evidence that histamine is involved in the headache mechanism in man.

Classification. A useful classification of vascular headache of the migraine type has been made recently by a panel on Headache under the auspices of the United States Public Health Service:

A. Vascular headache with sharply defined, transient visual, other sensory and/or motor prodromes (classic migraine).

B. Vascular headache without striking prodomes and less often unilateral than Types A and C (common migraine). Synonyms are "atypical migraine" or "sick head-

FIG. 27. Relation of amplitude of pulsations of temporal artery to intensity of headache after administration of ergotamine. The sharp decrease in amplitude of pulsations following injection closely paralleled rapid decrease in intensity of headache. Representative sections of photographic record are inserted. Average amplitude of pulsations before and after administration of ergotamine was ascertained by measuring individual pulsations from photographic record. Points on heavy black line represent these averages, as percentages. Initial or "control" amplitude was taken as 100 per cent. Interrupted line represents intervals of one second. (Wolff, H. G.: Headache and Other Head Pain, New York, Oxford)

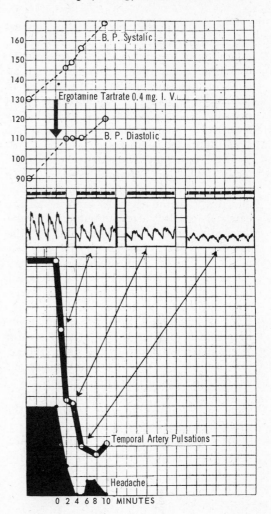

ache." Calling attention to certain relationships of this type of headache to seasonal, environmental, occupational, menstrual or other variables are such terms as: tropical, summer, Monday, weekend, relaxation, premenstrual, and menstrual headache.

C. Vascular headache, predominantly unilateral; associated on the same side with flushing, sweating, rhinorrhea and increased lacrimation; brief in duration and occurring in closely packed groups separated by long remissions (cluster headache). Identical or closely allied are: erythroprosopalgia (Bing); ciliary or migrainous neuralgia (Harris); erythromelalgia of the head or histaminic cephalgia (Horton); and petrosal neuralgia (Gardner et al.).

D. Vascular headache featured by sensory and motor phenomena which persist during and after the headache (hemiplegic migraine and ophthalmoplegic migraine).

E. Headache of possible vascular mechanism centered primarily in the lower face (lower-half headache). In this group are atypical facial neuralgia, sphenopalatine ganglion neuralgia (Sluder), and vidian neuralgia (Vail).

THE PATHOPHYSIOLOGY OF MIGRAINE HEADACHE

Vasodilation. Changes in the intensity of these vascular headaches of the migraine type are related to changes in the amplitude of pulsations of the cranial arteries,

chiefly the branches of the external carotid arteries. Reduction in amplitude of pulsations of the temporal artery by digital pressure on the carotid artery on the affected side is accompanied by reduction in intensity of the headache. Conversely, experimental distention of extracranial arteries by increasing the intravascular pressure results in pain. It has also been shown by means of observations and photographs, made both before and during action of *ergotamine tartrate* and of *norepinephrine,* that these agents *reduce the amplitude of pulsations* of the aforementioned arteries by about 50 per cent, and concurrently diminish the intensity of or terminate the migraine headache (Fig. 27).

There is considerable evidence against the view that the headache is due chiefly to dilatation of the dural and the cerebral arteries, since not even extremely severe attacks of migraine headache are reduced in intensity by raising the cerebrospinal fluid pressure as high as 800 mm. of water by means of a manometer system attached to a needle in the lumbar sac.

The internal and the external carotid arteries and the vertebral arteries have branches both in the subcutaneous tissue and in the meninges. The branches of the external carotid artery predominate numerically, both superficially and on the dura. On the other hand, the anterior meningeal artery arises from branches of the internal carotid artery, as do the superficial frontal and the supraorbital artery. Since the area supplied by the latter structures is commonly involved in migraine headaches, branches of the internal carotid artery may contribute to the pain. Therefore, it is obvious that it would be arbitrary to contrast these arteries too sharply.

Although most attacks of migraine headaches are limited to the temporal, the frontal or the occipital region, some patients have pain elsewhere. In the face, below the eye and behind and below the zygoma, severe throbbing pain, which seems to emanate from the back teeth of the upper jaw, occasionally occurs. Another variant is facial pain, which spreads behind the angle of the jaw, down the neck and into the shoulder. The aching sensations in the shoulder sometimes are associated with the awareness of unusual throbbing in the neck.

The pains described can and probably do result from dilatation and distention of the extracranial portion of the middle meningeal artery, between its origin and the point of entrance into the skull, the internal maxillary artery and the trunks of the external and the common carotid artery. It has been shown that the latter structures are sensitive to pain, and the sites in which pain is felt are the face, the neck and the shoulder.

The effect on migraine headache of reducing cranial intravascular pressure is demonstrated by a patient with migraine headache who was the subject of investigation on the human centrifuge. The headache in this 22-year-old female dental technician was either right frontal or generalized and had been recurring frequently for four weeks, in a setting of dissatisfaction with her work and increasing tension. The

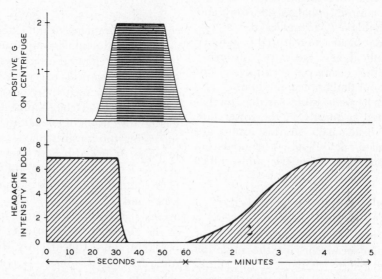

FIG. 28. Effect of centrifugation (positive G) on migraine headache in a woman, aged 22.

dominant stress centered about her inability, due to circumstances beyond her control, to maintain her usual high standards of performance. During exposure to centrifugal force of 2.0 G in the head-to-seat direction it was possible to eliminate the headache completely (Fig. 28).

It is likely, therefore, that for the *fever* headache and that experimentally induced by *histamine,* the cerebral branches of the *internal carotid,* the *basilar* and the *vertebral* arteries at the base of the brain are primarily responsible. To the migraine headache, however, the extracranial, and possibly the dural, branches of the *external carotid* artery are the chief contributors.

Muscle Spasm. An ancillary mechanism of pain during the migraine headache attack involves the sustained *contraction of the muscles* of the head and the neck. Pain in the head from any cause induces secondary contractions of these muscles, which, when maintained, become in themselves a source of pain. Though present in all, the amount of muscle spasm varies greatly from patient to patient.

Such painful contractions may persist for some time longer than the primary cause of the contraction, i.e., pain arising from cranial vasodilatation. This affords an explanation of the failure to obtain relatively prompt relief after ergotamine tartrate administration in some patients who have a major muscle component in their headaches.

Arteritis. There is still another factor in the failure to achieve prompt relief from migraine headache after the administration of ergotamine tartrate. After several hours of migraine headache, involving, for example, the temporal artery, this artery may appear prominent and distended and become more easily palpable through the skin. Instead of being easily collapsible, it becomes rigid, pipelike and less readily compressible by the palpating finger. Also, the artery may be tender when compressed. Patients so affected report that after the first hour or two of a migraine headache attack the quality of the headache changes in that the initial pulsating or throbbing is less conspicuous or even absent and the pain becomes a steady ache. Under such conditions, ergotamine tartrate fails to

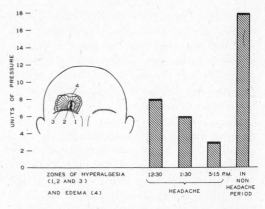

FIG. 29. Demonstration of the progressively lowered thresholds of deep pain during a vascular headache of the migraine type in the supraorbital region.

eliminate headache promptly or even to reduce its intensity appreciably.

To account for such changes, it was postulated that following the sustained dilatation of a local artery of the head there occurs a transient change in the structure of the artery wall, namely, *thickening or edema of the muscular and the adventitial structures.* To lend validity to this concept experiments were done in which the arteries of cats' ears were studied following prolonged vasodilatation by infusion for 2 hours of 10 ml. of mammalian Ringer's solution containing a vasodilator agent (0.05 mg. acetylcholine). The dilated artery walls were compared with the arterial walls of a control ear by means of serial sections. Measurements demonstrated thickening of the arterial walls of the infused ear. Also, the vasoconstrictor agent, ergotamine tartrate, was found to be less prompt and less effective in constricting arteries with such thickened or edematous walls, as compared with its action on vessel walls early in a headache.

Hyperalgesia. Contributing to the migraine headache attack is the heightened tenderness of tissues located in and about the painfully dilated large cranial arteries, associated with local edema. *Deep-pain-thresholds* of affected scalp tissues have been found to be *lowered greatly* during headache (Fig. 29), and the lowered thresholds persisted for hours or days after spontaneous ending of the headache. Furthermore, it was demonstrated that the onset of certain migraine headaches is preceded by a lowering of the jolt threshold. In some instances this lowered threshold also persists for some hours after headache has subsided.

Humoral Factors. Sterile isotonic saline (2 ml.) was injected subcutaneously, and as much fluid as possible withdrawn under gentle negative pressure during a 2-minute interval (1) from the tender regions of the heads of persons during headaches of a wide range of intensity, (2) from the tender region of the scalp following headache attacks, (3) from the nontender regions of the heads of persons subject to headache but during headache-free periods, and (4) from persons not subject to headache attacks. (Fig. 30).

It was found that specimens of tissue fluid collected from the head during the headache attacks contain a substance that could be distinguished from serotonin, potassium, ATP, substance P, acetycholine and histamine, although these and other substances may also have been present. The active substance relaxed the isolated rat duodenum, contracted the rat uterus and depressed the blood pressure of the rat. A constant ratio of activity on these several assay preparations among several specimens of tissue fluid indicated that the observed activity of the specimens was probably due to a single substance.

The activity of the specimens could be stabilized by boiling. Incubation with chymotrypsin inactivated the stabilized specimens, indicating that the active substance remaining after stabilization is a polypeptide. The heat-stabilized substance had many of the properties of bradykinin, kallidin, or plasma kinin. However, when analyzed quantitatively using several assay procedures, including electrophoresis, it was evident that the substance is not identical to any of these, although it closely resembles them and is a polypeptide of the same general type. This polypeptide has been labeled neurokinin and has been found by Wolff and his associates to appear during neuronal excitation. It appears in tissue fluid of the skin of man during antidromic dorsal root stimulation and during axon reflex flare. It is not the result of vasodilatation alone since it is not released during reactive hyperemia. It has also been found in the cerebrospinal fluid of patients during vascular headache of the migraine type.

The neurokinin content of specimens collected during headache averages 8 times as much and in rare instances may be 35 times as much as that of control specimens, and the amount is closely related to the intensity of the headache attack (Fig. 31). Following administration of ergotamine tartrate in subjects with headache, the intensity of headache, amplitude of cranial artery pulsations, local tenderness, and neurokinin activity all decrease concurrently. Lowered deep pain thresholds return to normal.

In addition to the polypeptide, headache fluid contains a proteolytic enzyme, cap-

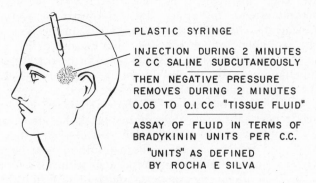

PLASTIC SYRINGE

INJECTION DURING 2 MINUTES
2 CC SALINE SUBCUTANEOUSLY

THEN NEGATIVE PRESSURE
REMOVES DURING 2 MINUTES
0.05 TO 0.1 CC "TISSUE FLUID"

ASSAY OF FLUID IN TERMS OF
BRADYKININ UNITS PER C.C.

"UNITS" AS DEFINED
BY ROCHA E SILVA

FIG. 30. Method of obtaining fluid from painful tissues for bioassay of "headache stuff."

able of forming neurokinin (presumably by cleavage of a plasma globulin present in subsurface extracellular fluid).

The increased content of polypeptide (neurokinin) and protease found locally can account for many of the features of vascular headache of the migraine type. Neurokinin is an extremely powerful vaso-dilator. When injected intradermally, tissue fluids containing mixtures of neurokinin and protease induce pain and erythema, lower pain threshold and increase capillary permeability.

Since the release or activation of neurokinin-forming enzyme and subsequent formation of neurokinin have been observed during neuronal excitation in man in a variety of circumstances, the potent hypotensive and vasodilator action of neurokinin and its formation during neuronal excitation suggest that it contributes to local vasomotor control in the central nervous system.

The Migraine Headache Attack as the Outcome of Central Nervous System Activity. Migraine headache attacks are linked to activity of the central nervous system since they often occur following a long period of alertness, striving, extraordinary effort or major frustration usually associated with feelings of anger and resentment. They may begin with vasoconstriction affecting the cerebral cortex and the retina. The painful local reaction in the extracranial vessels may thus be an epiphenomenon of the excessive operation of the normal mechanisms for functional vasodilatation within the central nervous system. A common innervation of the branches of the external and internal carotid arteries could lead to a simultaneous release of vasodilator substances both intracranially and extracranially. Thus, the pain of vascular headache of the migraine type can be seen as the outcome of the combined effects of *large artery dilatation* plus the action of *pain threshold-lowering substances* accumulating in the blood vessel walls and perivascular tissue. These substances are implicated in local vasomotor control. Their accumulation, neurogenically induced, results in a *sterile inflammatory reaction*.

Craniovascular Instability and Vascular

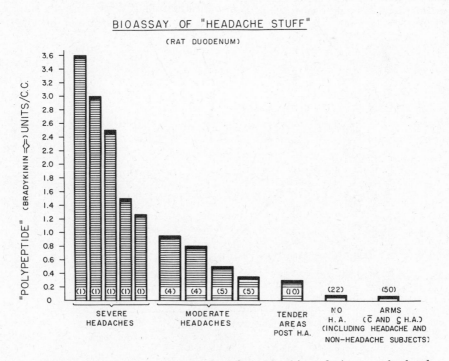

Fig. 31. Results of bioassay of tissue fluid from 23 subjects during vascular headaches of the migraine type.

Headache. Repeated measurements over several days of the amplitude of pulsation of the cranial arteries by Marcussen and Kunkle, and later by Tunis, indicated that in many subjects who have vascular headaches, the variation in tone of the artery walls during headache-free periods is far greater than in those who do not have recurrent headaches, and is greatest in the days preceding an attack (Fig. 34). These observations gave support to the concept that the cranial vasomotor apparatus of patients with vascular headaches is more labile than is that of persons who are not subject to headache.

Pharmacodynamic Properties of l-Methyl-D-Lysergic Acid Butanolamide Bimaleate Relevant to Vascular Headache of the Migraine Type. Recently, the possibility of shedding further light on the pathophysiology of vascular headache of the migraine type was suggested by the reports of a number of investigators that 1-methyl-d-lysergic acid butanolamide bimaleate,* while lacking the capacity to terminate an existing headache, is often effective in reducing the number and severity of headache attacks

*Supplied as UML-491 methysergide or "Sansert" for these investigations by the Sandoz Pharmaceutical Company.

when the agent is maintained at adequate blood levels. Although it does not by itself induce vasoconstriction, it does enhance the vasoconstrictor action of norepinephrine.

1. ANTI-INFLAMMATORY ACTION OF 1-METHYL-D-LYSERGIC ACID BUTANOLAMIDE BIMALEATE. This agent is effective in diminishing edema formation induced by the injection of serotonin in the rat's paw. In order to show that this phenomenon was not specific to inflammation induced by serotonin, areas of sterile inflammatory response were produced through the subcutaneous administration of manganese butyrate to seven human subjects. The flare responses induced during UML-491 therapy were significantly smaller than those induced either before or several weeks subsequent to its administration (Fig. 32). A verification of this study was made in animal experiments by Zileli where the volume of inflammatory exudate in croton oil pouches was significantly less after pretreatment with UML-491.

2. INHIBITION OF VASOMOTOR REFLEXES. Dampening of the pressor reaction to carotid occlusion is a well recognized property of many of the ergot alkaloids. In the anesthetized cat, this pressor response can be abolished by infusion of UML-491 at

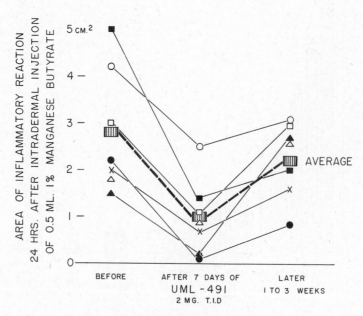

FIG. 32. The anti-inflammatory action of UML-491 in 7 human subjects.

a rate of 1.0 mg./kg./hour, suggesting a moderate depressing action on the vasomotor centers, thus damping vasoconstrictor reflexes. Although the amounts of the agent required to *abolish* these reflexes in the cat are many times more than the amounts that are effective in the prevention of migraine attacks, it is possible that damping of vasoconstrictor reflexes may also be induced by UML-491 in patients with migraine.

Evidence relevant to such a modifying effect on the sensitivity of vasomotor centers was afforded by a study of a series of persons subject to vascular headaches of the migraine type regarding the effect of this alkaloid on the carotid sinus reflex, the cold pressor reflex and the breath-holding reflex. These were selected as samples of vasomotor reflexes that could be tested in man, although it is recognized that they represent different reactions than those implicated in vascular headache of the migraine type. The magnitude of these reflexes was studied before, during, and in some instances after the daily administration of 8 to 12 mg. amounts of UML-491 Methysergide in divided doses. It was observed that those subjects experiencing the most striking reduction or elimination of

headache also exhibited the greatest inhibitory effect on their vascular reactions to noxious and painful stimulation.

3. Inhibition of Changes in Responsivity of Cranial Vessels Associated with Shifts of Body Fluid. The migraine attack is characterized by initial vasconstriction followed by vasodilatation. When effective, UML-491 prevents both the preheadache (visual loss) or vasoconstrictor phase and the headache or vasodilator phase. Of its two actions, inhibition of central vasoconstrictor reflex effects and augmentation of peripheral vasoconstriction produced by catecholamines, the former could be significant in inhibiting the initial vasoconstrictor phase of the attack, and the latter in minimizing the subsequent painful dilatation of the vasodilator phase. On the other hand, it is conceivable that the prevention of the initial vasoconstriction makes the subsequent vasodilatation unlikely to occur.

Since initial fluid retention and subsequent diuresis are part of the migraine attack and changes in the reactivity of the bulbar conjunctival blood vessels occur during such periods of fluid shift, the effects of UML-491 on these phenomena were studied. Fluid shifts were experimentally

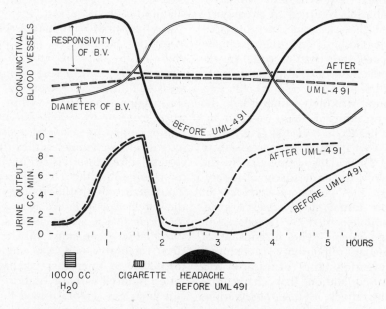

Fig. 33. Schema of damping effect of UML-491 methysergide on blood vessel responsivity.

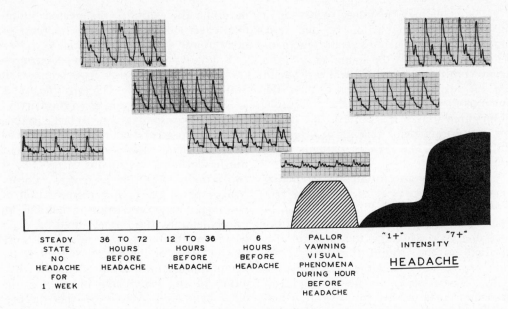

FIG. 34. Record of the variations in temporal artery pulsations in a subject having recurrent vascular headaches of the migraine type.

induced by evoking diencephalic reactions through nicotine. It was observed that concurrently with the oliguria the bulbar conjunctival vessels dilate and become less responsive to serial dilutions of norepinephrine. During the subsequent diuresis, all conjunctival vessels constricted and the response of these vessels to serial dilutions of norepinephrine returned to preoliguric levels. Headache was sometimes initiated during the vasodilator and oliguric phase and terminated shortly after with the beginning of the vasoconstriction and diuresis. Prior administration of UML-491 during 48 hours strikingly diminished the magnitude of both of these vascular responses; no headache occurred (Fig. 33).

4. VASOMOTOR INSTABILITY AND VASCULAR HEADACHE. These data suggest that in the prophylaxis of vascular headache of the migraine type the peripheral actions of UML-491 on cranial blood vessels are significantly supplemented by its effects on the nervous system. The magnitude of cranial vascular responsivity is reduced, thereby preventing crises of vasoconstriction and vasodilatation that characterize the migraine attack. These observations further support the thesis that *the migraine attack is the symptomatic manifestation of recurrent heightened reactivity of cranial blood vessels.* Moreover, the modification of vasomotor reflexes, concurrent with a period of reduction in the intensity and frequency of headache attacks, adds further support to the inference that *unstable cranial vasomotor functions* are a prime factor in the pathophysiology of this variety of headache.

Mechanism of Scotomata Associated with Migraine Headache. The preheadache phase of the migraine attack is sometimes featured by scintillating scotomata and areas of blindness. These result from vasoconstriction—sometimes within the retina, where constricted vessels can be seen and photographed by means of a slit lamp and microscope, sometimes within the calcarine cortex, where vasoconstriction is indicated by changes in the electroencephalogram. To demonstrate further that dysfunction of the cerebral vasculature is responsible for the preheadache symptoms of scotomata, a vasodilator agent, amyl nitrite, known to effect cerebral vessels, was employed. It is justifiable to infer that cerebral vasodilatation induced without a fall in blood pressure increases cerebral blood flow, whereas a sharp drop in blood pressure, regardless of the state of the cerebral arteries, decreases the cerebral blood flow. Symptoms due to cerebral vasoconstriction should be overcome by cerebral vasodilatation in the presence of a sustained normal level of blood pressure, but they should be augmented by a fall in blood pressure with accompanying decrease in cerebral blood flow. Experiments based on these two potential actions of the vasodilator drug amyl nitrate were performed by a subject having preheadache scotomata who was skillful in observing his own visual fields.

It was apparent from such experiments that cerebral vasodilatation associated with a sustained normal level of blood pressure caused symptoms to disappear, whereas a procedure that decreased cerebral blood flow caused the symptoms to become worse. From this it may be deduced that cerebral vasoconstriction was responsible for the visual defect in this patient with migraine. It is also likely that the cause of the visual defect was not in the retina or the orbit, but within the cranial cavity.

The preheadache phenomena of migraine, i.e., visual disturbances, paresthesias and dysarthria, associated with (and probably due to) cranial vasoconstriction, can be modified or abolished by certain agents which produce cranial vasodilatation. A series of patients was given a mixture of 10 per cent carbon dioxide and 90 per cent oxygen by face mask during the preheadache or early headache phase. This mixture abolished the preheadache phenomena and aborted the headache in most of the trials. Ten per cent carbon dioxide in air was less effective, having a shorter and more transient effect.

Pharmacodynamics of the Urine of Patients with Migraine. Water and electrolyte balance studies of persons with the migraine type of vascular headaches indicate that in about half of those having migraine headache there is retention of water, sodium, potassium and steroids in the period just preceding the headache attack. During the retention phase the creatinine output in the urine is reduced, suggesting that the renal vessels also participate in the vasoconstriction occurring about the head. With the onset of the headache and during the subsequent hours there is a diuresis of water, sodium, potassium and steroids. The described changes are not related causally or mechanistically to the onset, the intensity or the duration of the migraine attack. Instead, they are manifestations of the widespread bodily changes accompanying adaptive reactions during and after stressful periods. The migraine attack is a concurrent but independent feature.

Formulation of the Dynamics of the Migraine Attack. For a period of several hours to several days preceding the headache there is increased variability of the contractile state of the cranial arteries, indicated by facial flushing or pallor due to dilatation or constriction of extracranial vessels and by other transient cranial vasomotor phenomena, such as vertigo. In the hour preceding the headache, visual and other nonpainful sensory phenomena due to local constriction of cerebral arteries or, sometimes, retinal vessels occur in about 10 to 15 per cent of the instances. These may take the form of scintillating scotomas or visual field defects, such as unilateral or homonymous hemianopsia. As the vasoconstrictor preheadache phenomena recede, vasodilator headache manifestations commence, sometimes overlapping the last traces of preheadache phenomena, sometimes beginning after a short symptom-free interval. The pain is throbbing and aching in quality, is appreciably reduced by pressure on the common carotid and superficial artery, and is characteristically modified by the action of vasoconstrictor agents.

The migraine attack is but one aspect of a diffuse disturbance in function occurring episodically during or shortly after a stressful period of which resentment, fatigue and prolonged tension are features. In certain circumstances, even during intervals of stress, the migraine headache or preheadache phenomena may diminish or actually fail to recur. However, other bodily or mood disturbances may be accentuated and become the basis of the dominant complaint. These other phenomena, referred to as migraine equivalents, include a variety of abdominal, thoracic and extremity pains and nonpainful attacks of vomiting, diarrhea, diffuse edema, transient mood disorder and fever.

Individuals with migraine headache are, in most instances, tense, driving people who are rigid, ambitious and perfectionistic. They have found that doing "more than and better than" their fellows brings many rewards. Nevertheless, this is accomplished at great cost in energy. They strive continually to do a flawless job at whatever they attempt, disregarding their own bodily demands for rest. The outcome of this pernicious way of life is resentment, tension, fatigue and exhaustion. In this seting headache makes its appearance.

A person with migraine deals with his life situations in a way which excessively depletes his reserve of energy. The rate at which this energy is expended is dependent on his reactions to the circumstances. Beyond a certain point he is no longer able to continue the costly and extravagant adjustment he has been making. He exhausts his bodily capacity to continue to deal effectively with his situation. When he reaches this point there is a collapse of his adaptive or protective apparatus. At that time, vasomotor instability supervenes, characterized by a cranial vascular reaction which becomes painful, and he usually withdraws from his frustrating and threatening life situation. During the period of retreat there is apparently a restoration of the energy reserves which then permits a repetition of the whole pernicious cycle of excessive striving.

In reaction to threats, the human organism may use devices which are inappropriate, but the setting in motion of an integrated pattern of reaction devised to deal with threats appears to afford a measure of relief from anxiety and tension. Many patients with migraine, although prostrated during and perhaps immediately after a headache, have after the attack feelings of increased energy and effectiveness which persist until accumulations of tension, hostility and resentment again begin to build up.

Thus the migraine attack may be considered one of the phases of an inappropriate protective or adaptive reaction involving cranial circulatory apparatus which is manifest when the subject has reached the limit of his capacity to tolerate tension, hostility, frustration and fatigue.

Protocols of a series of carefully studied patients with migraine with particular reference to the events of the 24 hours preceding a given headache, revealed that in many instances there occurred an episode to which the patient reacted with rage and resentment, to which he was unable to give full expression. This type of blocked reaction took place during a short period of a high degree of anxiety and tension, or following a longer period of gradually accumulating tension. In many instances the precipitating event was in itself trivial and would not have disturbed these individuals under other circumstances. In the setting in which it did occur, it was "the straw that broke the camel's back," the final insult. Each had been accumulating hostility, resentment and tension for varying periods before he was exposed to the event which precipitated the headache. The following protocol is representative.

A 30-year-old Italian housewife had a history of almost daily unilateral headache of varying intensity and duration for about two months. Prior to this series of attacks she had had typical migraine headaches every few weeks since adolescence. The present series of headaches paralleled the development of a progressively severe feeding problem in her 4-year-old daughter. The patient stated that her headaches followed meals with monotonous regularity. The child refused to eat, despite the patient's every effort to induce her to do so. At this persistent refusal, the mother would become angry and berate the child violently. Often she would attempt to force food between the child's clenched teeth. Failing this, the mother became so enraged several times that she assaulted her daughter so violently that the child was left stunned and bruised. Within an hour after such an encounter the patient would develop a high-intensity headache, usually unilateral, which required ergotamine tartrate or opiates for relief. Later this woman realized that she might seriously injure her daughter during one of these assaults and would therefore storm out of the room before she gave way to physical violence. Under such circumstances the subsequent headache would be more intense. The mother felt extremely guilty about her failure as a parent and was humiliated by the comments of neighbors who overheard her outbursts and observed the child's progressive loss of weight.

During her first clinic visit, the patient confessed her story to a friendly and sympathetic physician. She displayed considerable emotion during the interview and felt appreciably relieved at the end. She had no further headache during the following week, the first remission in months. At her next visit, the same physician adopted a stern and unsympathetic attitude. He scolded the patient for her behavior and criticized her for her failure to control herself in dealing with the child, pointing out the damage which she was doing to the child and to herself. All this the patient seemed to accept well, smiling and agreeing with the physician. The interview terminated after an hour and the patient left the clinic. Ten minutes later she developed a high intensity bitemporal and frontal throbbing headache accompanied by some blurring of vision and nausea. The headache was abolished within 30 minutes after the intramuscular injection of ergotamine tartrate (Fig. 35).

MECHANISM OF HEADACHE ASSOCIATED WITH ARTERIAL HYPERTENSION

Studies made of the headache associated with hypertension have revealed that essentially the same mechanism is operative in producing this pain as in producing the migraine headache. It is to be emphasized that this statement applies not to the so-called hypertensive encephalopathy of Fishberg, "hypertensive crisis," but rather to the frequent, severe and often incapacitating headaches suffered by hypertensive patients who may otherwise be free of symptoms. The term hypertensive headache is misleading, since it implies that the frequency and the severity of the headache are directly related to the level of the blood pressure.

Almost all the patients with hypertension and associated headaches in this series had had headaches for many years. In numerous instances the headache was known to have preceded the onset of the hypertension and, in some patients, changed only in intensity with the rise in blood pressure.

The following data indicate that the pial and the cerebral arteries are not the prime contributors to the headache and that the headache associated with *hypertension,* like that of migraine, arises chiefly from the dilatation and distention of certain branches of the *external carotid artery:*

1. The headache was not relieved by increasing the cerebrospinal fluid pressure.

2. There was no increase in the amplitude of pulsations of the intracranial arteries during the headache, and the amplitude of pulsations of these arteries did not become less as the headache diminished in intensity.

3. Ergotamine tartrate, which in the head acts chiefly on the branches of the ex-

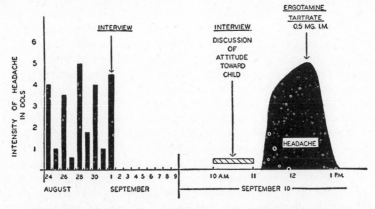

FIG. 35. Experimental precipitation of a migraine headache attack in a setting of mounting tension by the introduction of a topic arousing conflict, anger and guilt. Attack terminated by the intravascular administration of ergotamine tartrate. Initial interview on September 1, by dispelling guilt and conflict, reduced the frequency and intensity of attacks. The subsequent interview, intensifying these feelings, precipitated the headache.

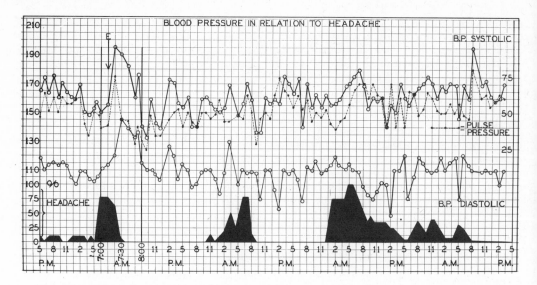

Fig. 36. Relation of blood pressure to headache in a patient with hypertension and associated headache. The fluctuations of the blood pressure and the incidence and severity of the headache vary independently. Thus, headache occurred with a B.P. of 140/75 on one occasion, whereas headache disappeared as the B.P. rose from 145/90 to 195/110 at another time. At E, to the left of the chart, is shown the record of a headache terminated by ergotamine tratrate.

ternal carotid artery, reduced the intensity of the headache.

4. Manual pressure on the temporal, frontal, supraorbital, postauricular or occipital artery decreased or abolished the headache.

5. Ligation of the middle meningeal or the temporal artery, especially the latter, decreased the intensity of the headache for some months.

That the headache in subjects with hypertension bears no direct relationship to the level of blood pressure or pulse pressure has also been observed. The headache may be present when the blood pressure is relatively high, moderate or low. By pressing the thumb upon the common carotid artery the intensity of the headache is reduced with an accompanying decline in the amplitude of the pulsations. Decrease in the intensity of headache in the temporal region followed similar pressure upon the corresponding temporal artery. Furthermore, when ergotamine tartrate did succeed in decreasing appreciably the amplitude of pulsations of the cranial arteries for a shorter or longer period, the intensity of the hypertensive headache decreased

despite the fact that the ergotamine tartrate considerably increased the already elevated systolic and diastolic pressures. If little or no reduction of the amplitude of pulsation of the arteries occurred there was no reduction in the intensity of the headache.

The fact that the high level of blood pressure among hypertensive subjects is not a sufficient condition for headache does not justify the assumption that these phenomena are entirely unrelated. This would be contraindicated by the facts of common experience, since some persons with hypertension never had headache until the hypertension became established. It seems reasonable to postulate that a cranial artery only slightly relaxed for whatever reason would not distend as much, and possibly not to the point of producing pain, if the blood pressure were low. If, however, the sustained level were raised, distention would be greater and therefore pain might readily follow. In other words, a degree of change in the contractile state of the arterial wall, compatible with comfort when blood pressure is average, would be associated with pain when the blood pressure is elevated. During an average or normal contractile state of the arterial walls, distention does not occur and, correspondingly, there is no headache. Should this contractile state be impaired, as by stress, fatigue, or other conditions, distention and headache follow (Fig. 36). In brief, high blood pressure is a necessary, but not a sufficient condition for this type of headache. There is a significant relation between headache associated with hypertension and the contractile state of the cranial arteries.

This conception is supported by analogy with the experimental evidence described for histamine headache.

Headache of Temporal Arteritis

In the syndrome of arteritis of the temporal vessel, and sometimes of other cranial arteries, the associated headache is the main feature (Kilbourne and Wolff, 1946). Furthermore, when the inflammatory na-

ture of the disorder is relatively inconspicuous, the localization of the headache and, the associated tenderness of the temporal artery may lead to the erroneous diagnosis of atypical migraine. The headache is of high intensity, throbbing and persistent. It is felt as a deep ache and is also often burning in quality. Other features of the syndrome are not pertinent to this discussion.

Pain from Nasal and the Paranasal Structures

Quality and Intensity. The headache associated with frontal sinus disease is localized diffusely over the frontal region, and with antral disease over the maxillary region. The headache associated with sphenoid and ethmoid disease is experienced between and in back of the eyes and over the vertex. Commonly, when sinus

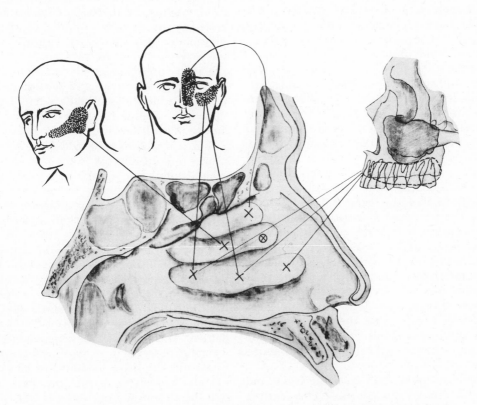

Fig. 37. The points stimulated on the turbinates are indicated by crosses, from which lines lead to the indicated areas in which pain of 4 plus to 6 plus intensity was felt. (Wolff, H. G.: Headache and Other Head Pain, New York, Oxford).

disease is of sufficient duration, there is pain in the back of the head, the neck and the shoulders, in addition to the headache experienced in the front and the top of the head.

Headaches are less frequent when the patient has been for some time in the recumbent position, or resting, and are less often present at night than during the day. Moreover, the pain associated with maxillary sinus disease gradually diminishes when the patient assumes the recumbent position with the diseased side uppermost. Relief in the recumbent position is not prompt, usually requiring about 30 minutes to be achieved.

The headache associated with frontal sinus disease commonly begins about 9 A.M., gradually becomes worse and ends toward evening or on retiring. The pain associated with maxillary sinus disease often has its onset in the early afternoon.

In all instances the pain is of a deep, dull, aching, nonpulsatile quality. It is seldom, if ever, associated with vomiting or nausea. The headache that accompanies chronic sinus disease is of a low order of intensity. The headache associated with acute sinus disease is sometimes of greater intensity, but seldom very severe. Pain does not achieve the intensity noted in some instances of migraine, or of the headache associated with ruptured cerebral aneurysm, meningitis or certain febrile illnesses, or of that induced by certain drugs.

The headache associated with disease of the nasal and the paranasal structures is commonly reduced in intensity or abolished by aspirin or codeine. The intensity of pain is increased by shaking the head or by the head-down position. The headache is intensified by procedures that increase the venous pressure, such as straining, coughing, or a tight collar. Also, it is intensified by states that increase the engorgement of the mucosa, such as anxiety and resentment, menstruation, cold air, sexual excitement or the effects of alcohol.

Mechanism of Pain from the Nasal and the Paranasal Structures. The mucosa covering the approaches to the paranasal sinuses is found to be the most pain-sensitive of the nasal and the paranasal struc-

tures and cavities, whereas the mucosa lining the sinuses is of relatively low sensitivity.

On a 1 (minimum pain) to 10 (maximum pain) scale a given faradic stimulus will produce pain of the indicated intensities at the following sites: tongue 1, septum 1 to 2, turbinates 4 to 6, nasofrontal duct 5 to 7, ostium of the maxillary sinus 6 to 9, lining of frontal or maxillary sinus 1 to 2 (see Fig. 37).

Most of the pain from faradic, mechanical and chemical stimulation of the mucosa of the nasal and the paranasal cavities is referred pain, i.e., it is felt at a site other than that stimulated. It is diffuse, sustained, of a deep, aching nature, and nonpulsatile. It is associated with lacrimation, photophobia, erythema and hyperalgesia. The pain and its associated effects outlast the period of stimulation.

The pain thus produced experimentally is referred chiefly to those regions of the head supplied by the 2nd division and, to a less extent, to those supplied by the 1st division of the 5th cranial nerve. When severe enough, or of sufficient duration, the pain spreads over most of the region supplied by that division of the 5th cranial nerve to which it is initially referred, and sometimes spreads from the region of the 2nd to that of the 1st division.

The stimulation of several different sites results in pain referred to the same region. Thus, stimulation of the nasal structures near the midline results in the same area of referred pain as does stimulation of the ostium and the more lateral wall of the maxillary sinus.

A thin rubber balloon was inserted into the maxillary sinus of a subject through a fistulous opening so that pressure could be applied to the walls of the sinus by inflating the balloon. When a pressure of 50 to 80 mm. Hg was maintained for $2\frac{1}{2}$ hours, pain of low intensity was experienced. It was also observed that sustained pressure within the sinus was accompanied by swelling and reddening of the turbinates and that the pain in the face could be abolished by procainization of the swollen, reddened turbinates, even while maintaining pressure.

Negative pressure within the sealed sinus resulting from applying suction of 100 to 150 mm. Hg for periods of a few minutes elicited a feeling of drawing in the face, which the patient described as the feeling that "her face would collapse." When the negative pressure was rapidly increased to 250 mm. Hg, however, an immediate intense pain was experienced on the side of the nose and in the teeth.

Pain in the back of the head or neck never results directly from stimulation of the mucosa of any of the nasal or paranasal structures. Such pain is due to the secondary effects of prolonged contraction of the cervical and head muscles.

Section of the 5th cranial sensory nerve root in most instances causes the mucosa of the aforementioned areas to be insensitive, with the exception of the pharynx, the tonsils, the fossa of Rosenmuller, the eustachian tubes, the external auditory canal and the ear drum.

Inflammation and engorgement of the turbinates, ostia, nasofrontal ducts and superior nasal spaces are responsible for most of the pain emanating from the nasal and the paranasal structures. If a headache is not associated with turbinate engorgement and inflammation, it is in all probability not the result of disease of the nasal or the paranasal structures. Furthermore, if a zygomatic, frontal, temporal, or vertex headache is not greatly reduced in intensity or eliminated by shrinking or local anesthetization of the nasal structures, it is also in all probability not due to disease of the nasal or the paranasal structures.

Alterations in Nasal Function Occurring as Part of the Individual's Pattern of Adjustment to his Environment and Their Relevance to Headache. An example of this relationship is given in the following case history.

A young male subject who was a junior physician on a hospital staff made daily notes about his activities, his interpersonal relations and feeling states. In addition, his nasal function was observed each day, and records were made of the color of the nasal mucosa, the amount of secretion and of swelling of the nasal structures, and the degree of obstruction to inhaling air.

During a period in which the subject was exposed to serious threats to his independence, he was also subjected to threats to his career by an inefficient intern and to danger of losing the approval of his superiors.

He first tried to cope with the situation by suggesting a plan to maintain the ward's efficiency. When this failed, the subject began, in addition to his own work, to per-

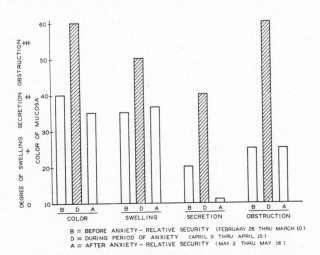

FIG. 38. Sustained hyperemia, swelling, hypersecretion and obstruction in the nose during 12 days of anxiety and resentment compared with control periods before and after.

form the neglected duties himself. At this time, because of his wife's pregnancy, it was necessary to give up his apartment and go to live in the home of a relative.

In this setting of threat to his career and the fear of loss of the approval of his senior colleagues, as well as the conflict arising from his being forced to sacrifice those symbols of independence which his own home represented, the subject developed an anxiety state with feelings of insecurity, guilt, resentment and hostility.

Figure 38 demonstrates the increase in redness of the nasal mucosa associated with a significant increase in the amount of secretion, swelling and obstruction sustained throughout this 12-day period.

DEVELOPMENT OF PAIN. During the entire period of conflict the subject was aware of a constant "irritation" in both nostrils which, at times, developed the quality of a burning pain of low intensity. This was increased by forced inspiration, and associated with it there occurred a dull, aching pain which spread from the bridge of the nose into the orbit and along the zygoma

to the ear on each side of the swollen nasal structures. When the swelling shifted to the opposite nostril the pain correspondingly changed position. The pain, which also involved the teeth, especially those of the upper jaw, alternated with a "feeling of fullness," was worse during the working hours of the day, especially during periods of stress, and was minimal in the early morning and the late evening. When pain was relatively intense, local deep tenderness also was noted. Photophobia occurred, especially on the painful side, with injection of the sclerae and the skin of the cheek. Distribution of headache is shown schematically in Figure 39.

COMMENT. The data of this episode indicate that together with sustained conflict there may occur prolonged nasal hyperfunction accompanied by obstruction, facial pain and tenderness. Such symptoms often are attributed to acute sinusitis. However, in this case no infection of the sinuses was demonstrated, and the disturbance with accompanying symptoms subsided completely when the subject's conflicts were resolved.

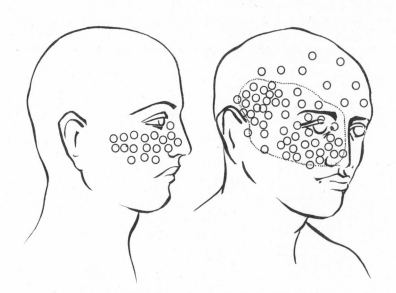

FIG. 39. Distribution of pain during nasal hyperfunction associated with emotional conflict: *(Left)* transitory reaction; *(Right)* sustained reaction during prolonged, intense conflict. This was associated with photophobia, lacrimation, congestion of the conjunctiva on the right, intense erythema and "hyperalgesia" over the zygoma.

GENESIS OF PAIN FROM THE EYE

Headache associated with various ocular disorders has long been recognized as a clinical entity. Errors of refraction (hypermetropia, astigmatism), anomalies of accommodation, disturbances of muscular equilibrium and glaucoma are universally described as causing headache. In addition refractive errors are said to give rise to such other symptoms as aching of the eyes, sandy feeling in the eyes, pulling sensations in and about the orbit and congestion of the conjunctivae.

Investigations have been made on the pain-sensitive structures, both superficial and deep, of the eye; on the headaches and the eyeaches associated with refractive errors and extraocular muscle imbalances; and on photophobia.

Using persons with normal eyes as experimental subjects, the modalities of touch, pain and temperature were investigated on both the conjunctiva and the cornea. Cotton wisps applied to the conjunctiva produced the sensation of touch without pain, and localization of the area touched was fairly accurate. Applicators cooled to below 30° C. were recognized as cool or cold, whereas above this temperature, up to 70° C., they were recognized only as touch. Sharp or pinching stimuli produced pain. On the cornea only pain and cold sensations were recognized.

Patients with increased intraocular pressure described a sharp pain which at first remained localized in the eyeball, then extended as a "bad ache" along the rim of the orbit and finally throughout most of the area supplied by the ophthalmic division of the trigeminal nerve. Nausea and vomiting sometimes accompanied such headaches. In patients having operations for strabismus under local anesthesia, pinching, sticking, or cutting the extraocular muscles caused no sensation, but traction produced prompt exclamations of pain. The pain was described as an aching sensation felt in the eye on the same side as the muscle stimulated and deep in the orbit. There was no consistent radiation of pain from traction on the extraocular muscles, and no pain was felt in the back of the head or the neck.

Traction on the iris tissue with a small toothed forceps or by chemical agents (mydriatics or miotics) caused varying degrees of pain in the eyeball which in some instances was accompanied by radiation to the area supplied by the ophthalmic division of the trigeminal nerve on the same side.

It is recognized that hyperopia, astigmatism and marked extraocular muscle imbalances can produce such symptoms as a sensation of ocular discomfort and aching, a feeling of heaviness in the head, and actual headache, which usually starts around and over the eyes subsequently radiates to the occiput and the back of the head.

The explanations of these symptoms are (1) that they are the result of the *sustained contraction of intraocular muscles* associated with excessive accommodative effort; and (2) that they are secondary to the unusually great and *sustained extraocular muscle contraction* resulting from the effort to produce distinct retinal images and single binocular vision with fusion.

Simple myopia, in contrast with the ocular defects just mentioned, usually does not produce headache. The reason for this is found in the fact that the myope, in attempting to improve his vision by the contraction of his eye muscles, actually makes his vision worse and hence soon abandons the attempt.

Furthermore, it was found that experimentally induced hyperopia and astigmatism caused headaches, while induced myopia did not. Induced extraocular muscle imbalance caused tenseness and irritability, and if prolonged, headache developed with abnormal electromyograms from the muscles of the head and the neck. Spontaneously occurring muscle imbalances produce the same symptoms and the same type of myograms.

Any severe headache may be accompanied by photophobia, which may be of two varieties. In the diseased eye, in which inflammation of the iris and the ciliary body exists, light may cause intense pain felt in the eye and over the area supplied by the ophthalmic division of the 5th nerve, when the light stimulus is accompanied by movement of the inflamed iris. When the latter structure is immobilized, pain is allayed.

Another type of photophobia occurs in persons with healthy irides. It can be elicited by abnormally large amounts of light, or by normal amounts of light under certain conditions, such as surface irritation of the conjunctiva by chemical (2 per cent ethylmorphine hydrochloride) or by mechanical (a foreign body) means. Vascular congestion can be abolished without affecting such experimentally induced photophobia. On the other hand, the photophobia can be diminished by surface anesthesia, but not by midriasis or cycloplegia. Surface anesthesia also reduces the normal winking responses to a bright light. This is probably due to abolition of the normal sensory impulses from air currents, lid pressure, etc. Photophobia may be absent in the presence of the Argyll Robertson pupil.

MUSCLES OF THE HEAD AND THE NECK AS SOURCES OF PAIN

Pain and tightness in the back of the head and the neck are frequent complaints. The sensations are variously described as a stiff cap, viselike, a weight, pressure, a tight band, a cramp, drawing, aching or soreness. Tenderness throughout the trapezius muscles is commonly associated with these complaints and is most intense along the top of the shoulders and in the upper neck. Another common complaint is that of pain, pressure, or paresthesia over the vertex of the head. Here, tension in the neck is less obvious, but pain usually can be elicited by palpation of the trapezius muscles.

The effect of pain in the head upon the head and the neck muscles was studied in several series of observations. Muscle potentials were recorded on a 2-channel ink-writing oscillograph by means of solder electrodes applied over the frontal, the temporal, the occipital and the neck muscles.

Headaches of short duration were induced by spinal drainage and by the in-

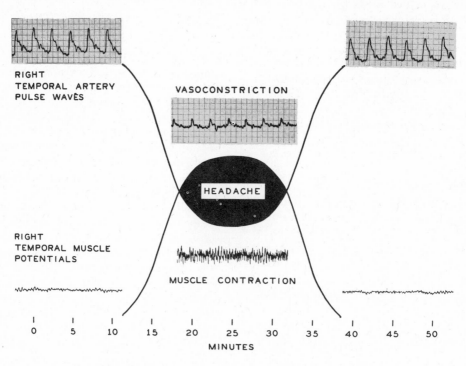

RIGHT TEMPORAL ARTERY PULSE WAVES

VASOCONSTRICTION

RIGHT TEMPORAL MUSCLE POTENTIALS

HEADACHE

MUSCLE CONTRACTION

| | | | | | | | | | | |
| 0 | 5 | 10 | 15 | 20 | 25 | 30 | 35 | 40 | 45 | 50 |

MINUTES

FIG. 40. Muscle contraction headache, right temporal region.

travenous injection of histamine. Contraction of the head and the neck muscles was observed in association with the pain, but no pain arose from the muscles themselves, probably because of the short duration of the induced head pain.

In another series prolonged pain in the head was induced by means of repeated injections of 6 per cent saline into the right temporal muscle. This continuous pain in the head caused marked muscle contraction and secondary pain in the back of the head and the neck (Fig. 40).

An irritant introduced into and left in the conjunctival sac sometimes reflexly caused contraction of the head and the neck muscles and gave rise to secondary pain and paresthesia in the scalp and the neck.

Abnormally sustained contraction of the external ocular muscles brought about by placing a +3D vertical prism in front of the dominant eye caused a sustained contraction in the neck muscles, followed by pain in the neck and the shoulder.

Observations made in patients with pain in the occiput and the neck associated with inflammation or other dysfunction about the head (pansinusitis, migraine headache and caplike, vise, or pressure sensations), revealed sustained contraction of neck and head muscles. The intensity of the pain in the neck and over the back of the head could be modified by hot packs and massage.

These studies demonstrate that noxious stimulation in any part of the head, or emotional tension, lead to sustained contraction of the head and the neck muscles, secondarily giving rise to pain from the shoulders, the neck and the head.

Moreover, such muscles were tender on palpation. Injection with physiologic saline solution of especially tender areas caused an increase in head sensations and pain, whereas injection of 1 per cent procaine solution into such areas eliminated untoward head sensations.

The exceedingly common "tension headache" found in tense, aggressive and frustrated, anxious people also was associated with electromyographic evidence of prolonged contraction of the muscles of the head and the neck, and with evidence from pulse wave records of constriction of the nutrient vessels to the muscles involved. Bilateral pulse waves recorded from the supraorbital, the temporal and the occipital arteries during muscle-contraction headache intervals exhibited evidence of greater vasoconstriction than did records made in headache-free intervals. During such headaches there was as much as a 10-fold increase in amplitude of action potentials from the involved muscles. Furthermore, reduction or elimination of tension through change in the subject's emotions and attitudes by modification of the life situation and by administration of phenobarbital for a few days reduced muscle contraction and vasoconstriction, and eliminated pressure, tight sensations and headache.

TEETH AS A SOURCE OF HEADACHE

In a series of experiments in which electrical stimulation was applied to defective teeth it was demonstrated that when an upper tooth was stimulated pain was experienced at first locally, then diffusely in tissues supplied by the second division of the 5th cranial nerve. Noxious impulses arising from the lower teeth caused pain to be felt at first locally and then diffusely in tissues supplied by the 3rd division of the 5th cranial nerve. If stimulation was sufficiently intense and prolonged, regardless of its site of origin, homolateral spread of the pain into all 3 divisions of the trigeminal nerve occurred. Homolateral hyperalgesia, both superficial and deep, and vasomotor reactions of tissues in the head remote from the site of the stimulated tooth were common.

Injections of procaine locally into the tissues involved in the area of headache associated with noxious impulses from a tooth, reduced in intensity but failed to eliminate pain and the sensation of fullness and tightness in areas adjacent to the region of anesthesia. However, blocking the noxious afferent impulses from stimulated teeth by peridontal infiltration with procaine completely and immediately relieved head pain.

Thus, it seems likely that the diffuse headache associated with disease of the teeth results from afferent impulses from the teeth, causing excitatory processes in the brain stem which spread to exert their effects on many other structures innervated by the 5th cranial nerve. Furthermore, when pain in the teeth is prolonged or severe, sustained contraction of the muscles of the head and the neck may occur, and in these patients pain and "tightness" may persist in the occiput and the neck for a short period, even after blocking the afferent impulses from diseased teeth.

Chronic or Recurrent Post-Traumatic Headache

A series of patients with headache following head injury was studied. The headaches were found to be of three varieties: (1) severe pain or circumscribed tenderness in a scar or site of impact; (2) a steady pressure sensation or aching pain in a circumscribed area or in a caplike distribution; (3) a throbbing and aching pain occurring in attacks usually unilateral and in the temporal or frontal region.

The first type was represented by those patients who had tender areas in the scalp. These persisted sometimes for as long as 6 years after the trauma. Such tender spots were often related to visible scars and were often at or near the site of injury. Injection of the tender areas with isotonic saline accentuated the pain, while injection with procaine predictably eliminated it. It is inferred that the pain comes from stimulation of pain endings caught in the locally damaged tissue.

The second type resulted from sustained skeletal muscle contraction. It was demonstrated by means of electromyograms in these patients that pain in any part of the head induced a sustained contraction of the head or neck muscles sometimes remote from the original site of noxious stimulation, which in turn gave rise to steady pressure or aching pain in the head or the neck, the exact site depending on the locus of the contracted muscles. However, such sustained and often painful contraction occurred even without tender scars or circumscribed areas of tenderness and was associated with tension and apprehension. In some instances these contractions represented unconscious protective immobilization of the head and the neck.

The third type of headache was caused by recurrent episodes of dilatation of cranial arteries. Such pain was reduced by compression of the painful arteries. Headache was eliminated by intramuscular injection of ergotamine tartrate. Such headaches were also associated with tension, anxiety, resentment and fatigue.

Sometimes the same patient exhibited more than one mechanism of headache. Thus, in this series, post-traumatic headache and other sensations arose from structures on the outside of the head. Nearly all patients studied harbored resentment related to the circumstances of the accident, or fear that they had sustained permanent damage to their brains. Such emotional reactions and attitudes were intimately related to the above-mentioned mechanisms of post-traumatic headache.

The mechanisms of the pain following head trauma (excepting epidural and subdural hematoma and subarachnoid hemorrhage) are therefore of three types: (1) pain due to local tissue damage; (2) pain due to sustained neck or head muscle contraction; (3) pain due to dilatation of the branches of the external carotid arteries.

DISCOVERY OF THE CAUSE: IMPORTANT CONSIDERATIONS IN DIAGNOSIS

Incidence

The most commonly encountered headaches are vascular headaches of the migraine type and the headaches from sustained muscle contraction accompanying vasoconstriction and associated with anxiety and emotional tension. The headaches associated with fever and septicemia probably rank next in frequency and then come those due to nasal and paranasal and eye disease. The headaches of meningitis, aneurysm, brain tumor and brain abscess, though important and dramatic, are much less common.

Intensity

The most intense headaches are those due to ruptured intracranial aneurysm, meningitis, fever, migraine, and those associated with arterial hypertension. The subarachnoid hemorrhage resulting usually from ruptured intracranial aneurysm produces a headache that is sudden in onset, reaches great intensity in a very short time and may be associated with feelings of faintness or with unconsciousness. The onset of pain is soon followed by the development of a stiff neck and the presence of blood in the lumbar spinal fluid. The very intense headache of meningitis is accompanied by a very stiff neck which prevents passive flexion of the head on the chest. The spasm of the muscles of the neck associated with the intense headaches of migraine permits flexion of the neck.

The intensity of the headaches associated with brain tumors, brain abscesses, sinus disease and eye disease is usually only moderately severe. Hemorrhage into the parenchyma of the brain seldom causes headaches unless the hemorrhage breaks through into the ventricular or subarachnoid spaces; then, intense headache may result. Also, hemorrhage into a brain tumor causing additional and serious displacement of the brain may result in a moderately severe headache.

Brain abscess may be a painless disorder unless associated with circumscribed meningitis or periostitis. However, when of long standing, brain abscess may produce headache because of generalized brain displacement and traction on pain-sensitive structures.

One rare form of very intense headache is encountered in patients in the terminal phase of brain tumor. This headache is generalized, paroxysmal and agonizing and often ends in stupor. The pain may last for 30 seconds to 30 minutes and then disappear as quickly as it came, leaving the patient exhausted. With such headache the patient may pass into coma and die.

QUALITY OF HEADACHE

The headaches of fever, migraine, hemangiomatous tumors and those associated with arterial hypertension are characteristically throbbing or pulsating in quality. Headache from secondary muscle spasm associated with emotional tension or with eye or sinus disease has the quality of tightness or external pressure, and may be band-like, caplike, or viselike. The headache of brain tumors and of meningitis, though occasionally pulsating, is usually of a steady aching quality.

SITE

Vascular headaches of the migraine type may occur anywhere in the head and the face and may involve the neck. The most common site is the temple, usually on the right side. The migraine headache at some time involves both the right and the left sides, although any one attack may be strictly unilateral. The headache of sinus or eye disease, shortly after its onset, is usually in the front of the head, roughly in the region near the site of stimulation; subsequently, the pain may be predominantly in the back of the head and the neck due to secondary muscle contraction. Headaches associated with pituitary adenomata and parasellar tumors are often bitemporal.

The headaches of posterior fossa tumors, early in the development of the tumor and before the beginning of general brain displacement, are usually over the occiput or behind the ear. Headaches from supratentorial tumors, before serious brain displacement occurs, are usually in the front or on the top of the head. Occasionally, if the tumor involves the dura and the bone, the headache may be near or over the site of the lesion. Early in the course of the tumor or before general displacement of the brain has occurred, the headache is usually on the side of the tumor.

Subdural hematoma produces a headache of considerable intensity, usually localized over or near the site of the lesion, most commonly over the frontoparietal areas. The headache may be intermittent but is present, usually, some time each day, for weeks, months, or longer. A history of almost continuous headache from the date of injury is characteristic; there is no long "silent period" immediately after the injury.

The headaches associated with tumors of the cerebellopontile angle and acoustic neurinoma are often localized in the postauricular region. Like other brain-tumor headaches, they are intermittent, and of moderate intensity. They are associated with hyperalgesia of the postauricular region on the same side as the tumor. Headache is one of the earliest manifestations of acoustic neurinoma. Headache is a later manifestation of cerebellopontile angle tumors.

The muscle-contraction headaches or pressure sensations associated with emotional tension are usually first evident and most intense in the neck, the shoulders and the occiput, but later spread to include the frontal region. They may be unilateral or bilateral.

Disease involving the dome of the diaphragm or the phrenic nerve causes pain high in the shoulder and the neck. Similarly in rare instances coronary occlusion and myocardial insufficiency cause pain in the lower jaw, high in the neck and in the occiput. Disease and dysfunction of structures below the diaphragm do not ordinarily induce headache except indirectly through fever, sepsis or bacteremia.

However, in special circumstances headache may occur with excessive distention of the urinary bladder or rectum. It has been demonstrated in paraplegics whose level of cord transection is T-6 or higher, that excessive distention of the bladder or rectum results in a vascular pressor response in the segments below the level of the lesion. Prompt rise in blood pressure occurs, and cranial blood vessels not involved in the pressor response become dilated, causing headache.

TENDERNESS

During migraine headaches and often for some hours thereafter there is hyperalgesia or tenderness near the large arteries on the outside of the head in the affected region. As mentioned above, it has been demonstrated that deep-pain thresholds are lowered. Also, there may be tenderness of the skin of the face as a result of inflammation of the nasal and the paranasal spaces. Muscle in a state of sustained contraction, secondary to pain anywhere in the head, may become tender on palpation. Thus, brushing and combing the hair may be a painful experience during or after muscle tension or migraine headache. With myositis and myalgia there may be tender areas in the muscles of the head and the neck. Because of the hyperalgesia, percussion of the head may cause pain over or near an underlying brain tumor.

Periostitis secondary to frontal, ethmoid, or sphenoid sinus disease or mastoiditis produces a pain of moderate to severe intensity associated with local tenderness at the site of disease. If the pain is sufficiently severe and continuous it may become generalized. If the mastoid or sinus disease is limited to the bone (osteomyelitis) it is usually completely painless. The tenderness or hyperalgesia associated with mastoid disease with periostitis is far greater than the hyperalgesia associated with posterior fossa brain tumor.

Tenderness at a site of head injury, and often associated with a scar, may persist for many years. Also, in post-traumatic headache there often occur tender muscles or nodules in parts of the head remote from the site of injury. Headache of the vascular type akin to migraine with tenderness over the arteries may be initiated by head injury.

EFFECT OF MANUAL PRESSURE

Pressure upon the temporal, frontal, supraorbital, postauricular, occipital and common carotid arteries often reduces the intensity of migraine headache and that associated with arterial hypertention. No other type is so definitely modified by manual pressure, although supporting the head makes any patient with headache feel more comfortable.

The headache or pressure sensations associated with emotional tension and resulting from sustained muscle contraction are intensified by firm pressure upon tender muscles or regions of tenderness.

EFFECT OF POSITION OF THE HEAD

In many instances migraine headache is made worse by assuming a horizontal position and is relieved by an erect position. It is often made worse by ascending stairs, by moving about rapidly, or by lifting objects. Sitting quietly in an upright position often proves to be most comfortable. The recumbent position may at first make the headache associated with nasal and paranasal disease more intense, but subsequently the headache subsides. A sudden change in position, usually from the recumbent to the sitting and less frequently from the sitting to the recumbent, may make the headache of brain tumor more intense. Unlike the migraine headache, the headache of brain tumor is often worse when the patient is in the upright position. The head-down position aggravates some headaches, except those due to spinal drainage and occasionally those associated with brain tumors. Shaking the head tends to augment the intensity of intracranial vascular headache and brain-tumor headache, but may reduce that due to muscle spasm from tension or that secondary to sinus and eye diseases. Muscle contraction headache is usually reduced in intensity by movements of the head and the neck which extend the contracted muscles. Straining at stool and coughing increase all but muscle headaches. Sharp flexion or over-extension of the head reduces the intensity of post-puncture headache.

DURATION OF HEADACHE

Headache of the migraine variety may be as brief as 20 or 30 minutes, or it may last for days, or, rarely, for weeks. The usual headache is terminated within 24 hours. A striking feature of migraine is the complete freedom from headache between prostrating attacks. The headaches of brain tumor are intermittent, but usually occur during part of every day and vary in intensity from time to time. Headache associated with chronic sinus disease is intermittent but quite predictable; it may occur during the working hours of each day for weeks or even months.

Muscle contraction headache or pressure sensations associated with sustained tension and anxiety may persist for days, weeks, or even years.

TIME OF DAY

Headaches associated with hypertension and migraine most commonly have their onset in the early hours of the morning so that the patient awakens with the pain.

Such migraine headaches characteristically diminish in intensity with the "setting of the sun" or in the evening. The headache of brain tumor, if it be connected in any way with the time of day, is more severe in the early part of the day, though not in the early hours of the morning. The headache associated with nasal and paranasal disease usually occurs in the morning and improves toward the late afternoon or when the patient retires. Headache associated with eye disease usually begins in the latter part of the day or evening.

Muscle contraction headache or pressure sensations are usually worse at the end of the working day.

DAY OF THE WEEK AND THE MONTH

Migraine headaches are common during week-ends, during the first period of vacation holidays and immediately after vacation. They are very common just before the onset of menstruation. Patients with migraine often have fixed days of the week when their headaches occur.

SEASON OF THE YEAR

Headache associated with nasal and paranasal disease is usually more common during periods when the upper respiratory infections prevail, namely, the darker months of the year. Migraine headache occurs during periods of increased conflict, tension or stress for the individual; for example, during early fall for the school teacher, during "rush" or "holiday" seasons for the merchant, during very hot or humid weather for those who feel ineffective and prostrated during such climatic states.

MUSCLE SPASM

Contractions of the muscles of the head and the neck occur with all headaches. If the contractions are of sufficient duration, they themselves become a cause of headache. Headache and a very stiff neck accompanied by Kernig's sign are associated with widespread meningitis. The Kernig sign may be absent even late in the course of a carcinomatous invasion of the meninges at the base of the brain. Headache and stiff neck are common with tumors of the posterior fossa, but the stiff neck may be overcome by persuasion and passive movement of the head by the examining physician. Neck stiffness may sometimes occur with prolonged postpuncture headache.

Spasm of the muscles of the neck, the head and the back may become so great with meningitis that it cannot be relaxed and the patient assumes the position of opisthotonos. With posterior fossa tumors muscle spasm may cause tilting of the head or lifting of the shoulder. The muscle spasm headache associated with prolonged anxiety and tension may cause backward tilting of the head and half closing of the eyes. Muscle spasm is always an accompaniment of migraine headache and is one explanation of the slow relief afforded by ergotamine tartrate to some patients in whom this component is major.

PHOTOPHOBIA

Photophobia is associated with any headache experienced chiefly in the front or the top of the head. It is commonly noted in patients with meningitis, migraine, nasal and paranasal disease, eye disease, braintumor and muscle-spasm headache. Congestion of the sclera and the conjunctiva may accompany such photophobia. If the intensity of the pain is very great, photophobia, lacrimation and sweating of the homolateral forehead and side of the face also occur.

PERIODICITY

Headaches which begin in childhood or at puberty and occur especially with menstruation and at certain fixed intervals during many years are in all likelihood of the migraine variety. Migraine headaches often stop at menopause. On the other hand, they may occasionally begin at this time.

MUCOUS MEMBRANE INJECTION

Redness and swelling of the mucous membrane of the nose with or without nosebleeds may occur with migraine. Also, injection of the conjunctiva may be seen. Headache caused by disease of the nasal and the paranasal sinuses is always accompanied by obvious congestion of the turbinates and the nasal mucous membranes.

GASTROINTESTINAL AND VASOMOTOR DISTURBANCES

Anorexia, nausea and vomiting, though most commonly associated with migraine headaches, may be associated with any headache, and the more intense the headache the more likely they are to occur. Vomiting without nausea may occur with brain tumors, especially those of the posterior fossa. Nausea and vomiting with little or no headache may occur in persons with migraine. The headache associated with sinus or eye disease is seldom associated with vomiting. Constipation often is associated with migraine, although diarrhea also occurs. Distention and flatulence are common in migraine and tension headaches, but are seldom associated with other headaches.

Excessive pallor, also cold hands and feet, are characteristic prodromal accompaniments of the migraine attack. Tachycardia and extrasystoles frequently are noted.

POLYURIA

Polyuria is commonly associated with migraine headache attacks and, with the exception of the headache associated with 3rd ventricle tumors, seldom occurs with other headaches. Weight gain of several pounds preceding the migraine attack is common, but not invariable. It usually develops some hours before, but sometimes occurs well in advance of the headache (7 to 10 days). During subsidence of the headache, weight loss occurs with increased rates of excretion of water, sodium and potassium. However, these fluid and electrolyte changes are not related causally or mechanistically to the onset, the intensity or the duration of the migraine attack. Instead, they are manifestations of the widespread bodily changes accompanying adaptive reactions during and after stressful periods. Thus the migraine attack is a concurrent but independent feature. Tension states with headaches may be linked with frequency of urination.

VISUAL DISTURBANCES

Both scintillating scotomata and visual field defects such as unilateral or homonymous hemianopsia may occur with migraine headaches. Such defects in vision may occur with brain-tumor headaches when the tumor is due to a lesion of the occipital lobes or is adjacent to the visual pathways. The visual disturbances of migraine, with the exception of blurred vision and diplopia, seldom occur with the headache but usually precede it. The visual disturbance is usually of short duration, persisting for less than an hour. Enlarged pupils and lacrimation may cause dimness of vision during a migraine headache, but when visual defects outlast the headache attack it is likely that one is dealing with cerebral vascular accident or a brain tumor. Defects in color vision and colored rings around lights may occur with the headache associated with glaucoma. Ptosis of the eyelid may be an accompaniment of the brain-tumor headache and occasionally that of migraine. It occurs with a rare variety of migraine called ophthalmoplegic migraine, in which case it is probably due to an aneurysm of the circle of Willis. Partial closure of the eyes due to muscle spasm may accompany any headache and give the impression of faulty vision.

VERTIGO AND OTHER SENSORY DISTURBANCES

Vertigo may be a forerunner of a migraine headache attack. Vertigo is sometimes associated with the headaches of brain tumors, although feelings of unsteadiness are more common. Fleeting vertigo with sudden movement or rotation of the head often accompanies the posttraumatic headache. Ménière's syndrome is frequently associated with headache. Other sensory disturbances, such as paresthesias of the hands and the face, may occur as a forerunner of the migraine headache. However, paresthesias that persist during or outlast the headache attack are more common in patients with brain tumors and in those with certain types of cerebral seizure.

MOOD

The wish to retire from people and responsibilities, a dejected, depressed, irritable, or negativistic mental state bordering on prostration or stupor is a dominant aspect of the migraine attack and in some instances may be more disturbing than the pain in the head. Apathy, listlessness or even euphoria may be associated with brain-tumor headache. Depression is not a feature, although obviously a depressed person may also have brain tumor.

The headache associated with muscle contraction may occur in a tense, irritable person, but the patient is usually more willing to accept attention, massage, or medication in contrast with the patient with a migraine headache attack who commonly expresses the wish to be left alone. Exaltation or feelings of especial well-being are common sequels to the migraine headache attack. The suffering experienced with the headache of fever, meningitis, or ruptured aneurysm may be very great, and the mental state is that of reaction to intense pain.

SLEEP

Migraine headaches, even of the most severe type, do not disrupt sleep entirely, except for short periods. Those of brain tumor, sinus disease and muscle spasm permit sleep. Therefore, when an individual complains of long periods of sleep loss because of headache, it is well to consider anxiety or depression as the dominant aspect of the illness. The headache of meninigitis usually interrupts sleep.

EYEGROUNDS

When headache is linked with papilledema, it is in most instances due to an expanding intracranial mass. However, in patients with brain tumor, headache often occurs without papilledema, and papilledema without headache. In the advanced phase of hypertensive encephalopathy, headache and papilledema are usual. Aneurysm and subdural hematoma may cause intense headache without papilledema. Meningitis does not affect the eye-grounds except possibly to induce slight suffusion. During migraine headache arterial and venous dilatation in eyegrounds is usual. Albuminuric retinitis may not be associated with headache; when headache is present the two phenomena are not directly related.

FAMILY HISTORY

The headache of migraine and that associated with arterial hypertension are the only familial headaches. Evidence permits the assumption that inheritance of the migraine headache trait is through a recessive gene with a penetrance of approximately 70 per cent.

LEUKOCYTOSIS

The headaches of meningitis and subarachnoid hemorrhage are usually accompanied by leukocytosis; the headache of typhoid fever, by leukopenia. There may be leukopenia with the headache associated with influenza or grippe. Headache and stiff neck with slight if any leukocytosis is noted in luetic meningitis and sometimes in tuberculous meningitis.

The headache following severe convulsions or a series of convulsions may be associated with leukocytosis. The headache associated with brain tumor, particularly if it be in the frontal region, is sometimes accompanied by leukocytosis. Leukocytosis coupled with fever is most commonly associated with brain abscess.

CEREBROSPINAL FLUID

Headache and pleocytosis may be associated with meningitis, whereas the headache associated with the onset of acute infections outside the cranial cavity usually is accompanied by only a slight increase or no increase in the number of cells in the spinal fluid. Intracranial pressure may be increased with headache associated with brain tumor, but often no increase occurs.

The headache of brain abscess is commonly associated with a slight increase in the number of cells. The Wassermann test of the spinal fluid is positive if luetic meningitis or gumma is responsible for the headache. The cerebrospinal fluid is normal during the headache of migraine, hypertensive vascular disease or fever, and usually normal in meningismus. When a headache results from a brain tumor in contact with the arachnoid space, there may be an increase in protein and cells in the spinal fluid.

Blood in the spinal fluid or xanthochromia not due to spinal cord injury or disease is almost always accompanied by headache. This combination commonly occurs with head injury, carcinomatosis (especially of the meninges), subarachnoid hemorrhage and ruptured cerebral aneurysm. It less commonly occurs with subdural hematoma, meningioma and glioma.

ELECTROENCEPHALOGRAMS

When electroencephalography is performed in a large series of patients with the complaint of headache, without reference to the type of headache, the number of abnormal records is not much different from that found in a similar group of headache-free individuals. However, the incidence of abnormal electroencephalographic records increases significantly when patients with vascular headache of the migraine type are studied. Patients having focal motor, sensory or mental disturbances during one phase of a migraine attack are those most likely to have focal electroencephalographic abnormalities. These abnormalities may be separated into three broad categories:

1. Transient focal electroencephalographic changes that appear only very briefly along with a focal neurological sign, and then disappear almost simultaneously with the dwindling of the neurological defect (as with scotomata).

2. Transient focal abnormalities lasting hours or days. These are exemplified by the infrequent occurrence of hemiparesis accompanying and sometimes outlasting the migraine attack.

3. Persistent focal and/or generalized slow activity seen during headache-free intervals. This accounts for only a small percentage of the electroencephalographic changes.

ROENTGENOGRAMS

X-ray pictures of the head in patients with migraine or the headaches of hypertension, meningitis, ruptured aneurysm, brain abscess, show nothing unusual. Aneurysm can sometimes be demonstrated by arteriograms. Moreover, x-ray examinations reveal nothing in at least half of the patients with brain tumor. Frontal hyperostosis is not in itself a cause of headache. Calcification of the falx, of the cerebral arteries, of the pineal body, or of the choroid plexus, does not cause headache. A small sella turcica is in itself no cause of headache.

Long-standing osteosclerosis of the mastoid region and increased density of the sinuses do not in themselves cause headache.

Disease of the nasal and paranasal sinuses can cause headache without enough change to be evident in x-ray plates. On the other hand, there may be serious disease of the sinuses with osteomyelitis without headache.

FACTORS THAT MODIFY HEADACHE

Decompression of the skull and removal of brain tumors very commonly afford relief of headache due to such tumors. This is not universally true, since headaches caused by pituitary adenomata often persist after the tumor has been removed.

Ligation or obliteration of the middle meningeal artery will sometimes relieve headache due to brain tumor even though the latter has become inoperable. Such procedures often fail, however, since traction upon other pain-sensitive structures may continue to cause pain.

Ligation of the superficial temporal artery or other superficial scalp arteries may reduce or eliminate migraine headaches in certain patients.

The evacuation of pus from beneath the periosteum and from the adjacent paranasal sinuses and mastoid cells often affords prompt relief of the headache associated with empyema of these regions. However, the persistence or development of frontal headache after simple sinusotomy is evidence of the presence of extradural infection and possibly of subdural infection. Similarly, the persistence or development of postauricular or preauricular headache after simple mastoidectomy is good evidence for the existence of adjacent extradural and possibly subdural infection.

CHEMICAL AGENTS THAT MODIFY AND THAT PREVENT HEADACHES

The effectiveness of analgesics is dependent entirely upon the intensity of pain and not at all on the site or origin or the particular mechanism inducing the pain. Thus, 60 mg. of codeine sulfate or 15 mg. of morphine sulfate may be necessary for the high-intensity headaches of meningitis, migraine, ruptured aneurysm and of certain fevers such as typhus and typhoid fever, whereas agents such as acetylsalicylic acid in 0.3 to 0.6 Gm. doses are effective against other types of headache. Fortunately the headache of brain tumor is seldom so intense as to require opiates. Ergotamine tartrate if given parenterally and in sufficient amounts will modify or abolish the headache of migraine. It does not affect other types except those associated with arterial hypertension. Norepinephrine, in a dilution of 4 ml. of a 0.2 per cent solution in a liter of 5 per cent dextrose in water, can be administered intravenously at an average rate of 4 drops per second or sufficient to raise the systolic blood pressure 20 to 40 mm. Hg. Mild headaches of migraine type have been eliminated in 30 minutes with infusion of norepinephrine; severe headaches, in 45 to 160 minutes. Phenobarbital, given over a period of days or weeks (0.015 to 0.030 Gm., t. i. d.), by inducing relaxation may reduce or eliminate muscle-contraction headache.

While not useful in therapy of a headache already established, nevertheless, the administration of 1-methyl-d-lysergic acid butanolamide bimaleate (Methysergide Sansert, Sandoz) in 2 mg. amounts from 2 to 6 times a day is often effective in diminishing the frequency and intensity, or in preventing the occurrrence, of vascular headaches of the migraine type. Because of its occasional serious side effects, patients receiving this medication should be under the continuous supervision of a physician.

LIFE SITUATIONS AND REACTIONS

Migraine headaches commonly occur when hereditarily susceptible persons attempt to control feelings of anxiety, tension, anger, or resentment by means of organized and intense activity. No amount of therapeutic or preventive medication alone can take the place of helping the patient to understand himself and whatever pernicious attitudes he may have and to recognize those factors in his life that may be causing him to go in the wrong direction, or at the wrong pace. Two out of three patients with vascular and/or muscle tension headache can thus be greatly helped.

BIBLIOGRAPHY

Camp, W. A., and Wolff, H. G.: Studies on headache. Electroencephalographic abnormalities in patients with vascular headache of the migraine type, A.M.A. Arch. Neurol. 4:475-485, 1961.

Chapman, L. F., Goodell, H., and Wolff, H. G.: Augmentation of the inflammatory reaction by activity of the central nervous system, A.M.A. Arch. Neurol. 1:557-582, 1959.

Chapman, L. F., Ramos, A. O., Goodell, H., Silverman, G., and Wolff, H. G.: A humoral agent implicated in vascular headache of the migraine type, A.M.A. Arch. Neurol. 3:223-229, 1960; Trans. Amer. Neurol. Ass., 85:42-45; 200-202, 1960.

————: Definition of a biochemical agent implicated in the mechanism of vascular headache of the migraine type, Trans. Ass. Amer. Physicians 73:259-271, 1960.

Clark, D., Hough, H. B., and Wolff, H. G.: Experimental studies on headache, observations on headache produced by histamine. A.M.A. Arch. Neurol. Psychiat. 35:1054, 1936.

Dalessio, D. J., Camp, W. A., Goodell, H., and Wolff, H. G.: Studies on headache. The mode of action of UML-491 and its relevance to the nature of vascular headache of the migraine type, A.M.A. Arch. Neurol. 4:235-240, 1961.

Dalessio, D. J., Chapman, L. F., Zileli, T., Cattell, M., Ehrlich, R., Fortuin, F., Goodell, H., and Wolff, H. G.: Studies on headache. The responses of the bulbar conjunctival blood vessels during induced oliguria and diuresis, and their modification by UML-491, A.M.A. Arch. Neurol. 5:590-593, 1961.

Dalessio, D. J., Camp, W. A., Goodell, H., Chapman, L. F., Zileli, T., Ramos, A. O., Ehrlich, R., Fortuin, F., Cattell, M., and Wolff, H. G.: Studies on headache. The relevance of the prophylactic action of UML-491 in vascular headache of the migraine type to the pathophysiology of this syndrome, World Neurol. 3:66, 1962.

Eckardt, L. B., McLean, J. M., and Goodell, H.. Experimental studies on headache: the genesis of pain from the eye, Proc. Assn. Res. Nerv. Ment. Dis. 23:209, 1943.

Goodell, H, Lewontin, R. and Wolff, H. G.: Familial occurrence of migraine headache. A study of heredity, Arch. Neurol. Psychiat. 72:325, 1954.

Graham, J. R., and Wolff, H. G.: Mechanism of migraine headache and action of ergotamine tartrate, Proc. Assn. Res. Nerv. Ment. Dis. 18:638, 1937; Arch. Neurol. Psychiat. 39:737, 1938.

Grimes, E.: The migraine instability, Med. J. Rec. 134:417, 1931.

Holmes, T. H., Goodell, H., Wolf, S. G., and Wolff, H. G.: The nose; an experimental study of reactions within the nose in human subjects during varying life experiences, Springfield, Ill., Thomas, 1950.

Kilbourne, E. D., and Wolff, H. G.: Cranial arteritis: a critical evaluation of the syndrome of "temporal arteritis" with report of a case, Ann. Int. Med. 24:1, 1946.

Kunkle, E. C., Ray, B. S., and Wolff, H. G.: Studies on headache. The mechanism and significance of the headache associated with brain tumor, Bull. New York Acad. Med. 18:400, 1942.

————: Studies on headache: An analysis of the headache associated with changes in intracranial pressure, Arch. Neurol. Psychiat. 49:323, 1943.

Kunkle, E. C., Lund, D. W., and Maher, P. J.: Analysis of vascular mechanisms in headache by use of the human centrifuge, with observations upon pain perception under increased positive G, Arch. Neurol. Psychiat. 60:253, 1948.

Kunkle, E. C., Pfeiffer, J. B., Wilhoit, W. M., and Hamrick, L. W.: Recurrent brief headache in "cluster" headache, Trans. Am. Neurol. Ass: 77:240, 1952.

Kunkle, E. C., Hernandez, R. R., Johnson, W. T., and Baumann, J. A.: Adaptive responses of cranial vessels in the head-down position, Trans. Am. Neurol. Ass. 87:151, 1962.

Marcussen, R. M., and Wolff, H. G.: A formulation of the dynamics of the migraine attack, Psychosom. Med. 11:251, 1949.

————: Studies on headache. 1. Effects of carbon dioxide-oxygen mixtures given during preheadache phase of the migraine attack; 2. Further analysis of the pain mechanisms in headache, Arch. Neurol. Psychiat. 63:42, 1950.

Ostfeld, A. M., Reis, D. J., Goodell, H., and Wolff, H. G.: Headache and hydration. The significance of two varieties of fluid accumulation in patients with vascular headache of the migraine type, A.M.A. Arch. Int. Med. 96:142-152, 1955; Trans. Amer. Physicians 68:255, 1955.

Ostfeld, A. M., and Wolff, H. G.: Arterenol (norepinephrine) and vascular headache of the migraine type. Studies on headache, Arch. Neurol. Psychiat. 74:131-136, 1955; Trans. Amer. Neurol. Ass., p. 142, 1954.

————: Studies on headache: reactivity of bulbar conjunctival vessels during the migraine type of headache and muscle contraction headache (abstract), (Am. Fed. Clin. Res.) Clin. Res. 4:1956; Arch. Neurol. Psychiat. 77:113, 1957.

Ostfeld, A. M., Chapman, L. F., Goodell, H., and Wolff, H. G.: Studies in headache. Summary of evidence concerning a noxious agent active locally during migraine headache, Psychosom. Med. 19:199-208, 1957.

Ostfeld, A. M., and Wolff, H. G.: Studies on headache: participation of ocular structures in the migraine syndrome, Modern Problems in Ophthalmology 1:634-647, 1957.

Pickering, G. W.: Experimental observations on headache, Brit. M. J. 1:907, 1939.

Pichler, E., Ostfeld, A. M., Goodell, H., and Wolff, H. G.: Studies on headache. Central versus peripheral action of ergotamine tartrate and its relevance to the therapy of migraine headache, Arch. Neurol. Psychiat. 76:571-577, 1956.

Ray, B. S., and Wolff, H. G.: Experimental studies on headache. Pain-sensitive structures of the head and their significance in headache, A.M.A. Arch. Surg. 41:813, 1940.

Robertson, S., Goodell, H., and Wolff, H. G.: Headache; the teeth as a source of headache and other pain, Arch. Neurol. Psychiat. 57:277, 1947.

Robertson, S., and Wolff, H. G.: Studies on headache: distension of the rectum, sigmoid colon and bladder as a source of headache in intact humans, Arch. Neurol. Psychiat. 63:52, 1950.

Schottstadt, W. W., and Wolff, H. G.: Studies on headache. Variations in fluid and electrolyte excretion in association with vascular headache of the migraine type, Arch. Neurol. Psychiat. 73:158-164, 1955.

Schumacher, G. A., and Guthrie, T. C.: Mechanism of headache induced by distention of bladder and rectum in patients with spinal cord injuries, Trans. Am. Neurol. Ass., 74:205, 1949.

Schumacher, G. A., Ray, B. S., and Wolff, H. G.: Experimental studies on headache. Further analysis of histamine headache and its pain pathways, Arch. Neurol. Psychiat. 44:701, 1940.

Schumacher, G. A., and Wolff, H. G.: Experimental studies on headache. (A) Contrast of histamine headache with the headache of migraine and that associated with hypertension. (B) Contrast of vascular mechanisms in preheadache and headache phenomena of migraine, Arch. Neurol. Pyschiat. 45:199, 1941.

Simons, D. J., Day, E., Goodell, H., and Wolff, H. G.: Experimental studies on headache; muscles of the scalp and neck as sources of pain, Proc. Ass. Res. Nerv. Ment. Dis. 23:228, 1943.

Simons, D. J., and Wolff, H. G.: Experimental studies on headache: the mechanism of chronic or recurrent post-traumatic headache, Psychosom. Med. 8:293, 1946.

Sutherland, A. M., and Wolff, H. G.: Experimental studies on headache. Further analysis of the mechanism of headache in migraine, hypertension and fever, Arch. Neurol. Psychiat. 44:929, 1940.

Thompson, C. E., and Witham, A. C.: Paroxysmal hypertension in spinal cord injuries, New England J. Med. 239:291, 1948.

Torda, C., and Wolff, H. G.: Experimental studies on headache. The pharmacodynamics of the urine of patients with migraine headache, Fed. Proc., Am. Soc. Pharmacol. Exp. Therap. 2:44, March, 1943.

————: Experimental studies on headache: Transient thickening of walls and cranial arteries in relation to certain phenomena of migraine headache and action of ergotamine tartrate on thickened vessels, Arch. Neurol. Psychiat. 53:329, 1945.

Tunis, M. M., and Wolff, H. G.: Studies on headache. Cranial artery vasoconstriction and muscle contraction headache, Arch. Neurol. Psychiat. 71:425, 1954.

————: Studies on headache. Long-term observations of the cranial arteries in subjects with vascular headache of the migraine type, Arch. Neurol. Psychiat. 70:551, 1953.

Whitteridge, D., Gilliatt, R. W., and Guttmann, L.: Inspiratory vasoconstriction in patients after spinal cord injuries, J. Physiol. 107:67-75, 1948.

Wolff, H. G.: The cerebral circulation, Physiol. Rev. 16:545, 1936.

Wolff, H. G.: Personality features and reactions of subjects with migraine, Arch. Neurol. Psychiat. 37:895, 1937.

Wolff, H. G.: Headache and Other Head Pain, ed. 2, New York, Oxford, 1963.

Wolff, H. G.: Stress and adaptive patterns resulting in tissue damage in man, M. Clin. N. Amer. 39:783, 1955.

Wolff, H. G., and Tunis, M. M.: Analysis of cranial artery pressure pulse waves in patients with vascular headache of the migraine type, Trans. Ass. Am. Phys. 65:240, 1952.

Wolff, H. G., Tunis, M. M., and Goodell, H.: Studies on headache. Evidence of tissue damage and changes in pain sensitivity in subjects with vascular headaches of the migraine type, A.M.A. Arch. Int. Med. 92:478, 1953.

Wolff, H. G.: Stress and Disease, Springfield, Ill., Thomas, 1952.

Zileli, T., Chapman, L. F., and Wolff, H. G.: Anti-inflammatory action of UML-491 demonstrated by granuloma pouch technique in rats, Arch. Int. Pharmacodyn. 136:463, 1962.

Zileli, T., Goodell, H., Hinkle, L. E., and Wolff, H. G.: Studies on headache: the modifying effect of UML-491 on the sensitivity of vasomotor centers and its relevance to vascular headache, in press.

5

Sore Tongue and Sore Mouth

RICHARD W. VILTER

Since the earliest day of medicine, the tongue has been a barometer of health. Hippocrates[1] correlated the dry, heavily coated, fissured tongue with fever and dehydration, and he associated a poor prognosis with the red, ulcerated tongue and mouth of the patient with protracted dysentery.

With the medical renaissance of the eighteenth and the nineteenth centuries, observations on the state of the tongue and the mouth became as important as the taking of the pulse. Indeed, by 1844 glossology had become so important a part of the medical art that a Dr. Benjamin Ridge proposed the fantastic theory that the viscera were represented by definite areas on the tongue and that an abnormality in a viscus was reflected in this predetermined area. The physician was not alone in holding the tongue in high regard. The patient and his family often considered it the only sure indicator of health or disease and regarded that physician poorly who did not greet his patient with the request, "Stick out your tongue, please." Such aphorisms as "raw red tongue—raw red gut" or "coated tongue—constipation" stem from this period.

During the first half of the twentieth century, the science of medicine rapidly outstripped the art, and many reputable physicians, aware that the beliefs of previous centuries were frequently "old wives'

tales," preferred to confine their observations to such newly developed instruments as the fluoroscope and the electrocardiograph. Observation of the tongue and the mouth was so simple that it was frequently neglected and, in fact, often considered as the mark of the "old-timer."

In recent years, however, observations of the condition of tongue and mouth have begun to assume new diagnostic importance. Interpretations have been based on controlled clinical observations rather than on empiricism. The change began about 1900 with William Hunter's description of the glossitis of pernicious anemia.[2] Later, hematologists such as Minot and Murphy[3] substantiated Hunter's observations and made use of them as diagnostic measures; but the present emphasis on the significance of oral lesions is due, primarily, to the work of nutritionists such as Spies,[4,5] Jolliffe,[6] Sydenstricker,[7,8] Sebrell,[9] and Kruse,[10,11] who have stressed the importance of tongue and mouth lesions in the early diagnosis of nutritional deficiency diseases. The complicated mechanisms whereby the tongue and the mouth mirror the abnormalities of the body as a whole have only begun to be unraveled, but knowledge of metabolic diseases is increasing rapidly. Already the importance of questioning the patient concerning soreness or burning of the tongue and of careful examination of the tongue have been re-established.

125

This chapter is concerned with the description, the interpretation and the differential diagnosis of *painful* abnormalities of tongue and mouth which reflect metabolic disease. Wherever possible the altered physiology responsible for the abnormalities provides the background for the discussion.

NORMAL MORPHOLOGY AND PHYSIOLOGY OF TONGUE AND MOUTH

Under normal conditions the ventral surface of the tongue is covered by smooth, pink, mucous membrane and lymphoid follicles. On its dorsal surface the filiform, fungiform and circumvallate papillae, containing the end organs of taste, produce a rough grayish-red appearance. The twelve large mushroomlike circumvallate papillae are arranged in an inverted V-shape at the base of the tongue. The hairlike filiform papillae, the most numerous type present, are fine projections of mucous membrane capped by tufts of squamous epithelial cells and usually are arranged in rows parallel to the row of circumvallate papillae. These inverted V-shaped rows gradually merge into parallel straight lines on the anterior surface of the tongue, and finally at the tip this regular arrangement is lost. The fungiform papillae are conical or mushroom-shaped and are covered by smooth, thin epithelium. They are larger than the filiform papillae among which they are scattered and usually occur in greatest abundance at the tip and the sides of the tongue. The thick epithelial tufts of the filiform papillae give the tongue its characteristic gray-white coating, while the globular, pale-red fungiform papillae give the tongue a speckled-pink appearance.

The tongue is usually not furrowed except for a mid-line groove. A common variant is the scrotal tongue, which appears more bulky than usual and many irregularly placed grooves and furrows transect it. However, the general arrangement and the appearance of the papillae are unaffected.

In health the buccal mucous membrane has an even grayish-red color and may be crossed by fine grayish ridges where it settles between the rows of teeth when the mouth is closed. By close inspection, particularly if a small magnifying glass is used, one can distinguish a meshwork of tiny blood vessels just under the epithelium from which this color is derived. The mucous membrane covering the gums has a somewhat lighter red color. The gingival margins and the interdental papillae (the projections of gum between the teeth) have the same appearance as the rest of the gum.

The exposed portions of the lips are dry, vermilion in color, and usually are marked by slight superficial vertical wrinkling. Inside "the line of closure" the lips are moist and of the same even grayish-red color as the rest of the oral mucous membrane. The hard palate is usually a pale pink and shades gradually into the deeper pink and red color of the soft palate and the uvula.

This highly vascularized mucous membrane, like the skin, is constantly shedding its outermost layers. Metabolic changes, particularly those affecting capillaries and the formation of new cells, may easily alter this process and thereby alter its appearance. Like the skin, the mucous membrane has many highly differentiated appendages (papillae of the tongue, interdental papillae and teeth) which react in predictable fashions under abnormal conditions. The oral cavity is dark, moistened by saliva and traumatized by the acts of chewing and smoking. Food which collects in crevices and is attacked by bacterial saprophytes, ferments and forms the nidus for growth of pathogenic organisms. Such points of irritation have decreased tissue resistance and are frequently the first areas visibly affected by metabolic disturbances.

MEDICAL HISTORY AND PHYSICAL EXAMINATION

The physician may be approached by his patient primarily because of sore burning tongue and mouth "as though scalded by hot coffee," or this complaint may be uncovered only after careful history-taking in a patient who has some apparently unrelated difficulty such as shortness of breath, weakness or anxiety.

A careful investigation of the complaint of sore tongue and mouth is essential if the history is to be helpful. Such investigation should be directed toward establishing the onset, the duration and the relationship of the sore tongue to seasons of the year, to types, quantity and quality of food, to smoking, alcohol ingestion, therapy with drugs, such as heavy metals, and to emotional disturbances. The relationship to other symptoms, especially those of the gastroenteric tract, is of great importance. Frequently an extremely accurate impression of the pathologic process responsible for the complaints can be gained by such a search. Even in the absence of a specific complaint referable to the oral cavity, this area deserves close scrutiny, for some patients with well-defined pathology, either have no referable complaints or are so inured to them that they are ignored. Conversely, symptoms of sore tongue and mouth may be present and clinically significant even though no gross morphologic change is visible.

In most instances a careful gross examination of the oral cavity will give the internist as much useful information as he could gain from biomicroscopic examination and the use of other technical refinements. Occasionally a small hand lens is helpful in studying detail of very early lesions.

In considering the *pathologic physiology* or *mechanisms* that may lead to *sore tongue* or *sore mouth,* a division into (1) systemic and (2) local conditions may be made. The systemic disorders include those of nutritional origin and a large and varied miscellaneous group.

SYSTEMIC DISEASES THAT MAY CAUSE SORE TONGUE AND SORE MOUTH

Nutritional Deficiency Diseases—Vitamin B Complex, Vitamin C and Related Deficiency States

Etiology. Nutritional deficiency diseases usually occur for one of the following reasons: (1) deficient intake of essential nutrients because of poverty, ignorance, anorexia, food fads or diets prescribed or self-imposed; or because alcohol or vitamin-free carbohydrate is substituted for foods rich in essential nutrients; (2) deficient absorption of essential nutrients because of gastroenteric tract diseases, such as chronic ulcerative colitis and the steatorrheas; (3) failure of utilization of essential nutrients as may happen when the liver is damaged; (4) requirements increased beyond the normal dietary intake as may occur in pregnancy, lactation, chronic febrile states and hyperthyroidism; (5) increased elimination of essential nutrients in urine, feces or vomitus as may occur in chronic diarrheal states; (6) decreased production of certain essential nutrients by colon organisms following prolonged oral administration of antibiotic drugs, especially sulfonamides; (7) blockade of chemical reactions by which essential nutrients are converted into biologically active compounds, competition of metabolically inactive analogues with their biologically active relatives for a locus on a protein apoenzyme, or destruction of the completed coenzyme. An example of blockade is the inhibiting effect of aminopterin (4 amino pteroylglutamic acid) on folic acid reductase, preventing the conversion of folic acid to its active form, tetrahydrofolic acid. An example of competition can be found in the inhibitory effect that 4 desoxypyridoxine (a vitamin B_6 antagonist) has on enzymatic reactions, such as transamination, in which pyridoxal phosphate serves as a prosthetic group. Finally irradiation may destroy coenzymes or apoenzyme—coenzyme complexes, or drugs like isonicotinic acid hydrazide may conjugate with pyridoxal to form an inactive isonicotinic acid hydrazone. Should the history indicate that one of these situations may pertain, a close search should be made for symptoms and signs of nutritional deficiency disease.

Incidence of Nutritional Deficiency Diseases. Nutritional deficiency diseases tend to occur in the spring and to a lesser degree in the autumn. This seasonal variation holds true whether the deficiency is due to inadequate diet or is secondary to one of the other etiologic factors listed above.[12] These diseases are most common in women during the childbearing period, in children during the period of rapid growth and development, and in men after their most productive years have passed. Bachelors and widowers who cook for themselves or eat in restaurants are prone to develop these diseases. Since wheat flour enriched with niacin, thiamin, riboflavin and iron has been generally available throughout the United States of America, and with the improvement of the general standard of living of most American families, the incidence of full-blown nutritional deficiency disease has been reduced nearly to zero.

The diet may still be inadequate in very low income families, food faddists, chronic alcoholic addicts, or persons under the stresses of adolescence, pregnancy, lactation, chronic infections, hypermetabolic diseases, malabsorption and old age. Less than 5 per cent of the robust people in the United States eat diets that are marginal in essential nutrients. Enough food is available so that no one need eat a deficient diet.[13] Only through continued elevation in the standard of living and repeated efforts at nutritional education for all the people will nutritional deficiency diseases be eliminated. Until this millenium is reached, the physician must be on the alert constantly for the symptoms and signs suggestive of the disordered metabolism resulting from insufficient essential nutrients.

Pathologic Physiology and Chemistry. A patient's sore tongue and mouth may be the only grossly visible sign that he has nutritional deficiency disease. Yet he is sick in every cell of his body and, indeed, has been biochemically sick for a variable period of time (the prodromal period of the deficiency state) prior to the appearance of the first gross or microscopic lesion. The vascularity, constant moisture, bacterial flora, foci of infection and recurring slight traumatization which are characteristics of the oral cavity account for the frequency with which the earliest morphologic changes occur here. The deficiency diseases do not induce changes in resting tissues as quickly as in tissues undergoing constant regeneration and repair.

The abnormalities that occur in the mouth and tongue as a result of two different deficiency states may be identical. Conditions unrelated to deficiency disease may also produce the same changes in these organs. Although these observations have always puzzled students of nutrition, it is probable that the explanation lies in the rather restricted spectrum of changes possible in the tongue and mouth. One possible change is vasodilation causing hyperemia and redness. Atrophy or hypertrophy of the epithelium, capillary rupture with submucous hemorrhage and infarction, ulceration and necrosis are still others. When one considers these limits on the possibilities of reaction and the close chemical relationships of the nutritional deficiency diseases, it is not surprising that they frequently cause very similar changes in the tongue and the mouth. These oral lesions are the readily visible manifestations of gross or microscopic cellular damage, tissue inflammation and hyperemia occurring in the esophagus, the stomach and the intestine,[14] of lesions of the skin which may at this time be visible only under the microscope,[15] and of chemical changes in muscle, liver and other viscera[16] which may be detected with the aid of highly specialized biochemical and bacteriologic technics.[17,18]

These chemical abnormalities of which we have some slight knowledge are the primary causes for the visible structural changes. Information gained from investigations in the respiration of yeast cells, bacteria and various animal tissues indicate that many of the vitamins, particularly the vitamins of the B complex and probably vitamin C, are integral parts of complex respiratory enzymes or catalysts.[19-22] These vitamins, after undergoing certain changes in the body, enter into and implement oxidation-reduction reactions which allow the cell to breathe, perform work and liberate energy. In the process, the catalyst is inactivated and then is regenerated although the body is constantly incurring some loss of the catalyst or its progenitors through excretion. When these substances are absent, the cells lose their ability to utilize oxygen and die. When there is a deficiency of these substances, the body utilizes whatever stores of these essential substances may be available for such emergencies. Alternate and possibly less efficient reactions that do not require the deficient substance may also be called into play. Only after these protective mechanisms break down does the essential respiration of the cell suffer and illness occur. Thus the process of depletion is usually a long one, and all possible homeostatic mechanisms are utilized to protect vital cell functions.

Many of the B-complex vitamins are essential for certain biochemical chain reactions, each vitamin being responsible for the normal completion of one or more stages. The vitamins influence these processes after being chemically incorporated into coenzymes.

These coenzymes are organic compounds which, in the presence of specific protein enzymes, catalyze oxidation, reduction, transamination, decarboxylation, phosphorylation and many other critical cellular reactions. Without either the coenzyme or the protein apoenzyme, the reaction stops. For instance, niacin, thiamin, riboflavin and adenylic acid are essential for normal carbohydrate metabolism of yeast cells and probably of animal tissues also.

Figure 41 represents a simplification of the many reactions that may be involved in carbohydrate metabolism. It is included in this schematic form to facilitate visualization of the interrelated functions of many of the B-complex vitamins.

Niacin is an essential part of diphosphopyridine nucleotide (DPN), triphosphopyridine nucleotide (TPN), and a third coenzyme, pyridine ribose phosphate.

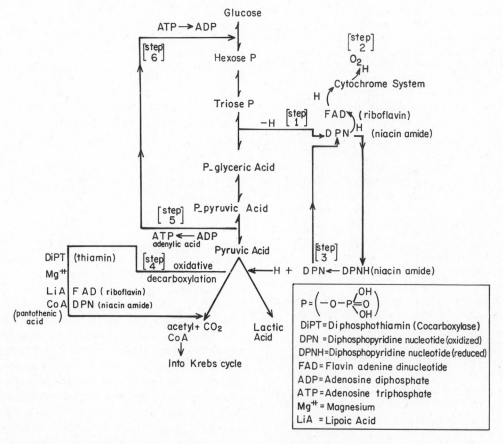

Fig. 41. A schematic representation of the Emden-Myerhof Pathway of carbohydrate oxidation illustrating the probable mechanism through which B-complex vitamins control and implement these reactions and the chemical interrelationships of these vitamins.

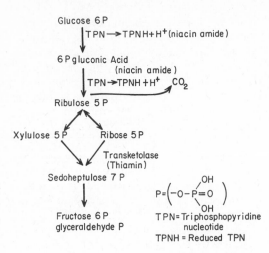

Glucose 6 P

6 P gluconic Acid
(niacin amide)

Ribulose 5 P

Xylulose 5 P   Ribose 5 P

Transketolase
(Thiamin)

Sedoheptulose 7 P

Fructose 6 P
glyceraldehyde P

$P = \left(-O - P = O \right)$ with OH, OH

TPN = Triphosphopyridine
nucleotide
TPNH = Reduced TPN

Fig. 42. Direct oxidative pathway for glucose or the hexose monophosphate shunt. The roles played by niacin and thiamin are indicated in this diagram.

Thiamin is a component of cocarboxylase (diphospho thiamin) and transketolase. Riboflavin, also a precursor of several coenzymes, combines tightly with specific protein enzymes to form flavoproteins. It can fulfill its coenzyme role only when it is phosphorylated (riboflavin 5-phosphate) or when it is in the form of a nucleotide (flavin adeninedinucleotide). Adenylic acid may act as a means for carrying phosphate through reversible phosphorylation to adenosine diphosphate and adenosine triphosphate.

Diphosphopyridine nucleotide (DPN), in conjunction with its specific protein enzyme, catalyzes the conversion of a "triose phosphate" to phosphoglyceric acid (Fig. 41, Step 1). In this oxidation reaction, it accepts a hydrogen ion (it acts as a dehydrogenase), and temporarily is reduced (to DPNH) having oxidized the substrate, "triose phosphate." However, it may be regenerated by donating its excess hydrogen ion to flavin adenine dinucleotide, and in this manner it regains its original oxidized form (DPN). The flavin adenine dinucleotide is reduced when it receives this hydrogen ion, but is reoxidized when it transfers the hydrogen ion through the cytochrome system to oxygen (Step 2). On the other hand, DPNH may donate its hydrogen ion to pyruvic acid, thus implementing the reduction of pyruvic acid to lactic acid (Step 3). In either case, DPN is made available again for the primary dehydrogenating reaction. Energy released in this DPN ⇆ DPNH reaction is utilized for the phosphorylation of adenosine diphosphate to form the triphosphate (ATP).

Cocarboxylase, in conjunction with its specific protein enzyme, catalyzes the decarboxylation and oxidation of pyruvic acid through intermediate metabolites to carbon dioxide and water. It is regenerated when lipoic acid accepts the carbon remnant of pyruvic acid (acetate) from it. The acetate finally is shifted to coenzyme A and thence into the Krebs tricarboxylic acid cycle, while lipoic acid is regenerated through the action of diphosphopyridine nucelotide and flavin adenine dinucleotide (Step 4). Adenylic acid after having been converted into adenosine diphosphate acts as a phosphate carrier by accepting phosphate ion from phosphopyruvic acid. It becomes adenosine triphosphate (ATP), and in turn transfers its energy-rich phosphate to hexose (Step 6). Through this reaction hexose phosphate and adenosine diphosphate are formed.

The B-complex vitamins are involved also in the direct oxidative pathway, which is frequently called the hexose monophosphate shunt (see Fig. 42). Glucose-6-phosphate is oxidized to 6-phosphogluconic acid by the enzyme glucose-6-phosphate dehydrogenase, for which TPN (triphosphopyridine nucleotide) is the coenzyme. Further TPN-dependent oxidation occurs when phosphogluconic acid is converted to 3-keto gluconic acid 6-phosphate. Carbon dioxide is lost from the first position and ribulose-5-phosphate is formed. After some internal rearrangements, a 2-carbon ketone from xylulose-5-phosphate is transferred to ribose-5-phosphate to form sedoheptulose-7-phosphate. This transketolase reaction is catalyzed by thiamin diphosphate. Further rearrangements occur, leaving ultimately glyceraldehyde phosphate and fructose-6-phosphate.

It is probable that these and other vitamins of the B complex are essential for similar reactions in protein, fat, steroid and nucleic acid metabolism. Pyridoxal phosphate, the coenzyme form of vitamin B_6, acts as a decarboxylase,[20] transaminase,[21] desulfurase,[22] and racemase[22] for certain amino acids. It is also essential for the conversion of tryptophane to nicotinamide derivatives (DPN),[23] and for the interconversion of the essential fatty acids,[24] linoleic, and arachidonic acids. Pantothenic acid takes part in an enzyme system concerned with acetylation,[25] and folic acid and vitamin B_{12} are intimately connected with the formation of nucleotides and nucleic acid.[26,27]

A strong reducing agent, vitamin C, is probably essential to many oxidation-reduction systems and phosphatase activity, though its exact chemical function has not yet been defined. It is essential to the normal metabolism of tyrosine and phenylalanine.[28] When vitamin C is deficient in animals, premature infants, or adult humans, intermediate phenolic products of the metabolism of these two amino acids appear in the urine in large amounts. A similar abnormality occurs when there is insufficient folic acid,[29] and it seems likely that a close biochemical relationship exists between ascorbic acid and folic acid. Ascorbic acid or other reducing agents are essential for the protection of the folic acid coenzymes (tetrahydrofolic acid and related compounds) from oxidative influences. This is another example of vitamin interdependency.

The biochemical abnormalities attendant upon vitamin C depletion probably lead to the basic pathologic changes of the scorbutic state, the failure of normal formation of collagen and intercellular cement substance. These fundamental abnormalities result in increased fragility of capillaries and decreased strength of fibrous tissue and other tissues of mesenchymal origin—the basic abnormalities of clinical scurvy.[30]

A discussion of all the possible chemical aspects of nutrition and nutritional deficiency diseases is beyond the scope of this chapter. Actually, biochemists have only scratched the surface of this very important subject. The chemical reactions cited, though they be incomplete and possibly may be inaccurate in the light of future developments, illustrate most clearly the chemical relationships of the vitamins and in turn of the vitamin-deficiency diseases. These reactions show why nutrition must be adequate in all essential nutrients before health can be optimum.

Multiple Deficiency States. Deficiency diseases seldom occur as single clinical entities, although for didactic clarity they will be described as though they did. Under natural circumstances they almost always occur as multiple deficiency states. Deficient diets seldom if ever are lacking in only one essential nutrient. For instance, food deficient in one of the vitamins of the B complex is apt to be deficient in all of these vitamins and probably in minerals and protein also. In addition, many of the vitamins and minerals are essential for closely related biochemical reactions in the cells (Fig. 41), for the release of energy through the Krebs Cycle and for the formation of the active coenzyme forms of other vitamins.

Niacin Deficiency (Pellagrous Stomatitis and Glossitis). As the niacin concentration in the tissues decreases, the deficient person may become aware of burning sensations in the tongue following the intake of hot or spicy foods. The continuous burning resembles the sensation commonly experienced following the ingestion of extremely hot coffee. This complaint may come and go; it is usually most intense during spring and fall seasons and is associated with mild anorexia, fatigue, nervousness, irritability, alternating periods of constipation and diarrhea and burning sensations in the epigastrium. As the deficiency becomes severe, or a complicating disease develops which increases the body requirement for niacin, the mouth and the tongue may become so sore that it is impossible for the patient to ingest or swallow anything but liquid food. Concomitantly other symptoms and signs may develop such as severe watery diarrhea, burning erythematous skin eruptions, cheilosis, angular stomatitis, seborrhea or dyssebacea in the nasolabial folds, mental confusion, delirium, and occasionally spastic paraplegia.

While the deficiency is mild, there may be no gross abnormalities visible in the tongue and the mouth even though these structures may be hyperesthetic. If the deficiency continues or increases in severity, the fungiform papillae become increasingly vascular and prominent, imparting a distinctive redness to the tip and the sides of the tongue where these papillae are most numerous. At this stage these papillae stand out as swollen red globules on a background of apparently normal filiform papillae. However, the filiform papillae may be affected later. Those at the tip and the lateral margins are affected first, and from these areas the process usually spreads backward toward the circumvallate papillae. The filiform papillae become swollen, denuded of epithelial tufts, hyperemic and fused in certain areas, giving the tongue an edematous, slick, fissured, fiery scarlet-red appearance. All coating is absent, and the teeth leave indentations along the margins of the swollen organ. Minute ulcerations may appear which enlarge and become infected with staphylococci, hemolytic streptococci, Vincent's organisms or fungi. These ulcers frequently are covered with a white or gray membrane. Occasionally only one portion of the tongue, usually an area located at the tip or the side, is involved. This involved area may move from place to place on the tongue, leaving atrophic spots behind. This type of localized painful excoriation of the tongue has been called "Moeller's Glossitis" in older literature.

The same fiery redness observed on the dorsal surface of the tongue occurs on the ventral surface and in the smooth mucous mebrane of the cheeks, the gums and the soft palate. The mucous membranes of the stomach, the rectum, the vagina and the anterior urethra are similarly affected. The nasal mucous membrane frequently remains pallid in contrast with its boggy blue-red appearance in virus diseases such as influenza. Often superficial ulcerations may occur particularly where the sharp edges of broken teeth irritate contiguous buccal mucous membrane. At this stage, the mouth and the tongue are extremely painful, and saliva may drool from the mouth and over the pillow and the bed clothes. All types of food are shunned by the patient because of the pain.

Remissions and exacerbations in this clinical picture may be anticipated even though the patient receives no crystalline vitamin or diet therapy. Morphologic changes that tend to be permanent occur as the deficiency state continues over months or years. In point of time this may be called a chronic deficiency state. The hyperemic, swollen vascular papillae, both fungiform and filiform, become flattened, atrophic, and gradually disappear, leaving a ridged or furrowed "bald" tongue. This bald tongue during periods of remission may be quite pallid, but during periods of exacerbation may again become fiery red. Frequently, even at this stage, the hyperemic rudiments of the papillae can be seen with the naked eye as small pinpoint red dots, especially along the tip and the sides of the tongue. The mucous membranes of the buccal cavity are affected by the same atrophic process, the interdental papillae of the gums recede, and secondary pyorrhea and other infections of the gums are common. Patients with chronic vitamin B complex deficiency diseases frequently lose their teeth at an early age because of these gum changes.[31]

The syndrome just described has been shown to be the result of niacin and tryptophane lack. Such a deficiency state has been induced in human beings by corn diets deficient in these substances but fortified with the other essential nutrients.[32] Glossitis occurred when the deficiency state was acute, whereas dermatitis was more likely when the deficiency state was induced more slowly. Whitish plaques and ulcerations developed under the tongue, cheilosis and angular stomatitis were observed as were diarrhea, irritability, restlessness, and weakness. This clinical picture developed when the niacin and tryptophane intakes were 4 mg. and 180 mg. respectively each day. Slightly more niacin and tryptophane provided by a "wheat diet" appeared to be protective.

With adequate therapy, acute pellagrous glossitis clears rapidly, frequently within 24 to 48 hours. In those patients with more chronic disease and glossal atrophy, regeneration of papillae may occur in time, usually after weeks of therapy. Much of the apparent regeneration observed early in the course of therapy is due to the disappearance of edema. The longer the period of deficiency, the slower and more incomplete the process of regeneration. Papillae may never regenerate on chronically scarred tongues even after the most adequate therapy.

Riboflavin Deficiency (Ariboflavinosis). Riboflavin deficiency once was the most common deficiency disease in the southern part of the United States.[33] Symptoms related to the tongue and the mouth are usually mild. It is difficult to be sure that the usual burning sensations in the tongue experienced by the patient with riboflavin deficiency are caused by a lack of riboflavin or an associated deficiency of niacin. Tenderness and soreness at the corners of the mouth and along the lips are usually caused by cracking of the surface epithelium and secondary infection. In some patients moderate or severe morphologic changes in the tongue and the mouth due to riboflavin deficiency may produce no symptoms at all. The eyes, however, may burn, itch or feel as though sand has found its way into them, and the patient usually is weak, irritable and lacking in appetite.

As a rule, the first oral lesion is a painless grayish papule.[9] This lesion occurs at one or both of the angles of the mouth. The papule enlarges and gradually breaks down, resulting in a fissure, secondary infection, ulceration, and yellowish heaped-up crusts—angular stomatitis or perlèche (to lick).[34] The lips become red and fissured (cheilosis). Remissions are common as in all deficiency diseases, but unless the diet is improved, relapse is almost certain. The process is extremely indolent, and remissions or relapses may persist for months. After several relapses the angles of the mouth may be scarred permanently.

The buccal mucosa of the cheeks is usually affected along with the angles of the mouth.[35] At first, the fine reticulated vascular pattern previously described as normal for this area is obliterated by engorgement, and the mucous membrane has a flat, dull-red color. With progression, the mucous membrane becomes edematous, grayish and pebbly. It tends to exfoliate in sheets, causing a distinctive mottled or moth-eaten appearance, some areas are gray-pink and others dull red. Because of the swelling, the occlusal line becomes prominent, and individual tooth imprints may be visible. The lips are involved in the same process. That part of the lips within the line of closure has the same pebbly, moth-eaten, dusky-red appearance as the rest of the buccal mucous membranes. The vermilion borders of the lips exfoliate, dry, fissure and crack (cheilosis). The line of closure is usually well demarcated and exhibits a striking dusky-red color. The end stage of this stomatitis is an atrophic moth-eaten mucous membrane.

The tongue is affected less frequently in riboflavin deficiency. The fungiform papillae enlarge and become hyperemic, followed by a similar process affecting the filiform papillae. However, they do not lose their shape or surface epithelium as in niacin deficiency. In contrast, the epithelium thickens and becomes edematous, which produces the rows of bulbous hyperemic papillae of the so-called "cobblestone tongue." (This term has been applied to syphilitic glossitis with leukoplakia in the older literature.) Since thickened edematous mucous membrane covers the hyperemic vascular tuft of each papilla, the tongue is a diffuse dusky red or magenta color. This magenta tongue contrasts sharply with the brilliant scarlet red tongue of niacin deficiency.[7] The magenta color of the tongue may be deepened by the sluggish circulation in the dilated vessels of the papillae, essentially stagnation cyanosis.

Concomitantly, other grossly visible tissue changes due to riboflavin deficiency may occur. Conjunctival injection and diffuse superficial keratitis[36] are common findings. Erosions similar to cheilosis may occur at the ocular canthi, in the nasolabial folds or at the mucocutaneous junction of the anus and of the vagina. Hypertrophy of the sebaceous glands over the bridge of the nose associated with plugging of the ducts of the glands may lead to a rough "shark skin" effect. This process frequently affects the skin in the nasolabial fold at well as on the nose and has been called dyssebacea. Seborrhealike dermatitis may occur in the nasolabial fold as well. Pure riboflavin deficiency induced in human beings by a diet containing 0.55 mg. of riboflavin daily caused angular stomatitis and cheilosis, and seborrhealike lesions of the scrotum and the external genitalia, but the magenta tongue, lesions of the oral mucosa, and of the eyes were not reported.[37]

After repeated episodes of acute riboflavin deficiency, scars may be found at the angles of the mouth and less commonly in the corneae. The mucous membrane of the mouth is thin and mottled. The tongue and the lips are fissured and dry. It is possible that some of the senile changes in conjunctivae, corneae, lenses and skin, such as fatty and hyaline deposits, pingueculae, arcus senilis, cataracts, atrophy of the skin, senile hyperkeratoses, etc., are in part the result of chronic riboflavin and other longstanding vitamin deficiency states.

Other B-Complex Deficiency States. No specific oral lesions in human beings can be related to a deficiency of thiamine, pantothenic acid, para-amino benzoic acid, choline, or inositol. Rosenblum and Jolliffe[38] described a lesion characterized by irregular desquamation of the mucous membranes of tongue and buccal cavity leading to small whitish patches on a dull reddish-purple background suggestive of riboflavin deficiency. The lesion, however, responded to pyridoxine after niacin and riboflavin had failed to induce healing. Smith and Martin[39] reported cheilosis typical of riboflavin deficiency which responded to pyridoxine after riboflavin had failed. Vilter and his associates[40] have described oral lesions in 50 patients with vitamin B_6 deficiency induced by desoxypyridoxine, a Vitamin B_6 antagonist.* The deficiency state could be induced most readily when the patient was on a diet poor in the vitamin B complex, but, with larger doses of the antagonist, it occurred in patients on a normal hospital diet. Erythema and

* A vitamin antagonist is usually a chemical analogue of the essential nutrient, so similar in structure that the cell cannot differentiate between the two. The antagonist, or "antimetabolite," as it is sometimes called, is biologically inactive and induces deficiency of the active metabolite by replacing the active substance in biologic reactions, bringing the reaction to an end.[41]

atrophy of the tongue occurred in 14 patients, cheilosis and angular stomatitis in 3. The oral mucosa was involved, also, in either a diffuse or spotty erythematous process. A much more common lesion was seborrheic dermatitis beginning in the nasolabial folds and spreading over the cheeks, the chin, the eyebrows, the forehead, down the neck and over the shoulders. Peripheral neuritis occurred also. Patients with this deficiency state excreted abnormally large amounts of xanthurenic acid in the urine after a test dose of tryptophane, suggesting that the conversion of tryptophane to nicotinamide coenzymes was impaired. All of these lesions failed to respond to niacin, thiamin, and riboflavin, but improved within 48 hours after the administration of any of the vitamin B_6 group (pyridoxine, pyridoxal or pyridoxamine). Patients studied by Sydenstricker, Singal and Briggs[42] developed manifestations of biotin deficiency on a diet poor in B-complex vitamins but supplemented with the available crystalline members of this group, except biotin. The absorption of biotin from the gastroenteric tract was limited sharply by including desiccated egg white, containing the protein avidin (which combines with biotin and prevents its absorption), in an amount equivalent to 30 per cent of the total calories. The changes in the tongue varied from the geographic type to general atrophy of the lingual papillae or marginal atrophy. Cure resulted in 3 to 5 days after the administration of from 150 to 300 μg. of biotin per day.

Acute folinic acid deficiency induced by aminopterin or amethopterin, antagonists of the reaction which converts folic acid to folinic acid, may cause very severe soreness and ulceration of the mouth and the tongue. These lesions usually begin as erythematous patches on the buccal mucosa or gums; the superficial epithelium sloughs and ulcers appear. These spread and may involve the entire oral cavity. Since the drugs mentioned above are used in persons with acute leukemia, the lesions frequently become purpuric, and infected with all varities of organisms. If antibiotics and cortisone have been administered also, fungal infections are frequent. The lesion cannot be differentiated with assurance on morphologic grounds from the purpuric secondarily infected ulcerating lesions of the acute leukemic process. However, lesions due to acute leukemia come and go irrespective of the drug being administered, and improve as a clinical remission is induced, while the lesions due to aminopterin toxicity usually respond rapidly when folinic acid is given.[41]

Such observations illustrate the morphologic counterpart of the biochemical interrelationships of the B-complex vitamins which have already been stressed. The fact that deficiencies of different vitamins should induce similar morphologic changes in the tongue and mouth is not surprising when one recalls these chemical interrelationships, and the probability that the tongue and the mouth can respond in only a few ways to damage. These observations also illustrate the lack of specificity of a morphologic oral lesion for a deficiency of one member of the vitamin B complex. The lack of specificity of these lesions will be discussed in subsequent sections.

Atrophic Glossitis (Hunter's Glossitis; Beefy Tongue). As this chapter is written,

atrophic glossitis cannot be considered as a disease entity. The acute glossal lesions of many systemic diseases (including those already described) may lead to atrophy of the glossal mucous membrane if adequate treatment is not given (see Fig. 43). We can only describe the lesion, catalogue the disorders that may be responsible, and speculate on their clinical similarities and probable metabolic interrelationships.[43-49]

The following are conditions with which atrophic glossitis frequently is associated:

1. Vitamin B_{12} deficiencies

a. Addisonian pernicious anemia, due to a genetically-conditioned lack of the mucoprotein substance called "the intrinsic factor," without which physiologic amounts of vitamin B_{12} cannot be absorbed from the intestinal tract[50,51] (See Table 10.)

b. Postgastrectomy pernicious anemia, due to surgical removal of the stomach and elimination of intrinsic factor[52]

c. Fish tapeworm infestation, which interferes with the activity of the intrinsic factor[53]

d. Intestinal blind loop syndromes and other mechanical gastrointestinal ab-

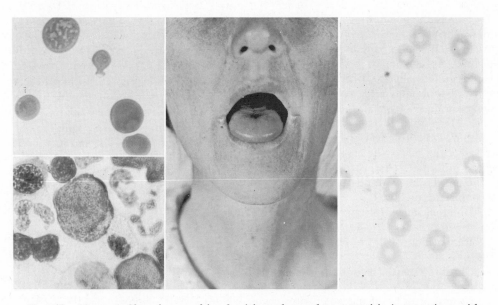

FIG. 43. *(Center)* Chronic atrophic glossitis and angular stomatitis in a patient with mixed vitamin B-complex deficiency disease. Similar lesions of tongue and mouth occur in patients with macrocytic megaloblastic anemia. *(Left, top)* Macrocytic erythrocytes. *(Left, bottom)* Bone marrow megaloblast. Patients with microcytic hypochromic anemia of chronic blood loss and iron deficiency also develop this lesion of tongue and mouth. *(Right)* Microcytic hypochromic erythrocytes.

normalities which allow proliferation of microorganisms that interfere with absorption of vitamin B_{12}[54]

e. The Vegans syndrome, or pure vegetarianism, which results in dietary deficiency of vitamin B_{12}[55]

2. Folic Acid deficiencies

a. Megaloblastic anemia of pregnancy, due to metabolic demands of the fetus for folic acid, maternal dietary inadequacy, vomiting and a theoretical metabolic abnormality which interferes with the conversion of food folic acid to the folic acid coenzymes[56]

b. Vitamin B_{12}-refractory megaloblastic anemia, due, it is thought, to failure of the metabolic processes responsible for the conversion of food folic acid to the coenzyme forms[57]

c. Megaloblastic anemia of cirrhosis, due to dietary lack of folic acid and to possible increased demands for folic acid as a result of liver failure[58]

3. Combined deficiencies of folic acid, vitamin B_{12} and ascorbic acid

a. Nutritional macrocytic anemia[47]

b. Megaloblastic anemia of malabsorption syndromes, particularly sprue,[59-61] a disease of obscure etiology, which results in deficiencies of all the hematopoietic vitamins, but especially folic acid. Diseases of the small bowel, such as idiopathic steatorrhea, regional ileitis, intestinal lipodystrophy, lymphoma and tuberculosis are other examples[62]

c. Megaloblastic anemia of infancy,[63] a combined dietary deficiency of folic acid and ascorbic acid due to an unsupplemented milk diet. (Ascorbic acid deficiency in the adult may result occasionally in megaloblastic anemia.[70])

4. Iron-deficiency (microcytic hypochromic) anemia[64]

5. Idiopathic atrophic gastritis with achlorhydria

6. Chronic vitamin-B-complex deficiency disease

7. Glossal atrophy of unknown cause.

Symptomatically, the tongue and the mouth feel dry, and there are exacerbations and remissions of burning and tingling sensations and paresthesias of taste. Atrophy is the most prominent morpho-

logic feature. In a quiescent phase the tongue is small, slick and glistening. All vestiges of papillae except the circumvallate are absent, and the mucous membrane is thin. It is usually ridged and furrowed where the atrophic process has involved muscle underlying mucous membrane. If the patient is very anemic, the color of his atrophic tongue will usually be a faint pink. If he is moderately anemic, the color will be a dull red.

With exacerbations of the pathologic process which may occur at any time before adequate therapy is administered, the mouth is extremely sore so that only liquid foods can be tolerated. Diffuse swelling may occur, and the color may become the raw, bluish-red, shiny hue of rare beefsteak. Anemia must be severe (usually red blood cell count under 1.5 million or hemoglobin under 4 gm.) before the tongue remains pallid.

If the tongue is examined closely during these periods of pathologic activity, multiple small pinpoint red dots corresponding with the hyperemic capillaries of the atrophied papillae will usually be visible. Small superficial ulcerations, erosions and hemorrhages may occur in the mucous membrane. The ulcerations may become secondarily infected with any of a number of pathogenic or saprophytic bacteria or molds. In periods of remission and exacerbation the buccal mucous membranes have essentially the same appearance as does the tongue. Erosions at the angles of the mouth similar to those seen in riboflavin deficiency occur frequently, especially in association with chronic iron deficiency.

Periods of exacerbation usually correspond with or immediately precede periods of activity in the causative disease, e.g., a relapse in the anemia of pernicious anemia, although occasionally they occur while the anemia is under control or many years before anemia or other signs of the fundamental disease appear. Acute or atrophic glossitis may also appear as a manifestation of sprue before the appearance of steatorrhea.[65]

Each of the diseases with which atrophic glossitis is associated is usually character-

PLATE 1

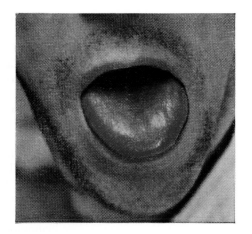 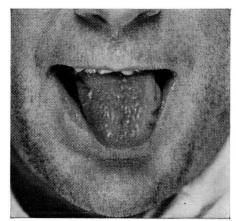

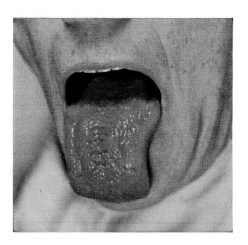 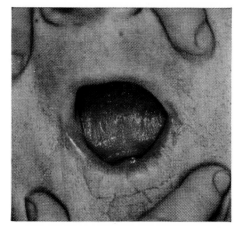

(*Upper left*) Acute pellagrous glossitis in a patient with pancreatic insufficiency and steatorrhea. The tongue is scarlet red, swollen and uncoated. Discrete hyperemic papillae are obscured by the swelling. Healing fissures are visible at the angles of the mouth. These are due to associated riboflavin deficiency.

(*Upper right*) Acute pellagrous glossitis superimposed on chronic pellagrous glossitis in a chronic alcoholic addict. The tongue is red, smooth, slick and deeply furrowed. No papillae are visible.

(*Lower left*) Magenta tongue of riboflavin deficiency in a patient with long-standing congestive heart failure and anorexia. The blue-red color is distinctive. There is moderate papillary atrophy which is probably the result of an associated chronic niacin deficiency.

(*Lower right*) Cheilosis of riboflavin deficiency in a patient with hepatic cirrhosis. These are superficial fissures and erosions at the mucocutaneous junctions of the angles of the mouth. The tongue is magenta.

PLATE 2

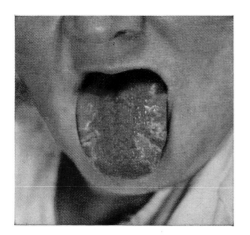 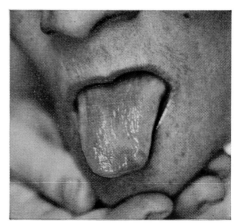

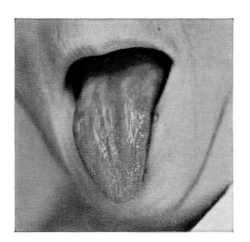 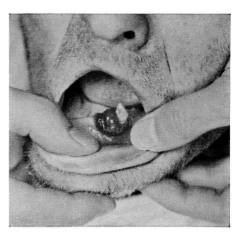

(*Upper left*) Geographiclike tongue in a patient with uncontrolled diabetes mellitus and neurotic vomiting. The bulbous papillae at the tip are of the "cobblestone" variety. This lesion cleared when diabetes mellitus was controlled and an adequate diet was supplemented with niacin and riboflavin.

(*Upper right*) Atrophic glossitis in a Negro patient with microcytic hypochromic anemia. The tongue is extremely smooth, pale and devoid of papillae.

(*Lower left*) Atrophic glossitis with leukoplakia. The posterior portion of the tongue is atrophic and streaked with thin whitish keratotic epithelium.

(*Lower right*) Acute scorbutic gingivitis. The gum surrounding the one remaining tooth snag is swollen and blue-red. The edentulous portion of the gum is normal.

TABLE 10. SYNDROMES CHARACTERIZED BY ACUTE GLOSSITIS OR GLOSSAL ATROPHY
AND MACROCYTIC ANEMIA CLASSIFIED ACCORDING TO PRESENT CONCEPTS
OF ETIOLOGY AND THERAPY

TYPE OF MACROCYTIC ANEMIA	CLINICAL CHARACTERISTICS					PROBABLE DEFICIENCY	INDICATED THERAPY
	FREE HYDRO-CHLORIC ACID	COM-BINED SYSTEM DISEASE	DIAR-RHEA	STEATOR-RHEA	RESPONSE TO PARENTERAL VITAMIN B_{12}		
Pernicious anemia	0	+	±	0	++++	Vitamin B_{12} due to intrinsic factor lack	Parenteral vitamin B_{12}
Nutritional macrocytic anemia	±	0	+	0	++++	Vitamin B_{12} and folic acid	Vitamin B_{12} Folic acid
Sprue	±	0	+	+	++	Folic acid and vitamin B_{12} due to malabsorption	Folic acid
Vitamin B_{12}-refactory megaloblastic anemia	±	0	±	0	±	Folic acid coen-zymes due to metabolic error	Folic acid
Megaloblastic anemia of pregnancy	±	0	±	0	±	Folic acid coen-zymes due to fetal demands, vomiting, dietary lack and metabolic error	Folic acid
Megaloblastic anemia of infancy	±	0	±	0	±	Folic acid, ascorbic acid due to dietary lack	Folic acid Ascorbic acid

ized also by gastrointestinal disturbances, hypochlorhydria, achylorhydria or achylia gastrica, anemia which is macrocytic and megaloblastic (except in iron deficiency states) and by multiple vitamin deficiency diseases. Among the macrocytic anemias with glossitis, separation can be made on the basis of one or more distinctive clinical or laboratory manifestations or by demonstrating that a specific therapeutic agent will induce a remission of the glossal atrophy and the anemia (Table 10).*

In addition to the data given in Table 10, iron will relieve the anemia, glossitis and cheilosis of iron deficiency; niacin and riboflavin will relieve the glossitis and cheilosis of pellagra. Idiopathic atrophic gastritis and glossitis is sometimes benefited by oral liver extract or stomach preparations, folic acid, vitamin B_{12} or parenteral liver extract, or B-complex vitamins. Only too often no effective therapeutic agent can be found.

There is no explanation that is entirely satisfactory for the morphologic similarity of the acute and the chronic glossal changes

* The use of vitamin B_{12} labeled with radioactive cobalt has improved the accuracy with which some of the conditions resulting in glossal atrophy and megaloblastic anemia can be differentiated. When vitamin B_{12} is given orally to a patient with pernicious anemia, only a minute amount is absorbed. However, when the same dose is given with intrinsic factor, vitamin B_{12} is absorbed as effectively as in normal persons. Patients with sprue absorb vitamin B_{12} poorly whether or not intrinsic factor is given. Patients with dietary deficiencies of vitamin B_{12} or folic acid absorb Vitamin B_{12} normally without added intrinsic factor. The physiologic defect of patients with intestinal lesions such as blind loops or pouches may be clarified by showing that aureomycin will frequently improve vitamin B_{12} absorption under these conditions.[86-88]

that occur in these apparently different deficiency states.

Deficiencies of the folic acid coenzymes and vitamin B_{12} interfere with the transfer of single carbon units, the former in a direct manner, the latter indirectly. Vitamin B_{12} seems to be necessary for certain reduction reactions of biological importance. Through these functions, both vitamins are involved in chemical chain reactions which culminate in the synthesis of nucleic acids. These reactions are blocked by a deficiency of either of these vitamin systems.[27] Studies of the growth requirements of certain microorganisms have suggested that the formation of thymine deoxyribotide is blocked by deficiencies of both vitamins. The formation of other purine and pyrimidine nucleotides may be blocked also but such deficiencies are not so rate-limiting as is a deficiency of the thymine derivative. Since thymine,[66] uracil[67] and orotic acid[68] (a precursor of pyrimidines) given in large doses will induce remissions in persons with pernicious anemia, it is probable that the same relationship holds in human metabolism.

The megaloblast, which is characteristic of the bone marrow cytology in persons with pernicious anemia and related macrocytic anemias, may be a primitive erythroblast with abnormal or deficient nucleoprotein.[27] Cytologic changes similar to those seen in the megaloblast have been observed in the cells of the stomach and other mucosal surfaces, indicating the widespread involvement of tissues in these deficiency states,[69] the tongue no less than other parts of the gastroenteric tract. Since ribose nucleic acid (the cytoplasmic and nucleolar type) controls the formation of protein, and deoxyribose nucleic acid (the nuclear type) governs the processes of cell division, one can readily see that fundamental aspects of cellular growth and multiplication are involved when folic acid or vitamin B_{12} are lacking.

The B-complex vitamins, niacin, riboflavin, vitamin B_6 and biotin (see preceding sections) have many different functions, most of which are concerned with the release of energy; iron is essential for the oxygen transport capacity of hemoglobin, and for the activity of the respiratory enzymes, catalase, and the cytochromes. A deficiency of any of these substances adversely affects the metabolism of all the cells of the body, but certain areas, because of local conditions and demands, show the deficiency effects most strikingly. The tongue and the mouth are such areas and react to all these deficiency states in essentially the same way—with vasodilatation, inflammation and edema, followed eventually by atrophy of the papillae and the surface mucosa. It is true that there are few other ways in which these tissues can react to injury, and this may be the real explanation for the similarity of appearance. On the other hand, all these essential nutrients are chemically dependent on each other and control fundamental reactions involved in the release of energy and the regeneration of cells. This, too, may be a common denominator.

Vitamin-C Deficiency (Scurvy). The principal complaints referable to the oral cavity in clinical scurvy are soreness, swelling and bleeding of the gums. In advanced cases the distress may be so great that the patient is unable to chew food. Lesions usually occur late in the development of the clinical disease. Pyorrhea and other diseases of the gums seem to be predisposing factors favoring earlier occurrence. Gross lesions occur seldom, if ever, in edentulous scorbutic patients.

The first oral lesions of scurvy usually occur in the interdental papillae,[11] spread to the gingival margins and finally to the alveolar mucous membrane. They do not ordinarily extend beyond the alveolar-labial junction. Capillary dilatation and congestion are the earliest visible changes. The interdental papillae and then the gum itself become a deep blue-red color as blood extravasates into these tissues. Swelling occurs and the interdental papillae and the gingival margins may become so edematous that collars of swollen blue-red friable mucous membrane surround the teeth and in advanced cases may almost cover them. Debris and microorganisms collect or are already present in pockets along the gingival margins. Infection and ulceration may spread from these areas to involve and destroy much of the gum. Infarction and gangrene of the interdental papillae may occur. Only in the most severely affected cases does one observe spontaneous oozing of blood or frank hemorrhages. Usually trauma is necessary to induce bleeding. When bleeding does occur, it is seldom excessive or exsanguinating. The breath is fetid, and salivation is increased.

As the process subsides, atrophy of the interdental papillae and retraction of the gums from about the teeth occur. With repeated exacerbations and remissions of the scorbutic process there may be extreme recession of the gums from about the teeth. The net result may be the same as that following long-standing pyorrhea. The teeth loosen, rotate, or fall out in advanced cases due to rarefaction and reabsorption of alveolar bone. The gum becomes pale and scarred. Should an acute deficiency of vitamin C supervene, the gum may again become so blue-red and swollen that the atrophic phase is completely masked.

Other characteristic lesions of scurvy are: (1) follicular hyperkeratoses and perifollicular hemorrhages, especially on the extremities; (2) larger confluent ecchymoses, especially around the joints and the poplitial spaces or at sites of slight trauma; (3) painful, tender, sometimes swollen joints (hemarthroses); and (4) in children subperiosteal hemorrhages may occur before the gum changes are visible. In adults, normocytic or moderately macrocytic anemia usually occurs only after a prolonged period of severe vitamin-C depletion.[70] The anemia responds to the administration of vitamin C and seems to be due to interference with blood formation by the vitamin-C deficiency as well as by deficiencies of other essential nutrients, especially folic acid. Infants and children who have scurvy may develop more severe anemia, sometimes quite rapidly, due to loss of blood into the extensive subperiosteal hemorrhages.

OTHER SYSTEMIC DISEASES

Many systemic diseases or local irritative processes may produce lesions which at some stage are morphologically similar to those that occur in the vitamin-deficiency states.

These various conditions must be recognized and understood in order to avoid mistakes in determining the mechanism producing the sore tongue or sore mouth.

Cirrhosis, Nutritional or Postnecrotic. Vitamin deficiency diseases are common in patients with cirrhosis, particularly in those with the nutritional (alcoholic addict) type. Anorexia or vomiting may bring about deficiency states in persons with postnecrotic cirrhosis, too. When dietary deficiency disease is responsible, dietary improvement or supplementation of the diet with B-complex vitamins will overcome the lesion. However, very frequently one finds a very red tongue, sometimes with papillary atrophy, sometimes with papillary hypertrophy, but always with dilated, engorged capillaries in the papillae or their remnants. Usually the oral mucosa is spotted with erythematous lesions also. These lesions usually do not cause pain, and they do not respond to any of the B-complex vitamins, to liver or to yeast. As the liver disease improves, these glossal and stomal lesions improve also. The reverse is true when liver failure ensues. Soreness may then appear due to superimposed moniliasis, which can be recognized by the white patches which appear on lips, tongue or soft palate.

Inability of the damaged liver to form coenzymes from the B-complex vitamins is usually considered to be the cause for this type of glossitis and stomatitis. However, this is an unproved hypothesis.

Leukemia, Hypoplastic Anemia, Idiopathic and Drug-Induced Neutropenia and Idiopathic Thrombocytopenia. Sore, swollen gums from which blood constantly oozes may be found in patients with any type of acute or subacute leukemia, severe hypoplastic anemia, malignant neutropenia or thrombocytopenia. Thrombocytopenia and capillary damage are responsible for the bleeding into the tissues, and the breakdown of the barriers against infection is responsible for the redness, ulceration, and swelling. Secondary infection and ulceration may make the mouth extremely sore and foul. Particularly in neutropenic states when no polymorphonuclear neutrophiles can be found in the blood, the mouth, the pharynx and the tonsils may be severely inflamed, swollen, ulcerated, and necrotic (agranulocytic angina). So much tissue may be destroyed by the necrotic ulcers or noma that a sinus tract may form, and the lesion may present itself externally on the cheek.

In acute monoblastic leukemia,[71] particularly, infiltration of the tissues of the gums with leukemic cells may account for some of the swelling and necrosis. Careful hematologic studies, with particular emphasis on the differential white blood cell count, platelet count and bone marrow examination will establish the diagnosis in these cases.

The Erythemas and "Collagen" Diseases. Certain diseases of obscure etiology such as erythema multiforme, disseminated lupus erythematosus and periarteritis nodosa may produce painful oral lesions.

Erythema multiforme, when severe, may affect the mouth as well as the skin, eyes, genitalia, lungs and joints (Stevens-Johnson Syndrome).[72] The lesions may be of any type. In severe cases, bullae or purpuric vesicles may form. Secondary infection usually is superimposed and the mouth, the gums and the tongue rapidly become extremely sore and foul. The oral lesions seldom occur in the absence of the skin eruption. One variant called Behçet's syndrome, is characterized by arthritis, conjunctivitis, urethritis, keratodermia blennorrhagica and erosive mucocutaneous vesicles. The oral and dermal bullae of these conditions must be differentiated from pemphigus and pemphigoid.

Disseminated lupus erythematosus may produce areas of purpura on the buccal mucosa which progress to infarction, secondary infection and necrotic sloughs and shaggy, grayish ulcers.[73] The diagnosis will depend on finding one or more of the other protean manifestations of the disease: (1) disseminated erythematous skin lesions, (2) serous pleural, pericardial and peritoneal effusions, (3) arthralgia and arthritis, (4) nephritis, (5) myocardosis, (6) leukopenia and (7) the lupus cell phenomenon.

A diffuse orange-red discoloration of the tongue associated with burning sensations in the organ has been noted in persons with fulminating periarteritis nodosa. None of the vitamins of the B-complex or liver extract improve this glossitis. The etiology of the glossitis is as obscure as the primary disease.

Lichen Planus. This dermatologic condition is associated frequently with oral lesions, plaques scattered irregularly over the tongue of a whitish cast, and pearly lacelike or spider-weblike threads on the oral mucous membrane. Occasionally, these occur without typical skin lesions. The etiology is unknown, but one usually finds strong psychogenic factors in affected patients.

Systemic Infections, Scarlet Fever, Syphilis. In the early stages of scarlet fever the tongue is coated and dry. After 2 or 3 days, however, epithelial exfoliation begins. At first, only the swollen, red fungiform papillae can be seen which on the gray background of the coated filiform papillae give the tongue a "raspberry" appearance. The exfoliation continues until all papillae, filiform and fungiform alike appear to be swollen red knobs. This is the so-called strawberry tongue. The oral mucous membranes and the lips may partake in the same process and appear redder than normal. This enanthem is seldom painful; at least any soreness is obscured by the highly inflamed sore throat and cervical lymphadenitis so characteristic of the disease.

Secondary syphilis also produces oral lesions, the mucous patches, which are painless unless secondarily infected. These lesions may appear anywhere in the oral cavity. They are usually circumscribed, flat, superficial white or gray patches which bleed easily when scraped. If they are widespread over the tongue and if secondary infection occurs, the tongue may become fiery red, painful and flecked with white patches. Under these conditions secondary syphilitic glossitis may easily be confused with acute pellagrous glossitis. At times differentiation will depend upon a careful history and search for other signs of primary and secondary syphilis or deficiency disease.

Tertiary syphilis usually does not produce painful lesions of the mouth. Solitary or multiple gummata may destroy large areas of tongue, palate and gingiva without causing soreness or burning sensations. An obliterative endarteritis in the tongue during the secondary stage of syphilis may lead in the tertiary stage to atrophy of epithelium and muscle (glass tongue or sclerosing glossitis). This condition may be confused with atrophic glossitis, but in syphilitic glossal atrophy, the extensive replacement fibrosis can be determined by palpation. It is frequently the precursor of keratoses and leukoplakia. The rhagades or scars about the angles of the mouth and the lips in congenital syphilitics must be differentiated from scars in the same areas due to chronic riboflavin and iron deficiencies.

Exogenous Intoxications, Heavy Metals. Subacute or chronic poisoning with mercury or one of its salts may cause severe swelling, redness, erosion and ulceration of the mouth, the tongue and the gums. Mercuric sulfide formed in the mouth from mercuric salts excreted by the salivary glands acts as the tissue irritant. Salivation is excessive and the salivary glands may be tender and swollen.

Bismuth and lead poisoning usually lead to deposition of bismuth or lead sulfide in a black line along the gingival margins when teeth are present—the bismuth or lead line. The pigment may be deposited in any part of the mouth, the pharynx or the gastroenteric tract where infection or putrefaction of food and debris liberate hydrogen sulfide. Stomatitis of varying degrees of severity may occur in either case but more commonly with bismuth poisoning, since bismuth sulfide is a more potent tissue irritant than is lead sulfide.

Dilantin Gingivitis. An occasional patient who is taking Dilantin (diphenylhydantoin) for the control of epilepsy may develop hypertrophy of the gums, particularly when his oral hygiene is poor. The gums become sore, swollen and bleed easily. As the condition progresses, the swollen gums may almost cover the teeth. Drug hypersensitivity is generally believed to be the cause.

Endogenous Intoxication, Uremia. Ulcerated, bleeding, and necrotic lesions of the gums and oral mucous membranes may occur in the terminal stages of renal insufficiency, but are only rarely the presenting symptoms. Usually these lesions occur only when nitrogen retention is profound and when there is a high degree of metabolic acidosis. The lesion may be single and located at a point where a broken tooth has irritated the oral mucosa or the tongue, or may be diffuse and involve large areas of the mouth. When the gums are principally involved and are swollen and oozing blood, a mistaken diagnosis of scurvy may be entertained. It is probable that these lesions are similar to the mucosal erosions that may occur throughout the gastroenteric tract in uremia, principally in the stomach, the duodenum and the colon. The exact pathogenesis is unknown, but is probably related to capillary damage and tissue infarction.

Allergy. Local contact, inhalation or ingestion of various allergens may cause localized or diffuse erythema, swelling and ulceration of the buccal mucosa, the gums and the tongue with sensations of itching and burning.[74] It is reported that allergy to amalgam tooth fillings or minute galvanic currents induced between several types of metal fillings in the moist oral cavity may produce localized areas of irritation, erythema and burning sensations. Local contact testing with the suspected allergen or the therapeutic test of elimination of the suspected allergen will aid in differential diagnosis.

Antibiotics. Penicillin hypersensitivity has been implicated as a cause of the burning sensations of the tongue and the mouth which occur in many patients given this drug, particularly in the form of lozenges or troches.[75] More commonly, however, a different mechanism is responsible. Suppression of the normal bacterial flora of the oral cavity by the antibiotic allows uninhibited growth of other organisms, particularly fungi.[76,77] Moniliasis of the tongue, the mouth, the esophagus and in fact, any part of the gastroenteric, the tracheobronchial or the genitourinary tracts has been found, particularly in debilitated patients given penicillin for long periods. The tongue and the mouth may become sore and inflamed, ulcers may form, and usually the physician will see small white patches on the mucous membrane from which monilia can be obtained in smear or culture. Similar lesions occur in patients receiving Aureomycin, Terramycin, tetracycline, and chloramphenicol.[76] Usually in these cases the tongue is swollen, the papillae edematous, and in some areas fused, producing a cobblestone, fissured appearance. The color most frequently is orange-red, but occasionally the scarlet red of niacin deficiency or the magenta color of riboflavin deficiency is so closely mimicked that it is impossible to differentiate the lesions by appearance alone. Diarrhea, itching and burning about the anus and the vagina, flatulence, and intestinal discomfort occur even more commonly that the oral symptoms and have the same cause.[76] There is no evidence that any of these lesions are due to interference by the antibiotics in the metabolism of any of the vitamins, though this suggestion has been made.

Persons taking penicillin, particularly by the oral route, have occasionally developed a painless, black hairy tongue.[77] The papillary tufts are much elongated, thickened and fused, and pigment deposited on these unsloughed papillae gives the tongue a yellowish-brown or black appearance. This type of tongue lesion may occur and remit spontaneously in persons who have not had contact with antibiotics. In either case, the cause is usually overgrowth with a fungus such as *Aspergillus niger*.

These lesions do not respond to any of the vitamins, but disappear within a few days or several weeks after the antibiotic is discontinued.

The Menopause. Burning sensations in the tongue and mild glossal atrophy may occur as manifestations of decreased production of estrogens after the menopause. These changes are probably similar to those which occur in the vagina—senile vaginitis. Improvement is prompt when estrogens are administered.

Neurologic Lesions. Hypoglossal nuclear lesions occurring in amyotrophic lateral sclerosis, syringomyelia and related conditions may lead to glossal atrophy. The atrophy of the muscle is much more striking than the atrophy of mucous membrane. The tongue is smooth, deeply furrowed and

paretic. Fibrillary twitchings may be present, and inadvertent trauma from the teeth may lead to soreness and pain. Supranuclear lesions involving sensory and motor tracts may lead to contralateral parasthesias, numbness and tingling sensations, as well as slight paresis. Such lesions are seldom, if ever, the only cause for the patient's visit to the physician. Associated neurologic abnormalities will suggest the correct diagnosis and interpretations.

Psychoneuroses. Sensations of burning, dryness, stinging, itching, soreness or taste disturbance (metallic) in the tongue and the mouth without any related objective evidence of inflammation or lack of salivation may occur as a manifestation of anxiety neurosis which is said to be related to lack of sexual gratification and similar frustrations. Women in the postmenopausal period are affected most commonly. Men have this symptom only occasionally. Cancerophobia seems to be a commonly associated factor also.[78] Usually patients with neurotic glossodynia have had their symptoms for long periods of time with exacerbations and remissions related to emotional upsets rather than to seasons of the year, periods of dietary insufficiency, anemia, or local irritative factors. Frequently such patients date the onset of the symptom to the administration of an antibiotic. Occasionally tooth imprints may appear on the tongue of tense, anxious persons who speak very infrequently and who press the tongue forward against the teeth. This may occur in the absence of true glossal swelling. The underlying emotional factors must be clear before such a diagnosis is made. It must be remembered that in the prodromal period of niacin deficiency burning of the tongue is common without change in gross morphology. During this prodromal period the patient is usually emotionally unstable, irritable and anxious. In the absence of a history suggestive of a psychoneurosis, a therapeutic test with niacin may be necessary. The physician also must be aware that a patient with a psychoneurosis manifesting itself by faulty function of the gastroenteric tract may not eat an adequate diet and therefore may develop niacin deficiency as a secondary disorder. Only through careful interpretation of all available historical data can the physician hope to understand the true sequence of events.

LOCAL ORAL LESIONS

The following types of local lesions of the oral cavity must be considered in differential diagnosis: acute and chronic oral sepsis, pyorrhea, granulomas, lesions due to local trauma and irritation, certain conditions thought to be developmental abnormalities and lesions of unknown etiology.[79-82]

Vincent's Stomatitis. Of the acute infections, Vincent's stomatitis (trench mouth) is probably most common. This disease caused by Vincent's spirochetes and fusiform bacilli is highly contagious and may reach epidemic proportions. The acute inflammation may involve any or all structures of the oral cavity and the throat. Painful ulcers form on the gingiva, the buccal mucosa or the tongue. They are deep and may destroy considerable tissue. Fever and leukocytosis are common. There is considerable evidence that this disease usually attacks previously devitalized oral mucous membranes. The organisms are common secondary invaders of pellagrous lesions. Though the infection may be acquired by persons with no aparrent underlying disease, the careful physician will always search for evidence of nutritional deficiency or other devitalizing processes when he is confronted by a patient with Vincent's stomatitis.

Herpetic Gingivostomatitis and Aphthous Stomatitis. Herpes zoster and herpes simplex may attack the tongue and the mouth and lead to very painful vesicular eruptions. Herpetic gingivostomatitis due to the herpes simplex virus (the common cold sore) tends to remain localized on the lips and around the nose in adults unless they are severely debilitated. Rather commonly in children and rarely in adults, these painful vesicles, which rapidly form shallow whitish ulcers with a red areola, involve the entire oral cavity and tongue. There may be fever and lymphadenopathy associated with this infection, and occasionally the virus attacks the skin over parts or all of the body. Children may have

several attacks of this very painful disabling condition.

When similar ulcers occur singly or in groups of two or three, within the mouth, at the base of the tongue or on the lips, the condition is usually called aphthous stomatitis or canker sores. They, too, are suspected of being due to viral infection. Frequently they may become secondarily infected with staphylococci and streptococci. They may last for a few days or a few weeks and are prone to recur. When they heal, they leave no scar due to the very superficial epithelial involvement. These ulcers occur commonly in adolescent youths, and in malnourished adults. They tend to occur also in persons with poor oral hygiene. No clear-cut etiology for the recurrence of these lesions has been discovered. Deficiency disease, allergy, local trauma and psychoneurotic mechanisms have been suspected. Since etiologic mechanisms are unknown, a multiplicity of therapeutic agents has been recommended, none of which is of proven value. Improvement in oral hygiene and diet, elimination of such habits as thumb-sucking, repeated vaccination with vaccinia virus, hyposensitization to bacterial invaders and psychotherapy are only a few of the therapeutic methods which have been proposed.[83]

Isolated simple papillitis of the tongue is extremely common—the single swollen exquisitely tender papilla on the tip or the sides of the tongue which appears suddenly, lasts a day or so, then disappears, leaving the tongue apparently normal. Occasionally under magnification, such an involved papilla appears as though it has burst and extruded a yellowish content. The cause of this phenomenon is unknown.

Enteritis. A virus type of enteritis in infants described by Dodd and Buddingh may cause painful vesicles on the tongue and in the mouth.[84] Infections with yeasts and molds, such as thrush, do not ordinarily cause pain.

Chronic Granulomas. Of the chronic granulomas, tuberculosis, actinomycosis and blastomycosis may produce painful inflamed ulcerations of the tongue, the lips and the mouth. Primary syphilitic chancre is usually nonpainful. Secondary syphilitic lesions, tertiary gummata and sclerosing glossitis have already been described.

Hyperplasia of the deep epithelial layers of the mouth and tongue may frequently follow long-standing metabolic, infectious or irritative glossitis. When such hyperplasia results in hyperkeratosis of the surface epithelium and the formation of white translucent plaques, we call the lesions *leukoplakia*.

Leukoplakia is usually asymptomatic. It frequently appears on a background of syphilitic or metabolic atrophic glossitis and commonly occurs in those who use tobacco excessively. Its chief importance lies in the fact that it is a precarcinomatous lesion.

Tumors. Benign and malignant tumors of the tongue and oral mucosa are rare. They are usually nonpainful unless secondarily infected.

Local trauma caused by poorly fitted dentures, sharp broken teeth, excessively hot coffee, or caustic and irritative medications may produce inflammatory changes and burning sensations lasting several days or as long as the trauma persists. Pipe smokers are acquainted with burning sensations in the tongue after excessive smoking.

An interesting lesion morphologically similar to the angular stomatitis of B-complex deficiency diseases may occur in edentulous patients or those whose dentures no longer are satisfactory because of shrinking of the alveolar ridge.[85] Due to malocclusion, the closed mouths of such patients often have deep crevices at the angles. Saliva and debris collect in these crevices, irritate and erode skin and the mucous membranes and eventually cause deep, secondarily infected fissures. These perlèchelike lesions do not respond to vitamins of the B complex alone, but heal when the creases are eliminated by adequate dentures. It is probable that dietary deficiency in the beginning is often a contributory factor, but B-complex vitamins will not induce healing until the local traumatic factors of stagnant saliva and secondary infection are removed by mechanically opening the "bite."

Pain or burning sensations in the tongue and the mouth may occur in trifacial neuralgia, xerostomia (particularly in mouth breathers) and has been described in Costen's syndrome (auriculotemporal nerve disturbance due to temporomandibular joint displacement). The appearance of the mucous membranes is not altered in these conditions.

Certain other conditions of the tongue of developmental or unknown etiology must also be considered in differential diagnosis. Median rhomboid glossitis, a congenital anomaly possibly arising from remnants of the tuberculum impar, appears as a plaque on the dorsum of the tongue just anterior to the circumvallate papillae. The surface is smooth and glistening and covered with stratified squamous epithelium. It is painless and harmless.

Geographic tongue (glossitis areata exfoliativa—wandering rash of the tongue) usually appears at an early age. The surface of the tongue is divided into irregular zones by zigzag white lines which are formed from thickened hypertrophic filiform papillae. Within these lines the filiform papillae have atrophied, and isolated fungiform papillae appear larger and redder than normal. These "hills and valleys" give the tongue the appearance of a relief map—the geographic tongue. These areas of atrophy and hypertrophy may migrate or remain stationary. Usually the condition is painless, although at times the patient may experience sensations of burning. The etiology is not established. In some cases it may be a manifestation of vitamin B-complex deficiency disease. In others it seems to be related to neurogenic disturbances; in still others it seems to be congenital.

SUMMARY

A burning sensation or soreness in the tongue and the mouth may be more commonly a manifestation of systemic disease than of local pathology. This chapter attempts to correlate these symptoms and the hyperemic, swollen or atrophied mucous membrane of vitamin B-complex deficiency diseases, scurvy, pernicious anemia and related erythrocyte maturation factor deficiency states, iron-deficiency anemia, achlorhydria and atrophic gastritis and to explain these changes in the light of deranged cellular biochemistry. Other systemic and local diseases are considered which may produce the same general complaints. A burning tongue and mouth evaluated by careful history and physical examination, frequently provide the key leading to the solution of an otherwise obscure diagnostic problem.

REFERENCES

1. Adams, F.: The Genuine Works of Hippocrates, New York, William Wood & Co., 1886. 2 vol.

2. Hunter, W.: Further observations on pernicious anemia (seven cases): A chronic infective disease, Lancet 1:221-224, 296-299, 371-377, 1900.

3. Minot, G. R., and Murphy, W. P.: A diet rich in liver in the treatment of pernicious anemia; study of 105 cases, J.A.M.A. 89:759, 1927.

4. Spies, T. D., and Cooper, C.: The diagnosis of pellagra, Internat. Clin. 4:1, 1937.

5. Spies, T. D., Vilter, R. W., and Ashe, W. F.: Pellagra, beriberi and riboflavin deficiency in human beings, diagnosis and treatment, J.A.M.A. 113:931, 1939.

6. Joliffe, Norman, Fein, H. D., and Rosenblum, L. A.: Riboflavin deficiency in man, New England J. Med. 221:921, 1939.

7. Sydenstricker, V. P.: The clinical manifestations of nicotinic acid and riboflavin deficiency (pellagra), Ann. Int. Med. 14:1499, 1941.

8. ———: Clinical manifestations of ariboflavinosis, Am. J. Pub. Health 31:344, 1941.

9. Sebrell, W. H., and Butler, R. E.: Riboflavin deficiency in man, preliminary note, Public Health Reports 60:2282, 1938; 64:2121, 1939.

10. Kruse, H. D.: The lingual manifestations of aniacinosis with especial consideration of the detection of early changes by biomicroscopy, The Milbank Memorial Fund Quart. 20:262, 1942.

11. ———: The gingival manifestations of avitaminosis C, with especial consideration of the detection of early changes by biomicroscopy, The Milbank Memorial Fund Quart. 20:290, 1942.

12. Bean, W. B., Spies, T. D., and Blankenhorn, M. A.: Secondary pellagra, Medicine 23:1, 1944.

13. Wells, O. V.: Current food trends, Nutr. Rev. 17:161, 1959.

14. Spies, T. D., Bean, W. B., and Ashe, W. F.: Recent advances in the treatment of pellagra and associated deficiencies, Ann. Int. Med. 12:1830, 1939.

15. Moore, R. A., Spies, T. D., and Cooper, Z. K.: Histopathology of the skin in pellagra, Arch. Derm. Syph. 46:100, 1942.

16. Axelrod, A. E., Spies, T. D., and Elvehjem, C. A.: Effect of nicotinic acid deficiency upon coenzyme I content of human erythrocyte and muscle, J. Biol. Chem. 138:667, 1941.

17. Evans, E. A., Jr., ed.: The Biological Action of the Vitamins, A Symposium, Chicago, Univ. Chicago Press, 1942.

18. Baumann, C. A., and Stare, F. J.: Coenzymes, Physiol. Rev. 19:353, 1939.

19. Devlin, T. M.: The relation of diet to oxidative enzymes, in Wohl, M. G., and Goodhart, R. S., eds.: Modern Nutrition in Health and Disease, ed. 2, p. 446, Philadelphia, Lea & Febiger, 1960.

20. Bellamy, W. D., Umbreit, W. W., and Gunselus, I. C.: Function of pyridoxine; conversion of members of vitamin B_6 group into codecarboxylase, J. Biol. Chem. 160:461, 1945.

21. Schlenk, F., and Snell, E. E.: Vitamin B_6 and transamination, J. Biol. Chem. 157:425, 1945.

22. Snell, E. E.: Summary of known metabolic functions of nicotinic acid, riboflavin and vitamin B_6, Physiol. Rev. 33:509, 1953.

23. Chiun-Tong Ling, Hegsted, D. Mark, and Stare, F. J.: The effect of pyridoxine deficiency on the tryptophane-niacin transformation in rats, J. Biol. Chem. 174:803, 1948.

24. Witten, W., and Holman, R. T.: Polyethenoid fatty acid metabolism. VI. Effect of pyridoxine on essential fatty acid conversion, Arch. Biochem. 41:266, 1952.

25. Lipman, F., Kaplan, N. O., Novelli, G. D., Tuttle, L. C., and Guirard, B. M.: Coenzyme for acetylation, a pantothenic acid derivative, J. Biol. Chem. 167:869, 1947.

26. Stokes, J. L.: Substitution of thymine for "folic acid" in the nutrition of the lactic acid bacteria, J. Bact. 48:201, 1944.

27. Vilter, R. W., Will J. J., Wright, T., and Rullman, D.: Interrelationships of vitamin B_{12}, folic acid, and ascorbic acid in the megaloblastic anemias, Am. J. Clin. Nutr. 12:130, 1963.

28. Woodruff, C. W., Cherrington, M. E., Stockell, A. K., and Darby, W. J.: The effect of pteroylglutamic acid and related compounds on tyrosine metabolism in the scorbutic guinea pig, J. Biol. Chem. 178:861, 1949.

29. Govan, C. D., and Gordon, H. H.: The effect of pteroylglutamic acid on the aro-

matic amino acid metabolism of premature infants, Science 109:332, 1949.

30. Wolbach, S. B., and Bessey, O. A.: Tissue changes in vitamin deficiencies, Physiol. Rev. 22:233, 1942.

31. Mann, A. W.: Nutrition as it affects the teeth. Med. Clin. N. Amer. 27:545, 1943.

32. Goldsmith, G. A., Sarett, H. P., Register, V. D., and Gibbens, J.: Studies of niacin requirements in man. I. Experimental pellagra in subjects on corn diets low in niacin and tryptophane, J. Clin. Invest. 31:533, 1952.

33. Spies, T. D., Bean, W. B., Vilter, R. W., and Huff, N. E.: Endemic riboflavin deficiency in infants and children, Amer. J. Med. Sci. 200:697-701, 1940.

34. Stannus, H. S.: Problems in riboflavin and allied deficiencies, Brit. M. J. 2:103-105, 140-144, 1944.

35. Sandstead, H. R.: Deficiency stomatitis, Supplement No. 169 to U. S. Public Health Reports, 1943.

36. Cleckley, H. M., and Kruse, H. D.: The ocular manifestations of ariboflavinosis; progress note, J.A.M.A. 114:2437, 1940.

37. Horwitt, M. K., Hills, O. W., Harvey, C. C., Liebert, E., and Steinberg, D. L.: Effects of dietary depletion of riboflavin, J. Nutr. 39:357, 1949.

38. Rosenblum, L. A., and Jolliffe, N.: The oral manifestations of vitamin deficiencies, J.A.M.A. 117:2245, 1941.

39. Smith, S. G., and Martin, D. W.: Cheilosis successfully treated with synthetic vitamin B_6, Proc. Soc. Exper., Biol. Med. 43:660, 1940.

40. Vilter, R. W., Mueller, J. F., Glazer, H. S., Jarrold, T., Abraham, J., Thompson, C., and Hawkins, V. R.: The effect of vitamin B_6 deficiency induced by desoxypyridoxine in human beings, J. Lab. Clin. Med. 42:335, 1953.

41. Schoenbach, E. B., Greenspan, E. M., and Colsky, J.: Reversal of aminopterin and amethopterin toxicity by citrovorum factor, J.A.M.A. 144:1558, 1950.

42. Sydenstricker, V. P., Singal, S. A., Briggs, A. P., DeVaughan, N. M., and Isbell, H.: Observations on "egg white injury" in man, J.A.M.A. 118:1199, 1942.

43. Oatway, W. H., Jr., and Middleton, W. S.: Correlation of lingual changes with other clinical data, A.M.A. Arch. Int. Med. 49:860, 1932.

44. Manson-Bahr, P.: Glossitis and vitamin B_2 complex in pellagra, sprue and allied states, Lancet 2:317, 356, 1940.

45. Abels, J. C., Rekers, P. E., Martin, H. E., and Rhoads, C. P.: Relationship between dietary deficiency and occurrence of papillary atrophy of tongue and oral leukoplakia, Cancer Res. 2:381, 1942.

46. Harris, S., and Harris, S., Jr.: Pellagra, pernicious anemia and sprue; allied nutritional diseases, South. M. J. 36:739, 1943.

47. Moore, Carl V., Vilter, R. W., Minnich, V. M., and Spies, T. D.: Nutritional macrocytic anemia in patients with pellagra or deficiency of the vitamin B complex, J. Lab. Clin. Med. 29:1226, 1944.

48. Castle, W. B., and Townsend, W. C.: Observations on etiological relationship of achylia gastrica to pernicious anemia: the effect of the administration to patients with pernicious anemia of beef muscle after incubation with normal human gastric juice, Amer. J. Med. Sci. 178:764-777, 1929.

49. Schieve, J. F., and Rundles, R. W.: Response of lingual manifestations of pernicious anemia to pteroylglutamic acid and vitamin B_{12}, J. Lab. Clin. Med. 34:439, 1949.

50. West, R., and Reisner, E. H.: Treatment of pernicious anemia with crystalline vitamin B_{12}, Am. J. Med. 6:643, 1949.

51. Herbert, V., Castro, Z., and Wasserman, L. R.: Stoichiometric relation between liver-receptor, intrinsic factor and vitamin B_{12}, Proc. Soc. Exp. Biol. Med. 104:160, 1960.

52. MacLean, L. D., and Sundberg, R. D.: Incidence of megaloblastic anemia after total gastrectomy, New England J. Med. 254:885, 1956.

53. Nyberg, W.: The influence of *Diphyllobothrium latum* on the vitamin B_{12}-intrinsic factor complex. I. In vivo studies with Schilling test technique. Acta. Med. Scand. 167:185, 1960.

54. Doscherholmen, A., and Hagen, P. S.: Absorption of CO^{60} labeled vitamin B_{12} in intestinal blind loop megaloblastic anemia, J. Lab. Clin. Med., 44:790, 1954.

55. Wokes, F., Badenock, J., and Sinclair, H. M.: Human dietary deficiency of vitamin B_{12}, Amer. J. Clin. Nutr. 3:375, 1955.

56. Gatenby, P. B., and Lillie, E. W.: Clinical analysis of 100 cases of severe megaloblastic anemia of pregnancy. Brit. M. J. 2:1111, 1960.

57. Mueller, J. F., Hawkins, V. R., and Vilter, R. W., Liver extract-refractory megaloblastic anemia, Blood 4:1117, 1949.

58. Jandl, J., and Lear, A. A.: The metabolism of folic acid in cirrhosis, Ann. Int. Med. 45:1027, 1956.

59. Darby, W. J., and Jones, E.: Treatment of sprue with synthetic *L. casei* factor (folic

acid, vitamin M), Proc. Soc. Exp. Biol. Med. 60:259, 1945.

60. Butterworth, C. E., Nadel, H., Perez-Santiago, E., Santini, R., and Gardner, F. Folic acid absorption, excretion and leukocyte concentration in tropical sprue, J. Lab. Clin. Med. 50:673, 1957.

61. Althausen, T. L., DeMelendez, L. C., and Perez-Santiago, E.: Role of nutritional deficiencies in tropical sprue, Am. J. Clin. Nutr. 10:3, 1962.

62. Vilter, R. W.: Treatment of macrocytic anemias, A.M.A. Arch. Int. Med. 95:482, 1955.

63. May, C. D., Nelson, E. N., Lowe, C. V., Salmon, R. J.: Pathogenesis of megaloblastic anemia in infancy; an interrelationship between pteroylglutamic acid and ascorbic acid, Amer. J. Dis. Child. 80:191, 1950.

64. Moore, C. V.: Iron and the essential trace elements, *in* Wohl, M. G., and Goodhart, R. S., eds.: Modern Nutrition in Health and Disease, ed. 2, pp. 235-273, Philadelphia, Lea & Febiger, 1960.

65. Joliffe, N., and Fein, H. D.: Some observations on acute and chronic glossitis, Rev. Gastroenterol. 15:132, 1948.

66. Spies, T. D., Frommeyer, W. B., Jr., Vilter, C. F., and English, A.: Thymine; antianemic properties, Blood 1:185, 1946.

67. Vilter, R. W., Horrigan, D., Mueller, J. F., Jarrold, T., Vilter, C. F., Hawkins, V., and Seaman, A.: Studies on the relationships of vitamin B_{12}, folic acid, thymine, uracil and methyl-group donors in persons with pernicious anemia and related megaloblastic anemia, Blood 5:695, 1950.

68. Rundles, R. W., and Brewer, S. S., Jr.: Hematologic responses in pernicious anemia to orotic acid, Blood 13:99, 1958.

69. Klayman, M. I., and Massey, B. W.: Further observations on gastric cytology of pernicious anemia, J. Lab. Clin. Med. 44:820, 1954.

70. Vilter, R. W.: Vitamin C (ascorbic acid), *in* Wohl, M. G., and Goodhart, R. S., eds.: Modern Nutrition in Health and Disease, ed. 2, pp. 337-392, Philadelphia, Lea & Febiger, 1960.

71. Forkner, C. E.: Clinical and pathological differentiation of the acute leukemias, A.M.A. Arch. Int. Med. 53:1, 1934.

72. Soll, S. N.: Eruptive fever with involvement of the respiratory tract, conjunctivitis, stomatitis and balanitis, etc., Arch. Int. Med. 79:475, 1947.

73. Harvey, A. McG.: Systemic lupus erythematosus, *in* Cecil and Loeb: Textbook of Medicine, ed. 10, p. 641, Philadelphia, Saunders, 1959.

74. Goldman, L., and Goldman, B.: Contact testing of buccal mucous membrane for stomatitis venenata, Arch. Derm. Syph. 50:79, 1944.

75. Goldman, L., and Farrington, J.: Contact testing of the buccal mucous membrane with special reference to penicillin, Ann. Allergy 4:457, 1946.

76. Woods, J. W., Manning, I. H., Jr., and Patterson, C. N.: Monilial infections complicating the therapeutic use of antibiotics, J.A.M.A. 145:207, 1951.

77. Wolfron, S.: Black hairy tongue associated with penicillin therapy, J.A.M.A. 140:1206, 1949.

78. Karshan, Maxwell, Kutscher, A. H., Silvers, H. F., Stein, George, and Ziskin, D. E.: Studies in the etiology of idiopathic orolingual paresthesias, Amer. J. Dig. Dis. 19: 341, 1952.

79. Rogers, A. M., Coriell, L. L., Blank, H., and Scott, T. F. McN.: Acute herpetic gingivostomatitis in the adult, New England J. Med. 241:330, 1949.

80. Thoma, K. H.: Oral Pathology: A Histological, Roentgenological, and Clinical Study of the Diseases of the Teeth, Jaws, and Mouth, ed. 2, St. Louis, Mosby, 1954.

81. McCarthy, F. P.: A clinical and pathological study of oral disease based on 2,300 consecutive cases, J.A.M.A. 116:16, 1941.

82. Jeghers, H.: Medical progress; nutrition; the appearance of the tongue as an index of nutritional deficiency, New England J. Med. 227:221, 1942.

83. Ship, I. I., Merritt, A. D., and Stanley, H. R.: Recurrent aphthous ulcers, Amer. J. Med. 32:32, 1962.

84. Buddingh, C. J., and Dodd, K.: Stomatitis and diarrhea of infants caused by a hitherto unrecognized virus, J. Pediat. 25:105, 1944.

85. Ellenberg, M., and Pollack, H.: Pseudo-ariboflavinosis, J.A.M.A. 119:790, 1942.

86. Schilling, R. F.: Intrinsic factor studies. II. The effect of gastric juice on the urinary excretion of radioactivity after the oral administration of radioactive vitamin B_{12}, J. Lab. Clin. Med. 42:860, 1953.

87. Halstead, J. A., Swendseid, M. E., Lewis, P. M., and Gasster, M.: Mechanisms involved in the development of vitamin B_{12} deficiency, Gastroenterology 30:21, 1956.

88. Jerzy-Glass, G. B.: Intestinal absorption and hepatic uptake of vitamin B_{12} in diseases of the gastrointestinal tract, Gastroenterology 30:37, 1956.

6

Thoracic Pain

JOHN R. SMITH AND ROBERT PAINE

Pain arising in the chest, in common with pain originating elswhere, may occur in the presence of local lesions of no seriousness, or may indicate important somatic or visceral disease. Thoracic pain may be difficult to evaluate, particularly when it is of visceral type. Chest pain may be the only presenting indication of disease.

Information regarding many types and mechanisms of thoracic pain is fragmentary. Other forms of chest pain, such as that from the heart and the pleura, have been more extensively investigated. In the short space of this chapter it will not be possible to include detailed descriptions of all the types of thoracic pain. The mechanisms of the common and important forms will be presented briefly.

ORIGIN OF PAINFUL STIMULI

There is now convincing evidence that there are nerve fibers specifically concerned with the transmission of pain impulses.[1,2] Further evidence indicates that tissue damage from trauma, bacterial invasion or other disease stimulates pain nerve endings by tissue tension or by chemical factors present in the injured tissue, or by both these factors together.[1] It is clear that a wide variety of pathologic changes may lead to tension or chemical irritation to provoke pain; on the other hand, extensive tissue damage may be incurred, without pain, if these factors are absent.

Tissue Tension. That tissue tension will provoke pain is seen readily when a single hair is plucked. The pain is undoubtedly produced by direct tension exerted on the nerve endings.[3] Tension, applied to a wide area of normal skin, must be considerable before pain occurs; but tension (and chemical factors) in inflamed skin may produce exquisite pain. Inflammatory reactions are intensely painful when associated with much exudation ("as in the painful boil before pus issues from it")[3] or with edema. Throbbing pain occurs with the rise of tension from each pulse wave into inflamed areas. Distention of the adventitia of blood vessels is said to be painful,[62,89] perhaps reaching a peak of severity in dissecting aneurysm of the aorta. Some workers have considered the pain of angina pectoris and myocardial infarction to arise from tension on the sheaths of the coronary arteries, although this explanation is now not widely accepted. Abnormal dilatation of hollow viscera has been shown to be painful.[5] The role of tissue tension in pain stimulation is therefore important. The above examples are only a few.

Chemical Factors. The nature of the chemical excitants of pain in tissue injury is not known with certainty. It has been suggested that the liberation of potassium ions stimulates pain endings.[3] Moore *et al.*[4] demonstrated that pain nerve endings are sensitive to potassium ions in certain concentrations. Acid changes in certain tissue (i.e., ischemic muscle) may be adequate to produce pain.[4] Lewis[3] speaks of a "pain-producing substance" present in normal tissue, which is liberated when injury to the tissue is sustained. It is well known that the contraction of muscle when the blood supply is impaired (ischemia) may give rise to intolerable discomfort. Such a condition may occur, for instance, following an arterial embolus where a limb may become ischemic. It is seen to a lesser extent in the course of Raynaud's disease. Lewis and his co-workers[63] and others[64] suggested that the pain of muscle ischemia results from the accumulation of "metabolites" in the tissue with widespread irritation of pain nerve endings (cf. Cardiac Pain). It is further possible that such metabolites may accumulate in tissue in infections or other diseases in sufficient concentration to provoke pain.

Whatever such chemical factors may be, they operate, often together with tension within the tissue, to cause discomfort.

With these fundamental pain stimuli in mind, many painful symptoms find reasonable explanations when considered in relation to the known, or to the suspected pathology in a given clinical problem.

Pathways of Pain. The impulses of all painful sensations below the level of the cranial nerves enter the spinal cord by fibers traversing the posterior ganglia and the dorsal roots and are transmitted to neurones in the posterior horns. The somatic and the visceral pain fibers share these pathways. Therefore, impulses from visceral nerve endings arrive at the same re-

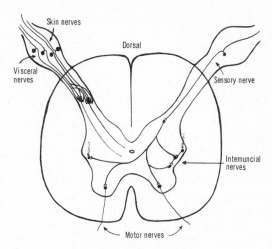

FIG. 44. Diagrammatic sketch of a cross section of the spinal cord illustrating certain nervous connections to explain the reference of pain. It is generally believed that visceral pain fibers may synapse in the spinal cord with certain neurones transmitting pain sensation from the skin. When these visceral pain fibers come under intense stimulation, the stimuli may affect the cutaneous neurones because of the crossed synapses, so that a sensation of cutaneous pain is simultaneously experienced. Referred pain may be due in part to reflex muscle spasm, also mediated through intraspinal nerve connections as shown at the right of the diagram.

ception point among the posterior horn cells as do impulses of somatic origin. An appreciation of this merger into a common path is essential to the understanding of the distributions of pain in visceral disease. *Visceral pain will be noted in that somatic area with which it shares a final common path.*

The precise localization of somatic pain differs from the wider distribution of visceral pain because, in general, visceral pain is transmitted to several segmental levels while somatic pain is transmitted to a single level. However, it is important to realize that the intensity and the duration of painful stimuli also influence the extent of spread of pain to adjoining segments, whether the reception is visceral or somatic. For instance, a traumatic injury to one digit may, after a time, be followed by discomfort in the entire arm and shoulder.

Extension of pain to other levels demonstrates the existence of intermediate neurones connecting the posterior horn cells with other areas in the cord. These include the spinothalamic tract, the intermediolateral nuclei and the anterior horn cells as well as internuncial cells connecting with the higher and lower segments of the cord. Impulses transmitted to the spinothalamic tract result in thalamic and cortical action in the awareness of pain. Impulses transmitted to the intermedio-lateral (sympathetic) nuclei may call forth the sympathetic discharges responsible for causalgic states, and impulses transmitted to the motor cells of the anterior horn produce the reflex muscular spasm associated with pain.

PAIN ARISING IN THE CHEST WALL

The integument and the muscles of the chest wall are subject to essentially the same diseases as similar tissues elsewhere. The pain-sensory innervation of these tissues is conveyed to the dorsal roots through the cutaneous and the intercostal nerves. Generally, pain arising from the thoracic integument and other superficial tissues is sharply localized. Furuncles and other infections, contusions, and abrasions of varying severity may produce superficial, well-localized pain. Owing to the anatomic peculiarities of the thorax, pain of distinctive nature may arise from involvement of muscles, nerves and bone. These will be considered separately.

Intercostal Nerve Pain

Irritation of the intercostal nerves may arise from a *neuritis* of those nerves, resulting from trauma, systemic or upper respiratory infections or other toxic cause, or pressure upon the nerve.[7] The neuritis is often aggravated by exposure to cold. The onset of the pain is usually sudden. The pain is localized in the intercostal space, the patient being readily able to identify the exact site of tenderness. The nature of the pan may be stabbing, lancinating, burning, and, in severe cases, occurring in paroxysms when the patient breathes deeply, coughs, or moves suddenly. We have been interested in the frequency with which intercostal neuritis is localized about the precordium, leading the patient to believe that he has heart disease. However, in intercostal nerve irritation, localized tenderness may be found along the course of the inflamed nerve, and slight pressure elicits paroxysms of pain. Pressure points where tenderness is maximum may be located near the vertebrae, in the axillary lines, or near the parasternal lines.

Herpes zoster is a distinctive form of dorsal root irritation producing an acute inflammatory dermatosis. The disease occurs more frequently in persons who are chronically ill, or in malnourished individuals.[7] The sensory root ganglia and corresponding peripheral nerves may be involved in any region, although the process is usually restricted to a few successive roots and nerves. The formation of herpetic lesions is generally heralded by intense burning, or knifelike pain along the nerve course. When the intercostal nerves are affected, the patient may be aware of pain extending from the spine along the lateral thoracic wall to the anterior midline. The movements of the trunk and of respiration may be restricted because of the pain. The pain is continuous and is usually punctuated by paroxysms of increased severity. Frequently the pain of herpes zoster is incapacitating and continues for many weeks, even after the herpetic lesions have healed. During the disease, hypesthesia of the skin occurs; hyperesthesia is rare. The nature of herpes zoster is imperfectly understood. It appears to arise from irritation and intense hemorrhagic inflammation of the sensory root ganglia; the peripheral nerves show degeneration of fibers and occasionally evidence of active inflammation. Stern[8] has obtained a virus from the lesions which, is similar to that of varicella. Antibodies have been demonstrated in patients convalescing from herpes zoster capable of neutralizing the virus present in the lesions. Others, however, have suggested[9] that while there is a specific viral etiologic agent in herpes zoster[100,101] the lesions may be precipitated by bacteria, by neoplasms, by chemical agents and by other noninfectious, irritating agents.

Holmes[10] has called attention to *slipping rib cartilages* as important causes of chest pain. He notes that the costal cartilages of the 8th, the 9th or the 10th ribs, on either side, may loosen from their fibrous attachments; this is followed by deformity—a curling upward of the end of the cartilage on the inner aspect of the rib, in close relation to the intercostal nerve. The condition is of traumatic origin. The manifestations of pain are varied. Usually the pain is a dull ache, often tolerated for years. Occasionally the pain is acute, stabbing, paroxysmal in type, incapacitating in severity. Localized tenderness to pressure over the lesion is present. The usual chronicity of the disease, together with location of the pain and the tenderness, ordinarily makes the diagnosis clear.

MYALGIA

Irritation of muscles is a frequent cause of somatic pain. Apparently muscle is a tissue from which only one sort of pain is produced; the discomfort is aching in nature.[6] The intense aching pain occurring during exercise of ischemic muscle is well known.[63] Muscle pain of the same nature was noted by Lewis[6] when isotonic acids or hypertonic solutions were injected directly into the tissue. Firm squeezing of a muscle will likewise produce the pain. Muscle pain, if sufficiently intense, may be referred to other dermatomes common to the muscle itself, though often the pain is well localized at the site of muscle injury.

Inflammation of muscles and pain may occur in a great variety of pathologic processes.[12,13] These processes may be local (e.g., trauma, hematomas) or diffuse (e.g., systemic infections, trichinosis, myositis ossificans, etc.). Perhaps the commonest conditions provoking muscular pain about the chest result from exercise of "untrained" muscles of the shoulder girdle. Incessant or paroxysmal severe cough may render the intercostal muscles painful. Fibromyositis involving the shoulder muscles may occur; it presents no particular problem of identification, for the shoulder and the arms may be tender on motion, and the muscles are readily palpated for tenderness. Myositis involving the intercostal muscles may give rise to marked discomfort, and nodules and induration in the muscles[12] may be present. Another form of myalgia has been emphasized by Mendlowitz.[14] He noted in a large group of soldiers that strain of the pectoralis minor muscle may cause marked discomfort in the anterior chest wall. The pain was aching in character and was confined, in general, to the area of the muscle, including the corresponding shoulder. The pain did not radiate to the arms. Involvement of the left pectoralis minor muscle produced symptoms superficially resembling cardiac pain. Curiously enough, Dixon[12] found that pain of muscular origin may be partially relieved by the use of nitrites. This fact should be borne in mind lest the condition be confused with smooth-muscle pain.

OSTALGIA

The source of pain from bone is the numerous sensory nerve endings in the periosteum and, to a lesser extent, in the endosteum. Therefore, bone disease may be present without pain until these structures are involved. Affections of the periosteum give rise to intense pain, usually well localized, whereas chronic disease, often affecting the bone marrow and endosteum, may result in poorly localized pain of varying severity. Reference of the pain to corresponding body segments may occur by the mechanism already described. Trauma (with or without fracture) resulting in periostitis and acute osteomyelitis may affect the bony thorax or the spine. Exquisite tenderness occurs over the affected point.[7] The pain is sharp and severe. In osteomyelitis the pain may be continuous for many hours.

Bone pain in syphilitic aortitis may be continuous and so severe as to be incapacitating. We have recently observed a number of cases of aortitis and aneurysm with gradual erosion of the sternum and contiguous costal cartilage. In these cases there was unremitting, well-localized pain, boring or burning in type. The usual analgesics provided little or no relief.

Intense, aching, boring back pain may occur in malignant metastases to the thoracic vertebrae[15] as from carcinoma of the prostate or hypernephroma; often it is referred to the corresponding dermatomes. The pain is constant and usually requires continuous narcotization. Frequently, in our experience, the metastatic vertebral lesions cannot be seen roentgenographically, but their presence may be suspected from the intense symptoms and the finding of carcinoma elsewhere. Mediastinal tumors, other than aortitis, may provoke chronic aching or dull chest pain (often substernal) by pressure against the spine or the ribs. Hodgkin's disease and lymphosarcoma are common examples. Leukemia has long been known to produce costal pain in its advanced stages, particularly producing areas of point tenderness in the sternum.[16] Multiple myeloma, osteitis deformans and sarcoma, involving the ribs or the thoracic spine, may likewise cause ostalgia.

POSTERIOR ROOT PAIN

The clinical and the pathologic features of dorsal root pain and its differentiation from underlying visceral pain have been repeatedly emphasized.[102] Dorsal root pain

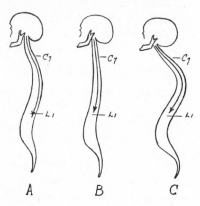

Fig. 45. Diagram showing position of the spinal cord with respect to abnormal degrees of vertebral flexion and extension. A illustrates normal spinal curvature. The end of the cord lies at the level of L-1 or L-2, indicated by arrow point. B and C show abnormal dorsal straightening and kyphosis occurring in spinal osteoarthritis. In both instances the neural canal is lengthened and the cord is relatively displaced cephalad. Tension is exerted on the spinal nerves.

refers to irritation, mechanical or otherwise, of the dorsal radicles in the proximity of the spinal cord. As with the other forms of somatic pain described before, root pain may be felt at the point of irritation, but is frequently referred to points along the peripheral course of a nerve. Root irritation of the thoracic spinal segments is often referred to the lateral and anterior chest wall.[17]

The lesions producing dorsal root pain may be toxic or infectious (*radiculitis*), but the pain is more frequently the result of mechanical irritation of the root due to *spinal disease* or *deformity*. Bony spurs about the intervertebral foramina in hypertrophic osteoarthritis may irritate the nerves on motion of the spine.[19] Narrowing of the intervertebral spaces by compression of the intervertebral disks may bring pressure on the nerve trunks. Cervical ribs and apposition of the anterior scalene muscle to the brachial plexus have been noted to produce root pain referred to the chest wall.[19]

Smith and Kountz[17] observed that dorsal root pain may be caused by *thoracic deformity* alone. They reasoned that in early osteoarthritis, swelling and thickening of the intervertebral disks straightens and lengthens the spine so that the spinal cord is drawn cephalad. This exerts tension on the spinal nerves in their exit through the intervertebral foramina, and they are irritated upon motion. As the spinal arthritis progresses, the vertebral bodies are thinned anteriorly with final anterior collapse to produce kyphosis (the characteristic hump). In this way, the spinal canal is even more lengthened, the spinal nerves are constantly taut, and irritation of nerves occurs on motion of the column.

The pain of dorsal root irritation is often stabbing, or there may be twinges of sharp aching pain localized in the spinal region. The pain is accentuated on motion, such as bending, use of the arms, or torsion of the trunk. Patients with spinal osteoarthritis commonly awaken at night in pain, presumably because relaxation in sleep allows the spine greater flexion and irritation of nerves by osteophytes or tension. Reference of the pain to the lateral and anterior chest wall is common: it may be sharp, but is often dull and aching in nature. Occasionally the discomfort is projected to one or both arms through branches of the brachial plexus. Referred pain occuring about the sternum and the shoulders, often paroxysmal, may closely resemble angina pectoris and sometimes is confused with it.[17,18] The confusion may be heightened by the partial relief obtained by the use of nitroglycerin.[18] Careful study of these patients will reveal a history of back pain; the pain is more superficial than heart pain (cf. Cardiac Pain), is only indifferently relieved by nitrites and is usually associated with exertion involving the upper part of the body.

Upper anterior and posterior chest pain can result not only from dorsal root irritation but also from cervical disorders, because the distribution of nerves originating as high as C_3 and C_4 may extend as far caudally as the nipple line. The pectoral, the suprascapular, the dorsal scapular and the long thoracic nerves originating in the lower cervical level can, upon irritation, cause pain in the chest, the midscapular and the postscapular areas.

While the anterior or ventral roots are motor in type, they can be productive of a dull deep boring type of discomfort when stimulated and can, therefore, produce a form of discomfort different from that attributed to posterior root disturbance. The anterior roots also play a role in the production of somatic echoes of visceral pain.

BREAST PAIN

With the accumulation of extensive data concerning disease of the mammary tissue, particularly carcinoma, increasing importance has been attached to the prompt investigation of the symptoms or signs of breast disease.

The sensory nerves of the breast are gathered into the 2nd, 3rd, 4th, 5th and 6th intercostal nerves through the terminal brachial and medial antebrachial cutaneous twigs of the lower four of these nerves.[20] In addition, pain fibers in the second intercostal nerves have a common connection with the intercostobrachial nerve of the brachial plexus. A few pain fibers may

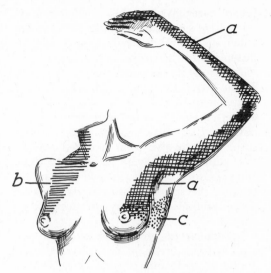

FIG. 46. Diagram illustrating diffusion of pain arising from the breasts. Crosshatching (*a*) shows reference of mammary pain into axilla and along medial aspect of the arm. Pain (*b*) may be projected to supraclavicular level and into the neck. Breast pain may diffuse around the thorax (*c*) through the intercostal nerves (see text). Pain may be referred to the back and to the posterior aspects of the shoulder girdle (not shown).

ascend in the 2nd and 3rd cervical nerves from the region of the clavicles. Furthermore, sensory impulses from the medial brachial and medial antebrachial cutaneous nerves, as well as from the ulnar, may enter the spinal cord in the same segments as sensory impulses from the breast tissue innervated by the upper intercostal nerves. Diffusion of pain from the breasts passes around the chest and into the back, along the medial aspects of the arms and occasionally over the neck.[21]

The integument of the breasts, including the nipples and areolae, shows accurate localization of painful superficial stimuli in common with integumentary structures elsewhere. Pain from cutaneous incisions, furuncles, contusions of the surface, and similar lesions is superficial and is generally readily identified by the patient. Fissuring of the nipples and inflammation in the papillary ducts and areolae will often produce intense, well-localized pain. The breast parenchyma seems to be peculiarly insensitive to painful stimuli[20] except when the stimulus occurs as the result of distention of the stroma. Such stromal distention may be confined to a small segment of the parenchyma (e.g., in some cases of carcinoma), or may involve large portions of the glandular tissue. Furthermore, it is possible that invading, malignant tumor tissue may involve pain nerve endings so that pain may be severe and even constant. Inflammatory lesions, in addition to distending the stromal tissue, irritate sensory nerve endings and may produce severe pain.[22]

Inflammatory breast disease is a common cause of breast pain. The citation of a case of acute puerperal mastitis will exemplify certain types of mammary pain. We observed a young woman with bilaterally fissured nipples, two weeks postpartum. Localized pain in the nipples was so intense that nursing became almost impossible. There was intense pain to palpation of all of the breast tissue, which was engorged and grossly nodular. The pain, sharp, cutting and aching, was referred to the axillae and along the medial aspects of the arms to the little and the ring fingers. There was a fever of 104° F. With infections of lesser severity, the symptoms may be misleading. Veil[23] studied a case of cellulitis of the breast displaying intermittent precordial pain and radiation of the discomfort to the left arm. Angina pectoris was considered to be present; however, with clearing of the cellulitis all symptoms disappeared.

Benign and malignant tumors of the breasts are common causes of painful symptoms. It seems possible that a tumor which is situated so as to produce distention of the mammary parenchyma, or involves pain nerve endings, may account for the pain.[20] However, large tumors may be present without necessarily provoking the symptom. The position and the nature of the neoplastic tissue would therefore appear to be primarily concerned in determining the presence of pain.

Mastodynia is one of the commonest conditions producing mammary pain. The onset of pain is gradual, during months or years; frequently it is intensified in the premenstruum. The discomfort is present particularly in the upper outer quadrant of the breast, which is firm, thick and tender to palpation. The pain, at first, may be intermittent, occurring only at the premenstrual period, but later may be persistent. Jarring or movement of the breasts may accentuate the pain. It may radiate to the inner aspects of the arms as a dull (or intense) ache and is aggravated by motion of the arms. These breasts show imperfect lobular development with increased periductal stroma, epithelial proliferation and changes tending toward cyst formation and adenosis.[21]

Other tumors and chronic inflammatory disease cause mammary pain which resembles mastodynia. Or there may be an aching within the breast, a prickling sensation, or lancinating pain projected along the side of the breast and into the axillae and the arms.[22,24] Cheatle and Cutler[25] state that the pain of carcinoma may be lancinating or stabbing, radiating to the characteristic places. The breast may ache incessantly, and the patient attempts to support it to prevent jarring. Cheatle and Cutler[25] further state that localized nodularity, tumor and stabbing pain (if present) occurring in the same place in the breast calls for immediate investigation as to the presence of carcinoma. Pain in neoplastic breast disease is not uniformly present.

PAIN ARISING FROM THE TRACHEA, THE PLEURA AND THE DIAPHRAGM

TRACHEOBRONCHIAL PAIN

The symptom of substernal pain from acute tracheitis is familiar to most persons. The discomfort is usually felt under the upper portion of the sternum and it is frequently described as a burning sensation. Coughing accentuates the discomfort. This pain is often accompanied by similar pain lateral to the sternum at points corresponding to the positions of the major bronchi. Sharp foreign bodies, such as fishbones, in the wall of the upper trachea may cause continuous pain in the anterior aspect of the neck.[26] Some patients with irritating foreign material, carcinoma,[28] or inflammatory lesions in the major bronchi will localize pain with accuracy in the right or left anterior chest, corresponding to the particular bronchus involved. Because of this, it is generally assumed that tracheo-bronchial pain is referred to sites in the neck or anterior chest at the same levels as the points of irritation in the air passages.

Although lower respiratory tract pain is common, the symptom has received scant attention. Investigation[27] indicates that stimuli applied directly to the tracheal or bronchial mucosa, in patients *under bronchoscopy,* are construed as painful sensations in the anterior cervical or anterior thoracic area. In addition, the pain is on the homolateral side of the neck or chest to the point of stimulation. The sites of pain are consistent and symmetrical. Morton *et al.*[27] further showed that section of the vagus nerves (below the recurrent laryngeal branches but superior to the pulmonary plexus) abolished the pain on the side of the vagus section. The cough reflex was also abolished. In a few instances, pain of tracheobronchial origin was referred to the contralateral side following vagotomy. These observations reaffirm the older suggestions that the pain-sensory innervation of the trachea and large bronchi is carried entirely in the vagus trunks. On the other hand, the finer bronchi and the lung parenchyma appear to be free of pain inner-

vation.[26] Graham[26] has frequently cauterized the mucosa of small open bronchi through openings in the chest wall, the patient being unaware of the procedure except for cough from the smoke of searing tissue. Likewise, extensive disease may occur in the periphery of the lung without the occurrence of pain until the process extends to the parietal pleura. Pleural irritation then results in pain.

PLEURAL PAIN

It seems well established that the parietal pleura is amply supplied with pain endings, and that the visceral pleura is insensitive. These facts were brought out in the interesting experiments of Capps and Coleman.[29] They introduced a large trochar and cannula into the pleural space in patients with pleural effusion, and stimulated various places on the pleural surfaces by means of a silver wire passed through the cannula. They found that the visceral pleura and the lung parenchyma were insensitive to such stimuli, but that stimulation of the parietal pleura gave rise to sharp pain. The pain could be well localized by the subject. It seemed clear, therefore, that pain arising from pleural irritation depends upon involvement of the parietal pleural

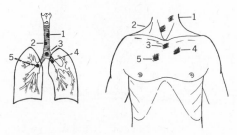

FIG. 47. When a bronchoscope is introduced into the tracheobronchial tree and when faradic stimulation is applied at points 1, 2, 3, 4 and 5, the patient may recall pain occurring at the corresponding points marked on the figure of the thorax. Note that the points of pain are homolateral to the areas of stimulation. Diagram based on the observations of Morton and his co-workers.[27]

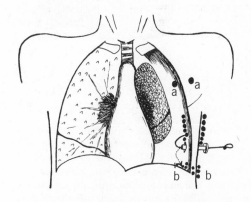

FIG. 48. Stimulation of the parietal pleural membrane by means of a silver wire produces sharp pain. Such stimuli to the parietal pleura of the anterior, lateral and posterior chest wall is referred to the superficial tissue at corresponding points in the wall (*a* and *b*) as shown in this sketch. Pain from pleural irritation is usually well localized.

membrane. Pain fibers, originating in the parietal pleura, are conveyed through the chest wall as fine twigs of the intercostal nerves. Irritation of these nerve fibers results in pain in the chest wall—usually construed as arising in the skin—which may be sharply localized, knifelike and cutting in nature and accentuated on any respiratory movement. Arising in the most inferior portions of the pleura, the pain may be referred along the costal margins or into the upper abdominal quadrants. The discomfort is often dramatically relieved by anesthetization of the skin.[30]

The mechanism by which painful stimuli are initiated in an inflamed parietal membrane has been the subject of some discussion. It has been generally held that friction between the two pleural surfaces, when the membranes are irritated and covered with fibrinous exudate, produces the sharp pain. Other theories suggest that intercostal muscle spasm due to the pleurisy, or stretching of the parietal pleura, causes the characteristic pain. The latter theory is consistent with Bray's observation[31] that during inspiration the superior excursion of the ribs widened the intercostal spaces appreciably. The widening of the spaces, he reasoned, stretches the parietal pleural membrane; when the pleura is inflamed, such stretching irritates the pain fibrils, and sharp cutting inspiratory pain results. While pleural stretching may be concerned in the production of pleural pain, other mechanisms have been suggested. There is evidence that pulling or tugging upon the membrane causes severe pain. Goldman[32] observed that patients with artificial pneumothorax often devel-

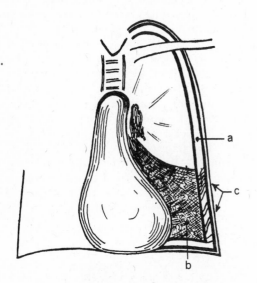

Fig. 49. Schematic diagram showing lobar consolidation and acute fibrinous pleurisy. The pleural space (a) is drawn in exaggeration, beneath which the consolidated lung lobe (b) is shown. Multiple fibrinous strands are represented by the small lines (c). Movement of the pleural surfaces in respiration will exert tension upon the fibrinous strands, pulling upon the parietal pleural membrane. Such tension upon the parietal pleura probably produces the exquisite pain which characterizes the disease, in addition to tension caused by widening of the interspaces on movement and friction of the inflamed surfaces. Actually, the fibrinous deposit is dense so that individual strands are not visible, and the pleural membranes show acute inflammation.

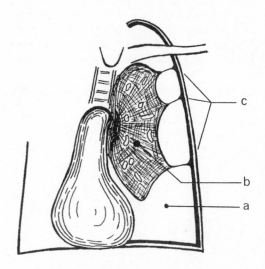

Fig. 50. Schematic diagram, showing partial collapse of the left lung by air in the pleural cavity (a) (pneumothorax). Complete collapse of the lung (b) is prevented by a number of "string" adhesions (c). It is readily understood how forcible collapse of a lung may produce tension upon the parietal pleural membrane when adhesions are present (as illustrated here); such tension explains the pain of pneumothorax when pleural adhesions are present.

oped pain when adhesions between the pleural surfaces are present. He believed that if adhesions are present when a lung is forcibly collapsed in pneumothorax therapy, traction on the parietal pleura by the adhesions results in pain. This suggestion affords an interesting explanation for the pain of acute fibrinous pleurisy. The paroxysms of pain may be due to many points of traction upon the irritated parietal pleura by countless fibrinous strands, as well as by stretching of the membrane on costal movement. It also seems probable that irritation is further augmented by simple friction (clinically manifested by a friction rub) between the roughened surfaces of the pleural membranes.

Pleural pain is frequently encountered in acute fibrinous pleurisy complicating pulmonary inflammatory disease. Pneumonic processes reaching the extreme periphery of the lung cause a visceral pleuritis which quickly involves the contiguous parietal pleura. Pulmonary infarction may give rise to pleurisy if the infarcted tissue extends to the pleural surface. Krause and Chester[33] found that pain was one of the commonest symptoms in their series of cases of pulmonary infarction. Tumor, especially bronchiogenic carcinoma[34] may be attended by severe, continuous pain when the tumor tissue, extending to the pleurae through the lung, constantly irritates the pain nerve endings in the pleura. The occurrence of spontaneous pneumothorax is often signalized by severe pain, usually in the upper and lateral thoracic wall, and is aggravated exquisitely by any movement and by the slight cough and dyspnea which accompany it.[35] It is probable that adhesions, brought under tension by rapid recession of the lung, cause such pain. Spontaneous pneumothorax may occur without pain.

As stated before, pleuritic pain is knife-like or "stabbing" in nature and its position is usually easily defined by the patient. Laughing, coughing, or even normal respiratory movement will produce paroxysms of exquisite pain. The notable exception is invasion of the parietal pleura by tumor, where pain endings are constantly irritated.

DIAPHRAGMATIC PAIN

The diaphragmatic pleura receives a dual pain innervation through the phrenic and the intercostal nerves. Capps and Coleman,[29] using the technic described before, found that stimulation of the central portion of the diaphragmatic pleura with a wire resulted in sharp pain referred to the region of the superior ridge of the trapezius muscle (the somatic segmental area innervated by nerves of common origin to the phrenic). The peripheral rim, anteriorly and laterally, and the posterior third of the diaphragmatic pleura have pain fibers reaching the 5th and the 6th intercostal nerves.[36] Stimulation of the peripheral portions of the diaphragmatic pleura results in sharp pain felt along the costal margins. The latter pain may be projected to the epigastrium, subchondral regions, or lumbar regions, by the lower thoracic somatic nerves. The peritoneal surface of the diaphragm is apparently supplied by the same pain-sensory innervation, for stimulation of the central diaphragmatic peritoneum results in pain along the upper border of the

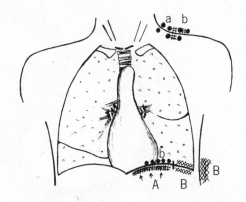

FIG. 51. Irritation of the pleura of the central area of the diaphragm (solid cirles) causes pain along the superior ridge of the trapezius muscle and supraclavicular fossa (solid circles); stimulation of the marginal diaphragmatic pleura (xx) provokes pain at corresponding points in the thoracic wall (xx). Similarly, irritation of the central diaphragmatic peritoneal surface produces pain in the shoulder and neck of the same side and stimulation of the marginal peritoneal surface results in pain referred to the abdominal wall (xx).

trapezius.[29,37] Stimulation of the periphery of the diaphragmatic peritoneum causes pain reflected along the costal margins.

It is easy to understand, therefore, how affections of the diaphragm may be clinically localized by the position of the referred pain. *Diaphragmatic pleurisy*, secondary to pneumonia or pericarditis, is common, and sharp pain along the trapezius or costal margins, accentuated on diaphragmatic motion in coughing or deep breathing, occurs. *Subphrenic abscess* may produce painful symptoms which are similar to diaphragmatic pleurisy. There may be tenderness to palpation about the costal margins with sharp pain occurring on marked excursion of the diaphragm. Irritation of the central portion of the diaphragmatic peritoneum produces sharp pain in the shoulder on the affected side.

Herniation of abdominal viscera through a diaphragmatic hiatus may give rise to lower chest or upper abdominal pain.[38] It is often difficult to decide whether the pain originates in the diaphragm or from the anatomic distortion and disturbed function of the herniated viscus. Diaphragmatic hernias may provoke mild epigastric distress or pain simulating that of peptic ulcer. Reference of discomfort to the lower sternal area may closely resemble seizures of cardiac pain.[39] The overlapping of symptoms appears to depend on pain reference mechanisms of common distribution.

An interesting type of lower chest pain, attributed to the diaphragm, is "stitch"—a sharp pain occurring about the costal margin on exertion. It was attributed by Moor[40] to interference with diaphragmatic motion. Capps[41] has recently studied the

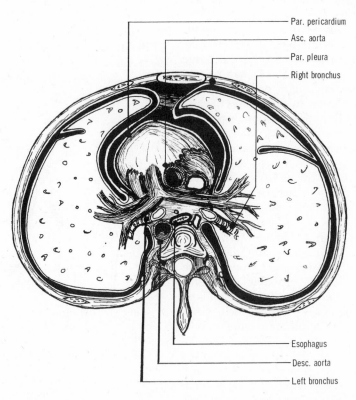

Par. pericardium
Asc. aorta
Par. pleura
Right bronchus

Esophagus
Desc. aorta
Left bronchus

Fig. 52. Diagram of a transverse section through the thorax at a level immediately superior to the heart. The mediastinum and its contents are shown, together with the pleural and pericardial membranes. The pleuropericardial space is particularly exaggerated to accentuate its relationships clearly. (Based on an illustration in Gray's Anatomy of the Human Body, ed. 22, Philadelphia, Lea & Febiger.)

sideache occurring on strenuous exertion at the right costal border in normal persons. He reasoned that diaphragmatic anoxemia might precipitate the pain. It seems reasonable that pain originating in the muscle of the diaphragm may be referred to the level of diaphragmatic attachment and the corresponding intercostal nerve.

PAIN ARISING FROM ORGANS CONTAINED IN THE MEDIASTINUM; MEDIASTINAL PAIN

Pain arising from the mediastinum or its contained organs is frequently difficult to evaluate. Regardless of its origin, pain arising from various mediastinal structures has much in common and is frequently referred to identical peripheral sites. The subject is as difficult to present as such pain may be to interpret at the bedside. As an approach, it is well to recall that the mediastinum is a *space* bounded by structures which can give rise to pain in themselves. Disease of the thoracic spine, affections of the esophagus, the pericardium, the pleurae and other structures produce pain which may be referable to the mediastinum. On the other hand, inflammatory lesions and tumors within the mediastinum may provoke pain if extensive or critically located. A few of the commoner forms of pain arising from the mediastinum and mediastinal organs will be considered briefly.

PERICARDIAL PAIN

The mechanism of pain arising in pericardial disease is puzzling. One might think of the acute pain of pericarditis as occurring from the movement of opposed, inflamed pericardial membranes, or that pain may be produced by marked distention of the sac by fluid. However, the experiments of Capps and Coleman[29] indicate that there are very few pain fibers in the pericardium. Using their cannula and silver-wire technic, they stimulated the endothelial surfaces of the pericardium in patients with pericardial effusion. No pain resulted from scratching the visceral surface. With the same stimulus no pain occurred in the parietal layer except when the *parietal membrane* was stimulated opposite the *5th and the 6th* intercostal spaces. Such stimulation resulted in sharp pain about the superior

border of the trapezius as in central diaphragmatic stimulation (see Fig. 53). From these findings it seemed probable that a few pain fibers in the lower parietal pericardium, adjacent to the diaphragm, are carried in the phrenic nerves, but that elsewhere the pericardial membranes are devoid of pain sensation.

It remains to be explained why pain, usually substernal or immediately to the left of the sternum, occurs in some cases of *acute pericarditis*. Since the pericardium is largely insensible to pain, it seems probable that irritation of contiguous structures must occur to cause the pain of pericarditis. The parietal pleura and the pericardium are in close apposition (see Fig. 52) in the mediastinal enclosure. Inflammation from an acute pericarditis might then easily spread to the neighboring pleura, producing pain,[29] or even to other mediastinal tissues. The situation of the pain (substernal or to the left of the sternum) is in keeping with the segment of pleura which may be involved. Barnes and Burchell,[42] studying pain in apparently benign pericarditis, noted that difficulty in swallowing, deep breathing, or torsion of the trunk frequently accentuated the pain, suggesting that an associated inflammation of the esophagus and other mediastinal structures was present.

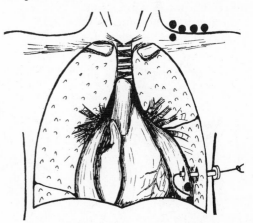

FIG 53. Diagrammatic sketch of cannula and silver wire in the pericardial sac. Most of the pericardial surface is insensitive to pain, but stimulation of the sac at the level of intercostal spaces 5 to 6 produces pain referred to the superior border of the trapezius muscle and supraclavicular fossa.

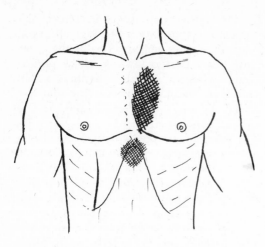

FIG. 54. Crosshatching illustrates the common sites of pain in pericardial disease. The pain may be substernal or to the left of the sternum and may be felt in the epigastrium. In some instances, pain may be more extensively referred (see text).

As noted, acute pericarditis may be accompanied by pain, which is substernal, along the left sternal border, and occasionally epigastric. The pain is often sharp, lancinating and paroxysmal; it may be continuous. The pain of pericarditis may be severe, closely resembling that of myocardial infarction[42] (cf. Cardiac Pain), although it is less agonizing and usually requires no narcosis for relief.

Pericardial effusion, often massive, is usually not accompanied by painful symp-

toms; however, in the series studied by Camp and White,[43] pain occurred not infrequently. Pericardial effusion may be manifested as a feeling of fullness within the chest, or as intermittent or continuous frank substernal pain, or ill-defined pain.[44] Distress of essentially the same nature may occur in tuberculous pericarditis.

ESOPHAGEAL PAIN

Esophageal pain, occurring as the only symptom, may be confusing because of its similarity to other visceral thoracic pain. Such pain presents itself as deep thoracic pain, or it is referred to corresponding somatic segments, conforming with visceral referred pain in general. However, other symptoms, such as progressive dysphagia, regurgitation of freshly eaten solid food, together with persistent pain or pain on swallowing, suggest esophageal disease.

The esophageal mucosa appears to be more sensitive to pain in its upper portion than in the middle and the cardiac regions. Acid, regurgitated from the stomach, produces an unpleasant burning sensation in the upper thoracic, cervical and nasopharyngeal regions, with no sensation referable to the lower esophagus.[47]

Pain arising from the muscular portion of the tube is clearly demonstrated in the experiments of Paine and Poulton.[45] They introduced tubes, to the ends of which balloons were affixed, into the esophagus. When the balloons were inflated in the

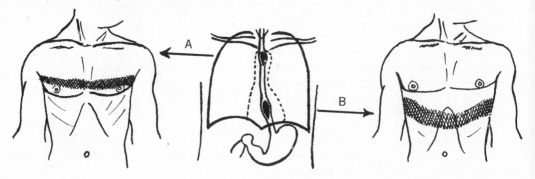

FIG. 55. Esophageal pain may be projected around the chest at the level of the spinal segment corresponding to the esophageal lesion. Schematically, pain from a lesion in the esophagus corresponding with the 4th thoracic spinal nerve (represented by arrow A in the central figure) may be referred as a band of pain about the thorax. An esophageal lesion at the level of the 7th or the 8th spinal nerves may manifest itself in pain about the chest following the course of those nerves (arrow B).

lower esophagus, a burning pain was induced, becoming "gripping" in character when the subject swallowed. Paine and Poulton reasoned that distention of the organ is painful, and that muscle contraction, attempting to overcome distention, results in paroxysmal cramping pain. These observers further noted that pain from the distended esophagus may be substernal or epigastric or may be referable to the back, but that the level of the referred pain corresponds closely to the level of the distended portion of the esophagus through successive spinal segments. Thus, the higher the pain in the esophagus, the higher the level of pain felt about the sternum and the back.

Heartburn. Probably the commonest symptom involving the esophagus is "heartburn." Heartburn is a vague term, and there is considerable difference of opinion as to the exact nature of the symptom. It may best be described as a "hot" or burning sensation occurring substernally or about the heart following a meal. It disappears within a short time. Heartburn has been attributed to regurgitation of acid gastric content into the esophagus, reversed esophageal peristalsis, or failure of the cardia to open promptly on deglutition. Alvarez is of the opinion that, whatever the cause, it may be initiated by reversed gastric peristalsis.

Acute esophagitis may be caused by the swallowing of foreign bodies, such as bones or other sharp objects, spicy foods and as a complication of acute infectious disease. The mucosa as well as the muscle may be involved. Paroxysmal pain on deglutition is one of the most constant symptoms, the pain being substernal and radiating to the back. There is often no discomfort when the esophagus is quiescent, although dull discomfort frequently persists. Chronic esophagitis, often seen in chronic alcoholics and heavy smokers, or following acute disease, may produce essentially the same symptoms. In phlegmonous esophagitis, painful symptoms are accentuated markedly,[15] accompanied by fever, chills, nausea and vomiting and great fetor of the vomitus. There may be constant substernal and back pain, so accentuated on swallowing

that taking food is nearly impossible. Carcinoma of the esophagus, in itself, provokes no pain, though pain occurs with the esophagitis which frequently complicates it.

Cardiospasm (spasticity of the cardia) may not be accompanied by distress.[46] However, pain on deglutition often occurs, which is substernal, epigastric or along the left border of the lower thoracic spine.

Esophageal pain, therefore, is referred to the sternum or back at the level of the lesion. While the type and location of pain per se may be inconclusive, the occurrence of painful dysphagia and regurgitation of undigested food material, necessitating a liquid diet, and weight loss at once suggest esophageal disease.

MEDIASTINAL PAIN

Extensive mediastinal distortion from tumors or other disease may occur without producing painful symptoms. Indeed, enormous mediastinal tumors may be present with no discomfort to the patient other than cough, dyspnea and moderate wheezing. Mediastinal lymph nodes involved by Hodgkin's disease,[53] neurofibromata or other tumors may not give rise to pain unless nervous structures are involved. In explanation of such clinical phenomena it seems possible that the mobility of the mediastinum, together with the resiliency of the tissues which bound it, may allow for considerable distortion without necessarily irritating pain-sensitive structures. However, many mediastinal tumors do provoke pain, usually in association with dyspnea and cough.[51] The pain may first be manifest by a sensation of substernal weight or "oppression" which is ill-defined. Over a period of weeks or months the pain may become severe. The discomfort usually remains substernal, but varies greatly in intensity. Involvement of the esophagus by tumor in the posterior mediastinum may produce pain on swallowing. Certain tumors, such as carcinoma of the lung apex (Pancoast),[54] may be accompanied by sharp axillary, shoulder and subscapular pain radiating along the medial aspects of the arms. Large aneurysms of the aorta may produce symptoms particularly when they exert pressure upon the chest wall, although vague discomfort appears to arise from the aneurysms themselves in some instances[55] (cf. Aortic Pain).

Spontaneous mediastinal emphysema is frequently accompanied by agonizing pain. The syndrome has been vividly described by Hamman,[50] who believes it to be more common than is generally thought. From his observations, it appears that rupture of the lung may occur through an attenuated alveolus; the air then dissects along fascial planes to the mediastinum. Pneumothorax occasionally complicates mediastinal emphysema, and it has been suggested that some cases of pneumothorax may result from unrecognized mediastinal emphysema. The condition often occurs when the individual is making no effort and is sitting or lying quietly. The accident is generally heralded by intense, agonizing substernal pain, radiating to the nape and to the shoulders. It seldom radiates to the arms. Such pain may persist for hours; indeed, a needle may have to be inserted into the mediastinum to permit the escape of air before relief is secured. In some instances the pain is milder, though it is "oppressive" and is substernal in location. Frequently a distinctive crepitus is heard synchronous with the heartbeat indicating the presence of air about the heart.

Mediastinal pain may be caused by acute inflammatory disease, or by traumatic rupture of the esophagus, or disintegration of the esophageal wall from carcinoma.[15,48] Occasionally inflammation may be caused by the passage of infection through lymphatics or by burrowing along the fascial planes of the neck.[48,49] Under such conditions the complaint of constant substernal pain is common, but the site of the pain is difficult to localize. The pain may seem to be present in the back, particularly if the vertebrae are involved, and percussion of the dorsal spine may elicit paroxysms of pain. Tenderness of the sternum has occasionally been noted. Pain may be accentuated on swallowing if the esophagus is affected by the inflammatory process. Sudden motions of the trunk may be accompanied by severe discomfort. Painful symptoms of this nature should raise the question of mediastinitis, particularly if there are indications of infection in the neck, esophageal disease, or other lesions such as retroperitoneal infection or pneumonia.

Chronic mediastinitis may arise as the result of tuberculosis, or following other chronic infections.[51] Occasionally, mediastinitis occurs for which no cause can be elicited, as described by Pick.[52] Chronic mediastinal inflammation may give rise to pain (together with dyspnea). The discomfort may be a severe, unremitting substernal oppression, or a burning and aching sensation substernally or in the precordium. Some cases may run their course with little or no pain. Frequently, striking physical signs occur which point to the underlying disease.

CARDIAC PAIN

ORIGIN OF CARDIAC PAIN

In 1768 William Heberden accurately described the symptomatology of angina pectoris.[56] As Osler aptly put it, Heberden said little about the cause of the disease and had the "good fortune to get very close to the truth in what he did say." Herrick's[57] classic description of acute coronary occlusion in 1912 gave impetus to the study of the recognition and cause of coronary insufficiency and cardiac pain. One consideration was almost immediately apparent, namely, that cardiac pain results from diminution or cessation of blood flow to the myocardium.[58,59,60] How such diminution of flow causes pain has remained a controversial question to date. Some authors have held that anoxemia of the myocardium provoked pain.[60] Others believed that important vasomotor reflexes or spasm of the vessels accounted for paroxysms of heart pain, the painful impulses arising from the vessels themselves. Others postulated that pain is provoked by distention of the walls of the coronary vessels. Wenckebach[61] suggested that sudden distention of the coronary arteries proximal to a point of occlusion or sudden distention of the aortic wall might provoke paroxysmal pain, a view which subsequently was amplified by Gorham and Martin.[62] However, these viewpoints have remained largely speculative for lack of conclusive support from animal experiments[60] and clinical observation.

At present, the conception most widely held in explanation of cardiac pain is that heart pain results from an *accumulation of metabolites* within an ischemic segment of the myocardium. The theory had its inception in the work of Lewis, Pickering and Rothschild.[63] They applied pressure to an arm by a blood-pressure cuff and noted the occurrence of intolerable pain a short time (70 seconds) after exercise of the arm was begun. Similar occlusion of the resting arm was not followed by pain despite the development of intense cyanosis. The conclusion was reached that during ischemic muscular contraction a substance is produced which causes pain, but that anoxemia alone does not produce such discomfort. Katz *et al.*[64] pursued this idea further and presented striking evidence that a substance, or substances, produced during muscular contraction, accumulates in the presence of ischemia and anoxia and provokes intolerable pain; angina pectoris and inter-

mittent claudication were thought to be due to this mechanism. Thus, it seems possible that ischemia of the myocardium, whether it be transient (causing angina pectoris) or prolonged (producing the pain of myocardial infarction), may set off pain impulses by causing rapid accumulation of metabolites within the heart muscle.

RESTRICTION OF CORONARY FLOW

From the foregoing discussion, it seems probable that the inception of cardiac pain results from *myocardial ischemia*. Furthermore, the evidence indicates that failure of myocardial nutrition occurs most frequently from insufficiency of the coronary circulation. The anatomic and physiologic factors governing the coronary blood flow have been extensively investigated and are of importance to the understanding of the genesis of ischemia of the heart muscle. These principles will be considered briefly.

The blood supply to the myocardium may be retarded or arrested by obstruction or distortion of the lumen of the arteries, and by changes in dynamics of flow from

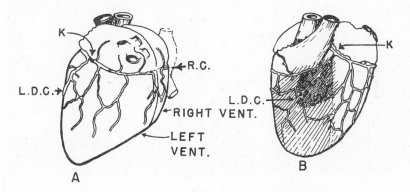

FIG. 56. (A) Diagrammatic sketch of a heart in which a theoretically *slow* occlusion has developed in the left circumflex coronary artery (at point K), and a second partial occlusion farther along the course of the vessel. Collateral channels from the left descending coronary artery (L.D.C.) and from the right coronary artery (R.C.) are shown in exaggeration, permitting circulation about the point of occlusion. Establishment of such collateral blood supply may be important in sustaining anatomic and functional integrity of the myocardium following obstruction of major vessels. (B) Sketch of a heart in which the left descending coronary artery is theoretically occluded *suddenly* at point K. Wide crosshatching indicates general area of ischemia distal to the obstruction. Although blood vessels near the point of occlusion may be filled, thorough irrigation of these vessels is lacking and an infarct forms in the area indicated by dense shading.

valvular disease, heart failure or other mechanical disturbances. Another consideration is the reflex effect upon the coronary vessels which reduces the caliber of the arteries.

Obstructive lesions of the coronary vessels are encountered frequently at necropsy in the hearts of patients who have suffered attacks of cardiac pain.[65] The lesions are usually atherosclerotic. Less commonly, the coronary ostia may be critically narrowed in syphilitic aortitis, or the arteries may be occluded by emboli from endocardial disease within the left cardiac chambers. Atherosclerotic narrowing of the lumina may be so marked that adequate coronary flow is maintained only at rest. Therefore, a rise in work load of the heart

brought about by exertion or emotional stimulation may result in myocardial ischemia because of the failure of the vessels to provide the increased amounts of blood required. Under these conditions, the patient may suffer attacks of heart pain on effort. During rest, the coronary circulation is again adequate to meet the minimum requirements of the heart muscle; the attacks of pain cease.

The sudden obstruction of a major coronary vessel (usually by thrombosis) and the occurrence of frank myocardial infarction may be attended by violent pain. Fortunately, in many of these patients the remainder of the coronary circulation is sufficiently intact to assure cardiac function until the infarct heals. There is further

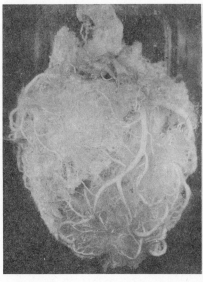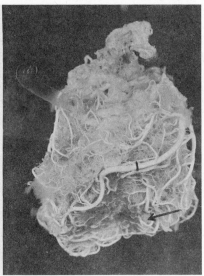

Fig. 57 (*Left*). Cast of the coronary arterial system of a dog heart filled with Neoprene latex. The heart muscle and blood vessels have been removed by digestion in concentrated hydrochloric acid. Delicate tracery of fine arteries and capillaries are preserved in the casting, which is suspended in water.

Fig. 58 (*Right*). Neoprene latex casting of the coronary arteries of a dog heart. The left descending coronary artery is prominently displayed on the surface of the cast. Previous to injection of the arteries with Neoprene, the left descending coronary vessel was ligated at the point shown by the small black line. After injection with latex, the left descending coronary distal to the ligation (black line) was filled from collateral vessels. The area below this artery (indicated by arrow) failed to fill with latex, leaving a depression in the casting. The specimen indicates that an abundance of anastomoses exist between the major coronary arteries and that the vessels which were not injected occupy a smaller area than would be expected from ligation of a large artery. (Figs. 57 and 58 from Smith and Henry: J. Lab. Clin. Med. 30:462)

evidence that collateral circulation may occur about the periphery of an infarct so that the area of resultant necrosis may be much smaller than would be expected from occlusion of the vessel.

It is interesting that some patients may have extensive coronary artery disease, without infarction and without having suffered pain or impairment of cardiac function. Blumgart and his associates[65] have pointed out that gradual occlusion of the principal coronary vessels may be accompanied by the development of extensive anastomoses between the branches of the right and left coronary arteries. An effective collateral circulation is then established to enhance the circulation around points of obstruction (Fig. 56). Such enhancement of the circulation may sustain myocardial function for many years. The devious networks of vessels which bridge the occlusions of large arteries have been shown in various ways.[65,66] Smith and Henry[66] ligated major coronary vessels in the extirpated hearts of dogs. Subsequent perfusion of the vessels with an opaque material indicated that the twigs included in the obstructed area were readily filled by the rich anastomoses derived from neighboring arteries (Figs. 57 and 58). Prinzmetal and his co-workers[67] were able to demonstrate that red blood cells labeled with radioactive phosphorus readily penetrated areas distal to the obstruction in the beating hearts of dogs and man, because of the rich collateral blood supply. They suggested that blood flow through collateral channels operates to limit the size of infarcts, thereby lessening the danger of cardiac rupture as well as promoting the process of healing. On the other hand, it is evident that further occlusions of arteries of the collateral system may again increase myocardial ischemia, or result in infarction of the muscle, possibly with attacks of cardiac pain.

Convincing experimental evidence has also been evolved to show that other mechanisms may operate to increase the coronary flow. Gregg et al.[68] observed marked increases in coronary arterial inflow when the right ventricle was placed under increased work by constriction of the pulmonary artery. The increased flow was evident even when the aortic blood pressure diminished. They considered the augmented flow to be due to dilatation of the coronary arteries by metabolites present in the working cardiac muscle. Similar observations were made by Smith and Jensen[69] in experimental acute heart failure. They demonstrated that when the hearts of heart-lung preparations were made to fail by the administration of a toxic substance, there was a sharp increase in coronary inflow— even as the systemic blood pressure and cardiac output diminished. The phenomenon could be explained only by coronary dilatation. Therefore, it seems possible that any increase in work load for the heart muscle will result in greater blood flow from dilatation of the vessels. These experiments offer no clue as to the possible duration of coronary dilatation in hearts placed under chronic strain. Nevertheless, it is likely that the effects of coronary dilatation, and even of increased anastomotic circulation, may be largely neutralized by extensive narrowing and hardening of the vessel walls or by progressive occlusion of essential collateral channels. The flow may be insufficient to correct ischemia resulting from increased work, and exertional attacks of heart pain occur. Furthermore, it is often observed that drugs administered for the purpose of causing coronary dilatation appear to be ineffective, possibly because of previous continued dilatation of all of the vessels.

Interference with the dynamics of the coronary flow may be more difficult to understand. Passage of blood through the coronary vessels is dependent upon the head of pressure, the resistance to flow through the vascular bed and the pressure existing at the venous end of the circuit. It must be assumed also that an optimum quantity of blood is available for irrigation of the system. The resistance of the vascular bed is further modified by the compression and relaxation of intramural vessels by myocardial motion. Certain alterations of any of these factors may be detrimental. Aortic valvular disease (stenosis or insufficiency) may modify pressures at the aortic openings of the arteries, reducing the net flow into the system. In addition, it is possible that *dilatation* of the myocardium impedes the flow. When the inflow of blood is measured into an *atrial branch* of the coronary system, dilatation of the atrial chamber inhibits the inflow into the artery even when a high perfusion pressure is maintained.[70] Other evidence indicates that most of the blood which passes through the coronary arteries is returned to the right cardiac chambers through the coronary sinus, the anterior cardiac veins and the thebesian system of veins. Therefore, the elevation of right intraventricular pressure and right atrial tension (increased venous pressure) of sufficient degree may reduce the effective pressure gradient between the pressure head (in the aorta) and the escaping venous blood, with consequent diminution of flow through the capillaries.[71] It is easy to visualize that in congestive heart failure or in other conditions tending to *raise tensions in the right cardiac chambers,* the coronary flow may be impeded.

It has been postulated for many years that reflex coronary vasopasm may occur transiently, provoking myocardial ischemia and attacks of angina pectoris. However, coronary spasm has been difficult to produce in experimental animals, and the concept must be considered unproved.[60] It is notable that patients with attacks of angina pectoris frequently observe an increase in the severity and the frequency of the seizures when they are chilled and exercising. Riseman and his associates[72,73] exercised patients with angina pectoris in heated and cold rooms. These patients did not tolerate exertion in the cold room as well as in the warm air, and attacks of cardiac pain were definitely more frequent. In addition, a greater incidence of anginal attacks was noted by patients who were exercising in a warm environment when their hands were chilled by immersion in ice water or when they were holding ice cubes. These workers considered their findings as evidence that *reflex coronary constriction* may be an important factor in the precipitation of anginal seizures. This viewpoint and the alternate contention (that the angina of exertion occurs because of sudden increase in cardiac load and a disproportionately small coronary circulation)

have not been completely reconciled. In the light of the physiologic evidence now at hand, it is possible that both mechanisms of reducing coronary blood flow may operate to produce cardiac pain.

Occasionally, cardiac pain may be precipitated when the dynamics of the coronary circulation are normal. It is not uncommon for patients suffering from *pernicious anemia* to have attacks of angina on exertion, presumably due to the primary lack of nutrition to the myocardium. Large doses of *epinephrine* may augment the work of the myocardium, beyond the existing coronary flow, and cause pain.[74,109]

In some instances the administration of digitalis in cardiac failure has been noted to produce angina pectoris or to intensify the frequency and severity of attacks;[75] fortunately, this is not the usual occurrence with the use of digitalis.[76]

With reference to any of these mechanisms, it appears to be basically important that *attacks of cardiac pain occur when critical myocardial ischemia is produced, either by an absolute diminution of the coronary blood flow or by increased demand on the heart out of proportion to the available blood supply.*

CHARACTERISTICS OF HEART PAIN

For convenience of discussion, cardiac pain will be considered as (1) paroxysmal (angina pectoris) and as (2) the pain of myocardial infarction.

Angina Pectoris. Typically, angina pectoris is characterized by the occurrence of substernal pain on exertion. Patients describe the pain as an "oppression," a tightness or crowding within the chest, or a heaviness substernally. Occasionally the sensation is said to be that of a viselike gripping of the sternum and the lateral chest, and less commonly it is described as burning. The pain is rarely severe; more often it is of moderate intensity. It is never stabbing, never precipitated by coughing or respiratory movements. As the pain radiates to the upper extremities and elsewhere, the sensation is characterized as an ache, a numbness, tingling or other vague discomfort. The location of the pain is usually under the upper portion of the sternum, but it may be felt beneath the entire extent of the sternum. Anginal pain is usually, but not always, substernal. It may occur to the left of the sternum, in the precordium.[77] Under such conditions, the pain must be carefully studied, as pain in the precordium or in the region of the apical impulse is common to other disorders. Therefore, the occurrence of precordial pain must be interpreted with great care.[11]

The discomfort of angina pectoris commonly radiates from the substernal region. Frequently, the sensation is projected over the left pectoral region to the left shoulder and along the medial aspect of the left arm to the elbow.[77] The pain may be further projected through the forearm to the hand along the distribution of the ulnar nerve. Less commonly, the pain radiates to the right shoulder and arm with or without concomitant left-sided projection. Reference of the pain to the shoulders and to the inferior part of the neck has been described; these patients may have the sensation of a portmanteau clasped about the neck.[78] Occasionally, the pain is referred to the neck as a constriction, or as a pain in the left side of the neck and face. We observed a patient whose substernal pain radiated through the neck and localized as

a severe ache in the left temporomandibular joint; movement of the mandible intensified the pain. Radiation of the substernal discomfort to the epigastrium and the right costal margin may also occur, but such pain always has a thoracic component as well.[77]

Attacks of angina pectoris are often precipitated by excitement or exertion. They may occur at night as in aortic valve disease, or after meals. The paroxysms usually last a few minutes to a half hour and usually disappear quickly when the patient rests;[77] frequently the subject is forcibly halted by the severity of the attack. The administration of nitroglycerin or other powerful vasodilating drugs dispels the attack, so many sufferers are taught to carry nitroglycerin or amyl nitrite with them to allay the seizures.

The pain of acute myocardial infarction is similar to that of angina, though generally more severe and more prolonged. It is variously described. To some, it is an intolerable crushing or clutching, substernally or over the precordium; to others, it is a viselike gripping of the chest, or a pain the awfulness of which defies description.[79] The agony may be extreme. It often diffuses widely through the chest. Strong

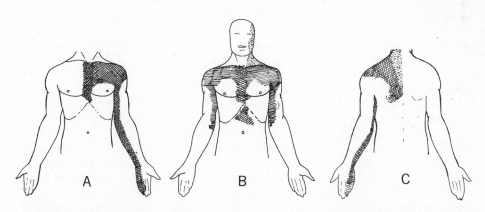

FIG. 59. Positions and common points of reference of cardiac pain. (A) Area of substernal discomfort projected to the left shoulder and arm over the distribution of the ulnar nerve. Reference of pain may be confined only to the left shoulder, or to the shoulder and along the arm only to the elbow. Less frequently pain may be referred to the right shoulder and arm (B) or to both shoulders, arms and hands simultaneously. Occasional radiation to the epigastrium and right upper abdominal quadrant may take place. Projection of anginal pain to the back is also encountered less frequently (C); reference is usually to the area of the left scapula or the interscapular region.

persons sometimes toss, pace the floor and tear at the breast in anguish. In some patients the pain is moderate, or may be only slight. Unlike angina, the pain continues for hours and often is controlled only by large doses of morphine.

Radiation of the pain is similar to that of angina. When the pain is referred to the upper abdomen and is of explosive severity, the resulting upper abdominal symptoms may resemble acute hemorrhagic pancreatitis, perforation of a peptic ulcer or other forms of acute abdominal conditions requiring surgery.[80,81] There may be muscle guard or even abdominal rigidity, which, together with fever and leukocytosis, frequently causes confusion. When the heart pain is referred to the right upper quadrant and back the condition is likely to be confused with cholecystitis.[81] In some patients the onset of myocardial infarction is signalized by a sensation of distention in the epigastrium, so that the patient believes himself to have "acute indigestion."

Myocardial infarction is followed not infrequently by a *painful disability of the shoulders and hands,* characterized initially by mild to severe pain in one or both shoulders.[103,104] Pain may arise immediately, or weeks or months after the infarction. There may be tenderness and limitation of motion of the shoulder, suggestive of periarthritis. Later the hand may become swollen, glossy, stiff and painful on motion.[82,83]

The etiology of the "shoulder-hand syndrome" is uncertain. It may be in part the result of persistent stimulation of the intermedio-lateral nuclei of the sympathetic nerves by internuncial transmission from the posterior horn cells. It is thought that chronic sympathetic stimulation can produce changes in blood flow to these somatic areas and contribute to musculoskeletal changes in the extremity.

Similarly, prolonged reflex stimulation of the anterior horn cells may provoke chronic spasm of somatic muscles, and subsequently inflammation of muscle and related cartilaginous structures. A mechanism seems evident which causes the tender spots on the chest wall and arm in the presence of myocardial disease. The basic similarity of this thoracic muscle spasm to the muscular rigidity in acute abdominal disease should be noted. It is also clear that the presence of similar tender, trigger areas does not necessarily relate *specifically* to a *visceral* disease because it could result from any long-standing posterior horn cell stimulation regardless of its origin. Once the tender area has developed, it is often self-perpetuating, supplying its own afferent pain sensation to maintain the reflex sensory motor arc. Not infrequently, one observes patients who, after a myocardial infarction, complain of persistent anterior chest pain with the fear that the symptom results from continuing active myocardial ischemia. However, the myocardium may be healed and the pain stimuli may originate in the spastic muscles at the site of somatic referral; the somatic pain may be now both the cause and the result of the persisting muscle and joint irritation.

It is possible that operative procedures for the relief of "intolerable angina pectoris" are often effective because they do, in fact, involve incision of the sensory or motor nerves of this somatic-somatic sensory-motor cycle. Ligation of the internal mammary artery, a procedure formerly used in such cases, was occasionally effective possibly because of interruption of the anterior intercostal nerves at the site of incision. Similarly, injection of procaine into the painful areas of the chest wall may result also in the interruption of the self-sustaining cycle and incur the permanent relief of pain.

After myocardial infarction and following operative procedures upon the heart, one or more episodes of chest pain, fever and perhaps cough and dyspnea may occur.[105,106,107,108] There is often evidence of pericarditis, pleurisy and pneumonitis in such instances. The pain is usually of a pleuritic or pericarditic type and can be distinguished from the pain of myocardial ischemia. The pathogenesis of these post-infarction and postcardiotomy syndromes may relate to the demonstrated presence of *antiheart antibodies* in the serum of these patients. It may be postulated that infarction, or incision, of the heart releases previously bound substances into the circulation to which the individual reacts with the production of antibodies. It has been postulated that the autoantibodies then attack the antigen in the pleura, pericardium or myocardium, and incite an inflammatory reaction at these sites.

Precordial ache and tenderness. Functional precordial pain has occasionally been confused with cardiac pain.[11] Patients become alarmed at the occurrence of pain about the heart, and the physician should not be led into the pitfall of hasty or superficial consideration of these symptoms. White[11] has carefully described the "heart pains which are not angina."

Many persons complain of an aching about the heart when they are fatigued at the day's end. Others may notice sharp twinges of pain in the area of the apex beat, and the chest wall at that point is tender to pressure. Tense, hyperkinetic, easily fatigued persons frequently suffer from heartache. Such patients are often in good health and show no evidence of disease anywhere. In neurocirculatory asthenia and in some other types of neurosis, intense precordial aching or stabbing pain is often the principal complaint; a few of these patients are semi-invalids because of the pain and the belief that they are suffering from a fatal illness. On the other hand, precordial pain not infrequently occurs in the presence of marked cardiac enlargement. While the discomfort may be transient, it often persists for days and requires large doses of analgesic drugs. Because of its association with heart disease, the symptom may be confused with true cardiac pain. We observed a 19-year-old girl with acute rheumatic myocarditis and heart failure. The heart was greatly enlarged. She complained bitterly of sharp pain localized about the apex impulse, and palpation of the area revealed rather exquisite tenderness on light pressure.

It is often difficult to find an explanation for precordial ache, particularly in persons of good mental and physical health. Possibly the constant impact of the heart against the chest wall irritates the intercostal muscles and nerves locally; fatigue may then translate the local irritation into symptoms of pain. This explanation would also seem to hold when such pain occurs with marked cardiac enlargement.

TRACTS AND REFERENCE OF CARDIAC PAIN

It seems well established that pain fibers from the heart pass from the cardiac plexus, enter the upper five or six thoracic sympathetic ganglia (through which they pass without interruption) and thence on through the rami communicantes to the corresponding spinal (or dorsal root) ganglia. The cell bodies of these fibers lie in the spinal ganglia.[111] Afferent pain neurones also pass through the inferior, middle and superior cardiac nerves through the cervical sympathetic ganglia and over rami communicantes to the cervical spinal ganglia.[111] There is also some evidence that a few pain neurones are conveyed from the superior cervical ganglion to the trigeminal ganglion. However, the majority of pain fibers from the heart course through the inferior cervical sympathetic and upper two or three thoracic ganglia. Elsewhere, they are much fewer in number. The pain neurones synapse with neurones of the second order in the posterior gray columns of the spinal cord (cf. Physiology of Pain). (See Fig. 60.)

Consideration of the anatomic transmission of cardiac pain immediately suggests the mechanism of reference of heart pain. It seems probable that the greater part of pain impulses reaching the upper dorsal ganglia are projected as pain in one or both pectoral regions; pain occurring along the inner aspects of the arms may result from common connections through the brachial plexus. In some individuals, predominating pain impulses may flow into the cervical dorsal roots provoking neck pain; in a few, pain impulses appear to reach the ganglion of the 5th cranial nerve. It has been suggested that the common anginal symptom of substernal oppression may be reflex muscular contraction of the anterior intercostal muscles. If the pain barrage is severe, mass excitation of visceromotor reflexes such as sweating, lowered blood pressure, ashy cyanosis and other evidence of vasomotor disturbance, and nausea and vomiting may become prominent.

The relation between cardiac pain and pain in the upper abdominal region is less readily explained. Miller[84] points out that difficulty in diagnosis arises when pain is referred to distant areas not directly related to the organ involved. In most persons, visceral afferent fibers converge upon a limited number of dorsal roots which come into relation with a restricted number of afferent somatic fibers. Therefore, in diseases of the heart, the gallbladder, the stomach and other viscera, pain is usually referred to characteristic localities. With respect to the gallbladder, the visceral afferent pathways are numerous (extending from T_1 to T_{12}), and while the pain impulses are carried predominantly in the lower thoracic nerves, they may be included in many more segmental levels. In this way gallbladder pain may be referred to segments commonly reserved for cardiac pain; acute heart pain may, in turn, be projected to the right upper quadrant and flank. Miller further notes that cardiac pain is occasionally transmitted over accessory afferent fibers. These are generally too few to carry impulses in any quantity, though in some individuals they may be in sufficient concentration to refer pain to divergent sites. Possibly such a mechanism ac-

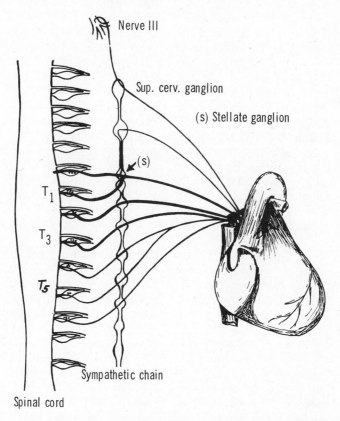

Nerve III

Sup. cerv. ganglion

(s) Stellate ganglion

(s)

T_1

T_3

T_5

Sympathetic chain

Spinal cord

Fig. 60. Course of cardiac-aortic pain fibers. Pain fibers from the cardiac and aortic plexuses pass directly through the sympathetic trunk and over the rami communicantes to the dorsal root ganglia. A few afferent fibers traverse the middle cervical ganglion, from which they probably course inferiorly in the sympathetic trunk to the stellate ganglion, thence to the corresponding spinal roots. A few fibers may course through the superior cervical ganglion to the trigeminal ganglion, accounting for the occasional radiation of cardiac pain to the face.

counts for the radiation of pain to the upper abdomen in cardiac infarctions and for the pain that resembles heart pain in acute abdominal accidents. In this connection, it is interesting that Wertheimer[85] and Leriche[86] observed the occurrence of severe anginal symptoms on stimulation of the central end of the severed greater splanchnic nerves in patients at operation.

AORTIC PAIN

Mechanisms of Aortic Pain

Clinical and experimental evidence indicates that the lesions of the aorta or of the smaller arteries in general may produce pain. The painful dilatations of the cranial arteries in migraine and the pain produced by arterial punctures for clinical studies are common examples. It is generally held that the adventitia of large blood vessels contain pain fibers.[89] Spiegel and Wassermann[90] found that acute stretching of the wall of the aortic arch produces pain. They demonstrated also that coating the aorta with irritating substances had profoundly painful effects. These authors concluded that aortic pain results from stimulation of the adventitia.

Afferent aortic pain fibers appear to run in close relation to those from the heart. White[88] has observed that the intractable pain of angina pectoris or aneurysm is abated by resection of the upper 5 thoracic ganglia, or the rami communicantes, or by interruption of the corresponding dorsal roots proximal to the root ganglia. Aortic pain neurones pass to the sympathetic chain ganglia from the aortic plexus, traverse the rami communicantes and reach their cell bodies in the dorsal root ganglia (Fig. 60).

It has been suggested that the pain of dissecting aneurysm of the aorta occurs because of marked distention of the adventitial coat.[88] On the other hand, syphilitic aortitis may lead to aneurysms of great size without discomfort to the patient. Syphilitic aortitis may give rise to attacks of angina pectoris by reducing the coronary flow through involvement of the mouths of the coronary arteries. Occasionally aortitis may provoke substernal discomfort that is dull,

burning and continuous. Mills and Horton[55] have suggested that such pain in some cases of aortic aneurysm results from sudden distention of the aneurysmal sac. They observed that the pain was frequently aggravated by recumbency, by exercise, by cough or upon deep breathing. In our experience aortitis and aneurysms due to syphilis have rarely been observed to produce painful symptoms, unless saccular dilatation had become so large as to impinge upon the chest wall or spine.

It is difficult to understand how the marked dilatation of syphilitic aortic aneurysm occurs with so little pain. Possibly in the slowly dilating aorta, adventitial distortion is gradual, and forceful stimuli to adventitial pain endings are not present. A further possibility is that afferent nerve endings may be largely destroyed by extensive syphilitic involvement of the vasa vasorum and the adventitia.

Quite in contrast to syphilitic aneurysms are the sudden disruptions of the aortic coats frequently accompanied by agonizing pain. *Dissecting aneurysms* apparently usually result from changes which first occur in the media. The pathologic changes in the medial coat lead to a rent in the intima, often just superior to the aortic valves. Blood enters under pressure from the lumen and splits apart the layers of the arterial wall. In the process of dissection, the muscle coats are torn apart, and the adventitia, in places, may be lifted from the underlying media. Intense distention of the portions of the wall outside of the burrowing column of blood occurs. We[91] have frequently observed dissecting aneurysms in open-chest experimental dog preparations. If the blood pressure is normal or high, and the aortic intima is then torn by a blunt instrument, blood burrows into the aortic wall so that the adventitia and a few strands of the medial coat are raised as a huge, bulbous purplish swelling which creeps distally along the aorta. The aneurysmal sac becomes thin and tenuous in places where there is subadventitial dissection; elsewhere the sac may be firmer from support of underlying dissected layers of the media. Seepage from the thinner parts of the sac usually occurs, terminating in rupture. Pathologic evidence indicates that a similar mechanical rending of the vessel may occur in patients.[92] The basic lesion leading to aortic dissection appears to be medial cystic necrosis[93] of the wall of the vessel.[94,95] The evidence offered by Bauersfeld[97] indicates that cystic disease of the media causes a rupture of the vasa vasorum with the formation of medial hematomas; the hematomas may split the aortic wall. Tension of the intima then tears the membrane and dissection is extended from pressure within the lumen. Most patients with dissecting aneurysms have had pre-existing arterial hypertension. Marked elevation of blood pressure may facilitate rapid disruption and final rupture of the aortic wall when a small tear in the intima has occurred.

CHARACTERISTICS OF AORTIC PAIN

Clinically, aortic pain is most clearly recognized when dissecting aneurysms occur. Such pain may be dramatic; it is sudden in onset and quickly becomes severe and agonizing. When the aneurysm is confined to the aortic arch, the pain is substernal or diffuses over the upper anterior chest. It may be projected to the shoulders.[92,96] Projection into the arms is infrequent. As dissection proceeds over the arch and into the descending aorta, extreme pain may be felt at the base of the neck and along the back —particularly in the interscapular area. The agony is continuous and requires heavy narcotization. Although grayish cyanosis and other signs of visceromotor reflex disturbances appear, the blood pressure is usually sustained. In the grip of such pain, some patients may be distraught: they may climb in and out of bed, roll about, assume grotesque postures, or press their chests against chairs or walls in an effort to obtain relief.[98] This behavior is in contrast with that of individuals with myocardial infarction, who may lie quietly, and often exhibit signs of collapse. Cases of dissecting aneurysm are described[92] in which symptoms have been transient or mild, suggesting angina pectoris. In some cases (usually found unexpectedly at necropsy) no pain has occurred, though the aorta may be extensively damaged.

Peery[99] has drawn attention to incomplete rupture of the aorta. This lesion is produced by an intimal tear without dissection of the vessel wall. It may provoke severe substernal pain of a "stabbing" or "tearing" quality, but it is not as severe as that of dissecting aneurysm. This pain may be confused with that of coronary occlusion. Incomplete rupture of the aorta can give way to dissection of the aortic wall at any time.

SUMMARY

The essential clinical features of thoracic pain have been briefly presented, and the painful symptoms interpreted in the light of the underlying, known pathologic physiology. Pain arising from the chest wall, thoracic respiratory system, mediastinum, esophagus, and cardiovascular system is discussed.

REFERENCES

1. Heinbecker, P.: Heart pain, J. Thoracic Surg. 10:44, 1940.
2. Heinbecker, P., Bishop, G. H., and O'Leary, J.: Pain and touch fibres in peripheral nerves, Arch. Neurol. Psychiat. 29:771, 1933.
3. Lewis, T.: Pain, New York, Macmillan, 1942.
4. Moore, R. M.: Stimulation of peripheral nerve-elements subserving pain-sensibility by intra-arterial injections of neutral solutions, Amer. J. Physiol. 110:191, 1934.
   Dennis, J., and Moore, R. M.: Potassium changes in functioning heart under conditions of ischemia and of congestion, Amer. J. Physiol. 123:443, 1938.
5. Hamilton, J. B.: The pathways and production of pain, Yale J. Biol. Med. 9:215, 1936-37.
6. Lewis, T.: Suggestions relating to the study of somatic pain, Brit. M. J. 1:321, 1938.
7. Behan, R. J.: Pain, New York, Appleton, 1920.
8. Stern, E. S.: Mechanism of herpes zoster and its relation to chicken-pox, Brit. J. Dermatol. 49:263, 1937.
9. Goeckerman, W. H., and Wilhelm, L. F. X.: Herpes zoster and herpes simplex, Arch. Dermatol. Syphilol. 35:868, 1937.
10. Holmes, J. F.: Slipping rib cartilage, with report of cases, Amer. J. Surg. 54:326, 1941.
11. White, P. D.: Diseases of the Coronary Arteries and Cardiac Pain, New York, Macmillan, 1936.

12. Dixon, R. H.: Cure or relief of cases misdiagnosed "angina of effort," Brit. M. J. 2: 891, 1938.

13. Schmidt, R.: Pain: Its Causation and Diagnostic Significance in Internal Diseases (Translation by Vogel and Zinsser), Philadelphia, Lippincott, 1911.

14. Mendlowitz, M.: Strain of the pectoralis minor muscle, an important cause of precordial pain in soldiers, Amer. Heart J. 30: 123, 1945.

15. Graham, E. A., Singer, J. J., and Ballon, H. C.: Surgical Diseases of the Chest, Philadelphia, Lea, 1935.

16. Craver, L. F.: Tenderness of the sternum in leukemia, Amer. J. Med. Sc. 174:799, 1927.

17. Smith, J. R., and Kountz, W. B.: Deformities of the thoracic spine as a cause of anginoid pain, Ann. Int. Med. 17:604, 1942.

18. Davis, D.: Spinal nerve root pain (radiculitis) simulating coronary occlusion; a common syndrome, Amer. Heart J. 35:70, 1948.

19. Reid, W. D.: Pressure on the brachial plexus causing simulation of coronary disease, J.A.M.A. 110:1724, 1938.

20. Fitzwilliams, D. C. L.: On the Breast, St. Louis, Mosby, 1924.

21. Geschickter, C. F.: Diseases of the Breast, Philadelphia, Lippincott, 1943.

22. Labbé, L., and Coyne, P.: Traité des Tumeurs Bénignes du Sein, Paris, Masson, 1876.

23. Veil, P.: Cellulite du sein et engine de poitrine, Arch. d. mal. du cœur 25:703, 1932.

24. de Cholnoky, T.: Benign tumors of the breast, A.M.A. Arch. Surg. 38:79, 1939.

25. Cheatle, G., and Cutler, M.: Tumors of the Breast, Philadelphia, Lippincott, 1931.

26. Graham, E. A.: Personal communication.

27. Morton, D. R., Klassen, K. P., and Curtis, G. M.: The effect of high vagus section upon the clinical physiology of the bronchi, in 1949 Proc. of Central Soc. Clin. Research, J. Lab. Clin. Med. 34:1730, 1949.

28. Bonner, L. M.: Primary lung tumor, J.A.M.A. 94:1044, 1930.

29. Capps, J. A., and Coleman, G. H.: An Experimental and Clinical Study of Pain in the Pleura, Pericardium and Peritoneum, New York, Macmillan, 1932.

30. Dybdahl, G. L.: The control of pleuritic pain by the use of cutaneous anesthesia, Permanente Med. Fdn. Bull. 2:30, 1944.

31. Bray, H. A.: The tension theory of pleuritic pain, Am. Rev. Tuberc. 13:14, 1926.

32. Goldman, A.: Personal communication.

33. Krause, G. R., and Chester, E. M.: Infarction of the lung; clinical and roentgenological study, A.M.A. Arch. Int. Med. 67:1144, 1941.

34. Carlson, H. A., and Ballon, H. C.: The operability of carcinoma of the lung, J. Thoracic Surg. 2:323, 1933.

35. Ornstein, G. G., and Ulmar, D.: Clinical Tuberculosis, vol. II, G-21, Philadelphia, Davis, 1941.

36. Kiss, F., and Ballon, H. C.: Contribution to the nerve supply of the diaphragm, Anat. Rec. 41:285, 1928-29.

37. Hinsey, J. C., and Phillips, R. A.: Observations upon diaphragmatic sensation, J. Neurophysiol. 3:175, 1940.

38. Master, A. M., Dack, S., Stone, J., and Grishman, A.: Differential diagnosis of hiatus hernia and coronary artery disease, A.M.A. Arch. Surg. 58:428, 1949.

39. Jones, C. M., and Chapman, W. P.: Studies on the mechanism of the pain in angina pectoris with particular relation to hiatus hernia, Tr. A. Amer. Physicians 57:139, 1942.

40. Moor, F.: The cause of "stitch," Brit. M. J. 2:282, 1923.

41. Capps, R.: Cause of the so-called side ache that occurs in normal persons, A.M.A. Arch. Int. Med. 68:94, 1941.

42. Barnes, A. R., and Burchell, H. B.: Acute pericarditis simulating acute coronary occlusion, Amer. Heart J. 23:247, 1942.

43. Camp, P. D., and White, P. D.: Pericardial effusion; a clinical study, Amer. J. Med. Sc. 184:728, 1932.

44. Harvey, A. M., and Whitehill, M. R.: Tuberculous pericarditis, Medicine 16:45, 1937.

45. Paine, W. W., and Poulton, E. P.: Experiments on visceral sensation: I, The relation of pain to activity in the human eosophagus, J. Physiol. 63:217, 1927.

———: Visceral pain in the upper alimentary tract, Quart. J. Med. 17:53, 1923-24.

46. Hurst, A. F., and Rake, G. W.: Achalasia of the cardia, Quart. J. Med. 23:491, 1929-30.

47. Alvarez, W. C.: An Introduction to Gastroenterology, New York, Hoeber, 1941.

48. Neuhof, H., and Rabin, C. B.: Acute mediastinitis; roentgenological, pathological and clinical features and principles of operative treatment, Amer. J. Roentgenol. 44:684 1940.

49. Furstenburg, A. C.: Acute mediastinal suppuration, Trans. Amer. Laryng., Rhin. & Otol. Soc., p. 210, 1929.

50. Hamman, L.: Spontaneous mediastinal emphysema, Johns Hopkins Hosp. Bull. 64:1, 1939.

51. McLester, J. S.: Diseases of the Mediastinum, *in* Oxford Medicine, New York, Oxford Univ. Press.

52. Pick, F.: Ueber chronische unter dem Bilde der Lebercirrhose verlaufende Perikarditis (perikarditische Pseudolebercirrhose) nebst Bemerkungen ueber die Zuckergussleber (Curschmann), Ztschr. f. klin. Med. 29:385, 1896.

53. Middleton, W. S.: Some clinical caprices of Hodgkin's disease, Ann. Int. Med. 11:448, 1937.

54. Pancoast, H. K.: Superior pulmonary sulcus tumor. Tumor characterized by pain, Horner's syndrome, destruction of bone and atrophy of hand muscles, J.A.M.A. 99:1391, 1932.

55. Mills, J. H., and Horton, B. T.: Clinical aspects of aneurysm, A.M.A. Arch. Int. Med. 62:949, 1938.

56. Heberden, W.: Pectoris Dolor, *reprinted in* Classic Descriptions of Disease (Major), Baltimore, Thomas, 1932.

57. Herrick, J. B.: Clinical features of sudden obstruction of the coronary arteries, J.A.M.A. 59:2015, 1912.

58. Sutton, D. C., and Lueth, H. C.: Pain, A.M.A. Arch. Int. Med. 45:827, 1930.

59. Pearcy, J. F., Priest, W. S., and Van Allen, C. M.: Pain due to the temporary occlusion of the coronary arteries in dogs, Amer. Heart J. 4:390, 1928-29.

60. Keefer, C. S., and Resnik, W. H.: Angina pectoris; A syndrome caused by anoxemia of the myocardium, A.M.A. Arch. Int. Med. 41:769, 1928.

61. Wenckebach, K. F.: Angina pectoris and the possibilities of its surgical relief, Brit. M. J. 1:809, 1924.

62. Gorham, L. W., and Martin, S. J.: Coronary occlusion with and without pain, A.M.A. Arch. Int. Med. 62:821, 1938.

63. Lewis, T., Pickering, G. W., and Rothschild, P.: Observations upon muscular pain in intermittent claudication, Heart 15:359, 1931.

64. Katz, L. N., Lindner, E., and Landt, H.: On the nature of the substance(s) producing pain in contracting skeletal muscle; its bearing on the problems of angina pectoris and intermittent claudication, J. Clin. Invest. 14:807, 1935.

65. Blumgart, H. L., Schlesinger, M. J., and Davis, D.: Studies on the relation of the clinical manifestations of angina pectoris, coronary thrombosis, and myocardial infarction to the pathological findings, Amer. Heart J. 19:1, 1940.

66. Smith, J. R., and Henry, M. J.: Demonstration of the coronary arterial system with neoprene latex, J. Lab. Clin. Med. 30:462, 1945.

67. Prinzmetal, M., Bergman, H. C., *et al.*: Studies on the coronary circulation. III. Collateral circulation of beating human and dog hearts with coronary occlusion, Amer. Heart J. 35:689, 1948.

68. Gregg, D. E., Pritchard, W. H., Shipley, R. E., and Wearn, J. T.: Augmentation of blood flow in the coronary arteries with elevation of right ventricular pressure, Amer. J. Physiol. 139:726, 1943.

69. Smith, J. R., and Jensen, J.: Observations on the effect of theophylline amino-isobutanol in experimental heart failure, J. Lab. Clin. Med. 31:850, 1946.

70. Smith, J. R., and Layton, I. C.: The flow of blood supplying the cardiac atria, Proc. Soc. Exper. Biol. Med. 62:59, 1946.

71. Visscher, M. B.: The restriction of the coronary flow as a general factor in heart failure, J.A.M.A. 113:987, 1939.

72. Riseman, J. E. F., and Brown, M. G.: The duration of attacks of angina pectoris on exertion and the effect of nitroglycerine and amyl nitrite, New England J. Med. 217:470, 1937.

73. Freedberg, A. S., Spiegl, E. D., and Riseman, J. E. F.: Effect of external heat and cold on patients with angina pectoris: Evidences for the existence of a reflex factor, Amer. Heart J. 27:611, 1944.

74. Herrick, J. B.: The coronary artery in health and disease, Amer. Heart J. 6:589, 1930-31.

75. Fenn, G. K., and Gilbert, N. C.: Anginal pain as a result of digitalis administration, J.A.M.A. 98:99, 1932.

76. Gold, H., Otto, H., Kwit, N. T., and Satchwell, H.: Does digitalis influence the course of cardiac pain? A study of 120 selected cases of angina pectoris, J.A.M.A. 110:895, 1938.

77. Harrison, T. R.: Clinical aspects of pain in the chest; I, Angina pectoris, Amer. J. Med. Sc. 207:561, 1944.

78. Gallavardin, L.: Syndromes angineux anormaux, Médecine 18:193, 1937.

79. Levine, S. A.: Coronary thrombosis, its various clinical features, Medicine 8:245, 1929.

80. Levine, S. A., and Tranter, C. L.: Infarction of the heart simulating acute surgical abdominal conditions, Amer. J. Med. Sci. 155:57, 1918.

81. Breyfogle, H. S.: The frequency of coexisting gallbladder and coronary artery disease, J.A.M.A. 114:1434, 1940.

82. Ernstene, A. C., and Rinell, J.: Pain in the shoulder as a sequel to myocardial infarction, A.M.A. Arch. Int. Med. 66:800, 1940.

83. Askey, J. M.: The syndrome of painful disability of the shoulder and hand complicating coronary occlusion, Amer. Heart J. 22:1, 1941.

84. Miller, H. R.: Interrelationship of disease of the coronary arteries and gallbladder, Amer. Heart J. 24:579, 1942.

85. Wertheimer, P.: A propos des doleurs provoquées par l'excitation des grands splanchniques, Presse méd. 45:1628, 1937.

86. Leriche, R.: Des doleurs provoquées par l'excitation dés grands splanchniques, Presse méd. 45:971, 1937.

87. White, J. C., Garrey, W. E., and Atkins, J. A.: Cardiac innervation; Experimental and clinical studies, A.M.A. Arch. Surg. 26:765, 1933.

88. White, J. C.: The neurological mechanism of cardio-aortic pain, A. Research Nerv. Ment. Dis., Proc. 15:181, 1935.

89. Singer, R.: Experimentelle Studien über die Schmerzempfindlichkeit des Herzens und der grossen Gefässe und ihre Beziehung zur Angina Pectoris, Wien. Arch. f. in. Med. 12:193, 1926.

90. Spiegel, E. A., and Wassermann, S.: Experimentelle Studien über die Entstehung des Aortenschmerzes und seine Leitung zum Zentralnervensystem, Ztschr. f. d. ges. exper. Med. 52:180, 1926.

91. Smith, J. R., and Paine, R.: Unpublished observations.

92. Flaxman, N.: Dissecting aneurysm of the aorta, Amer. Heart J. 24:654, 1942.

93. Erdheim, J.: Medionecrosis aortae idiopathica cystica, Virchows Arch. f. path. Anat. u. Physiol. 276:187, 1930.

94. Sailer, S.: Dissecting aneurysm of the aorta, A.M.A., Arch. Path. 33:704, 1942.

95. Niehaus, F. W., and Wright, W. D.: Dissecting aneurysm of the aorta, J. Lab. Clin. Med. 26:1248, 1941.

96. Kountz, W. B., and Hempelmann, L.: Chromotrophic degeneration and rupture of the aorta following thyroidectomy in cases of hypertension, Amer. Heart J. 20:599, 1940.

97. Bauersfeld, S. R.: Dissecting aneurysm of the aorta: A presentation of fifteen cases and a review of the recent literature, Ann. Int. Med. 26:873, 1947.

98. Tillman, Clifford: Personal communication.

99. Peery, T. M.: Incomplete rupture of the aorta; heretofore unrecognized stage of dissecting aneurysm and cause of cardiac pain and cardiac murmurs, A.M.A. Arch. Int. Med. 70:689, 1942.

100. Weller, T. H., Whitton, H. M., and Bell, J. E.: The etiologic agents of varicella and herpes zoster: Isolation, propagation and cultural characteristics in vitro, J. Exper. Med. 108:843-868, 1958.

101. Wesselhoeft, C.: Chicken pox and herpes zoster, R. I. Med. J. 40:387-395, 1957.

102. Davis, D.: Radicular Syndromes With Emphasis On Chest Pain Simulating Coronary Disease, Year Book Pub., 1957.

103. Steinbrocker, O.: Shoulder-hand syndrome, Amer. J. Med. 3:402, 1947.

104. Edeiken, J.: Shoulder-hand syndrome, Circ. 16:14, 1957.

105. Dressler, W., Yurkoksky, J., and McStarr, M.: Amer. Heart J. 54:42, 1957.

106. Dressler, W.: A post-myocardial infarction syndrome, J.A.M.A. 160:1379, 1956.

107. Weiser, N. J., Kantor, M., Russell, H. K.: Posterior myocardial infarction syndrome, Circ. 20:371, 1959.

108. Gregg, D. E.: Physiology of the coronary circulation, Circ. 27:1128, 1963.

109. White, J. C.: Cardiac pain, anatomic pathways and physiologic mechanisms, Circ. 16:644, 1957.

7

Abdominal Pain

STEWART WOLF

Abdominal pain is probably responsible for more requests to the physician for house calls during the night than any other single symptom. Intense pain in any portion of the abdomen may result from a wide variety of conditions, some benign, others demanding immediate attention. The differential diagnosis of abdominal pain calls for the physician's keenest perception and nicest judgments.

MECHANISMS

As pointed out in the discussion of pain in Chapter 3, pain receptors are distributed widely but in varying concentration throughout the body. To produce the sensation, an adequate stimulus of some sort is required. Most often this involves a mechanical distortion of the nerve structure constituting the pain-ending or an alteration in the chemical composition of the surrounding tissue. Recent work has established *neurokinin*, a polypeptide resulting from local proteolytic action, as a substance which lowers the threshold for pain. Whether or not neurokinin is implicated in the pain mechanism as a transmitter substance or neurohumor is not clear as yet, but it has been shown to be produced locally in response to stimulation of nerve roots. See the discussion under The Stimulus in Chapter 3 and under Humoral Factors in Chapter 4.

Between the diaphragm and the pelvis,

the region generally designated as the abdomen, the following mechanisms for pain production may be encountered: (1) Distension of tubes, vessels and viscera; (2) Vigorous contraction of smooth muscle; (3) Peritoneal inflammation; (4) Peritoneal stretching; (5) Vascular distention; (6) Ischemia; (7) Irritation or inflammation of spinal roots and peripheral nerves; (8) Stress on vertebral bodies or periosteum; (9) Sustained contraction of skeletal muscle or other processes in the abdominal wall; (10) Probably other unknown processes.

The larger arteries of the mesenteries themselves and the parietal peritoneum are pain-sensitive as noted in the earlier chapter on pain. With respect to structures derived from the endoderm, including the gut, however, some confusion has existed. Pains occurring from disturbances along the course of the gastrointestinal tract are commonly met with in medical practice, but efforts to induce them by deliberate stimulation have not always been successful. Thus, because it has been cut, burned, and crushed in the conscious subject without complaint of pain, the wall of the gut itself has been thought to be insensitive to pain. More recent evidence indicates that such a conclusion is premature, and that under appropriate circumstances both the mucosa and deeper structures of the gut are as sensitive to pain as are the urethra, the bladder, the ureters, and the kidney pelves.

176

Such structures are relatively insensitive when there is no engorgement or inflammation. However, in the presence of hyperemia the pain threshold is lowered and ordinarily non-noxious stimuli produce pain. It is likely that *hyperemia* and *inflammation* are important determinants of pain in the abdomen from whatever structure.

PATHWAYS

Pain felt in the abdomen must be either transmitted through spinal roots T-6 through T-12 or referred to these segments because of impulses traveling from neighboring structures in the chest, the extremities or the pelvis by the mechanisms outlined below under referred pain. Some structures within the chest are innervated from segments as low as T-9. Therefore, the location of the sensation of pain in chest or abdomen or even elsewhere in the body hardly establishes the site of the disease.

Impulses resulting in pain travel mainly in neurons which accompany the sympathetic trunks. However, there is evidence that some pain fibers travel in the vagus, and certainly some pain sensations from within the abdomen are transmitted via the intercostal nerves. All afferent nerves have their cell bodies in the dorsal root ganglia whether they travel in autonomic trunks or in segmental nerves.

The neurons themselves are mainly of the small unmyelinated variety, Gasser's Class C. They mediate an aching sort of pain, poorly localized.

REFERRED PAIN

Deep pains characteristically spread to be felt in areas other than those stimulated. The spread may involve deep or superficial pathways or both. This effect has been called referred pain. It is attributable to the spread of excitation in the neuraxis to other portions of the same segment or to segments adjacent to those into which the noxious impulses are conducted. This gives rise to pain experienced in parts innervated by deep and superficial branches of the affected segments and also causes a variety of motor effects.

The phenomenon of "spread" has been demonstrated in a man who had undergone a unilateral interruption of the spinothalamic pathways below T-1. Noxious stimulation of the anesthetic half of his body induced pain felt diffusely on the opposite side. This finding illustrates the way in which spread of excitation occurs within the cord from noxious impulses entering it, even though the pathways which bring to consciousness the pain from the side stimulated have been severed. In general, the more intense the noxious stimulation, the more widespread is the area of reference. The spread of excitation occurs by way of the neurons of the dorsal horn and the association pathways, usually more readily toward the head but also caudad when the stimulus is intense. There arise in turn impulses on the same side and on the opposite side of the cord or brain stem. Some of these ascend to suprasegmental structures where neural activity is ultimately felt as pain.

The central spread of excitation also appears to give rise to a state in which sensory impulses, coming in over the segment at their usual threshold values, seem more intense and more persistent than they otherwise would. For example, noxious stimulation of an area of referred pain is often productive of more discomfort than similar stimulation of an uninvolved region. Its actual threshold for cutaneous pain, however, is not altered. This phenomenon is included in the term *hyperalgesia*. Such hyperalgesia follows noxious stimulation of either superficial or deep structures. When it involves the latter it is usually spoken of as *local tenderness*. In an area of skin involved in a process of referred pain, not only do pain sensations arising from noxious stimulation appear intensified, but so do all sensations arising from other sensory stimuli.

The hyperalgesia and hyperesthesia due to accentuation of the effects of sensory impulses arising in the tissues of a segment involved in a process of referred pain may constitute the principal element of discomfort from a given visceral disease. If that is the case local anesthetization of the superficial tissues by procaine would greatly reduce the patient's discomfort by blocking impulses arising *in the skin*. This effect has been noted by many investigators but has been accorded undue importance as an explanation of the phenomena of referred pain. Procainization of superficial tissues is capable of blocking stimuli arising in the anesthetized area, but not of interrupting the central spread of excitation within the cord.

Not only is *receptor* activity involved in the spread of excitation in the nervous sys-

tem, but *effector* activity as well. as illustrated by the skeletal muscle spasms, the smooth muscle and the gland effects shown in Figures 61 and 62. Modified activity involving motility which occurs during painful states is also involved. For example, the occurrence of muscle spasms may additionally complicate the proper localization of deep pains. Noxious stimulation of the ureter has been shown to result in contraction of abdominal muscles which, when sustained, may become a source of fresh

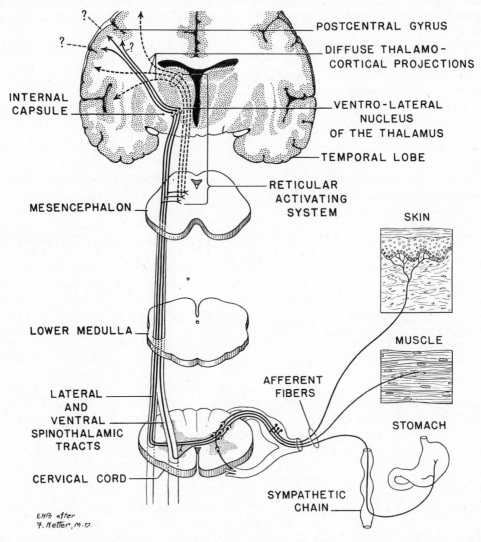

FIG. 61. Diagrammatic representation of pathways for pain. The question marks represent as yet undefined but doubtless vast numbers of connections for impulses from a single pain fiber at the highest integrative level. (Drawn by E. H. Broedel, adapted with permission from the Ciba Collection of Medical Illustrations by F. Netter, M.D.)

noxious impulses. At length the pain from the contracted muscles may overshadow that from the ureter.

Such *secondarily contracted muscles may* also give rise to *local rigidity and tenderness* occurring in addition to the local tenderness attributable to the central modification of sensory impulses from an area of referred pain described above. This *dual mechanism,* which provides for pain and tenderness at a site remote from that of original noxious stimulation, thus includes another (muscular) peripheral source of noxious impulses similar to that referred to above in the skin. It, too, has given rise to confusion and controversy. In this case the controversy has largely concerned whether or not the pain and tenderness in areas of referred pain can be abolished by local infiltration of muscles with procaine. It now appears clear that pain and tenderness induced by secondary muscle spasm are modifiable by locally infiltrated procaine. When such effects predominate in the pain experience, infiltration of muscles with procaine may be effective in virtually

abolishing the discomfort of visceral disease. When considerable pain is felt *in situ,* however, or when referred pain and tenderness are induced by a central spread of excitation involving sensory neurons, local infiltration of muscles with procaine would not be expected to modify the central effects although it would block fresh impulses arising in the periphery whose effects would become enhanced upon reaching the cord.

TYPES OF DEEP PAIN

To epitomize, it may be said that there are three categories of deep pain:

1. True Visceral and Deep Somatic Pain. Such pain is felt at the site of primary stimulation and may or may not be associated with referred pain. It is eliminated by infiltration of procaine into the site of noxious stimulation or by blocking its afferent nerves, but it is not altered by infiltration of procaine into other structures supplied by the same or adjacent neural segments.

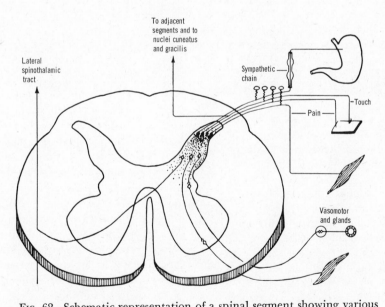

Fig. 62. Schematic representation of a spinal segment showing various effects of excitatory spread of noxious impulses from a primary noxious stimulus in the stomach. The skin becomes hyperalgesic and hyperesthetic and muscle becomes tender. Effector structures innervating blood vessels and glands (sweat and sebaceous) are involved, as well as those innervating skeletal muscles, causing contractions which may in themselves become painful.

2. Referred Pain. Such pain may occur in addition to or in the absence of the true visceral and deep somatic pain described above. It is experienced at a site other than that of stimulation but in tissues supplied by the same or adjacent neural segments. It may occur either with or without associated hyperalgesia and hyperaesthesia.

A. *Without Superficial and/or deep Hyperalgesia.* In this case pain depends only on the central effects of the spread of excitation of the original noxious impulses to the same and adjacent segments of the cord, whence they are relayed to higher centers for perception and interpretation. Injection of procaine into superficial or deep regions of referred pain does not reduce the intensity of pain due to this mechanism.

B. *With Superficial and/or Deep Hyperalgesia.* Referred pain may be accentuated in intensity by virtue of the effects of ordinarily non-noxious stimuli from zones of reference. Impulses from such sources, normally inadequate to produce pain, may do so upon reaching the cord in a segment involved in central spread of excitation. Procaine injected into superficial or deep hyperalgesic structures will abolish this element of the referred pain phenomenon, resulting in more or less reduction of the subject's discomfort, depending on the amount of hyperalgesia. Often, when superficial hyperalgesia is a leading feature of the deep pain experience, the patient may be substantially relieved by spraying ethyl chloride on the affected area of skin.

3. Pain due to Secondary Skeletal Muscular Contractions which Provide a Fresh Source of Noxious Impulses. Pain may result from secondary effects of the central spread of excitation on the effector structures, including painful contractions of skeletal muscles. Such disturbances may be widespread and the pains may be experienced in situations remote from the original source of noxious stimuli. Local infiltration of the contracted muscles with procaine abolishes this type of pain by disrupting its peripheral mechanism.

LOCATION OF DEEP PAIN

A major source of confusion among those concerned with identification of various pains has been failure fully to realize the fact that a referred pain need not involve the whole segment of reference. In fact referred pain usually does not. Most pains arising from disease in abdominal viscera are felt anteriorly on the abdomen in the ventral part of the segment concerned. Ureteral pain is first felt anteriorly, and posteriorly in the flanks only when the stimulus is intense. Pain from the kidney pelvis a few millimeters away, however, is characteristically first felt at the costovertebral angle. Pain from noxious stimulation of the gallbladder may be felt only posteriorly at the angle of the scapula in a portion of the 9th thoracic segment. Thus pains from deep structures may be:

1. Felt *in situ* and often fairly well localized.

2. *Referred* (A) along the *deep* distribution of spinal nerves or (B) along their *cutaneous* distribution or both. Reference occurs most readily (a) first to other parts of the same segment; (b) next to adjacent segments higher in the cord; (c) next to adjacent segments lower down; and (d) finally to corresponding segments on the opposite side of the cord without ever involving the whole of the original segment.

Disease of specific organs of the body often gives rise to a pattern of distribution of pain which is characteristic of that organ. Why noxious impulses from several structures innervated by the same segments are referred along more or less characteristic pathways involving specific parts of the segments is not clear, but it is probably related to experience. We are generally more conscious of the front (ventral) half of our bodies than the rear (dorsal) and we are especially conscious of parts which customarily receive noxious stimuli from the outside such as the precordium and epigastrium. It is logical to expect that these parts of the thoracic segments would be most involved in painful experiences.

ETIOLOGIC CLASSIFICATION OF ABDOMINAL PAIN

The common conditions and the diseases that can cause abdominal pain are (1) those involving structures within the abdominal cavity and (2) those involving structures outside the abdominal cavity.

Etiologic classification of abdominal pain:

1. Pain originating within the abdomen
   A. Disease of hollow organs
      Bowel, gallbladder, ducts, etc.
   B. Peritonitis
      Chemical or bacterial
   C. Vascular
      Mesenteric thrombosis; dissecting aneurysm, etc.
   D. Tension on supporting structures
      On mesenteries; distention of capsules (spleen, liver, lymph nodes)
2. Pain originating outside the abdomen
   A. Referred pain
      From thorax, spine, spinal cord, pelvis, genito-urinary tract, etc.
   B. Metabolic pain
      (a) Endogenous
         Toxic: uremia, diabetic acidosis, porphyria, etc.
         Allergic: food hypersensitivity
      (b) Exogenous
         Toxic: drugs, lead, etc.
         Biologic: bacterial toxins, insect and snake venoms, etc.
   C. Neurogenic pain
      Spinal cord or root pain; tabes, causalgia, etc.
   D. Psychogenic pain.

STRUCTURES RESPONSIBLE FOR PAIN

Esophagus. The commonest pain from the esophagus is heartburn, a burning pain felt substernally and fairly well localized over the site of stimulation. This pain has been shown by Jones to be due to spasm of the cardiac end of the esophagus. The spasm may be induced by mechanical, thermal, chemical or electrical stimuli. The commonest mechanism of heartburn in man is thought to include the regurgitation of highly acid gastric juice into the esophagus which has already had its pain threshold lowered by the presence of engorgement or inflammation.

The pain of peptic ulcer which arises from the stomach or duodenum is also frequently described as burning. It is of special interest that burning pain, ordinarily associated with noxious stimulation of the skin, can be elicited from the upper gastrointestinal tract and from other mucous membranes, as, for example, in the nose.

Stomach and Adjacent Structures. The sensibility of the stomach has been explored in a subject with a large gastric stoma. When the mucosa *in its normal state* was pinched between the blades of a forceps *no pain* resulted. Likewise the application of 50 or 95 per cent alcohol, 1.0 N HCl or 0.1 N NaOH or 1:30 suspension of mustard failed to induce pain in the healthy mucosa. However, when the *mucosa was inflamed,* congested and edematous from whatever cause, local mechanical and chemical stimulation *evoked pain* of considerable intensity. Thus, although the number of nerve fibers and endings subserving pain may be relatively small, it has been conclusively shown, by virtue of the fact that pain occurred upon noxious stimulation of the inflamed gastric mucosa, that *true visceral pain* exists. These observations have since been confirmed on the mucosae of the bladder and large bowel.

Not only do gastric pains arise from the mucosa but also from *deeper structures* in the stomach as well. There is considerable evidence to suggest that the muscular layers may be capable of initiating noxious impulses. In experiments on the fistulous subject already referred to it was found that contractions of the stomach in its normal state of a magnitude of 30 mm. Hg pressure against an indwelling balloon induced pain. When the stomach was engorged and hyperemic, however, contractions of only 20 mm. Hg pressure induced pain. This pain could hardly come from stretching of mesenteric attachments since there is less traction as the result of 20 mm. Hg pressure that of 30 mm. It seems likely, therefore, that some of the pain emanates from the structures deeper than the mucosa, namely from the muscularis, the serosa, or the visceral peritoneum. When the stomach was stretched by glass rods it was found that when the contractile state of the stomach was average the pressure necessary to produce pain was 100 Gm. per sq. cm. However, when the stomach wall was strongly contracted, pressure of 50 Gm. per sq. cm. (half that originally applied) was found sufficient to produce pain. On the other hand, when the stomach was relatively relaxed, 150 Gm. per sq. cm. were necessary to induce pain. These observations suggest that either the muscularis or serosa may contribute to pain experienced from the stomach.

The Pancreas, the Liver, and the Biliary Tract. Noxious impulses from the pancreas, the liver and the biliary tracts appear to travel in the same pathways as do those from the stomach. These facts explain in part the difficulties encountered in the differential diagnosis of epigastric pain. Not only may pain felt in the epigastrium arise from the structures named but also from the retroperitoneal tissues, from the skeletal muscles, or from lesions of the nervous system such as herpes zoster or cord tumors which involve dorsal roots. Epigastric pains may even be referred from the heart or other thoracic structures as mentioned above, or from impulses arising in the lower bowel, including the transverse colon and appendix. The hepatic parenchyma has not been shown to be sensitive, but noxious stimulation by rapid distention of its capsule does give rise to pain. The capsule is apparently able to accommodate to very slow distension without the occurrence of pain. The same generalizations apply to other solid organs including the spleen and possibly the kidneys. Pain from the gallbladder has been found to be commonly localized in the distribution of T-9 either anteriorly beneath the right costal margin or posteriorly at the angle of the scapula.

The Small and the Large Intestines. Noxious impulses from the small intestine travel in splanchnic pathways, but enter the cord slightly lower than do those from the stomach, from T_9 to T_{11}. The afferent innervation of the colon above the sigmoid is also carried in the sympathetic trunks. Below this level it is probably mainly supplied by afferent fibers through its mesenteries from the lower thoracic and upper lumbar segmental nerves without involvement of sympathetic or parasympathetic pathways. The rectum, however, does receive afferent nerves through the parasympathetic rami from S_2 to S_4.

Urinary Tract Pain. In the urogenital tract, renal and ureteral pain arises from noxious impulses reaching the cord via the lower splanchnic trunks and the lower 2 thoracic and 1st lumbar segments. Painful distention of the detrusor muscles initiates noxious impulses which, like those from the lower colon and rectum appear to travel in segmental nerves in the peritoneum.

From the trigone and structures below the bladder noxious impulses reach the cord over the sacral parasympathetic rami from S-2 to S-4. Noxious stimulation of the bladder trigone and region of the urethral origin causes pain to be felt at the distal tip of the urethra.

The Prostate and the Testes. Prostatic pain may be felt in the perineum or referred to the lower lumbar region, where it may be confused with skeletal, muscular, nerve, rectal or renal pain. Pains arising from noxious stimulation of the spermatic cords and testicular structures are felt largely *in situ* but may be referred up into the hypogastric region, where they may be mistaken for colonic or other pains. Down into the testes and along the groin and inner aspects of the thighs the pains of renal colic are commonly referred, where they may appear to arise from the spermatic channels or from local vascular lesions such as thrombophlebitis.

The Uterus, the Tubes, and the Ovaries. In the female, noxious impulses arising in the fundus uteri reach the central nervous system by way of the superior hypogastric plexus, entering the cord from T-10 to L-1. However, impulses from the cervix travel in the 2nd and the 4th sacral nerves with impulses from the bladder neck. Noxious impulses from the Fallopian tubes and the ovaries reach the cord at the 10th thoracic level, travelling in the plexus of nerves which accompany the ovarian vessels. Closely contiguous structures including the broad ligaments, other mesenteries and retroperitoneal structures are innervated by branches of the lumbosacral plexus and segmental nerves. Thus to relieve the pain of ovarian carcinoma it is necessary to sever a wide extent of pathways in order to denervate structures almost invariably invaded by the growth.

The commonest pains arising from the female genital structures are the pains of dysmenorrhea and labor. It is likely that most dysmenorrhea is related to the subject's reaction to contractions of the uterine musculature. Other pains associated with menstruation or uterine contraction may occur, however, from traction on adherent structures involved in an inflammatory, fibrotic or neoplastic process. The pains of labor doubtless arise from the muscular activity of the fundus uteri.

Disorders in the Chest

Intrathoracic diseases that may give rise to pain in the abdomen must be kept in mind, particularly rheumatic fever, lobar pneumonia and coronary artery disease. More often than not in these instances the abdominal pain is the result of some involvement of the diaphragmatic surface. Confusion of intrathoracic with intra-abdominal disease is encountered more often in children than in adults and certainly the patient's age is very important in evaluating pain in the abdomen and elsewhere. In old persons, for example, there may be very serious intra-abdominal disturbance, including peritonitis, without any substantial pain.

CLINICAL ANALYSIS

The correct diagnosis of the basis for abdominal pain depends more on a shrewd history than on any other single factor, although physical examination and laboratory findings are sometimes of decisive importance. Not only is a thorough description of the characteristics of the pain important, but so also is the past history. For example, in the diagnosis of common duct stone or some of the various complications of peptic ulcer, a history of typical biliary or ulcer pain years before may provide a useful lead. The history must be taken from the patient with special attention to points which would allow application of data that are known. The most useful description of the pain is likely to be available while the patient is actually experiencing the sensation. Hence, if the original history was obtained during a painless interval, it is profitable to ask the patient to recapitulate his experience while the pain is going on. The following are the most pertinent questions:

1. Locality. The site of pain must first be reliably determined together with its extent and whether or not there are secondary areas of reference. For example sharply circumscribed pain is characteristic of peptic ulcer, while colonic pain is likely to be more diffusely spread over the abdomen.

2. Quality. Whether the noxious impulses originate in the superficial or deep structures may often be determined from the quality of the pain. The patient's own words are useful in conveying information regarding the significance of the pain and in indicating the degree and nature of his reaction to the experience, but quality should be expressed in standard terms, which are known to relate distinguishable aspects of pain. Thus bright, pricking, burning or itching pains come from the skin while dull aching pains characteristically arise in deeper structures. Burning pain, as already pointed out, may arise from the mucous membrane of the upper gastrointestinal tract.

3. Temporal Factors. It is important to know whether pain is intermittent, continuous, pulsatile, or characterized by wavelike rise and fall in intensity. Knowledge of the duration of a painful experience is also essential. Gallbladder pains are likely to be intermittent. The pain of pancreatic tumor is characteristically persistent and unchanging. The pain of abdominal aneurysm may occasionally pulsate. Those from the digestive tube come and go in waves. From the upper gastrointestinal tract pains are likely to bear some relation to meals, while those from the lowermost portion are more apt to be related temporally to defecation. Other pains are related to special times of the day or seasons of the year.

4. Circumstances Under Which Pain Occurs or Is Aggravated. Pleuritic pain is ordinarily associated with breathing, heart muscle pain with exercise, peptic ulcer pain with an acid-containing stomach empty of food, and rectal pain with urgency to defecate. The pain from lesions involving spinal roots is likely to be accentuated by coughing, straining or sneezing, while pain from hernia is likely to be modified by changes in the position of the body. Most pains may be noted to occur or be aggravated under certain specific circumstances and this characteristic is often highly useful in diagnosis.

5. Factors Which Reduce Pain. The pains of peptic ulcer may be relieved by eating. Those of gallstones are usually made worse by eating, especially by ingestion of fat. Certain positions of the body or pressure on the abdomen may reduce the pain of a pancreatic cyst or tumor. Those suffering from gut pains may writhe or lie in a jack-knife position. The coronary patient is usually immobile and on his back. Locally applied heat often reduces the intensity of pain from muscle tension. Analgesics reduce the intensity of pains in general. Knowledge of whether or not a given pain can be obliterated by the threshold-raising effects of a certain analgesic provides the physician with a rough index of its intensity.

6. Intensity. Biliary and renal colic and the pains of herpes zoster are usually of high intensity, while those of chronic pancreatitis, for example, are of lower intensity but because of their immutability and persistence may induce even greater anguish, or pain reaction. Intensity is likely to be the most difficult aspect of the pain for a patient to describe and for the physician to recognize. This may be partly due to confusion in the minds of both regarding the distinction between pain perception and reaction. Since it is known to be possible to distinguish and recall, with reasonable accuracy, various grades of pain intensity, it is useful to ask the patient to compare in terms of "plusses" his own estimate of intensity using 10 plus for the most intense pain he has ever experienced. Another method whereby the intensity of a patient's pain may be roughly calibrated by the physician is as follows: He first pinches with moderate force his patient's biceps indicating that such pain is of approximately 2 plus intensity. A pinch of roughly twice that force is then administered and designated as 4 plus. Finally, an extremely forceful pinch is administered and designated as 8 plus. The patient is then asked

to evaluate the intensity of his own pain in terms of these standards.

7. Examination. In the examination of the patient special features to be noted are the presence or absence of local, deep tenderness or surface hyperalgesia, other sensory and motor phenomena and vascular disturbances such as changes in sweating and skin temperature and muscle spasm. Carefully observing the patient during a painful episode may also be of great help. It may be possible to see, feel, or hear movements of the gut. In general, a careful analysis of a patient's painful experience by well-directed questioning and examining for relevant features greatly increases the likelihood of accurate diagnosis. As mentioned above under Factors Which Reduce Pain, the position assumed by the patient may have diagnostic value. Strict immobility with a facial expression of anguish characterizes the patient with generalized peritonitis, while the patient with biliary colic writhes. The legs may be pulled up against the abdomen in intestinal colic, especially in children. Flexion at the hip may indicate a psoas abscess, whether related to appendicitis, perinephric abscess or tuberculous spondylitis. Patients with pericarditis are said to prefer to support themselves on their knees and elbows.

THE ACUTE ABDOMEN

Use of the term acute abdomen is usually reserved for a situation in which the patient is suddenly incapacitated by a very intense abdominal pain which may or may not be associated with fever, nausea, vomiting, and shock. The special feature on examination is the finding of spasm of the abdominal muscles, sometimes amounting to a boardlike rigidity. In such situations a surgical consultation is imperative although the situation may not necessarily require operative intervention. Appendicitis is the commonest reason for an acute abdomen and still one of the most difficult conditions to diagnose precisely. Most often the acute abdomen is the result of intestinal obstruction, perforation of a viscus, or peritonitis. The acute abdomen may well present an emergency and yet more errors are made through failure to take time to question and examine the patient than from delay occasioned by a careful analysis of the problem. When the parietal peritoneum is an important source of the pain, unusual or abnormal position of an organ such as a retrocecal appendix or a rotated sigmoid may cause confusion. So may also the failure to take into account the complex peritoneal gutters through which pus may travel to a site distant from its origin. Thus, the corrosive fluid from a perforated ulcer may spread down the right pericolic gutter to produce intense pain and muscle spasm in the right lower quadrant. Conversely, fluid from a ruptured appendix may spread upward to the suprahepatic or infrahepatic spaces. The same principles apply to the diagnosis of the acute abdomen as to other less dramatic situations involving abdominal pain. Again, intrathoracic conditions must be thought of; careful examination of the chest is indispensable.

Laboratory Procedures. Among the laboratory tests which are particularly helpful in differential diagnosis are the white blood cell count and the serum amylase determination. In appendicitis, the white blood cell count is usually elevated but rarely above 25,000. Pneumonia, however, which may produce a confusing picture of abdominal pain, is often associated with a very high white blood cell count. On the other hand tabes dorsalis or acidosis associated with diabetes or renal disease may be accompanied by abdominal pain and a normal white blood cell count, by the presence of ketonemia and ketonuria in the case of diabetes and an elevated blood urea nitrogen level in the case of renal failure. The serum amylase is most characteristically elevated in acute pancreatitis. Here, a level of higher than 600 mg. per cent is usually achieved. In an acute exacerbation of chronic pancreatitis, however, the serum amylase may be normal. Here a lowered amylase in the urine may provide a lead. The perforation of a peptic ulcer near to and involving the tissues near the pancreas may produce elevation of serum amylase to levels around 400 mg. per cent.

Other procedures which may be helpful in differential diagnosis include sickle cell preparations, examination of the blood for hemoglobinopathies and Ehrlich's test for urinary porphobilinogen. In lead intoxication and other forms of porphyrinuria abdominal pains are said to be associated with spasm of the stomach and duodenum demonstrable on roentgenography. Roentgenologic examination of the abdomen is often helpful, particularly if there is free air in the abdominal cavity indicating an intestinal perforation or air-fluid levels within the lumen of the gut indicating intestinal obstruction. Gallstones may, of course, be visualized, and also occasionally calcification of the pancreas or blood vessels. The introduction of barium into either end of the intestinal tract may increase the possibility for diagnosis. Another procedure which some physicians have found to be of substantial help is the peritoneal tap. Fluid so obtained when stained, or cultured or tested for pancreatic enzymes may establish the diagnosis in a puzzling instance of acute abdominal pain.

BIBLIOGRAPHY

Chapman, L. F., Ramos, A., Goodell, H., Silverman, G., and Wolff, H. G.: A humoral agent implicated in vascular headache of the migraine type, A.M.A. Arch. Neurol. 3:223-229, 1960; Trans. Am. Neurol. Assn., p. 42-45; 200-202, 1960

Hardy, J. D., Wolff, H. G., and Goodell, H.: Pain Sensations and Reactions, Baltimore, Williams & Wilkins, 1952.

Head, H.: On disturbances of sensation with especial reference to the pain of visceral disease, Brain 16:1, 1893.

Jones, C.: Digestive Tract Pain, Diagnosis and Treatment. Experimental Observations, New York, Macmillan, 1938.

Lennander, K. G.: Abdominal pains especially in ileus, J.A.M.A. 49:836, 1907.

Lewis, T., and Kellgren, J. H.: Observations relating to referred pain, viscero-motor reflexes and other associated phenomena, Clin. Sci. 4: 47, 1939.

Lim, R. K.: Visceral Receptors and Visceral Pain, Annals N. Y. Acad. Sci. 86:73-89, 1960.

Menaker, G. J.: The Physiology and Mechanism of Acute Abdominal Pain, Surg. Clin. No. Amer. 42:241-248, 1962.

Ross, J.: On the segmental distribution of sensory disorders, Brain 10:333, 1888.

Ryle, J. A.: Visceral pain and referred pain, Lancet 1:895, 1926.

Weiss, S., and Davis, D.: Significance of afferent impulses from skin in mechanism of visceral pain; skin infiltration as useful therapeutic measure, Am. J. Med. Sci. 176:517, 1928.

Wolff, H., and Wolf, S.: Pain, ed. 2, Springfield, Ill., Thomas, 1958.

Zollinger, R., Maddock, W. G., and Wolf, S.: Evaluation of the acute abdomen, (Symposium presented before 44th Annual Assembly of Interstate Postgraduate Medical Assoc. at Chicago), Postgrad. Med. 28:51, 1960.

Editorial: Visceral Pain, Lancet 2:1084, 1961.

8

Back Pain

R. H. FREYBERG

ANATOMIC AND PHYSIOLOGIC CONSIDERATIONS

Pain in the back is one of the most commonly encountered complaints in the practice of medicine. The frequency of back pain and backache can readily be appreciated if one understands the structures and the functions of the human back. The major structures making up the back are the vertebral column with its stabilizing ligaments, the muscles and their fascia, the spinal cord with its coverings and segmental spinal nerves, and the nutrient blood vessels.

The spinal cord is enclosed within a column of vertebrae, each possessing an anterior weight-bearing body and a posterior arch which surrounds the spinal canal. The bodies of the vertebrae are separated one from the other by intervertebral disks which act as cushioning devices to minimize the shock of trauma and movements of the spine. Each disk is composed of a central expansile portion (the nucleus pulposus) surrounded by strong fibrous connective tissue (the annulus fibrosus). Each intervertebral disk, by the force of its expansile center, tends to be spherical in shape, but the compression of the vertebrae forces it into a flat ovoid mass. The body weight is balanced on these intervertebral disks (Fig. 63).

Movement of the spine between its ver-

tebral segments is accomplished through diarthrodial joints located in pairs between the posterior arches of the vertebrae. The stability of the spine is provided by strong ligaments which span the spinal column from segment to segment; some pass longitudinally connecting many vertebrae through the length of the spinal column, others cross obliquely between two or three segments.

The spine articulates with the pelvis through the sacro-iliac joints, composed of cartilage-covered surfaces of the upper three segments of the sacrum which oppose the cartilage-covered surfaces of the adjacent iliac bones. Strong strands of fibrous tissue bind together the nonarticulating opposing surfaces of the spine and the pelvis. Ribs which surround and protect the thoracic vital organs articulate with the dorsal spine.

An important portion of the back is its musculature composed of three layers of muscles which support the trunk and produce its movements (Fig. 64). All of the muscles of the dorsal and lumbar back are covered and surrounded by the three layers of the lumbo-dorsal fascia; some muscles attach directly into this strong fascia.

Within the canal of the spinal column the spinal cord extends downward from the brain to its termination in the lowermost nerves and the ligaments which anchor its caudal end to the coccyx. From the spinal cord, pairs of nerves emerge at each vertebral segment to innervate the trunk and extremities (as described in a subsequent section of this chapter).

The back serves several important functions. It provides the body's principle support and stability, but at the same time provides for mobility of the trunk in all planes of motion. Movements of the head and of the extremities in relation to the trunk are accomplished largely by muscles located in the back. All movements involved in locomotion, standing and sitting depend upon the motion and the stability of the joints in the spine, and are accomplished by the back muscles. The spinal curves strengthen the spine, add to its flexibility, minimize jarring of the brain and stretch of the spinal cord. The dorsal kyphotic curve favors lodgement of the thoracic organs. The springy intervertebral cartilaginous disks buffer the jolts of locomotion on the brain and the spinal cord.

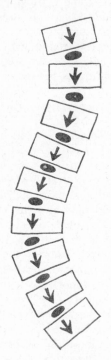

Fig. 63. This sketch illustrates the way in which the weight of the trunk of the body is balanced on the nuclei of the intervertebral disks.

The two important functions of the spinal muscles are to supply postural tone and to provide movement to the trunk and the structures attached to it. Postural tone, which is controlled by the autonomic nervous system, is normally maintained without effort or fatigue. In the erect position the strong flexor and extensor muscles are kept in a balanced state of contraction by a static, postural, autonomic reflex mechanism. Should this function of the muscles fail, voluntary contraction of the muscles is required to supplement the autonomic function. This quickly leads to fatigue, faulty posture and back pain. Maintenance of a normal motor system of the back depends upon functional integrity of bones, joints, tendons, muscles and nerves. These components of the back also form the physiologic system which provides motion. Accurate knowledge of the anatomic and biomechanical features of this system is required in order to understand many of its disorders.

Sensory, motor and autonomic nerves to the supporting structures of the torso and the extremities and many nerves to the viscera pass through the back. Abdominal and pelvic organs are maintained in their respective positions largely by suspending ligaments attached to the back.

It is not surprising, therefore, that back pain may be produced by diverse lesions involving these many structures. The analysis of backache depends upon recognition of the nature and the location of the underlying illness. This requires complete and systematic examination of the entire body and shrewd evaluation of all of these findings in relation to the patient's complaints. In the discussion which follows no effort will be made to define all the lesions that may cause pain in the back, nor will the method of examination be discussed; instead, in so far as possible, the objective will be to explain the reason for back pain characterizing various illnesses. Differential diagnosis of specific lesions will not be outlined; rather, the mechanism of production of back pain by various causes will be emphasized, knowledge of which provides the logical basis for accurate diagnosis and proper therapy.

FIG. 64. The muscula-
ture of the back. On the
left are shown the super-
ficial layer of muscles;
on the right the deeper
paraspinous muscles are
sketched. Note the
strong attachments of
the back muscles to the
pelvic and shoulder gir-
dles.

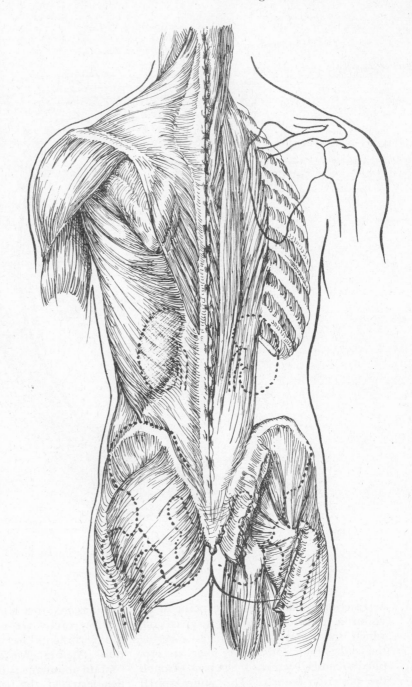

NEUROLOGIC CONSIDERATIONS

In this analysis of the pathogenesis of
back pain, it is important to give special
consideration to the innervation of the
structures of the back. Pairs of nerves
emerge from the spinal cord through foramina in the column at each vertebral segment (Fig 65). These nerves derive from
the cord through two roots: the anterior
root is composed solely of motor fibers,
the posterior root contains only sensory
fibers. Just distal to the foramen the two
roots unite into one nerve which divides
near the spinal column into an anterior and

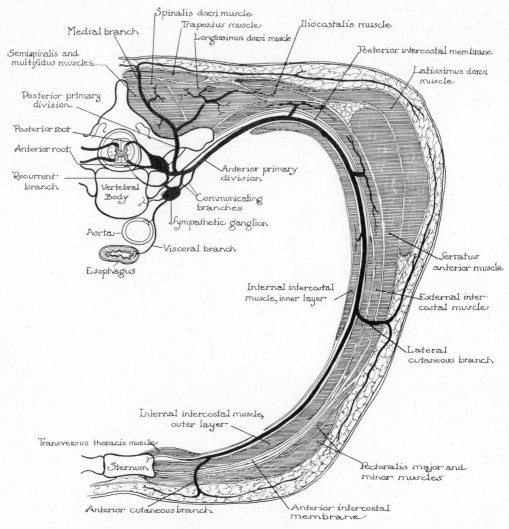

Fig. 65. A spinal nerve at the midthoracic level.

a posterior branch. Near the point of division a recurrent branch is given off, which innervates the meninges covering the cord. Motor and sensory fibers are supplied to most structures of the back through the posterior branch. The upper spinal nerves group themselves to form much of the plexus innervating the arms; the lower spinal nerves form other plexuses from which large bundles of fibers constitute important nerves to the lower extremities.

Smaller branches of regional nerves follow close along blood vessels to reach their termination. The vertebrae are innervated much as are other bones: the cortex and the marrow cavity are poorly supplied, while the periosteum has rich sensory innervation. The numerous spinous ligaments also contain abundant pain fibers. Kellgren[1] has demonstrated the sensitivity of many of these ligaments. Muscles, fascia and tendons in the back are innervated as they are elsewhere. At their bony attachments the regional periosteum shares the nerve distribution. The posterior articulations of the spine have a nerve supply comparable to that of joints in the extremities (discussed in Chapter 9).

The parietal pleura, parietal peritoneum and ligaments of the abdomen and pelvis which attach to the back are abundantly supplied with sensory nerves. In these structures the mechanism of initiating painful stimuli depends chiefly upon stretching, distending, tearing or severing the membranes containing terminal nerve fibers and end organs and by chemical irritation (explained in Chapter 9). Lesions affecting cartilage and bone without distorting the periosteal covering or irritating the soft structures attached thereto are relatively indolent. Discomfort arises chiefly when the periosteum, the ligaments, the fascia and the other richly innervated structures are affected.

Within the spinal canal, painful stimuli may arise from irritation of sensory nerves which are abundant in the meninges, from stretching or pressure upon the sensory roots of spinal nerves, or from stimulation of pain fibers in the spinal cord.

CAUSES OF BACK PAIN

The foregoing discussion makes it clear that many different types of lesions affecting one or another tissue in the back may cause pain. The mechanism of production of pain in the back will now be considered.

BACK PAIN ARISING FROM LESIONS OF THE SPINAL COLUMN

Most disorders of the spine cause pain. The spine is frequently injured. If trauma is sufficient to *fracture* the spine, the resulting irritation of the periosteum, the stretch of ligaments, pressure from edema and hemorrhage, and spasm of muscles produce pain in the region of the fracture. Spasm of the numerous large back muscles may increase the discomfort greatly. Displacement of bone fragments may be sufficient to cause pressure on the meninges, on the pain tracts in the spinal cord or on the spinal nerve roots and so produce pain. *Dislocation* or *fracture-dislocation* of the spine causes pain in a manner similar to that of a simple fracture. Traumatic lesions are more apt to occur in the cervical and lumbar portions of the spine where there is normally more flexibility and less protection.

Spondylolisthesis (displacement of a portion of the spine on the remainder) occurs most often in the lumbar spine. This lesion develops at the site of a congenital spinal anomaly where weakness or instability of the supporting structures allows displacement at times of physical strain such as lifting heavy objects or pushing with strong force. The bony displacement causes strain on adjacent ligaments and articulations, protective muscle spasm develops and all of these changes contribute to produce pain. Seldom is there difficulty in recognizing this condition. There is usually a suggestive history, plus certain physical abnormalities including a palpable "shelf" at the site of the malposition, painful flexion and extension of the back with limitation of these motions and characteristic findings in the roentgenogram.

Various metabolic disorders may cause *osteoporosis* of the spine. Mild decalcification may be asymptomatic. However, the degree of pain and disability cannot always be correlated with the severity or extent of radiographic findings. Some patients with severe pain show only minor changes in the roentgenograms; others with extensive radiographic changes may have little or no pain.[2] If vertebrae become markedly osteoporotic, they may mold under the expansile pressure of the intervertebral disks, and produce strain on regional tissues, which causes backache. Minor injuries to such osteoporotic bone may cause compression fracture of one or more vertebrae, usually in the lumbar or dorsal portion.[3] When this happens there is usually sudden, severe, regional back pain. Radiculitis may add another type of severe pain.

The most common *infections* that cause back pain are acute hematogenous osteomyelitis (staphylococcal) and tuberculosis of the spine (Pott's disease). However, effective antimicrobial therapy has reduced greatly the incidence of all infections of bone. Osteomyelitis in vertebrae has characteristics of osteomyelitis elsewhere, including the development of suppuration, abscess formation, bone destruction, sequestration, involucrum formation, periosteal elevation, penetration and dissection along muscle or fascial planes, soft tissue abscesses and sinus formation. The type and the intensity of the pain depend upon the degree of stretching of the periosteum, the amount of irritation from the products of inflammation, and the stimulation of nerve endings or compression of fibers caused by edema and muscle spasm.

Tuberculosis of the spine is always a metastatic process resulting from hematogenous dissemination of tubercle bacilli. It may begin in a vertebra or in an intervertebral disk, whence it involves adjacent structures. In the early stages, pain and tenderness may be confined to a relatively small portion of the back in the region of the infection. As the tuberculous process advances one or more vertebral bodies may collapse, causing an angular kyphosis (gibbus), which produces altered weight-bearing and strain of ligaments, muscles and fascia. Muscle spasm may become extensive and cause more widespread back pain. If a paraspinous tuberculous abscess develops it may press upon nerve roots or fibers, causing pain in the distribution of the nerve. An abscess may dissect between fascial planes to produce pain quite remote from the original lesion, or it may point into the spinal canal and cause irritation of the meninges. Purulent meningitis may develop if infection is liberated within the spinal canal. Sometimes spinal cord compression causes transverse myelitis. A diagnosis of Pott's disease is usually readily proved by characteristic roentgenograms and the demonstration of tuberculous infection.[4]

A vertebra may be the site of *primary sarcoma*. More often, vertebrae are invaded by *metastatic carcinoma* or *multiple myeloma*. Whatever the nature of the neoplasm, if tumor formation is small and does not stretch or irritate the periosteum there may be no discomfort. When the tumor enlarges so that it erodes the cortex and stretches or tears the periosteum, or when it so weakens the support in the back that strain of ligaments or joint capsules and muscle spasm result, or when there is direct pressure on nerves, back pain may be agonizing. It is often described as "expansile" or "boring" pain. It is usually constantly present but intensified by weight-bearing and movement. Opiates often fail to give relief. Vertebral fractures may result from neoplastic destruction of the bone. Roentgenograms usually clarify the diagnosis.

PAIN ARISING FROM LESIONS OF THE JOINTS AND INTERVERTEBRAL DISKS

The apophyseal joints, which are true joints with articular cartilage, joint capsule and synovial membrane, may become inflamed, just as do extremity joints. The most common form of joint inflammation to affect the apophyseal joints is *ankylosing spondylitis* ("rheumatoid spondylitis," Marie-Strumpell disease, von Bechterew's disease, spondylitis adolescens). Recently much doubt has arisen regarding the classification of this form of spinal arthritis as rheumatoid, because of many dissimilarities from classical rheumatoid disease affecting extremity joints, including absence of the rheumatoid factor in the serum in this form of spondylitis. However, the pathologic features in the spinal joints in this disease are comparable to those of classical rheumatoid arthritis of extremity joints. The additional features of extensive spasm of regional back muscles and the paraspinous calcification underneath spinal ligaments contribute to stiffness, immobility and pain, and the irritation of spinal nerve roots may produce radiculitis. Consequently, this is usually a very painful disease.

The disease usually begins with arthritis in the sacro-iliac joints and slowly spreads to involve apophyseal joints in an ascending manner. Over the course of years, the sacro-iliac joints usually become anklyosed, and the posterior articulations that have been affected may become fused. Permanent stiffness of the spine may result from intra-articular ankylosis, but more often it is due to subligamentous calcification, a pathologic change peculiarly characteristic of this disease. During preanklyosing stages pain is the most troublesome symptom and it usually begins in the lumbosacral region. The mechanism of production of pain in this type of spondylitis is the same as for extremity joint rheumatoid arthritis (discussed in Chapter 9).

Arthritis of the hips may complicate ankylosing spondylitis. However, the pain which characteristically occurs in the early stages of this disease usually results from irritation of the fascia, the ligaments and the tendons that attach to the low back. The back pain spreads upward as the inflammation ascends in the spine, and the parts earlier affected become less painful as stiffness and ankylosis develop. When spondylitis affects the dorsal spine, costovertebral articulations are usually involved in the inflammatory process so that chest expansion becomes painful and restricted. Radiculitis may result from spinal nerve root irritation. Sneezing, coughing and other movements that suddenly jar the back or increase the intraspinal pressure produce severe neuralgia in the back or along the thoracic or the abdominal segmental nerves.

Whenever a teen-age or young adult male complains of pain in the lower back or legs, ankylosing spondylitis should be suspected, and a roentgenogram of the pelvis and lumbar spine should be made.[5] Although sacriiliac arthritis may exist without the development of spondylitis, it is wise to consider roentgenographic evidence of bilateral sacro-iliac arthritis indicative of early ankylosing spondylitis because of the frequency with which rheumatoid spondylitis begins in these joints. A few erroneous diagnoses may be made by following this policy, but much more often the correct diagnosis will be made sufficiently early to allow much better treatment of this terribly crippling disease.[6]

Tuberculosis may affect one sacro-iliac joint, seldom both simultaneously. Disease of one sacro-iliac joint causes unilateral, regional back pain with or without muscle spasm. Tenderness is usually present only over the affected joint. Gaenslen's and Lasegue's maneuvers are useful diagnostic procedures to determine whether the lesion is in the sacro-iliac joint, and roentgenograms often identify the lesion.

Low back pain which occurs after lifting or other vigorous activities which strain the lower back is often considered by patients to be due to a *sacro-iliac disorder*. The once popular terms "sacro-iliac strain" or "throwing the sacro-iliac out" are based on fallacious reasoning.[7] Mechanical lesions of the sacro-iliac joints are indeed rare.

The junctions between the vertebral bodies are not true articulations; motion is not accomplished by gliding or hingelike action between vertebral bodies. However, the segmental bony construction of fibrocartilaginous disks between vertebrae allows flexibility of the spine. Because it shares so extensively in almost all physical activities, the spine commonly undergoes changes due to wear and tear, manifested in later years as degeneration of the cartilaginous intervertebral disks and as hypertrophic lipping and spurring at the edges of the vertebrae. Complete bony bridging between vertebral bodies may result from osteophytic growths. These changes characterize *osteoarthritis* (hypertrophic arthritis) of the spine, more correctly labeled degenerative changes of the spine.[8] Irritation of ligaments, fascia, and other fibrous tissue about the spinal column accounts for the back pain, which is sometimes severely aggravated by standing and by movement of the spine. Pressure on nerve roots is a common cause for radicular pain along the irritated spinal nerve. This type of arthritis more commonly affects those parts of the spine where there is greater motion, i.e., the lumbar and cervical portions. Sacro-iliac joints are affected infrequently. Intra-articular ankylosis does not occur. Pain of an aching character (backache) is often present and sharp pain may occur with motion in the spine. Diagnosis is not difficult, for roentgenograms show the characteristic osteophytes and degenerative changes.

At the lumbosacral junction a flexible portion of the spine joins with the rigid pelvis at a place where there is considerable weight-bearing and where motion is important for lifting, stooping and the like. Consequently, *traumatic lesions* occur frequently at this site. With increased lordosis of the lumbar spine or excessive forward tilt to the pelvis there is widening of the lumbosacral angle sufficient to cause strain of the longitudinal ligaments, the tendons and the fascia, and in this way cause backache. This can be relieved by correcting the abnormal position. Often the 5th lumbar disk is traumatized and degenerates, leaving a thin lumbosacral space that may also cause strain or pressure on regional tissues sufficient to cause backache.

If the anatomy of the back is understood it should be expected that some lesions of the lower back may irritate the sciatic nerve roots. Low back pain and *sciatica* frequently occur simultaneously; sometimes sciatica is the only symptom of a lower back disorder. Usually it becomes necessary to interpret sciatic pain in relation to disorders arising in the spine.

Intervertebral disk disease is the most common cause of sciatic pain.[9,10] General features of the disk syndrome, its diagnosis and treatment, will not be reviewed here—attention will be focused upon the pain characterizing this syndrome. Quite often severe pain begins suddenly with a "slipping" or "snapping" which the patient experiences in the act of stooping, lifting, or arising from a sitting or lying position. This pain is usually in the midline, the patient may list to one side and often cannot straighten his back because of pain and muscle spasm. Sneezing and coughing aggravate the pain. These attacks are believed by some investigators[11] to represent the beginning of degenerative changes in the disk with softening and loosening of the nucleus pulposus and its posterior displacement within the disk, which then produces pain by stretching the posterior spinous ligament (Fig 66). The symptoms of the disk lesion in this stage (without actual herniation) may be relieved by maneuvers that will straighten the spine and readjust pressure so that the nucleus is returned to its normal central position, thereby relieving the pressure on adjacent ligaments and eliminating the irritation set up by the displacement.

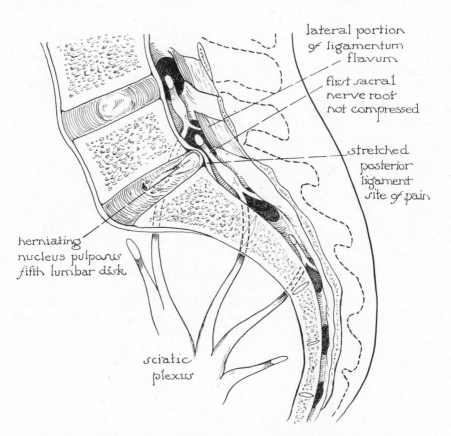

lateral portion of ligamentum flavum

first sacral nerve root not compressed

stretched posterior ligament site of pain

herniating nucleus pulposus fifth lumbar disk

sciatic plexus

Fig. 66. Posterior displacement of the nucleus pulposus without herniation may stretch the posterior spinous ligament and may not protrude sufficiently to compress nerve roots. (Keegan, J. J.: J.A.M.A. 126:868)

True herniation of the nucleus pulposus occurs when there is a tear of the annulus and a sufficient amount of the disk escapes underneath the posterior longitudinal ligament. There is then a tumor within the spinal canal that usually causes pressure on a nerve root (Fig. 67). Such a rupture may be sudden or gradual. Symptoms indicating unilateral nerve-root compression are the distinguishing characteristics. The patient usually complains of aching pain in the superior midgluteal region with sharper, more variable pain radiating down the posterior thigh and calf (sciatica).

Several factors are involved in the compression of a nerve root by herniation of an intervertebral disk fragment.[12,13] Usually the herniation is located to one side of the midline directly beneath an emerging nerve root. If the spinal canal is large the herni-ated fragment may displace the root and may not compress it. In such instances there may be several episodes of back pain without definite root symptoms. In most persons there is considerable flattening or narrowing of the spinal canal at the lumbosacral junction, so that herniation at this level usually compresses the nerve root against the ligamentum flavum and lamina. The nerve root is fixed laterally, and herniation of the disk usually occurs medial to it so that compression develops in the narrow lateral angle of the spinal canal beneath a portion of the ligamentum flavum.

The earliest and most common complaint of nerve root irritation from herniation of a disk in the lumbar region is superior midgluteal pain. This is best explained as resulting from compression of the posterior primary division of the nerve against the

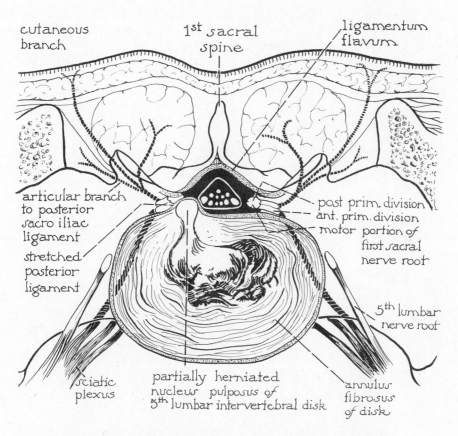

Fig. 67. Showing how herniation of the nucleus pulposus through torn annular tissue may produce an intraspinal tumor that will compress a nerve root and cause sciatica. (Keegan, J. J.: J.A.M.A. 126:868)

ligamentum flavum (Fig 67). In this division are the fibers that supply sensation to the gluteal region. The central portion of the medial half of the root contains the sensory fibers that form the anterior primary division of the nerve to the leg. Greater compression may involve the anterior primary division of the root that joins with other roots to form the great sciatic nerve which innervates most of the lower extremity below the knee.

Each of the roots forming the sciatic nerve has a segmental distribution, both motor and sensory (Fig. 68). The areas of the limb usually reported to be the sites of pain and paresthesia from disk lesions are the posterior thigh and the calf, the lateral portion of the ankle and the foot. These segments are supplied by the first sacral root. The portion of the limb innervated by L-5 is more lateral on the thigh and the leg, the front of the ankle, the top of the foot and the 2nd, the 3rd and the 4th toes. Since all nerve roots have different dermatomes, determining the location of pain by careful history taking and the demonstration of sensory changes in the limbs will indicate the nerve root involved and will locate the level of the disk lesion. If the roots supplying the heel or

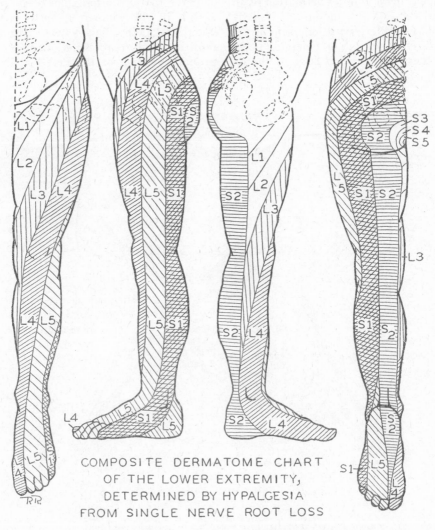

COMPOSITE DERMATOME CHART
OF THE LOWER EXTREMITY,
DETERMINED BY HYPALGESIA
FROM SINGLE NERVE ROOT LOSS

FIG. 68. Dermatome charts of the lower extremity.
(Keegan, J. J.: J.A.M.A. 126:868)

patellar areas are compressed, these deep tendon reflexes will be diminished, or absent, thus contributing important diagnostic and localizing information.

The majority of disk lesions occurs in the lumbar region at L-5 or L-4, accounting for the high incidence of lower back pain and sciatica. The nerve root commonly compressed by protrusion of disk L-5 is S-1; by disk L-4 it is L-5, etc. When unilateral nerve root pain, loss of reflex and dermatome hypalgesia exist as the chief characteristics of a patient's illness, the pathologic condition must be directly related to involvement of a nerve root on that side. The recognition of the 1st sacral root syndrome strongly suggests herniation of the L-5 disk and eliminates most other causes of back pain. If there is complete herniation of the nucleus pulposus through a tear of the annulus, tension on the annulus and longitudinal spinous ligament ceases, so there no longer is back pain. There may be only nerve root irritation, causing limb pain and sensory changes.[14]

Lesions of disks in the cervical portion of the spine will produce the same type of pain in the back and pain and altered sensation from nerve root pressure as described for the lumbar disk syndrome. The only difference is in the location of the back pain and the involvement of the upper extremities instead of the lower.[15] Movements of the head and neck aggravate the discomforts. "Whip-lash" injuries may cause the *cervical discogenic syndrome*.[16]

Lesions of the Ligaments, the Fascia and the Muscles

Although involvement of the ligaments, the fascia and the muscles contributes much to the discomfort of disease primarily affecting the spinal column and its articulations, these structures are subject to relatively few primary pathologic processes causing backache. All or any of these soft tissues may be injured in performing heavy work, especially when lifting, pushing or pulling in a stooped position. In sports or accidental injuries these structures alone may be traumatized. When there is no true joint dislocation so-called *back strain* or *sprain* is the result of incomplete tears or

stretching of the tendons at the site of their attachments or unusual use of muscles so that soreness and muscle spasm occur. The erector spinae, quadratus lumborum, latissimus dorsi and trapezius are the muscles commonly injured in these ways. Diagnosis of such injuries depends chiefly upon knowledge of the circumstances of the injury and upon elimination of dislocation-fractures, disk lesions, and other causes by careful studies, *including roentgenograms.*

Pain in the back frequently results from *spasm of the muscles,* which occurs as part of a protective mechanism for a lesion in the spinal column. Irritation of muscles may cause myalgia, tenderness and stiffness which are so commonly experienced following unusual exercise or exposure to dampness and cold. Suppurative myositis in the back is very rare. More often *myositis* exists as part of a generalized disease, such as trichinosis. Muscle biopsy may be required to establish the diagnosis.

A common clinical entity affecting the muscles and the fascia causing backache is that form of nonarticular rheumatism called *fibrositis, myofibrositis,* or *muscular rheumatism.* This condition is often incorrectly diagnosed as spinal arthritis, from which it needs to be differentiated. In fibrositis the posterior neck, the shoulders, the interscapular region and the lumbar region are the most frequently affected. The onset may be abrupt so that it causes an acute painful stiff neck or sore stiff lower back, (lumbago). Severe muscle spasm prevents motion of the involved part and produces much of the pain characterizing this condition. The neck becomes rigid in a position of partial rotation or tilt to one side when the cervical area is affected; a list or a stoop develops when the trouble is in the lumbar back. The jarring of walking may cause so much pain that the patient prefers to remain in bed. When the onset is acute its termination also usually is rapid and complete.

When this disorder has a more insidious onset it may persist as a chronic difficulty. Then the pain is usually a dull ache, and is worse after a night's rest or prolonged inactivity when a "jelling effect" is noted. With activity pain and stiffness lessen; consequently, through the middle of the day the patient is relatively comfortable, but toward evening, with fatigue, stiffness and aching become worse. The affected tissues are usually tender to pressure and squeezing. Pressure over "trigger points" may produce more widespread discomfort. Differentiation from spinal arthritis is established by normal roentgenograms and the absence of features of a systemic disease.

In this form of nonarticular rheumatism, characteristic histopathologic changes are not found. It is likely that the clinical features result from chemical or physicochemical alterations in the fibrous tissue. Studies of stiffness exhibited in many connective tissue diseases indicate that stiffness is accounted for by changes in the elasticity and the viscosity of the tendons more than by changes in the muscles or the joint capsules.[17]

Unless the adjacent soft tissues are irritated, osteoarthritis of the spine causes little or no discomfort; indeed, it is common to find degenerative changes when roentgenograms of the spine are made when no pain has been experienced in the region of the abnormalities. However, degenerative changes in the spine may produce pain, stiffness, and limited motion through the mechanism of irritation of the fibrous tissue structures adjacent to the affected spine. This is a syndrome often referred to as *secondary fibritis* (a fibrositis secondary to spinal osteoarthritis).

Degenerative changes in cervical vertebrae and disks frequently cause *irritation of the spinal nerve roots* entering the brachial plexus, thereby producing shoulder or arm pain. In such instances there is usually neckache, along with more severe pain in the dermatomes of the cervical nerves affected. Movement of the head and the neck increases the pain in the neck and intensifies the component of arm discomfort. Roentgenograms differentiate this from other conditions with which it might be confused.

LESIONS OF THE SPINAL CORD AND THE MENINGES

Trauma of sufficient violence to injure the spinal cord or the meninges almost invariably causes extensive injury to the structural tissues of the back, which is the chief cause of the resultant back pain. *Infection* of the spinal cord and its coverings sometimes is the cause of back pain. Anterior poliomyelitis, for example, usually is characterized in the early stages by posterior headache and stiff neck. In the invasive stage of the disease these symptoms appear to result from reflex phenomena caused by the inflammation, edema and irritation of the invaded nervous tissues. If there is localization of the virus in motor cells supplying spinal muscles, pain and tenderness of the corresponding muscles result.

Diseases which irritate the meninges cause back pain via the recurrent branch of the spinal nerve which carries sensory fibers from the meninges (Fig 65). The discomfort results chiefly from *reflex spasm* of back muscles causing stiff neck (meningismus) and leg signs (Kernig's, Lasegue's and others) characteristic of meningitis. However, back pain is not an outstanding symptom of meningitis. Study of the spinal fluid establishes the diagnosis.

Neoplasms which originate in the spinal cord or its coverings may produce regional back pain by stretch of, or pressure on the meninges, or by invasion of supporting structures of the back. Pain from spinal cord tumors is referred to the sites of distribution of the peripheral nerves affected more often than it exists in the back. When spinal cord tumors cause back pain or referred pain there are usually characteristic sensory or motor changes. Clinical examination, study of the dynamics and the characteristics of the spinal fluid, and roentgenograms of the spine usually indicate the nature of the trouble.

BACK PAIN FROM FAULTY BODY MECHANICS

Many people who have dull back pain do not have a disease localized in any structure of the back; rather, they have a postural defect which strains the back as a whole. In order to understand backache which results from faulty body mechanics it is only necessary to stand for several hours in an unnatural stooped position. Strain of the muscles, the tendon attachments, the

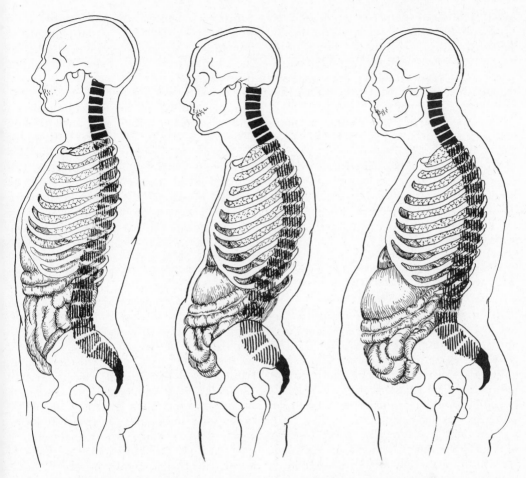

Fig. 69. The postural disorder of "slouch back" (center) and this abnormal posture combined with obesity (right) contrast sharply with normal posture (left).

fascia, the ligaments and the joints causes aching which may persist for days. In a like manner, defective posture may strain tissues that tend to compensate for a postural defect and thus produce continuous and prolonged pain.[18]

Inequality of leg length, arthritis of the hip, scoliosis and other lesions that cause imbalance of the paired structures of the back or alter the line of weight-bearing may cause back pain. The disturbance in the line of weight-bearing may be in the anteroposterior plane. Examples are dorsal kyphosis, increased lumbar lordosis and "sway-back" from disproportionate abdominal obesity or gravidity. Any abnormal posture causes strain on some of the ver-

tebral joint capsules, on the intervertebral ligaments, the tendon attachments and the muscles of the back. Postural tone of the back muscles, normally maintained without effort or fatigue by the autonomic nervous system, is then partly maintained by voluntary contraction of some of the muscles in the back in an effort to compensate. This quickly leads to fatigue and back pain. The discomfort is added to by the strain on the joint capsules and the ligaments in the spine where the increased curvature exists.[19]

The disturbed relationships of many parts affected by the "slouch" position of the back (with increased dorsal kyphosis, increased lumbar lordosis and a more horizontal position of the pelvis) are illustrated in Figure 69. Obesity with a protuberant abdomen adds to the harmful results. Forward displacement and ptosis of the abdominal viscera causes strain on the suspensory ligaments which attach to the back, thus producing aching pain in the back.

Proper supports for pes planus, exercises to correct postural defects caused by weak back muscles, restoration of good standing, sitting and sleeping postures, and correction of accentuated spinal curvatures are beneficial in properly selected cases.[20] The relief obtained from proper correction attests to the importance of faulty body mechanics as a cause for backache.

Back Pain Secondary to Lesions of Thoracic, Abdominal or Pelvic Organs

In other chapters, the mechanism of reflex pain originating in somatic structures and referred to viscera is explained. The converse of this, viscerosomatic referred pain, is another cause for aching or severe pain in the back. *Lesions in the peripheral portion of the lungs* which may irritate the posterior parietal pleura may cause back pain in the thoracic region. With this type of back pain there are usually important respiratory symptoms that do not accompany primary back pain. Mediastinal tumors (neoplasm and aortic aneurysm) may cause back pain. Saccular aneurysms may erode vertebrae or ribs, causing severe boring pain or radicular pain from irritation of spinal nerve roots. Dissecting aortic aneurysms commonly cause agonizing pain in the back.

Pain in the back is more apt to result from diseased viscera in the abdomen and the pelvis than from intrathoracic illness. The mechanism whereby *gallbladder disease, liver abscess* or *right subdiaphragmatic abscess* cause pain referred to the right shoulder is well known. Other abdominal lesions may also cause back pain. Backache or sharp pain in the back frequently results from *lesions of the gastrointestinal tract*. In most instances, visceral dysfunction causes prominent gastrointestinal symptoms, and backache is a lesser complaint, but Jones[21] and others[22,23,24] have reported instances of duodenal ulcer in which back pain was the only symptom. In most instances back pain from peptic ulcer is a dull ache in the midline (or slightly to either side) between D-5 and D-10. Frequently these patients have been studied by an orthopedist, neurologist, neurosurgeon, gynecologist and internist without finding cause for the pain until massive hemorrhage or roentgenograms indicate the existence of the gastrointestinal lesion. Ulceration is usually found on the posterior wall, in which case back pain seems logical, but occasionally it is found anteriorly.

Low back pain may be caused by disease of the colon or the rectum, especially when constipation exists. The classic balloon experiments of Jones[21] indicate a mechanical basis for the backache due to disorders of the intestine. A distended balloon in the duodenal cap sometimes caused pain in the back or pain that radiated from the xyphoid process through the abdomen to the back. When a balloon was distended in the second portion of the duodenum, pain often occurred in the back or around the margin of the thoracic cage. Distention of the colon frequently caused low backache; sometimes this was the *only* symptom. These studies showed that most, if not all, symptoms caused by these disturbances are fundamentally associated with local distention of the gut either above an area of spasm or above an area of organic disease which causes constriction of the bowel. The splanchnic nerves enter the cord from D-5 to D-12. Nerves to the stomach and the duodenum probably originate in the upper portion of this section of the cord. It has been shown that evulsion of the splanchnic nerves performed under local anesthesia causes severe pain. Often low backache is caused by spasm or dilatation of the colon, and promptly disappears when the bowel disorder is relieved. The fact that the lumbosacral pain due to distention of the sigmoid colon from feces or gas is relieved a few minutes after an enema indicates that the pain is on a mechanical basis.

Perforation of a peptic ulcer may cause pain referred to the back. An ulcer in the posterior wall of the stomach or the duodenum and *penetrating into the pancreas,* or a carcinoma of the pancreas, sometimes causes low dorsal back pain. Agonizing lumbar back pain may be produced by *acute pancreatitis* or *dissecting aneurysm* of the abdominal aorta.[25]

There are records of a number of instances in which lower back pain in the midline or slightly to the right side was caused by an inflamed and distended *retrocecal appendix*. Sudden onset of pain in this region should always make one suspicious of this lesion.

Painful disorders of the kidney parenchyma or capsule usually produce flank pain. Experimental evidence produced by Ockerblad[26] indicates that *obstructive uropathies* which produce stretching of the capsule of the kidney cause pain in the flank. The average area of pain was found to be small (8 to 10 cm. in diameter). If there are pain and tenderness in the costovertebral angle on one or both sides, the urinary tract should be investigated for a causative lesion.

Inflammation in the *prostate* and the *seminal vesicles* may cause low lumbar or sacral pain. Many references have been made to the frequency with which chronic lower back pain is caused by infection or other diseases of the pelvic organs. Chronic lower back pain due to pelvic disease rarely occurs in patients who do not have other more prominent symptoms that would lead to consultation with a urologist or a gynecologist.

Also, it should be emphasized that lower back pain in females is usually *not* due to pelvic disorders. Congestion at the onset of menses, the mechanical burden of the late stage of pregnancy and some pelvic tumors may cause backache for obvious reasons. Sometimes severe infection in the female pelvic organs may cause reflex pain in the low back. However, it has been the experience of most rheumatologists and gynecologists that uterine displacement and low-grade pelvic infection seldom cause backache.

Miscellaneous Causes of Pain in the Back

In the prodromal stages of various febrile illnesses backache may exist along with generalized aching (arthralgia, ostalgia and myalgia) in the extremities. Sometimes septicemia may be ushered in by severe back pain, but soon malaise, fever and other symptoms indicate the nature of the disease.

It is important to realize that some persons who complain of backache have no organic disease anywhere to cause it. Some of these persons are maliciously feigning pain which does not exist. Recent studies among the armed forces have revealed a high frequency of "psychogenic rheumatism" occurring as a somatic manifestation of psychoneurosis. Boland and Corr[27] reported that the lower back is the most frequent site of this manifestation and that, in the group of soldiers studied, back pain was much more often due to psychoneurosis than to intrinsic disease of the spine or to organic rheumatic disease. *Psychogenic backache* is very difficult to diagnose for there are few reliable characteristics. Careful study often reveals unusual localization of pain or bizarre radiation which does not conform to any anatomic pattern.[28] Usually it is uninfluenced by factors that intensity or relieve the pain of organic diseases. Other psychoneurotic manifestations are frequently present. Most difficult is the problem of proper evaluation of the psychogenic back pain co-existing with organic disease capable of producing backache.[29,30]

SUMMARY

Various causes of back pain are explained on the basis of underlying pathologic physiology. Back pain may be caused by disease in any of the many structures in the back. The responsible disease sometimes is evident immediately and in the majority of cases it can be determined through a thorough, systematic study. The complex structure of the back and the multiplicity of ailments to which the component tissues are subject make it imperative to approach the problem in each patient with an unprejudiced viewpoint and to carefully evaluate all evidence in an orderly fashion. Many mistaken diagnoses originate in the narrow viewpoint of specialists who fail to realize that the cause for back pain may lie outside their specialty. The orthopedist must realize that lower back pain may not be due to structural disease of the back, the gynecologist cannot account for all cases of low backache on the basis of pelvic disease, the neurologist can explain only some of the instances of back pain on lesions of the spinal cord or peripheral nerves, and the internist must realize that the different forms of arthritis or nonarticular rheumatism do not account for all instances of pain in the back. Perhaps in no other medical problem is it so important to consider all of the possibilities and to pursue a systematic study to a logical conclusion.

A carefully elicited and complete history of the manner of onset, the location, the radiation and the nature of the pain, the factors that aggravate it and those that relieve it, should be obtained. Thorough physical examination should include special back and leg maneuvers to allow recognition of disturbance of structure and function if they exist. Examination of the thorax should be made whenever pain is located in the upper part of the back. When there is lower back pain examination of the abdomen, the pelvis, and the rectum, including direct visualization of as many of these parts as can be seen, may be required. Roentgenograms of the spine and the pelvis are invaluable aids and in some instances special x-ray procedures (such as myelography) may be helpful. Studies of blood cytology and chemistry, erythrocyte sedimentation and urinalysis are usually indicated. Such a systematic investigation, supplemented by specialists' examinations and consultations, seasoned by experience, should correctly solve most problems of disease producing pain in the back. There are usually anatomic or physiologic disturbances to indicate a structural basis for back pain. Disturbances of posture can usually be recognized as a basis for faulty body mechanics. If back pain is referred from visceral disease, symptoms and signs of such disease will usually be found, if sought.

Pain in the back ranks among the most common problems of medical diagnosis. A thorough study based upon the knowledge of the structure and the function of the back and the lesions that produce pain, together with intelligent interpretation of all findings, will usually yield the solution.

REFERENCES

1. Kellgren, J. H.: On distribution of pain arising from deep somatic structures with charts of segmental pain areas, Clin. Sc. 4: 35-46, 1939.
2. Moldawer, M.: Senile osteoporosis. The physiologic basis of treatment, A.M.A. Arch. Int. Med. 96:202, 1955.
3. Freyberg, R. H., and Gascon, J.: The problem of pathologic fractures in patients with rheumatoid arthritis receiving prolonged corticosteroid therapy, Proc. X International Congress on Rheumatic Diseases, Ed. Minerva Medica, vol. 1, 378-382; Turin, Italy, 1961.
4. Harrold, A. J.: Tuberculosis of the spine, a reassessment of the problem and the results of conservative treatment, Post-Grad. M. J. 31:495, (Oct.) 1955.
5. Polley, H. F.: Symposium on rheumatic diseases; diagnosis and treatment of rheumatoid spondylitis, Med. Clin. of N. A., 39:509, (Mar.) 1955.
6. Hollander, J. H., et al.: Arthritis and Allied Conditions, Philadelphia, Lea & Febiger, 1960.
7. Cleveland, M., Aldridge, A. H., Bosworth, D. M., Ray, B. S., and Thomas, S. F.: Management of low back pain, Proc. N. Y. Acad. Med. 35:778-800, 1959.
8. Wilson, J. C., Jr.: Degenerative arthritis of the lumbosacral joint, the end-space lesion, J.A.M.A. 169:1437, 1959.
9. Rose, G. K.: Backache and the disc, Lancet 1:1143, 1954.
10. Gill, G. G., and White, H. L.: Mechanisms of nerve-root compression and irritation in backache, Clin. Orthop. 5:66, 1955.
11. Keegan, J. J.: Diagnosis of herniation of lumbar intervertebral disk by neurologic signs, J.A.M.A. 126:868-873, 1944.
12. Jacobs, J. E.: Neuralgia and backache, West. J. Surg. 64:202, 1956.
13. Bradford, F. K.: Low back and sciatic pain, J. Indiana Med. Ass. 50:559, 1957.
14. Morrell, R. M.: Herniated lumbar intervertebral disc—cutaneous hyperalgesia as an early sign, Milit. Med. 124:257, 1959.
15. Jackson, R.: The cervical syndrome, Clin. Orthop. 5:138, 1955.
16. Hackett, G. S.: Whiplash injury, Amer. Practit. 10:1333, 1959.
17. Wright, V., and Johns, R. J.: Physical factors concerned with the stiffness of normal and diseased joints, Bull. Johns Hopkins Hosp. 106:215, (Apr.) 1960.

18. Denny-Brown, D.: Clinical problems in neuro-muscular physiology, Amer. J. Med. 15:368-390, 1953.

19. Gaston, S. R., and Schlesinger, E. B.: Symposium on orthopedic surgery; low back syndrome, Surg. Clin. N. Am. 31:329, 1951.

20. Hauser, E. D. W.: Corrective cast for treatment of low back pain, J.A.M.A. 128:92-93, 1945.

21. Jones, C. M.: Back pain in gastro-intestinal disease, Med. Clin. N. Amer. 22:749-760, 1938.

22. Gilson, S. B.: Back pain in peptic ulcer, New York J. Med. 61:625-627, 1961.

23. Mixter, W. J.: Back pain in lesions of gastro-intestinal tract, with particular reference to duodenal ulcer, Am. J. Digest. Dis. Nutr. 4:736-739, 1938.

24. Compere, E. L.: Symptom-complex of visceral spinal pain, Illinois Med. J. 74:434-442, 1938.

25. Burt, H. A., Fletcher, W. D., and Mattingly, S.: Pitfalls in the diagnosis of backache, Ann. Phys. Med. 2:1, (Jan.) 1954.

26. Ockerblad, N. F.: Urological backaches, Kansas City Med. J. 21:22-24, 1945.

27. Boland, E. W., and Corr, W. D.: Psychogenic rheumatism, J.A.M.A. 123:805-809, 1943.

28. Levy, R. L.: Psychogenic musculoskeletal reactions, M. Bull. U.S. Army, Europe 12:175, 1955.

29. Wolff, H. G.: Stress and Disease, Springfield, Ill., Thomas, 1953.

30. Sundt, P. E.: Psychogenic rheumatism, Proc. Roy. Soc. Med. 48:66, 1955.

9

Joint and Periarticular Pain

R. H. Freyberg

ANATOMIC CONSIDERATIONS
PHYSIOLOGIC CONSIDERATIONS
PATHOGENESIS OF ARTICULAR AND
   PERIARTICULAR PAIN

DIAGNOSTIC CONSIDERATIONS
MONARTICULAR PAIN
POLYARTICULAR PAIN

Pain in and about the joints is one of the commonest complaints with which the physician is confronted. The first, and usually the major, symptom of most rheumatic diseases is pain in the region of the affected joints; it persists throughout the active disease. Arthralgia is also a prominent symptom of many nonrheumatic constitutional diseases. In addition to joint pain there is usually much discomfort in the periarticular connective tissues (the ligaments, the tendons, the muscles, the fascia and the periosteum); indeed these fibrous structures are importantly involved in most rheumatic diseases. Knowledge of the mechanisms of production of articular and periarticular pain is important in regard to diagnosis and as a basis for proper therapy.

ANATOMIC CONSIDERATIONS

Studies of the innervation of the joints and the periarticular connective tissues conducted prior to 1930 have been summarized by Gerneck.[1] Using more modern investigative procedures, this subject has been restudied by several investigators. Much of the following anatomic discussion is based upon studies done by the author and Dr. Charley J. Smyth while collaborating in the Rackham Arthritic Research Unit at the University of Michigan between 1938 and 1942.

Joints receive their nerve supply from mixed nerves which also innervate the muscles, the bones and the skin of the same area. Following along the blood vesels to the joints, the articular nerve branches richly supply the joint capsule, and the terminal branches of unmyelinated and some finely myelinated fibers distribute through the synovium and the subsynovial tissue, the adjacent ligaments and the periosteum. In the outer portion of the joint capsule, larger branches of the articular nerves divide to form a rich plexus from which finer branches course, usually along the arterioles, into the subsynovial tissue where a secondary plexus may form close to the synovial surface, or they may terminate individually in synovial and subsynovial cells.

Nerves terminate in the joint capsule and in the synovium in one of three ways:

1. In a fine network often surrounding an arteriole close to the inner lining of the capsule (Fig. 70, Parts 1, 2 and 5, and Fig. 71 top, right)

2. As free nerve endings which may be very close to or actually in the surface (synovial) cells (Fig. 70, Parts 3 and 4, and Fig. 71 top, left)

3. In a special end organ (infrequently). This special end organ is an oval, laminated structure (Fig. 71, bottom, l. and r.) usually found deep in the fibrous portion of the capsule. It appears to be a form of pacinian corpuscle, and very likely functions as a pressure sense end-organ, as this type of corpuscle is known to do when located in the fascia, the tendons and the muscles.

No nerves are found in articular cartilage or in compact bone. Usually nerves travel to articular structures alongside blood vessels; as joint cartilage is avascular, it is to be expected that this tissue should contain no nerves. The importance of this will be emphasized in connection with affections involving the articular cartilage primarily, such as degenerative disease of joints (osteoarthritis).

Periarticular tissues are abundantly innervated, and in all these structures the

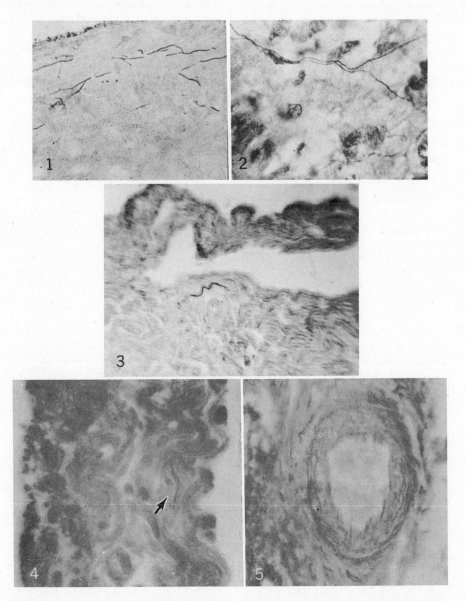

FIG. 70. Sections of human joint capsule, showing silver impregnated nerve fibers. (1) Very near the synovial surfaces at the top of the section there is a rich plexus of small unmyelinated nerves. (2) A higher magnification of subsynovial tissue, shows fine unmyelinated fibrils dividing, joining in a knotlike mesh and separating again. (3) A single unmyelinated nerve very close to the synovial surface near the base of a villus. (4) High-power magnification of a villus cut in longitudinal section, showing a single nerve fiber just beneath the surface. (5) High-power magnification of a synovial blood vessel, showing numerous unmyelinated nerve fibers in or near the adventitia.

nerves have endings like those found in the joint capsule.[2,3] The smaller fibers from these various tissues form larger bundles which become parts of the dorsal spinal nerve root of that segment. The constituent parts of these nerves synapse in similar spinal cord segments. Therefore it is clear why stimuli originating in structures *about* the joints may give rise to a type of painful sensation considered by some patients as originating *in* the joint tissue.

PHYSIOLOGIC CONSIDERATIONS

Lennander[4] found all the articular and the periarticular structures (articular capsule, the synovium, the muscle, the tendon, the fascia, the ligament, the cancellous bone and the periosteum) to be sensitive to pain; the articular cartilage and the cortical bone were insensitive. These results were found to be consistent in patients under different conditions including varying degrees and

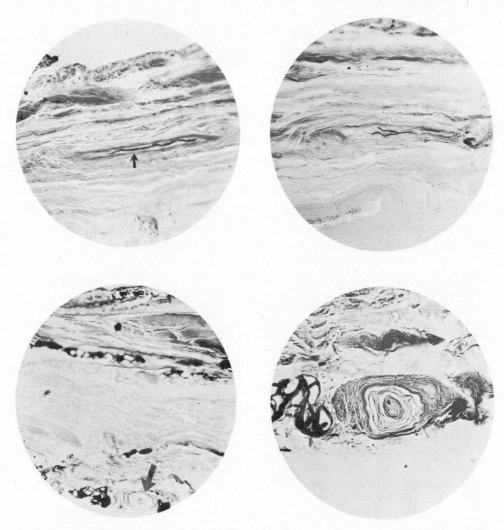

Fig. 71. Sections of human joint capsule stained with osmic acid. (*Top, left*) A subsynovial nerve containing myelinated fibers. Note its proximity to the surface synovial cells at the top of the section. (*Top, right*) Higher magnification of subsynovial tissue, showing a branching myelinated nerve alongside of an artery. (*Bottom, left*) Deep in a joint capsule (synovium at top) is a laminated nerve end-organ, a pacinian corpuscle. (*Bottom, right*) Higher magnification of a pacinian corpuscle located deep in the fibrous tissue of the joint capsule.

types of anesthesia and without anesthesia. Others[5,6,7] have subsequently confirmed these findings. The only structures about which there is doubt concerning sensitivity to pain are the fibrocartilaginous menisci of the knee joints. It has been reported[2] that direct stimulation of these menisci causes no pain, that displacement is painful, and that electrical stimulation causes pain, although in these studies[8] it is difficult to exclude the possibility that the impulses might have originated in surrounding tissue to which the stimuli might have spread.

The type, the localization and the distribution of pain arising from structures in and about the joints have been extensively studied by Lewis and Kellgren; their fundamental research will be reviewed here in some detail. Kellgren[9] injected muscles in various locations with hypertonic saline solution and observed that pain was always felt diffusely and was referred in a spinal-segmental pattern. Ligaments irritated in a like manner gave rise to pain similar in nature to the pain produced in muscle; it was a continuous ache felt *deep* in the limbs or the trunk. This pain was associated with tenderness of the deep structures, in a distribution corresponding to the location of the pain; its presence enabled the persons studied to localize the discomfort accurately to the areas stimulated. Experiments repeated in the same subjects gave remarkably constant results, even though weeks elapsed between observations. Charts of the distribution of pain produced by injection of intraspinous ligaments showed segmental areas of pain which did not correspond exactly with the dermatomes of skin tenderness; this variation suggests that distribution of *deep* pain and tenderness corresponds with the segmental innervation of the *deep* structures rather than of the integument. Pain which arose from the periosteum covering the tibia, the sternum, the vertebral spines, the acromion and the olecranon processes, or the phalanges, (bone structures all of which are close to the surface) was confined to the neighborhood of the point stimulated, whereas pain which arose from deeply situated periosteum was felt more diffusely. Stimulation of nerve endings in the deep fascia in the trunk and the limbs, in the subcutaneous ligaments and the tendon sheaths such as those in the wrists and ankles, and in superficially placed tendons (the patellar and the Achilles tendon), also caused more localized pain like that from superficial periosteum. Deeply situated intermuscular fascia and ligaments gave rise to pain over a larger area, as from deeply located periosteum. Whether pain arising from a given structure is felt as localized or more diffuse pain depends upon the location of that structure (superficial or deep) more than upon the nature of the tissue (periosteum, ligament, tendon or fascia).

Pain arising from muscles of the extremities usually was localized in the neighborhood of the joints which those muscles move, if these joints were in the segmental pain areas corresponding with the nerve supplying these muscles. Pain from smaller joints, such as those in the hands and the feet, tends to be more localized, whereas pain arising in larger joints (the hips and the shoulders) is usually more segmental in distribution. Thus pain arising from disease in the hip joint and the quadriceps femoris muscle is often felt in the knee, and pain arising in the tibialis anticus muscle may be localized in the ankle joint.

The extensive physiologic investigations of Gardner[10,11,12,13] indicate without doubt that the joint capsules and the ligaments are sensitive to painful stimuli. There is less clear evidence that the nerves shown in histologic specimens to terminate in the synovial lining of the joint capsules are pain receptors. Various methods used experimentally to stimulate nerve endings in the synovial lining may also have stimulated pain receptors in the deeper layers of the joint capsule. However, the studies of Kellgren and Samuel[7] conducted in the human knee joint indicated that although the synovial membrane is relatively insensitive, there are some areas of the synovia that are definitely pain-sensitive. The majority of the nerves in the synovial membrane are autonomic in origin and are contained in the blood vessel walls, whereas the fibrous joint capsule and articular ligaments are supplied with somatic nerves with a variety of specialized and unspecialized nerve endings, as shown also by the studies of Gardner.[13]

Lewis and Kellgren[14] studied referred somatic pain in relation to referred pain originating in a viscus. It was found that, at its height, somatic pain experimentally produced in the trunk was accompanied by muscle rigidity and deep tenderness. With induced pain in the extremities, muscle spasm and tenderness were less evident. These features of somatic pain are similar to corresponding abnormalities associated with visceral pain. The nature of somatic pain was found to be exactly like that known to have visceral origin: it was constant, of unvarying intensity and of a quality different from the burning pain originating from the skin or the mucous membranes. Induced somatic pain was frequently accompanied by paresthesia and subsequent hyperalgesia similar in type and location to such symptoms occurring with visceral pain. Lewis[15] states that pain of deep somatic origin cannot be distinguished from that of visceral origin, that deep somatic and visceral structures are supplied by a common set of afferent nerves, stimulation of which produces similar pain and reflex phenomena. It is not surprising, therefore, that observers[16] have called attention to the clinical resemblance of pains from various rheumatic conditions causing pain in the spine, the thorax, the shoulders and the arms to the syndrome of angina pectoris.

Until recently it was thought that pain fibers were carried only in the somatic nerves entering the spinal cord through the posterior roots. Recent reports of Herfort[17,18] indicate that at least a portion of the pain fibers from the lower extremities arrive at the cord centers through the autonomic pathways. Herfort has reported substantial relief of pain due to arthritis in the hip and knee joints by performing the operation of "extended lumbar sympathectomy." By severing the lumbar sympathetic chain along the retroaortic plexus and sectioning the decussating fibers in the prevertebral plexus relief of pain in the lower extremities was accomplished in the majority of arthritic patients operated upon. Herfort believes that this surgical procedure accomplishes this benefit by "the ablation of afferent pain pathways running from the articular surfaces of the lower extremities and traversing the lumbar paravertebral sympathetic trunks and the retroaortic plexus."[17] These observations appear to support the thesis that important sensory innervation of the articular structures of the hip, the knee and the ankle joints is derived from the lumbar *sympathic* ganglia. Support for this thesis is also provided by the report[19] that transient diminution of pain resulted from the administration of tetraethylammonium bromide to patients with rhematoid arthritis. Furthermore, neuropathic joint changes did not occur in any of the sympathectomized patients; this would indicate that the *peri*articular and *extra*capsular tissues are not denervated by section of the lumbar sympathetic trunks, and that there is preservation of the extracapsular protopathic sensation providing sensation of joint position.

PATHOGENESIS
OF ARTICULAR PAIN

The mechanism of excitation of pain-conducting nerve fibers in rheumatic disorders appears to differ in various diseases. Lennander[4] has shown experimentally that when sensitive tissues about joints are stimulated by pinching, tearing, cauterizing by acid or heat, cutting, sticking or use of electric currents the same type of pain results. Lewis[15] confirmed these observations and also has consistently initiated pain by injection of chemical irritants. Knowing that pain can be induced by such different types of stimuli, one can readily understand why most abnormalities of the joints and the periarticular tissues are accompanied by pain.

The nature of the stimuli differs in various types of disease. *Postural abnormalities* and *traumatic joint lesions* produce pain by stretching, pinching or tearing supportive tissues (the ligaments, the joint capsule, the tendons, the fascia and the periosteum). *Neoplastic diseases,* by reason of growth of the tumor and the resultant destructive changes, interrupt continuity, stretch, pinch or otherwise irritate pain nerves and their endings. *Inflammation* that characterizes so many rheumatic diseases (infectious arthritis, rheumatic fever, rheumatoid, arthritis, gouty arthritis, bursitis and tenosynovitis) excites pain by chemical irritation, stretching, tension, pinching and, if there are destructive changes of supporting tissues, by pressure upon nerve endings that are normally protected. *Swelling of the joint capsule* and periarticular tissue or *hydrops* of the joints produce pain by stretching the joint capsule as shown by the relief resulting from aspiration of excessive intra-articular fluid. Absence of discomfort when joint tissues are loosely distended by noninflammatory edema indicates that pain acompanying inflammation of articular structures must be produced by some stimulus other than mechanical irritation. *Chemical irritants* formed during the inflammatory reaction appear to act as important excitants of pain nerve endings but the nature of these chemical irritants is not known.

Traumatic or inflammatory joint disease often is accompanied by *spasm* of adjacent muscles; this contributes to the pain by adding the discomfort of muscle pain or by stimulation of nerve endings in the periosteum through fascial and tendinous attachments. Faulty body mechanics also adds to traction and strain.

DIAGNOSTIC CONSIDERATIONS

The diagnostic significance of joint pain will be considered from two aspects:

1. The evaluation of differences in articular and periarticular pain and the relation of these variations to definite causes.

2. The consideration of characteristics of rheumatic pain occurring in the more common forms of rheumatic diseases, and the correlation of this symptom with associated abnormalities, placing emphasis on practical considerations. It must be appreciated that joint pain may be influenced by many things other than the nature of the pain stimulus. Some persons complain bitterly of discomfort that others may consider trivial, indicating wide variations in the threshold and the tolerance for pain.

A detailed description of the pain is required for the correct interpretation of the symptom. It is important to know the *nature* of the pain, its *localization* or *distribution,* its *constancy* or *variability* and the *factors which accentuate or relieve it.* Different patients may describe pain quite differently as dull, aching, sharp, burning, tearing, pulling, boring, and the like. Even though the patient's intelligence, vocabulary and impressionability may influence his description, the nature of the lesion is a very important factor in accounting for true basic differences in type and severity of joint pain.

MONARTICULAR PAIN

Pain in only one joint may result from a number of different local disorders.

Trauma frequently affects only one articulation. When caused by a single injury, it is usually of sufficient severity that there is a definite history of recent trauma, making the etiologic diagnosis evident. Such trauma commonly originates from sports injuries, occupational injuries, violence or accidental injuries. Traumatic joint lesions are usually one of the following: strain, sprain, traumatic synovitis, fracture of bone extending into the joint, tear of ligaments, tendons or capsule (often resulting in internal joint derangements which thereafter cause recurrent joint pain following relatively minor injury) and joint dislocations. The pain resulting from traumatic joint lesions varies in character depending on the extent of the injury, the joint involved, the tissue reaction to the trauma and other factors.

Sometimes traumatic joint lesions heal in such a way as to disturb the patient's posture or to produce abnormal weight-bearing. During ensuing years degenerative lesions may develop in the damaged joint and thus account for monarticular pain. The hip, the knee, the ankle and the foot are more apt to exhibit such lesions, which are more common in older individuals who have led very active lives. This group of disorders overlaps the field of osteoarthritis and will be considered in more detail in the discussion of that disease.

Neoplastic disease affecting only one joint is rare and is usually a primary tumor (fibroma, fibrosarcoma or synovioma). A bone tumor adjacent to a joint may cause pain in the articulation or referred to it especially during motion of the joint. Neoplasms are likely to cause severe pain frequently described as "expansile" or "boring." Irregular joint swelling, and characteristic roentgenograms, usually indicate the correct diagnosis.

Degenerative joint changes resulting in osteoarthritis frequently cause joint pain in older adults. Although several joints usually are affected, a single weight-bearing joint (hip or knee) may be affected.

Septic Joint. This form of joint disease has decreased in frequency greatly since improved antimicrobial therapy has become available. Infection of articular structures by different microbial agents may result in the accumulation of pus within the joint cavity—a "septic joint." This disorder is usually characterized by severe throbbing pain, which increases as the joint capsule becomes more distended with pus. The patient keeps the affected part in the position of greatest comfort; this characteristic attitude is helpful in the diagnosis. Movement of the affected joint increases the pain due to the increased tension and stretching of the inflamed joint capsule. Unless promptly and adequately treated, there may be extensive destruction of articular cartilage and subchondral bone which is readily visualized by roentgenograms. Study of aspirated synovial fluid usually leads to the correct diagnosis. Culture of the pus reveals the nature of the infecting organism and indicates the proper specific therapy.

Tuberculosis commonly affects a single joint. Tuberculous infection may extend into a joint from a focus in an adjacent bone, or tuberculous joint synovitis may be a metastatic lesion. Characteristically, the disease progresses slowly and the pain is at first mild, but it is usually aggravated by weight-bearing and movement of the joint. Destruction of cartilage and bone usually intensifies the pain and the joint dysfunction. After destructive changes occur, the roentgenographic appearance may be diagnostic.[20] The low-grade nature of the inflammation accounts for the "cold" or "cool" joint. Since bone and joint tu-

berculosis is secondary to tuberculous infection elsewhere in the body, identification of the primary infection is helpful in diagnosis. Tuberculin tests should be made in suspected cases. Often the true nature of the infection is not learned until joint aspiration or biopsy is performed. The possibility of tuberculous arthritis should always be considered when a patient has painful monarticular joint inflammation.

Neuropathic joint disease is often painless. However, mild or moderate discomfort occurring at a joint that may exhibit much swelling and hypermobility should make one suspect a Charcot's joint. Special diagnostic studies usually clarify the diagnosis.

The sudden onset of severe monarticular pain, especially if it is located at the "bunion-joint" in an adult male, always should suggest an attack of *gouty arthritis* (to be described later).

Rheumatoid arthritis commonly affects many joints but in some atypical cases it may begin and persist for many months in only one joint. This possibility must be considered in evaluating monarticular pain.

Nonarticular Rheumatism. Frequently a bursa located near a joint becomes inflamed as a result of trauma, infection or other irritation. The swelling or distention of the sac with fluid may stimulate the pain nerve endings which are numerous in and about the bursa. Because movement of the adjacent joint adds to the irritation, the increased pain caused by the joint motion frequently is erroneously ascribed to disease in the articulation itself. However, bursal pain is elicited only by those motions that disturb the relationship of the bursa, whereas with joint inflammation usually all motions of the affected joint cause pain. The tendons, the tendon sheaths, the muscles and the fascia near a joint may be affected in a similar manner and give rise to "joint pain." When a periarticular disorder exists alone the location of the swelling and the tenderness, and the fact that pain is produced or accentuated only by certain motions of the adjacent joint, serve to differentiate such a lesion from an affection of the joint itself. It is important to distinguish nonarticular from articular rheumatism, for the treatment and the prognosis differ for the two disorders.

SINGLE JOINTS INVOLVED

The diagnostic significance of monarticular pain will now be considered as a symptom in various anatomic locations.

Finger Joint. Pain in a single finger joint is usually due to trauma. The nature and the severity of the pain vary according to the nature of the injury. Diagnosis is based on the history of recent injury, physical findings and roentgenographic findings. A typical example of such a lesion is the "baseball finger," which is traumatic arthritis produced by the extension of a fracture of a phalanx into the adjacent joint, usually the terminal interphalangeal joint.

Wrist. Sprains, strains and fractures of the wrist are common. One lesion characteristically located at the wrist is "ganglion," a localized swelling of one or more of the tendon sheaths which becomes filled with gelatinous fluid. This swelling may be painless but usually there is dull, aching pain. If the ganglion enlarges rapidly, pain may be severe. Diagnosis is readily made by recognition of the cystic swelling, accompanied by local signs of inflammation.

Elbow. Pain at this joint frequently results from trauma, for this articulation is readily injured. At the tip of the elbow the olecranon bursa is frequently traumatized. The pain is usually sharply localized to the inflamed bursa and there may be marked tenderness, crepitant fluctuation, and palpable increase in local heat. Swelling of the distended bursa may be considerable. The pain from acute bursitis usually subsides quickly with proper treatment. Chronic olecranon bursitis is common with rheumatoid arthritis and gout.

Another common cause of elbow pain is "tennis elbow" or *epicondylitis*, which results from severe and repeated pulling of the forearm muscle tendons at their insertion into the humeral epicondyle.[21] Foregoing physiologic and pathologic considerations of joint pain readily explain why pain produced by such a lesion would be considered by the patient as elbow joint pain. Tenderness sharply localized to the epicondyle, pain accentuated by forceful contraction of the muscles of the forearm and absence of pain and signs of inflammation at the elbow joint capsule distinguish this lesion.

Shoulder. Most shoulder pain is not due to arthritis! Besides *fractures* and *dislocations* that cause pain in this joint (concerning which there is usually no diagnostic problem) there are several forms of periarthritis of the shoulder.

One or another form of periarticular (nonarticular) connective tissue disease commonly causes the painful stiff shoulder.[22,23] The most common cause of the painful shoulder syndrome is *calcific tendonitis*.[24] What was usually called bursitis of the shoulder has been recently shown to be, in fact, an inflammation of one of the tendons inserting into the greater trochanter of the humerus, usually the tendon of the supraspinatous muscle.[25] This condition has an acute onset, characterized by severe pain localized in the subacromial region of the shoulder, where there is sharply localized tenderness. Restricted motion in abduction and in abduction combined with rotation makes it difficult or impossible to get the hand behind the back at the level of the waist or the neck. These features of the clinical syndrome make the diagnosis quite certain. Because of the proximity of the involved tendons to the deltoid muscle, pain may be referred to the humeral attachment of the deltoid muscle. Not infrequently calcium salts are deposited in the inflamed portion of the tendon and this condition is then referred to as *calcareous tendonitis*. If the calcium deposit ruptures through the peritendonous tissues, it may localize in the subacromial bursa, which lies over the supraspinatous tendon. Then the condition is complicated by *calcific bursitis*. Frequently calcific tendonitis and subacromial bursitis coexist. Infrequently bursitis exists alone, producing similar shoulder pain. From the character of the pain and its localization alone it is impossible to know whether the lesion is in the tendon, the bursa, or both.

Pain is produced, in part, by distention

of the tendon, or the bursa, or both, and is frequently promptly relieved by puncturing the surface of the distended structure, or aspirating the distended bursal space.

Calcareous tendonitis and calcific bursitis are often associated with pain on abduction and rotation of the shoulder, motions which stretch the inflamed tendon or bursal walls, but flexion and extension do not cause pain. This is in contrast with arthritis of the shoulder which produces pain on motion in all planes.

Tendonitis may develop insidiously; in such cases pain and tenderness are similarly localized, but less severe. Calcium salts may be deposited in the tendon, but often they are not. The character of the pain is the same, unless a firm calcium deposit develops, which may in itself cause or aggravate the pain started by the tendonitis.

Persistence of tendonitis and/or bursitis at the shoulder may cause irritation of other fibrous structures around the shoulder joint capsule and a chronic condition of *adhesive capsulitis* may develop, producing dull aching pain, diffuse minor tenderness which causes progressive limitation of all motions of the shoulder until the motion becomes almost nil. This is the so-called frozen shoulder, a poor, but descriptive term for the almost motionless, painful, stiff shoulder.

If trauma causes a tear in the tendons attaching to the humeral trochanter, or a tear in the musculotendinous cuff, abduction of the shoulder cannot be initiated, a helpful diagnostic characteristic of this lesion. Tears of the musculotendinous cuff of the glenohumeral joint capsule account for a large percentage of cases of shoulder pain. In this condition pain is sharply localized in the subacromial region.

Another form of periarthritis of the shoulder is *bicipital tenosynovitis*. This lesion is characterized by pain and tenderness over the bicipital groove and around the long head of the biceps tendon. The pain can be initiated by movement of the arm requiring contraction of the biceps muscle, and there is persistent tenderness over the lesser tuberosity of the humerus.

Brachial neuritis characteristically causes a more severe and sharp pain which radiates through the distribution of the involved nerves, and in this way it can be differentiated from shoulder joint or periarticular disease. Different associated abnormalities in these conditions also aid in diagnosis.[26]

Shoulder pain may be the principal or the only symptom of *osteoarthritis* involving cervical vertebrae 4, 5 or 6 as a result of osteophytic lesions causing pressure on those spinal nerves which innervate the shoulder. Production or accentuation of the pain by movement of the neck are characteristic of this condition, and roentgenograms confirm the diagnosis.

Since the nature of pain from visceral disease has been found by Lewis and Kellgren to be indistinguishable from that due to somatic disease, it is not surprising that the shoulder, which is in the somatic structure, and innervated by nerves from the same segment that supplies the heart, should be the site of pain after myocardial infarction.[27,28] Absence of aggravation by shoulder motion and detection of signs of cardiac or coronary artery disease help to establish the diagnosis.

Diseases of the gallbladder, the liver or the right basilar pleura may stimulate nerves in the right diaphragm and cause pain felt in the right shoulder. This pain may be sharp, stabbing and severe and may be followed by a dull ache. It can usually be differentiated from the discomfort of shoulder disease by its characteristic location in the scapular region and the absence of signs of shoulder joint abnormality.

Hip. This large, important weight-bearing joint, due to its deep location, cannot be examined directly as satisfactorily as can most other joints. To learn the cause of hip pain, it is often necessary to conduct extensive studies, employing indirect observations. During childhood, *aseptic necrosis* and *osteochondritis* of the femoral head,[29] *separation* and displacement of the capital femoral epiphysis, and *tuberculosis* frequently cause hip pain. Recalling the discussion concerning the reference of pain originating in deep structures to more superficial areas supplied by nerves from the same spinal segment, it is readily understood that persons with disease of the hip may complain of pain along the anterior aspect of the thigh or at the knee. Similarly, associated with hip pain from any cause, pain along the distribution of the femoral nerve is the rule. Such pain should suggest lesions at the hip rather than in the lower back, disorders of which are most frequently associated with leg pain of sciatic or obturator nerve distribution.

Sometimes hip pain and associated anterior thigh discomfort is caused by strain or tension of the hip-joint capsule. Such lesions may result from trauma sustained years before the pain begins. With these types of post-traumatic disorders pain may occur only at a certain point in a particular motion of the joint. No other abnormalities exist. The lesions are important only because of the discomfort.

Septic arthritis of the hip joint is usually very painful, chiefly because the capsule of this large articulation is so firm that it is relatively nonexpansile; consequently, a small amount of purulent intracapsular fluid causes great tension of the capsule, resulting in severe pain. The position of flexion, abduction and external rotation gives greatest relaxation of the capsule and explains the characteristic attitude of the patient afflicted with this lesion.

Osteoarthritis (malum coxae senilis) is a very common cause of hip-joint pain in an adult past middle age. The pain of this disorder is usually of the dull aching type, felt chiefly when bearing weight; it is accentuated by walking. It gradually grows more severe, and sometimes incapacitates the patient. The mechanism of production of this pain will be discussed in the section on degenerative joint changes. Very frequently anterior thigh or knee pain is a prominent feature of this disorder. Otherwise good health, absence of clinical and laboratory signs of inflammation, limitation of motion at the affected joint, and characteristic roentgenograms help establish this diagnosis.

Pain located at the greater trochanter may be due to underlying bone disease; more often it is caused by *trochanteric tendonitis* or *bursitis*. Although less common than similar lesions about the shoulder joint, tendonitis or bursitis should be considered when tenderness is localized in the region of the femoral trochanter and when the hip joint is normal. The pain is often described as being felt in the hip.

Knee. Pain occurs at the knee more often than at any other joint for several reasons. The knee joint is a large joint, important in locomotion and weight-bearing; it is a complex joint, the structures of which can readily be injured or inflamed; and it is situated in a vulnerable anatomic location.

Trauma is frequently responsible for knee pain. The numerous traumatic lesions common to other joints will not now be considered but the lesions peculiar to the knee deserve special mention.

Numerous intra-articular structures may be strained, torn, or otherwise injured so as to cause internal derangement of the joint, which usually produces severe pain. The manner of production of the injury and the localization of the pain may indicate the nature of the lesion. When the injured structure is rather superficial, sharp localization of tenderness may be diagnostic of the structure traumatized. For example, tenderness localized bilaterally adjacent to the patella at or below the level of the tibiofemoral joint line indicates injury of the infrapatellar fat pad; tenderness at a point midway between the patella and the internal collateral ligament is characteristic of tear of the anterior portion of the internal semilunar cartilage; and tenderness localized to the medial aspect of the knee at the joint line usually results from injury of the internal collateral ligament. Painful locking of the joint is usually the result of a movable fragment attached to an internal structure such as a semilunar cartilage or to the pressure of a loose body in the joint. All the lesions are painful because of stretching, pinching or tearing of sensitive joint structures.

Pain localized at the site of attachment of the patellar tendon, and produced by extension of the leg at the knee in an adolescent child, is characteristic of partial separation of the tibial tubercle (Osgood-Schlatter disease). The pain is due to tension on the sensitive, traumatized tissues of the epiphysis by contraction of the quadriceps muscle. Tenderness sharply localized at the tubercle and characteristic roentgenograms establish the diagnosis.

Massive hemorrhage into the knee joint cavity (which is frequent in hemophiliacs) causes diffuse, quite severe pain, accentuated by standing or by movement of the joint. History of injury, tender diffuse swelling of "doughy" consistency and discoloration from superficial hemorrhage suggest the nature of the lesion; aspiration of blood proves the nature of the swelling causing the pain.

The knee is frequently painful because of *osteoarthritic changes*. Pain from this disease is dull or aching in nature and is usually felt only with weight-bearing movement of the knee during climbing or descending stairs or hills, walking on uneven ground or arising from a sitting position. In large measure it is produced by irregularities of weight-bearing surfaces or osteophytic projections straining the sensitive tissues around the articular surfaces (the synovium, the fibrous capsule, the ligaments, the periosteum, etc.).

The knee is frequently the site of *neuropathic joint disease,* diagnostic features of which have been described.

Pain in the posterior aspect of the knee may be caused by *cystic swelling* of the joint capsule or the adjacent tendon sheaths. The cyst results from herniation of the synovial membrane through the posterior part of the joint capsule or from the escape of fluid through the normal anatomic connections of the knee joint into bursae or tendon sheaths (most commonly of the medial gastrocnemius or semimembranosus). In all these conditions swelling, producing tension or traction, accounts for the localized pain, which is relieved by aspiration or surgical removal of the hernial sac.

It is appropriate to caution again that dull, aching pain felt anteriorly at the knee may be caused by a hip-joint disorder, and if the knee and the surrounding structures are normal, disease of the hip should be suspected and searched for.

Ankle. This joint is particularly subject to sprain, which causes pain localized to the lateral or medial aspect of the joint,

depending upon whether the injury caused forced inversion or eversion of the foot. Other traumatic lesions common to many joints need no special mention here. Monarticular arthritis of the ankle is not common.

Foot. Injury or inflammation of the Achilles tendon or the Achilles bursa causes pain and tenderness localized at the sites of these structures. Foot strain frequently results from relaxation of the anatomic arches. The postural disturbance resulting from *pes planus* may be sufficient to cause posterior leg pain or even backache. Diffuse pain felt on the plantar aspect of the foot may be caused by strain or inflammation of the plantar fascia. Metatarsal pain may be due to pinching of the nerve between the 4th and the 5th metatarsal bones (Morton's metatarsalgia), to stretching of the capsule of a metatarsophalangeal joint or the adjacent periosteum (Freiberg-Kohler's disease), or to periosteal irritation from fracture of a metatarsal shaft (march fracture). The history of metatarsal pain existing months before other joints become affected with *rheumatoid arthritis* has been sufficiently frequent that one should suspect this disease whenever an adult complains of foot strain or metatarsal pain and tenderness. Clavus, callus or bunion formation usually can be readily identified as causes of local pain at the toes. Severely painful inflammation localized at the medial aspect of the bunion joint in male adults is characteristic of *acute gouty arthritis* of the first metatarsophalangeal articulation (podagra).[30]

POLYARTICULAR PAIN

Systemic Disorders. Aching in and about many joints is usually part of the symptomatology of a constitutional disease. Many acute systemic infections, during their prodromal or early clinical stages, cause diffuse aching, including multiple arthralgias. The mechanism of production of arthralgia in such diseases is not known. The nature of the disease causing such somatic pain usually becomes evident by the early development of characteristic features. The rheumatic symptoms lessen or disappear early in the illness. Severe joint pain may be a prominent symptom of a generalized non-rheumatic disease such as acute leukemia.

Arthralgia and periarticular pain occur frequently and may be prominent symptoms in *chronic brucellosis;* suppurative arthritis develops occasionally, but brucellosis seldom causes chronic nonsuppurative polyarthritis.[31]

Infectious Arthritis. Gonococcal arthritis, once a common form of specific infectious arthritis, is now relatively rare because antibiotic therapy is so effective for the initial infection. Between 10 and 20 days after the onset of gonorrhea, if there is systemic spread of the infection, the patient experiences marked malaise with aching throughout the body. A few days later the general aching and arthralgia subside and signs of inflammation appear in a few joints, in which pain becomes intensified. The pain of gonococcal arthritis is due to the effects of inflammation of the synovium and the joint capsule. If purulent arthritis develops, the characteristics of septic joint disease appear. Although rare, the possibility of gonococcal joint disease should be kept in mind, for adequate therapy is very effective in accomplishing cure. Unrecognized and inadequately treated, gonococcal infection in a joint may rapidly cause irreparable destruction of the articular cartilage and consequent crippling.

Other infections such as meningococcal and pneumococcal diseases, may be complicated by infectious arthritis involving multiple joints with clinical features similar to those described for gonococcal arthritis, but all forms of specific infectious arthritis are rare now that antimicrobial therapy is so effective. Culture of joint fluid aspirated from infected joints usually establishes the etiology of the joint disease.

Rheumatic Fever. This febrile disease occurs primarily in children and young adults. The joint pain of rheumatic fever is usually so characteristic that it is very helpful in diagnosis. The onset of the arthritis of rheumatic fever usually begins shortly after a hemolytic streptococcal infection, frequently in the tonsils or the pharynx. Several joints, often paired joints, become inflamed; the synovitis worsens rapidly so that within 24 hours the joints are markedly swollen, red, hot and exquisitely tender. Intense pain may be so severe that the slightest jarring of the bed or the weight of bed clothes on the joints causes the discomfort to be excruciating. After several days inflammation leaves the affected joints and moves to others; thus the disease is characterized by "migratory" arthritis. There are no anatomic or functional residua after the joint inflammation subsides.

If one knows these typical features, the diagnosis can usually be made correctly. The joint pain is due entirely to the inflammation, is quantitatively related to its severity and leaves as the synovitis subsides. Salicylates more quickly and completely relieve the joint pain and inflammation of acute rheumatic fever than that of any other disease. The existence of carditis or chorea, and normal appearance of the joint structures in roentgenograms, are other valuable diagnostic aids.

Gouty Arthritis. No discomfort produced by rheumatic disease is more characteristic than the pain of an acute attack of gout. The disease occurs almost exclusively in adult males. The sudden onset of severe pain of increasing intensity in one or more joints, often the bunion joint of the foot (podagra), is typical. After only a few hours the affected joints may be intensely inflamed and severely painful. There is exquisite tenderness at the inflamed joint. Without treatment the inflammation and the discomfort usually subside after several days, leaving no residual abnormality. The patient resumes normal activity and continues to feel entirely well for months or years until another similar painful bout of gouty arthritis may be experienced in joints previously affected or in other articulations.

Numerous provocative factors are known. These include overeating, irregular meals, purine-rich foods, alcoholic debauches, fatigue, exposure to severe cold or dampness, ill-fitting shoes, unusual physical activity and many other irregularities of life. The attacks tend to increase in frequency and severity, and residual changes may develop in the repeatedly affected joints due to tophus formation and destruction of joint tissues. Gout should be suspected from the history of a typical attack in an adult male. The clinical impression is strengthened by finding hyperuricemia, but the diagnosis is proved only by the demonstration of urate crystals in tophi or joint fluids.[32]

It is not known whether local concentration of urates in joint structures is a factor in production of the attack of gouty arthritis, but recently it has been shown by Howell and Seegmiller[33] that injection of urate *crystals* can produce synovitis simulating gouty arthritis. The discomfort of acute gouty arthritis is due entirely to the synovitis. In chronic tophaceous gout the structural changes in the joints add to the pain when the joints are moved or support weight.

In doubtful cases the diagnosis is aided by observing dramatic relief of inflammation and pain by the proper administration of colchicine. The fact that it is so dependably effective in gout and usually valueless in other rheumatic disorders makes the use of colchicine a helpful therapeutic test.[34]

Rheumatoid Arthritis. A very common cause of polyarticular pain is rheumatoid arthritis. The joint abnormalities of this diffuse connective tissue disease begin with inflammation of the synovium and the joint capsule. The joint inflammation becomes chronic and causes the pain at the affected joints, but since the inflammation is commonly not intense, the pain is usually described as dull or aching in character. The joint discomfort is usually quite constant, and is intensified by movement of the joint and by weight-bearing, which adds strain and tension on the joint capsule and the periarticular structures. When joint fluid accumulates, distention of the inflamed capsule adds to the joint pain and restricts motion.

As the disease progresses the synovitis causes cartilage destruction resulting in irregularities of joint surfaces. There may be a grating type of discomfort when the joint is moved. Additional discomfort may be caused by muscle spasm. As crippling results, the joint deformities are additional causes of pain. The paresthesia and the neuralgic and the myalgic pains which frequently occur in this disease are due, at least in part, to inflammatory infiltrations in the perineurium of peripheral nerves and in muscles,[35,36] or to the neuropathy due to vasculitis.[37]

Much discomfort from this disease is due to nonarticular abnormalities, especially irritation of the muscles and the periarticular connective tissue, as shown by the early beneficial response to corticotrophin and corticosteroids. Benefit from these hormones in the rheumatoid patient usually begins with relief of stiffness, allowing greater and easier motion, followed by significant improvement in the joint synovitis.

In the very early stage of the disease there may be nothing to differentiate rheumatoid arthritis from other diseases with polyarticular nonpurulent inflammation. As the disease progresses, the chronicity with remissions and relapses, the evidence of systemic illness with slight fever, the leukocytosis, the elevated erythrocyte sedimentation rate, the anemia, the malnutrition, the skin and muscle atrophy, the development of joint deformity and ankylosis and the characteristic roentgenographic changes, make diagnosis easy. Demonstration of the rheumatoid factor in serologic tests is confirmatory, but is usually not possible in early stages of the disease when help in diagnosis is most needed. Rheumatoid arthritis affects individuals of any age, but is much more frequent in young and middle-aged adults. Juvenile rheumatoid arthritis (Still's disease) usually has characteristics similar to the adult disease.[38] Chronicity, greater constitutional changes, muscle, skin and bone atrophy, joint deformities and the absence of cardiac abnormalities help to differentiate the disease from rheumatic fever, with which it may be confused.

Features clinically indistinguishable from classical rheumatoid disease frequently characterize the syndrome of systemic lupus erythematosus. Visceral inflammation and the demonstration of the lupus factor (L. E. cell, etc.) help to identify this syndrome.[39]

Degenerative Joint Changes. Osteoarthritis (hypertrophic arthritis, degenerative disease of joints) is about as common a cause of joint pain as rheumatoid arthritis. This disorder begins as a degenerative change of articular cartilage which slowly progresses to cause thinning of the cartilage, irregular joint surfaces and irritation of the periosteum covering the adjacent bone, with resultant osteophytic and hypertrophic changes. Since cartilage contains no nerves, as long as the disease is confined to that structure the degeneration may progress subtly and indolently. After articular cartilage becomes eroded and osteophytes develop, movement of the joint and its use in weight-bearing produce pain as a result of strain and tension on the sensitive supporting periarticular fibrous tissues. Joint pain in osteoarthritis is largely due to ligamentous or muscular strains or to mild synovitis.[40] When the affected joints are not being subjected to weight-bearing, the patient is usually comfortable.

The sharply contrasting pathology of the two common forms of chronic arthritis—rheumatoid and osteoarthritis—fully explains the differences in the joint discomfort accompanying these disorders. Osteoarthritis is a disease of older adults who are usually constitutionally healthy; it is a local joint disorder chiefly affecting the weight-bearing articulations. These characteristics, together with the absence of signs of inflammation usually clarify the diagnosis.

Because of the frequency of degenerative joint changes in older persons, it is not unusual for persons beyond middle age who develop joint inflammation due to rheumatoid arthritis to exhibit characteristics of each disease process, including both types of pain. Similarly gout or specific infectious arthritis may occur with osteoarthritis.

Nonarticular Rheumatism—Fibrositis. A painful disease that should be differentiated from common forms of chronic arthritis is the type of nonarticular rheumatism frequently called primary fibrositis, muscular rheumatism or periarthritis. This occurs frequently in adults of middle age or older. Joints are not affected, but the adjacent fascia, muscles, tendons and ligaments are involved. There is no characteristic histopathology in the affected nonarticular connective tissue. The abnormality appears to be due to chemical or physicochemical changes of undefined nature.

This disease may be quite widespread or localized to such parts as the neck, the lumbar spine, or one or both shoulders or hands. The discomfort is usually described as "not a pain but an aching soreness" associated with stiffness of the affected parts. Symptoms are usually worse in the morning after a night's rest, as though the muscles had congealed; with activity through the day the pain and stiffness lessen and may disappear. Toward evening, with fatigue, the discomfort tends to increase. Diagnosis must be based on the pattern of symptoms, the physical findings and the exclusion of other diseases. In differentiation, the absence of physical and roentgenographic signs of abnormality of the joint structures, the absence of fever, leukocytosis, anemia, and undernutrition and the presence of a normal erythrocyte sedimentation rate are all helpful.[41,42]

Unexplained Arthralgia. Sometimes patients complain of constant or oft-recurring pain involving many joints, when repeated physical examination and laboratory studies fail to reveal any evidence of joint disease. The pain is usually described as a "soreness" or "aching"; it may be constant or intermittent. Etiologic possibilities include psychogenic, allergic, or "toxic" factors. Present knowledge concerning the mechanism of such joint pain is so meager that further discussion would be futile. Often it is necessary to diagnose "arthralgia, unexplained." It is wise to observe these patients for a long time to eliminate the possibility that such pain is a prodromal manifestation of slowly developing chronic arthritis.

SUMMARY

Joint pain and periarticular discomfort are very common symptoms of many different diseases. For full understanding of joint and periarticular pain, and in order to interpret these symptoms most profitably in diagnosis, it is necessary to understand the anatomic and physiologic bases for articular pain; it is then necessary to analyze the mechanism of production of pain by different pathologic processes. This information, in conjunction with an understanding of the pathologic and clinical characteristics of various diseases, provides a basis for the utilization of the symptoms of joint pain to maximum advantage in diagnosis.

The nature of the discomfort of a few diseases of joints and periarticular structures is so characteristic that correct diagnosis can be suspected from the analysis of the pain alone. In most instances, however, pain calls attention to the fact that a disorder affecting the joints or periarticular structures exists, and its nature suggests the cause, but diagnosis can be made with confidence only after correlating all of the clinical and laboratory data with the symptoms.

REFERENCES

1. Gerneck, I.: Ueber die Nerven den Synovialmembran (Vorlansige Mitteilung), Arch. f. Orthop. 28:599-604, 1930.
2. Stilwell, D. L., Jr.: The innervation of tendons and aponeuroses, Amer. J. Anat. 100: 289, 1957.
3. ———: Regional variations in the innervation of deep fasciae and aponeuroses, Anat. Rec. 127:635, 1957.
4. Lennander, K. G.: Mitt. a. d. Grenzgeb. d. Med. u Clin. 15:465, 1906.
5. Lewis, T.: Suggestions relating to study of somatic pain, Brit. M. J. 1:321-325, 1938.
6. Kellgren, J. H.: On distribution of pain arising from deep somatic structures with charts of segmental pain areas, Clin. Sc. 4: 35-46, 1939.
7. Kellgren, J. H., and Samuel, E. P.: The sensitivity and innervation of the articular capsule, J. Bone and Joint Surg. 32B:84, 1950.
8. Raszeja, F., and Billewicz-Stankiewicz, J.: Sur l'innervation de la capsule articulaire du genou chez le lapin, Compt. rend. Soc. de biol. 115:1267-1268, 1934.
9. Kellgren, J. H.: Observations on referred pain arising from muscle, Clin. Sc. 3:175-190, 1938.
10. Gardner, E.: Nerve supply of muscles, joints and other deep structures, Bull. Hosp. for Joint Dis. 21:153, 1960.
11. ———: The innervation of the knee joint, Anat. Rec. 101:109-130, 1948.
12. ———: The nerve supply of diarthrodial joints, Stanford Med. Bull. 6:367-373, 1948.
13. ———: Physiology of movable joints, Physiol. Rev. 30:127-176, 1950.
14. Lewis, T., and Kellgren, J. H.: Observations relating to referred pain, viscero-motor reflexes and other associated phenomena, Clin. Sc. 4:47-71, 1939.
15. Lewis, T.: Pain, New York, Macmillan, 1942.
16. Ernstene, A. C., and Kinell, J.: Pain in shoulder as sequel to myocardial infarction, A.M.A. Arch. Int. Med. 66:800-806, 1940.
17. Herfort, R. A.: Extended Sympathectomy in Treatment of Chronic Arthritis, J. Am. Geriat. Soc. 5:904, 1957.
18. Herfort, R. A., and Nickerson, S. H.: Relief of arthritic pain and rehabilitation of chronic arthritic patient by extended sympathetic denervation, Arch. Phys. Med. 40: 133-140, 1959.
19. Howell, T. H.: Relief of pain in rheumatoid arthritis with tetraethylammonium bromide, Lancet 1:204, 1950.
20. Rose, G. K.: Tuberculosis of the knee joint, Brit. J. Clin. Pract. 13:241, 1959.
21. Tegner, W. S.: Tennis elbow, Postgrad. Med. J. 35:390, 1959.
22. Steinbrocker, O., Neustadt, D., and Bosch, S. J.: Painful shoulder syndromes, their diagnosis and treatment, M. Clin. N. Am. 39:563, 1955.
23. Albert, S. M., and Rechtman, A. M.: The painful shoulder, Am. Practit. 7:72, 1956.
24. Mosley, H. F.: Disorders of the shoulder, Clin. Symposia 11:75, 1959.
25. Smyth, C. J., et al.: Rheumatism and Arthritis, (Twelfth Rheumatism Review), Ann. Int. Med. 50:366-494, 634-801, 1959.
26. Bucy, P. C., and Oberhill, H. R.: Pain in the shoulder and arm from neurological involvement, J.A.M.A. 169:798, 1959.
27. Ernstene, A. C., and Kinell, J.: Pain in shoulder as sequel to myocardial infarction, A.M.A. Arch. Int. Med. 66:800-806, 1940.
28. Morgan, E. H.: Pain in the shoulder and upper extremity: visceral causes considered by the internist, J.A.M.A. 169:804, 1959.
29. Monnet, J. C.: Osteochondritis deformans, J. Okla. Med. Ass. 52:376, 1959.
30. Smyth, C. J.: Gout, in Hollander: Arthritis, 6th Ed. p. 859, Philadelphia, Lea & Febiger, 1960.
31. Green, M. E., and Freyberg, R. H.: Incidence of brucellosis in patients with rheumatic disease, Amer. J. Med. Sci. 201: 495-504, 1941.
32. McCarty, D. J., and Hollander, J. L.: Identification of urate crystals in gouty synovial fluid, Ann. Int. Med. 54:452, 1961.

33. Seegmiller, J. E., Howell, R. R., and Mala-
wista, S. E.: Inflammatory reaction to sodium urate; its possible relationship to genesis of acute gouty arthritis, J.A.M.A. 180:
469, 1962.

34. Freyberg, R. H.: Gout, Arth. and Rheum.
5:624, 1962.

35. Freund, H. A., Steiner, G., Leichtentritt, B.,
and Price, A. E.: Peripheral nerves in
chronic atrophic arthritis, J. Lab. Clin. Med.
27:1256-1258, 1942.

36. ————: Nodular polymyositis in rheumatoid arthritis, Science 101:202-203, 1945.

37. Johnson, R. L., Smyth, C. J., Holt, G. W.,
Lubchenco, A., and Valentine, E.: Steroid
therapy and vascular lesions in rheumatoid
arthritis, Arth. and Rheum. 2:224, 1959.

38. Grokoest, A. W., Snyder, A. I., and
Schlaeger, R.: Juvenile Rheumatoid Arthritis, Boston, Little, Brown, 1962.

39. Talbott, J. H., and Ferrandis, R. M.: Collagen Diseases, New York, Grune & Stratton,
1956.

40. Kellgren, J. H.: Some painful joint conditions and their relation to osteoarthritis,
Clin. Sci. 4:193-205, 1945.

41. Rosenberg, E. F.: Classification and management of fibrositis, Med. Clin. N. Am. 42:
1613-1627, 1958.

42. Graham, W.: Fibrositis and nonarticular
rheumatism, Phys. Ther. Rev. 35:128, 1955.

10

Pain in the Extremities

RAY DAVID WILLIAMS

PERSPECTIVE OF THE PROBLEM

The complexity of the problem and the variety of tissues involved in consideration of pain in an extremity are manifest in the reactions of the diagnostician who is confronted by a person complaining of pain in the foot. First of all, he listens to the uninterrupted description of the pain and then supplements pertinent points by cross-questioning, for he has learned that the history of the pain is perhaps the most important part of the examination. He looks at the foot for evidence of ulceration and discoloration of the skin; he palpates the foot for signs of heat, edema and point tenderness in the tarsal and the metatarsal joints. The quality of pulsations of the posterior tibial, dorsalis pedis, popliteal and femoral arteries is noted and, as the examination proceeds proximally, the characteristics of the veins, the joints and the muscles are observed. The joints of the ankle, the knee and the hip are extremely flexed, extended and rotated, and the joints of the lower back are carefully examined by palpation. The thigh is flexed on the abdomen, and the leg is extended to determine the effects of traction on the nerve trunks. The patient is caused to cough for evidence of aggravation of the pain by increase of fluid pressure in the spinal canal and to "bear down" for evidence of aggravation of pain by increase of pressure of the pelvic organs on the lumbosacral plexus and, if pain is produced by such manipulations, the pelvic plexuses are palpated by combined pelvic and abdominal routes. If examination up to this point has not provided a clue to the cause of pain, the examiner ponders the possibility of defect within the spinal canal and this prompts a detailed examination of reflexes and other tests of the central nervous system. If a clue to the cause of pain is not yet found he considers whether the defect might be in the brain or even in the psyche.

ANATOMIC BASIS OF PAIN

It is evident that a pain in the foot, for example, may arise distally from defects of the skin, the bones, the joints or the muscles of the foot, or the muscles and the bones of the leg and the thigh. It may arise medially from defects of the nerve plexuses secondary to disease of the pelvic organs. Pain may arise proximally from disorders of the spinal column which affect the dorsal ganglia and the nerve roots of the spinal cord. Defects of the spinal cord may cause pain in the extremity, especially when there is involvement of nerve fibers in the anterior commissure and the spinothalamic tract. Pain may arise most proximally from defects of the brain.

The reviews by Tower[1] on the receptive mechanism of pain and by Gasser[2] on the pain-producing impulses in the peripheral nerves indicate that the element or unit of the peripheral sensory receptive mechanism for pain is not a spot innervated by a particular nerve fiber but an area of terminal distribution of a unit neurone of variable extent but of much more than spot dimensions. In any area many such unit terminals overlap and interlock intricately, still there is no fusion. Bishop[3] has presented evidence concerning the nature of the unit pain area and has shown that it is composed of the terminals of several fibers derived from a nerve twig. It appears that pain impulses are carried in both myelinated and unmyelinated fibers, the fastest conduction velocity being in the myelinated fibers and the slowest being in the unmyelinated fibers. These nerve fibers are aggregated into peripheral nerves which subserve definite cutaneous areas. The nerves are rearranged into nerve plexuses and finally enter the spinal canal to form dorsal ganglia. The fibers are then reformed into the posterior root which enters the cord as a number of rootlets in the line of the posterior lateral sulcus. These rootlets break up on entering the cord into medial and lateral filaments. The fibers of the lateral filaments are small and are both myelinated and unmyelinated. They enter Lissauer's tract where they ascend for a short distance and then end in the gray matter of the posterior horn. At this point new neurones arise and cross through the anterior commissure of the spinal cord to be reformed in the lateral spinothalamic tract, where they ascend to the lateral nucleus of the optic thalamus. New neurones are formed which go to the sensory cortex. The anatomic elements in the transmission of impulses of pain are diagrammatically represented in Figures 72 and 73. Old and new contributions to the anatomy and physiology of pain were reviewed by Sweet.[4]

PSYCHIATRIC BASIS OF PAIN

It is recognized that seemingly identical degrees of trauma in two persons may produce quite different degrees of response. One person may react with more than usual overt signs of severe pain while the other exhibits evidence of only minor discomfort. In the former instance the threshold of pain is said to be low and in the latter instance the threshold is said to be high. However, it is known that deprivation, abuse and disease can convert the strong person into a state in which pain is poorly tolerated. In contrast, habituation to pain, with lessened response, may occur under certain circumstances. The factors affecting the threshold for pain must be evaluated in each clinical case.

METABOLIC BASIS OF PAIN

Pain arising in any tissue may represent a disturbance of its normal metabolic processes. The total quantity of metabolic derangement may vary independently of the total intensity of metabolic disorder. For example, a limb deprived of its arterial blood supply has easily demonstrable accumulation of intermediary carbohydrate metabolites such as pyruvic acid and lactic acid and a great disarrangement of extracellular and intracellular fluids and minerals. On the other hand, compression of a dorsal root by a tumor may cause little or no accumulation of intermediary metabolites in the spinal fluid and perhaps only by microhistochemical methods of analysis could one demonstrate accumulation of metabolites or derangement of intracellular and extracellular phases in the nerve root beneath and distal to the tumor. However, in the latter instance, although the quan-

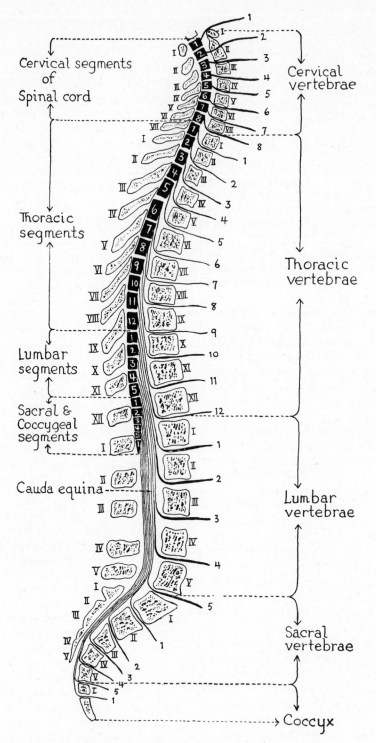

FIG. 72. Diagram of the position of the spinal cord segments with reference to the bodies and spinous processes of the vertebrae. Note also the place of origin of the nerve roots from the spinal cord and their emergence from the corresponding intervertebral foramina. (Modified from Tandler and Ranzi.) (Strong and Elwyn: Human Neuroanatomy, Baltimore, Williams & Wilkins)

tum of disturbance is small, the intensity of the local metabolic disorder may be high. The metabolic processes which support and condition the central and the peripheral nervous systems are as yet quite imperfectly understood. Certain facets of our current knowledge are reviewed by Brücke.[5]

The fundamental metabolic processes in all peripheral tissues are essentially the same, especially in the catabolic (breakdown) phase. It appears quite certain that the anabolic (buildup) phase is limited or absent in certain tissues, for example, ner-

vous tissues. Nervous tissues are parasitic in the sense that they depend on other tissues of the body for menstruum of carbohydrate substances which they use for energy. Therefore, all tissues are not equally susceptible to abnormal metabolic conditions. For example, deprivation of thiamine of a degree sufficient to produce neuropathy associated with pain and paralysis of muscles of the legs may not be sufficient to produce severe disturbance of muscles of the arm or of the heart.

We have considerable knowledge of the

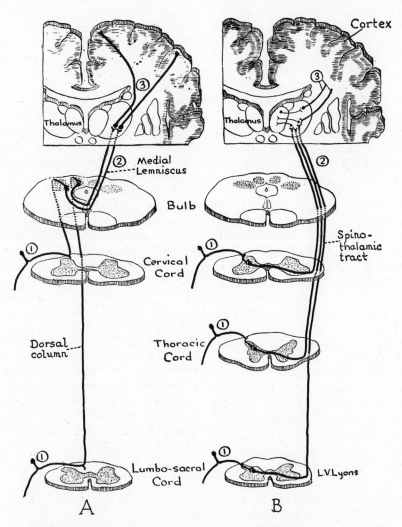

Fig. 73. Scheme of dorsal column (A) and spinothalamic tract (B) and the paths of which they are a part. (1) first neuron (spinal ganglionic); (2) second neuron (medial lemniscus in A, spinothalamic in B); (3) third neuron (thalamocortical). (Strong and Elwyn: Human Neuroanatomy, Baltimore, Williams & Wilkins)

variations in energy metabolism in healthy and diseased tissues, but we know much less of the disequilibrium of water and mineral phases in diseased tissues. Perhaps disorder of the mineral and water phases in traumatized tissues is of the greatest importance in causation of pain, for in traumatized tissue there is not only an increase of blood supply but there is also an accumulation of fluids and minerals. Pain-producing substances in human inflammatory exudates and plasma were demonstrated by Armstrong.[6] Lindahl[7] studied pain in the skin by jet injection of water-soluble substances. He tried varying the osmotic pressure, varying concentrations of inorganic ions, organic metabolites, histamine, serotonin and acetyl choline. All caused some pain. Pain was demonstrated by shift of hydrogen ion concentration above a pH of 9.1 or below a pH of 6.2, with maximal pain at a pH of 3.2.

NATURE AND CAUSATION OF PAIN IN THE EXTREMITIES

Skin

When the pain impulse originates in the skin it is sharply localized. It varies in intensity and duration, but it does not vary in essential quality or tone although it can be produced by pricking, by heat or by electrical stimulation. Stimuli of short duration, such as pricking, burning or plucking a hair, produce a pricking sensation, but stimuli of longer duration give rise to a burning sensation. Continued friction, abrasion and crushing of the skin and application of ultraviolet light or of irritant substances to the skin all give rise to a definite continuous pain. Long-continued stimuli apparently injure the skin and give rise to local redness and tenderness which may appear within a few minutes or be delayed for several hours. This delayed reaction is associated with a condition of increased responsiveness to stimuli, a condition which Sir Thomas Lewis designated *hyperalgesia*. The state of the skin in the hyperalgesic state is such that stimuli which are perceived merely as touch in adjacent areas are felt as painful stimuli in the sensitized area. The response is not only more intense, but it also has an unusual diffuseness. A single tug or brush of the skin of this area elicits unpleasant burning with the act, and after an interval of a few seconds there is a recurrence of similar pain which lasts several minutes. Warming the affected area of the skin to 40°C. or cooling it to from 5° to 15°C. may cause severe pain. An area of skin made hyperalgesic may exhibit spontaneous pain which is relieved by warming or cooling.

Tension upon hyperalgesic areas of the skin plays an important role in causing spontaneous pain. If the area is on the foot, the dependent position greatly aggravates the pain, and elevation of the foot decreases the pain. The aggravating effect can be produced by increasing the venous pressure in the leg with a tourniquet applied proximally to the hyperalgesic area with the pressure of the cuff somewhat above the venous pressure. However, the pain is relieved if pressure in the cuff is raised above the arterial pressure and venous filling is prevented. Lewis[8] has studied cutaneous hyperalgesia induced by crushing or faradization of the skin or faradization of the cutaneous nerves subserving areas of the skin. He observed that when the skin is faradized, after an interval of 6 minutes an area of soreness developed around the area of faradization and that within a few more minutes the size of the area had increased and spread up and down the arm. The soreness was detected when the skin was lightly rubbed. He also observed that when a cutaneous nerve was faradized an area of the cutaneous distribution of the nerve became hyperalgesic in ten or fifteen minutes and was maintained for a number of hours. If prior to the stimulation the nerve was blocked with procaine distal to the point of stimulation, hyperalgesia did not develop. He reached the conclusion that stimulation of the cutaneous nerve, which ordinarily is thought to carry impulses only from the periphery to the central nervous system, created impulses that traversed the nerve centrifugally and changed the skin supplied so that it liberated substances which acted on the pain receptors. On the basis of his observations he postulated a system of nerves which, belonging to the posterior root system, are associated with local defense against injury; he called them nocifensor nerves. The existence of a separate system of nerves is denied by Tower[1] and Wolff.[9]

Lewis and Pickering[10] have studied the trophic disturbances of the skin, the subcutaneous tissues and the underlying muscle arising from defects of the peripheral nerves. One of the most common clinical conditions is that of *causalgia* arising from injury but not transection of the median or the sciatic nerves. Within a few days or a few weeks pain develops in the territory of the nerve. The pain increases in severity and characteristically it is burning in quality. There is extreme tenderness of the corresponding area, and pain is elicited by friction rather than pressure, for pressure appears to relieve the pain. Extremes of temperature provoke the pain, and the patient guards the limb from all contacts. After a time the skin of the affected area assumes a red or purple tint; it is glossy or smooth and devoid of wrinkles. Such areas of the skin are often wet with sweat and are sites of herpetic lesions. It appears certain that initially there is no defect of the skin but that later definite defects of the skin are present. These gross disturbances of the skin apparently arise as a result of chronic *centrifugal impulses* from the injured cutaneous nerve. Armstrong *et al.*[6] have described the isolation of a substance from inflammatory exudates and fresh plasma which produced pain when applied to the base of a cantharidin blister. It is of considerable interest that sympathectomy of the region abolishes the pain. The mechanism of relief of pain by sympathectomy is not clear, but it has been observed that following removal of the sympathetic ganglia there is an increased flow of blood through the cutaneous areas and an improvement in the color of the skin.

Herpes zoster, degenerative disorders of the peripheral nerves secondary to arteriosclerosis and vasospastic disease and inflammatory or traumatic lesions of the peripheral nerves are common clinical causes of hyperalgesic states. Osteoarthritis of the cervical and lumbar vertebral joints is a frequent cause of irritation of the dorsal roots and the spinal nerves. Impulses passing centrifugally (antidromically) create areas of cutaneous hyperalgesia, and such areas may be sites of herpetic lesions.

The skin and the subcutaneous tissues are affected by disorders of the blood vessels.[7] Maintenance of normal vasomotor tone is a function of the sympathetic nervous system. Several vasotropic disorders, such as acroparesthesia, erythromelalgia, Raynaud's disease and scleroderma, are thought to be caused by primary defects of the blood vessels of a nature which results in a hyperdynamic response to their innervation. Sympathectomy in such derangements exerts a favorable effect. The trophic disturbance appears to be secondary to excessive *constriction* or *dilatation* of the blood vessels. The skin defects are, as a rule, the more superficial manifestations of trophic defect of the entire digit or limb.

Acroparesthesia occurs more frequently in women than in men, usually between the ages of 30 and 60 years, and it may be associated with naturally occurring or artificially induced menopause. Long-continued immersion of the hands in water appears to be a precipitating factor. The subject complains of unpleasant sensations in the hands or the feet. The sensations are crawling, tingling or swelling and they are more severe at night. The distribution is not according to the distribution of peripheral nerves, but the areas on the hands and the feet are of glove or stocking distribution. These areas may exhibit hyperesthesia or hypoesthesia. The hands and feet are cold and pale.

Erythromelalgia occurs more frequently in men than in women and in the group from 20 to 40 years of age. Exposures to extremes of temperature or to trauma from vibrating tools appear to be precipitating factors. The pain in the extremity is described as burning, sticking and tingling. The pain is usually intermittent and it is made worse by dependency of the extremity. The skin becomes red. Initially the pulsations of the arteries and the arterioles are quite forceful, but gradually arterial pulsations become less forceful and the color of the extremity becomes a dull red or violet. The subcutaneous tissues tend to become edematous. The palms of the hands and the soles of the feet are involved; touch and pressure become extremely painful and it is difficult for the subject to wear gloves and shoes. The skin becomes thick and tight and the nails grow thick and brittle. The underlying muscles become atrophic and tender.

Raynaud's disease occurs more frequently among females than among males, usually between the ages of 25 and 35 years. One or more fingers or toes, the border of the ear or the tip of the nose suddenly becomes white and cold. Cold sweat appears on the affected area and in the same area numbness, formication and some pain are felt, although perception of all types of stimuli may be lost. Pulsation of the local artery may be lost. This stage of cold pallor gives way to a stage of mottled cyanosis and vesicles containing blood or blue-black serous fluid may appear. When the vasospasm is long continued, the superficial layers of the skin become gangrenous. With the remission of the cold pallor stage and the return of blood flow to the affected areas of the skin, the subcutaneous tissues and the underlying muscles, the pain becomes excruciating and the type of pain is similar to that arising from asphyxiated muscle.

Scleroderma often follows or accompanies the Raynaud's syndrome. One first notices edema of the subcutaneous tissues. The skin becomes indurated and then brown and hard, and as the subcutaneous tissue atrophies the skin becomes attached to the underlying muscle or bone.

The fundamental defect in these several vasotropic disorders is *inadequate oxygen supply* to the tissues. The cold pallor of the area involved and the obliteration of pulsations of the larger arteries in Raynaud's syndrome indicate that there is spasm of the larger arteries and complete arrest of circulation. The relatively good pulsations of the larger arteries in the conditions of acroparesthesia and erythromelalgia indicate spasm of the smaller arterioles. Normally a portion of the blood in the peripheral tissues passes through arteriovenous shunts and a portion passes through the capillary bed. If the precapillary arteriole is involved in spasm one may have the paradox of inadequate peripheral circulation in the presence of a bounding pulse. One sees a somewhat analogous phenomenon in the leg which has a shunt between the femoral artery and the vein and in diseases such as thyrotoxicosis and thiamine deficiency in which there is a relative arteriovenous shunt and pooling of capillary blood in the extremity. In these disorders there is a dusky-red cyanosis of the extremity and relatively excellent pulsations.

If it could be demonstrated that in Raynaud's syndrome the vasospasm is more proximal and that in acroparesthesia and erythromelalgia the vasospasm is more distal, the occasional coexistence of these disorders in the same person would be explained and the frequently beneficial effect of sympathectomy in all of these disorders would have a logical basis. However, it would appear that in Raynaud's syndrome the blood vessels are unusually responsive to *vasoconstrictor* impulses and that in acroparesthesia and erythromelalgia the blood vessels are abnormally responsive to the *vasodilator* impulses. The several possible mechanisms of sympathectomy in relief of pain associated with Raynaud's disease, acrocyanosis, scleroderma, causalgia, and related disorders have been reviewed by Ross.[12]

MUSCLE

A detailed study of pain in muscle was reported by Kellgren.[13] All of the somatic muscles give rise to pain. Pain is slight when muscles are pricked with a needle or cut with a sharp knife, but it is severe when they are injected with an irritating substance. A characteristic pain is elicited when muscle is squeezed or when the muscle is exercised severely. The pain is diffuse and agonizing when the stimulus is strong, but it is mild and sharply localized when the stimulus is mild in degree. Diffuse pain appears to be projected to the region of those deep structures in which pain is well localized, which are innervated by the same spinal segments as the structures stimulated. In this way pain in muscle is given its segmental distribution. This segmental distribution of diffuse pain may simply be a form of false localization.

The spinal nerve, after emerging from the intervertebral foramen, immediately divides into two primary divisions. The posterior primary divisions of the spinal nerves are generally distributed to the skin of the back of the trunk, the back of the head, the shoulder and the buttock and to the longitudinal muscles of the back, but not to the muscles of the limbs. The anterior primary divisions of the spinal nerves are composed of elements of both dorsal and ventral roots and are distributed to structures of the lateral and the anterior aspects of the body including the limbs. Kellgren[14] made further observations on the effects of injecting hypertonic saline into the interspinous ligaments. He noted that in the thoracic area stimulation of the interspinous ligaments produced pain not only in muscles of the back but also in muscles of the lateral and anterior thorax. As he proceeded downward he observed that stimulation of interspinous ligaments of the lower thoracic spine produced pain in and phantom tumor of muscles of the abdominal wall. Stimulation of interspinous ligaments of the lumbar spine produced pain in muscles of the legs.

Kellgren concluded from his studies on injection of the interspinous ligaments and of muscles in the extremity that the segmental areas of pain produced by injection of muscles with hypertonic saline are determined by the nerve roots involved in supplying the corresponding muscle, so that different muscles supplied by a common root source will yield a common general field of pain distribution. In the arm there are some muscles the motor innervation of which is regarded as derived from single spinal segments (e.g., rhomboids C 5, flexor carpi radialis C 6, abductor pollicis longus C 7 and dorsal interossei C 8) and injection of these muscles produces pain in a fairly simple deep-pain segmental pattern. In the leg no muscles are supplied on the motor side from a single segment but, broadly speaking, the muscles supplied by the 2nd, the 3rd and the 4th lumbar segments give pain distributed over some part of the front of the thigh, the knee, the shin and the ankle while muscles supplied by the 5th lumbar and the first and the second sacral segments give pain distributed over the buttocks, the back of the thigh and the calf and the foot. The distribution of pain arising from muscles follows a spinal segmental pattern. The pain is deep and diffuse and the pattern does not correspond with the sensory segmental pattern of the skin as demonstrated by Foerster[15] and Head.[16] Pain in muscle secondary to irritation of nerve roots and posterior primary divisions of spinal nerves will be discussed again in the paragraphs on referred pain.

Lewis[17] has conducted extensive studies of ischemia of muscles as a cause of pain. His technic was that of arresting the blood flow of the limb with a sphygmomanometer cuff and working the muscles under relatively anerobic conditions. The muscles of the limb were exercised by rhythmic contractions. After from 20 to 60 seconds pain in the muscles of the limb increased quickly and reached such an intensity that exercise could no longer be performed. The pain was rather diffuse, but it was felt with greatest intensity in the region of the muscles used. It was continuous and did not come and go as the muscle contracted and relaxed. The pain was not caused by tension on nerve elements, for, when pressure was applied to the nerve by a special clamp, the characteristic pain was not produced. The pain in the muscles continued unabated until the circulation was restored and then it ceased in a few seconds. Arrest of circulation without exercising the limb caused within a few minutes a deep cyanosis but not pain, although the circulation was arrested for 15 to 20 minutes. Moreover, a preliminary arrest of the circulation did not materially expedite the onset of pain once exercise had begun. Apparently the immediate cause of pain was not arrest of blood flow and consequent lack of oxygen, but the cause of pain was related to the process of contraction of muscle. That the ultimate cause of pain in such circumstances was *lack of oxygen* has been demonstrated by Pickering and Wayne[18] in cases of anemia and in subjects who had been breathing gases of low oxygen tension.

Horisberger and Rodbard,[31] after recent studies similar to those of Lewis, concluded that their results support the concept of Lewis that a P factor produced in contracting ischemic muscle diffuses to the extracellular space where it stimulates pain fibers. Fatigue appears to share the same mechanism. On resumption of blood flow, P factor is presumptively washed from the site: it may persist as "latent pain," for up to about 10 minutes, becoming manifest as a decrease in the number of contractions which can be performed before pain during a subsequent ischemic period.

Working muscle has a high energy turnover, and in the process of its contraction intermediary products of carbohydrate metabolism are formed. Among the several intermediary metabolites formed in the process of contraction *pyruvic acid* and *lactic acid* have been extensively studied. These substances are known to be formed in large quantities normally in contracting muscle. It is known that they accumulate rapidly in muscles exercised under relatively anerobic conditions. A source of energy is ultimately necessary in the contraction process and this substance is *glycogen* or *glucose*. There are, however, other substances, the *coenzymes* made from thiamine, niacin and riboflavin and *oxygen,* that are necessary for continuation of the process of contraction. In normal muscle there are adequate stores of carbohydrate and coenzymes and, therefore, in relatively short periods of exercise the limiting nutrient when the flow of blood is stopped appears to be the supply of oxygen. However, it must be kept in mind that deficiency of any one of these substances, glycogen, coenzymes or oxygen, might be the cause of pain in clinical cases. The writer has repeatedly encountered muscular aches and pains associated with extreme muscular tenderness in cases of *thiamine deficiency* induced among young subjects who did not have evidence of defective oxygen supply in the limbs.[19]

The cause of muscular pain (myalgia) in acute *virus infections* such as dengue fever, influenza, smallpox, poliomyelitis and encephalitis is not known. In many of such cases there is some evidence of central nervous system involvement (headache, meningism, changes of reflexes and peripheral neuritis) and in such instances one might assume that the dorsal ganglion cells are involved and give rise to pain directly or that the central nervous system becomes more responsive to ordinary stimuli from the periphery (lowered threshold for pain). However, the virus of these generalized infections might also invade the cells of the muscles and interfere with their normal metabolic processes. In the latter instance the pain would be of peripheral origin and somewhat analogous to limitation of oxygen supply or interference with action of the respiratory enzymes. The mechanism by which viruses kill cells is not known, although it is assumed that they inactivate biochemical reactions or compete with the cell for substrate.

One of the commonest causes of pain in muscles is overexercise, particularly among persons unused to strenuous exercise. The muscular pain and soreness comes hours or days after the exercise. Overextension of muscles and resultant strain of muscle sheaths and tendons must be an important contributing cause. The cause of pain in tendons and fascia is discussed under separate heading. It is quite probable that severe and long-continued rises of cellular metabolites associated with excessive exercise cause changes of intracellular and extracellular phases of minerals and water and that these disorders stimulate pain nerve endings. The overexercised muscle has a tense and firm consistency which suggests an increase of volume secondary to increase of extracellular or intracellular fluid.

The invasion of muscle by parasites such as *Trichinella spiralis* produces an intense myositis. In many areas of the muscle there are not only local inflammatory processes, but there is also thrombosis of many of the smaller blood vessels. The pain could be caused either by the local inflammatory processes or by ischemia of isolated groups of muscle fibers. Edema about the eyes, the nose and the face and eosinophilia are evidence of more specific reactions of the body of allergic nature and the relation of these reactions to the muscular pain is not known.

Muscular pain is commonly found among persons who have *defective blood supply* to the limb. The artery may become gradually obliterated as a result of arteriosclerosis or as a result of progressive obliterative arteritis (Buerger's disease). The veins may become obliterated as a result of thrombophlebitis or phlebothrombosis or edematous fluid may interfere with venous return. Under conditions of impaired arterial supply or venous return the muscles of the limb (most often the legs) do not receive sufficient oxygen supply to permit performance of continuous work and after a few steps the characteristic pain of *intermittent claudication* appears. This is the pain of ischemic muscle.

Causes of Muscular Pain

Muscular pain is commonly due to the following causes:

1. Interference with blood supply
   A. Progressive occlusion of the arteries as in arteriosclerosis
   B. Progressive obliteration of the arteries as in Buerger's disease
   C. Recurrent vasospastic disease, such as Raynaud's disease
   D. Defective venous return, as in venous thrombosis
   E. Acute occlusion of arteries
2. Nutritional deficiency disease such as thiamine and niacin deficiency
3. Invasion of muscle by specific organisms such as trichinella spiralis
4. Overstrain of untrained muscle fibers, fascia and ligaments associated probably with changes of intracellular and extracellular phases
5. In association with acute infectious diseases of virus origin
6. Gross hemorrhage into muscle

Fasciae, Subcutaneous Ligaments, Tendon Sheaths and Bursae

The deep fasciae are sensitive to painful stimuli. Kellgren[13] has examined them in detail. He used the method of injection of hypertonic saline and observed that the subcutaneous ligaments and tendon sheaths gave rise to local pain, although the pain may be felt over a wide area when it is severe. The intermuscular fascia and deeply situated periosteum and ligaments do not give rise to local pain but to diffuse pain. Whether pain arising from a given structure is felt diffusely or is confined to the region of the site stimulated depends more on whether the point stimulated lies deeply or superficially than on its anatomic nature (whether fascia, ligament or periosteum). Beneath the skin there is apparently a second sensitive layer in which pain is localized with fair accuracy. This consists of the deep fascia encasing the limbs and any periosteum, ligament or tendon sheath that is situated superficially. All of the structures in this layer give rise to diffuse pain of more or less segmental distribution. Thus the quality of pain derived from all of these deep-lying somatic structures is similar to that derived from muscle, although the pain derived from muscle is likely to waver in intensity, and that from fascial sheaths, tendon and periosteum is generally an aching pain. The mechanism of pain production in these relatively avascular structures is not known. Their metabolic processes have not been extensively studied. It would appear that pain arises in them when their nerve fibers or endings are disrupted by trauma. These structures are relatively inelastic and resist pressure from underlying inflammatory processes. The pain of subcutaneous abscesses is likely to be quite severe and to be sharply localized.

Progressive myositis ossificans is a disease of unknown etiology which is characterized by proliferative inflammation in portions of the fibrous tissues of muscles, tendons, aponeuroses, fasciae and ligaments. Calcium is deposited in the involved structures and ultimately leads to formation of bone and destruction of involved muscles. *Intramuscular fibrositis* appears to be a variant of interstitial myositis. *Primary fibrositis* consists of an inflammatory hyperplasia of white fibrous tissue anywhere in the body, that is, in fasciae, aponeuroses, sheaths of muscles and nerves, tendons, ligaments, articular capsules, subcutaneous tissues and periosteum. These various forms of fibrositis tend to affect muscles and tendons of the spine, but they also affect muscles and tendons of the extremity. Since there is greater degree of movement of muscles and tendons of the extremity, minor degrees of disorder of the fascia and tendons of the limbs lead to severe pain.

Primary fibrositis of the subacromial bursa (subdeltoid bursitis) is an inflammation of the subacromial bursa, adjacent tendons and the capsule of the shoulder joint. Pain is elicited when the shoulder is abducted or the arm internally rotated. Pressure on the bursa causes pain.

The common clinical conditions in which pain arises from fasciae, tendons, aponeuroses and bursae are:

1. Rupture of tendinous insertions in overstretch of tendons.

2. Inflammatory processes within the spaces bounded by tendons and fasciae.

3. Generalized inflammatory hyperplasia of fibrous tissues, that is, interstitial myositis, intramuscular fibrositis, perineural fibrositis (neuralgia) and primary fibrositis of bursae.

BONE AND PERIOSTEUM

Stimulation of bone does not cause pain if the periosteum has been anesthetized. Compact bone can be bored without pain, but when cancellous bone is reached a vague and poorly localized pain is felt. This type of pain is encountered when bone marrow is aspirated or when fluids are injected under pressure into the marrow cavity. In these circumstances sudden *changes of pressure within the marrow cavity* appear to be the cause of pain.

Although bone is relatively insensitive to ordinary stimuli such as boring and cutting, several common disorders of bone are associated with severe pain. It is generally recognized that the periosteum is extremely sensitive to many types of stimuli and especially to stretching or disruption of continuity. It is probable that traction-tension of the periosteum is the cause of pain in expanding lesions of bone such as acute abscesses (osteomyelitis), bone tumors (primary and metastatic), expanding bone cysts, tuberculosis of the bone and gumma of the bone. It is frequently observed that when the abscess, gumma or tumor of the bone breaks through the periosteum, the pain may cease in a dramatic manner.

Pain in rachitic bone might be caused by expansile overgrowth of the soft matrix which exerts traction-tension on the periosteum or by failure of the soft matrix to give adequate support, thus putting the periosteum under tension. A similar mechanism may be operative in the production of pain in bone when it is the site of nonexpansile cystic change (bone cysts of hyperparathyroidism).

Hemorrhage beneath the periosteum, as in scurvy or inflammatory disease of the periosteum (periostitis), causes severe pain and in these instances tension on the periosteum appears to be the cause of pain.

Fracture of bone is associated with pain apparently caused by disruption of the pain-sensitive periosteum of the bone, plus trauma of the soft tissues about the bone, associated with hemorrhage and accumulation of interstitial fluid and spasm of muscles about the site of fracture.

Hypertrophic pulmonary osteoarthropathy causes pain in the long bones which may be secondary to proliferation of the inner layer of the periosteum, a process that has some of the characteristics of a periostitis. However, in this disease there is always considerable edema of the soft tissues about the bone which may be secondary to a low-grade anoxemia of the soft tissues.

Osteitis deformans (Paget's disease) may be accompanied by pain, especially when the process involves the tibia, the femur and the humerus. If the process involves the pelvic bones, the lumbosacral and the dorsal spine, the pain may be severe and of the referred type (that is, pain may be experienced in the trunk, the abdomen or the legs). The cause of pain is not known, but in most instances there is traction-tension on the periosteum either by formation of cysts in the bone or by lack of support of the periosteum by the bony structures.

The common disorders of bone and periosteum associated with pain are:

1. Abscesses of bone (osteomyelitis, tuberculosis)

2. Tumors of the bone (primary and secondary neoplasms; gumma)

3. Hemorrhage beneath the periosteum

4. Periostitis

5. Metaplasia of the bone (rickets; bone

cysts; osteitis deformans; hypertrophic pulmonary osteoarthropathy)

6. Fracture of bone

Joints of the Extremities

Pain originating from joints of the limbs is fairly accurately localized. Pain from the joints of the hand and the foot is quite accurately localized, while pain from the shoulder and the hip joints is less accurately localized and has a more segmental distribution. Pain in a joint tends to be a continuous ache that is aggravated by movement. Movements tend to be limited, and one or more acutely tender spots can be found in the ligaments about the joint. Anesthesia of these tender areas relieves the pain and diminishes the muscular spasm that contributes to the discomfort. The procedure of anesthetizing painful points about joints is extremely useful in differentiating pain arising from the joint and pain arising elsewhere and referred to the joint. The mechanism of pain in joints is discussed in other chapters.

Arteries and Veins

Pain is often, but not always, felt when a needle already through the skin and the subcutaneous tissues is pushed through the coats of an artery. Apparently the intimal layers of arteries are somewhat sensitive to pain. However, the periarterial tissues are quite sensitive to pain, and traction on them or injection of irritating substances about an artery causes severe pain. Apparently the local pain that occurs at the site of an infected thrombosed artery or at the site of an organizing *thrombus* arises from inflammatory and mechanical tension exerted primarily on the periarterial tissues. Lewis[20] reached the conclusion that in *embolism* of an artery of a limb, pain may occur in the region of the clot as a late symptom. The early pain is, in his opinion, not due to the impact or to any other physiologic change stimulating nerves or nerve endings at the site of the clot. The pain is felt in the limb distal to the obstruction, and an interval elapses between the arrest of circulation and the onset of pain. Pain occurs after obstruction of an artery of sufficient size to produce ischemia of the limb,

and the pain is for the most part the result of *ischemia of muscle*. Exceptions to this rule are rare, although occlusion of arteries to the skin as in subacute bacterial endocarditis or cerebrospinal meningitis may cause areas of necrosis of the skin that can cause pain. Embolism or thrombosis of an artery that supplies muscular tissue such as the limb, the bowel or the heart causes pain in contrast with occlusion or thrombosis of nonmuscular tissues such as the brain, the lung or the spleen which does not directly cause pain.

Traction on or distention of the walls of a vein as in thrombophlebitis or phlebothrombosis may cause pain locally. If venous occlusion impairs return of blood from the muscle or the skin of the limb, pain is felt distally to the site of occlusion. Venous distention and accumulation of edematous fluid in the limb may cause some discomfort even at rest, especially when the limb is dependent; but considerable pain is felt only when the muscles of the limb are exercised.

It is apparent that vascular diseases cause pain when they *interfere with metabolic processes* of pain-sensitive tissues such as, the muscle or the skin or when *inflammatory reactions* involve the adventitial tissues of the vessel. The larger vessels have a considerable musculature of the wall, and an occlusion of the vasa vasorum would cause local necrosis and local inflammatory reaction. Periarteritis nodosa is characterized by infiltration of the adventitia, vasa vasorum and loose connective tissue by polymorphonuclear leukocytes, lymphocytes and eosinophils with resulting necrosis of the media and elastic fibers and formation of multiple aneurysms and thromboses with resulting infarctions not only in the peripheral tissues but also in the walls of the arteries themselves.

It is evident that pain almost never arises in the arteries themselves except under conditions of disruption of coats of the artery by aneurysm, thrombosis of the vasa vasorum or inflammatory reactions within the walls of the arteries. The pain so commonly associated with disease of the arteries is secondary to ischemia of pain-sensitive tissues supplied by the artery. Arteriosclerosis, progressive obliteration of arteries

(Buerger's disease), recurrent compression of arteries and veins (compression of the subclavian artery by the scalenus anticus muscle—Haven's syndrome) and recurrent vasospastic disorders (Raynaud's syndrome) cause pain *because they create ischemia* of pain-sensitive tissue.

PERIPHERAL NERVES; NEUROPATHY AND NEURITIS

Affections of peripheral nerves are variously classified as neuropathy or neuritis. In general, neuropathy is applied to disorders in which *degeneration* of nervous tissue is the pathologic process, and neuritis is applied to affections in which *infection* of the nerve or the nerve cell is the primary pathologic process. A clear clinical distinction cannot always be made, for the two pathologic processes may coexist. For example, a nerve that has been undergoing degeneration as a result of thiamine deficiency is much more susceptible to trauma and inflammatory processes than is the normal nerve. Compression of the common peroneal nerve when one crosses one's knees does not ordinarily cause neuropathy; but if a person has thiamine deficiency and crosses his knees, he may develop paralysis of the peroneal muscles. Pressure-traction on a nerve or a nerve plexus may cause neuropathy during ether anesthesia as a result of pressure and the lipoid solvent effect of ether on the sheath of the nerve.

The peripheral nerves are exceedingly attenuated processes of trophic cells. The cells of the nervous system depend on carbohydrate substances for their energy. *Defects of carbohydrate metabolism* (such as thiamine and niacin deficiency and diabetes mellitus) and *defects of oxygenation of tissues* (such as exist in arteriosclerosis, anemia and carbon monoxide poisoning) so impair the metabolic processes of the trophic cell that it cannot sustain the neuron, and the response of the trophic cell is to "cast off" the peripheral process which can be reformed under favorable circumstances.

A distinction must be made between the peripheral nerves, the nerve plexuses and the nerve radicles. Affections of either or all three of these components may exist simultaneously. However, affections of nerve plexuses and nerve radicles are to be discussed under separate headings as a matter of convenience.

Mononeuritis. One nerve may be affected (*mononeuritis* or *mononeuropathy*) by trauma, extension of inflammation or in association with activity of a focus of infection. Direct trauma either causes discontinuity of the nerve or causes inflammatory reaction of the nerve or the perineural tissues which in turn creates pressure on the nerve and thus effects discontinuity of function. Indirect trauma may be caused by prolonged traction-pressure on the nerve. For example, plasterers who work with their hands above their heads have pressure-traction on the long thoracic nerve by the scalenus medius muscle; floor layers, berry pickers and garden workers have pressure on the common peroneal nerve by the peroneal muscles. The effects of mild repeated blows or severe single blows on nerve trunks are evident in the reactions of the ulnar nerve to the blows of an air-compression hammer or the reaction of the same nerve to use of the palm of the hand as a hammer. The cause of the nerve defect in these circumstances is not at all clear, but it is significant that the paralysis of muscles or the pain follows the trauma by a number of days. It is probable that the interstitial tissues of the nerve are contused, and the subsequent organization of these areas results in compression of the axon, although it is possible that the vasa nervorum become occluded and ischemia of the nerve trunk is then the cause of failure of function.

Another large group of defects of single nerves is secondary to disease of adjacent structures such as inflamed joints, myositis, fibrositis, abscesses and tumor. Very rarely the organisms of leprosy, tuberculosis and syphilis actually invade nerves. It is quite probable that disease of tissues adjacent to the nerve interferes with nutrition of the axon.

Defects of single nerves are manifest as paralytic and irritative phenomena. Spasm and fibrillary twitching of muscles and pain in the cutaneous distribution of the nerves are the symptoms. The pain is a constant burning or scalding sensation interspersed with stabbing sensations. Formication, itching and mistaken sensations are common. In lesions of the ulnar and the median nerves the pain spreads up and down the arm from the site of injury and is distributed to the cutaneous area of the nerves (Figs. 74 and 75). The pain (causalgia) is hot and burning, with extreme hyperesthesia; the skin of the area subserved by the nerve becomes glossy and blue and it sweats profusely; the nails may cease to grow. Usually there is tenderness along the course of the nerve. Another peripheral nerve lesion associated with pain is that of the lateral cutaneous nerve of the thigh. This nerve arises from the 2nd and 3rd lumbar segments and appears in the thigh several inches below Poupart's ligament. As it emerges from the fascia lata it is relatively fixed in position and it is vulnerable to the pressure of girdles and belts.

THE COMMON CAUSES OF MONONEURITIS are, therefore, direct trauma, indirect trauma with organization of contused tissues about the nerve, traction-pressure on nerves with interruption of vascular supply, extension of inflammatory processes of adjacent tissues and invasion of the nerve by specific organisms or by tumor.

Polyneuritis. Several nerves may be affected simultaneously (*polyneuropathy* or *polyneuritis*), but the cause of multiple nerve involvement is usually a systemic disease. The systemic disorders associated with multiple defects of nerves are:

1. Vitamin deficiencies. The deficiencies may be primary (lack of intake) or secondary to vomiting, diarrhea, carcinoma or alcoholism. The tissues of the body are fairly well balanced foodstuff and may supply the needs of the body for some time. Therefore, vitamin deficiency disease does not necessarily accompany partial or complete starvation.

2. Metabolic and degenerative disease. Diabetes mellitus, uremia, anemia, arteriosclerosis and Buerger's disease frequently have associated polyneuropathy.

3. Toxins and poisons. Bacterial exotoxins, carbon monoxide poisoning, poisoning with heavy metals, such as lead, arsenic and mercury, lipoid solvents such as chloro-

form and benzene, aniline dyes and triorthocresyl phosphate.

4. Primary infections, such as anterior poliomyelitis, acute infectious polyneuritis (neuronitis) and vaccinal polyneuritis.

Polyneuropathy has been reported following nearly every acute infectious disease and after ingestion or injection of nearly every heavy metal. In many such instances there is often a predisposing factor of nutritional deficiency disease which has impaired the metabolic processes of the cells. Cells that are poorly nourished do not well withstand further stress whether infectious agent, heavy metal or anoxia. However, among the many cases of carbon monoxide poisoning only a few develop polyneuropathy, and among the thousands of persons who develop influenza only an occasional one develops polyneuritis.

THE CHIEF SYMPTOMS of polyneuropathy or polyneuritis are paresthesiae, pain, muscular weakness and atrophy of muscles. Since the longest neurons suffer first and are the first to undergo degeneration, the first symptoms refer to the feet and then progress upward in a stocking type of distribution. The fingers often are not affected until the lower limbs are involved to the middle of the thigh, but once the paresthesiae are detected in the fingers they progress upward in a glove type of distribution. Numbness or "pins and needles" sensations are followed later by development of areas of hyperesthesia or even anesthesia. As units of the deep tendon reflexes are irritated, the reflexes become *hyperactive,* but when the reflex arcs are interrupted, the tendon reflexes *disappear.* Weakness and atrophy of muscles may become severe. When the motor nerves are involved and lose function, the distal muscles are the first involved, and as a rule the extensor muscles fail before the flexor muscles. Pain is a variable symptom of polyneuritis; the discomfort may be as mild as a numbness, tingling or formication or it may be lancinating in nature during the late irritative phase of nerve degeneration. An area of the extremity may be extremely painful in the irritative phase and be totally anesthetic in the subsequent phases of degeneration. However, the muscles are extremely sensitive to pressure during all phases of peripheral polyneuropathy.

THE PATHOLOGIC PROCESS in the nerves in polyneuritis is essentially that which follows section of the nerve. The external layer of myelin is broken up. The sheath of Schwann swells; the perinuclear zone of cytoplasm becomes condensed and these processes envelop the broken-up myelin. The axis cylinder becomes granular and breaks up into small particles. Degeneration of the peripheral nerve appears to be a nonspecific reaction of the trophic cell to any disorder that seriously impairs its metabolic activity. It is obvious that there is biochemical disturbances of the trophic

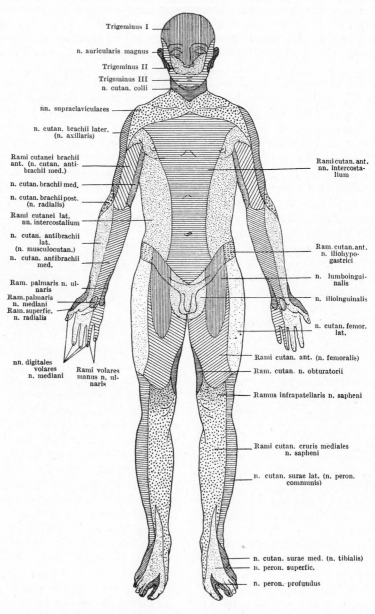

FIG. 74. Diagram of superficial skin innervation on the ventral surface of the body. (After Flatau.) (Grinker, Roy R.: Neurology, ed. 3, Springfield, Thomas)

cell and axon in states of anoxemia (anemia, arteriosclerosis and carbon monoxide poisoning), thiamine and niacin deficiency and of uncontrolled diabetes mellitus. The heavy metals inactivate sulfhydryl (—SH) groups with formation of mercaptans. The sulfhydryl group is found in compounds such as glutathione. These compounds are known to be integral parts of oxidation-reduction systems, to be involved in intermediary protein metabolism and to be used in detoxification of heavy metals. The lipoid solvents either destroy cell membranes or interfere with reactions at the cell membrane. The mechanism by which viruses kill cells is not known, but they prob-

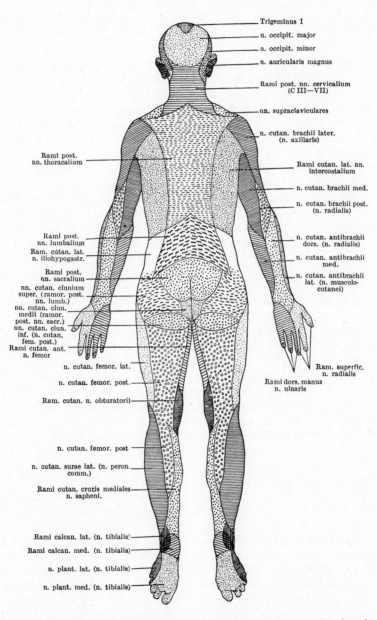

FIG. 75. Diagram of the superficial skin innervation on the dorsal surface of the body. (After Flatau.) (Grinker, Roy R.: Neurology, ed. 3, Springfield, Thomas)

ably act as competitors for substrate or enzymes of the menstruum of the cell.

There is considerable discussion about the causes of polyneuropathy in systemic diseases such as vitamin deficiency, alcoholism, diabetes mellitus and arteriosclerosis. It must be reiterated that *polyneuropathy is a nonspecific reaction* of the trophic cell and axon to any condition that is unfavorable to the metabolic activity of the cell. Polyneuropathy has been described in deficiencies of thiamine[19] (beriberi), niacin (pellagra), pyridoxine and pantothenic acid.[21] Thiamine and niacin are known to be required in certain phases of carbohydrate metabolism, and nerve cells depend on carbohydrate for energy. Deficiency of thiamine is associated with accumulation of pyruvic acid and other intermediary metabolites in the tissues, and there is some evidence that these substances are toxic to the cell in high concentration, although it is more likely that a high level of pyruvic acid only mirrors the general failure of the cell to convert food to energy.

Wintrobe[21] has described degenerative changes in nervous tissues of swine during restriction of pyridoxine and pantothenic acid. The role of pyridoxine in human nutrition has been reviewed by Wayne *et al.*[22]

The association of polyneuropathy and *alcoholism* has been frequently observed. Some observers believe that alcoholism leads to nutritional deficiency which in turn leads to neuritis, while others believe that alcohol is a neurotoxin that can be the sole cause of neuropathy. However, in most cases degeneration of nervous tissue is associated with both chronic nutritional deficiency and chronically excessive levels of alcohol. The writer has repeatedly observed that ingestion of alcohol materially lowers the elevated pyruvic acid levels in the circulating blood of subjects having thiamine deficiency and, for a short time, lessens the constitutional signs and symptoms of thiamine deficiency. Alcohol increases the metabolic activity of cells, and it is quite probable that neuropathy associated with chronic alcoholism may be secondary to abnormally increased metabolic activity of the nerve cells. The neuropathy associated with *febrile states* and *thyro-*

toxicosis may have a similar origin. It is for this reason perhaps that maintenance of adequate nutrition is the most important factor in the prevention of neuropathy in these conditions.

Diabetic neuropathy has been extensively reviewed by Rundles.[23] Histopathology of the central nervous system after exposure to high altitudes, hypoglycemia and other conditions associated with central anoxia has been presented by Hoff, Grenell and Fulton.[24] Peripheral neuropathy is encountered among persons who have diabetes mellitus, who do not have evidence of vitamin deficiency or of defective circulation. Under these conditions it would appear that a defect of metabolism of the nerve cell is the cause of the neuropathy. Neuropathy is more commonly found among older diabetics who have *vascular disease* and have had *inadequate supply of insulin*. On the other hand it may also be found among younger diabetic persons who have chronically taken excessive doses of insulin and have been subjected to long-continued states of *hypoglycemia*. This paradox is difficult to explain unless one assumes that in both excesses and deficits of insulin the metabolic activity of the nerve cell is impaired. This is not difficult to accept, for the coma of the untreated diabetic and the state of collapse of the person in hypoglycemia are simply extremes of underinsulin and overinsulin therapy. When insulin is supplied in excessive doses glucose is taken up by the peripheral tissues, and the level of blood sugar falls. It is possible that adequate amounts of glucose are not made available to the nerve cell. It is not generally known that when large doses of insulin are administered and the blood sugar falls to low levels, there are abnormally high levels of pyruvic acid and lactic acid in the blood and presumably in the cells of the body. It is probable that under these conditions certain tissues are metabolizing glucose at abnormally high rates, but it is not known that the nerve cells are participating in this abnormally increased rate of carbohydrate metabolism. One must conclude that an excessive dose of insulin either lowers the amount of glucose made available to the nerve cell for its energy or that it increases the metabolic activity of the nerve cell to an abnormal degree, thus causing abnormal accumulation of metabolites such as pyruvic acid and lactic acid in the nerve cell. On the other hand, inadequate doses of insulin might cause neuropathy if sufficient glucose was not made available to the cell, if the metabolic activity of the cell was not maintained at an adequate level or if metabolites such as acetone, diacetic acid and betahydroxybutyric acid increased in the cell to an abnormal degree. The phenomena of neuropathies following long-continued insulin excess or insulin deficit may simply be evidences of nonspecific interference with metabolic processes of the nerve cells.

The mechanism by which progressive *obliteration of the vascular supply* to a limb causes pain and neuropathy is generally believed to be a failure of nutrition of the trophic cell or neuron. The principal nutritional deficit is of oxygen supply, not only to nerves but also to other pain-sensitive tissues of the limbs. In many instances the pain is not a manifestation of neuropathy but it is a symptom of ischemia of pain-sensitive tissue. In certain cases provision of additional supplies of thiamine and niacin appears to ameliorate the neuropathy. Perhaps in these cases there is also a failure of supply of nutrients other than oxygen which are required by the cell, and the provision of these extra nutrients enables the tissue to respire adequately with somewhat lower tensions of oxygen.

Patients who have *pernicious anemia* with spinal cord involvement (subacute combined degeneration of the spinal cord, combined system disease) complain of numbness and tingling of the feet and the hands. The extremities may become painful and hyperalgesic, and there may be diminished tactile acuity and atrophy of small muscles of the hands and the feet. These symptoms are evidences of inadequate supply of oxygen, not only to the trophic cell and the neuron but also to other tissues of the extremities. If the pernicious anemia is untreated, evidence of defect of trophic cells of the dorsal ganglia and the anterior horn cells becomes apparent. The histochemical defect in pernicious

anemia may not be specific, for long-continued severe anemias from other causes may give evidences of defects in both peripheral nerves and structures within the spinal canal. Much of the numbness and tingling encountered in both pernicious anemia and secondary anemia are caused by defective metabolism of tissues about the nerve endings, that is, muscle and skin. Later they may be caused by defects of the nerves or central nervous system. Patients who have severe anemia also may have the typical pain of intermittent claudication, that is, the pain of intermittent ischemia of muscle.

Neuritis of the nerve plexuses (plexus neuritis, neuralgia) is etiologically, clinically and pathologically a mononeuritis. Inflammatory disturbance of the plexus is likely to spread upward with involvement of the nerve roots (radiculitis) or downward to involve the peripheral nerves (peripheral neuritis). In all cases of plexus neuritis there is tenderness over the plexus. The cervical plexus is behind muscles, and tenderness of the nerves is difficult to elicit; but the brachial plexus is more superficial, and tenderness can be elicited above and below the clavicle. Tenderness of the lumbar plexus can be elicited by pressure deep in the lower abdomen. Tenderness of the sacral plexus can be elicited by rectal and vaginal routes. In both lumbar and sacral neuritis straining (as at stool or as in lifting a load) causes pain; the pain is distributed in the areas of cutaneous distribution of nerves involved in the plexus (Figs. 74 and 75). Causative agents are legion, but trauma and infection are the most common.

CERVICAL PLEXUS NEURITIS frequently follows carrying heavy loads on the shoulder and against the neck. The *brachial plexus* is injured by falling on the shoulder and the side of the head or by jerking the arm. The *scalenus anticus syndrome* (Naffziger syndrome) is that of pain radiating from the neck down the arm and the forearm beginning at about the seventh cervical spinal process and passing down over the shoulder. The nerves involved are those of the brachial plexus which are compressed by the scalenus anticus muscle or by a cervical rib. Compression of the subclavian artery by the scalenus muscle (Haven's syndrome) produces pain in the arm, but the pain in this instance is caused by ischemia of the muscles of the arm and not by compression of the nerve. Irritation of the lowermost fibers of the brachial plexus by tumors in the apex of the lung or tumors in the axilla causes pain in the distribution of nerves of the plexus.

THE LUMBAR AND THE SACRAL PLEXUSES are less often injured by trauma, but they are more often involved in disease of the pelvic organs such as: infections of the rectum, the sigmoid and the low-lying appendix, infection of the prostate, the Fallopian tubes and the broad ligament and tumors of the uterus, the prostate, the colon and the ovaries. The pain is an ach-

ing in the thighs, the buttocks and about the rectum; the pain is aggravated by straining, by rotation of the thighs or flexion of the thigh on the abdomen and extension of the leg—movements that stretch the nerves of the lumbosacral plexus. Palpation of tissues about the plexus by rectal, vaginal and abdominal routes elicits tenderness of the plexus.

FALSE LOCALIZATION OF PAIN (REFERRED PAIN)

Affections of the spinal nerves, the posterior roots, the posterior ganglia, the dorsal radicles, the posterior horn, the anterior commissure, the spinothalamic tract (lateral), the thalamus and the sensory cortex

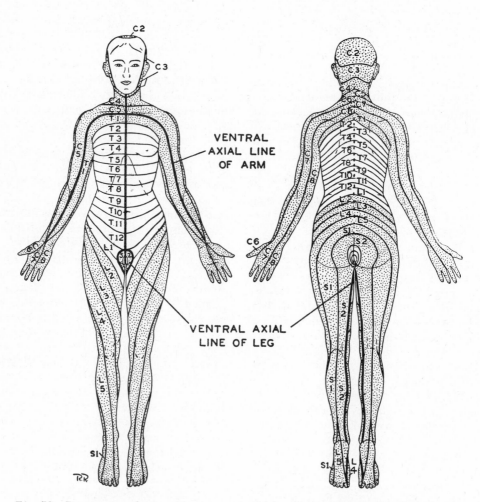

Fig. 76. Dermatome chart, with new patterns in the extremities based on single nerve-root syndromes. (Keegan and Garrett: Anat. Rec. 102:411)

of the brain may give rise to pain felt in the extremities. However, depending on the somatic level of the affection of the nervous pathway, the pain may be felt over the heart, over the gallbladder or over other visceral structures. In the above instances neither the extremity nor the visceral organ is the site of the abnormal stimulus, but the pain has been falsely localized, that is, referred falsely to these structures. For example, hypertrophic osteoarthritis of the cervical 5th and 6th vertebral joints with associated irritation of the 6th cervical radicle may cause pain in the thenar eminence of the hand. In the sense of this example, the term referred pain is used in

LOWER CERVICAL

SIXTH CERVICAL

PAIN Upper Medial Scapula
TENDERNESS over Transverse
 Process of Vertebra
Pain RADIATION to Lateral Arm
NUMBNESS of Thumb
HYPOALGESIA as outlined
REFLEX of Flexor Carpi Radialis
 & Biceps Tendons Reduced
MOTOR WEAKNESS of Thumb
 Biceps & Scapular Muscles

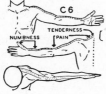

SEVENTH CERVICAL

PAIN Upper Medial Scapula
TENDERNESS over Transverse
 Process of Vertebra
Pain RADIATION to Postero-
 Lateral Arm
NUMBNESS of 2nd & 3rd Digits
HYPOALGESIA as outlined
REFLEX of Triceps Tendon
 Reduced (?)
MOTOR WEAKNESS of 2nd
 and 3rd Digits

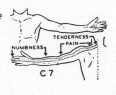

EIGHTH CERVICAL

PAIN over Medial Scapular Spine
TENDERNESS Over Transverse
 Process of Vertebra
Pain RADIATION to Postero-Medial Arm
NUMBNESS of 4th & 5th Digits
HYPOALGESIA as outlined
REFLEX No Changes Recognized
MOTOR WEAKNESS of 4th and
 5th Digits

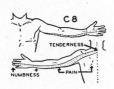

SCALENUS ANTICUS SYNDROME
(EIGHTH CERV. - FIRST THORACIC)

PAIN in Axilla & Medial Arm
TENDERNESS over Scalenus
 Anticus Insertion
NUMBNESS of 4th & 5th Digits
 and Medial Forearm
HYPOALGESIA as outlined
 (Posterior Primary Divisions of
 C8-T1 Not Involved)
REFLEX No Changes Recognized
MOTOR WEAKNESS of 4th & 5th Digits
ATROPHY Small Muscles
 of Hand

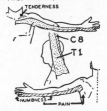

LUMBO SACRAL

FOURTH LUMBAR

PAIN in Gluteal (Hip) Region below Iliac Crest
TENDERNESS over Transverse Process of Vertebra
Pain RADIATION to Anterior Thigh and Leg
NUMBNESS of Anterior Leg, Great Toe
HYPOALGESIA as outlined
REFLEX of Patellar Tendon Reduced
 or absent
MOTOR WEAKNESS of Dorsiflexors of
 Great Toe

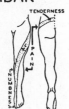

FIFTH LUMBAR

PAIN in Gluteal (Hip) Region between
 Ischial Tuberosity and Femoral Trochanter.
TENDERNESS over Transverse Process
 of Vertebra
Pain RADIATION to Lateral
 Thigh and Leg
NUMBNESS of Lateral Leg, 3 Middle
 (or gt.) Toes
HYPOALGESIA as outlined
REFLEX: Usually No Alteration
MOTOR WEAKNESS of Dorsiflexors
 of ankle and Toes
ATROPHY of Peroneal Muscle Group

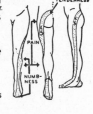

FIRST SACRAL

PAIN in Medial Gluteal (Hip) Region
 (over Ischial Tuberosity)
TENDERNESS over Transverse Process of Vertebra
Pain RADIATION to Posterior Thigh and Leg
NUMBNESS of Posterior Leg, Little Toe
HYPOALGESIA as outlined
REFLEX of Achilles Tendon Reduced or
 Absent
MOTOR WEAKNESS of Plantar Flexors

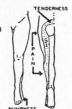

SECOND SACRAL

PAIN in Medial Gluteal Fold
TENDERNESS over Upper Lateral
 Sacrum
Pain RADIATION to Postero-Medial
 Thigh, Leg and Heel
NUMBNESS of Postero-Medial Thigh
 and Labium Majus
HYPOALGESIA as outlined
REFLEX Plantar Flexion
 Response Reduced
MOTOR WEAKNESS
 None Recognized

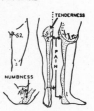

FIG. 77. Common single nerve-root syndromes. (Adapted from Keegan and Garrett: Anat. Rec. 102:415, 417, 419 and 420)

this discussion. The confusion and the disagreement in the use of this term is extensively reviewed by Lewis.[25]

Pain arising in the heart and referred to the neck and the left arm (angina pectoris) and pain arising in the diaphragm and referred to the neck and the shoulder (diaphragmatic pain) are discussed in other chapters.

RADICULAR SYNDROME

The spinal cord fits loosely in the canal and rises slightly when the spine is flexed and sinks slightly when the spine is extended. In the cervical region the nerve roots run almost transversely, while in the lumbar area they run vertically. Although the cord is fairly movable, the nerve roots are rather firmly attached by the meninges. The first pair of cervical nerves (motor) leave behind the articular processes of the first two vertebrae, but all other nerves pass out through the intervertebral foramina, the second leaving behind the first vertebra and the eighth dorsal root leaving behind and below the seventh vertebra. Therefore, in the cervical region if the 6th vertebra is crushed against the 7th, symptoms will refer to the 7th dorsal root. It must be kept in mind that the rootlets are spread out as they enter the cord and that the lowest filament of one root approximates or overlaps the highest filaments of the next lower root.

Each dorsal nerve root relays impulses arising from superficial (skin, superficial periosteum and ligaments) and deep (intermuscular fascia, muscle and bone) structures. The superficial areas have been extensively studied by Head,[16] Foerster[15] and Keegan[26] and the cutaneous dermatomes diagrammatically represented in Figures 76 and 77 are based on the data of Keegan; however,

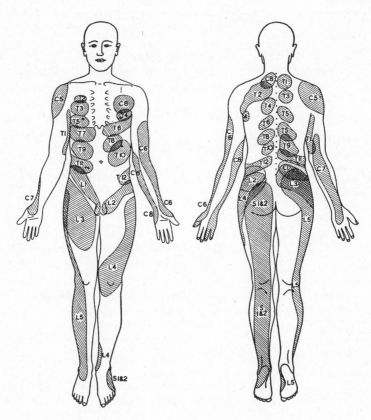

Fig. 78. The segmental areas of deep pain. Kellgren developed the segmental areas of deep pain by injection of the corresponding interspinous ligaments. (Lewis, Thomas: Pain, London, Macmillan)

the segmental areas of deep pain, as might be expected, are somewhat higher and more limited. The segmental areas of deep pain were studied by Kellgren[14] and are represented in Figure 78. It will be recalled that Kellgren injected hypertonic saline solution into the interspinous ligaments and elicited pain and tenderness in the deep structures of the limbs, and the pain lasted for several minutes. The pain was produced by disturbance of nerve endings in the interspinous ligaments, but the pathway of transmission of the impulse is not clear unless one assumes that the interspinous ligaments are innervated by filaments of the posterior primary division of the spinal nerve (Figs. 72 and 73). The distinction between the superficial and the deep dermatomes is important from the standpoint of accurate localization of pain.

A considerable extension of Kellgren's study of the patterns of pain which follow the stimulation of paravertebral and limb muscles was reported by Inman and Saunders[27] and ten years later from the same school Schiller *et al.*[28] made additional observations on autonomic repercussions and cutaneous sensory changes in the skin overlying areas of deep pain and on the influence of somatic and sympathetic nerve block. Their patterns of referred pain after intervertebral injection of a 6 per cent saline solution differ somewhat from those of Kellgren and are given in a series of excellent diagrams in their article.

The pains of sensory radicular distribution are highly characteristic: they are *sharp, lancinating, burning and intermittent* and are referred to cutaneous areas; however, deep aching and tenderness of muscles is present during the intervals between the shooting pains. The superficial area becomes quite *hyperesthetic,* and even light touch is painful. Deep pressure, on the other hand, is not painful, and patients use deep pressure in an attempt to relieve the pain. Coughing, straining and sneezing cause exacerbation of pain. Various manipulations cause pain, for example, with the patient supine, raising the leg more than 45° (Lasegue's procedure) or extension of the knee with the thigh flexed on the abdomen (Kernig's procedure) or flexion of the neck on the sternum (Brudzinski's procedure) produce pain in the superficial or deep areas of segmental distribution because such procedures exert pressure, traction or tension on the affected nerve roots.

The common causes of the radicular syndrome are: herpes zoster, meningitis, tabes; osteoarthritis of the spine, hypertrophy of the ligamentum flavum, dislocation and fracture of vertebral bodies; herniation of the nucleus pulposus, extramedullary tumors of the spinal cord, tumors of the dorsal roots, metastatic carcinoma of the vertebral bodies; syphilis, syringomyelia, hematomyelia, myelitis. A few of these conditions occur with great frequency.

Herpes zoster is an inflammatory process of the dorsal ganglion associated with pain in the cutaneous distribution of the spinal segment and appearance in some cases of herpetic lesions. However, apparently pain in and appearance of herpes on the area of cutaneous distribution of the root may follow root irritation by osteophytes, herniation of a nucleus pulposus and tumor of the cord or meninges. The recurrence of herpes zoster in the same area suggests local predisposing factors.

Fracture-dislocation of vertebral bodies, herniation of the nucleus pulposus and calcification of the ligaments of the spine (hypertrophic osteoarthritis of the spine) are extremely frequent causes of pain in the arm and the leg. The mechanism of production of the last type of pain has been demonstrated by Kellgren, and it appears to arise from irritation or disruption of nerve fiber endings in the ligaments about the vertebral joints. Apparently the interspinal ligaments are innervated in a segmental manner; irritation of them stimulates the posterior division of the spinal nerve, and pain is produced in the extremity as a manifestation of referred pain. In many instances there are peripheral areas of severe hyperalgesia and hyperesthesia associated with skin changes highly suggestive of antidromic effect, that is, impulses passing peripherally over the sensory nerve.

This group of affections cannot be overemphasized, for trivial injuries of the intervertebral disks and ligaments about the vertebrae may cause abnormal calcifications of these structures. Calcification of the ligaments of the vertebral joints may begin at a very early age (25 to 30 years) and give rise to symptoms of pain in the trunk or the extremities.

Keegan[26] studied many clinical cases in which herniation of an intervertebral disk compressed a single nerve root intraspinally and was operated on for relief. On the basis of his many observations, Keegan developed a new dermatome chart (Figs. 76 and 77).

Defects of the leptomeninges, such as acute and chronic adhesive leptomeningitis, may cause pain by traction on the dorsal roots to which they are closely applied. The adhesive process may be circumscribed and simulate a cord tumor or it may be disseminated. It appears probable that the nerve is directly injured and also suffers impairment of its vascular supply.

SPINAL CORD SYNDROME

The dorsal roots enter the spinal cord in the form of root filaments; some of the filaments are medial and some are lateral to the midline. The lateral filaments, which carry pain and temperature, many of them unmyelinated, enter the marginal zone of Lissauer, which is a white column and here secondary connections are made which cross in the anterior commissure to reform and enter the lateral spinothalamic tract of the opposite side to ascend to the lateral nucleus of the thalamus. The incoming fibers push the existing ones laterally; consequently, the lower part of the body is represented by the lateral half of the spinothalamic tract. Tumors in the spinal canal external to the cord gradually fill the space, crowding out the subarachnoid fluid and interfering with local circulation. The area of the cord nearest the tumor suffers most; hence the ipsilateral spinothalamic tract is compressed. The outer fibers are compressed first, and these are from the lower part of the body. Therefore, *disorders of perception of pain and temperature in the legs are frequently caused by tumors in the spinal canal.* The disorder may be a loss of appreciation of

painful and thermal stimuli rather than pain, although pain is sometimes quite severe, especially in tumors of the cauda equina and nerve roots.

Any defect of the central gray matter destroys or irritates fibers crossing in the anterior commissure. Therefore, defects of the cord involving the anterior commissure (central myelitis, syphilis, arteriosclerosis or other disorders associated with thrombosis of the anterior spinal artery) cause defective perception of pain and temperature and, in some instances, pain. The pain is at the level of the lesion, but not above or below it. Pain, if present, is a dull ache or a burning and is referred to the deep and cutaneous distribution subserved by the neuron.

Spinal cord tumors cause motor defects and pain, paresthesia or loss of sensation. If the tumor is near a nerve root, a typical radicular syndrome is the result; for example, tumor at the level of C-1, 2, 3 and 4 causes pain in the neck and the postauricular region and the top of the shoulder; tumor at the level of C-5, 6, 7 and 8 causes pain in the arm; tumor at the level of L-1, 2 and 3 compresses both cord and roots and causes pain in the back, the anterior aspect of the thigh and the upper part of the leg; lumbosacral tumors cause pain in the back, the sciatic region or the perineum; tumors of the filum terminale and the cauda equina cause pain in the small of the back, the sciatic region or the perineum.

CEREBRAL CORTEX SYNDROME; THALAMIC SYNDROME

Subjective disturbance of the sense of pain from lesions of the cerebral cortex was reviewed by Michelsen,[29] who presented cases of lesions of the parietal area and the thalamus associated with spontaneous pain, hyperpathia and epileptic seizures not associated with muscular spasticity or secondary joint, bursa and muscle changes.

Defects of appreciation of ordinary stimuli have long been associated with lesions of the thalamus. Pinprick, heat and cold when applied to the affected side of the body are appreciated only if fairly intense, and there is a delay in the appreciation of the stimulus.[30] Once a sensation is elicited, it evokes a feeling that is far more intense and disagreeable than normal. Scraping, scratching and rubbing cause greater discomfort on the affected side. Spontaneous pains characteristic of the thalamic syndrome may be caused by slight normally unappreciated stimuli of the periphery or by irritative scars of the thalamus following glial organization after vascular accident. Apparently in the thalamic syndrome sensory disturbances of a painful nature can arise as a result of irritation of the nervous pathways anywhere from the periphery to the cortex. The exact mechanism of production of pain in thalamic and cortical lesions is not known.

EVALUATION OF PAINFUL SENSATION

In analysis of pain in the extremity the most important step is obtaining adequate history. Physical examination, although it be done with the greatest care, cannot compensate for inadequate reconstruction of the onset and the development of the painful sensation. Sir Thomas Lewis emphasized the following characteristics in the anamnesis of painful sensation: severity, quality, localization, duration or time-intensity curve of pain, circumstances in which pain develops and duplication of pain.

SEVERITY

If the pain threshold of the individual patient is kept in mind, determination of severity of pain is helpful. Mere statement of severity is not sufficient, for one must elicit collateral signs and symptoms. For example, if the pain was associated with pallor, cold sweat, prostration or syncope, or if the pain was followed by vomiting or assumption of abnormal or unusual positions or if movement was restricted during the pain, one can assume that the pain was relatively severe.

QUALITY

The subject may variously describe the pain as burning, stabbing or twisting. His statements will be clearer if he recalls the types of pain that he has experienced. Most persons have experienced the bright pain of burned or excoriated skin, pinprick or pulled hair. The pain of muscle cramp, squeezed muscle or fatigued muscle is a common experience. Not everyone is familiar with the sensations derived from tendons, periosteum or joint, although a similar dull pain is elicited by squeezing the web of the hands. The pains of a sprained ankle, knee or back are fairly common experiences. The quality of pain derived from stimulation of nerves is familiar and is likened to the "foot going to sleep" or "hitting the crazy bone."

LOCALIZATION

Localization of pain is rarely neglected by the patient and, if the experience is not too remote in time, he is able to state with fair accuracy the location of the pain as being in the skin, the muscle, the bone or the joint. However, it is particularly important to elicit all of the painful areas. For example, pain in the arm may be dominant in the patient's mind, but specific inquiry may reveal that he also had pain in the neck. Pain in the calf of the leg and the heel may be dominant, for example, but eliciting history of pain in the back is important in determining the presence or absence of a herniated nucleus pulposus as the cause of the pain.

DURATION OF TIME-INTENSITY CURVE

Most persons have experienced the sharp pain of a needle prick, the pulsating pain of an abscessed tooth or headache, the long and less rhythmic pain of intestinal colic or distended urinary bladder, the continuous ache of a fatigued muscle or the shooting, tingling sensation of striking the "funny bone."

DUPLICATION OF PAIN, CIRCUMSTANCES UNDER WHICH PAIN DEVELOPS

The patient may recognize that a pain in the calf of the leg is associated with walking and that cessation of walking relieves the pain, that a pain in the leg is associated with bending or twisting the back, that a pain in the arm is associated with movements of the neck or with putting the hands above the head, that numbness and tingling of the ulnar side of the hand is associated with resting the elbows on the arm of the chair or that coughing, sneezing or straining at stool causes pain in the legs.

BREAKING SENSORY NERVE CHANNELS

The effect of anesthetizing peripheral nerves, nerve plexuses, bursas and joints should be determined more frequently than it is, for only in this way can the site of pain be accurately localized in many cases and the pain demonstrated to be central or peripheral in origin.

SUMMARY

Pain in the limbs may be caused by disorders involving any of the structures or tissues of the extremities, or by disturbance elsewhere with the sensory phenomena referred to the limbs. Pain originating in the various sites tends to reveal the point from which it arises by certain qualities and by its location. The nature of the pathologic process resulting in pain may be mechanical, chemical, thermal, toxic, nutritional, metabolic, circulatory, or may involve combinations of these categories. The type of pain, its distribution and the associated clinical phenomena yield important clues as to its cause.

REFERENCES

1. Tower, S. S.: Pain: definition and properties of the unit for sensory reception, Proc. A. Res. Nerv. Ment. Dis. 23:16, 1943.
2. Gasser, H. S.: Pain-producing impulses in peripheral nerves, Proc. A. Res. Nerv. Ment. Dis. 23:44, 1943.
3. Bishop, G. H.: Responses to electrical stimulation of single sensory units of skin, J. Neurophysiol. 6:361, 1943; The structural identity of the pain spot in human skin, J. Neurophysiol. 7:185, 1944.
4. Sweet, W. H., Ch. 12, Handbook of Physiology: Neurophysiology 1, American Physiological Society, Washington, D. C., 1959.
5. Brücke, F., ed.: Proceedings of the Fourth International Congress of Biochemistry: Part III, Biochemistry of the Central Nervous System, New York, Pergamon Press, 1958.
6. Armstrong, D., Jepson, J. B., Keele, C. A., and Stewart, J. W.: Pain-producing substances in human inflammatory exudates and plasma, J. Physiol. 135:350, 1957.
7. Lindahl, O.: Experimental skin pain, Acta Physiol. Scand. 51, Suppl. 179, 1961.
8. Lewis, T.: Pain, Ch. 6, New York, Macmillan, 1942.
9. Wolff, H. G., Hardy, J. D., and Goodell, H.: Experimental studies on the nature of hyperalgesia, Arch. Neurol. Psychiat. 63:188-189, 1950.
10. Lewis, T., and Pickering, G. W.: Circulatory changes in the fingers in some diseases of the nervous system with special reference to digital atrophy of peripheral nerve lesions, Clin. Sci. 2:149, 1936.
11. ———: Observations upon maladies in which the blood supply to digits ceases intermittently or permanently and upon bilateral gangrene of digits; observations relevant to so-called Raynaud's disease, Clin. Sci. 1:327, 1934.
12. Ross, J. P.: Some unsolved problems in the surgery of the sympathetic nervous system, Ann. Roy. Coll. Surg. Eng. 13:356-368, 1953.
13. Kellgren, J. H.: Observations on referred pain arising from muscle, Clin. Sci. 3:175, 1938.
14. ———: On the distribution of pain arising from deep somatic structures with charts of segmental pain areas, Clin. Sci. 4:335, 1939.
15. Foerster, O.: The dermatomes in man, Brain 56:1, 1933.
16. Head, H.: On disturbances of sensation with especial reference to the pain of visceral disease, Brain 16:1, 1893.
17. Lewis, T.: Pain, Ch. 8, New York, Macmillan, 1942.
18. Pickering, G. W., and Wayne, E. J.: Observations on angina pectoris and intermittent claudication in anemia, Clin. Sci. 1:305, 1934.
19. Williams, R. D., Mason, H. L., Smith, B. F., and Wilder, R. M.: Induced thiamine (Vitamin B_1) deficiency and the thiamine requirement of man, Arch. Int. Med. 69:721, 1942; Williams, R. D., Mason, H. L., Power, M. H., and Wilder, R. M.: Induced thiamine (Vitamin B_1) deficiency in man, relation of depletion of thiamine to development of biochemical defect and of polyneuropathy, Arch. Int. Med. 71:38, 1943.
20. Lewis, T.: Pain as an early symptom of arterial embolism and its causation, Clin. Sci. 2:237, 1936.
21. Follis, R. H., and Wintrobe, M. M.: A comparison of the effects of pyridoxine and pantothenic acid deficiencies on the nervous system of swine, J. Exper. Med. 81:539, 1945.

22. Wayne, L., Will, J. J., Feldman, B. I., Becker, L. S., and Vilter, R. W.: Vitamin B$_6$ in internal medicine, Arch. Int. Med. 10: 143-155, 1958.

23. Rundles, R. W.: Diabetic neuropathy, Medicine 24:111, 1945.

24. Hoff, E. C., Grenell, R. G., and Fulton, J. F.: Histopathology of the central nervous system after exposure to high altitudes, hypoglycemia and other conditions associated with central anoxia, Medicine 24:161, 1945.

25. Lewis, T.: Pain, Chaps. 10, 11, 12, New York, Macmillan, 1942.

26. Keegan, J. J., and Garrett, F. D.: The segmental distribution of the cutaneous nerves in the limbs of man, Anat. Rec. 102:409-438, 1948.

27. Inman, V. T., and Saunders, J. B. de C. M.: Referred pain from skeletal structures, J. Nerv. Ment. Dis. 99:660-667, 1944.

28. Feinstein, B., Langston, J. N. K., Jameson, R. M., and Schiller, F.: Experiments of pain referred from deep somatic tissues, J. Bone Joint Surg. 36 A (Oct.) 1954.

29. Michelsen, J. J.: Subjective disturbances of the sense of pain from lesions of the cerebral cortex, Pain, Proc. A. Res. Nerv. Ment. Dis. 23:86, 1943.

30. Walker, A. E.: The Primate Thalamus, Chicago, U. Chicago Press, 1941.

31. Horisberger, B., and Rodbard, S.: Relation between pain and fatigue in contracting ischemic muscle, Am. J. Cardiol. 8:481-484, 1961.

11

Clubbed Fingers and Hypertrophic Osteoarthropathy

BERNARD S. LIPMAN AND EDWARD MASSIE

Clubbing is a physical sign characterized by bulbous changes and diffuse enlargement of the terminal phalanges of the fingers and toes.

Hypertrophic osteoarthropathy is generally considered a further extension of the clubbing process. A chronic proliferative subperiosteal osteitis involves the distal ends of the extremities and is manifested by the digital clubbing and in addition by swelling, pain, and tenderness over the larger involved bones and over the accompanying joints. However, some authors still believe that real differences in clinical significance exist between clubbing and osteoarthropathy and that the etiology and the pathogenesis of these two conditions are different. It is important to define the terms separately.

Many different names have been proposed for what we now know as clubbing and hypertrophic osteoarthropathy. The phenomenon of clubbing has been called *Hippocratic fingers, drumstick fingers, parrot-beak nails, watch-glass nails* and *serpent's head fingers.*

Hypertrophic osteoarthropathy has been called *pulmonary hypertrophic osteo-arthropathy* (originally by Marie[1]), *secondary hypertrophic osteo-arthropathy, hyperplastic osteo-arthropathy, toxigenic ossifying osteoperiostitis, Marie-Bamberger syndrome* and numerous other names. As informa-

tion accumulated, it became apparent that the bone lesions were characterized by the deposition of new-formed periosteal bone and that sometimes there were also joint manifestations; moreover, it became apparent that such changes were not limited strictly to an association with diseases of the lung.

The terms now generally accepted are *hypertrophic osteoarthropathy* for the changes in the larger bones and joints and *clubbing* for the distal extremity changes in toes and fingers.

RELATIONSHIP OF CLUBBING TO HYPERTROPHIC OSTEOARTHROPATHY

At first there was thought to be no relationship between clubbing and hypertrophic osteoarthropathy. They were described separately and considered to be independent entities. Under the unified theory, they have been considered as variations of the same process: hypertrophic osteoarthropathy being the more advanced stage with manifestations not only in the fingers but also in the more proximal parts of the extremities. This relationship is supported by the following facts: (1) The two conditions, either separately or together, occur in association with the same diseases. (2) Clubbing of the fingers is a constant characteristic finding in hypertrophic osteoarthropathy although varying in degree. (3) The osseous changes in simple clubbing resemble those of hypertrophic osteoarthropathy.

As would be expected of the milder, earlier manifestation, clubbing is seen much more frequently than the more advanced state called hypertrophic osteoarthropathy.

As early as the 5th century b.c., Hippocrates[2] described curving of the fingernails in a case of empyema. In the latter part of the nineteenth century von Bamberger[3] and Marie[1] drew attention to distinctive changes in the extremities associated with certain diseases of the lungs and heart. Since these early reports, numerous publications have appeared dealing with the intriguing physical evidences in the extremities of more serious internal disease and with the problem of how they are related. Mendlowitz[4] in his review (1942) gave 337 references. Much remains obscure, particularly concerning the pathologic physiology. As Samuel West[5] stated in 1897, "clubbing is one of those phenomena with which we are so familiar that we appear to know more about it than we really do."

RECOGNITION

CLINICAL FEATURES

The symptoms of clubbing are almost entirely objective, particularly in cases which are developing slowly; usually the patient is not aware of the deformity until it is brought to his attention. Recognition is not difficult if one keeps the possibility in mind and observes the extremities carefully. Occasionally, especially in cases secondary to lung tumors, the more rapid onset of changes in the pulp and nail bed attract the patient's or his manicurist's attention and should alert the physician to the necessity of a chest roentgenogram. In cases of acute clubbing, a feeling of warmth, a burning sensation, sweating, and rarely pain in the finger tips may occur. It is important to detect early clubbing.

Because of its diagnostic implications the condition in its early stages may at times be confused with other abnormalities of the fingers. Early clubbing should be differenti-

ated from: (1) simple curving of the nail, which is seen normally—especially in the Negro; (2) chronic paronychia, in which the soft tissues at the base of the nail are swollen and no change occurs in the nail bed itself; (3) Heberden's nodes, which lie more proximally and rarely cause diagnostic difficulty; (4) chronic infectious arthritis, in which the swelling is periarticular and no change is apparent in the nail bed; (5) epidermoid cysts of the bony phalanges; and (6) felons, where there is associated pain and absence of changes in the other fingers. Early in the process of clubbing, thickening of the fibroelastic tissue of the nail bed produces a definite firm transverse ridge at the root of the nail, best observed on the dorsal aspect of the finger. Lovibond[6] noted this "profile sign." When one views a normal finger from the side, one sees an obtuse angle of about 160° between the base of the nail and the adjacent dorsal surface of the terminal phalanx. This angle is referred to as the "base angle" and is clearly demonstrated in the normal thumb. In early clubbing the base angle is obliterated and it becomes 180° or greater. This "profile sign" is one of the best means of detecting the beginning stage of true clubbing.

Figure 80A illustrates the normal base angle of approximately 160°; Figure 80B shows curving, an alteration that may be present in many normal finger nails. Notice that the base angle is not interfered with, in spite of the fact that the distal nail is considerably curved downward. If the original nail is curved, the clubbing will accordingly be accompanied by curving. Figure 80C illustrates the characteristic base

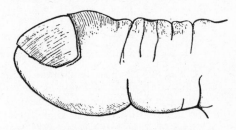

Fig. 79. Drawing of a clubbed finger from Marie's classic report. (Marie: Rev. de méd. 10:1)

angle obliteration in early clubbing; Figure 80D shows advanced clubbing (the base angle is greater than 180° and projects dorsally). In Figures 80E and 80F, illustrating chronic paronychia and Heberden's nodes respectively, the base angle persists undisturbed.

Clubbing usually occurs first in the thumb and index finger, spreading to the other digits later. In the advanced stage there is an increase in all tissues of the finger tips, the soft tissues as well as the nails, so that the ends of the fingers assume a bulbous appearance. In Figure 81, note the typical clubbed fingers in a girl with congenital heart disease. The overlying skin as well as the volar pads are smooth, shiny and bright pink in color. The vascular bed gives a lilac or cyanotic hue to the nails. Witherspoon[7] pointed out that the return of color following slight pressure on the finger nail is characteristically slower than normal. The base of the nail may be elevated so that its outline is seen beneath the skin's surface. Furthermore the nail can be rocked back and forth as if it were floating on a soft edematous pad. Patients may complain of *excessive sweating,* a feeling of *warmth,* or a *burning sensation* in the finger tips; pain is rare but may occur in cases of very acute clubbing. Abnormally frequent filing or clipping of the finger nails is often necessary because of the *accelerated* rate of growth, and longitudinal striations in the nail may appear. Hangnails form readily, due to the rapid growth of the cuticle, resulting often in acute and chronic paronychia. In long-standing cases, particularly in congenital heart disease, dorsiflexion with hyperextensibility of the dis-

tal phalangeal joints may be present. Figure 82 illustrates the appearance of clubbed fingers in a man with carcinoma of the lung.

Various forms of clubbing ("drum-stick," "watch-glass," "parrot-beak" and "serpent's head") have been described, and these variations are now known to be attributable to the duration and the degree of the process as well as to differences in the initial anatomy of the digits. Clubbing of the toes nearly always develops in association with clubbing of the fingers but is more difficult to recognize because of the wide range in the shape of normal toes. The early stage may be best recognized in the large toe. Successive measurements of the nail surface are at times necessary to confirm the diagnosis. Several authors, Mendlowitz,[4] Angel,[78] Buchman and Hrowat,[79] report the presence of clubbing (swelling, thickening, and furrowing of the skin) over the nose, the molar region, the eyelids and the ears.

Hypertrophic osteoarthropathy should always be sought for in the presence of clubbing. Locke[8] stated, "Every case of hypertrophic osteoarthropathy so far recorded has shown well-developed clubbing of the fingers and toes, and it is regarded as an absolutely constant sign of the disease." On the other hand, review of the literature[69,75,77] reveals that clubbing may occasionally be absent in an otherwise typical case of pulmonary osteoarthropathy or that clubbing manifests itself later than the bone changes. Locke reported 39 cases of "simple" clubbing in which 12 (30 per cent) showed roentgen evidence of periosteal proliferation of the long bones indicative

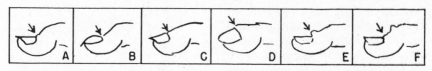

FIG. 80. Characteristic profile configurations of the finger. (A) Normal finger, illustrating the base angle of the nail (usually about 160°). (B) "Curving" of the nail, a variation of the normal. The base angle is undisturbed. (C) Early clubbing, with the base angle obliterated—positive "profile sign." (Club finger nails may also be curved.) (D) Advanced clubbing, with base angle greater than 180°. Base of nail projects upward. Over-all area of nail is increased. (E) Chronic paronychia, with fundamental base angle unaltered. (F) Heberden's node, with normal base angle. (Lovibond: Lancet 1:363)

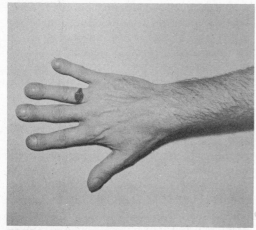

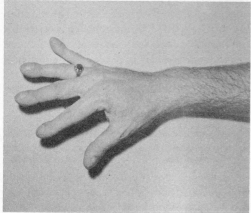

FIG. 81. Eleven-year-old girl with cyanosis from congenital heart disease (tetralogy of Fallot).

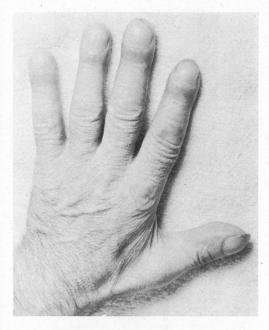

FIG. 82. Clubbed fingers in a 59-year-old man with carcinoma of the lung.

of hypertrophic osteoarthropathy. Such findings bear out the close association of these two conditions. Hypertrophic osteoarthropathy in its early stages may be asymptomatic and detectable only on roentgenograms; on the other hand, the onset may be heralded by *aching pains* in the joints and *tenderness* along the shafts of the involved bones. The pain may be severe, aggravated by movement, and may precede detectable roentgenographic changes. It may vary in intensity from a slight discomfort to a deep, dull aching pain which is transient. The skin over the involved areas may be warm, reddened, and thickened by a brawny nonpitting edema. In some series, pain in the bones has been the only presenting complaint in as high

as 40 per cent of the cases, the underlying more serious disease having caused less evident symptoms or none at all. Such bone and joint symptoms warrant careful search for evidence of clubbing and osteoarthropathy and search for the underlying cause (chest roentgenograms, etc.). Craig[9] and others have implicated *arthralgia* as one of the earliest clinical manifestations of intrathoracic lesions, the hypertrophic osteoarthropathy in such cases being an early complication. Symptoms of pulmonary osteoarthropathy may precede by 1 to 18 months the detection of localized lung lesions, particularly neoplastic disease of the chest, in contrast with suppurative lung processes in which the onset of symptoms of osteoarthropathy tends to lag behind respiratory and systemic manifestations.[70,71,72,76] Early diagnosis of cancer of the lung may be hastened by early detection of hypertrophic osteoarthropathy. The pains in the extremities are occasionally mistaken for rheumatoid arthritis or hypertrophic osteoarthritis. A moderate degree of joint *effusion* may be seen along with some limitation of motion. Partial or complete ankylosis has been reported in advanced cases. *Edema and hypertrophy of*

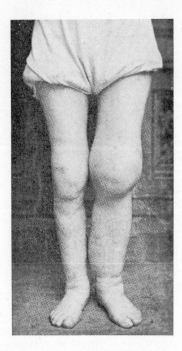

FIG. 83. Enlargement of both legs, particularly the left, in a case of hypertrophic osteoarthropathy. Note the large effusion in the left knee joint. (Norris and Landis: Diseases of the Chest, ed. 6, Philadelphia, Saunders)

the subcutaneous tissue of the limbs are observed (Fig. 83).

Osteoarthropathy may occur at any age. Gottlieb *et al.*[80] reported clubbing and osteoarthropathy in a 2-year-old infant with chronic pyopneumothorax. Kennedy reported similar findings in a 7½-month-old infant with multiple lung abscesses from birth.

Hypertrophic osteoarthropathy was at one time confused with acromegaly, in which enlargement of the hands and feet is characteristic. There may be awkwardness of gait and clumsiness of movement in the hands and fingers due to the increased size and weight of the limbs in advanced stages of hypertrophic osteoarthropathy. The diagnosis may also be confused with thrombophlebitis, venous stasis, congestive heart failure, nutritional edema, or peripheral neuropathy. Several reports mention the presence, in association with osteoarthropathy, of muscular weakness; bone pain, which is deep-seated, burning

in character and aggravated by lowering of the extremities; dusky discoloration of the fingertips; stiffness of the fingers; increased sweating; skin lesions, characterized by redness, glistening appearance, and warmth over the affected areas; increased hair growth; and broadened or cylindrical appearance of the distal thirds of the extremities produced by thickened skin and a firm, hard, pitting edema.[69,74] Spontaneous fractures may occur, apparently due to extreme osteoporosis.

The changes associated with clubbing are *usually gradual* in onset, taking place over a period of many weeks, months or years. However, they have been noted to appear *within one week* of the onset of the underlying disease.[11] Similarly, hypertrophic osteoarthropathy may be evident in a few weeks or not until a period of as much as 20 years after the onset of the associated malady. Clubbing and hypertrophic osteoarthropathy may disappear and reappear synchronously with remissions and exacerbations of the underlying disorder. Changes in the degree of clubbing have been used as a gauge of the activity of the concomitant disease. Disappearance of the phenomena in the extremities has been reported following successful medical or surgical treatment of chronic pulmonary infections, subacute bacterial endocarditis, mediastinal and pulmonary tumors, cyanotic congenital heart disease, ulcerative colitis, regional ileitis, amebic dysentery and sprue. Improvement, and even disappearance, have occurred also after collapse therapy in pulmonary tuberculosis, following antiluetic therapy in syphilis of the lung, and in subjects with chronic mountain sickness after descent to sea level.[4,12] In fact, failure of improvement in the osteoarticular manifestations following successful management of chronic lung infections should arouse suspicion of an underlying malignant process.[73] Vogl *et al.*[69] reported a case in which the general downhill course and the intractability of the pulmonary infection and of the symptoms of osteoarthropathy led to surgical exploration and detection of an underlying lung cancer.

A remarkable occurrence confirmed by many observers is the very rapid disappearance of pain in the bone which may occur following removal of a pulmonary tumor or other etiologic factor. Pain may disappear in 24 to 48 hours, thus suggesting the importance of circulatory or toxic (perhaps chemical) factors in the causation of the pain rather than the bone changes themselves being directly responsible. Flavell,[81] believing that the manifestations of osteoarthropathy were caused by a neural reflex from the lung, reported 5 inoperable cases of carcinoma of the lung in which vagotomy on the affected side provided immediate relief of symptoms. Steroid therapy and phlebotomies have also been suggested as therapy for symptomatic relief in inoperable cases;[82] the value of these measures is unproven.

Laboratory Tests

The most common abnormal laboratory finding is an elevated sedimentation rate. In addition, various other altered laboratory tests may occur as a result of the underlying disease processes. Since the concentrations of phosphorus and of alkaline phosphatase in the blood may be elevated during destruction and repair of bone, these values may also be changed in hypertrophic osteoarthropathy. This aspect bears further study.

X-Ray Findings

The roentgenologic changes are variable and depend upon the intensity and the duration of the pathologic process. In early clubbing there is usually no radiologic evidence of alteration. Somewhat later, a burr-like proliferation of the tuft of one or more of the terminal phalanges may appear. In long-standing cases of clubbing, atrophic changes occur ranging from simple osteoporosis to complete resorption (see terminal phalanx, 5th digit, Fig. 84). Erosion of the terminal tufts is rare; not infrequently, however, there is atrophy and spindling (narrowing of the shafts) of the terminal, and sometimes of the other, phalanges and of the metacarpals and metatarsals (Fig 84). The phalanges may show considerable elongation and prominent tufts when the clubbing occurs in childhood prior to cessation of growth. The development of newly

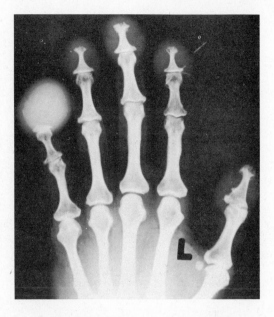

Fig. 84. Roentgenographic appearance of hand in patient also exhibiting changes in many other bones. Note resorption of terminal phalanx of the fifth digit, also narrowing of shafts and osteoporosis of other phalanges of this digit. In some of the phalanges of the other fingers osteoporosis predominates, in others there is thickening of the cortical bone. (D. C. Weir, St. Louis)

formed periosteal bone in the terminal phalanges has been reported only rarely.

Fully developed hypertrophic osteoarthropathy produces distinctive roentgenographic alterations. These are generally extensive and involve earliest and most frequently the tibia, the fibula, the radius, the ulna, the femur, the humerus, the metacarpal and the metatarsal bones. Later the phalanges, the clavicles, and the pelvis may be implicated and, very rarely, the tarsals, the carpals, the vertebrae, the ribs, the scapulae and the skull.[4,14,15] Some authors state that the skull and the mandible are never involved. Characteristically roughened, uneven, linear densities which represent the newly formed periosteal calcium deposits are observed along the shafts of the involved bones; the appearance suggests that of chronic periostitis (Fig. 85). The periosteal reaction is usually most evident along the distal half of the long bones. The den-

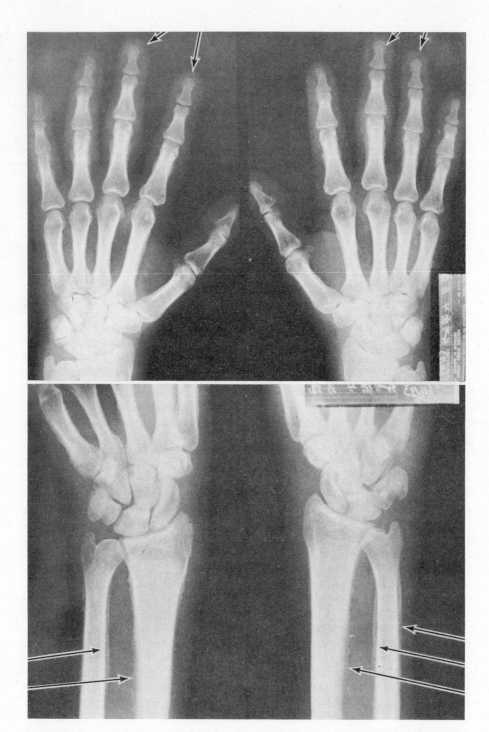

FIG. 85. Roentgenogram of hands and distal forearms in a case of clubbing and hypertrophic osteoarthropathy. Note the periosteal proliferation (noted by arrows) along the shaft of the radius, the ulna, the metacarpals and the phalanges. Burrlike proliferation of the distal phalanges is also present as indicated by arrows.

sities are thickest in the region of the peripheral epiphyses and at the points of muscular insertions. With remissions and exacerbations of the underlying disease, the repeated layered calcification in the periosteum may give a laminated x-ray appearance. The periosteal new bone may vary from the simple, smooth, parallel type of normal new bone to the rough, irregular, lacelike appearance of abnormal periosteal proliferation. In advanced cases, osteoporosis of the cancellous portion and thinning of the cortex of the original bone are found. Pathologic fractures may occur. Occasionally osteoporosis of the newly formed periosteal bone is seen. It should be pointed out that the roentgenographic diagnosis of hypertrophic osteo-arthropathy is doubtful in the absence of definite periosteal proliferation. The new bone may be from 1 to 10 mm. in thickness. Gall et al.[73] noted that in the early stage of development, the periosteum showed signs of inflammation, thickening, and early division into two layers. The outer layer showed an accumulation of inflammatory cells. The inner layer consisted of a fibrillary intercellular substance that was soon replaced by an osteoid matrix. The new subperiosteal bone layer fused with the original cortex and numerous osteoclasts appeared and caused focal areas of bone resorption. A thickened spongy shaft with a rarefying osteitis of the older bone resulted.

The new subperiosteal bone is formed chiefly near the epiphyses and at the points of musculotendinous insertions. It tends to progress to the proximal ends of the bones, but these changes are seldom seen in areas covered by the articular capsule. If the new subperiosteal bone displaces the thickened periosteum rapidly, pain and tenderness may occur, but if the process progresses slowly there may be no discomfort. Various parts of the skeleton may show different stages of the disease, which may advance rapidly in one area while regressing in another.

MEDICAL IMPORTANCE

Clubbing and hypertrophic osteoarthropathy, although often relatively innocuous in themselves, owe their importance to the fact that usually they are associated with significant underlying diseases. However, these conditions may be absent even in the severe forms of the diseases with which they are often associated. Furthermore, clubbing may occur as an isolated condition, unassociated with any known systemic disorder, an example being hereditary clubbing.

The frequent association of these pathological changes in bones with chronic pulmonary diseases is well recognized. Of the 144 cases of hypertrophic osteoarthropathy reported by Locke,[8] 113 (78%) were associated with diseases of the respiratory tract. Review of more recently published reports indicates that between 75 and 80 per cent of cases with clubbing and hypertrophic osteoarthropathy are associated with diseases of the pulmonary system; 10 to 15 per cent occur with diseases of the cardiovascular system; 5 to 10 per cent are associated with lesions of the gastrointestinal tract, including the liver, and another 5 to 10 per cent fall into a miscellaneous group. Of the associated pulmonary diseases reported by Locke,[8] tuberculosis (20%), bronchiectasis (19%), malignancy (7%) and empyema (5%) occurred most recently. However, the great recent progress of thoracic surgery has brought the realization that the precentage of persons who develop clubbing and hypertrophic osteoarthropathy which is secondary to bronchiectasis or pulmonary malignancy is higher than was thought. Poppe[16] reviewed 129 cases in which lobectomy was done at Barnes Hospital for bronchiectasis or chronic lung abscess. Of these, 103 patients (79%) had clubbing in varying degrees. Of 276 tuberculous patients at Koch Hospital in St. Louis surveyed by Poppe,[16] 71 (25%) revealed evidence of clubbing.

Skorneck and Ginsburg[83] emphasize a distinction between clubbing and osteoarthropathy. In a 3-year roentgenologic study of 390 patients with pulmonary tuberculosis they found no cases of osteoarthropathy; in 3 patients who were misdiagnosed as tuberculous and where osteoarthropathy was found, the final correct diagnoses were lung cancer in 2 and pyogenic abscess in 1. The authors went so far as to state that the finding of osteoarthropathy, but not clubbing, militates against a diagnosis of tuberculosis. In the presence of hypertrophic osteoarthropathy intrathoracic neoplasm is the most important condition to be excluded. In the cardiovascular group of diseases, clubbed fingers were present in association with cyanotic congenital heart disease in 132 (13%) of Abbott's[17] 1,000 cases. Friedberg[18] noted clubbing in about 66 per cent of fatal cases of subacute bacterial endocarditis, whereas Blumer[19] reported the incidence of clubbed fingers in subacute bacterial endocarditis to be 18 of 48 cases (36%). Trever[95] described 2 cases of congenital cyanotic heart disease with long-standing clubbing and hypertrophic osteoarthropathy, emphasizing the distinction between simple clubbing and osteoarthropathy. In congenital cyanotic heart disease the literature shows a high incidence of clubbing but a low incidence of osteoarthropathy and no case of osteoarthropathy occurred earlier than the age of 11.

The various diseases which should be suspected in the presence of clubbing or hypertrophic osteoarthropathy are:

Pulmonary Group. Bronchiectasis;[20] primary and secondary tumors of the lung,[21,22] bronchus,[9,23] mediastinum,[4] thymus,[24] and chest wall;[25] chronic empyema;[1,26,27] lung abscess;[28,29] fibroid pulmonary tuberculosis with excavation;[30,31] chronic pneumonitis;[2,8] emphysema associated with chronic suppurative conditions;[32] pneumoconiosis;[2] neurogenic tumor of the diaphragm;[98] atelectasis;[10] cystic disease of the lung;[33] chest deformities;[26] syphilis of the lung;[34] actinomycosis;[35] Hodgkin's disease involving the lung or mediastinum;[36] pulmonary hemangioma;[37,38] and aortic aneurysm with compression of the lung.[39]

Cardiac Group. Cyanotic congenital heart disease with a venous-arterial shunt (right to left flow)[6,16,40,41,42] subacute bacterial endocarditis[17,18,48] (rare in bacteria-free stage);[4] chronic congestive heart failure;[44] and cardiac tumors.[4]

Hepatic Group. Cholangiolytic or Hanot's type of cirrhosis; obstructive biliary cirrhosis secondary to bile duct obstruction; cirrhosis associated with chronic malaria; hepatomegaly with amebic abscess; and, rarely, in portal cirrhosis.[45]

Gastrointestinal Group. Chronic ulcerative colitis; regional enteritis; intestinal tuberculosis; chronic bacillary and amebic dysentery; sprue; ascaris infestation; multiple polyposis of the colon; abdominal Hodgkin's disease; pyloric obstruction and gastrectasia associated with carcinoma of the pylorus or duodenal ulcer; and, rarely, in carcinoma of the colon.[4,46,47,48]

Mixed Group. Idiopathic; hereditary; post-thyroidectomy; nasopharyngeal tumors; pituitary gland abnormality; myxedema due to I[131]; generalized lymphosarcomatosis; chronic mountain sickness (Monge's disease); chronic osteomyelitis with amyloidosis; and pseudohypertrophic muscular dystrophy.[4,10,49,50]

Miscellaneous Group. *Unilateral clubbing* may be present in aneurysm of the subclavian artery, the innominate artery or the arch of the aorta; lymphangitis; brachial arteriovenous aneurysm; and superior sulcus tumor (Pancoast tumor).[51,52,53]

PATHOLOGY

The pathology of clubbing and hypertrophic osteoarthropathy has received comparatively little consideration because of the difficulty in securing postmortem finger specimens for study, the inability to obtain suitable preparations for examination, and our inadequate knowledge of the normal histology of the finger tips. However, on the basis of various reports in the literature, the pathologic changes appear to consist chiefly of hypertrophy and hyperplasia.[2,8,12,54,55,56,57,58] There is increased proliferation of all tissues of the finger tip, especially in the fibrous elastic portion of the nail bed and in the fatty connective tissue of the ball of the finger. Corresponding with an increase in the underlying substance, there is an increase in the cross-sectional area of the nail. Newly formed capillaries have been observed, as well as dilatation and increased thickness of the walls of the small blood vessels in the end of the finger. The terminal phalanx may show increased thickness of its periosteum and of the ungual process itself or, in advanced cases, complete resorption of the bone. Bigler[84] stated that the shape of the clubbed digit is the result of the increased thickness of the nail bed. He stated that the nail bed is loosely textured, with large fibroblasts in a reticular network. The glomera are increased as are extravascular lymphocytes and eosinophils. In chronic clubbing the increased thickness is due to increased collagen deposition in the nail bed with no evidence of edema.

In hypertrophic osteoarthropathy there is calcification of the periosteum, and islands of newly formed periosteal bone may be found along the shaft of the long bones, thickest in the region of the peripheral epiphysis and at the points of musculo-tendinous insertions. There is thinning of the cortex of the original bone and osteoporosis of the cancellous portion. Bone resorption may extend to the new periosteal bone, leaving a thin trabeculated space between the cortex and the periosteum. In patients with exacerbations and remissions, one sees multiple laminations suggestive of tree-trunk layers. Pathologic fractures may occur if thinning and osteoporosis exceed the capacities of the reparative processes. With joint involvement (which occurs in approximately one third of the cases), the joint capsule and the synovial membrane occasionally are thickened and there may be fluid collection within the joint capsule. Proliferation of the subsynovial granulation tissue associated with lymphocytosis and fibrinoid degeneration of the synovial membrane has been reported, resulting in pannus formation. Pressure from the pannus can produce degeneration of the cartilage with erosion; if this occurs, the process may terminate in ankylosis.

PATHOGENESIS

The pathogenesis of clubbing and hypertrophic osteoarthropathy has been in dispute since the time when these conditions were first recognized. Because of their diagnostic significance, they have engaged the interest of many clinicians, and numerous theories have been proposed—none of which has to this date been proved. In the eighteenth century it was thought that clubbing was due to emaciation, as described in the works of Laennec.[59] Pigeaux[59] in 1832 advanced the theory that circulatory alterations caused edema and increased cellularity of the connective tissue of the finger tip, resulting in clubbing. In the latter part of the nineteenth century, following the classic papers of Marie[1] and von Bamberger,[3] the theory that chronic infection might be responsible was widely accepted. The popularity of this theory was soon shared by the toxic hypothesis. (Circulating toxins were believed to act on susceptible peripheral capillaries and thus produce the characteristic changes.) However, the association of clubbing and hypertrophic osteoarthropathy with pulmonary neoplasms and congenital heart disorders provided evidence that these theories were inadequate. Verrusio[60] and others later postulated the mechanical theory, which proposed that clubbing was due to capillary stasis resulting from back pressure. The fact that clubbing was rarely seen in patients with heart failure and the fact that actual pressure measurements[61] failed to substantiate the presence of stasis were cited as evidence against this hypothesis. Numerous additional theories have been suggested, such as vitamin deficiency,[57] malfunction of the endocrine glands (pituitary,[62] thyroid,[60] parathyroid,[60] and gonads[60]), nerve injury,[32] lymph stasis,[63] change in blood volume,[64] increased intracranial pressure,[60] and reflex nerve impulses from peripheral pulmonic nerve fibers influencing the formation of arteriovenous anastomoses in the limbs.

Many attempts have been made to study clubbing and hypertrophic osteoarthropathy in animals. A number of unsuccessful methods were tried to reproduce these conditions in rabbits, guinea pigs, dogs, cats and monkeys.[2,28,65,66] It was not until 1940 that Mendlowitz and Leslie[67] successfully induced hypertrophic osteoarthropathy experimentally in one of three dogs by anastomosing the left and adjacent main pulmonary artery to the left auricle, resulting in a right-to-left heart shunt, simulating congenital heart disease with cyanosis. By this method they were able to produce the gross and microscopic evidences of periosteal proliferation seen in hypertrophic osteoarthropathy (Figs. 86 and 87). Careful studies revealed no change in the venous pressure, ether circulation time or oxygen consumption. The main experimental find-

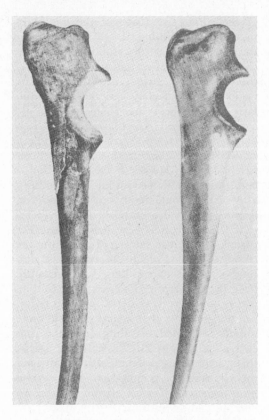

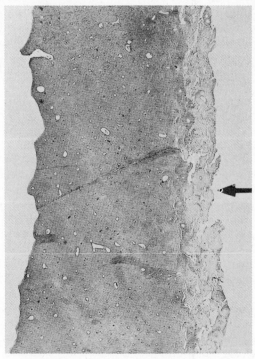

FIG. 87. Photomicrograph of transverse section of tibia of the dog with experimentally induced hypertrophic osteoarthropathy showing new-formed periosteum. (Mendlowitz and Leslie: Am. Heart J. 24:141)

FIG. 86. Comparison of the ulna of a dog with experimentally induced hypertrophic osteoarthropathy (left) with ulna of a normal dog (right). Note the roughened, irregular, elevated areas of the new-formed periosteum on the left. (Mendlowitz and Leslie: Am. Heart J. 24:141)

ing was an increase in the cardiac output; the blood flow through the lungs remained relatively unchanged. Mendlowitz[61] also demonstrated the presence of increased peripheral blood flow in patients with acquired clubbed fingers by means of calorimetric and brachiodigital arterial blood pressure gradient methods. Furthermore, he was able to show that the accelerated finger tip blood flow waxed and waned with exacerbations and remissions of clubbing and the underlying disease. In 1959, Wilson confirmed Mendlowitz's findings of increased blood flow in clubbed fingers. He concluded that the increased flow passed largely through numerous arteriovenous anastomoses and was in excess of physiologic requirements, resulting in accelerated growth due to

"forced feeding." Wilson noted that clubbing on the left hand regressed after ligation of the left subclavion artery in patients with tetralogy of Fallot who underwent surgical correction by the Blalock technique.

Blood flow and temperature regulation of the distal phalanges is a function of the glomus, as observed by Wilkins,[86] Grant[87] Bland, Popoff[88] and others. The glomus is a highly specialized arteriovenous anastomosis present in the digital nail beds and pads. It consists of an afferent artery joining the so-called Sucquet-Hoyer canal, from which 2 to 5 arterioles arise which subdivide into capillaries supplying the canal and related structures. The venous portion consists of a large receptacle forming a cape around the glomus and emptying into the subcapillary and deep veins of the digit. Reports concerning the influence of age on the number of glomera and the distribution of glomera vary according to the different counting techniques utilized. The fact that the glomus is a chief regulator of blood flow in the distal phalanx is established; its role is therefore inferred, but not proved, to be of major importance in the genesis of clubbing.[89]

Hall[90] in 1959 postulated that clubbing may be caused by a substance which is normally inactivated by the lungs and which dilates the digital glomera. He suggested that this substance might be ferritin. Shorr[91] described a vasodepressor material (VDM) produced by ischemic skeletal muscle, spleen, and liver, which caused dilatation of the arteriovenous anastomosis in the mesentery and intestines of animals. The VDM material produced by the liver was identified as ferritin. Ferritin, in its *oxidized* form, was inert against epinephrine; but in its *reduced* form blocked the vasoconstrictive action of epinephrine. Crismon[92] reported that *rutin,* a flavonoid, blocked the vasodepressor effect of ferritin. Utilizing the reported findings on ferritin and rutin, Hall[90] performed a study on subjects with and without clubbing. The capillary blood flow through the finger tips was evaluated by a radiosodium (Na^{24}) clearance technic before and after the intravenous injection of rutin. Hall concluded from his findings that one of the possible causes of clubbing was the long-term result of dilatation of the glomera in the nail-beds by the reduced ferritin which had evaded oxidation. In view of the fact that there is controversial evidence in the literature on rutin and its effect on vasodepressor materials (VDM) such as ferritin,[93] Hall's concept is stimulating but needs confirmation, particularly in regard to determination of the amount of reduced ferritin as opposed to oxidized ferritin in subjects with clubbing.

Mauer[68] again raised the hypothesis that local tissue anoxia is the predisposing factor leading to clubbing. His thesis is based upon the fact that in patients who have a disease associated with clubbing, the erythrocytes are altered physically as evidenced by the elevated sedimentation rate. The delivery and uptake of oxygen by the tissues are thus hindered by the altered physical state of the red blood cells and local anoxia results. It is known, however, that tissue anoxia alone does not cause clubbing, since clubbing does not occur with the slow rate of flow and cold finger tips of Raynaud's syndrome. Mauer postulates that the increased blood flow present in clubbing is secondary to the anoxia and that the rapid flow, the associated tissue warmth, and the rouleaux formation are all factors in the pathogenesis of clubbing.

More recently it has been considered that the derangement of peripheral circulation may be dependent upon some pathologic intrathoracic reflex which is promptly abolished by surgical removal of the primary lesion.[69] Flavell[81] reported prompt relief of pain due to osteoarthropathy by vagotomy on the side of the affected lung cancer in 5 cases. Trevor reported a similar response of joint pains to atropinization. The validity of this concept could be investigated by preoperative and prompt postoperative capillary bed studies. Such studies may greatly contribute to the solving of the problem of hypertrophic osteoarthropathy.

Barnes *et al.*[94] showed that widespread vascular hypoplasia existed in arteriovenous aneurysm of the lung. Cudkowicz[96] and Armstrong[97] believed that a similar vascular abnormality might be present in hypertrophic osteoarthropathy. They examined the lungs of 15 cases with clubbing due to intrathoracic pathology. When they injected a radiopaque medium into the diseased lungs, they found occlusion of the major branches of the pulmonary artery in almost all cases. They demonstrated precapillary bronchopulmonary anastomoses which diverted bronchial blood into the low-pressure pulmonary artery bed distal to the occlusion. Since these anastomoses did not occur in normal, healthy lungs, and resembled the anastomoses found in clubbed fingers, the authors postulated that the resulting ischemia of the lung set up antidromic impulses in the peripheral pulmonic nerve fibers which reflexly influenced the formation of the arteriovenous anastomoses in the limbs.

The fact that hypertrophy and hyperplasia may result from circulatory changes often has been observed clinically. Arteriovenous fistulas, for example, are known to lead to myocardial hypertrophy as well as to abnormal increases in growth of single limbs. The increased growth of limbs has been stated to be common if the fistula is acquired before the closure of the epiphyses. Sir Thomas Lewis indicated that the accelerated growth results from the more rapid flow of blood distal to the arteriovenous shunt, although the details of how the rapid blood flow produces increased growth in the face of diminished oxygen tension are lacking. Lovell postulated that increased blood flow in excess of tissue requirements produced accelerated growth due to "forced feeding." In the light of this theory one may speculate that neurogenic, toxic, anoxic, endocrine, and other factors may be associated with the pathogenesis of clubbing and osteoarthropathy. The exact mechanism by which circulatory changes produce the definite hypertrophy and hyperplasia seen pathologically is still unexplained. Thus, in spite of extensive study and voluminous literature, the pathogenesis of clubbing and hypertrophic osteoarthropathy remains conjectural.

SUMMARY

Clubbing is characterized by bulbous deformity of the fingers and toes. As a diagnostic sign it is of great significance, since it suggests the presence of underlying diseases affecting certain organs and systems—particularly the lungs and the heart, and less often the liver and the gastro-intestinal tract.

Hypertrophic osteoarthropathy represents a more advanced stage of the same process and is associated with the same disease conditions. Its presence should be considered particularly in those patients with clubbing who develop pain, tenderness and swelling about the joints and along the shafts of the bones. The roentgenographic finding of periosteal proliferation and other characteristic bone changes confirms the diagnosis.

Recognition of these conditions is not difficult if one keeps the possibilities in mind and if one observes the extremities carefully. *Early* recognition can be a clue to the *early* diagnosis of intrathoracic malignancy.

REFERENCES

1. Marie, P.: De l' osteo-arthropathie hypertrophiante pneumique, Rev. de méd. 10:1, 1890.
2. Hippocrates, with English Translation by W. H. S. Jones, London, Heinemann, Loeb Classical Library, Prognostic Number 17, 2:35, 1923.
3. von Bamberger, E.: Ueber Knochenveranderungen bei chronischen Lungen- und Herzkrankheiten, Ztschr. klin. Med. 18:193, 1890.
4. Mendlowitz, M.: Clubbing and hypertrophic osteoarthropathy, Medicine 21:269, 1942.
5. West, S.: Two cases of clubbing of the fingers developing within a fortnight and four weeks respectively, Tr. Clin. Soc. London 30:60, 1897.
6. Lovibond, J. L.: The diagnosis of clubbed fingers, Lancet 1:363, 1938.
7. Witherspoon, J. T.: Congenital and familial clubbing of the fingers and toes, with a possibly inherited tendency, Arch. Int. Med. 57:18, 1936.
8. Locke, E. A.: Secondary hypertrophic osteoarthropathy and its relation to simple clubfingers, Arch. Int. Med. 15:659, 1915.
9. Craig, J. W.: Hypertrophic pulmonary osteoarthropathy as the first symptom of pulmonary neoplasm, Brit. M. J. 1:750, 1937.
10. Locke, E. A.: Clubbing and Hypertrophic Osteoarthropathy (Revised by A. Grollman), Oxford Medicine, vol. 4, p. 447, New York, Oxford, 1943.
11. Lipman, B.: Personal observations.
12. Blalock, A., and Taussig, H. V.: The surgical treatment of malformations of the heart in which there is pulmonary stenosis or pulmonary atresia, J.A.M.A. 128:189, 1945.
13. Weens, H. S., and Brown, C. E.: Atrophy of terminal phalanges in clubbing and hypertrophic osteoarthropathy, Radiology 45:27, 1945.
14. Temple, H. L., and Jaspin, G.: Hypertrophic osteoarthropathy, Am. J. Roentgenol. 60:232, 1948.
15. Holt, J. F., and Hodges, F. J.: Significant skeletal irregularities of the hands, Radiology 44:23, 1945.
16. Poppe, J. K.: Diagnostic significance of clubbed fingers, Dis. of Chest 13:658, 1947.
17. Abbott, M. E.: Atlas of Congenital Heart Disease, New York, Am. Heart Ass., 1936.
18. Friedberg, C. K.: Diseases of the Heart, Philadelphia, Saunders, 1949.
19. Blumer, G.: Subacute bacterial endocarditis, Medicine, 2:105, 1923.

20. Whiteside, L. C.: A case of bronchiectasis with hypertrophic pulmonary osteoarthropathy, U. S. Naval Med. Bull. 8:658, 1914.

21. Pulmonary hypertrophic osteoarthropathy in adenocarcinoma of the lung (Mass. Gen. Case 31281), New England J. Med. 233:44, 1945.

22. Pulmonary hypertrophic osteoarthropathy in fibrosarcoma of the lung (Mass. Gen. Case 31271), New England J. Med. 233:18, 1945.

23. Paterson, R. S.: Pulmonary osteoarthropathy, Brit. J. Radiol. 32: 435, 1927.

24. Miller, F. R.: Carcinoma of thymus, with marked pulmonary osteoarthropathy, Radiology 32:651, 1939.

25. Konschegg, T.: Uber die Bamberger-Mariesche Krankheit, Virch. Arch. 271:164, 1929.

26. Symes-Thompson, H. E.: Two cases of hypertrophic pulmonary osteo-arthropathy, Lancet 1:385, 1909.

27. Springthorpe, J. W.: Case of hypertrophic pulmonary osteo-arthropathy, Brit. M. J. 1:1257, 1895.

28. Phemister, D. B.: Chronic lung abscess with osteo-arthropathy, Surg. Clin. Chicago 1:381, 1917.

29. Kerr, J.: Pulmonary hypertrophic osteoarthropathy, Brit. M. J. 2:1215, 1893.

30. Zesas, D. G.: An den Osteoarthropathien bei Lungentuberculose, Med. Klin. 5:1480, 1909.

31. Kaplan, R. H., and Munson, L.: Clubbed fingers in pulmonary tuberculosis, Am. Rev. Tuberc. 44:439, 1941.

32. Shaw, H. B., and Cooper, R. H.: "Pulmonary hypertrophic osteo-arthropathy" occurring in a case of congenital heart disease, Lancet 1:880, 1907.

33. Montuschi, E.: Clubbing associated with congenital lung cyst, Brit. M. J. 1:1310, 1938.

34. Munro, W. T.: Syphilis of the Lung, Lancet 1:1376, 1922.

35. Wynn, W. H.: Case of actinomycosis (streptothrichosis) of lung and liver successfully treated with a vaccine, Brit. M. J. 1:554, 1908.

36. Parkes Weber, F., and Ladinghaus, J. C. G.: Uber einen Fall von Lymphadenoma (Hodgkinsche Krankheit) des Mediastinums verbunden mit einer hochgradigen hypertrophischen Pulmonalosteoarthropathie, Deutsches Arch. klin. Med. 96:217, 1909.

37. Rodes, C. B.: Cavernous hemangiomas of the lung with secondary polycythemia, J.A.M.A. 110:1915, 1938.

38. Plaut, A.: Hemangioendothelioma of the lung, Arch. Path. 29:517, 1940.

39. Lang, H. B., and Bower, G. C.: A report of a case of hypertrophic osteoarthropathy, Psychiat. Quart. 4:277, 1930.

40. Means, M. G., and Brown, N. W.: Secondary osteoarthropathy in congenital heart disease, Am. Heart J. 34:262, 1947.

41. White, P. D., and Sprague, H. B.: The tetralogy of Fallot, J.A.M.A. 92:787, 1929.

42. Wahl, H. R., and Gard, R. L.: Aneurism of the pulmonary artery, Surg. Gynec. Obst. 52:1129, 1931.

43. Cotton, T. F.: Clubbed fingers as a sign of subacute infective endocarditis, Heart 9:347, 1922.

44. Thorburn, W.: Three cases of "hypertrophic pulmonary osteo-arthropathy" with remarks, Brit. M. J. 1:1155, 1893.

45. Rolleston, H. D., and McNee, J. W.: Diseases of the Liver, Gall-bladder, and Bileducts, London, Macmillan, 1929.

46. Schlicke, C. P., and Bargen, J. A.: "Clubbed fingers" and ulcerative colitis, Am. J. Digest. Dis. 7:17, 1940.

47. Bennett, I., Hunter, D., and Vaughan, J. M.: Idiopathic steatorrhoea (Gee's disease); nutritional disturbance associated with tetany, osteomalatia, and anaemia, Quart. J. Med., N. S. 1:603, 1932.

48. Preble, R. B.: Gastrectasis with tetany and the so-called pulmonary hypertrophic osteoarthritis of Marie, Medicine 4:1, 1898.

49. Camp, L. J. D., and Scanlon, R. L.: Chronic idiopathic hypertrophic osteoarthropathy, Radiology 50:581, 1948.

50. Rynearson, E. H., and Sacasa, C. F.: Hypertrophic pulmonary osteoarthropathy (acropachy) afflicting a patient who had postoperative myxedema and progressive exophthalmos, Proc. Staff Meet. Mayo Clin. 16:353, 1941.

51. Smith, T.: A case of aneurysm of the right axillary artery. Ligature of the subclavian; pyemia. Death on the twenty-second day. With remarks on clubbing of the fingers and toes, Tr. Path. Soc. London 23:74, 78, 1872.

52. Baur, J.: De l' hippocratisme dans les affections cardiovasculaires, Rev. de méd. 30:993, 1910.

53. Poland, A.: Statistics of subclavian aneurism, Guys' Hosp. Rep. 15:47, 1870.

54. Campbell, D.: The Hippocratic fingers, Brit. M. J. 1:145, 1924.

55. Charr, R., and Swenson, P. C.: Clubbed fingers, Am. J. Roentgenol. 55:325, 1946.

56. Parkes Weber, F.: The histology of the new bone-formation in a case of pulmonary hypertrophic osteoarthropathy, Proc. Roy. Soc. Med. 2:187, 1908.

57. Crump, C.: Histologie der allgemeinen Osteophytose (osteoarthropathie hypertrophiante pneumique), Virchows Arch. path. Anat. 271:467, 1929.

58. Thorburn, W., and Westamacott, F. H.: The pathology of hypertrophic pulmonary osteoarthropathy, Tr. Path. Soc. London 47:177, 1896.

59. Laennec, R. T. H., and Pigeaux, D. M., *cited by* Mendlowitz, Medicine 21:269, 1942.

60. Verrusio, M., Massalongo, R., Danuco, I., and Sirshew, P., *cited in* discussion by Charr and Swenson: Am. J. Roentgenol. 55:325, 1946.

61. Mendlowitz, M.: Measurements of blood flow and blood pressure in clubbed fingers, J. Clin. Invest. 20:113, 1941.

62. Fried, B. M.: Chronic pulmonary osteoarthropathy; dyspituitarism as a probable cause, Arch. Int. Med. 72:565, 1943.

63. Bryan, L.: Secondary hypertrophic osteoarthropathy following metastatic sarcoma of the lung, Calif. West. Med. 23:449, 1925.

64. Pritchard, E.: Familial clubbing of fingers and toes, Brit. M. J. 1:752, 1938.

65. Compere, E. L., Adams, W. E., and Compere, C. L.: Possible etiologic factors in the production of pulmonary osteoarthropathy, Proc. Soc. Exper. Biol. Med. 28:1083, 1931.

66. van Hazel, W.: Joint manifestations associated with intrathoracic tumors, J. Thoracic Surg. 9:495, 1940.

67. Mendlowitz, M., and Leslie, A.: The experimental simulation in the dog of the cyanosis in hypertrophic osteoarthropathy associated with congenital heart disease, Am. Heart J. 24:141, 1942.

68. Mauer, E. F.: Etiology of clubbed fingers, Am. Heart J. 34:852, 1947.

69. Vogl, A., Blumenfeld, S., and Gutner, L. B.: Diagnostic significance of pulmonary hypertrophic osteoarthropathy, Am. J. Med. 18:51, 1955.

70. Berg, R., Jr.: Arthralgia as a first symptom of pulmonary lesions, Dis. Chest 16:483, 1949.

71. Deutschberger, O., Maglione, A. A., and Gill, J. J.: An unusual case of intrathoracic fibroma associated with pulmonary hypertrophic osteoarthropathy, Am. J. Roentgenol. 59:738, 1953.

72. Fischl, J. R.: Severe hypertrophic pulmonary osteoarthropathy. Report of a case due to carcinoma of the lung with operation and recovery, Am. J. Roentgenol. 64:42, 1950.

73. Gall, E. A., Bennett, G. A., and Bauer, W.: Generalized hypertrophic osteoarthropathy, Am. J. Path. 27:349, 1951.

74. Holmes, H. H., Bauman, E., and Ragan, C.: Symptomatic arthritis due to hypertrophic osteoarthropathy in pulmonary neoplastic disease, Ann. Rheumat. Dis. 9:169, 1950.

75. Pattison, J. D., Beck, E., and Miller, W. B.: Hypertrophic osteoarthropathy in carcinoma of the lung, J.A.M.A. 146:783, 1951.

76. Robinson, W. D., *et al.:* Rheumatism and arthritis. Review of American and English literature of recent years, part II. Ann. Int. Med. 39:498, 1953.

77. Shapiro, L.: Ossifying periostitis of Bamberger-Marie, Bull. Hosp. Joint Dis. 2:77, 1941.

78. Angel, J. H.: Pachydermo-periostosis (idiopathic osteoarthropathy), Brit. M. J. 2:789, 1957.

79. Buchman, D., and Hrowat, E. A.: Idiopathic clubbing and hypertrophic osteoarthropathy, Arch. Int. Med. 97:355, 1956.

80. Gottlieb, C., Sharlin, H. S., and Feld, H.: Hypertrophic pulmonary osteoarthropathy, J. Pediat. 30:462, 1947.

81. Flavell, G.: Reversal of pulmonary hypertrophic osteoarthropathy by vagotomy, Lancet 1:260, 1956.

82. Shapiro, M.: Hypertrophic osteoarthropathy, A.M.A. Arch. Int. Med. 98:700, 1956.

83. Skorneck, A. B., and Ginsburg, L. B.: Pulmonary hypertrophic osteoarthropathy (periostitis) : its absence in pulmonary tuberculosis, New England J. Med. 258:1079, 1958.

84. Bigler, F. C.: The morphology of clubbing, Am. J. Path. 34:237, 1958.

85. Wilson, G. M.: Local circulatory changes associated with clubbing of the fingers and toes, Quart. J. Med. 21:201, 1959.

86. Wilkins, R. W., Doupe, J., and Newman, H. W.: The rate of blood flow in normal fingers, Clin. Sci. 3:403, 1938.

87. Grant, R. T., and Bland, E. F.: Observations on arteriovenous anastomosis in human skin and in the bird's foot with special reference to reaction to cold, Heart 15:385, 1931.

88. Popoff, N. W.: Digital vascular system, with reference to the state of glomus in inflammation, arteriosclerotic gangrene, diabetic gangrene, thrombo-angiitis and supernumerary digits in man, A.M.A. Arch. Path. 18:295, 1934.

89. Ribot, S.: Unilateral clubbing following traumatic obstruction of the axillary vein, A.M.A. Arch. Int. Med. 98:482, 1956.

90. Hall, G. H.: The cause of digital clubbing, Lancet 1:750, 1959.

91. Shorr, E.: Intermediary and biological activities of ferritin, Harvey Lectures 50:112, 1954.

92. Crismon: Rutin and other flavonoids as potentiators of terminal vascular responses to epinephrine and as antagonists of vasodepressor materials, Am. J. Physiol. 164:391, 1951.

93. Williams, J.: The etiology of digital clubbing, Am. Heart J. 63:139, 1962.

94. Barnes, C. G., Fatti, L., and Pryce, D. M.: Arteriovenous aneurysm of the lung, Thorax 3:148, 1948.

95. Trever, R. W.: Hypertrophic osteoarthropathy in association with congenital cyanotic heart disease, Ann. Int. Med. 48:660, 1958.

96. Cudkowicz, L., and Wraith, D. G.: A method of study of the pulmonary circulation in finger clubbing, Thorax 12:313, 1957.

97. Cudkowicz, L., and Armstrong, J. B.: Finger clubbing and changes in the bronchial circulation, Brit. J. Tuberc. 47:227, 1953.

98. Trivedi, S. A.: Neurilemmoma of the diaphragm causing severe hypertrophic pulmonary osteoarthropathy, Brit. J. Tuberc. 52:214, 1958.

12

Generalized Vasospasm and Arterial Hypertension

HENRY A. SCHROEDER

DEFINITION

By vasospasm* is meant a condition in which the total effective luminal cross-sectional area of an arterial bed is diminished. In other words, the caliber of the arteries available for the flow of blood is less than that required for circulation at a normal flow and a normal pressure. By generalized vasospasm is meant a condition of lessened caliber throughout all vascular beds of more or less equal degree. Although veins may take part in the reaction, this chapter is concerned primarily with vasospastic states involving the arterial side of the circulation; states of vasodilatation exist less frequently and often are unassociated with secondary vascular phenomena.

---

* The term vasospasm is used in this chapter in preference to vasoconstriction for the following reasons: (1) The circulation is normally in a state of vasoconstriction, or tonus, as is obvious to anyone dealing with anesthetized or pithed animals. (2) This discussion deals with *excessive* vasoconstriction resulting from and causing disorders and disease. (3) When prolonged constriction of vascular smooth muscle occurs, the muscle may be considered spastic.

CIRCULATION, LOCAL AND GENERAL

Because the flow of blood is dependent upon pressure and volume, a reduction in the caliber of the arteries in only one circulatory area would cause ischemia unless systemic pressure rose compensatorily; in that event hyperemia in the rest of the body would result, until cardiac or volume adjustments occurred. On the other hand, generalized vasospasm would cause hypertension unless cardiac output fell or circulating blood volume decreased. Intermittent changes in the caliber of local vessels are constantly taking place, giving rise to minor or major variations in flow, a readily adjustable but eventually stable system derived from the checks and the balances of homeostatic mechanisms designed to meet the changing nutritive requirements of tissues through their capillaries.

Vasospasm of itself increases *resistance* to blood flow. The concept of peripheral resistance is often confusing to the student, depending as it does on the ratio of two measurable functions, pressure and flow. Actually, this relationship is the analogue of Ohm's law: $E = IR$, where E is voltage or pressure, I is amperage, current or flow, and R is resistance (ohms). Thus, resistance is a ratio and can be expressed in arbitrary units.

The Poiseuille equation for flow of homogeneous viscous fluids flowing through pipes states:

$$\text{fluid flow} = \frac{\text{(pressure difference) (radius)}^4}{\text{(vessel length) (fluid viscosity)}} \left(\frac{\pi}{8} \right)$$

Substituting this equation to indicate resistance:

$$\text{resistance} = \frac{\text{pressure}}{\text{flow}} = \frac{\text{(length) (viscosity)}}{\text{(vessel radius)}^4} \left(\frac{8}{\pi} \right)$$

Because the length of muscular vessels probably does not alter much, this formula shows that resistance varies inversely as the fourth power of the radius. Halving the radius would increase the resistance 16 times and blood pressure would double if the radii of all vessels were reduced about 16 per cent, if blood were a homogeneous fluid, which it is not. Obviously, rapid changes of peripheral resistance are determined by changes in the radii of all blood vessels* rather than by altering vessel length or viscosity, the latter varying only when the major constituents of blood are changed.

Fortunately, both blood and blood vessels have "built-in" physical characteristics in respect to effective blood viscosity, dampening major circulatory changes. The blood is viscous enough to prevent turbulence in large vessels but as it passes through very small arteries its effective viscosity decreases. In the capillaries, viscosity increases, probably due to distortion of red blood cells.

---

* The terms vasomotor tone or vascular tonus are used to refer somewhat vaguely to some of the dynamic forces influencing cross-sectional areas of vessels, i.e., distending pressure and stiffness. If vessels were gum rubber these forces would dominate, as they may in the elastic aorta. In small terminal arteries and arterioles the pressure is fairly low (Fig. 88) but the ratio of radius to thickness of wall is large. Therefore, the force tending to stretch the vessel walls becomes greater as the lumina narrow.[1] Muscular activity or tension in the smooth muscle of the small vessel wall probably dominates in determining the radius or the total cross-sectional area.

As the rate of flow becomes greater, effective viscosity lessens to a point at which it becomes constant. At low levels of pressure, effective viscosity increases, thereby tending to maintain peripheral resistance. In glass tubes, blood is 4 to 5 times as viscous as water, but in the circulation it is only 2.2 times as viscous as water. Therefore, both the pipes and the fluid flowing through them are ideally constituted for the purpose, a truly efficient system so far not imitated by hydraulic engineers.

The fallacy of using either absolute or percentage changes in evaluating variations of blood pressure caused by stimulatory or depressant measures becomes obvious from a few simple calculations based on the assumption that Poiseuille's law in general holds for blood and that blood flow is constant. Let us say that a certain procedure (cold pressor test, breath holding, Valsalva's maneuver) raises diastolic blood pressure from 80 to 100 mm. Hg. The degree of change in the total caliber of vessels would be roughly 6 per cent. If a similar procedure raised pressure from 100 to 125 mm. Hg, the change in caliber would approximate 5.8 per cent, from 125 to 156 mm., 5.4 per cent, and from 156 to 195 mm., 5.1 per cent, as the vessels initially had a smaller caliber. Therefore, the stimulus was somewhat less effective at the higher pressures, although the absolute change in each case was 25 per cent greater and the relative change the same.

This characteristic probably partly accounts for the usual variability of blood pressure in the severely hypertensive patient. To double the pressure requires that the caliber be reduced by about one sixth. Shorter (already constricted) smooth muscle fibers may be less sensitive to ordinary nervous and chemical stimuli in terms of changes in their lengths than their more relaxed counterparts.

Adequate blood flow at optimal capillary pressure can be maintained at a wide range of central arterial pressures as long as cardiac output is normal. The determining factor is not the level of blood pressure nor wholly the cardiac output; it is the fall of pressure from major artery or aorta to capillary (Fig. 88).* Thus, a widely dilated vascular bed with a low blood pressure and adequate flow may provide plenty of capillary blood at normal intracapillary pressure and flow, with filtration and reabsorption of blood fluids and solutes proceeding normally. Likewise, adequate capillary pressure and flow may be maintained at very high pressures with intense vasoconstriction, the fall of pressure from aorta to capillary being great. The capillaries probably cannot distinguish between blood forced at high pressure through small pipes and the same amount of blood flowing at low pressures through large pipes. If a greater than normal part of the arterial pressure were transmitted to the capillary, its in-

---

* Green[2] has calculated the average pressure fall in various segments of the circulation of the dog as follows (mm. Hg): Aorta and large arteries, 2.8; main branches, 4.6; secondary branches, 4.8; tertiary branches, 13.4; terminal arteries, 4.5; terminal branches, 4.0; arterioles, 8.6. The greatest drop therefore occurs in arteries, not in arterioles.

creased pressure would cause congestion, increased filtration of fluids and eventually rupture at a point where venous limbs could not carry the increased load. If a less than normal part of the arterial pressure were passed on to capillaries, lessened filtration, greater reabsorption of fluids and finally ischemic stasis and dehydration would result. Therefore, an intrinsic local mechanism for controlling pressure and flow probably exists. The purpose of the circulation, the heart, the lungs and the blood vessels is to provide capillaries with adequate blood at an optimal pressure for filtration and reabsorption. It is in this light that we must view the question of vasospasm.

Because the circulation is composed of a series of shunts or resistances in parallel (Fig. 89), it is relatively easy to diminish the blood flow to one organ and increase that to another. Such large shifts occur constantly, during exercise when muscular flow is increased; during digestion when splanchnic flow is increased; during sleep when muscular flow may be low. These shifts are brought about by changes in the caliber of the arteries supplying the parts. Controlling factors are not well understood. Somehow the intrinsic needs of tissues for oxygen and food or for getting rid of metabolites determines the caliber of these vessels. Therefore we can postulate the

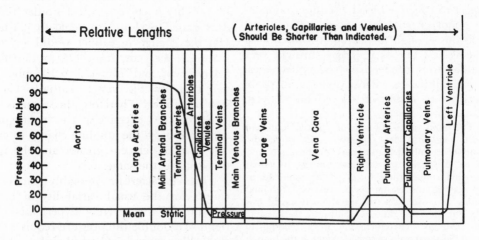

FIG. 88. The fall of pressure in the circulation through various anatomic divisions of the vascular system (after Green[2]). The relative length of each segment is indicated. Notice that most of the fall in pressure occurs in the smaller arteries and the arterioles. The static pressure is that which would be present during circulatory arrest.

presence of local regulatory mechanisms which in some way have general manifestations and affect other organs.* These may be concerned with chemical agents produced at the site of need, although not too much is known about them.

* The term reflex, as used in this article (and by most physiologists), often denotes an expression of ignorance and an intellectually satisfying semantic refuge therefrom. In most cases the sensory, motor, nervous and chemical components are unknown.

FACTORS INFLUENCING VASOSPASM

A knowledge of the anatomy and physiology of vascular smooth muscle aids in understanding some of the various factors which can influence the caliber of the arterial and arteriolar bed—for smooth muscle fibers can be affected directly by certain chemical substances applied to them from the blood, by other substances acting on

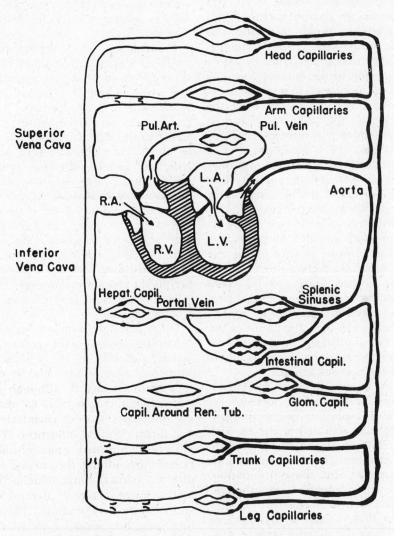

Fig. 89. Schematic diagram of the major parallel circuits in the body (from Green[2]). Each circuit contains a number of resistances in series, being the resistances offered by arteries and their branches, arterioles, capillaries, and veins; and a number in parallel, being collateral circuits. The kidney represents a special case with two in series; the portal circulation has two major ones in series and one in parallel (the spleen).

nerves supplying the muscle fibers, by the nerves themselves through the formation and release of chemical substances at their end organs, and indirectly from sensitization or desensitization of their structures by outside influences. These various factors are considered separately.

NEUROGENIC FACTORS

The sympathetic portion of the autonomic nervous system has its origin in the posterior hypothalamus where it receives connections from the cerebral cortex. Fibers pass through the spinal cord and out through the sympathetic chain of ganglia. The medullary vasomotor center probably supplies a portion of the outflow or acts as a synaptic junction for afferent fibers responsive to changes in pressure from the carotid artery and the aorta (moderator or buffer nerves) which pass through the glossopharyngeal and the vagus nerves. The various sympathetic ganglia contain synapses mediated by quaternary ammonium compounds, notably acetyl choline; from these synapses there is, in most areas, a direct communication of uninterrupted pathways to vascular smooth muscle. However, the splanchnic area forms an exception; the three splanchnic nerves enter other peripheral ganglia (celiac, aorticorenal) where further synaptic transmission takes place. The adrenal medulla also may be considered as a ganglion in the largest sense of the term, nervous stimulation causing release into the blood stream of chemical mediators for sympathetic nervous action.

Insofar as is known, there are two chemical mediators for sympathetic nervous activity, and both contain trivalent nitrogen.

Norepinephrine, released at the nervous end-organ, has been shown to be the substance which stimulates vascular smooth muscle to constrict after nerve stimulation. It is apparently Cannon's sympathin E. First described pharmacologically by Barger and Dale in 1910,[3] it has been shown to constrict all vascular smooth muscle relatively evenly when injected intravenously; the renal and the cerebral vascular beds, however, are a bit more sensitive to its action, especially the former. Therefore, peripheral resistance is increased through-

out the body and blood pressure rises, *provided* the heart is adequate to pump against the increased pressure and there is enough blood to pump. Just why the heart responds to the increased work demanded is not known, but the reflex mechanisms which respond to the change of pressure (moderator nerves) may in some way affect myocardial metabolism.* Because all vascular beds are constricted fairly evenly, no pronounced hyperemia or ischemia in any one circuit occurs. For a clear-cut discussion of this subject, the reader is referred to Barcroft.[4]

Epinephrine. The other known chemical mediator is epinephrine, which differs structurally from norepinephrine only in that one hydrogen on the tertiary nitrogen is replaced by a methyl group. This minor replacement alters the action of the substance drastically. Its potency is weakened to about five eighths that of norepinephrine, and instead of acting as a vasoconstrictor in all areas, it now predominantly dilates, with constrictor effects upon the skin and the kidneys.[4] The net result is a rise of cardiac output, an increased systolic and a lowered diastolic pressure and a shunting of blood from the constricted to the dilated area. Ordinary amounts lessen peripheral resistance; however, larger than "physiologic" doses give predominant constrictor effects.

Other trivalent nitrogenous compounds containing primary amine groups have vasoactivity (see below). While these chemical substances may or may not be considered as neurogenic factors, although classed as sympathomimetic amines, no sharp dividing line exists between chemical mediators and direct chemical influences. There is in vitro evidence that some synthetic compounds may inhibit the enzyme which oxidizes the natural sympathetic mediators, allowing longer action of natural catecholic amines at the nerve endings. These metabolites must be considered in all conditions involving localized functional vascular changes.

* For an excellent discussion of the reflexes dependent upon stretch receptors, the student is referred to the review by Aviado and Schmidt.[5]

Nephrogenic Factors

Renal Ischemia. Neurogenic vasospasm involves the renal vascular bed, which apparently is unique in that renal ischemia invokes the formation and release of humoral vasoconstrictor substances. The specialized circulation of the nephron, which has two arterioles, responds both to nervous stimulation and to the injection of catecholic amines by a relative decrease in caliber of the efferent arteriole, although both efferent and afferent arterioles can be affected. The net result is an increase in glomerular capillary pressure, an increased rate of filtration of blood, and a decreased total renal blood flow.

Just how and why this change calls forth "renal pressor mechanisms" is not understood. It depends upon reduction of renal blood flow by any means and is associated, perhaps, with diminished oxygen supply or with acidity of the cortex.[7] At any rate, a proteolytic enzyme, *renin*, acts upon an α_2-globulin substrate, *hypertensinogen*, to produce a vasoconstrictor polypeptide, *hypertensin*, *angiotonin* or *angiotensin*.[8] Why this happens can only be answered teleologically; the renin pressor system is one, and perhaps a major, protective mechanism against loss of blood flow through vital organs. Interestingly enough, angiotensin also appears to be antidiuretic.[9a] Other possible renal mechanisms set in motion by ischemia will be considered later.

Partial constriction of the renal artery of dogs is followed by a slow return of flow[9b] at a reduced pulse pressure, indicating "autonomous" control of the renal circulation. Renin may be released by diminution of the pulse pressure in the face of normal flow. A renal baroceptor which releases renin from the cortex has been suggested as a normal mechanism for controlling arterial pressure.[9c]

Local Metabolites

Not much is known of the local metabolites which affect vascular smooth muscle. Certainly, they may exist as distinct chemical substances produced in ischemic or hyperemic tissues, which can affect the caliber of blood vessels and cause stasis or further ischemia. Some of the amines derived by decarboxylation of amino acids show varying degrees of potency to affect vascular smooth muscle. Derivatives of imidazole (histamine) and indole (tryptamine, serotonin) as well as other phenolic compounds (tyramine, phenethylamine) and even aliphatic ones (isoamylamine, guanidine) have vascular activity. There are 6 basic types and 18 compounds derived from naturally occurring amino acids which are vasoactive. Many more synthetic analogues are available, which stimulate or block. The basic group for activity is the amine, often substituted by carbon or ring structures. In Table 11 are listed the simpler vasoactive substances derived from materials known to be present in blood or tissues, both free and as a constituent of proteins. Their vascular actions vary considerably in potency.[10] Derivatives and more complex products of protein breakdowns are also known but poorly investigated. The recent development of specifically acting drugs has provided a beginning to their study.

Most of these substances are tertiary nitrogenous compounds or purine derivatives. The former arise from decarboxylation of amino acids, either in the free state, possibly when in polypeptides or proteins, or from specific proteolysis. The latter come from nucleoproteins or exist in a relatively free state. In nature, vasoactivity, especially constriction, always is associated with *trivalent nitrogen;* vasodilatation with *synthetically blocked nitrogen,* with *aldehyde,* or with *purine derivatives.* Certain compounds (histamine, for example) have dual actions, both dilating capillaries and constricting arterioles. Several of them act upon the brain, especially the hypothalamus, affecting both sympathetic activity and mood.

An understanding of these metabolites which have demonstrated vasoactivity will help immeasurably in the synthesis of new drugs to combat their actions. Primary amines are present in both blood and urine.[11] From their known pharmacological actions, both on blood vessels and on cerebral activity, many of these amines must perform other as yet undetermined functions, in both normal and pathologic states.

TABLE 11. SOME NATURALLY OCCURRING VASOACTIVE SUBSTANCES

PRIMARY AMINES, ETC.	SOURCE	DECARBOXYLASE KNOWN	PRESSOR RATIO	ACTED ON BY MONOAMINE OXIDASE
l-Norepinephrine	Dihydroxyphenylalanine	+*	1640	+
l-Epinephrine	Dihydroxyphenylalanine	+*	1000	+
3-Dihydroxytyramine	Dihydroxyphenylalanine	+*	20	+
Tyramine	Tyrosine	+*	10	+
5-Hydroxytryptamine	5-Hydroxytryptophan	+*	10	+
Phenethylamine	Phenylalanine	+*	7	+
Tryptamine	Tryptophan	+*	3	+
n-Amylamine	Norleucine		2	+
n-Butylamine	Norvaline		2	+
Isoamylamine	Leucine		1	+
Ethanolamine	Serine		0.5	+
Histamine	Histidine	+	−	0
Putrescine	Arginine	+	−	0
Cadaverine	Lysine	+	−	0
Pyrrolidine	Proline		+	0
3-Hydroxypyrrolidine	Hydroxyproline		+	0
Taurine	Cysteine		0	0
Cysteamine	Cysteine	+	−	?
Guanidine	Arginine	+	40	0
Adenosine phosphates			−	0
Aldehydes			−	−
Acetyl choline			−	0

+ = pressor: The pressor ratio was evolved by Barger and Dale[58] with epinephrine as a standard.[3]
− = depressor.
*Aromatic l-amino acid decarboxylase.

TABLE 12. KNOWN BACTERIAL AND MAMMALIAN DECARBOXYLASES*

	BACTERIAL	MAMMALIAN Decarboxylase	Amine Oxidation	SPECIES OF ANIMAL
Histidine → Histamine	+	+†	+	Guinea pig, rabbit, mouse, kidney and liver
Tryptophan → Tryptamine	+	+†	+	Guinea pig kidney
Tyrosine → Tyramine	+†	+†	+	Guinea pig and rabbit kidney
DOPA → Hydroxytyramine		+†	+	Kidney and liver
Cysteic Acid → Taurine		+†		Liver
Serine → Ethanolamine		?	+	Indirect evidence in brain
Ornithine → Putrescine	+†	?	+	Indirect evidence in liver
? Amino Acid → Spermine		?	+	By analogy; no evidence
Lysine → Cadaverine	+†		+	Indirect evidence
Arginine → Agmatine	+†		?	
Glutamic Acid → α-Aminobutyric Acid	+	+†		Brain
Leucine → Isoamylamine	+			
Kynurenine → Kynuramine		+†	+	Plasma

Note: No other bacterial decarboxylases are known in some 800 strains tested. Other mammalian ones may occur.

* After Blaschko: Advances Enzymol. 5:67, 1945, and Gale: Advances Enzymol. 6:1, 1946.
† These are usually considered to contain pyridoxal phosphate.

Primary amines are generally oxidized by monoamine oxidases, of which two types are known. A tissue enzyme found in the liver, the kidney, the brain and other organs removes the amine group on most of the amines shown in Table 11. The liver probably accounts for oxidation of those amines formed in the gut by bacterial decarboxylases, which are absorbed in portal venous blood, the ammonia released being synthesized into urea. A plasma enzyme affects such substances as butylamine, amylamine, heptylamine, spermine, spermidine and kynuramine; it has been crystallized.[12] In addition, the copper protein, ceruloplasmin, has enzyme activity of a condensing nature on catecholic and phenolic amines (copper itself is a strong catalyst for catechols and is a cofactor in tyrosinase).* Undoubtedly other enzymatic systems contribute to the destruction of these active substances.

Primary amines are formed in the bowel by bacterial decarboxylases; presumably they are oxidized in the wall of the gut or, under some conditions, absorbed. They are also formed in the kidney under conditions of hypoxia by anaerobic decarboxylation, for monoamine oxidase is quite sensitive to oxygen tension. Some amino acids contribute a sizeable part of total urinary ammonia; in hypertension with renal ischemia urinary ammonia is reduced and arterial amine content increased.[13] It is an attractive hypothesis that hypoxic tissues in other parts of the body may fail to deaminate primary amines formed by local decarboxylases, thus accounting for some of the local vasomotor changes, but this remains to be proved. Too little is known about these probably prevalent and variously active products of partial metabolism of amino acids, although both decarboxylases and amine oxidases are relatively widespread in tissues. (Table 12).

ADRENOCORTICAL FACTORS

Insofar as is known, the natural hormones of the adrenal cortex have no direct activity upon vascular smooth muscle. How-

* Plasma monoamine oxidase contains copper as a cofactor.[12b]

ever, some of them do exhibit indirect effects which can be profound. Probably the vascular actions of steroids are confined to those which exhibit salt-retaining properties. *Desoxycorticosterone acetate* (DCA) has a prolonged pressor effect in hypertensive persons[14]; the glucoside has not. The response of the blood pressure to intravenously administered norepinephrine is enhanced by giving human beings DCA and salt and is depressed by giving them a low salt diet.[15] Likewise, chronic arterial hypertension can be produced in some animals given DCA and salt.[16] Hypertension usually, but not always, accompanies adrenal cortical hyperfunction in man. Salt alone may produce an effect in the experimental animal, but DCA alone will not. The most logical explanation for these findings is that salt and certain steroids together sensitize vascular smooth muscle to normally occurring vasoconstrictor substances; intracellular alterations in electrolytes, particularly sodium, potassium and magnesium occur. The functions of constriction and relaxation are accompanied by, and are probably dependent on, cationic shifts across the membrane of the muscle. It is also possible that electrolytes can profoundly affect nervous transmission, especially through autonomic (unmyelinated) nerves.[17]

Aldosterone appears to be the major salt-retaining hormone of the adrenal cortex. One, perhaps a major, mechanism for its release involves the renin-angiotensin system; angiotensin stimulates its production or movement into the circulation.[16b] The interaction of kidney and adrenal to maintain circulating homeostasis is thus clarified. The role of this steroid in sensitizing vascular smooth muscle, however, apparently may not include angiotensin. In the rabbit, aldosterone lessens the pressor activity of angiotensin.[16c]

PHYSIOLOGIC CONSIDERATIONS

In spite of a vast experience over a period of 50 years with natural vasoactive agents and with their synthetic derivatives, the exact mechanism and the locus of action of most of them is not known; about all that is known is whether blood pressure is raised, lowered, or affected in both directions by each agent. Newly discovered compounds are no exception. Consequently the student finds himself confused by the data although much of it was understood by Dale and his co-workers many years ago.[10] The actions of epinephrine and norepinephrine are definite. Norepinephrine is an over-all vasoconstrictor with local vasoconstrictor effects. Epinephrine is an over-all vasodilator with local constrictor effects.[4]

The known sources of various other natural substances are summarized in Table 11. Different animals respond differently to each; different human beings also probably have responses of varying degrees. For example, histamine constricts vascular smooth muscle in spite of its depressor activity caused by capillary dilatation. Because different areas of the body respond in different ways to these simple substances, the sum total of their actions, manifested by the level of blood pressure and the cardiac output, in no way delineates the specific local action of each. Without bearing in mind these local alterations, there is no way to ascertain their relative effects on each organic vascular bed.

Most of the arterial and arteriolar bed is composed of smooth muscle and all major arteries are strong muscular organs, with the relative amount of elastic tissue decreasing with lessening diameter from aorta to arterioles. A question arises, therefore, as to the relative part arteries of various sizes

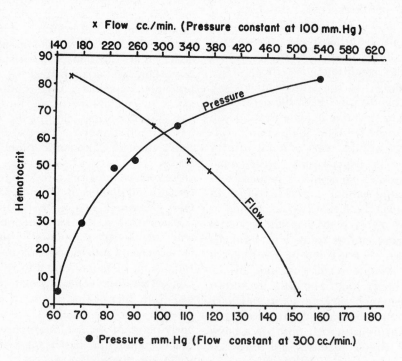

Fig. 90. The effect of viscosity of blood on peripheral resistance and on blood flow. Circles: the change in pressure necessary to maintain a constant flow at different hematocrits. Crosses: change in flow at a constant pressure. Curves were constructed from the experimental data of Whittaker and Winton, as redrawn by Lamport,[18] taken from perfusion experiments on the hind limb of a dog; they probably do not apply exactly for other organs. An assumption was made that pressure and flow were straight line functions. During anemic states the resistance falls moderately and during polycythemic states it increases markedly.

play in contributing to the resistance to flow and especially to its changes. Contrary to the prevalent belief that the arterioles are the "stopcocks of the circulation," Green's calculations[2] show that the major fall in pressure occurs at the smaller arterial branches. Therefore, all of the arteries, whatever their sizes, offer resistance to flow and the greater resistance is offered by the smaller vessels. It is likely that the whole arterial smooth muscular bed participates in vasospasm, whether by neurogenic vasoconstriction or by humoral vasoconstrictor and dilator substances. That the most pronounced effect will be seen in the smallest vessels may be inferred from the diminishing thicknesses of the walls of the arteries from larger to smaller vessels, their much greater numbers, and especially their vastly greater cross-sectional areas.*

Blood Pressure. As discussed previously, the blood pressure is a resultant of *cardiac output, volume, viscosity, elasticity* and *cross-sectional area*. Therefore, the student will do well to bear in mind that five factors are operating every time he measures blood pressure. A high blood pressure can be caused by a high cardiac output, by increased blood viscosity, or by peripheral vasospasm; a high systolic pressure results from hardened pipes. A low blood pressure can be caused by cardiac weakness or low cardiac output from other causes, by low blood volume, by low blood viscosity or by vasodilatation. Measurement of the blood pressure, without taking into account other clinical signs, can be misleading and tells us little about the actual state of the circulation.

Rapid and repeated fluctuations in blood pressure occur normally and must be borne in mind. Janeway was well aware of these spontaneous variations due to respiratory or Traube-Hering waves.[19] They can be as great as 25 mm. Hg systolic and 20 mm. Hg diastolic in some cases. Figure 91 shows examples. Normally, they are not to be re-

* Cross-sectional areas calculated by Green[2] for the dog are as follows (sq. cm.): Aorta, 0.8; large arteries, 3.0; main branches, 5.0; secondary branches, 5.0; tertiary branches, 11.7; terminal arteries, 19.6; terminal branches, 91; arterioles, 125; capillaries, 600.

garded as anything more than manifestations of the essential lability of a system designed to meet rapidly changing conditions rapidly, which is the resultant of 4 or 5 variables, each dependent upon the others.

The effects of one function upon another can be readily understood. Arterial elasticity, which helps determine systolic and pulse pressure, is decreased in high pressure (stretched) states and increased in low (relaxed) states[20] (Fig. 92). The effective viscosity of blood decreases in the smallest arterial vessels. Increased volume of blood available to the heart (increased venous pressure) results in a greater cardiac output, as Starling first showed. An increased volume output into the same sized arterial bed causes a rise in blood pressure. A smaller peripheral bed evokes a cardiac response.

CHEMICAL CONSIDERATIONS

As discussed above, certain chemical substances are the effectors for smooth muscle contraction, just as others are essential for nerve transmission across synapses. It is of basic interest that tetracovalent (quaternary) nitrogen (substituted ammonium), is required for nerve transmission; the brain, the ganglia and the nerve endings contain abundant amounts of nitrogen in this form.[17] Likewise, primary amine (tertiary) nitrogen appears to act differently upon sympathetic nervous end-organs or smooth muscle, although it also influences cerebral function. The mode of action is at present unknown.

Some alteration in metabolism of nitrogenous compounds is apparently set in motion by ischemia. The kidney is most vulnerable in this respect, perhaps because its metabolic rate and oxygen consumption are very high and considerable nitrogen metabolism must take place there in order to provide sufficient ammonia to conserve inorganic base. At any rate, ischemia appears to cause the release of vasoactive substances into the renal venous blood. There is no evidence that hyperemia causes a counteracting series of reactions.

The first change may lie in the insufficient deamination of certain primary amines (other than glutamine), because of oxygen lack. Decarboxylation can be an anaerobic process, deamination aerobic. This metabolic pathway is not the usual one for nitrogen metabolism. The second change appears to be the activation of the "renin pressor mechanism" with the pro-

duction of *angiotensin*. When ischemia is sustained, this mechanism apparently is active for 2 to 3 weeks, evidences for its activity having been discovered in several acute hypertensive and renal ischemic conditions, such as acute nephritis, toxemia of

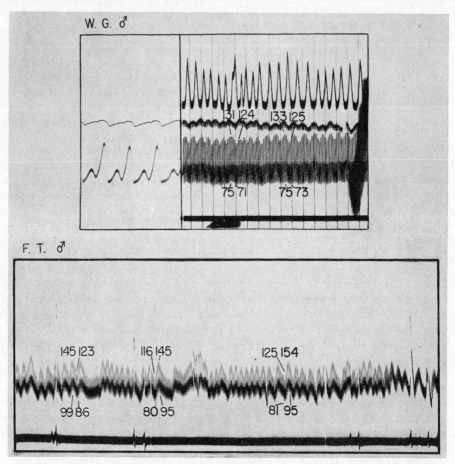

FIG. 91. Examples of variations of blood pressure in man recorded by a Hamilton optical manometer with a needle in the brachial artery at slow camera speeds right to left (1.25 mm./sec.). *First two curves:* W. G. was a 34-year-old normal white man suffering from primary syphilis. Upper tracing, respiration; middle, photoelectric plethysmograph of finger volume and pulse; lower, blood pressure. The variations in systolic pressure were at the most 9 mm. Hg, in diastolic 4 mm. F. T. was a 28-year-old man convalescent from a severe attack of paralytic poliomyelitis. Systolic variations were as much as 38 mm. Hg. diastolic, 19 mm. Note the wide swings occurring with respiration (which appeared normal). Presumably in this instance there was either profound neurogenic vasomotor derangement at a medullary level or wide variations in cardiac output; from the nature of his disease the former explanation is more tenable. This tracing illustrates well the fallacy of considering a single determination of blood pressure as a true reading.

Second two curves: W. D. was a 42-year-old man with hypertension associated with old healed pyelonephritis: Upper tracing, blood pressure; middle, photoelectric plethysmogram of finger; lower, (faint) respirations. Maximal variations

pregnancy and congestive failure. The third change may involve the production of long-acting vasopressor substances, which will be discussed in a later section. How this mechanism is called into play is unknown.

Angiotensin I, formed by renin from its substrate, is a decapeptide which is activated by a peptidase in blood which splits off two terminal amino acids. The resulting octapeptide, angiotensin II, is a very powerful vasoconstrictor; it probably contains terminal amine nitrogen, for it is

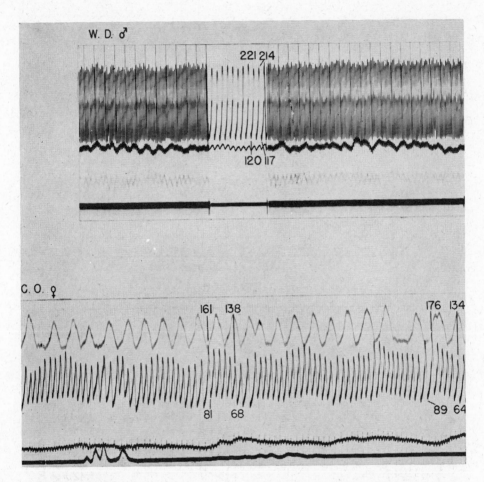

Fig. 91 (*Continued*)

are only about 7/3 mm. Hg. There is little "neurogenic" change. Camera speed 1.5 mm./sec. (middle 5 mm./sec.). C. O. was a 39-year-old woman with neurogenic hypertension without organic change, of 20 years' duration. Upper curve, respirations; middle, blood pressure; lower, lead II electrocardiogram. The maximal regular variations were as great as 42/25 mm. Hg and bore little relation to respiration. These variations are undoubtedly neurogenic in origin. Patient always exhibited hypertension when her blood pressure was taken by the auscultatory method. Her systolic pressure measured frequently by several physicians varied from 240 to 180 mm. Hg and her diastolic from 150 to 100; a well-trained nurse usually obtained it at 20 to 30 mm. lower. Direct arterial puncture varied from normotensive to slightly hypertensive levels. Obviously an erroneous impression of the severity of her hypertension was given to a physician by the indirect sphygmomanometer. The fallacy of a single reading is obvious. (Schroeder, H. A.: Hypertensive Diseases, Philadelphia, Lea & Febiger)

oxidized by monoamine oxidase in vitro which inhibits its action in vivo.[6e]

DISEASES ASSOCIATED WITH GENERALIZED VASOSPASM

Because homeostatic mechanisms keep various essential functions of the body in a state of balance, forces are called into play when balances are disturbed which tend to restore them to the optimal function possible. Since adequate blood flow is essential for life, many powerful forces must be available as emergency mechanisms. Some of these are beginning to be under-

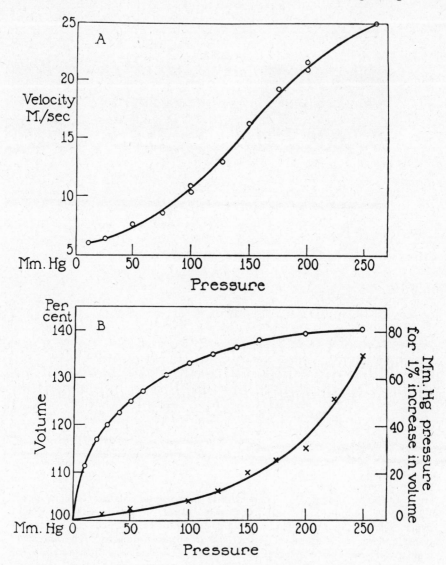

FIG. 92. The relation of pressure to velocity of the pulse wave in the normal brachial artery excised from the arm of a man, 40 years of age, 18 hours after death. The curve would be steeper if the artery were sclerotic. *Upper curve:* The progressively declining increase in arterial volume with each successive increase in pressure. As the pressure rises the arterial volume approaches the elastic limits of the artery until further increase of pressure causes little change in volume. *Lower curve:* The relation of arterial pressure to the amount of pressure necessary to produce a given increase (1 per cent) in arterial volume. At higher pressures the elastic limits of the artery are approached (Steele, Am. Heart J. 14:252)

stood. When, for a variety of reasons, effective circulating blood volume is lessened, a sequence of events is set in motion designed toward restoring that volume. The events do not depend upon the cause of the loss, which may be the result of hemorrhage, trauma, dehydration, cardiogenic disturbances in output, severe chemical and physical stresses and the like. Probably the first reaction is one of neurogenic vasospasm, which takes place following small reductions in cardiac output and which helps to maintain blood pressure. In fact, many of the stimuli which initiate generalized edema (Chap. 31) may begin with a vasospastic reaction the purpose of which is to protect certain vital organs, especially the heart, the coronary arteries and the brain, from ischemia by shifting available blood from less crucial areas, such as the skin, the splanchnic, the muscular and the renal areas. This reaction may operate under normal conditions to some degree; for example, it may protect blood flow to the brain in the upright position and during mild exercise.

If neurogenic vasoconstriction with its concomitant mobilization of blood is insufficient to restore adequate blood flow, the second reaction is evoked. Nephrogenic mechanisms depend upon circulating vasoconstrictor substances other than epinephrine and norepinephrine. It is likely that renal participation in neurogenic vasoconstriction initiates the production of these vasoactive materials. The release of renin allows this proteolytic enzyme to split its globulin substrate to angiotensin, which initiates the third reaction, release of aldosterone by the adrenal cortex. The net results are two: retention of sodium chloride by the kidney and sensitization of vascular smooth muscle to circulating vasoconstrictor substances. These three reactions, stated simply, but which are undoubtedly much more complex, appear to make up the body's primary defenses against diminished flow of blood.

Diseases and disorders may invoke one or all of these primary defenses and be dependent thereon. When all of them are active, edema can be the late result (see Chap. 31). When the third is relatively inactive, arterial hypertension may occur. Hypertension differs from the usual type of vasospastic reaction in that it is not initiated by a reduction in total effective circulating blood volume. Hypertension is to be considered a specialized form of vasospasm, in that nervous factors and local ischemic areas occur in the presence of a normal cardiac output. Therefore, the peripheral manifestations of hypertension are different in terms of blood flow to most areas of the body, although the mechanisms concerned are the same.

SHOCK

Shock, or vasomotor collapse, is probably the most typical of the acute vasospastic conditions resulting from loss of effective circulating blood volume. When blood is lost, trapped or collected in a congested area, a characteristic chain of reactions sets in. It has been suggested that volume receptors initiate the stimuli leading to vasospasm after blood loss.[21] Cardiac effects, i.e., tachycardia, may accompany the vasospasm. These reactions may be so gradual as to be barely perceptible, as is usually the case when a healthy adult loses a pint of blood.

After bleeding, constriction of the arterial vessels in the splanchnic areas, the kidneys, and the skin occurs; muscles are less affected.[22] Venous constriction may decrease the effective venous volume and promote cardiac filling.[23] Pulmonary vascular resistance rises.[24] The renal effects can be profound, with barely measurable rates of blood flow and filtration. Bacterial endotoxins will set off a similar series of vascular reactions;[25] since they can be checked by phenoxybenzamine, they may be humoral or nervous in mediation and possibly operate through stimuli from the brain itself. Cardiogenic shock leads to similar peripheral vasoconstriction. The peripheral resistance is increased, although the cardiac output may be very low.[26]

More profound or sustained losses are accompanied by the second reaction mediated by the kidneys.* Significant depression of blood pressure may or may not be present. When renal blood flow is lessened

* Wiggers does not accept wholly the participation of renal pressor mechanisms in shock;[26] the evidence is indirect in man and inconclusive in dogs.

angiotensin is formed and it then affects the kidneys. Angiotensin has been detected in peripheral blood during acute renal ischemic states. Oliguria, which may be the result of the renal vasospasm and antidiuretic hormones, also occurs in an attempt to restore losses of water.

The third mechanism is also brought into play, mediated through or by the adrenal cortex. Other mechanisms, including the release of stored red blood cells and the maturation of young ones, the synthesis of plasma proteins and repletion of lost colloids and crystalloids in blood, also take place during recovery. The end result is restoration of more normal circulatory hemodynamics. The reactions are listed here in order to form a coherent pattern. Actually each is little understood. Except in the case of neurogenic vasospasm rates of reaction are not known; probably their mechanisms are set in motion rapidly, but their end results are slow to develop. For example, retention of salt and water will cause no increase in body fluids unless water and salt are introduced into the body.

A continuation of the stimuli set in motion in shock (bleeding, cardiac damage, loss of protein-rich fluid into a traumatized area, endotoxins, gastrointestinal losses of salt and water) continues the vasospasm, which may be intense in the face of a low blood pressure. The shock is still reversible. Finally, at some point, possibly through prolonged tissue anoxia with its metabolic alterations leading to hemorrhagic necrosis of the bowel, shock becomes irreversible.* Vessels no longer seem to respond to vasoconstrictor substances, vast quantities of blood can be transfused without causing much more than capillary congestion, and general circulatory failure with death is the inevitable outcome. The transition point between reversible and irreversible shock is difficult to determine clinically and is of unknown chemical nature.

The cause of the intense vasoconstriction which occurs in shock is not known. Some

suggest, because of the increased coronary vasodilatation,[29] that it is due to epinephrine, norepinephrine or autonomic nervous stimulation. Norepinephrine infused in both hemorrhagic and normovolemic shock will raise the blood pressure and restore a markedly depressed renal blood flow toward normal.[30] The effect of this agent is opposite to that seen in normal renal states, where it decreases blood flow. Interestingly enough, the survival rates in animals are considerably improved in hemorrhagic shock when phenoxybenzamine and other adrenolytic agents are used.[31] They are now being tried in human cases.

The cause of irreversible shock has been variously attributed to cellular damage from vasoconstriction and ischemia, toxic production from bacteria, and sludged blood with agglutination and thrombosis.

Lillehei[32] has presented evidence that the irreversible stage is caused by endotoxins from gram-negative bacteria having profound vasoconstrictive properties, especially on the vessels of the splanchnic area. Gram-negative septicemia is said to be the most common cause of clinical irreversible shock among hospital patients. These endotoxins possibly are amines or are aminelike compounds (Table 12).

Apparently failure of response of smooth muscle to vasoconstrictor substances is usually a result, rather than the cause, of irreversible shock. Occasionally, when norepinephrine is infused for long periods of time, larger and larger amounts are required to maintain blood pressure. We have observed this phenomenon in such diverse disorders as coronary occlusion, surgical removal of a pheochromocytoma, bulbar poliomyelitis and disseminated chicken pox. Reactivity of vasoconstriction can be restored by mineralocorticoids, and presumably is dependent upon the status of the adrenal cortex.

Whether shock should be treated by adrenergic substances (norepinephrine) or by adrenergic blocking agents (phenoxybenzamine) as adjunctive measures to restoration of blood volume has not been decided. Apparently both methods have saved lives. It is entirely possible that certain types of

---

* Hamilton and Collins showed that depletion of the globulin substrate of renin, possibly through failure of hepatic synthesis, accompanied this stage.[27] By providing plasma protein, a temporary restoration of the renin pressor mechanism occurs.[28]

shock or certain stages of shock require vasoconstrictive measures while other types or stages require blocking agents. Certainly adequate capillary blood flow is the goal of therapy, but tests to ascertain whether a higher head of arterial pressure or a larger arteriolar cross-sectional area will achieve this end are unavailable.

The signs and symptoms of severe shock are those to be expected from ischemia with the resultant subnormal metabolism dependent upon hypoxia. *Cerebral ischemia* causes apathy, slow depressed cerebration, listlessness, restlessness, muscular hypotonia and weakness with involuntary movements, depressed tendon reflexes and sensation and depressed visual and auditory reflexes. The relative *dehydration* due to the loss of effective circulating blood volume accounts for the pale, livid and ashen color which may show cyanosis in some areas, the loose inelastic skin, the sunken eyeballs, the dry tongue, the thirst and the feeble heart sounds. The *intense vasoconstriction* is reflected by the pallor of skin and mucous membranes, the cold extremities, the collapsed superficial veins, the oliguria, the narrowed retinal vessels and the small pulse pressure. Prolonged renal ischemia may so damage the kidneys through hypoxia that renal shutdown from hypoxic nephrosis may persist and even be fatal after the peripheral circulatory collapse has been controlled.[33] Profound metabolic alterations occur in most organs and systems. While the blood pressure is low in advanced stages and may become imperceptible, and tachycardia is present, in incipient shock it may be normal with only a rapid heart rate and signs of vasoconstriction to define the state.* In fact, a wide variation of symptoms and signs may be present in individual cases.

CONGESTIVE HEART FAILURE

Evidence for generalized vasoconstriction in congestive circulatory failure is accumulating. At first glance, vasospasm might be expected to put an added strain on the left ventricle by increasing peripheral resistance in the face of a low cardiac output and a high blood volume. In that event, release of the vasospasm might promote greater flow with less cardiac work per unit of blood pumped. However, the high blood volume may be a protective mechanism against ischemia. Some workers believe that the failing heart activates the sympathetic nervous system, as do other circulatory emergencies, giving rise to increased peripheral resistance and increased venous tone.[34] Others have suggested that the venous constriction is mediated through the sympathetic nervous system, from centers in the brain, presumably the hypothalamus.[35] The presence, in failure, of venoconstriction, with arterial constriction as well, indicates that all vascular smooth muscle is involved. In severe valvular incompetency, the peripheral signs may be those of shock, with almost bloodless extremities.†

The nature of the vasospasm in congestive heart failure is not well understood. Renal vasoconstriction is profound, renal plasma flow seriously reduced and filtration fraction elevated. The renal hemodynamic picture is similar to that seen in shock and, to a much lesser extent, in hypertension. There is some evidence that spinal anesthesia and sympathetic ganglionic blockade diminish the vasospasm.[36,37] The finding of increased amounts of vasoexcitor material (VEM) in the blood of patients is suggestive of renal participation;[38] angiotensin can sometimes be found in renal venous blood.[39] Pherentasin has been demonstrated in a crude form.[40] Furthermore, there is increasing evidence that either excessive secretion or insufficient metabolism of adrenocortical steroids contributes strongly to the edema; potentiation of the action of normal or abnormal humoral vasoconstrictor substances may therefore occur. In that event, all of the three known vasospastic mechanisms may operate in this condition. The fact that arterial hypertension occa-

* For an excellent discussion of this subject, the reader is referred to Wiggers.[26]

† The author has seen intense peripheral venoconstriction in spite of the high venous pressure of tricuspid stenosis and insufficiency, to the point that puncture of veins in the arm was impossible and only the jugular was accessible.

sionally accompanies congestive failure and regresses when failure is controlled is evidence for generalized vasospasm in these cases.

PULMONARY VASOSPASM

The caliber of arteries and arterioles in the pulmonary vascular bed is apparently under neurogenic control through autonomic fibers, just as is peripheral vascular musculature. Ganglionic blocking agents decrease pulmonary vascular resistance[41]; anoxia or hypoxia increases it.[42] Sudden occlusion of a sizable section by embolus can initiate spasm of the whole bed, presumably through a nervous reflex. Norepinephrine raises pulmonary pressure just as it does systemic pressure; angiotensin, on the other hand, while raising pressure by increasing volume, lowers pulmonary vascular resistance.[43]

One characteristic of the lungs is their ability to "strain" out or destroy some vasoactive metabolites found in venous blood. For example, serotonin apparently is oxidized or conjugated in the pulmonary circuit.[44] Vasoconstrictors and dilators released from shed blood can be removed by passage through the lungs of experimental animals, a phenomenon long known to physiologists; how they are destroyed, whether by direct oxidation or by enzymatic action, is not known.

Chronic pulmonary vasospasm leads to increased right ventricular work, just as chronic peripheral vasospasm affects the left ventricle. The end result is *cor pulmonale*. Pulmonary hypertension is found in hypoxic states, insufficiency of the left ventricle with increased pulmonary venous pressure, and in severe disease of the parenchyma of the lungs, such as emphysema.

LOCAL VASOSPASTIC STATES

Chronic Hypoxia. Apparently, chronic hypoxia of several local areas is accompanied by vasospasm. The cause is unknown but obviously either neurogenic reflex mechanisms or locally produced metabolites must be operating. A certain amount of circulatory relief is obtained by an ischemic part—a limb, for example—when strong vasodilators are infused into

the artery supplying the part or when antimetabolites, surgical sympathectomy and blocking agents are used. These measures not only open up spastic areas, but more especially open collateral channels allowing greater blood supply to the part.[45] Unfortunately, the pharmacology of some of the effective agents, derivatives of imidazole, indole or phenylalanine, is not exactly known. The general principle that hypoxia produces vasospasm holds for lung, skin and extremity insofar as direct local circulatory effects are concerned; renal and cerebral hypoxia produce generalized vasospasm. In other areas of the body, the coronary,* splanchnic, hepatic, adrenal and thyroid circulations, for example, little is known about vascular reactivity to low oxygen states.† Because deamination is usually oxidative, it is possible that failure to deaminate could lead to accumulation of vasoactive primary amines, which can dilate capillaries or constrict arteries, venules and arterioles either directly or through the mediation of local reflexes.

Histamine is liberated from the skin by irritative procedures and heat, as are other primary amines (serotonin).[46] Certain synthetic substances liberate histamine and even deplete the skin of this substance.[47] Local vasoactive substances released in hypoxia deserve further study; their importance in causing symptoms is not known.

ARTERIAL HYPERTENSION

Chronic elevation of diastolic blood pressure is only a sign common to a variety of conditions, just as is chronic elevation of blood sugar, or acute and chronic elevation of body temperature and pulse rate. Blood pressure is one of the "vital signs," and an alteration from normal is no more to

---

* The coronary circulation appears unique, in that sympathetic stimulation increases flow, as do epinephrine, histamine and acetylcholine. No vasoconstrictor control can be demonstrated.[29b]

† While it is generally assumed that hypoxia is the initiating stimulus, this has not yet been proved and there is some evidence to the contrary, in brain and kidney, for example. Perhaps hypoxia is a factor locally and reflexes dependent on pressure receptors or biochemical alterations are the main factors in specialized organs concerned with vascular homeostasis.

be considered indicative of a specific disease than is fever. Unfortunately, one variety, loosely called essential hypertension (meaning of unknown cause), is so common in Western civilization that there is a tendency partly to neglect the remainder, which account for about ⅕ of all cases.

From the preceding discussion, it is apparent that one or more factors constantly operating could produce the special variety of generalized vasospasm which is found in chronic arterial hypertension. This seems to be true, since if we list the varieties of known diseases with which hypertension is associated, they fall in general into 3 major categories, diseases involving the autonomic nerves, the kidneys or the adrenals.[59]

Nonvasospastic Elevated Blood Pressure. High blood pressure may be associated with a number of conditions not secondary to chronic generalized vasospasm. Usually only the systolic pressure is elevated. Increased cardiac stroke volume, as in complete heart block, aortic insufficiency and marked bradycardia, may elevate the systolic pressure. Arteriovenous aneurysms or patent ductus arteriosus of large size raise the output and may sometimes elevate the systolic pressure. Loss of aortic elasticity through arteriosclerosis is probably the commonest cause. Hyperthyroidism is associated with vasodilatation, a high output and a high pulse pressure. Coarctation of the aorta may cause elevated systolic and diastolic pressures in the upper part of the body without vasoconstriction, due to the relatively large proportion of blood from each cardiac ejection being partly and temporarily trapped in that area. Increased blood viscosity in polycythemia vera can elevate the blood pressure, arteriolar run-off being slowed by the thickened blood. Tachycardia may appear to elevate the diastolic pressure falsely, as the diastolic slope of the pressure curve is interrupted by a succeeding beat before arterial run-off has progressed. These conditions must not be confused with vasospastic states. In general, elevation of the diastolic pressure with a normal heart rate, output, and blood

TABLE 13. CHRONIC EXPERIMENTAL
NEUROGENIC HYPERTENSION

STIMULUS CAUSING HYPERTENSION	ANIMAL	REMARKS
Psychogenic Alterations:		
Noise due to wind blast............	Rat	
Hereditary nervous temperament	Dog and ? Rat	(Esp. terrier)
Brain Lesions:		
Kaolin induced lesions of base...........	Dog, rat	
Hypothalamic injury..	Dog	
Increased intracranial pressure..........	Dog	
Decreased cerebral blood flow........	Dog	
Peripheral Neurogenic Mechanisms:		
Moderator nerve removal..........	Dog	
Repeated splanchnic stimulation	Dog	Temporary only
Increased Amounts of Chemical		
Effector substances: epinephrine, nor-epinephrine	Dog, rabbit	Acute only

viscosity is indicative of increased peripheral resistance.

Hypertension Involving Disorders of Autonomic Nerves. It is possible to produce chronic hypertension experimentally by provoking disorders of sympathetic nerves or by affecting cerebral centers (Table 13). Clinical analogues of most of these conditions exist (Table 14). While the evidence for sympathetic nervous overactivity in most cases of essential hypertension is indirect,[48] the use of newer specific drugs has established the fact that reduction of sympathetic tone can favorably affect the condition. However, the degree of hypertension produced by definite lesions of the nervous system is usually moderate, unless other factors come into play.

Benign neurogenic hypertension, not dependent upon specific lesions of nervous tissue, is believed to be an hereditary disorder associated with certain traits of personality; the somatic outflow is apparently

TABLE 14. CLINICAL NEUROGENIC HYPERTENSION

	REDUCED RENAL BLOOD FLOW	"ESSENTIAL" HYPERTENSION MIMICKED	FLUCTUATING B. P. FOUND	REMARKS
Pathologic Lesions in Brain				
Diminished blood flow due to creased intracranial pressure (tumors, trauma, infection)	Yes	No	Yes	Primary disease relatively acute and severe
Occlusion of carotid artery.........	Yes	Yes	Yes	From atherosclerosis
Altered function due to local inflammatory or degenerative states:				
Bulbar poliomyelitis.............	?	Yes	Yes ⎫	Chronic hypertension,
Basal encephalitis..............	?	Yes	Yes ⎬	usually mild
Hypothalamic injury...........	Yes	Yes	Yes	Hypertension may be severe
Pathologic Lesions Elsewhere				
Altered function due to general hypoxia:				
? Cardiac failure..............	Yes	No	Yes	Cardiac disease primary
Ascending paralysis............	?	No	Yes	Generally acute
Low oxygen tensions...........	Yes	No	Yes	Generally acute
Carbon monoxide posioning......	Yes	No	Yes	Generally acute
Functional Alterations in Hypothalamus with Similar Signs and Symptoms				
Diencephalic syndrome of neurogenic hypertension.......	Yes	Yes	Yes ⎫	Most have or develop
Anxiety states—chronic...........	Yes	Yes	Yes ⎬	"essential" hypertension
Increased Amounts of Chemical Effector Substances of Autonomic Nerves				
Pheochromocytoma..............	Yes	Yes	Yes	Epinephrine = high cardiac output. Norepine-epinephrine = normal cardiac output
Nicotine........................	Yes	Yes?	Yes	Usually a transient effect
Porphyrins in acute porphyria?.....	?	Yes	Yes	Usually a transient effect

through the sympathetic nervous system.[49] It is not known why the somatic manifestations are those of neurogenic vasospasm; perhaps hereditary, developmental or constitutional factors determine this method of reaction, rather than through the parasympathetic system. The vasospasm is readily reversed by sedation and by drugs which act upon hypothalamic autonomic centers or the cortical pathways leading to them during the mild or earlier stages of the disorder. Therefore, the disease represents a functional alteration in hemodynamics which can be mimicked by the slow infusion of norepinephrine. Pheochromocytomata releasing norepinephrine (usually extra-

adrenal ones) also produce a similar picture when the tumor is discharging. Those releasing epinephrine are associated with symptoms seen in epinephrine-induced hypertension. Most medullary tumors release both substances.

The hypertension caused by sympathetic discharges and that produced by norepinephrine can be considered examples of reversible neurogenic vasospasm, which possibly might remain so were it not for the presence of some renal or other mechanism which converts a reversible reaction into an irreversible one.

Hypertension Involving Disorders of the Kidneys. There appear to be two types of

TABLE 15. NEPHROGENIC HYPERTENSION IN MAN AND ANIMALS[13]
(WITHOUT RENAL INSUFFICIENCY)

	% HYPER-TENSIVE	RENAL BLOOD FLOW REDUCED	EXPERIMENTAL COUNTERPART
"Primary" Nephrogenic Hypertension			
Affections of renal parenchyma:			
Pyelonephritis and other infections.................	64	Yes	Rat
Hydronephrosis..........................	25	Yes	Rat
Polycystic kidneys........................	64	Yes	
Trauma and scarring.......................	Occ.	Yes	Rat
Tumors of certain variety only..............	Occ.	?	
Infarction, special types...................	Occ.	Yes	
Congenital hypoplasia and other lesions............	48	Yes	
Perinephritis..........................	Occ.	Yes	Rat, dog, rabbit
Gouty nephritis.........................	37	Yes	Rat
Ureteral obstruction......................	+	Yes	
Affections of renal capillaries:			
Glomerulonephritis.........................	35*	Yes	Rat
Disseminated lupus.......................	12	Yes	
Glomerulosclerosis (diabetic)..................	90†	Yes	
Embolic nephritis........................	+	Yes	
Affections of intrarenal arteries:			
Collagen disease (polyarteritis, dermatomyositis, scleroderma)...........................	53	Yes	
Thromboangiitis obliterans..................	+	Yes	
Certain metallic poisons....................	+	?	Rat
Affections of main renal arteries:			
Thrombosis, partial.......................	+	Yes⎫	Dog, monkey, rabbit, goat, rat, etc. (Goldblatt clamp)
Arteriosclerotic plaques....................	86	Yes⎬	
Aneurysm, dissecting......................	+	Yes⎭	
Coarctation of aorta......................	12	Occ.	Rat
Secondary Nephrogenic Hypertension			
Affections of renal arterioles:			
Secondary arteriolar nephrosclerosis.............	+‡	Yes	
Secondary Nephrogenic Vasospasm without Hypertension			
Generalized conditions leading to reduction in renal blood flow:			
Low cardiac output.......................	0	Yes	Dog
Congestive heart failure....................	Occ.	Yes	Dog
Shock and other hypovolemic states..............	0	Yes	Dog, etc.

* Systolic > 200 mm.
† Estimated.
‡ Present eventually in almost all cases.

nephrogenic hypertension, one dependent upon azotemia and one dependent upon renal ischemia. A large variety of renal disorders will produce arterial hypertension in *susceptible* animals; such lesions produced in certain unsusceptible animals cause no hypertension.[50] In man, the coexistence of renal parenchymal diseases and neurogenic vasospasm may cause severe arterial hypertension, while either influence alone may not do so. In Table 15 are shown some of the associated lesions. In fact, hypertension is not a universal accompaniment of any organic renal disease

Table 16. Endocrine Hypertension, Clinical Types

	Central Obesity	Menstrual Abnormalities	Cushinglike Findings	Hypertension Sometimes Found	Masculinization in Female	Feminization in Male	Remarks
Primary Adrenocortical Pathology with Hyperfunction							
Adenoma	+++	Yes	Yes	+	±	Rare	Cushing's syndrome
Carcinoma, some cases	0-+++	Usually	Usually	+	0-++++	Yes	Cushing's syndrome
Hyperplasia	+++	Yes	Yes	+	±	?	Cushing's syndrome
Hyperfunction	+++	Yes	Yes	+	±	?	Endocrine hypertensive syndrome
Specific adenoma or hyperplasia	0-+	No	No	+	0	0	Primary aldosteronism
Other Endocrine Pathology Simulating Hyperfunction of Adrenal							
Adrenallike ovarian tumor	Often	Yes	Often	+	±	—	May simulate several syndromes
Arrhenoblastoma	Occasionally	Yes	Occasionally	+	±	—	May simulate several syndromes
Chorionepithelioma	Occasionally	Yes	Occasionally	+	±	—	May simulate several syndromes
Thymic tumors	?	Yes	?	?	0	?	Rare and poorly described
Pineal tumors	?	Yes	?	?	0	?	Rare and poorly described
Pituitary Disturbances Leading to Adrenal Hyperfunction							
Basophilism	++++	Yes	Yes	+	±	±	Cushing's syndrome
Some cases of acromegaly	++	Yes	Yes	+	+	0	Mixed pituitary disease
Some cases of menopause	+++	Yes	Yes	+	+	—	Vaguely Cushinglike
Administration of ACTH	++	Often	Yes	+	0	Yes	Cushinglike
Hyperfunction	++	Yes	Yes	+	±	?	Endocrine hypertensive syndrome
Hormone Administration							
Cortisone and hydrocortisone	+	Yes	Yes	++	0	?	Vaguely Cushinglike
Aldosterone, DCA and salt	0	0	0	++	0	0	Hypertension only
Unknown Endocrine Disturbances							
Pre-eclampsia	0	—	0	+	0	—	Possibly due to steroid hormone aberrations
Eclampsia	0	—	0	+	0	0	

without azotemia; it is absent in 40 to 70 per cent of patients with organic renal lesions, according to various analyses.[13]

Long-sustained chronic hypertension on a neurogenic basis causes nephrogenic hypertension. Some change takes place in the kidney, or the kidney has already become susceptible, so that renal influence is added to the neurogenic. Later in the course of the disease, sclerosis of the renal arterioles and arteries develops and produces mechanical ischemia by narrowing the vessels supplying the nephrons. It is this change which makes hypertension a difficult problem to treat and leads to its fatal outcome. It does not matter, apparently, whether the hypertension originates with nervous impulses, or with secretion of adrenal medullary or cortical hormones from a tumor—the end result is the same. Failure to appreciate this secondary effect of chronic hypertension has led to many and varied interpretations of therapeutic results and prognoses.

Azotemic hypertension appears concurrently with renal insufficiency; it is usually of moderate degree and unassociated with marked cardiovascular changes. The chemical mediators may involve excessive retention of catecholic amines, found in higher blood concentrations, or other nitrogenous waste products not excreted by the kidney. It must be differentiated as sharply as clinical deductions allow from nonazotemic renal ischemic nephrogenic hypertension. The former condition is not well understood.

Hypertension Involving Disorders of the Adrenal Cortex. Certain disturbances of the adrenal cortices themselves, or the pituitary-adrenal axis, are associated with hypertension. While the exact hormones involved are not known, by analogy with experimental animals given desoxycorticosterone and salt, the salt-retaining hormones are believed to be involved. Some of these disorders cause other changes (Cushing's syndrome) (Table 16); others appear to induce only central obesity and hypertension associated with a low sodium concentration in sweat (a sign of excess of salt-retaining hormone).[51] There is little evidence for the adrenal being overactive

in neurogenic or nephrogenic hypertension, save in the end stages.

The "Irreversible" Stage of Hypertension. Regardless of the cause, late stages of chronic hypertension are irreversible insofar as their reaction to heavy sedation, anesthesia, specific nerve-blocking drugs, chemical and surgical sympathectomy and the like are concerned.* It is presumed that a variable but often progressively severe nephrogenic component, acting through humoral vasoconstrictor substances, enters the picture and maintains the hypertension in spite of almost total inhibition of neurogenic influences. The humoral substances present in such a situation have not been chemically delineated; several have been found. Pherentasin is apparently a polypeptide with an aliphatic linkage and primary amine, possibly containing sulfur and probably needing a trace metal for its action. It has a long, sustained, pressure-elevating effect in the rat and acts directly on rabbit aortic smooth muscle, even when opposed by such potent nerve blocking agents as phenoxybenzamine.[52] It is found in hypertensive arterial blood (and in a few people with congestive failure). A protein pressor principle has a similar action in animals.[53] Other unidentified substances have been detected in hypertensive blood and urine (Table 17). Angiotensin has not been found in excess in the chronic stage of hypertension, although pherentasin and angiotensin may be similar.

THE RESULTS OF CHRONIC VASOSPASM

Chronic generalized vasospasm associated with a normal or low blood pressure apparently does little more than reduce the amount of oxygen and nutrients to tissues. Serious secondary physical effects are not seen unless the condition becomes severe; that is, the predisposing influences, whether cardiac, volume or oxygen-lack, progress to a point incompatible with life. However, profound metabolic alterations may occur which may continue indefinitely or cause death of the organism. The

* The use of the word irreversible is hardly fair since the newer drugs, used properly, will reverse the condition eventually.[54,55,56]

TABLE 17. HUMORAL PRESSOR SUBSTANCES POSSIBLY INVOLVED IN HYPERTENSION AND OTHER VASOSPASTIC STATES

NAME	SOURCE	NATURE	SITE OF ACTION	DURATION OF ACTION	REMARKS
Angiotensin.......	Renin + substrate	Peptide	Smooth muscle	Acute	In acute renal ischemic states
Sustained Pressor Principle........	Ischemic kidney	Protein	?	Very long	In shock
Vasoexcitor Material (VEM)	Ischemic kidney	?	?	Long	Sensitizes vessels to epinephrine
Pherentasin........	Arterial blood	Peptide	Smooth muscle	Long	Chronic hypertension

body has extraordinary powers to adjust. Chemical alterations associated with local hypoxia and vasospasm, however, can produce tissue changes. In the fingers and the hands, when there is repeated neurogenic vasospasm (Raynaud's phenomenon), the skin becomes thickened and trophic changes develop. A combination of vasospasm and organic ischemia, or merely the latter, can cause gangrene. Pain is a frequent symptom of ischemia of muscle. Fibrosis, atrophy, alerations in smooth and striated muscle, thromboses and edema may be found.

Generalized vasospasm associated with elevated blood pressure causes certain physical effects which lead to diseases of vital organs. There are three main effects of vasospastic hypertension: (1) The work of the heart is increased in direct proportion to the pressure. This leads to hypertrophy, dilatation of the left ventricle and eventual failure. About half of all untreated hypertensive patients who die of this disease, do so in congestive failure.[57] (2) The sustained pressure, or a metabolic association thereof, causes arteriolar sclerosis. In the kidneys, this leads to nephrosclerosis and may involve azotemia. (3) The most serious effect is to increase the rate of progression of atherosclerosis; for atheromata are prone to develop at sites of high pressure. These three secondary effects constitute the hazard of chronic hypertension.

SUMMARY

Vasospasm is a fundamental reaction of the vascular smooth muscle to a number of stimuli, the common denominator of which appears to be a reduction in the blood flow required for essential metabolic processes or a diminution in the supply of oxygen to certain tissues. In acute conditions, it appears to preserve blood flow, insofar as possible, in certain organs at the expense of others. The known organs and systems which take part in the production of vasospasm are sympathetic nerves, the kidneys and the adrenal glands. Many metabolic alterations can occur, some of which enhance the vasospasm.[60] Hypoxia in certain local areas also will produce either local or general vasospasm, depending upon the area involved. Chronic arterial hypertension can be considered as a specialized form of generalized vasospasm.

REFERENCES

1. Peterson, L. H.: Vascular Tone, Mod. Conc. Cardiov. Dis. 33:725, 1962.
2. Green, H. D.: Circulatory system, physical principles, in Glasser, O., ed.: Medical Physics, vol. 2, Chicago, Yr. Bk. Pub., 1950.
3. Barger, G., and Dale, H. H.: Chemical structure and sympathomimetic action of amines, J. Physiol. 41:19, 1910.
4. Barcroft, H., and Swan, H. J. C.: Sympathetic Control of Human Blood Vessels, London, Arnold, 1953.
5. Aviado, D. M., Jr., and Schmidt, C. F.: Reflexes from stretch receptors in blood vessels, heart and lungs, Physiol. Rev. 35:247, 1955.
6a. Blaschko, H.: Amine oxidase and amine metabolism, Pharmacol. Rev. 4:415, 1952.
6b. Smith, D. J. and Alperi, S.: Amine oxidase and adrenergic vasoconstriction of dog and swine arteries, Fed. Proc. 13:140, 1954.

6c. Schroeder, H. A.: The effect of a preparation of amine oxidase on experimental hypertension. Science 95:306, 1942.

7. Olsen, N. S., and Schroeder, H. A.: Oxygen tension and pH of the renal cortex in acute ischemia and chronic hypertension, Am. J. Physiol. 163:181, 1950.

8a. Braun-Menendez, E., Fasciolo, J. C., Leloir, L. F., and Munoz, J. M.: The substance causing renal hypertension, J. Physiol. 98: 283, 1940.

8b. Page, I. H., and Helmer, O. M.: A crystalline pressor substance resulting from the reaction between renin and renin-activator, J. Exper. Med. 71:29, 1940.

9a. Nickel, J. F., Smythe, C. McC., Papper, E. M., and Bradley, S. E.: A study of the mode of action of the adrenal medullary hormones on sodium, potassium and water excretion in man, J. Clin. Invest. 33:1687, 1954.

9b. Schroeder, H. A., and Steele, J. M.: The behaviour of renal blood flow after partial constriction of the renal artery. J. Exper. Med. 72:707, 1940.

9c. Skinner, S. L., McCubbin, J. W., and Page, I. H.: Renal baroceptor control of renin secretion. Science 141:814, 1963.

10. Dale, H. H.: Adventures in Physiology, London, Pergamon Press, 1953.

11. Schroeder, H. A., and Olsen, N. S.: Humoral pressor substances and their relation to arterial hypertension, Am. Chemical Soc. Advances in Chemistry, Series No. 2, May 23, 1950.

12a. Yamada, H., and Yasunobu, K. T.: Monoamine Oxidase, J. Biol. Chem. 237:1511, 1962.

12b. Yamada, H., and Yasunobu, K. T.: Monoamine oxidase. II. Copper, one of the prosthetic groups of plasma monoamine oxidase, J. Biol. Chem. 237:3077, 1962.

13. Schroeder, H. A.: Hypertensive Diseases, Causes and Control, Philadelphia, Lea & Febiger, 1953.

14. Goldman, M. L., and Schroeder, H. A.: Immediate pressor effects of desoxycorticosterone acetate in arterial hypertension, Am. J. Med. 5:33, 1948.

15. Raab, W.: Hormonal and Neurogenic Cardiovascular Disorders, Baltimore, Williams & Wilkins, 1953.

16a. Selye, H., Hall, C. E., and Rawley, E. M.: Malignant hypertension produced by treatment with desoxycorticosterone acetate and sodium chloride, Canad. M.A.J. 49:88, 1943.

16b. Ganong, W. F., Mulrow, P. J., and Boryczka, C. G.: Evidence for a direct effect of angiotensin II on adrenal cortex of the dog. Proc. Soc. Exp. Biol. Med. 109:381, 1962.

16c. Katz, Y. J., Moore, R. S., Velasquez, A. M., and Tamosaitis, I. T.: Angiotensin pressor inhibition by aldosterone in the rabbit. Science 141:725, 1963.

17. Lorente de No, R.: On the effect of certain quaternary ammonium ions upon frog nerve, Parts I and II, J. Cell. & Comp. Physiol. 33: (Supplement) July, 1949.

18. Lamport, H.: Hemodynamics, in Fulton, J. F., ed.: Howell's Textbook of Physiology, ed. 15, Philadelphia, Saunders, 1946.

19. Janeway, T. C.: The Clinical Study of Blood-Pressure, New York, Appleton, 1904.

20. Steele, J. M.: Interpretation of arterial elasticity from measurements of pulse wave velocities. I. Effect of pressure, Am. Heart J. 14:452, 1937.

21. Gauer, O. H., Henry, J. P., Sieker, H. O., and Wendt, W. E.: The effect of negative pressure breathing on urine flow, J. Clin. Investigation 33:287, 1954.

22. Eckstein, R. W., Liebow, I. M., and Wiggers, C. J.: Lymph blood flow and vascular resistance changes in dogs during hemorrhagic hypotension and shock, Am. J. Physiol. 147: 685, 1946.

23. Edholm, O. G.: The Effects of Haemorrhage on the Cardiovascular System in Man, in: British Postgraduate Medical Federation Lectures on the Scientific Basis of Medicine, vol. 1, pp. 79-95, 1951-52, London, University of London, The Athlone Press, 1953.

24. Henry, J. P., Gauer, O. H., Sieker, H. O., and Wendt, W. E.: Pressure-volume relationship in the low-pressure side of the cardiovascular system, Am. J. Physiol. 171: 735, 1952.

25. Delauney, A., Lebrun, J., Delauney, M., and Foucquier, E.: Lésions et réactions du tissu lymphoide, Ann. Inst. Pasteur 76:314, 1949.

26. Wiggers, C. J.: Physiology of Shock, New York, Commonwealth Fund, 1950.

27. Hamilton, A. S., and Collins, D. A.: Role of the kidney in the maintenance of arterial blood pressure in hemorrhage, Am. J. M. Sc. 202:914, 1941.

28a. Sapirstein, L. A., Ogden, E., and Southard, F. D., Jr.: Renin-like substance in blood after hemorrhage, Proc. Soc. Exper. Biol. Med. 48:505, 1941.

28b. Sapirstein, L. A., Southard, F. D., Jr., and Ogden, E.: Restoration of blood pressure by renin activator after hemorrhage, Proc. Soc. Exper. Biol. Med. 50:320, 1942.

29a. Opdyke, D. F., and Foreman, R. C.: Study of coronary flow under conditions of hemorrhagic hypotension and shock, Am. J. Physiol. 148:726, 1947.

29b. Winbury, M. M., and Green, D. M.: Studies on the nervous and humoral control of coronary circulation, Am. J. Physiol. 170:555, 1952.

30. Moyer, J. H., and Morris, G.: Vasopressor agents for severe hypotension and shock, Postgrad. Med. 16:287, 1954.

31. Wiggers, H. C., Ingraham, R. C., Roemhild, F., and Goldberg, H.: Vasoconstriction and the development of irreversible hemorrhagic shock, Am. J. Physiol. 153:511, 1948.

32. Boch, K. D., ed.: Shock, Pathogenesis and Therapy, von Euler, U. S., Chairman, Berlin, Springer, 1962.

33. Dunn, J. S., Gillespie, M., and Niven, J. S. F.: Renal lesions in two cases of crush syndrome, Lancet 2:549, 1941.

34. Fejfar, Z., and Brod, J.: The mechanism of general haemodynamic changes in heart failure, Acta Med. Scandinav. 148:247, 1954.

35. Halmágyi, D., Felkai, B., Ivánzi, J., and Hetényi, G., Jr.: The role of the nervous system in the maintenance of venous hypertension in heart failure, Brit. Heart J. 14: 101, 1952.

36. Mokotoff, R., and Ross, G.: The effect of spinal anesthesia on the renal ischemia in congestive heart failure, J. Clin. Invest. 27:335, 1948.

37. Burch, R. R.: The effects of intravenous hexamethonium on venous pressure of normotensive and hypertensive patients with and without congestive heart failure, Circulation 11:271, 1955.

38. Mokotoff, R., Escher, D. J. W., Edelman, I. S., Grossman, J., Leiter, L., Weston, R. E., Zweifach, B. W., and Shorr, E.: Studies on vasotropic principles in blood (VEM and VDM) and renal hemodynamics in chronic heart failure, Fed. Proc. 8:112, 1949.

39. Merrill, A. J., Morrison, J. L., and Brannon, E. S.: Concentration of renin in renal venous blood in patients with chronic heart failure, Am. J. Med. 1:468, 1946.

40. Schroeder, H. A., and Olsen, N. S.: Pressor substances in arterial hypertension. II. Demonstration of pherentasin, a vasoactive material procured from blood, J. Exper. Med. 92:545, 1950.

41. Gilmore, H. R., Koppelman, H., McMichael, J., and Milne, I. G.: The effect of hexamethonium bromide on cardiac output

and pulmonary circulation, Lancet 2:898, 1952.

42a. Hall, P. W.: Effects of anoxia on post-arteriolar pulmonary vascular resistance, Circulation Res. 1:238, 1953.

42b. Harvey, R. M., Ferrer, M. I., Richards, D. W., and Cournand, A.: Influence of chronic pulmonary disease on the heart and circulation, Am. J. Med. 10:719, 1951.

43. Chimoskey, J. E., Blaquier, P. C., Taquini, A. C., Jr., and Bohr, D. F.: Effects of angiotensin on pulmonary and systemic hemodynamics. Am. J. Physiol. 202:690, 1962.

44. Page, I. H.: Serotonin (5-hydroxytryptamine), Physiol. Rev. 34:563, 1954.

45. Dixon, J. A., Scott, W. J. M., and Epstein, M. A.: Intra-arterial histamine in the treatment of occlusive peripheral arterial disease, Circulation 5:661, 1952.

46. Malméjac, J., Neverre, G., and Poulain, R.: Réactions cutanées à l'hyperthermie. Manifestations vasculaires. Compt. rend. Soc. de biol. 145:1512, 1951.

47. Feldberg, W., and Talesnik, J.: Reduction of tissue histamine by compound 48/80, J. Physiol. 120:550, 1953.

48. Goodall, McC., and Bogdonoff, M.: Essential hypertension with an elevated noradrenaline excretion. Am. Heart J. 61:640, 1961.

49. Schroeder, H. A.: Pathogenesis of hypertension, Am. J. Med. 10:189, 1951.

50. Schroeder, H. A., and Goldman, M. L.: Arterial hypertension in dogs. I. Methods, Circulation 5:730, 1952.

51. Schroeder, H. A., and Davies, D. F.: Studies on "essential" hypertension. V. An endocrine hypertensive syndrome, Ann. Int. Med. 40:516, 1954.

52. Schroeder, H. A., Perry, H. M., Jr., Dennis, E. G., and Mahoney, L. E.: Pressor substances in arterial hypertension. V. Chemical and pharmacological characteristics of pherentasin, J. Exper. Med. 102:319, 1955.

53. Shipley, R. E., Helmer, O. M., and Kohlstaedt, K. G.: The presence in blood of a principle which elicits a sustained pressor response in nephrectomized animals, Am. J. Physiol. 149:708, 1947.

54. Schroeder, H. A.: Management of arterial hypertension, Am. J. Med. 17:540, 1954.

55. Wilkins, R. W.: The management of essential hypertension, J. Chronic Diseases, 1:563, 1955.

56. Boch, K. D., and Cottier, P. T., eds.: Essential Hypertension, An International Sym-

posium Sponsored by Ciba, Ltd. Reubi, F. C., Chairman, Berlin, Springer, 1960.

57. Goldring, W., and Chasis, H.: Hypertension and Hypertensive Disease, New York, Commonwealth Fund, 1944.

58. Lovenberg, W., Weissbach, H., and Udenfriend, S.: Aromatic l-amino acid decarboxylase, J. Biol. Chem. 237:89, 1962.

59. Schroeder, H. A.: Mechanisms of Hypertension. Springfield, Ill., Thomas, 1957.

60. Dahl, L. K.: Metabolic aspects of hypertension, Ann. Rev. of Medicine 14:69, 1963.

13

Palpitation and Tachycardia

EDWARD MASSIE

PALPITATION

The word palpitation is a derivative of the Latin *palpitare,* which means to throb. Palpitation is usually a less direful heart symptom than pain and dyspnea and is extremely common. It consists of an unpleasant sensation of the heart's action, whether slow or fast, regular or irregular. It is more frequently the result of the less important disturbances of cardiac rhythm, namely, premature beats and atrial paroxysmal tachycardia, or of forceful regular heart action, either rapid or slow, resulting from effort, excitement, toxins (as from tobacco, caffeine, or alcohol), or infection. Minor degrees of disturbance more easily produce palpitation if the subject is a nervously sensitive person. Less frequently it may be caused by a more important disorder of heart rhythm such as atrial fibrillation, atrial flutter, or ventricular paroxysmal tachycardia.

It should be emphasized that palpitation and tachycardia often do not indicate a primary physical disorder but rather a psychic disturbance. They are the most important symptoms of cardiac neurosis. If such symptoms are analyzed critically it is seen that subjectively they result in what is termed heart consciousness and that they may be only manifestations of enhanced normal function. Various associated symptoms sometimes occur which are largely the result of more appreciative sensibilities. It is well known that when a person becomes nervously exhausted or hyperirritable his sense of values and judgment are often somewhat distorted, especially in matters concerned with his physical and psychic well-being. If at such a time the patient has occasion to lift some object or walk up up an incline, he may instantly notice rapid and forceful beating of his heart. This symptom usually disappears rapidly, but if similar experiences are repeated, he may become convinced that something serious has happened to his heart. The patient's nervous condition has brought about sufficient introspection, anxiety and uncertainty to produce an increase of cardiac irritability and a decrease of the threshold at which palpitation, tachycardia and the associated symptoms of cardiac neurosis become evident. Often the threshold of consciousness of the heart's action is so lowered that palpitation may be complained of when the rate and the rhythm are perfectly normal.

Palpitation is one of the most characteristic symptoms of neurocirculatory asthenia. In this condition it results, along with other symptoms of the disease, probably from an imbalance of the autonomic nervous system. Such an imbalance may be more or less constant in certain nervously hypersensitive individuals, but may also be precipitated in relatively normal persons by emotional or physical upsets acting reflexly on the autonomic nervous system.

The functional aspect of the symptom complex of palpitation was beautifully described in 1836 by John C. Williams* of Edinburgh who wrote a book on "Practical Observations on Nervous and Sympathetic Palpitation of the Heart, Particularly As Distinguished from Palpitation the Result of Organic Disease." He criticized the practice, usually followed up to that time, of attributing functional derangement of the heart to true heart disease. He taught that palpitation was

frequently, by a careless observer, regarded as symptomatic of some serious organic or structural change being established either in the coverings of the heart, its muscular texture, or in some of its natural valvular appurtenances. A careful and deliberate inquiry, however, will, in the generality of cases, enable us to strip them of their apparent obscurity and danger and reduce them to their place in nosological arrangement. Latterly there has been too great a rage for tracing diseases almost exclusively to vascular derangement. I deprecate this, because I am convinced of the increasing influence of the nervous system, both in health and in disease. A deservedly popular writer on medicine of the present day says, "The longer we live, the more we see; and the deeper we study, so much the more shall we become convinced, that not only are the primary impressions of morbific causes sustained by the sentient system of the human fabric, but it is here the primary morbid movements first begin, and are thence propagated to the vascular apparatus, which from that movement reacts upon, and is again influenced by the nervous system. No man, I am satisfied, can ever be a sound Pathologist, or a judicious practitioner, who devotes his attention to one of these systems in preference or to the exclusion of the other; through life they are perpetually acting, and inseparably linked together."

Williams goes on to quote a Dr. Baille as follows:

There are in truth few phenomena which puzzle, perplex, and lead to error the inexperienced (and sometimes the experienced) practitioner, so much as inordinate action of the heart.

* Quoted in the third edition of "Heart Disease" by Dr. Paul D. White.

He sees, or thinks he sees, some terrible cause for this tumult in the central organ of the circulation and frames his portentous diagnosis and prognosis accordingly. In the pride of his penetration he renders miserable for the time the friends and by his direful countenance damps the spirits of his patient. But ultimate recovery not seldom disappoints his fears and the Physician is mortified at his own success.

Neurocirculatory Asthenia. Palpitation is one of the most characteristic symptoms of neurocirculatory asthenia. This condition, first described during our Civil War, was very prevalent in World War I and again in World War II; therefore, it certainly merits detailed discussion. Among the current synonyms for this disease are "effort syndrome," "disorderly action of the heart," "soldier's heart" and "Da Costa's syndrome." The last term is derived from Da Costa's classical article on the irritable heart, published in 1871 and based upon his experiences as surgeon in the Northern armies in the Civil War. The incidence of this disease has since been found to increase sharply in wartime and to vary greatly from only a few cases among soldiers in military training to a considerable number under the strain and the hardship of combat. Although this condition came into prominence in World War I, it appears to have been even more of a problem in World War II.

Neurocirculatory asthenia of a pronounced degree is not too common in civilian life, primarily because those likely to develop the condition are usually able to avoid the factors of effort and nervous strain that help precipitate the undesirable symptoms. There is, however, no way to determine its frequency, for in the slight, and much more commonly unrecognized form, it is not likely to be recorded as a specific diagnosis. As a matter of fact, White and his associates were able to study a group of patients who had what was diagnosed in Army hospitals as neurocirculatory asthenia, and listed their various symptoms. Then, when a similar survey was made of the symptoms of patients on whom the diagnosis of *anxiety neurosis* had been made in the psychiatric wards, the similarity in symptoms was striking. Thus it would seem that two patients with the same complaints and symptoms might have different diagnoses, depending entirely upon whether they were seen by a psychiatrist or an internist.

CLINICALLY neurocirculatory asthenia is characterized by such prominent symptoms as palpitation, chest pain, weakness, dyspnea, sighing respiration, sweating, tremulousness, dizziness, nervousness, headache and faintness, all of which are aggravated by excitement or effort and accompany or follow periods of anxiety, nervousness, or physical strain and infection. This symptom complex may occur as the only manifestation of illness or it may be a complication of many diseases, including structural disease of the heart or of other organ systems. The disease appears to be a result of fundamental imbalance of the autonomic nervous system. Such imbalance may be more or less constant in certain nervously hypersensitive or constitutionally inferior individuals, but may also occur in relatively normal persons after psychic or physical upsets which act reflexly on the autonomic nervous system. The patient may be acutely aware of the most minor variations in the heart rhythm or rate. Palpitation may be so severe as a result of an occasional extrasystole or even mild exertion that the patient becomes more or less incapacitated. In contrast with the characteristic symptoms listed above, there are no prominent physical signs in neurocirculatory asthenia. Tachycardia is often present, although the cardiac rate may be normal when mental and physical rest are established—only to increase again with slight exertion or with a disturbing thought. Such physical findings as cold, moist hands, excessive perspiration, tremor of the fingers, dermatographism and variable and slightly elevated blood pressure are frequently encountered. The heart itself, in the great majority of cases, is structurally normal and shows no significant murmurs. In addition, no characteristic laboratory findings have been identified in neurocirculatory asthenia.

Relationship of Palpitation to Organic Heart Disease. Persons with normal hearts may complain of palpitation whenever the force or the rate of the cardiac beat is increased to more than a moderate degree. On the other hand, patients with actual cardiac disorders as a rule are fortunately somewhat less sensitive than normal individuals to the force and the rate of the cardiac beat. Perhaps this is a result in part of habituation, so that even in the presence of irregular rhythms or of undue increases in rate, the abnormal stimuli do not penetrate the patient's consciousness and the reflex phenomena at the basis of palpitation are not produced. Atrial fibrillation often is present when the patient has no sensation of any heart disorder. Occasionally such patients temporarily have palpitation after restoration to normal rhythm, although none was experienced when atrial fibrillation was present. In cardiac decompensation with profound disturbances of rate and rhythm, palpitation is not infrequently absent even when dyspnea and orthopnea are severe.

Quite frequently extrasystoles are discovered of which the patient has no knowledge. Consciousness of an extrasystole is apt to be the awareness of a sudden premature forceful beat followed by a longer than usual pause. In contrast, patients with aortic valve disease including the lesions of stenosis or insufficiency, in which the cardiac beat may be extremely forceful and heaving, usually experience no palpitation. Sometimes the sensations that develop from benign extrasystoles can be very disturbing as well as peculiar and distinctive, and it is well to be familiar with them since the description of the symptoms given by the patient may establish the diagnosis without further examination. The sensations are described in such varied ways as "a flop of the heart," "twisting or skipping of the heart," "sinking or fading away of the heart," "a sudden lump or choking feeling in the throat," "the heart turns a somersault" and "like the sensation of a fish turning in water." There may be fleeting lightheadedness or transient pain in the precordial or substernal area. These disturbances usually appear when the patient is relaxing or about ready to fall asleep, since at this time he is apt to become more conscious of any sensation occurring inside his body and since at rest the heart rate is slower and the opportunity is greater during the longer diastolic pauses for premature beats to arise. The sensations are generally absent while the patient is active, walking or busily engaged in his affairs.

Although it has been said repeatedly that extrasystoles are usually of no serious significance and that normal people may have them, it was the animal experiments by Beattie and Brow which have made it possible to ascribe a definite neurogenic origin to them. They showed that if certain nerve tracts coming from the hypothalamic region were cut in the animals with experimentally produced extrasystoles, the irregularity disappeared. They also found that if these tracts were cut beforehand, the extrasystoles could not be produced by the same technic that always produced them in animals not subjected to this treatment. Thus it appears that there is a center in the brain that can initiate, or that is ultimately connected with, the formation of premature heart beats. This demonstration points to a structural neurogenic basis for conditions that have long been regarded as functional.

Relationship of Palpitation to Tachycardia. Palpitation, as previously stated, is a normal sensation when the force of the heart beat and its rate are considerably elevated, and the subject may not only say he "feels his heart pounding" but that it is beating "too hard," "too fast" or both. Slight exertion in normal persons may cause only a little shortness of breath. When the activity is a little more strenuous, one is apt to become aware of the thumping of the heart against the chest wall. After rest the thumping sensation may persist for a while after the rate has returned to normal, showing that one may be aware of a "harder beat" (greater systolic contraction and cardiac output) when the rate is not increased. Persistence of tachycardia with greater cardiac activity beyond a normal or physiologic range of time suggests impaired cardiac reserve. Many of the physical fitness tests employed by the armed services are based upon accurate, graded observations of these phenomena in response to standard amounts of muscular effort.

Fortunately, persistent tachycardia is usually not accompanied by continual palpitation, or at least not to the degree one might expect. Patients with cardiac decompensation with pulse rates of over 100 per minute even at rest may have little or no palpitation. Although palpitation is a common symptom in thyrotoxicosis there is often comparatively little consciousness of heart action. Persons with chronic infections resulting in long-standing fever and tachycardia often have no palpitation in spite of pulse rates that may be very rapid. It seems that in many of these instances physiologic readjustment takes place so that the subject becomes accustomed to the greater rate and often the greater force of the cardiac contraction. A *sudden* alteration in rate or rhythm or in the force of the beat is apt to be perceived promptly whether the heart is normal or diseased. This is true whether the change is toward a slower, more orderly beat or toward rapid, irregular contraction. Static conditions, even though quite abnormal, may not be accompanied by palpitation.

TACHYCARDIA

The term tachycardia is derived from the Greek words meaning quick and heart. Rapid action of the heart is the most common and obvious cardiac manifestation; accordingly, it is often the first to be discovered by the patient himself and by the physician. The rate of the heart beat is the expression of the property of rhythmicity (automaticity) inherent in all parts of the heart muscle, but most highly developed in the specialized muscle cells that constitute the normal pacemaker. This pacemaker in the right atrium can keep the heart beating rhythmically independently of all extracardiac factors, as, for example, in the excised heart. However, in the body this inherent rhythm is always being modified. A great number of physiologic control mechanisms are capable of influencing the rate of the heartbeat. Practically all of these can be included under two headings, *chemical control* and *nervous control*.

Chemical control of the heart is effected by certain ions and also by the more complex substances, hormones, secreted by the endocrine glands. The integrity of the living cell is dependent on a constant osmotic pressure of the surrounding extracellular fluid which the body guards by various homeostatic mechanisms. The concentration of the *sodium* ion in extracellular fluid is responsible for almost all the osmotic pressure due to cations, and its constancy may be regarded as a measure of the constancy of the osmotic pressure. When the concentration of sodium in the blood increases, the posterior pituitary gland is stimulated to secrete the antidiuretic hormone, water is retained by the kidney and the normal concentration of sodium and the normal osmotic pressure is restored. It is assumed that this is the general manner in which the primary abnormal retention of sodium leads also to abnormal retention of water in congestive failure. Other mechanisms are probably also concerned in the regulation of water balance in congestive failure, for water may be retained even when the sodium ion is below normal and the extracellular fluid is hypotonic.

Potassium is the predominant intracellular electrolyte. A normal concentration of intracellular and extracellular potassium is essential for normal myocardial contraction. In the isolated heart, potassium antagonizes the tendency of calcium to cause systolic standstill (calcium rigor). When present in excess, potassium prolongs diastole and may cause complete inhibition with arrest of the heart. Various observations have suggested an intimate relationship between the action of the potassium ion and the action of acetyl choline, the humoral effector agent produced by vagal stimulation. Potassium may participate in nerve stimulation and muscular contraction by altering cell permeability. Changes in the concentration of potassium may produce clinical symptoms due to impairment of muscular activity and/or changes in the cardiac mechanism and in the electrocardiogram. *Calcium* ions (with sodium and potassium) are essential to proper cardiac contraction. The perfused isolated heart will stop in diastole if there is no calcium; an excess of calcium causes systolic arrest (calcium rigor). Like digitalis, calcium increases systolic contraction. Fear of a dangerous potentiating effect is a basis for the purported contraindication to the injection of calcium in digitalized patients. Injected *parathormone* produces effects which are somewhat similar to those of calcium: an early increase in heart rate, followed by slowing and by cardiac arrhythmia characterized by premature beats and shifting of the pacemaker. The *adrenal* gland, when stimulated by its sympathetic nerve supply, secretes a mixture containing 80 per cent *l*-epinephrine and 20 per cent norepinephrine. The direct effect of *l*-epinephrine on strips of myocardium is to increase the speed, vigor and power of myocardial contraction and to produce acceleration of the heart by acting on the pacemaker. In men, norepinephrine introduced into the bloodstream is reported to have a powerful vasoconstrictor effect on the peripheral vascular system but less effect on myocardial contraction. Increased contractile properties of the myocardium are noted but the heart rate slows.

The circulatory response to *hyperthyroidism* resembles that of a normal person to strenuous exercise. The cardiac impulse is diffuse and forceful. The heart is accelerated. There is good evidence that the tachycardia from excess thyroid hormone (*thyroxin*) represents a direct effect on the pacemaker activity of the myocardium. Hyperthyroidism imposes a heavy load on the myocardium, which must put out more useful work to supply the augmented metabolic requirement of the body while the efficiency of its contraction is diminished by tachycardia and by direct action of thyroid hormone on the myocardial fibers. When a patient with hyperthyroidism undertakes physical exertion, the circulatory reaction is exaggerated when compared to that of normal individuals performing the same task. In young persons the heart may compensate for this excessive load but, in older individuals, cardiavascular reserves may become exhausted and heart failure supervenes. If coronary sclerosis is present, angina pectoris may become evident. Atrial fibrillation is also likely to occur because of increased myocardial irritability. *Hypothyroidism* with its decrease in thyroxin may result from spontaneous thyroid atrophy, surgical excision of thyroid tissue or as the result of thyroid irradiation. Its principal cardiac effect is the development of a slow heart rate. The thyroid hormones act primarily and directly upon the heart itself and may also affect it through the mediation of its autonomic nerve supply. The hormone control of the heart comes into play slowly, after a significant latent period following the original stimulus initiating the cardiac response. In contrast, cardiac responses evoked by nervous influences usually occur promptly, the latent period between the stimulus and the effect being short. Furthermore, the response by way of the nervous system is of relatively short duration, the effect disappearing promptly when the stimulus ceases, whereas effects produced by hormones tend to persist, outlasting the stimulus for some time.

Nervous control of the heart is effected through the vagus and the sympathetic nerves. Figure 93 is a diagrammatic representation of the cardiovascular reflex mechanisms. The vagus may be considered the more important of the two nerves. It is tonically active at all times and exerts a continuous restraining influence upon the heart, keeping it beating at a slower rate than that which it would have if its intrinsic pacemaker, the sinoatrial node, were unchecked. This normal vagus tone is quite strong, and its removal leads to a marked and prompt increase in heart rate. Such removal or inhibition of the normal vagus tone is largely responsible for the tachycardia in nearly all the clinical conditions associated with acceleration of the heart. Viewing the vagus nerve as the efferent limb of a reflex arc and the vagus center in

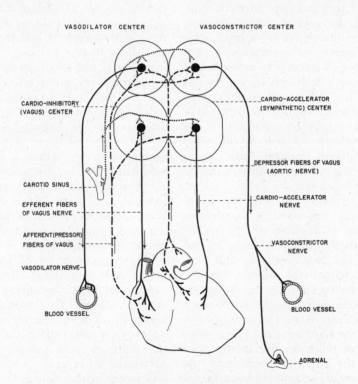

FIG. 93. Diagrammatic representation of the cardiovascular reflex mechanisms. Afferent vagal fibers are shown by broken lines; sinus nerve fibers, by a dotted line; efferent fibers to the heart and to the blood vessels, by a continuous line. The afferent fibers are represented as causing reciprocal effects upon the medullary centers. (Best, C. H., and Taylor, N. B.: The Physiologic Basis of Medical Practice, ed. 3, Baltimore, Williams & Wilkins)

the medulla as the center of the arc, the question arises as to what are the paths of the afferent impulses which reach the center and, by stimulating it, cause the heart to beat slower or, by inhibiting it, cause the heart to beat faster. Generally speaking, the potential afferent pathways capable of affecting the vagus center are all the afferent nerve fibers in the body. This concept means that all types of sensation from all parts of the body can affect the heart rate via the vagus center though they may or may not do so according to circumstances. All afferent nerve impulses are conducted into some part of the central nervous system (spinal cord or brain), and, once within it, there is at least the possibility of a pathway to every center within the central nervous system. The actual flow of impulses from afferent to efferent paths is regulated by the very complex functional organization of the central nervous system. Thus, sudden distraction by a loud noise (8th cranial nerve) or immersion in hot water (cutaneous nerves) may precipitate a change in pulse rate (vagus nerve) by this reflex mechanism. Obviously not every type or intensity of sensation is uniformly potent in this respect, and the cardiac rate is not continuously interfered with by the usual sensations. Afferent impulses from certain regions are especially predominant in influencing the heart rate.

It is not surprising that the more important afferent impulses for controlling the heart arise in portions of the circulatory system itself, especially those regions from which the heart receives and into which it discharges the blood. On the venous or receiving end, the Bainbridge reflex causes acceleration of the heart when the venous return is so excessive that it overdistends the *right atrium*. The sensory endings of this reflex arc are in the right atrium and the adjacent portions of the venae cavae and are stimulated by increased tension. The resultant nerve impulses course along the afferent fibers in the vagus and *inhibit the vagus center* so that the heart beats faster, thus tending to raise the heart output to balance the inflow.

On the arterial side is the *depressor reflex* whose afferent fibers arise from the root and the arch of the aorta and run to the medulla within the vagus nerve. The initiating stimulus for these fibers is *tension* within the aorta; the higher the tension, the greater the stimulus. With elevation in the aortic pressure, afferent impulses ascend to and *stimulate the vagus center* so that the heart beats more slowly, and this action tends to reduce the blood pressure to its proper level. The reverse occurs also in that lowered aortic pressure gives rise to afferent nerve impulses that inhibit the vagus center and so accelerate the heart by diminishing the vagus tone. A similar depressor reflex dependent primarily upon the pressure within the carotid artery for its activity has its afferent nerve endings in the *carotid sinus* which is a specially innervated part of the arteries and the adjacent tissues located at the bifurcation of the common carotid artery. The afferent fibers from the carotid sinus reach the medulla by way of the glossopharyngeal and the vagus nerves and the sympathetic trunk. The initiating stimulus is either increased or decreased intracarotid pressure tending to slow or accelerate the heart by affecting the vagus center in a similar fashion to the aortic depressor fibers already described. The highly developed nerve endings located in the *carotid body,* which is situated at the bifurcation of the common carotid artery, are *chemoreceptors* and are sensitive to oxygen lack and carbon dioxide excess. When either of these conditions is present, impulses from the carotid body aid in accelerating the heart.

The higher centers of the brain itself may also be considered one of the special regions for initiating afferent impulses for cardiac control, for *emotion* may cause nerve impulses to descend to the medulla where they may affect the vagus center sufficiently to cause a change in heart rate. *Increased intracranial pressure* is usually associated with slowing of the heart, brought about by overstimulation of the vagus center. The stimulation may be due both to direct mechanical effect on the vagus center cells in the medulla and to ischemia of the center from the adverse effect of the pressure upon its blood supply. Furthermore, *ischemia,* when not too severe, stimulates practically all the medullary centers, including the vasomotor centers; therefore, increased intracranial pressure causes peripheral constriction and consequent elevation of blood pressure. The vascular hypertension thus produced in turn acts upon the aorta and the carotid sinus so as to stimulate the depressor reflexes already described and is therefore a secondary reason for cardiac slowing in increased intracranial tension.

The sympathetic and the vagus centers in the medulla together form a functional unit referred to as the *cardiac center*. The quantity and the quality of the blood reaching this center affect the heart rate. Slight hypoxia of the cardiac center causes increased cardiac rate, as does also a small excess of carbon dioxide; a high degree of oxygen lack causes slowing of the heart, and a large excess of carbon dioxide may lead to heart block. These effects occur by means of efferent impulses coursing along the vagus, or the sympathetic nerves, or both. Increased temperature of the blood going to the center increases cardiac rate. Increased intracranial tension from any local cause tends to decrease the blood flow to the cardiac center and results in heart acceleration.

The sympathetic nerve control of the heart is subordinate to the vagus control because under normal resting conditions it is quite inactive and on stimulation the acceleration of the heart begins only after a definite latent period and develops gradually. If the normal sympathetic accelerating influence is entirely removed, the resultant cardiac slowing is usually negligible. In addition, the latency of the response on stimulation of the sympathetic trunk renders it relatively ineffective when there is need of prompt increase in the activity of the heart. However, since its effect manifests itself later than that wrought by the vagus, it persists longer and so maintains the responses initiated via the vagus. Usually increased sympathetic tone simultaneously induces secretion of adrenalin which further prolongs the acceleration of the heart. The sympathetic efferent nerve center is in the medulla. The afferent paths by which impulses may reach and affect it are identical with those already mentioned in conection with the vagus cardiac center. Similarly, the cardiovascular sensory areas

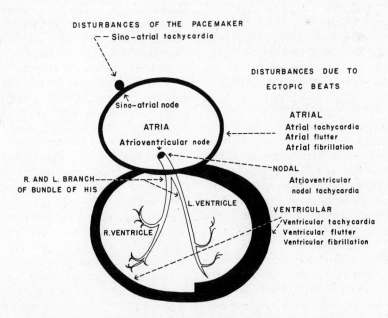

Fig. 94. Schematic diagram of arrhythmias associated with tachycardia. (Levine, S. A.: Clinical Electrocardiography, Oxford Loose-Leaf Medicine, vol. 2, New York, Oxford Univ. Press)

of the right atrium, the root of the aorta and the carotid sinus which are related to vagus control have an *analogously intimate relation* with sympathetic control. Consequently, cardiac acceleraton from an over-distended atrium, though predominantly brought about by inhibition of the vagus center, is partially produced by sympathetic nerve stimulation, and slowing of the heart by the vagus in the depressor reflex is enhanced by concomitant decrease in sympathetic tone. In most instances, however, the chief portion of the total response is effected through the vagus and to a much lesser extent through the sympathetic.

TYPES OF TACHYCARDIA

The varieties and the causes of tachycardia are so numerous that a classification is necessary. The most common type of tachycardia is that originating in the sino-atrial node. This is called sino-atrial tachycardia or simply sinus tachycardia. Next in frequency is paroxysmal atrial tachycardia, followed by rapid heart action associated with atrial fibrillation and atrial flutter. A relatively rare, but more serious, form of tachycardia is that arising from the ventricles called ventricular tachycardia; this may in turn predispose the heart to ventricular flutter and fibrillation. An infrequent form of paroxysmal tachycardia is that originating from the atrio-ventricular node. Figure 94 illustrates schematically the arrhythmias associated with tachycardia.

SINUS TACHYCARDIA

Sino-atrial tachycardia, sinus tachycardia or simple tachycardia, as it is otherwise known, is defined by Herrmann as a "sustained increase in the heart rate beyond the normal limits of the individual." Usually a rate of 100 beats or more per minute in a person over the age of 18 years is evidence enough to justify a diagnosis of sinus tachycardia. Although there is a wide range of the normal pulse rate at rest, a rate of over 100 beats per minute in the heart of a normal resting adult is infrequent. In contrast, the upper range of normal in children is about 120, while in infants it is 150.

Etiology. Sino-atrial tachycardia occurs in persistent form in many healthy individuals and is found normally as a trait in certain families. Transient sinus tachycardia is of daily occurrence in all individuals as a physiologic response to physical exertion, ingestion of food, emotion, pain and the application of heat to the body. It is particularly apt to appear when alcohol, tobacco, coffee or the like are used to excess. Caffeine, for example, acts by direct stimulation of the myocardium. Rarely, an individual will be found who can accelerate his pulse at will and then usually because he has learned how to arouse an intense emotion. This ability has been used by malingerers to simulate heart disease. The effect is mediated through the sympathoadrenal system. Pathologic causes of sino-atrial tachycardia include especially *infections* and *fever;* the pulse rate in general rises about 9 beats per minute for each degree Fahrenheit of temperature elevation. This increase is partly due to the direct effect of the high temperature on the heart, for the beat of the excised heart has been shown to be accelerated by warming.

Another abnormal cause of tachycardia includes a group of noninfectious noxious disturbances, prominent among which is *thyrotoxicosis.* Thyroxin accelerates the heart beat by direct action on the heart muscle fibers and also, indirectly, by increasing the metabolic rate.

Another pathologic cause of tachycardia is *infarction* of some part of the body in a sufficiently large area to give rise to reactions with fever and often leukocytosis. *Shock* and *hemorrhage* usually produce tachycardia as a compensatory reflex reaction to the lowered blood pressure.

Certain *drugs* particularly epinephrine (by direct effect on the myocardium and the conduction tissue), atropine (by blocking of vagal effects on the sino-atrial pacemaker) and the nitrites (through a carotid sinus reflex resulting in sympathoadrenal discharge) cause sinus tachycardia.

Episodes of *neurocirculatory asthenia* and *mental shock* often are associated with a rapid pulse. Sometimes the cause of the tachycardia cannot be definitely discovered.

The heart in *congestive failure* accelerates to a greater or less degree in an effort to maintain the volume of blood flow. Acceleration of beat, however, is not an intrinsic adaptation of the heart to increased work load for in the heart-lung preparation, accommodation to increased arterial resistance or greater venous return is accomplished without any change in the rate of the heart. It is not that the heart in such a preparation is unable to accelerate, for elevation in temperature is followed promptly by increase in rate. These observations on the isolated heart indicate that extrinsic mechanisms, nervous or chemical, are involved in the production of compensatory tachycardia in heart failure. Among the mechanisms that appear to be concerned are the Bainbridge and carotid sinus and aortic reflexes which have been discussed previously. It appears quite likely that, in the state of heart failure in which diminished cardiac output and elevated venous pressure are generally combined,

these various reflexes are primarily responsible for the production of tachycardia.

Symptoms. The symptoms displayed by an individual with sino-atrial tachycardia vary from little more than the objective sign of an increased pulse rate to a syndrome that may inhibit the normal activity of the patient. Palpitation is the most common of the symptoms encountered although restlessness, agitation, apprehension, anxiety and chest discomfort or pain may also be present, depending upon the symptom threshold and the nervous reactivity of the individual patient.

Diagnosis. As a rule, the diagnosis of sino-atrial tachycardia is obvious and clearly related to the exciting factor. The cardiac rhythm is usually regular, but shows fluctuations in rate in response to forced respiration and other physiologic stimuli such as emotion and effort. In differentiating it from other forms of tachycardia it

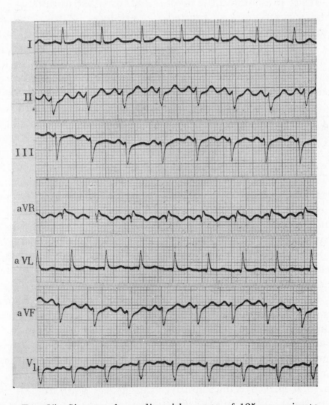

Fig. 95. Sinus tachycardia with a rate of 125 per minute. (Lipman and Massie: Clinical Scalar Electrocardiography, ed. 4, Chicago, Year Book Pub.)

should be remembered that sinus tachycardia has a gradual onset and a slight variation of the beat as compared with the abruptness and the marked regularity characterizing paroxysmal atrial or nodal tachycardia. Cases in which the increased pulse rate is due to psychogenic factors or an emotional imbalance generally exhibit a marked reduction in the pulse rate during sleep. Instances due to drug administration are easily singled out by a careful history. It would appear that many of the attacks called paroxysmal atrial tachycardia are really attacks of sinus tachycardia. Especially is this true when the heart rate is not above 150 to 160. The electrocardiographic findings in sinus tachycardia are illustrated in Figure 95.

Prognosis. The prognosis of sino-atrial tachycardia per se is good. In any given case it depends primarily on the fundamental cause of the tachycardia with the exception of those instances where serious heart disease is already present and the myocardial or coronary reserve is so limited that the tachycardia itself may precipitate heart failure.

Paroxysmal Atrial Tachycardia

In this arrhythmia a rapid series of impulses originates in an ectopic focus in either atrium. This is the most frequent of the abnormal or ectopic tachycardias. Its incidence is impossible to determine with any degree of accuracy because many persons may have short paroxysms of this type of tachycardia lasting seconds or minutes that are not interpreted as such either because they are not sufficiently troublesome to excite concern on the part of the person affected or because there is no opportunity to obtain an electrocardiogram at the time of the paroxysms.

Mechanism. The mechanism of atrial tachycardia consists of a rapid and regular sequence of abnormal heart beats originating in the atrium either from a given point outside the normal pacemaker or as a type of circus movement re-entering the atrial muscle which in turn is recovering rapidly from its refractory stage. The site of origin of a paroxysm of atrial tachycardia may be in any part of the atrial musculature. The

electrocardiographic picture resembles a series of premature atrial contractions occurring in quick succession. Electrocardiographically, the atrial complex differs from the normal P wave inasmuch as the origin of the impulse is abnormal and the course it takes through the atrium is likewise abnormal. The QRS complexes are similar in configuration to the QRS complexes of the basic mechanism unless aberration occurs. In such cases slurring, notching or widening of the QRS associated with defective conduction is present.

Atrial tachycardia may be confused with nodal tachycardia, particularly when the P waves are not identifiable. The two conditions, in such instances, are frequently grouped together under the term supraventricular tachycardia. Difficulty at times may be encountered in differentiating slow paroxysmal atrial tachycardia from rapid sinus tachycardia. Paroxysmal atrial tachycardia has a rate which varies from 150 to 250 beats per minute.

Etiology. Paroxysmal atrial tachycardia may occur at any age, but it is rare in infancy. It is found more often in the absence of heart disease than in its presence; yet if we compare the relative incidence in normal persons and in cardiac patients we find a higher incidence in the cardiac patients. It is frequently associated with indigestion, overexertion, fatigue, excess use of tobacco, alcohol or coffee. It may be psychogenic in origin and may start with a specific emotional reaction. It may be associated with various infections. Thyrotoxicosis should be suspected in every case until eliminated. Among the various forms of organic heart disease accompanied by paroxysmal atrial tachycardia, mitral stenosis probably has the highest incidence.

Symptoms. In most cases the patient is conscious of the disturbance of rhythm. The attack itself is instantaneous in onset and offset, and the patient is usually aware of this, describing it as coming on suddenly and stopping with a "thump." The patient complains of palpitation or fluttering of the heart, pounding in the chest, fulness in the neck; he becomes uneasy, nervous, dizzy and apprehensive and desires to lie down. Occasionally there is pain over the heart, and there may be typical anginal distress even with radiation to the arms. Sometimes nausea and vomiting occur and then attacks often cease. This experience suggests to the patient that it is all produced by indigestion or some recently eaten food. After a length of time, varying from minutes to hours and even days, the attack ends and the patient quickly recovers either in good condition or in a sufficiently weak state to remain inactive for a day or two. The distress experienced depends primarily on the duration of the attack, the cardiac rate and the condition of the heart before the attack occurred.

Diagnosis. The diagnosis of paroxysmal atrial tachycardia is simple in most cases. It is important to elicit evidence of an abrupt change in rhythm with an approximate doubling of heart rate. Usually the cardiac beat ranges from about 150 to 250 per minute. Although usually sudden cessation of the episode occurs, sometimes the attack does not appear to stop abruptly. This is due to the fact that in spite of the considerable drop in rate at the end of the

paroxysm, the sino-atrial rate when the heart resumes normal rhythm is elevated by excitement or otherwise, preventing the obvious sensation of marked change in the cardiac rhythm that occurred at the onset of the attack. Not only is the heart rapid and regular but its rate is very fixed for long intervals of time and cannot be altered by simple procedures like breathing or exercise which affect the rate of the normal heart. If repeated counts of the heart beat taken at the bedside several minutes apart show a significant difference in the rates, it speaks against the diagnosis of paroxysmal atrial tachycardia. The various methods that are used to stop an attack also serve as diagnostic procedures, for there is no other type of rapid heart action that can be made to return to a normal rate by such simple means and so quickly. *If vagus stimulation is produced by pressure* over the carotid sinus or the eyeball in this type of arrhythmia, the rate either remains unaltered or abruptly falls to the normal range With normal tachycardia or atrial flutter there is apt to be temporary slowing with

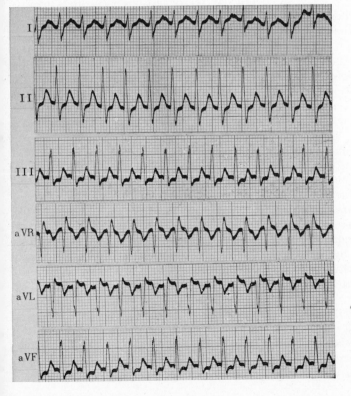

Fig. 96. Paroxysmal atrial tachycardia with a rate of 190 per minute. The P and T waves are superimposed. (Lipman and Massie: Clinical Scalar Electrocardiography, ed. 4, Chicago, Year Book Pub.)

gradual return to the previous rate, and when ventricular tachycardia is present vagus stimulation produces no effect. The electrocardiogram is almost invariably diagnostic (see Fig. 96), but there are a few puzzling records in which the tracing, unless it is taken at the beginning of the paroxysm, is not adequate to eliminate definitely a rare case of sinus tachycardia or atrial flutter.

Prognosis. The prognosis of paroxysmal atrial tachycardia is usually excellent as to life, but there are rare instances where the tachycardia is so excessive that cardiac failure results even in a normal person. It is always a more important disturbance, however, in the presence of serious heart disease. The cardiac conditions that are prone to be overburdened by this type of tachycardia include mitral stenosis, coronary insufficiency and cases of strain and enlargement of the left ventricle. The tendency to recurrence of attacks varies greatly from only a few attacks in a lifetime to almost daily paroxysms.

PAROXYSMAL ATRIAL TACHYCARDIA WITH
ATRIOVENTRICULAR BLOCK

There is another form of atrial tachycardia which is associated with varying degrees of atrioventricular block. The rising incidence of this arrhythmia and its significance with reference to digitalis intoxication has been gaining attention in recent years. Levine and Lown observed a number of instances of paroxysmal atrial tachycardia with atrioventricular block (PAT with block). In their series, only about 20 per cent of the patients had attacks in which digitalis intoxication could not be implicated as a causative factor. The remainder of the patients were thought to have developed PAT with block because of definite overdosage of digitalis or because digitalis intoxication was brought on by potassium loss during excessive mercurial diuresis.

The electrocardiographic features of PAT with block are as follows:

1. The onset is more gradual than that of supraventricular tachycardia without AV block. The normal P waves become progressively altered in appearance as the ectopic forces stimulate the atrium. Then the rate of this pacemaker speeds up with a 1:1 atrioventricular response initially, followed by the onset of variable atrioventricular block.

2. The differentiation of the atrial flutter pattern from PAT with block may be difficult at times, especially if the atrial rate is approximately 200 beats per minute. The atrial rate in the latter rhythm is usually between 150 and 190 beats per minute and seldom exceeds 200 beats per minute.

3. The AV block is a constant 2:1 in only 30 per cent of the patients, the remainder showing variable and often inconstant degrees of block. The degree of AV block can be increased by vagal stimulation and decreased by atropine or exercise.

4. Unlike the common form of supraventricular tachycardia, the atrial mechanism in PAT with block, with rare exceptions, cannot be converted to sinus rhythm by carotid sinus stimulation or other simple measures which increase the vagal tone. Generally, its response to various therapeutic agents more closely resembles that of atrial flutter than that of atrial tachycardia. When the P wave is superimposed on the QRS and T deflections, as is often the case, the diagnosis may easily be overlooked. Recognition of the mechanism often depends on a high degree of suspicion, as well as on vagal maneuvers which increase the degree of AV block and uncover the concealed P wave. Suspicion may be aroused by a knowledge of the clinical picture or by the appearance of a newly developed, unexplained, persistent deformity of the QRS complex, the ST segment, or the T wave. Figure 97 shows an example of paroxysmal atrial tachycardia with 2:1 atrioventricular block.

ATRIAL FLUTTER

A still higher degree of atrial disturbance is atrial flutter. It is relatively uncommon, its incidence being less than one-twelfth that of atrial fibrillation.

Mechanism. The mechanism producing atrial flutter (and also that causing atrial fibrillation) has been the subject of lively controversy for much of the last decade, and the divergence of opinion is just as marked now as ever. Although investigations in recent years have provided new and important information concerning the genesis of these two rhythms, none of these data incontestably prove or refute any of the theories currently favored. These theories are three in number—the concept of circus movement, the theory of multiple re-entry, and the theory of focal or multifocal impulse formation.

Atrial flutter is a very rapid regular atrial beat that replaces the normal atrial contraction. A rapid series of impulses is initiated in an ectopic area in either atrium. The atrial rate varies between 200 and 400 beats per minute, but following quinidine administration it may slow to less than 150. Usually the ventricular rate is only a fraction of that of the atria, as junctional tissue

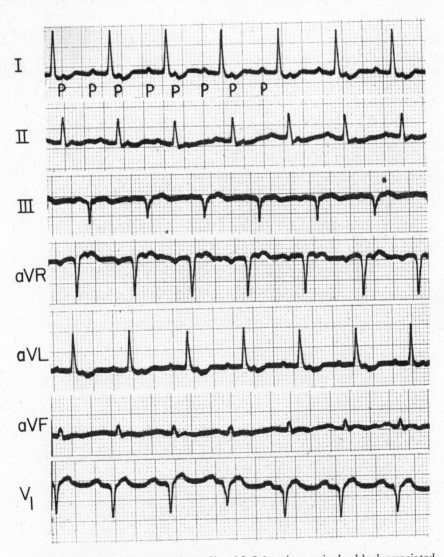

Fig. 97. Paroxysmal atrial tachycardia with 2:1 atrioventricular block associated with digitalis intoxication in a man 55 years of age. The rate of the paroxysmal atrial tachycardia is 200 beats per minute, while the ventricular rate is exactly one-half as fast. The symbol P indicates the ectopic atrial beats in lead I. (Massie and Walsh: Clinical Vectorcardiography and Electrocardiography, Chicago, Year Book Publishers)

cannot conduct impulses so rapidly and a certain degree of atrioventricular block results. In exceptional cases all atrial beats come through to the ventricles; then the heart rate is extremely rapid. Commonly the ratio of atrial to ventricular beats is 2:1 and less often 4:1 or even 5:1 or 6:1. Not infrequently the ventricular response is irregular as a result of a changing atrioventricular block.

Etiology. Unlike paroxysmal atrial tachycardia, which usually occurs in otherwise normal hearts, atrial flutter is apt to be *associated with organic heart disease,* either valvular or myocardial, although it can rarely occur as a purely functional disturb-

ance. Its incidence is probably highest in cases of mitral stenosis, hypertension and coronary heart disease. Occasionally one encounters it in patients with severe thyrotoxicosis. Atrial flutter occurs chiefly in adults, and the exciting factors are the same as those for paroxysmal atrial tachycardia.

Symptoms. Symptoms are produced when the rate of the ventricle is rapid, but are more common in the paroxysmal form of atrial flutter or if heart disease is advanced. The typical symptom is rapid, regular, forceful palpitation subjectively indistinguishable from paroxysmal tachycardia. Symptoms of congestive heart failure may be coincidental or may result from the rapid

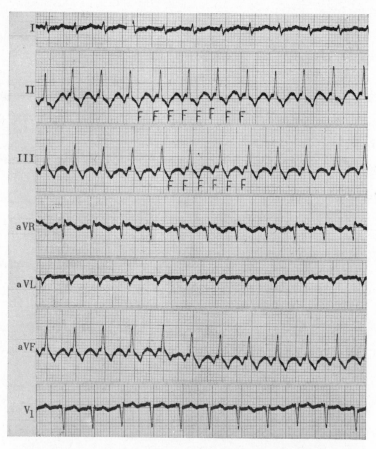

Fig. 98. Atrial flutter with 2:1 atrioventricular block. The atrial rate is 300 and ventricular rate 150 per minute. Note that the atrial waves (F) are represented by small notches in Lead I and by triangular form of P waves in Leads II, III and aVF. (Lipman and Massie: Clinical Scalar Electrocardiography, ed. 4, Chicago, Year Book Pub.)

ventricular action. Pain is rare, although precordial aching may occur. The patient may be made nervous and apprehensive from the alarm occasioned by the attack. If the ventricular rate is very rapid, as in 1:1 rhythm, and the heart rate approaches 300 per minute, dizziness, weakness and partial or complete syncope may result as a consequence of cerebral anemia and other effects of greatly reduced cardiac output.

Diagnosis. The diagnosis is easily made with the electrocardiogram but with diffi- culty in any other way. Atrial flutter is characterized at the bedside by long-con- tinued rapid beating at a precise rate. Tem- porary halving of the heart rate spontane- ously, by exercise, or by carotid sinus pressure is suggestive of this arrhythmia. Carotid sinus pressure slows the ventricle in "jumps" because it does not, as a rule, alter the atrial rate but only the ratio of atrial impulses conducted to the ventricle. On removal of the carotid sinus pressure the ventricular rate returns to its previous level, but often the return occurs in an ir- regular although rapid fashion. Severe exercise, on occasion, also causes a sudden change in the ventricular rate which reverts to its original level when the exertion is over. The neck veins always should be in- spected for the presence of the rapid regu- lar atrial waves. For this type of examina- tion the patient should be placed in such a position that the neck veins are only par- tially filled.

The electrocardiograms of atrial flutter are very peculiar and characteristic. In Lead I the atrial waves are represented by small notches. In Leads II and III the waves have a triangular form. The upstroke is sharp and smooth and the downstroke more prolonged and notched at its mid- point. The flutter waves are continuous, and as one cycle ends the next begins. They often resemble a tuning-fork record and at other times a picket fence. The rhythm of the atria is strikingly regular. The ven- tricular rate and rhythm will depend on the degree of heart block. With experience, one learns to detect flutter from the appear- ance of the electrocardiograms, but if there is any doubt as to the underlying mechan- ism, slowing of the ventricular rate by vagal

stimulation may allow the flutter waves to be more evident. Lead V_1 may be helpful in differentiating questionable cases since it often shows most clearly evidences of atrial activity if carefully examined. Figure 98 shows the electrocardiogram of a patient with atrial flutter and 2:1 atrioven- tricular block.

Prognosis. The prognosis is less favor- able than for paroxysmal atrial tachycardia because of the higher incidence of heart disease in association with flutter and be- cause of the longer paroxysms. Sometimes the flutter continues in more chronic form lasting for years.

ATRIAL FIBRILLATION

Atrial fibrillation is closely allied with atrial flutter and has about 12 to 15 times the clinical incidence. It is one of the com- monest and most important disorders of cardiac rhythm. It probably ranks fourth in frequency as a disturbance of rhythm, sino-atrial tachycardia, premature beats and paroxysmal atrial tachycardia ranking first, second and third respectively. Atrial fibril- lation, even of the paroxysmal type, rarely escapes notice and with rare exceptions comes eventually under the scrutiny of a physician.

Mechanism. Atrial fibrillation represents the highest degree of atrial disturbance. In this condition the number of atrial impulses per minute is very great, varying between 350 and 500. The mechanism is due to a circus motion in which the path is impure and irregular. The atria do not actually contract but rather remain distended in diastole and show fibrillary twitching. The speed of the atrial impulses is so great that areas of block or refractory points develop in the circuit, accounting for the irregu- larity of rate seen in the electrocardiogram. There is no constant pathologic finding in the atria to account for atrial fibrillation; accordingly, it is regarded as a functional derangement accompanying a number of conditions. This arrhythmia can be repro- duced in a dog's atrium by a rapid series of faradic stimulations. The number of atrial impulses is so great that only a por- tion of them can be conducted through the junctional tissue. Consequently, there is always some degree of atrioventricular block associated with this arrhythmia. The ventricular response occurs in a grossly irregular fashion. The peripheral pulse is necessarily irregular both in time and in force of contraction. The ventricles respond, usually at an average rate of 100 to 140 per minute in untreated cases, but rates above 200 sometimes occur.

Etiology. The condition occurs chiefly in adults of both sexes and is very rare in early childhood. The incidence of atrial fibrillation increases in frequency with increasing years; it is common in old age. The most common conditions with which this arrhythmia is associated are rheumatic valvular disease with mitral stenosis, hypertensive heart disease, coronary artery disease and hyperthyroidism. It may develop precipitously during acute infections such as pneumonia and in rheumatic fever. It

is seen not infrequently during the early stages of an acute coronary thrombosis. Rarely, it develops as a result of excessive digitalis therapy. In addition, there is the important group in which it is present either paroxysmally or permanently in otherwise healthy individuals and without any apparent cause such as organic heart disease or even excesses of tobacco or alcohol. It may follow excitement, trauma, operations or intoxications, particularly in nervously high-strung people.

Symptoms. Symptoms vary with the ventricular rate, the underlying functional state of the heart and the duration of the atrial fibrillation. In the chronic form atrial fibrillation may exist without symptoms. Usually, however, the patient is aware of the irregular heart action and has such sensations as fluttering, skipping, irregular beating or a pounding and heaving

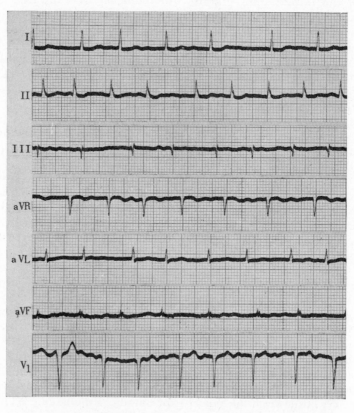

Fig. 99. Atrial fibrillation with an irregular ventricular rate of 75 to 110 per minute. (Lipman and Massie: Clinical Scalar Electrocardiography, ed. 4, Chicago, Year Book Pub.)

action. Palpitation is usually present and may be considered as the characteristic symptom of atrial fibrillation. Dyspnea and pain are much less common, but they may develop as a part of neurocirculatory asthenia if there is an associated marked psychic element. Although angina pectoris may appear, due to the extra work imposed by rapid heart action on a damaged myocardium, it is comparatively rare in atrial fibrillation, a fact that is best explained by the limitation of activity imposed by the arrhythmia itself and by medical advice. The entire symptomatic picture is particularly striking in the paroxysmal form, and there may also be the more general symptoms of anxiety, nervousness, pallor, cyanosis and collapse. The patient may even harbor feelings of impending death. Suc-

cessive attacks are apt to cause sufficient psychic trauma that chronic invalidism results even in the absence of signs of heart failure. Congestive failure may be coincidental with, precipitated by, or entirely caused by the rapid irregular ventricular action.

Diagnosis. The bedside recognition of this condition is generally simple. A rapid, apparently grossly irregular heart beat with an appreciable pulse deficit of 10 or more is due to atrial fibrillation in the great majority of cases. In addition, any tachycardia at a rate of over 120 that is grossly irregular is most likely the result of this arrhythmia. When the patient has a history of rheumatic fever and the signs of mitral stenosis, atrial fibrillation occurs frequently and should be suspected if an arrhythmia is

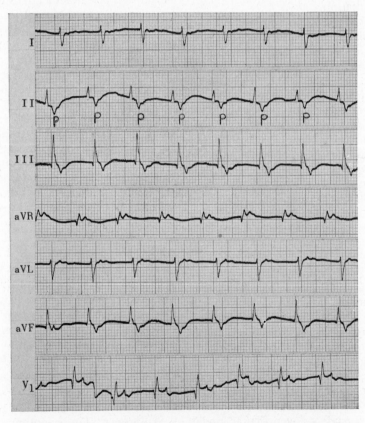

Fig. 100. Atrioventricular nodal rhythm with a rate of 108 per minute. The atrial complexes (labeled P in Lead II) are retrograde in nature and may be seen in all the leads. (Lipman and Massie: Clinical Scalar Electrocardiography, ed. 4, Chicago, Year Book Pub.)

found. The electrocardiogram gives immediate evidence of the condition and is of great diagnostic aid when there is a question as to clinical interpretation. The normal P wave in the tracing will be absent, and instead there will be found irregular, rapid undulations (F waves) of varying amplitude, contour and spacing. These F waves vary in form all the way from being clearly visible in most leads in coarse atrial fibrillation and impure flutter to being imperceptible in fine atrial fibrillation. There is a totally irregular ventricular spacing except in complete atrioventricular block, but, inasmuch as the course of impulses that succeed in reaching the ventricles travel down the normal atrioventricular conduction path, the ventricular complexes are normal in form. Figure 99 shows an example of the electrocardiographic finding in atrial fibrillation.

Prognosis. The prognosis in atrial fibrillation depends on the underlying heart condition and the treatment. In the absence of cardiac muscle or valve involvement the prognosis is excellent. The attack, even though subsiding spontaneously, may in some instances recur. In the presence of heart disease the result depends on the severity of the cardiac lesion and upon the ease of controlling the ventricular rate. It is possible to have recurrent episodes of atrial fibrillation over periods of many years in some patients, yet in those cases where the heart is seriously involved an attack may cause death in a matter of hours.

Paroxysmal Atrioventricular Nodal Tachycardia

This arrhythmia is a relatively infrequent variety of paroxysmal tachycardia. It may be diagnosed only by electrocardiographic means and even then the diagnosis is sometimes difficult. Because of the difficulty of distinguishing between this rhythm and paroxysmal atrial tachycardia, these arrhythmias are frequently grouped together under the term supraventricular tachycardia. Paroxysmal atrioventricular nodal tachycardia is due to rapid impulse formation in the atrioventricular node, both ventricles and atria being controlled from that center. The P waves of the electrocardiogram are inverted and just follow, precede, or occur simultaneously with the QRS complexes. An example is shown in Figure 100.

The etiology, symptomatology and prognosis of this arrhythmia are similar to those of paroxysmal atrial tachycardia.

Paroxysmal Ventricular Tachycardia

This arrhythmia is comparatively rare and occurs approximately in the ratio of 1:8 compared with paroxysmal atrial tachycardia.

Mechanism. Paroxysmal ventricular tachycardia may be regarded as a consecutive series of ventricular extrasystoles arising from an ectopic focus in the ventricle. There is much in the nature of this mechanism that resembles a circus motion. Since it starts from an abnormal focus in the ventricle and the impulse travels an abnormal course, the resultant complex will necessarily be unlike the normal configuration. Each individual complex resembles a ventricular extrasystole. The impulses may travel in a retrograde fashion up the junctional tissue and produce atrial contractions. Because the rate is rapid there may be a retrograde block so that only every other ventricular impulse produces an atrial contraction. At other times the atria contract independently and follow their own pacemaker in the sino-atrial node.

Etiology. This arrhythmia occurs in both sexes but, unlike paroxysmal atrial tachycardia, is much more limited to older persons. It appears but rarely in youth. It is a serious condition because of its much higher incidence among patients with important cardiac involvement or toxic states. Precipitating factors are as described above under paroxysmal tachycardia, but the underlying conditions are mainly acute myocardial infarction and very toxic doses of digitalis. Very rarely it may occur in normal people.

Symptoms. The symptomatology resembles that of paroxysmal atrial tachycardia with the exception that these patients are usually seriously ill with some underlying disease; consequently, the tachycardia pro-

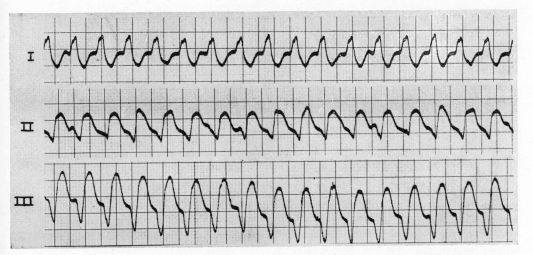

Fig. 101. Paroxysmal ventricular tachycardia with rate of 173 per minute. Note that the QRS complexes are widened and abnormally shaped. The P waves are hidden.

duces symptoms that are much more accentuated.

Diagnosis. The diagnosis can be made with certainly only by examining the electrocardiogram, which reveals abnormally shaped QRS waves resembling repeat ventricular premature beats, the heart rate usually is about 160 to 180 per minute and very rarely reaches the high levels of 220 or more that occur in atrial tachycardia. The atria beat independently, and the P waves may sometimes be clearly seen superimposed on the QRS and the T waves. Paroxysmal ventricular tachycardia is sometimes difficult to differentiate from paroxysmal atrial tachycardia with bundle branch block when the P waves are hard to identify. A typical electrocardiogram is shown in Figure 101.

There are some bedside methods that enable one to suspect the presence of paroxysmal ventricular tachycardia. When paroxysmal, the attacks begin and end suddenly. The rate is rapid but occasionally slight irregularities can be detected by auscultation, in contrast with atrial tachycardia. The condition may be suspected if the heart rate rises abruptly to a level between 140 to 160 per minute or if the rate is above 160 and the rhythm is slightly irregular. In addition, on careful examination, slight but suggestive differences in the intensity and the quality of the first

sound will be heard in some cases as a result of the different relationship between the ventricular and the atrial systoles in various cycles. Atrial pulsations as seen in the jugular vein are fewer in number than the ventricular rate, but this observation is especially difficult to make. Finally, this type of rapid heart action is not influenced by any of the methods that stimulate the vagus nerve. The duration of the attacks is somewhat like that of paroxysmal atrial tachycardia (that is, minutes or hours, and rarely days).

Prognosis. The prognosis is unfavorable because of the severe underlying heart disease or toxic condition. The occurrence of paroxysmal ventricular tachycardia usually indicates a short life, sometimes only a few hours and infrequently more than a few months or years.

Ventricular Flutter and Fibrillation

Ventricular flutter and fibrillation are related in the same way as are their analogous rhythms in the atria. Ventricular flutter is extremely rare. Ventricular fibrillation is, with few exceptions, an irreversible condition found in moribund patients and is one of the causes of sudden death. As in atrial fibrillation, the synergic contractions of the heart are replaced by an incoordinate quivering, each part of the ventricle beating independently. This incoordination directly suspends the pumping action of the heart, and fainting, coma, convulsions and death occur unless the attack quickly subsides. The pulse is absent, and the attack may resemble Adams-Stokes syndrome.

Diagnosis can be made only by electrocardiographic means. Ventricular flutter can be diagnosed in the electrocardiogram when regular continuous waves of large amplitude occur at a rate of over 250 per minute. In these deflections no distinction can be made between the QRS complex and the T wave. Ventricular fibrillation is diagnosed in the tracing by the absence of QRST complexes and the presence of irregular undulations of varying amplitude, contour and spacing. The rate of these may vary from 250 to 500 per minute. The waves are larger than in atrial fibrillation, and no ordinary QRST complexes are seen.

SUMMARY

Palpitation and tachycardia are among the most common complaints that cause patients to seek medical aid. Often, however, the complaint is the most grievous in the presence of the least serious organic disturbance. On the contrary, mild or moderate symptoms may indicate serious underlying disease. Palpitation often results from emotional or psychic disturbance and does not necessarily imply an organic cardiac condition. Increase in the force or the rate of the heart beat and the various cardiac arrythmias may cause palpitation. Tachycardia, strictly speaking, is a physical sign, but it is often a symptom, the subject complaining not so much of an awareness of the heart beat (palpitation) as of a consciousness that the rate is excessive. Frequent or persistent tachycardia may result from metabolic or hormonal disorders, emotional disturbances, psychic or nervous system disease, infections and other conditions affecting the total organism, as well as from cardiac disease. Every such complaint, therefore, deserves careful study until the mechanism is adequately understood. In this way the proper and logical therapeutic approach should become evident.

REFERENCES

Barker, P. S., Wilson, F. N., and Johnston, F. D.: Mechanism of auricular paroxysmal tachycardia, Am. Heart J. 26:435-445, 1943.

Beattie, J., Brow, G. R., and Long, C. N. H.: Physiological and anatomical evidence for existence of nerve tracts connecting the hypothalamus with spinal sympathetic centres, Proc. Roy. Soc., Series B 106:253-275, 1930.

Bellet, S.: Current concepts in therapy: Drug therapy in cardiac arrhythmias, II., New England J. Med. 262:979-981, 1960.

Best, C. H., and Taylor, N. B.: The Physiological Basis of Medical Practice, ed. 7, Baltimore, Williams & Wilkins, 1961.

Bristowe, J. S.: On recurrent palpitation of extreme rapidity in persons otherwise apparently healthy, Brain 10:164-198, 1887.

Burchell, H. B.: Cardiac manifestations of anxiety, Proc. Staff Meet. Mayo Clinic 22:433-440, 1947.

Campbell, M., and Elliott, G. A.: Paroxysmal auricular tachycardia, Brit. M. J. 1:123-160, 1939.

Cookson, H.: Aetiology and prognosis of auricular fibrillation, Quart. J. Med. 23:309-325, 1930.

Criteria Committee of the New York Heart Association: Nomenclature and Criteria for Diagnosis of Diseases of the Heart, ed. 4, New York, Little & Ives, 1940.

Ernstene, A. C.: Diagnosis and treatment of the cardiac arrhythmias, Cleveland Clin. Quart. 16:185-195, 1949.

Fishberg, A. M.: Heart Failure, ed. 2, Philadelphia, Lea, 1940.

Goodman, L., and Gilman, A.: The Pharmacological Basis of Therapeutics, ed. 2, New York, Macmillan, 1955.

Katz, L. N.: Electrocardiography, ed. 2, Philadelphia, Lea, 1946.

Katz, L. N., and Pick, A.: Clinical Electrocardiography, Part I., The Arrhythmias, Philadelphia, Lea, 1956.

Korth, C.: Production of extrasystoles by means of the central nervous system, Ann. Int. Med. 11:492-498, 1937.

Levine, S. A.: Clinical Heart Disease, ed. 5, Philadelphia, Saunders, 1958.

Levine, S. A., and Harvey, W. P.: Clinical Auscultation of the Heart, ed. 2, Philadelphia, Saunders, 1959.

Lewis, T.: The Soldier's Heart and the Effort Syndrome, ed. 2, London, Shaw, 1940.

————: The Mechanism and Graphic Registration of the Heart Beat, ed. 3, London, Shaw, 1925.

Lewis, T., Feil, H. S., and Stroud, W. D.: The nature of auricular flutter, Heart 7:191-243, 1920.

Lipman, B. S., and Massie, E.: Clinical Scalar Electrocardiography, ed. 4, Chicago, Yr. Bk. Pub., 1959.

Luten, D.: The Clinical Use of Digitalis, Springfield, Ill., Thomas, 1936.

Massie, E., and Walsh, T. J.: Clinical Vectorcardiography and Electrocardiography, Chicago, Yr. Bk. Pub., 1960.

Nash, J.: Surgical Physiology, Springfield, Ill., Thomas, 1942.

Oppenheimer, B. S.: Neurocirculatory asthenia and related problems in military medicine, Bull. New York Acad. Med. 18:367-382, 1942.

Prinzmetal, M., Corday, E., Brill, I. C., Oblath, R. W., and Kruger, H. E.: The Auricular Arrhythmias, Springfield, Ill., Thomas, 1952.

Prinzmetal, M., Corday, E., Brill, I. C., Sellers, A. L., Oblath, R. W., Flieg, W. A., and Kruger, H. E.: Mechanism of the auricular arrhythmias, Circulation 1:241-245, 1950.

Rushmer, R. F.: Cardiovascular Dynamics, Philadelphia, Saunders, 1961.

Sodi-Pollares, D., and Calder, R. M.: New Bases of Electrocardiography, St. Louis, Mosby, 1956.

Stroud, W. D.: Diagnosis and Treatment of Cardiovascular Disease, vols. 1 and 2, ed. 3, Philadelphia, Davis, 1945.

Waldman, S., and Moskowitz, S. N.: Treatment of attacks of sinus tachycardia with prostigmin, Ann. Int. Med. 20:793-805, 1944.

Weiss, E., and English, O. S.: Psychosomatic Medicine, ed. 3, Philadelphia, Saunders, 1957.

White, P. D.: Tachycardia and its Treatment, Modern Concepts of Cardiovascular Disease, New York, Am. Heart Ass., 9, No. 8, 1940.

———: Neurocirculatory Asthenia (Da Costa's Syndrome, Effort Syndrome, Irritable Heart of Soldiers), Mod. Conc. Cardiovas. Dis., New York, Am. Heart Ass., 11, No. 8, 1942.

———: Heart Disease, ed. 4, New York, Macmillan, 1951.

Wiggers, C. J.: Mechanism and nature of ventricular fibrillation, Am. Heart J. 20:399-412, 1944.

Willius, F. A.: Cardiac Clinics, St. Louis, Mosby, 1941.

14

Cough

ROGER S. MITCHELL

DEFINITION

Normal cough may be defined most simply as an explosive expiration. After a short inspiration the glottis is closed; the nasopharynx is also usually partially or completely closed off by the soft palate. A strong expiratory effort is then built up by the abdominal and thoracic muscles. At the end of this pressure build up, the normal airways are compressed to about 40 per cent of their inspiratory diameter. This narrowing is advantageous because velocity of air flow is increased and material to be removed is less able to escape the blast of air. At this point, the glottis is suddenly opened and air, plus any free material in the airways, will rush out through the mouth. Chest fluoroscopy at this time reveals a rapid contraction of the ribs and especially a rapid ascent of the diaphragm. Even a paralyzed hemidiaphragm shoots up at this time, an observation which indicates that the diaphragm has no *active* expiratory function.

MECHANISM OF COUGH

Cough in both normal and diseased subjects has been studied effectively by cinefluorobronchography. The normal trachea and bronchi, down to the smallest branches visible by this technic, show marked variations in caliber dependent upon the transluminal and hence, in part, upon the intrathoracic pressure. However, careful studies do not show any evidence in support of the old concept of true bronchial peristalsis. In chronic bronchitis, especially when it is accompanied by severe diffuse emphysema, the airways tend to collapse excessively on forced expiration. The collapse is greater in some portions of the bronchial tree than in others, and at the peak of expiratory effort, the collapse may be complete in advanced diffuse emphysema and in severe chronic bronchitis. This phenomenon is probably due both to airway (cartilage) damage and to the high positive extraluminal pressures in these pathologic states. Obviously, the expulsive advantages of a normal degree of airway narrowing are partially lost when any portion of the airway collapses either excessively or totally.

Cough is only one of the essential physiologic mechanisms for removal of normal bronchial mucus from the tracheobronchial tree. This mucus can be normal or abnormal in both quantity and quality; and it may or may not contain exudate, transudate, bacteria or foreign material. Other normal removal mechanisms are the ciliated epithelium, the subepithelial lymphatics and the phagocytes. The normal adult secretes about 100 ml. of bronchial mucus every 24 hours. It is estimated that usually it takes only about 30 to 60 minutes for mucus and/or foreign material to be swept from the levels of the respiratory bronchioles up to the mouth. Cilia do not ex-

310

tend below the respiratory bronchioles; foreign material which penetrates below this point is phagocytized and transmitted up to the cilia-bearing airways via the adjacent lymphatics.

Cough may occur either voluntarily or without conscious effort. Both *voluntary* and *involuntary* cough involve a *reflex arc*. Cough impulses may be stimulated in a number of different ways, including: irritation of the tracheobronchial or nasal mucosa; external pressure or pulling upon the trachea; pressure upon the carotid sinus, the liver, the spleen or the external auditory canal; pleural irritation; or lung congestion. The mucosa of the trachea and main bronchi is the most sensitive area; even a sudden inhalation of cold air may be a sufficient stimulus to induce coughing. Repeated uncontrolled coughing may itself irritate the airway mucosa and thus give rise to more cough stimuli. When cough occurs involuntarily, the stimuli usually must be especially strong, recurrent or cumulative. The afferent impulses travel via vagal or sympathetic trunks to an area near the olivary bodies in the medulla oblongata. The efferent impulses then descend to the various muscles of expiration and to the glottis.

One supposedly common cause of cough is *postnasal drip* arising from acute or chronic nasal or paranasal sinus inflammation. Pharyngeal and tracheal irritation can be induced in this way, but severe or chronic coughing is probably seldom thus caused. To attribute a severe chronic cough to nasal or sinus pathology is apt to encourage the overlooking of some more serious underlying disease.

The depth or effectiveness of a cough is partially the function of the depth of the initial inspiration. Cough is also obviously under some voluntary control; it can be suppressed, postponed, or made stronger or much weaker by the conscious effort of the individual whose medulla is receiving cough-initiating stimuli. Coughing is more effective in removing material from the large than from the small airways. This is because the smaller the *total* cross section of the airways at any point in the tracheobronchial tree, the more effective a sudden expiratory effort can be.

Repeated severe coughing may cause so-called cough syncope. This phenomenon is probably due to excessive stimulation of a hypersensitive carotid sinus.

A so-called nervous cough is also recognized. Such a cough probably begins with some customary pathology; it becomes chronic perhaps as a result of a subconscious desire for attention, plus the added factor of the chronic mucosal irritation caused by the cough itself. It is doubtful that these psychogenic coughs are due to some pathologic process involving a "cough center" in the brain. The evidence in support of such a center is quite meager.

When coughing is infrequent and not repetitive, when it occurs as part of a natural physiologic progression of events, and especially when it is productive of some material which needs to be removed from the airways, it may be regarded as normal or physiologic. When it is severe, repeated or uncontrolled, when it is ineffective for any reason such as excessively narrowed or collapsing airways, and especially when it is nonproductive or mostly nonproductive, it should be regarded as abnormal, unphysiologic and potentially harmful.

A therapeutic attack upon coughing can be directed at thinning bronchial secretions or at avoiding or removing abnormal irritation or suppressing the sensitivity of the sites of origin of afferent cough impulses. An intelligent attack upon cough thus requires an accurate knowledge of the cause or causes of the cough in the individual.

NATURE OF THE STIMULI THAT PRODUCE COUGH

The stimuli acting upon the endings of the vagus nerve in the pharynx, the larynx, the trachea, the bronchi (and occasionally in the esophagus) may be inflammatory, mechanical, chemical or thermal in nature.

INFLAMMATORY STIMULI

These include stimuli initiated by hyperemia or edema of the mucous membrane; by irritation from exudates upon the surface of the mucous membrane, as in diphtheria, Vincent's angina, or that seen in some cases of streptococcal infections of the respiratory mucous membranes. Ulcerations occurring in tuberculosis or syphilis of the larynx, through irritation of nerves or through contraction of scar tissue in the process of healing with resultant traction upon the nerve endings, often provoke coughing.

MECHANICAL STIMULI

The inhalation of dust, smoke or small foreign bodies is one of the commonest causes of cough. Cigarette smokers often have a chronic cough, produced sometimes by the foreign-body activity (inhaled smoke) present during the period of active smoking, but often present even when the subject is not smoking and resulting from chronic pharyngitis, laryngitis, tracheitis or bronchitis from prolonged inhalation of smoke. Small particles of any nature present in the inhaled air, or drawn in from the nose or the mouth and suddenly striking the sensitive mucous membranes of the air passages, may result in cough. The involuntary inhalation of oral or nasal secretions, or of food particles, or the presence of inflammatory exudates on the mucosal surface of the nasal passages, the pharynx, the larynx, the trachea or the bronchi may thus act as mechanical stimulants to coughing. The pressure or tension upon structures in the air passages that may result from mediastinal or bronchogenic tumors, aortic aneurysms, the enlarged peribronchial and mediastinal nodes in Hodgkin's disease, tuberculosis or neoplasms constitute other types of mechanical stimulation. Tension or pressure produced by distortion of the respiratory tract due to pulmonary fibrosis, atelectasis or pleural effusion may likewise be capable of initiating the stimulus for cough.

CHEMICAL STIMULI

Chemical stimuli that may result in cough are the inhalation of certain irritating gases such as chlorine, bromine, phosgene, chloropicrin, oxychlorcarbon, dichlorethyl sulfide, dichloromethyl ether and others. The fumes of certain strong chemicals—for example, iodine, sulfuric acid, nitric acid, ammonia—as well as the unpleasant odors of garlic, asafetida or

onion, are also capable of producing stimuli that sometimes result in coughing.

THERMAL STIMULI

Thermal stimuli include the inhalation of very hot or very cold air. However, it is rare for the sudden change in the temperature of the inspired air to be the sole cause of cough production; usually there is pathology somewhere in the respiratory tract that actually initiates the stimulus for coughing, and this is merely accentuated in its action by the temperature change.

PSYCHOGENIC COUGH

Psychogenic cough is not uncommon. It is found (1) in persons who have some organic basis for cough, but either consciously or unconsciously cough excessively. The cough may serve to gain attention and sympathy, to express hostile impulses, etc. It is also found (2) in persons with little or no organic basis for cough in whom it may serve as release of nervous tension during embarrassment, etc. When chronic it may assume the clinical characteristics of a tic, becoming an involuntary reflex.

CONDITIONS IN WHICH COUGH OCCURS

The conditions in which cough may be an important symptom can be classified as follows:

Inflammations
Cardiovascular disorders
Trauma and physical agents
Neoplasms
Allergic disorders
Other causes

INFLAMMATIONS

Acute pharyngitis may be bacterial or viral in origin. A diffuse redness, swelling and patchy exudate are common in most forms of this disease. In addition, a greyish membrane composed of pus cells, tissue debris, bacteria and fibrin is generally seen in the bacterial forms (diphtheritic, streptococcal and Vincent's anginal). While the characteristic appearance of the membrane in these three infections tends to differ slightly, bacteriologic examination of material obtained from the throat is the only reliable method of differentiating them. An acute necrotizing pharyngitis often appears during the course of agranulocytosis. The cough in all forms of acute pharyngitis is apt to be irritative and dry.

Acute laryngitis may occur separately or as a part of a viral or bacterial inflammation of the upper or lower respiratory tract. In addition to hoarseness and cough these patients often have a sore throat and, especially in *tuberculous laryngitis*, patients are apt also to suffer from very painful swallowing.

Laryngeal tuberculosis is nonspecific in appearance at the outset; as the process progresses, not only the true and false cords but also all adjacent structures become red, swollen, ulcerated and finally destroyed. Tuberculous laryngitis seldom occurs in the absence of active, infectious pulmonary and/or endobronchial tuberculosis. The diagnosis is best made by biopsy.

Acute tracheobronchitis, due to viral or bacterial agents, may occur as a separate illness or as a part or complication of an acute upper respiratory infection. This syndrome also occurs as a part of a number of specific infections, including influenza, measles, pertussis and occasionally typhoid fever. Symptoms include fever, dyspnea, substernal pain and a severe, irritative, often productive cough.

INFLUENZA is a virus infection characterized by an acute inflammation of the upper and lower respiratory tract, and often involving the gastrointestinal tract as well. It is characterized by sudden onset of fever, headache, myalgia, prostration and weakness. The acute symptoms usually subside in 3 or 4 days. Severe dry cough occurs in most cases. Abdominal pain with diarrhea and/or constipation may occur. The cough may become more prominent as the earlier systemic symptoms diminish. The cough, usually nonproductive, may be productive of small amounts of tenacious mucoid sputum.

Influenza is often complicated by a viral or bacterial pneumonia. It is caused by one of the strains of the influenza virus. If the causative virus belongs to one of the A strains (A, A prime or A-Asian) the disease is apt to be severe, to have a high incidence of complications and to occur in epidemic or pandemic waves. If the virus belongs to the B, C or D strains the influenza is apt to be much less severe and the epidemics are apt to be local rather than widespread.

PERTUSSIS is an acute infectious disease of the entire respiratory tract caused by the *Hemophilus pertussis*. It is called whooping cough because it is characterized by paroxysms of short efforts at coughing with little or no inspiration between them, followed by a sudden forceful "whooping" inspiration. Cough is such a predominant feature of pertussis because the organisms selectively attack the respiratory mucous membranes, where they cause an intense catarrhal inflammation and interference with ciliary action. The disease is also characterized by inflammatory swelling of the tracheobronchial lymph nodes, a fact which may also play a part in the genesis of the severe cough. Pertussis is frequently complicated by interstitial pneumonia or bronchopneumonia; if these complications are slow in resolving, patchy necrosis of the bronchi and adjacent tissues may lead to the late complication of bronchiectasis.

Chronic bronchitis is defined clinically as a chronic productive cough for at least 3 months of each year for at least 2 consecutive years. It is characterized pathologically by narrowed bronchial lumens due to thickened, inflamed bronchial walls, impairment of ciliary action, overproduction of excessively viscid bronchial mucus, and hypertrophy and increased numbers of bronchial glands and goblet cells. While its causes are not completely understood, the disease is closely associated with regular frequent inhaling of tobacco smoke, heavy industrial air pollution, cold damp climate and repeated deep viral and bacterial respiratory infections. It is also related at times to chronic episodic allergic bronchial asthma. Patients with chronic bronchitis tend to start their days with an episode of severe dry coughing culminating in the production of some sticky, often mucopurulent mucus. They frequently begin to notice dyspnea on exertion after some 10 to 30 years of coughing; by this time, the disease chronic bronchitis tends to merge into the disease diffuse pulmonary *emphysema* (alveolar wall destruction) and ultimately, in many cases, *cor pulmonale* develops. Repeated attacks of pneumonia are apt to occur during the evolution of these diseases. The attack of pneumonia, often complicated by pulmonary thromboses, frequently abruptly usher in further loss of exercise tolerance.

Bronchiectasis is, by definition, an irreversible destruction of the bronchial walls. It may result from an obstructive or slowly resolving pneumonitis, especially when due to necrotizing microorganisms. Bronchiectasis may also occur following the inhalation of a foreign body and following pertussis. A congenital or developmental form is recognized in which multiple epithelium-lined spaces, reminiscent of bronchogenic cysts, become acutely, and then chronically, infected. The cough in bronchiectasis is usually chronic and is typically worse in the morning. It is characteristically "loose" and relatively productive of large quantities of purulent, often foul, sputum. The sputum tends to settle into 2 or 3 layers upon standing. Patients with bronchiectasis often have severe hemoptysis because the necrotizing process has penetrated into a vessel and because the bronchial vasculature in bronchiectasis often gradually becomes hypertrophied. The diagnosis of bronchiectasis is confirmed by a bronchogram showing localized or widespread dilatation of bronchi and pooling of contrast medium. The dilatations are usually irregular or saccular and often interspersed with areas of narrowing. Smooth cylindrical dilatation, especially when only slight, is a feature of chronic bronchitis, rather than of true bronchiectasis.

Lobar pneumonia is usually caused by *D. pneumoniae,* less commonly by streptococci, staphylococci and other pus-forming bacteria. This disease occurs after exposure to cold, after an upper respiratory infection, after an alcoholic debauch or without any predisposing cause. Its onset is characteristically sudden, with severe prostration, a teeth-chattering chill, localized severe pleurisy, high fever and a slight but irritative cough. Within 1 to 2 days the cough tends to become productive of "rusty," frankly bloody or purulent sputum. The cough gradually becomes more severe and finally productive of copious amounts of purulent sputum as the process begins to resolve.

Bronchopneumonia may be caused by the pneumococci, the staphylococci, the streptococci, Klebsiella and various other bacteria or by various viral agents. Bronchopneumonia is apt to occur in the aged and infirm, following an alcoholic debauch, or in the very young. It is often a complication of influenza or some other severe infection involving the respiratory tract; it may follow the inhalation of food or other foreign material or various irritant gases. When due to one of several different viral agents, it is labelled *viral pneumonia* or *primary atypical pneumonia.* Cough in these pneumonias tends to be relatively dry and irritative at the outset, and only becomes severe and frankly productive as the process begins slowly to resolve.

Lung abscess is caused by the inhalation of foreign material (a piece of tonsil following tonsillectomy or a piece of tooth or food), by necrotizing inflammation behind an obstructive neoplasm, by necrosis within a malignant neoplasm or infarct, by blood stream dissemination of a suppurative process elsewhere in the body, by deep, penetrating chest trauma, or by the extension of a subphrenic or liver abscess through the diaphragm into the adjacent lung. During its early, formative phase a lung abscess behaves similarly to an acute severe pneumonia with dry, often relatively mild cough. As soon as necrosis has occurred in the center of the abscess and the fluid contents have gained access to a bronchus the cough becomes severe and productive of large amounts of foul, purulent, often blood-tinged material. The organisms most commonly involved are Klebsiella, the staphylococci and the pneumococci, but the infections are frequently mixed.

Pulmonary tuberculosis is a chronic inflammatory disease of the lungs often involving the bronchi as well. It is characterized by a recurring sequence of patches of acute pneumonic consolidation followed by necrosis, emptying of necrotic material into a bronchus, leaving an air-containing cavity, and the development of new areas of pneumonitis where the bacilli-laden necrotic material happens to lodge. Meanwhile, certain more favorable changes may take place, to a greater or lesser extent. The consolidation may resolve entirely or in part. As necrosis begins, the foci may begin to be walled off by a fibrous tissue reaction around them. Necrotic material may inspissate, become too thick to flow down a bronchus and ultimately calcify. These healing processes may cease without warning, with resumption of the emptying of necrotic foci into nearby bronchi and consequent spread of the disease to new areas. The factors most important in determining how a tuberculous process will behave are host resistance, the virulence of the individual infecting microorganisms, the presence of other diseases and conditions such as diabetes, silicosis and pregnancy, and the effectiveness of any chemotherapy which may be given. Cough in pulmonary tuberculosis may be due to the presence of exudate in the bronchi, to actual inflammation of the bronchi, usually near an area of parenchymal involvement, to complicating bronchial damage or bronchiectasis, to pleural irritation or to pressure upon bronchi caused by distortion, which is caused in turn by fibrous tissue contraction and/or atelectasis. Cough may be mild or severe, dry or nonproductive. The nature of the cough is dependent upon the status of the disease in the individual. Other symptoms commonly seen in tuberculosis are hemoptysis, pleurisy, weakness, easy fatigability, fever and weight loss.

Deep fungal infections which are apt to occur in the lungs include especially histoplasmosis and coccidioidomycosis; others are actinomycosis, nocardiosis, blastomycosis, cryptococcosis (torulosis), aspergillosis and mucormycosis. Pathologically these diseases attack the lung in much the same way as tuberculosis. Cough, caused by the same mechanism as that of tuberculosis, is frequently present. It will be dry or productive depending on whether a necrotic area has begun to slough into an open bronchus. The x-ray films of the pulmonary fungal diseases are usually not diagnostic and are often quite similar to or even indistinguishable from those of pulmonary tuberculosis. Skin tests and serologic tests are helpful in diagnosing histoplasmosis and coccidioidomycosis.

HISTOPLASMOSIS is endemic in the valleys of the Mississippi river and its tributaries. The acute form of the disease is commonly acquired by inhaling dried bat, pigeon or chicken dung (in caves, old buildings or especially in abandoned chicken yards). Despite the fact that 50 to 75 per cent of adults in the endemic area have been infected (they have a positive histoplasmin skin test), in most cases the primary infection is inapparent and both the acute and chronic active forms of the disease remain quite uncommon.

COCCIDIOIDOMYCOSIS is endemic in various hot arid parts of the world; southern California, New Mexico and Arizona and western Texas are the endemic areas in the United States. As is true of histoplasmosis, far more persons have the infection than the disease. The disseminated forms are more common in pregnant women and in Filipinos than in the rest of the population. In the acute nondisseminated form the disease is often manifested by a pulmonary nodule or a thin-walled cavity.

ACTINOMYCOSIS (caused by *Actinomyces bovis*) is apt to spread through natural tissue barriers and thus lead to chronic draining sinuses. Tissue sections and cultures will reveal the characteristic "sulfur granules."

NOCARDIOSIS (due to *Actinomyces asteroides*) usually attacks debilitated persons and those with other serious pulmonary diseases and is often fatal. The mycelia are faintly acid-fast and may· break up into rodlike forms which can be mistaken for tubercle bacilli.

NORTH AMERICAN BLASTOMYCOSIS behaves much like actinomycosis. About one third of cases have pulmonary involvement, usually with patchy pneumonia, cavitation and fibrosis. The skin and the lymph nodes are commonly involved.

PULMONARY CRYPTOCOCCOSIS commonly presents a solitary pulmonary nodule or cavity. A chronic low grade meningitis, which often ultimately proves fatal, is a common complication.

ASPERGILLOSIS occurs most commonly as a saprophytic "fungus ball" or mycetoma in an old inert pulmonary cavity caused by previous tuberculosis, fungus disease or lung abscess. A severe bronchitis often lasting for 2 or 3 months is occasionally seen.

MUCORMYCOSIS is a rare, terminal complication seen especially in older persons with severe uncontrolled diabetes.

Parasitic lung diseases may also cause cough due to bronchial irritation; these include paragonimiasis, schistosomiasis and ecchinococcal disease in particular.

Pleurisy with or without effusion, *pleurodynia* and *pleural empyema* may all cause cough by irritation of the afferent nerve endings in the pleura which are involved in the cough reflex arc.

CARDIOVASCULAR DISORDERS

Acute pulmonary edema is usually due to acute left ventricular failure. It may also follow the inhalation of smoke or noxious gases such as NO_2. It is characterized by intense vascular engorgement and by the transudation of fluid from congested capillaries into both the air spaces and interstitial tissues of the lungs. Cough in pulmonary edema is typically frequent, loose and productive of frothy, often pink, sputum. There is also severe dyspnea and orthopnea. An attack is often ushered in by an attack of paroxysmal nocturnal dyspnea (cardiac asthma). Fine crepitant rales can be heard throughout the lungs. The most common causes of acute left ventricular failure are hypertensive and arteriosclerotic heart disease and aortic regurgitation. A somewhat special form of pulmonary edema is seen in severe mitral stenosis. This form is more chronic and often less severe than others. It may be accompanied by frequent small hemoptyses and, in some cases, by crepitant rales at one or both apices. Other special forms of pulmonary edema are sometimes seen in uremia, in acute rheumatic fever with carditis, after hexamethonium therapy and rarely in normal persons when exposed to very high altitude and extreme cold. The roentgenographic picture of pulmonary edema is quite diagnostic and is characterized by small to large, symmetrical or asymmetrical patches of ill defined, cloudy infiltration, especially in the region around the lung roots.

Pulmonary infarction may cause mild to moderate cough which is usually dry, but sometimes productive of blood or blood-tinged sputum. The patient may or may not also have pleurisy with or without effusion and may or may not have some obvious source of pulmonary emboli.

Aortic aneurysm may cause severe cough by pressure on the trachea, the bronchi or the lung parenchyma, or by interference with one of the recurrent laryngeal nerves. When an aneurysm presses on the trachea, the cough is apt to have the brassy quality of major airway obstruction.

TRAUMA AND PHYSICAL AGENTS

Foreign bodies of all kinds may be aspirated into the airways. The resulting cough depends on the nature of the foreign material and the location and completeness of the resulting airway obstruction. An obstruction in the trachea or larynx is apt to cause an intense croupy or brassy cough, plus dyspnea, cyanosis and gagging. After the foreign body has become lodged the symptoms often tend to subside. A foreign body in one of the main bronchi is apt to cause a continuing irritative cough and wheeze. Obstruction farther down the bronchial tree is very apt to cause severe paroxysmal cough, often followed by pneumonitis, atelectasis or both. Atelectasis and pneumonia are particularly likely to occur when the inhaled object consists of vegetable matter, such as a peanut, which tends to incite an intense inflammatory reaction in the mucosa with which it remains in contact.

Irritant gases such as phosgene, chlorine, chloropicrin, NO_2, SO_2, ozone, nitro-olefins, tars, oxychlorcarbon, dichlorethyl sulfide, dichlormethylether and other organic solvents can cause intense inflammation of the respiratory mucosa, a severe irritative cough and ultimately acute pulmonary edema. Patchy pneumonia is a common complication. If the subject survives the initial insult, later changes such as bronchiolitis obliterans may prove fatal, especially following NO_2 inhalation. Intensely cold air may also act as a mild cough-inducing irritant especially in persons with some underlying chronic pulmonary pathology. Furthermore, any noxious or irritating gas is considerably more irritating when inhaled through the mouth than when inhaled through the nose, since the nose filters, warms, and moistens inhaled gases to a remarkable degree.

The **pneumoconioses** seldom cause cough unless complicated by extensive fibrosis, chronic bronchitis or some pulmonary infection. *Beryllium granulomatosis* is a rather special exception in that very intense paroxysmal dry cough, marked weight loss and alveolar capillary block without much impairment of ventilation are quite typical features. The roentgenographic appearance is very like miliary tuberculosis or miliary sarcoidosis.

NEOPLASMS

Primary bronchogenic carcinoma is a very common cause of cough, especially a severe and/or changing cough. The cough in bronchogenic carcinoma may be caused by partial airway obstruction and by bronchial mucosal irritation either directly or secondary to infection occurring distal to an obstructed bronchus. Cough, chest pain, and hemoptysis form the triad of symptoms so characteristic of this disease. The affected persons usually have been cigarette smokers for many years and often have long been accustomed to a chronic cough, especially in the mornings. When the malignant change takes place, the cough tends to change in some way, to become more or sometimes less productive, to become more persistent or severe, or to change in sound, often to become brassy. The associated chest pain may be pleuritic with or without a clear or bloody effusion, but often is vague and nonpleuritic.

Various other manifestations which should arouse suspicion of bronchogenic cancer in a person with a chronic or changing cough include personality change or Jacksonian epilepsy suggesting a metastatic focal brain lesion; evidence of involvement of the brachial plexus, or of a recurrent laryngeal, phrenic or cervical sympathetic nerve; recurrent pneumonitis, especially if in the same segment or lobe; or a wheeze which is either made worse or relieved by one or the other lateral recumbent positions. The diagnosis may be confirmed by roentgenologic examination of the chest (including fluoroscopy and tomography), bronchoscopy, and sputum cytology. A blind scalene node biopsy is only occasionally helpful, but biopsy of a palpable cervical node, especially when hard and located just behind the medial end of either clavicle, is much more apt to be diagnostic. Sometimes the diagnosis can be established only by open thoracotomy.

Metastatic lung tumors are not prone to cause cough except in two circumstances: when the metastasis occurs in a bronchus or when pulmonary metastasis takes the form of widespread lymphogenous or hematogenous involvement. In these widespread forms which cause marked alveolar-capillary (diffusion) block, cough is usually quite irritative, severe and dry.

Bronchial adenoma will compress or invade a bronchial wall and cause severe cough, often with severe hemoptysis.

Bronchiolar or alveolar cell carcinoma, also called **pulmonary adenomatosis,** usually causes chronic cough. Because this is a tumor of mucus-secreting tissues, affected persons may (but usually do not) expectorate large quantities of clear watery mucoid sputum. The roentgenographic picture frequently simulates an infiltrative process such as tuberculosis.

Primary mesothelioma of the pleura is usually malignant and may cause dry cough, although chest pain and an arthritis-like syndrome (severe pulmonary osteoarthropathy) are much more frequent and suggestive symptoms.

Leukemia may involve the mediastinal and lung root structures and cause a secondary pneumonitis or bronchitis with resultant cough.

Other primary lung tumors which may cause cough are primary *sarcoma,* a very rare tumor, and **bronchogenic cyst,** especially after it has become secondarily infected. Hamartoma, fibroma, lipoma, pulmonary sequestration and other rare benign tumors seldom if ever cause cough.

Mediastinal Tumors. Tumors of the thyroid or the thymus; teratomas, nerve tissue tumors, lymphomas, aneurysms, inflammatory enlargement of hilar or the paratracheal lymph nodes (due especially to tuberculosis, histoplasmosis or sarcoidosis) may all cause cough by pressure upon or invasion of the trachea or the bronchi.

ALLERGIC DISORDERS

Bronchial asthma may be defined as episodic expiratory dyspnea associated with wheezing, not necessarily associated with effort, often induced by contact with a specific substance (antigen), occurring in persons with a family history of allergy and accompanied by blood and sputum eosinophilia. Such patients are apt to show temporary relief after the administration of epinephrine, ephedrine or some other bronchodilator. While one may thus describe the so-called extrinsic type of asthma, the intrinsic variety may not exhibit all or even any of these features, but it often related to recurrent deep bronchial infections. The cough in asthma is dry, tight, wheezy and usually occurs in paroxysms. Chest examination during an attack reveals the suppressed breath sounds of small airway obstruction and musical rales or rhonchi. These signs may be present, but are less evident between attacks. Status asthmaticus is a protracted attack and is a late and critical phase of asthma in which response is no longer obtained with standard treatment. Death may occur in such an attack. Postmortem examination reveals extensive blocking of the finer airways with inspissated mucus plugs. Bronchial asthma should be carefully differentiated from cardiac asthma and from the various other conditions which cause cough and dyspnea with wheezing due to partial bronchial, tracheal or laryngeal obstruction.

Hay fever and vasomotor rhinitis may both cause a mild, usually dry cough because of the postnasal drip so frequently accompanying these conditions.

Other causes of cough include a wide range of conditions involving the lungs and tracheobronchial tree. Calcified parenchy-mal foci or lymph nodes may ulcerate their way into an adjacent bronchus (*broncholithiasis*) and in so doing cause an intense irritative cough until the material has sloughed out and the patient has expectorated a "lung stone" or chalky material. Hemoptyses frequently accompany this sequence of events. Primary *hemosiderosis* is a rare disease of unknown etiology characterized by cough, frequent small hemoptyses and progressive dyspnea.

Eosinophilic granuloma (Histiocytosis X) is characterized by diffuse roentgenographic involvement out of proportion to the mildness of symptoms which may include cough, episodes of spontaneous pneumothorax and occasionally diabetes insipidus.

Wegener's granulomatosis is a rare disease characterized by asymmetrical pulmonary infiltrates, often with large nodules which may cavitate, granulomatous involvement of the nasal septum and sinuses causing a severe catarrh, widespread necrotizing angiitis, and a focal glomerulonephritis which causes terminal renal insufficiency.

Sarcoidosis is a relatively common cause of hilar and paratracheal lymph node and/or lung parenchymal involvement which may cause dry cough and dyspnea.

Diffuse interstitial (Hamman-Rich) fibrosis is a rare disease of unknown cause usually presenting with evidence of diffuse bilateral pulmonary fibrosis, alveolar-capillary block and relatively little ventilatory impairment.

Alveolar proteinosis is a newly described disease of unknown cause in which the roentgenographic picture is reminiscent of a patchy pulmonary edema, in which the symptoms at the outset tend to be less severe than would be expected from the appearance of the infiltrate and in which death usually ensues with evidence of alveolar-capillary block.

Right middle lobe (compression) syndrome may also cause cough due to narrowing of the right middle lobe bronchus with associated atelectasis and pneumonitis. The right middle lobe bronchus is particularly vulnerable to compression by one or more enlarged lymph nodes situated at its origin from the right bronchus. Enlargement of the peribronchial lymph nodes at this site is most often caused by tuberculosis, but histoplasmosis and other infections and bronchogenic carcinoma may also cause this syndrome.

SUMMARY

Cough is essentially an explosive expiration. It may be involuntary or voluntary. When involuntary, the reflex arc responsible for cough consists of afferent impulses arising from irritation of the laryngeal tracheobronchial mucosa, pressure or traction on the trachea, pressure upon the carotid sinus, the liver, the spleen, or the external auditory canal, irritation of the pleura or congestion of the lung parenchyma. These impulses are transmitted by vagal or sympathetic trunks to an area in the medulla oblongata. The efferent impulses then descend to the various muscles of expiration.

The stimuli which can give rise to cough may be inflammatory, mechanical, chemical or thermal.

The specific diseases which may cause cough were discussed under the following headings: Inflammations, Cardiovascular Disorders, Trauma and Physical Agents, Neoplasms, Allergic Disorders, Other Causes.

BIBLIOGRAPHY

Bickerman, H. A., and Barach, A. L.: The experimental production of cough in human subjects induced by citric acid aerosols, Am. J. Med. Sci., 228:156-163, 1954.

Bucker, K.: Pathophysiology and pharmacology of cough, Pharmacol. Rev. 10:43-58, 1958.

Chakravarty, N. K., Matallana, A., Jensen, R., and Borison, H. L.: Central effects of antitussive drugs on cough and respiration, J. Pharmacol. 117:127-135, 1956.

Currens, J. H., and White, P. D.: Cough as a symptom of cardiovascular disease, Ann. Int. Med. 30:528-543, 1949.

Dawes, G. S., and Comroe, J. H.: Chemoreflexes from the heart and lungs, Physiol. Rev. 34:167-201, 1954.

Drinker, C. K.: The function of the nerves in lungs and thoracic wall, Amer. Rev. Tuberc. 58:1-14, 1948.

DiRienzo, S.: Physiopathologie des hustens, Fort. Rontgenstr. 78:1-14, 1953.

Ross, B. B., Gramiak, R., and Rahn, H.: Physical dynamics of the cough mechanism, J. App. Physiol. 8:264-268, 1955.

Sharpey-Schafer, E. P.: Effects of coughing on intrathoracic pressure, arterial pressure and peripheral blood flow, J. Physiol. 122:351-357, 1953.

————: The mechanism of syncope after coughing, Brit. M. J., 2:860-863, 1953.

Shane, S. J., Krzyski, T. K., and Copp, E. S.: Clinical evaluation of a new antitussive agent. Canad. M.A.J. 77:600-602, 1957.

15

Hemoptysis

ROGER S. MITCHELL

CAUSES OF HEMOPTYSIS
 TRAUMA
 FOREIGN BODIES
 INFLAMMATION

NEOPLASMS
VASCULAR AND CIRCULATORY CONDITIONS
MISCELLANEOUS CAUSES

Hemoptysis is the spitting of blood. The blood may originate from any portion of the respiratory tract, but especially from the main bronchi and the lung parenchyma. Blood spitting may also occur after inhaling blood originating in the nose, the throat or the upper gastrointestinal tract. A careful history and thorough examination of the nose and throat will usually enable the physician to localize the source of the bleeding in such cases. When blood originates in the nose, a bleeding point can usually be seen in one side of that organ. However, a severe gastrointestinal or pulmonary hemorrhage will occasionally be partly expelled through the nose. Bleeding from the deep respiratory tract usually recurs over a period of several hours or days and the blood is usually mixed to some extent with sputum.

Hemoptysis of blood from the trachea, the bronchi or the lungs occurs typically after cough.

It is important to determine if possible the side of origin of a pulmonary hemorrhage in cases with bilateral lesions or in those with no visible roentgenographic abnormality. Many patients insist that they can tell this by their feeling; such individuals are often, but not always, right. Bronchoscopy during a hemorrhage will sometimes permit the careful operator to determine the side of origin of a pulmonary hemorrhage. However, since blood from one lung can flow into the other, the bronchoscopist must see blood flowing actively from a bronchial orifice or must see the bleeding point in order to be sure of its location. Rales or rhonchi localized to one side or one area are helpful in establishing the origin of a pulmonary hemorrhage. In addition, it should be realized that blood may not be spit out until some time after it has escaped from a vessel, especially in cases with mild to moderate degrees of bleeding. Such a delay is suggested when the blood is partially clotted, is bright red, or is changed in some other way. A fresh hemorrhage from a pulmonary artery, the most common source, may be identified by its blue (unoxygenated) color.

The cause of a true hemoptysis may be ascertained in most subjects by means of a careful history and physical examination supplemented by standard posteroanterior and lateral chest roentgenograms. In the more difficult cases additional studies may be necessary, including Bucky and lordotic chest films, tomograms, chest fluoroscopy, bronchoscopy, bronchography, sputum bacteriology and cytology, tuberculosis and fungus skin tests, serology and finally, prolonged observation. However, it should be stressed that despite very complete studies, and even follow-up for several years, the cause cannot be ascertained in some 5 to 10 per cent of cases. This fact which implies that hemoptysis may often have a relatively benign origin, does not excuse the physician from making a thorough effort to determine the cause in every case. Bronchogenic carcinoma or pulmonary tuberculosis, for instance, may cause pulmonary hemorrhage *before* they can be diagnosed by any roentgenographic method.

It is important to determine the amount of blood being spit up. A little blood in the sputum is often sufficiently frightening to cause the patient to exaggerate. Knowledge of the alarm caused by hemoptysis may lead disturbed or dishonest persons to complain of blood-spitting which is nonexistent or self-induced. The actual coughing up of the blood should therefore always be observed by the physician whenever possible.

CAUSES OF HEMOPTYSIS

The causes of hemoptysis may be classified as follows:

Trauma
Foreign bodies
Inflammation
Neoplasms
Vascular and circulatory conditions
Miscellaneous causes

TRAUMA

Hemoptysis may result when the lungs are punctured by a fractured rib or are contused by severe blunt trauma to the chest or are inflamed by the inhalation of very noxious fumes or smoke. The tracheobronchial tree may be lacerated or fractured by such blunt trauma as a steering wheel delivers to the driver in an automobile collision. Stab or gunshot wound may injure any part of the lungs or airways. Very severe protracted coughing may lead to mucosal laceration and thus to hemoptysis or blood-stained sputum.

FOREIGN BODIES

Foreign bodies may cause bleeding by direct trauma to the airway mucosa or, indirectly, by causing bronchiectasis or simply by causing protracted severe coughing.

INFLAMMATION

Bleeding may come from infectious lesions in the pharynx, the larynx, the trachea, the bronchi or the lungs, especially when accompanied by severe coughing.

Bleeding is particularly apt to occur in necrotizing pulmonary infections such as tuberculosis, the deep fungal infections and pneumonia due to Klebsiella organisms and the staphylococci.

Hemorrhage in tuberculosis may be a very early sign, especially in persons with poor host resistance to tuberculosis; it is also common late in the course of the disease when the process has become predominantly fibrocaseous or has become complicated by bronchiectasis.

The appearance of the bloody sputum in Klebsiella pneumonia has been likened to currant jelly. In pneumococcus lobar pneumonia, the sputum may be faintly or grossly bloody, but, especially at the outset, is often characteristically rusty in appearance.

When an inflammatory process has gone on to abscess formation, bleeding is again common, but the blood is usually mixed with copious amounts of foul-smelling pus. Gangrene, another late manifestation of lung inflammation, is also accompanied by bleeding, often associated with the spitting up of necrotic lung tissue.

Bleeding may occur during deep fungus infections of the respiratory tract; as in tuberculosis, the bleeding may be an early sign of fresh lung necrosis or cavitation, or it may be a late manifestation of chronic ulcerative inflammation.

Parasitic diseases of the lung may also cause hemoptysis. One special type of bloody sputum, likened to anchovy sauce, occurs when an amebic abscess penetrates the right hemidiaphragm and lung from the liver, and causes a lung abscess.

Bleeding is a very common symptom of bronchiectasis. Bronchiectasis is, by definition, a necrosis of bronchial walls. The bronchial vasculature lining these walls often becomes relatively hypertrophied in chronic bronchiectasis. Because of this hypertrophy, and because of the systemic blood pressure within the bronchial arteries, hemoptysis in bronchiectasis is not only frequent but also is apt to be severe.

NEOPLASMS

The commonest cause of hemoptysis in persons past the age of 45 is primary bronchogenic carcinoma. Hemoptysis, together with severe and changing cough and nondescript chest pain, form the characteristic triad of symptoms of this very common neoplasm. Bleeding in primary bronchogenic cancer may occur because of mucosal ulceration, because of necrosis within the center of a tumor, or secondary to a pneumonic or bronchiectatic abscess formation process distal to an obstructing bronchial tumor.

Hemoptysis may be caused by metastatic cancer in the lung but this is rare.

Although primary bronchial adenoma is not common, when this lesion is present, bleeding is very common and is apt to be severe. If a bronchoscopist sees what he believes may be a bronchial adenoma, he should not attempt to biopsy it, as the danger of starting an uncontrollable hemorrhage is great.

Hemangioma is a rare tumor of the lung or tracheobronchial tree which may cause severe pulmonary hemorrhage. It may be benign or malignant.

Vascular and Circulatory Conditions

Left ventricular failure may cause acute pulmonary edema. The affected person may cough up large quantities of pink frothy material, and, occasionally, pure blood. In the special form of pulmonary edema which occurs in severe mitral stenosis pure blood is more commonly produced than pink froth. In pulmonary edema due to left ventricular failure, fine crepitant rales are heard throughout the lungs but especially at the lung bases. By contrast, in mitral stenosis the rales may be confined to, or more pronounced at, one or both apices. The reasons for the latter phenomenon are not known.

Pulmonary embolism and thrombosis are common causes of hemoptysis, especially when complicated by true lung tissue *infarction*. However, it should be stressed that many pulmonary vascular accidents occur without hemoptysis or pleurisy and without an obvious source of an embolus.

Aortic aneurysm may erode into some part of the tracheobronchial tree and cause an exsanguinating hemorrhage.

Arteriovenous fistulae may be acquired (usually through trauma) or congenital (usually part of a generalized Osler-Weber-Rendu's disease). In the latter disease they are often multiple, not only in the lung, but elsewhere in the body. Accompanying physical signs are clubbing, cyanosis and a bruit heard over the fistula. Bleeding may be severe.

Miscellaneous Causes

Various blood dyscrasias may lead to pulmonary hemorrhage with or without specific lesions located in the lungs or airways. These include *purpura, agranulocytosis* and *hemophilia.*

Leukemia or lymphoma may involve the lung parenchyma, usually late in the course of the disease, and cause hemoptysis.

Scurvy may cause bleeding from any organ, especially from a mucous membrane, and thus may be manifested by hemopytsis.

Primary hemosiderosis is a rare disease without known cause which usually occurs in young adults. It is characterized by protracted, frequent, recurrent small hemoptyses, dyspnea on exertion and a diffuse, almost miliary, infiltrate seen on the chest roentgenogram.

Pulmonary microlithiasis, cause unknown, may cause hemoptysis. Calcific foci either in the lung parenchyma or in lymph nodes may ulcerate into a bronchus *(broncholithiasis)* and in so doing cause hemoptysis. This process is usually accompanied by a severe irritative cough until the extrusion is complete.

The right middle lobe syndrome is due to a partial or complete obstruction of the rather long and narrow right middle lobe bronchus. This causes right middle lobe atelectasis, pneumonitis or both. The obstruction is usually due more to scar formation and/or inflammation than to physical compression of the lumen by an enlarged lymph node. While the cause may be primary malignancy, it is usually infectious and the infection is most commonly tuberculosis. Hemoptysis occasionally accompanies this syndrome.

Hemoptysis may rarely occur only during menstruation, the so-called *vicarious menstruation.* The cause is obscure.

SUMMARY

Hemoptysis is the term applied to the spitting of blood. It is very important to determine whether the blood originates in the nose, the throat, the gastrointestinal tract or the deep respiratory tract. The causes of bleeding from the deep respiratory tract are reviewed under the following headings: Trauma, Foreign Bodies, Neoplasms, Vascular and Circulatory Lesions, and Miscellaneous Causes.

BIBLIOGRAPHY

Barrett, R. J., and Tuttle, W. M.: A study of essential hemoptysis, J. Thoracic & Cardiovas. Surg. 40:468-474, 1960.

Boucot, K. R.: Hemoptysis in older men, J. Nat. M. Ass. 52:259-261, 1960.

Carr, D. T., and Douglass, B. E.: Hemoptysis, Med. Clin. N. Am. 38:945-948, 1954.

Chaves, A. D.: Hemoptysis in chest clinic patients, Am. Rev. Tuberc. 63:194-201, 1951.

Gale, D., and Lord, J. D.: Overgrowth of *Serratia marcescens* in the respiratory tract, simulating hemoptysis, J.A.M.A. 164:1328, 1957.

Heller, R.: The significance of hemoptysis, Tubercle 27:70-74, 1946.

Johnston, R. N., Lockhart, W., Ritchie, R. T., and Smith, D. H.: Haemoptysis, Brit. M. J. 5173:592-595, 1960.

Moersch, H. J.: Clinical significance of hemoptysis, J.A.M.A. 148:1461-1465, 1952.

Moersch, R. N., Devine, K. D., Woolner, L. B., Judd, E. S., Jr., and Schmidt, H. W.: Hemoptysis in cancer of the thyroid, J. Thoracic Surg. 31:329, 1956.

Parker, E. F.: Hemoptysis, its significance and methods of study, Dis. Chest 21:677-690, 1952.

Pursel, S. E., and Lindskog, G. E.: Hemoptysis. A clinical evaluation of 105 patients examined consecutively on a thoracic surgical service, Am. Rev. Resp. Dis. 84:329-336, 1961.

Sanders, C. R., and Smith, A. T.: The clinical significance of hemoptysis, New England J. Med. 247:790-793, 1952.

Segarra, F. O.: Bronchoscopy in hemoptysis, New England J. Med. 258:167-170, 1958.

16

Dyspnea

DANIEL S. LUKAS

The term dyspnea implies difficult or uncomfortable breathing. It is the sensation experienced when the act of breathing intrudes upon the conscious sphere as an unpleasant effort. The patient suffering from dyspnea is apt to say: "I'm short of breath"; "I can't catch my breath"; "I'm breathless" or "I feel like I'm suffocating."

Dyspnea is by no means always a symptom of disease. Normal individuals commonly experience this sensation with vigorous exertion. The level of physical activity provoking the symptom varies widely with age, sex, body size, the state of physical training, the altitude and the emotional motivation for the task being performed.

Dyspnea indicates disease only when it occurs at levels of activity below those expected to be normally tolerated. In this respect, since the normal range of tolerance for exertion is wide, it is very useful in taking the history to trace the development of the symptom in terms of diminishing ability to perform specific tasks. As an example: A patient may previously have been able to climb 3 flights of stairs at a moderately fast rate without discomfort but during the past year has noted progressive difficulty in performing this act and recently has been capable of climbing only one flight of stairs at a very slow rate because of shortness of breath.

Muscular fatigue very often accompanies dyspnea, and, particularly in patients with heart disease, the two symptoms may be inseparable. In some it may be overwhelming fatigue rather than dyspnea which brings activity to a halt. Therefore, an assessment of the tolerance for physical exertion is not complete without inquiry about the specific reactions that limit it. One cannot assume that the patient is dyspneic because he has a disease frequently provoking this symptom or because he manifests tachypnea or hyperpnea. These are *objective* signs of abnormality in breathing and suggest that shortness of breath may be one of his symptoms. Whether it is or not, however, can be answered only by the patient.

Dyspnea is a very important cause of disability in diseases of the lung and the heart. Although several attempts have been made to relate it to a single specific measurable abnormality in cardiac or pulmonary function none of these apply to all examples of this symptom. The results of many investigations over the years clearly indicate that many factors contribute to dyspnea, but there is no uniform agreement among interested investigators about the relative importance of each disturbance of function in its pathogenesis. A considerable part of the difficulty stems from the fact that the symptom is a subjective one and therefore susceptible to modification by emotional state and drive. It is unlikely on this basis alone that measurements of any single variable or even multiple variables of cardiopulmonary

324

function will correlate satisfactorily with the severity of dyspnea in *all* cases. Another aspect of the problem that is in great need of clarification is the nature of the stimuli, the sensory receptors and the nerve pathways that participate in the awareness of dyspnea. Little is known about the part played by visceral sensations arising from the pulmonary or cardiovascular structures as opposed to somatic sensations arising from the chest cage and the diaphragm.

The presently available information, which is the product of extensive investigation of cardiopulmonary function particularly in the recent past, indicates that dyspnea is primarily related to the *ventilatory component* of pulmonary function as opposed to the function of *gas exchange*.

THE VENTILATORY APPARATUS

The maintenance of an adequate flow of air to the alveoli of the lungs is essential to the normal performance of pulmonary function. The alternate expansion and relaxation of the chest bellows is responsible for this function.

The ability of the chest bellows to pump air into and out of the alveoli may be evaluated by measurement of the maximum breathing capacity *(ventilatory capacity)*. This is the maximum volume of air that can be breathed voluntarily in a minute. Maximum breathing capacity normally varies with body size, age and sex.[1] In young well-trained males it may attain values in the range of 200 liters per minute, whereas in small elderly ladies the normal level may be 60 liters per minute.

Ventilatory capacity measured in this way has been found to be greater than the ventilation attained during maximum exercise or maximum stimulation from carbon dioxide.[2] This clearly indicates that in the capacity of the normal chest bellows to perform there is a margin of reserve that is considerable under normal circumstances and that the ventilatory requirements of most human activities can be met quite adequately.

It is essential to recognize that the chest bellows is a complex apparatus. Its effectiveness in function depends on an intact and mobile rib cage, the health of the diaphragm and other respiratory muscles and their neural control and co-ordination. Of considerable importance is the patency of the various extrapulmonary and intrapulmonary airways. The elastic resistance of the pulmonary parenchyma and pleura (the resistance of these structures to stretching) is another significant determinant in performance. If the normal state or action of any of these components of the ventilatory apparatus are disturbed sufficiently, decrease in the maximum breathing capacity may ensue. Thus diaphragmatic paralysis, as in poliomyelitis, is associated with considerable impairment of ventilatory capacity.[3] Obstruction of the airways, particularly the small intrapulmonary segments of this system, as in asthma or emphysema, has a profound slowing effect on the volume rate of air flow in these passages and is a very common clinical cause of a diminished maximum breathing capacity.

Reduction in the ventilatory capacity is perhaps the most common disturbance in pulmonary function encountered among patients with various diseases of the lungs. The severity of dyspnea and the ease with which it is produced by exertion can be correlated fairly well with the degree to which the maximum breathing capacity is impaired. A very close approximation of dyspnea in physiologic terms is obtained when the levels of ventilation are compared with the ability to ventilate. Dyspnea is invariably experienced in normal individuals and in a variety of pulmonary diseases when the ventilation required by a particular activity or metabolic state occupies 30 to 40 per cent of the maximum breathing capacity or, to state the same thing in reverse, when only 60 to 70 per cent of the maximum breathing is not in use and is thus in reserve (breathing reserve).[4] From this relationship it is apparent that a very large ventilation, even though the maximum breathing capacity is normal, may cause dyspnea, and if the breathing capacity is low, relatively slight increases in ventilation from the resting state will produce this symptom. In many conditions not only is the ventilatory *capacity* reduced but also the ventilatory *requirements* during exercise are abnormally large.

Although it is widely applicable and clinically useful, the definition of the *dyspnea threshold* in terms of ventilation and maximum breathing capacity does not apply without reservation to all conditions provoking dyspnea. Two notable exceptions are pulmonary emphysema and cardiac disease. In emphysema the dyspnea threshold is very variable and the patient may have in use more than 50 per cent of his maximum breathing capacity during exertion without experiencing dyspnea. In heart disease the maximum breathing capacity may be normal and hyperventilation during exercise only mild, yet the patient may experience severe shortness of breath.[5]

MECHANICS AND WORK OF BREATHING

In seeking a physiologic common denominator for dyspnea considerable attention has been focused on the mechanics of breathing. The process of breathing is work. By the cyclic changes in intrapleural pressure produced by alternate contraction and relaxation of the respiratory muscles, the following forces must be overcome: the resistance of the lungs to stretch (elastic resistance), which depends on the physical properties of the lung tissues as well as on the surface tension acting at the interface between air and fluid lining the alveoli,[6,7] the resistance to the flow of gas in the airways, related to the geometric dimensions of the air passages, the velocity of gas flow within them, and the viscosity and density of the gas;[6,8] the resistance related to the friction of tissues as they slide over each other or are deformed. In addition, the respiratory muscles must overcome the elastic resistance of the chest wall and the frictional forces developed within the nonpulmonary tissues that are deformed or displaced during breathing. Of the total work expended by the normal subject in breathing at a rate of 15 times per minute, 63 per cent is spent on overcoming the elastic resistance of the lungs and chest wall, 29 per cent on overcoming airway resistance and only 8 per cent in deforming

tissues.[9] With faster rates, overcoming airway resistance requires a progressively larger percentage of the total work. Also, the balance between work in overcoming elastic resistance and that overcoming airway resistance is such that for any given level of alveolar ventilation there is an optimum rate of breathing. Decreasing or increasing the respiratory rate results in increased work expenditure.[9,10]

The work of quiet breathing during the course of a day involves an energy expenditure so small (0.4-0.5 Kg. M. per minute) that it can be supplied by 10 Gm. of sugar.[9] With increasing ventilation, the work performed by the respiratory muscles increases, and during maximum ventilation it is approximately 270 Kg. M. per minute.[9]

If the lungs are more than normally resistant to stretch (decreased pulmonary compliance) or if airway resistance is increased, the changes in intrapleural pressure and the work that are required to sustain a given level of ventilation are greater than normal. In patients with decreased compliance due to *pulmonary congestion,* the work expended on achieving a given minute volume during exercise may be 2 to 3 times normal.[11] In patients with *airway obstruction* due to emphysema, the force and work expended in overcoming resistance to airflow are increased considerably.[12] Disturbances in the chest bellows may also increase the work of breathing. In kyphoscoliosis, work done on moving the deformed chest cage in the process of breathing may be 5 or more times greater than normal.[13] In obesity, the decreased thoracic compliance produced by the encircling girdle of adipose tissue increases the mechanical work of breathing several fold.[14]

In order to perform their work the respiratory muscles require oxygen. The oxygen costs of breathing have been shown to increase disproportionately with increase in ventilation.[15] Thus at a ventilation 25 L. per minute greater than resting ventilation, the cost of each liter of ventilation is 1 ml. of oxygen per minute. At a ventilation in excess of 80 L. per minute, 3.2 ml. of oxygen are needed to support each liter of air breathed. And at 150 L. per minute,

1 L. of oxygen is consumed merely in the act of breathing.

The increased work of breathing in disease requires a greater oxygen supply to the respiratory muscles. A patient with severe pulmonary congestion may need more than 3 times the normal oxygen supply to support each liter of ventilation in excess of 15 L. per minute above the resting level.[15] A patient with emphysema may require 25 ml. of oxygen per minute to support each liter of ventilation above the resting level.[15] This exceeds the oxygen requirement for maintenance of more than 50 L. per minute in the normal. In kyphoscoliosis and in obesity, the oxygen costs of breathing are increased greatly.[13,16]

Although the data on work, oxygen requirements and the mechanics of breathing in both the normal state and in disease are far from complete, they do serve to emphasize in a more fundamental manner than otherwise possible the serious defects in the ventilatory apparatus produced by diseases involving the lungs. *Fatigue* of the respiratory muscles resulting from the increased work required of them in sustaining a given level of ventilation may play an important role in the sensation of dyspnea. In disease not only is the respiratory work for a given level of exertion greater than normal but the oxygen supply to the muscles of respiration is frequently disturbed by *hypoxemia* and a *restricted blood flow,* thus making them more susceptible to fatigue.

A critical level for the work of breathing at which dyspnea appears has not been found. Actually, in emphysema and mitral stenosis, dyspnea of sufficient severity to cause the patient to stop during exercise has been shown to occur at levels of breathing work considerably less than normal.[17] This may be related to poor oxygen supply to the muscles. Christie[17] has provided evidence that dyspnea severe enough to limit activity occurs when the intrapleural pressure changes required to effect ventilation are large (in the range of 30 cm. of water). He has suggested ". . . that dyspnea is conditioned not by the mechanical work of breathing but by the force which

has to be exerted on the lungs in order to increase ventilation in accordance with the demands of exercise." Of interest in this regard is the recent demonstration that the oxygen cost of breathing is more closely related to the total force exerted by the respiratory apparatus on the lungs and chest wall than it is to the mechanical work of breathing.[18] If Christie's concept is correct, then dyspnea is related primarily to stimuli arising from stretch receptors in the intrathoracic organs.

Thus, dyspnea is best interpreted as the subjective symptom which arises when the ventilatory apparatus is unduly taxed in meeting a certain requirement for ventilation. In the analysis of this symptom, factors which limit the capacity of the ventilatory apparatus to provide ventilation, or cause it to work excessively in meeting ventilatory requirements, as well as the demands for ventilation imposed on it must be taken into consideration.

VENTILATION

Relative constancy in the gas composition of the alveolar air is achieved by a cyclic flushing of the alveoli with air from the outside. The rate at which air is moved into and out of the lungs is termed ventilation and is conventionally expressed in liters per minute. At a constant tidal volume it is equal to the tidal volume times the respiratory rate.

Not all of each breath reaches the alveoli to participate in gas exchange. Some of it remains behind in the dead space in which no gas exchange occurs. Anatomically the dead space consists of the volume of air in the nasopharynx, the trachea, the bronchi and the nonrespiratory bronchioles. In the normal adult the dead space is from 100 to 150 ml. in size.[19]

Total ventilation is subdivided into two components: alveolar and dead space. The dead space component usually occupies less than 30 per cent of total ventilation.

The relationship between *alveolar ventilation* and carbon dioxide, and the rate at which carbon dioxide is manufactured and exhaled from the body is as follows:

Concentration of CO_2 in alveolar air =

$$\frac{CO_2 \text{ output per minute}}{\text{Alveolar ventilation per minute}}$$

A similar but more complicated relationship exists for oxygen with the notable difference that the concentration of oxygen in the alveolar air is related directly (rather than inversely) to alveolar ventilation.[20]

From these considerations it is apparent that alveolar ventilation, in relation to metabolic uptake of oxygen and release of carbon dioxide, ultimately determines the gas composition of both the alveolar air and blood flowing from the alveoli. At any given level of metabolism a decrease below normal in alveolar ventilation will cause the concentration of carbon dioxide in alveolar air to rise and that of oxygen to fall. Increase in the alveolar ventilation will have the opposite effect.

A decision about the appropriateness of ventilation in a given patient may be very difficult without knowledge of the relative sizes of the dead space and the tidal volume, the concentration of oxygen and of carbon dioxide in the arterial blood, and the metabolic rate.

Alveolar ventilation is regulated by complex homeostatic mechanisms,[21,22] and total ventilation may be modified by a host of factors. These mechanisms and factors can be subdivided into chemical, mechanical, physical, cortical and metabolic.

Chemical Factors. The respiratory center in the medulla is exquisitely sensitive to changes in the *concentration of carbon dioxide* in the arterial blood. An increment in carbon dioxide tension as small as 1.5 mm. Hg above the normal of 40 mm. Hg is enough to cause the alveolar ventilation to double.[23,24] Alveolar ventilation increases linearly with increase in arterial carbon dioxide tension but a limit is reached when carbon dioxide at a level of 9 per cent is inspired. Further increments in carbon dioxide concentration are associated with depression of alveolar ventilation and the mental manifestations related to the narcotic and anesthetic properties of the gas begin to appear.[22]

The respiratory center is also sensitive to changes in the *concentration of hydrogen ion* in the blood (pH). The increased ventilation that occurs on breathing carbon dioxide is partly due to the concomitant fall in pH of the blood.[22] For some time it was believed that the respiratory center was much less sensitive to change in hydrogen ion concentration than to change in carbon dioxide tension. This conclusion was based on the fact that the increase in ventilation during carbon dioxide inhalation is much greater than the increase occurring when the pH of the arterial blood is reduced to an equivalent degree by metabolic acidosis, such as may occur following ingestion of ammonium chloride. Thus inhalation of 5 per cent carbon dioxide which may be associated with a change in blood pH from 7.41 to 7.34 results in a 2.68-fold increase in alveolar ventilation. On the other hand, a metabolically induced acidosis with a pH of 7.34 may produce only a 1.09-fold increase in alveolar ventilation. However, Gray[22] has pointed out that in metabolic acidosis the concomitant decrease in carbon dioxide tension of the arterial blood definitely inhibits ventilation. The change in ventilation during metabolic acidosis is therefore the net effect of inhibition due to decrease of carbon dioxide tension and stimulation from increase in hydrogen ion concentration. The change observed on inhalation of carbon dioxide is due to the additive effect of increase of the two stimuli: carbon dioxide tension and hydrogen ion concentration.

Hyperventilation may become a conspicuous feature of metabolic acidosis. The very deep, usually rapid, respiration of acidosis forms a characteristic clinical picture called *Kussmaul breathing.* Such hyperventilation, often without dyspnea or consciousness of labored respiration, may accompany the ketoacidosis of diabetes, the acidosis of uremia or the formic acidosis of methyl alcohol poisoning.

At the present time it is not clear whether carbon dioxide tension or hydrogen ion concentration within the cells of the respiratory center is the chief stimulus to respiration. The problem has been complicated by the increasing evidence that the sensitivity of the respiratory center may be enhanced by prolonged hypocapnia. The hyperventilation which is a prominent feature of the acclimatization response to altitude has been found to persist on return to sea level.[22,25] Normal young men passively hyperventilated for 24 hours in a body respirator have been found to have a heightened ventilatory response to carbon dioxide inhalation persisting for as long as 11 days after removal from the respirator.[26]

Decrease in buffering capacity and bicarbonate concentration of the blood follows such prolonged hyperventilation and permits a greater fall in blood pH for a given increase of carbon dioxide tension. However, the phenomenon is not entirely dependent on decreased buffering capacity, since the response of ventilation to increase in hydrogen ion concentration in the blood is also greater.[27] This fact is directly applicable to patients who hyperventilate, since prolonged hyperventilation, regardless of cause, may be self-propagating by virtue of sensitization of the respiratory center. It may partially account for the severe hyperventilation observed in certain patients with pulmonary fibrosis and low blood bicarbonate levels.

On the other hand, prolonged exposure to high concentrations of carbon dioxide diminishes the sensitivity of the respiratory center. This has been observed in normal men after 4 to 6 days of exposure to 3 per cent carbon dioxide[28] and is a particularly striking and clinically important feature of patients with severe pulmonary disease and chronic elevations of their alveolar and arterial blood carbon dioxide levels (chronic respiratory acidosis). Again the diminished sensitivity has been definitely shown not to be entirely related to the concomitant increase in blood bicarbonate levels and the greater ability thereby to buffer the acid effect of increases in carbon dioxide tension, since the ventilatory response to change in arterial hydrogen ion concentration is impared also.[24]

Current evidence indicates that these alterations in the sensitivity of the respiratory center with prolonged hypocapnia or hypercapnia are related to changes in the buffering capacity of the brain.[29] It would appear that the activity of the respiratory center is conditioned by the concentrations within its cells of both carbon dioxide and buffer.[30,31]

Reduction in the oxygen tension of the arterial blood stimulates respiration. This effect is mediated by the cells in the carotid and the aortic bodies (peripheral chemoreceptors), which are sensitive to hypoxemia. The effect of hypoxemia on ventilation is not striking. It is not perceptible until the arterial oxygen has fallen to a level of about 65 mm. Hg from a normal of 95. The maximum response is only a 65 per cent increase in alveolar ventilation and occurs when the oxygen tension has dropped to 30 mm. Hg, a level which is attained at an altitude of 22,000 feet or by breathing 6 to 7 per cent oxygen at sea level.[22] However, the fall in blood carbon dioxide tension and rise in pH concurrent with such hyperventilation act to inhibit a further increase in ventilation. Gray[22] has calculated that an oxygen tension of 30 mm. Hg, allowed to act without opposition from a decrease in both carbon dioxide tension and hydrogen ion concentration, would evoke a 7-fold increased in alveolar ventilation.

The importance of hypoxemia in stimulating ventilation in patients with diseases of the lungs or heart is demonstrated by the decrease that occurs with administration of oxygen. This effect may be observed even though the hypoxemia is very slight.

Mechanical and Physical Factors. One of the most fascinating *regulatory mechanisms* of respiration relates to the *work of breathing*. For any given level of alveolar ventilation there is an optimum respiratory rate at which the muscular work of breathing is minimum. Change of breathing frequency in either direction results in the expenditure of larger amounts of work. Such an optimum frequency of breathing was originally predicted by Otis, Fenn and Rahn[9] from calculations based on the work involved in overcoming the elastic and the airflow resistances of the lungs. Christie and co-workers[32] have measured the work of breathing in normal subjects, have confirmed this optimum frequency (usually 15 per minute, as predicted by Otis, et al.) and have demonstrated that it was the frequency naturally chosen by their subjects. Moreover, when the elastic and the airway properties of the lung are modified by disease, as in mitral stenosis or pneumonia, the respiratory frequency at which minimum work is performed in sustaining a particular level of alveolar ventilation is different from normal. It is almost precisely this respiratory rate that the patient selects naturally.[11,33] This remarkable adjustment of respiratory frequency in the interests of body economy in both health and disease apparently is delicately controlled. The mechanisms involved have yet to be elucidated. Recently Meade has presented evidence that respiratory frequency is somewhat more closely adjusted to levels requiring minimum development of transpulmonary pressures and force by the respiratory muscles than it is to levels associated with minimum expenditure of work.[34] He has suggested that vagal afferent impulses arising from stretch receptors in the lungs, and of the type known since the work of Hering and Breuer in 1868, provide the signal for this control of respiratory rhythm.

Stimulation of any afferent nerve may bring about reflex changes. Pain fibers seem to be especially potent, and painful sensations from any source may cause hyperpnea. Occasionally this may be sufficiently prolonged and of sufficient intensity to produce severe hypocapnia and even tetany. Similar although less dramatic effects may be produced through cutaneous nerve fibers by exposure to heat and cold. Stimulation of abdominal viscera at the time of operation may cause moderate hyperpnea. There are numerous examples of the use of reflex stimulation of respiration for the accomplishment of practical clinical results. Mention may be made of spanking the newborn baby to initiate breathing, throwing on cold water or using aromatic spirits of ammonia to arouse a patient from syncope. There is evidence that reflexes originating in the muscle, the tendons or the joints of moving limbs increase ventilation and may play an important role in the ventilatory adjustments of exercise.[35]

Cerebral Cortical Factors. To a limited extent, normal breathing is under the control of cerebral centers. Gray[22] reminds us ". . . that innumerable daily acts require unconscious interference with the respiratory pattern. Eating, drinking, talking, singing, defecating and threading a needle all involve transitory interference with breathing."

By volition the alveolar ventilation can be increased to such an extent as to cause a profound fall in alveolar and arterial carbon dioxide tension with consequent fall in pH and tetany. Such voluntary hyperventilation may be continued by determined individuals to the point of unconsciousness. The unconsciousness is due to cerebral ischemia secondary to the decrease in peripheral vascular resistance, the consequent fall in blood pressure, and the constriction of the cerebral vascular bed that result from large, acute decreases in the carbon dioxide tension of arterial blood.[36]

The effect of emotion and of ideational stimuli upon respiration has long been known. Everyone is acquainted with the gasp of horror, the sobbing of grief, the hyperpnea of sexual excitement. On the other hand, the existence of pleasant, peaceful thoughts and of contentment may bring about in excitable, unstable individuals a slight diminution in pulmonary ventilation. Experiments of Finesinger have indicated some of the range of respiratory response to emotion and pain.[37,38] He has shown that unpleasant thoughts tend to augment both the volume and the rate of respiration; the resulting increases in ventilation amounting in some individuals to more than double the preliminary value. Such responses may occur independently of or at least out of proportion to the rate of oxygen absorption. They tend to be maximal in hysteria and in anxiety states. Similarly, painful stimuli produced by the injection of hypertonic saline, repeated pricking or electrical shock give similar results with maximal effects in hysterical and anxious subjects. Even recollection of painful stimuli in some individuals is sufficient to cause considerable increase in respiration.

Psychogenic dyspnea occurs as a manifestation of various types of psychoneuroses. The complaint is often of "smothering" and or being "unable to get a deep breath." Meanwhile, the patient is apt to exhibit periodic overbreathing, sometimes punctuated by deep sighing respirations. After the overbreathing there is of course a compensatory normal diminution in rate and depth of respiration. At such times the patient may become panicky because he "can't get his breath." In its extreme form these manifestations comprise *the hyperventilation syndrome.* The patient hyperventilates chronically. At irregular intervals ventilation is increased even further and the patient experiences sensations of "lightheadedness," dizziness, and numbness or cramping in the hands and feet (tetany). The blood carbon dioxide content, combining power and tension are low and the pH is alkaline.

It is wise to keep in mind two facts regarding this syndrome: (1) Once initiated and maintained for a period of time, hyperventilation tends to persist because of sensitization of the respiratory center (see above); (2) occasional patients, on recovery from encephalitis, may manifest involuntary hyperventilation over long periods of time.

Metabolic Factors. Increase in the *metabolic rate* requires an increase in the rate of exchange of oxygen and carbon dioxide by the lungs. In general, alveolar ventilation keeps pace with increased metabolic demands and the tensions of oxygen and carbon dioxide in the alveolar air and arterial blood are maintained within the normal range.

A considerable number of pathologic states and diseases may cause elevation of the metabolic rate. The presence of fever implies an increased demand for oxygen in accordance with van't Hoff's law which states that the velocity of chemical reactions is doubled or trebled with each temperature rise of 10° C. Measurements in the presence of fever have indicated an increase in oxygen requirement of approximately 13 per cent for each degree Centigrade rise in body temperature or 7 per cent for each degree Fahrenheit.[39] The increased ventilation that occurs on exposure to a hot environment has been shown to be proportional to an increase in oxygen consumption.

However, in the unsteady state that prevails immediately after the onset of thermal stress, the ventilatory response precedes the metabolic alterations and causes a fall in alveolar and blood carbon dioxide tensions. Immersion in a hot bath for 18 minutes has been shown to result in reduction of alveolar carbon dioxide tension to 25 mm. Hg.[40] In hyperthyroidism the basal metabolic rate may be increased by 10 to 100 per cent. Furthermore, all movements of the thyrotoxic patient are performed clumsily and inefficiently so that even at bed rest, the daily oxygen requirement of a moderately thyrotoxic patient may be more than twice normal. Among other diseases that are characterized by an increased oxygen utilization are leukemia (plus 20 to plus 80%), pernicious anemia (plus 7 to plus 33%), polycythemia (plus 10 to plus 40%). In each of these states, the increased ventilatory demand that accompanies the metabolic alterations may cause distress in otherwise ill or debilitated individuals.

The increase in ventilation in moderate exercise is directly proportional to the oxygen consumption. In severe grades of exercise, when the oxygen consumption increases beyond 2.0 to 2.5 L. per minute, ventilation rises out of proportion to the oxygen consumption. This has been attributed to the formation of lactic acid and consequent acidosis in severe exercise.[22] Arterial blood gas tensions are maintained at normal levels in moderate exercise but in severe exercise pH and carbon dioxide tension fall. Except in the most violent exertion, the arterial blood oxygen is not decreased.[41,42] In moderate exercise the total ventilation may reach 50 L. per minute; in the severest exercise, 120 L. per minute.

Despite many investigations and numerous reviews of the subject, agreement has not been reached concerning the factors responsible for the control of ventilation during exercise.[35,42,43] Recently interest has focused on the possible roles of the central blood volume, and of chemoreceptors located in the right heart or pulmonary arterial tree that are sensitive to the carbon dioxide tension of mixed venous blood.[42,44] It is of considerable clinical importance that the hyperventilation of exercise is greater in untrained individuals (such as patients whose activity has been restricted) than in individuals who are at the peak of athletic training.

DYSPNEA IN PULMONARY DISEASE

Acute and chronic diseases of the lungs are perhaps the most frequent clinical causes of dyspnea. Only 3 of the most common diseases are considered here in detail.

PULMONARY EMPHYSEMA

There is a growing accord among pulmonary physiologists that the fundamental defect in this disease is *chronic obstruction* of the small intrapulmonary airways.[45] Initially, obstruction may be due to congestion, edema and hypersecretion of the bronchial mucosa and spasm of the bronchial muscles. Later, as destruction of alveolar tissue occurs, the important dilating effect that the alveolar septae exert on the bronchioles is lost, thus adding another obstructive factor. When alveolar destruction is extensive the unsupported bronchioles may collapse completely during expiration.[45] The diminution in caliber of the airways during expiration increases the intrapleural and the alveolar pressures to high levels which in turn tends to collapse more bronchioles. Thus the rate of airflow, instead of increasing as it does normally with increase of intrapleural pressure, may actually decrease with increasing pressure.[45] The changes in pulmonary function that are characteristic of emphysema are readily understood if this fundamental obstructive defect is appreciated.

The disturbances in the ventilatory apparatus that result from such obstruction to airflow are frequently severe. The maximum breathing capacity is consistently impaired, and the severity of the dyspnea correlates very well with the reduction in this function. With advancing disease progressive impairment accompanied by increasing disability due to dyspnea is the rule. The maximum breathing capacity may reach such low levels (20 L. per minute) that the ventilatory requirements of even mild exercise cannot be met, and consequently the alveolar gas tensions deviate markedly from normal.

Improvement of the maximum breathing capacity after the administration of a nebulized bronchodilator is usual. The degree of improvement averages about 25 per cent of the prebronchodilator value, but is quite variable.[46]

A sudden increase in the severity of the dyspnea or progressive disability developing over a week or two is usually due to a superimposed bronchial or pulmonary infection with aggravation of airway obstruction. In view of the frequently precarious state of pulmonary function in these patients, such changes in symptoms deserve the utmost attention of the physician.

The work of breathing also is increased. At rest it may be only slightly greater than normal, but on exercise it is greatly increased. An emphysematous patient breathing 15 L. per minute may be doing as much work in effecting this ventilation as a normal individual breathing 30 to 40 L. per minute.[12] The greatest part of this work is spent on overcoming resistance to airflow in the airways, an act requiring active participation of the expiratory muscles.[12,45] Cournand and co-workers[15] recently have presented some data on the metabolic costs of such disordered breathing. A patient with emphysema and considerable bronchial obstruction manifested an increment in his oxygen consumption of 25 ml. for each liter increase in ventilation above the resting level (normal increase: 1 ml. of oxygen per L. of ventilation per minute). With relief of the reversible component of his bronchial obstruction the oxygen consumption required to support a liter per minute increase in ventilation fell to 6 ml.

Although in emphysema total ventilation at rest usually is increased slightly, it is only an occasional patient with early emphysema whose ventilation is greater than normal during exercise. Indeed, in those with severe hypoxemia and chronic respiratory acidosis, ventilation during exercise is usually less than normal, due perhaps to diminished sensitivity of the respiratory center. Therefore, the demands for ventilation made upon the crippled ventilatory apparatus in emphysema usually are not increased. But they require the use of a larger than normal fraction of the breathing capacity, and can be met only at the expense of large swings in intrapleural pressure and considerable muscular effort.

Clinically significant disturbances in gas exchange are common in emphysema and are related to obstruction in the intrapulmonary airways and consequent uneven distribution of air among the alveoli.[19,47] With progression of the disease an increasing number of alveoli are underventilated, which gives rise to progressive lowering of oxyhemoglobin saturation and eventually elevation of the carbon dioxide tension of the arterial blood. The physiologic dead space usually is expanded greatly by parenchymal areas in which the blood supply has been reduced or destroyed. Ventilation to these areas is wasted from the standpoint of gas exchange and may cause effectively functioning alveoli to be deprived of their share of ventilation. As a consequence of alveolar destruction, the area of alveolar capillary membrane available for gas exchange diminishes. The consequent decrease in diffusion capacity is partly responsible for the fall in arterial oxyhemoglobin saturation with exercise.[19,47]

The severe hypoxemia and perhaps the respiratory acidosis are responsible for the muscular fatigue which is a prominent symptom in such patients and may contribute to fatigue of the respiratory muscles. The intense, oppressive and alarming sensation of suffocation that they experience during and immediately after exertion is undoubtedly related to these alterations in the blood gases.

Cor Pulmonale. The development of cor pulmonale in emphysema is usually accompanied by intensification of dyspnea. The following factors contribute to this change: hypervolemia secondary to polycythemia with consequent alteration in pulmonary blood volume and increased elastic resistance of the lung; inability to increase cardiac output appropriately with exercise and therefore ischemia of the respiratory muscles; aggravation of pre-existing hypoxemia and respiratory acidosis; increase in the degree of pulmonary arterial hypertension with augmented respiratory reflexes arising from the pulmonary artery; and, perhaps most significantly, an underlying pulmonary infection, which is very frequently responsible for precipitating episodes of failure and which increases the disability of the ventilatory apparatus and elevates the rate of metabolic turnover of oxygen and carbon dioxide. The partial reversibility of these untoward developments is revealed by the striking improvement in dyspnea and over-all clinical and physiologic state that occurs with appropriate therapy.[48]

PULMONARY FIBROSIS

Because the nature and the extent of the fibrosis can vary widely, even if produced by the same etiologic agent, the type and the severity of disturbances in pulmonary function are variable.[49] In contrast to the *obstructive* defect present in emphysema, fibrosis produces a *restrictive* defect that is secondary to the marked decrease in pulmonary compliance. However, bronchial obstruction may complicate the basic disease process.

If fibrosis is extensive, it causes shrinkage of the total lung capacity, particularly of the vital capacity. The maximum breathing capacity, if at all disturbed, is decreased in proportion to, or less than, vital capacity. Hyperventilation is the rule and is particularly in evidence during exercise.

The increased muscular effort and the quite high intrapleural pressures required to hyperventilate the rigid lungs,[19] together with the hyperventilation, are probably the chief abnormalities responsible for the dyspnea.

Tachypnea and hyperventilation are often extreme in the *alveolar capillary block syndrome*.[50] Diseases such as Boeck's sarcoid, beryllium granulomatosis, scleroderma, lymphangitic carcinomatosis, and Rich-Hamman's pneumonitis, that produce a diffuse interstitial inflammatory and fibrotic reaction in the alveolar walls are common causes of this syndrome. The essential physiologic defect is a decrease in diffusion capacity that is due both to increased thickness of the alveolar-capillary membrane and to restriction of its total area. Characteristically, unsaturation of the arterial blood with oxygen is mild or absent at rest but becomes severe during exercise, since diffusion of oxygen at increased rates across the diseased membrane cannot occur without the development of a large oxygen pressure gradient between alveolar air and the blood leaving the alveoli. Because of the hyperventilation and the 20-fold greater diffusibility of carbon dioxide as compared to oxygen, the pressure of carbon dioxide in the arterial blood and, secondarily, the plasma carbon dioxide content and combining power, may be low (compensated respiratory alkalosis). Respiratory acidosis may appear in very advanced stages of the syndrome when alveolar ventilation becomes inadequate because of disturbances in the distribution of air among the alveoli.

The maximum breathing capacity is remarkably well preserved and may be greater than normal despite a reduction in vital capacity that is usually very severe. Disability is often out of proportion to the amount of pulmonary involvement visible in roentgenograms of the chest. Therefore, occasional patients with this syndrome have been suspected of being neurotic until studies of function have revealed the severity of the pulmonary insufficiency.

BRONCHIAL ASTHMA

Typical asthma results from contact of antibodies in the sensitized bronchial mucosa with antigens, either inhaled or carried in the blood. As the result of this immunologic reaction, cholinergic (vagus) fibers in the bronchi are stimulated. In response to this stimulus there occurs (1) *swelling* of the mucosa and the submucosa, (2) *contraction* of bronchial musculature and (3) *excessive secretion* of thick, tenacious mucus. All three of these functional derangements result in narrowing of the total bronchial lumen and even complete occlusion of the smaller bronchioles. The acute asthmatic paroxysm is characterized by obstruction to both inspiratory and expiratory phases of pulmonary ventilation. There is increased respiratory effort with use of the accessory muscles of respiration, which tend to aid inspiration more than

expiration. Wheezing and musical rales are heard over the lungs. Breathing is accomplished with the chest in a hyperinflated state in an attempt to overcome the obstruction to the airways. Expiration is prolonged, there is progressive distension of the lungs and residual volume increases acutely.

An attack terminates when the constricted bronchi widen, and the expectoration of mucus plugs is accomplished.

Repeated paroxysms may eventually produce two important changes: (1) hypertrophy of bronchiolar musculature, with increased tonus and permanent narrowing of bronchioles; (2) hypertrophy of bronchial mucous glands. These abnormal glands, instead of secreting small amounts of thin mucus, secrete large amounts of thick, tenacious mucus, which may plug so many bronchioles as to cause death.

Thus both structure and function may be altered in persistent asthma, with, at first, bronchiolar changes and later widespread pulmonary changes and chronic emphysema.

The actions of certain drugs gives insight into the mechanisms of asthma. *Iodides* thin mucous secretions, making cough more effective in clearing the airways. *Epinephrine* and ephedrine relieve bronchospasm and reduce bronchial edema. *Atropine* may reduce cholinergic effects. *Aminophylline* acts directly to relieve spasm of the bronchial musculature.

Since the essential disturbance in this condition is bronchiolar obstruction secondary to spasm of the muscle and edema of the mucosa of the bronchioles, many of the defects of pulmonary function characteristic of pulmonary emphysema occur with varying severity during the acute attack. With subsidence of the acute paroxysm, function improves greatly, although some depression of the maximum breathing capacity, increase in residual volume, hyperventilation and mild hypoxemia usually persist.[51,52] These residual defects, which are partially or completely reversed by administration of a bronchodilator,[51,52] are probably responsible for the decreased tolerance for exercise manifested between attacks by most asthmatics.

With repeated attacks of bronchiolar obstruction there is a general tendency over the years for all components of pulmonary function to decline and in many instances the physiologic pattern becomes indistinguishable from emphysema. However, this course is not invariable, particularly with effective therapy.

DYSPNEA IN CARDIAC DISEASE

Although dyspnea may occur in any of the various diseases of the heart, it is most prominent and most disabling in those associated with pulmonary congestion. Left ventricular failure from any cause and mitral stenosis are excellent examples. Hemodynamic studies in these conditions have revealed elevation of pressures in all segments of the pulmonary vascular bed consequent to increase in left atrial pressure.[53,54] The high pressures in the pulmonary veins and the capillaries are particularly noteworthy since they are responsible for the increased rate of transudation of fluid into the interstitial tissues and the alveoli of the lungs. In tight mitral stenosis the pressure at rest in the pulmonary capillaries is usually in the range of the plasma protein osmotic pressure.[55] This indicates that such patients live under the constant threat of pulmonary edema.

When such modifications of pulmonary circulation are longstanding, anatomic alterations characterized by fibrosis of the alveolar walls and pulmonary arteriolarsclerosis develop.[53,55] To these may be added the changes secondary to pulmonary infarction, a common complication of mitral stenosis.

These alterations in pulmonary hemodynamics and their secondary effects on the pulmonary parenchyma increase the resistance of the lungs to stretch up to three times normal.[11,56] This alteration in the viscoelastic properties of the lungs is mainly responsible for large swings in intrapleural pressure, increase in the work of breathing and the large oxygen requirement for each liter of ventilation.[11,15,56]

In a number of patients the resistance to airflow in the intrapulmonary airways is also greater than normal[56] and is responsible for a further increment in breathing work.

During exercise the pulmonary vascular pressures of patients with left ventricular disease, and particularly of those with mitral stenosis, rise considerably above the resting level.[53,54] Consequently, compliance of the lungs is less than in the resting state. This change in the elastic properties of the lungs is distinctly abnormal since normally pulmonary vascular pressures do not rise, and the compliance of the lungs increases with exercise.[32]

Hyperventilation of variable degree during both rest and exercise is usually present in patients with pulmonary congestion and serves to increase the burden imposed on the ventilatory apparatus. The degree of hyperventilation is not great and is therefore of itself not responsible for the dyspnea. The hyperpnea is out of proportion to metabolic demands since the arterial carbon dioxide tension is usually low or normal.[5] It is most likely caused by augmented stretch reflexes from the lungs. Hypoxemia may also contribute to the hyperventilation although it is usually mild in the absence of significant pulmonary edema.

Reduction of cardiac output and inability to increase output appropriately with exercise bear only a general relationship to the severity of dyspnea in patients with pulmonary congestion. In mitral stenosis the symptom may be quite disabling even though the cardiac output is normal. Early fatigue of exercising muscles is perhaps the most common symptom of an inadequate cardiac output. Since the respiratory muscles are performing two to three times as much as normal in achieving a particular level of ventilation, their early fatigue when blood flow is deficient may be an important contributing factor in the respiratory distress.

Orthopnea is a common symptom of pulmonary congestion. It is the term applied to the phenomenon of dyspnea which occurs at rest in the recumbent but not the upright or semivertical position. It is usually relieved by two or three pillows under the head and the back. Marshall and coworkers[11] have observed, in patients with mitral stenosis, considerable decrease in pulmonary compliance in the flat as compared to the upright position. The swings in intrapleural pressure during the respiratory cycle were consequently greater (over 40 cm. of water) and the work of breathing was two to three times greater in recumbency than in the upright position. The respiratory rate also increased to a frequency that corresponded strikingly to the frequency at which the work of ventilating the more rigid lungs was at a minimum.

The decrease in compliance on lying flat probably is related to the fact that more of the lung lies at or below the level of the heart. Thus the increased vascular pressures are distributed throughout a greater portion of the lungs and are augmented in the most dependent regions by the overlying column of blood. In the upright position a greater portion of the lungs lies above the heart. In these regions pulmonary venous and capillary pressures are lowered by hydrostatic effects.

Vigorous movements of the chest bellows are effected more readily in the upright position. This probably explains why some patients with chronic lung disease or bronchial asthma are intolerant of the recumbent position.

Paroxysmal nocturnal dyspnea may occur in mitral stenosis or in any condition that taxes the left ventricle sufficiently to cause it to fail (such as hypertension or aortic insufficiency). The attack may be severe, dramatic and terrifying.

The patient is aroused from his sleep gasping for air, and must sit up or stand to catch his breath. He may sweat profusely. Sometimes he throws open a window widely in an attempt to relieve the oppressive sensation of suffocation. The chest tends to become fixed in the position of forced inspiration. Both inspiratory and expiratory wheezes, often simulating typical asthma, are heard. In some cases overt *pulmonary edema* occurs, with many moist rales. The acute pulmonary edema rarely terminates fatally. Occasionally the attacks may recur several times a night, necessitating sleeping upright in a chair.

The mechanism of these attacks includes those factors which produce orthopnea as well as the hypervolemia that occurs during the redistribution of peripheral edema fluid when body position is changed from vertical to horizontal upon retiring[57] The hypervolemia constitutes an additional burden to the heart and of itself increases pulmonary venous and capillary pressures.[58] The actual attack may be "triggered" by coughing, abdominal distention, the hyperpneic phase of Cheyne-Stokes respiration, a startling noise or anything causing a sudden increase in heart rate and further acute elevation of pulmonary venous and capillary pressures. Usually the attack is terminated by assumption of the erect position and a few deep breaths of air. Cough, an important manifestation of pulmonary congestion, frequently occurs during the attack.

Cardiac Asthma. The asthmatic wheezes often heard in patients with pulmonary congestion have given rise to this term. The wheezes are a manifestation of pulmonary edema, and often are accompanied by other signs of this condition. Reduction in lumen of the small intrapulmonary airways by edema fluid and thickening of bronchiolar walls by edema is responsible for the wheezes. In addition, the high intrathoracic pressure required to overcome the obstruction during expiration tends to narrow the small bronchioles further and even collapse them.[56] Increased resistance to airflow during both inspiration and expiration has been measured in pulmonary congestion,[56] and found to be especially marked (4 times normal) in frank pulmonary edema.[59,60] The compliance of the lungs is reduced greatly in pulmonary edema with values as low as one tenth normal having been recorded. With recovery from edema, very significant reductions in airway resistance and increases in pulmonary compliance occur.[59,60]

Dyspnea Without Pulmonary Congestion. Dyspnea occurs in many forms of heart disease that are not associated with congestion of the lungs. Uncomplicated *pulmonic stenosis* is an excellent example. Probably the symptom is related to an inadequate cardiac output during exercise. In *tetralogy of Fallot* dyspnea may be severe and often is relieved by assuming a squatting position. In this and other forms of cyanotic heart disease, pre-existing hypoxemia is aggravated by exercise. It is of note that both dyspnea and fatigue appear during exertion when the arterial oxyhemoglobin saturation has fallen significantly below the resting level.

Cheyne-Stokes respiration, or periodic breathing, is a phenomenon that may occur in cardiac failure. It is characterized by alternating periods of hypoventilation and hyperventilation. In its typical form, there is an apneic phase lasting 15 to 60 seconds followed by a phase during which tidal volume increases with each breath to a peak level, and then decreases in decrescendo fashion to the apneic phase. At the onset of apnea, carbon dioxide tension in brachial or femoral arterial blood is at its lowest. As apnea persists, carbon dioxide tension gradually increases, and respiration is stimulated. Carbon dioxide tension continues to increase until maximum hyperventilation is attained, after which it and ventilation decrease until apnea again occurs.[61,62] The arterial oxyhemoglobin saturation varies in an inverse manner, being highest at onset of apnea and lowest during midhyperpnea. During the cycle, carbon dioxide tension may vary as much as 14 mm. Hg, and oxyhemoglobin saturation as much as 18 per cent.[61]

One of the factors fundamental to the production of such respiratory oscillations is the circulatory-induced delay in the feedback of information to the brain regarding the effects of ventilation on the pulmonary capillary blood. The circulation time from lung to peripheral artery has been shown to be one half the length of the Cheyne-Stokes cycle.[62] Thus the oscillating ventilatory pattern produces cyclic variations in the concentrations of respiratory gases in blood passing through the lungs; these cyclic variations eventually reach the respiratory control system but with a temporal phase shift of 180°.

Formerly it was believed that the respiratory center is depressed in Cheyne-Stokes respiration, but more recently it has been shown that respiratory alkalosis is frequently present, that the arterial carbon dioxide tension is lower than normal in both apneic and hyperpneic phases,[61,62] and that the respiratory response to inhalation of carbon dioxide is greater than normal.[61]

However, Plum and his associates[61,63] have called attention to supramedullary dysfunction of the brain in the pathogenesis of Cheyne-Stokes respiration. All patients they examined had signs of bilateral impairment of the descending motor pathways. The importance of supramedullary neuronal structures in controlling respiration was exemplified by the intense, metronomically regular hyperpnea (central neurogenic hyperventilation) they have observed in patients with destructive lesions of the central portion of the tegmentum of the pons.[63] In most of these patients, typical Cheyne-Stokes respirations preceded the development of continuous hyperventilation. Cyclic changes in cerebral blood flow also occur during Cheyne-Stokes respiration (flow being greater during hyperpnea), and may account for the fluctuations of mental state, electroencephalographic pattern, and signs of nervous system dysfunction during the cycle.[64]

Cheyne-Stokes respiration is sometimes seen in normal infants, in healthy elderly persons, and in normal individuals at high altitude. It also occurs when certain drugs (such as morphine) are administered; with increased intracranial pressure, in uremia, and in some forms of coma. It has been produced in dogs by prolonging circulation time from the heart to the brain.[65]

DYSPNEA IN ANEMIA

Exertional dyspnea is a common symptom of anemia, and is particularly marked in the more acute and the severe forms. Its pathogenesis is not completely understood.

The supply of oxygen to the tissues is dependent upon transport by hemoglobin. If the hemoglobin concentration and arterial oxyhemoglobin saturation are normal, the mixed venous blood in the resting state is about 75 per cent saturated with oxygen, since the mean extraction of oxygen by the tissues from each 100 ml. of blood is 4 ml. With reduction in hemoglobin concentration, and hence in the amount of oxygen in the arterial blood (normally 19.4 ml. per 100 ml.), the mixed venous blood saturation will decrease if extraction of oxygen from each 100 ml. of blood continues as usual. Tissue oxygen tension, which lies between the tension of the arterial and that of the venous blood, will therefore fall. This hypoxic effect is greatest in those tissues, such as contracting muscle, in which the extraction rate of oxygen is high.

The hypoxia is partially prevented by an increase in the cardiac output which permits tissue oxygen needs to be met at a lower extraction rate of oxygen from the blood.[66] In severe anemia the adjustment in output may fall short of the mark. If the hemoglobin concentration is 4 Gm. per 100 ml. of blood the cardiac output would have to be tripled to maintain tissue oxygen exchange at a normal level merely in the basal state.

The heart under these circumstances does not respond normally to stress[67] and may fail. In the production of dyspnea the roles played by the augmented blood flow through the lungs, and pulmonary congestion resulting from left ventricular failure or strain during exercise,[68] can only be speculated upon.

Although the arterial oxyhemoglobin saturation is within normal limits, the oxygen tension has been demonstrated to be decreased.[69] This may in part be responsible for the hyperventilation that is characteristic of anemia.

SUMMARY

Dyspnea is a subjective symptom related to the effort of breathing and as such must be regarded as originating in the ventilatory apparatus although the stimuli, the sensory receptors and the nerve pathways that participate in its appreciation are unknown.

Numerous acute and chronic diseases may affect the various components of the ventilatory apparatus—ribs, spine, respiratory muscles, their peripheral and central nervous control, the extrapulmonary and the intrapulmonary airways, alveolar tissue, pleura, and pulmonary vessels. Such disturbances, if sufficiently severe, decrease the capacity of the apparatus to ventilate and exaggerate the effort necessarily expended to make it function. Alterations in the parenchyma and the airways of the lung produced either by primary lung disease, or secondarily by heart disease, are the most common clinical causes of ventilatory dysfunction and dyspnea.

In many conditions the levels of ventilation required at rest and especially during exercise are greater than normal and serve to overtax a disabled ventilatory apparatus. Severe grades of hyperventilation, such as may occur during vigorous exertion, can provoke dyspnea even in a normal individual.

The rate of alveolar ventilation is adjusted to meet the wide fluctuations in metabolic needs for exchange of oxygen and carbon dioxide that occur in the course of human activity. These adjustments are initiated primarily by alterations in the gas composition and pH of the arterial blood and are designed to minimize such changes. Many additional reflex and emotional factors, which may assume importance in disease, are capable of modifying ventilation.

To appraise dyspnea adequately it is necessary to establish the severity of the symptom and the conditions under which it occurs. By the history and the physical examination all evidences of disability of the ventilatory apparatus and factors that increase the demands for ventilation must be sought. Detailed studies of pulmonary and cardiac function may be necessary, particularly in those individuals in whom adequate cause for the dyspnea cannot be found or in whom the symptom appears out of proportion to evidences of disease. In many instances simple studies such as observation of the patient during a simple exercise, fluoroscopy of the heart and the chest (with attention focused on the dynamics of the chest bellows), determination of blood carbon dioxide content and hematrocrit, a complete electrocardiogram, and measurement of vital capacity will suffice. However, the limitations of the last procedure as a measure of ventilatory capacity and index of dyspnea are considerable.

REFERENCES

1. Baldwin, E. de F., Cournand, A., and Richards, D. W., Jr.: Pulmonary insufficiency. I. Physiological classification, clinical methods

of analysis, standard values in normal subjects, Medicine 27:243, 1948.

2. Dripps, R. D., and Comroe, J. H., Jr.: The respiratory and circulatory response of normal man to inhalation of 7.6 and 10.4 per cent O_2 with a comparison of the maximal ventilation produced by severe muscular exercise, inhalation of CO_2 and maximal voluntary hyperventilation, Am. J. Physiol. 149:43, 1947.

3. Lukas, D. S., and Plum, F.: Pulmonary function in patients convalescing from acute poliomyelitis with respiratory paralysis, Am. J. Med. 12:388, 1952.

4. Cournand, A., and Richards, D. W., Jr.: Pulmonary insufficiency. I. Discussion of a physiological classification and presentation of clinical tests, Am. Rev. Tuberc. 44:26, 1941.

5. West, J. R., Bliss, H. A., Wood, J. A., and Richards, D. W., Jr.: Pulmonary function in rheumatic heart disease and its relation to exertional dyspnea in ambulatory patients, Circulation 8:178, 1953.

6. Mead, J.: Mechanical properties of lungs, Physiol. Rev. 41:281, 1961.

7. Pierce, J. A., Hocott, J. B., and Hefley, B. F.: Elastic properties and the geometry of the lungs, J. Clin. Invest. 40:1515, 1961.

8. Fry, D. L., and Hyatt, R. E.: Pulmonary mechanics: a unified analysis of the relationship between pressure, volume and gasflow in the lungs of normal and diseased human subjects, Am. J. Med. 29:672, 1960.

9. Otis, A. B., Fenn, W. O., and Rahn, H.: Mechanics of breathing in man, J. Appl. Physiol. 2:592, 1950.

10. Otis, A. B.: The work of breathing, Physiol. Rev. 34:449, 1954.

11. Marshall, R., McIlroy, M. B., and Christie, R. V.: The work of breathing in mitral stenosis, Clin. Sc. 13:137, 1954.

12. McIlroy, M. B., and Christie, R. V.: The work of breathing in emphysema, Clin. Sc. 13:147, 1954.

13. Bergofsky, E. H., Turino, G. M., and Fishman, A. P.: Cardiorespiratory failure in kyphoscoliosis, Medicine 38:263, 1959.

14. Naimark, A., and Cherniack, R. M.: Compliance of the respiratory system and its components in health and obesity, J. Appl. Physiol. 15:377, 1960.

15. Cournand, A., Richards, D. W., Jr., Bader, R. A., Bader, M. E., and Fishman, A. P.: The oxygen cost of breathing, Tr. A. Am. Physicians 67:162, 1954.

16. Kaufman, B. J., Ferguson, M. H., and Cher-

niack, R. M.: Hypoventilation in obesity, J. Clin. Invest. 38:500, 1959.

17. Marshall, R., Stone, R. W., and Christie, R. V.: The relationship of dyspnoea to respiratory effort in normal subjects, mitral stenosis and emphysema, Clin. Sc. 13:625, 1954.

18. McGregor, M., and Becklake, M. R.: The relationship of oxygen cost of breathing to respiratory mechanical work and respiratory force, J. Clin. Invest. 40:971, 1961.

19. Comroe, J. H., Jr., Forster, R. E., II, Du Bois, A. B., Briscoe, W. A.: The lung. Clinical Physiology and Pulmonary Function Tests, Chicago, Yr. Bk. Pub., 1955.

20. Pappenheimer, J. R., and others: Standardization of definitions and symbols in respiratory physiology, Fed. Proc. 9:602, 1950.

21. Pitts, R. F.: Regulation of respiration, in Fulton, J. F.: Textbook of Physiology, ed. 16, Philadelphia, Saunders, 1949.

22. Gray, J. S.: Pulmonary Ventilation and its Physiologic Regulation, Springfield, Ill., Thomas, 1950.

23. Haldane, J. S., and Priestley, J. G.: The regulation of the lung-ventilation, J. Physiol. 32:225, 1905.

24. Alexander, J. K., West, J. R., Wood, J. A., and Richards, D. W.: Analysis of the respiratory response to carbon dioxide inhalation in varying clinical states of hypercapnia, anoxia and acid-base derangement, J. Clin. Invest. 34:511, 1955.

25. Houston, C. S., and Riley, R. L.: Respiratory and circulatory changes during acclimatization to high altitude, Am. J. Physiol. 149:565, 1947.

26. Brown, E. B., Jr., Campbell, G. S., Johnson, M. N., Hemingway, A., and Visscher, M. B.: Changes in response to inhalation of CO_2 before and after 24 hours of hyperventilation in man, J. Appl. Physiol. 1:333, 1948.

27. Brown, E. B., Jr., Hemingway, A., and Visscher, M. B.: Arterial blood pH and pCO_2 changes in response to CO_2 inhalation after 24 hours of passive hyperventilation, J. Appl. Physiol. 2:544, 1950.

28. Schäfer, K.-E.: Atmung und Säure-Basengleichgewicht bei langdauerdem Aufenthalt in 3% CO_2, Pflüger's Arch. Ges. Physiol. 251:689, 1949.

29. Brown, E. B., Jr.: Changes in brain pH response to CO_2 after prolonged hypoxic hyperventilation, J. Appl. Physiol. 2:549, 1950.

30. Leusen, I. R.: Chemosensitivity of the respiratory center. Influence of changes in the H^+ and total buffer concentrations in the

cerebral ventricles on respiration, Am. J. Physiol. 176:45, 1954.

31. ———: Acid-base equilibrium between blood and cerebralspinal fluid, Am. J. Physiol. 176:513, 1954.

32. McIlroy, M. B., Marshall, R., and Christie, R. V.: The work of breathing in normal subjects, Clin. Sci. 13:127, 1954.

33. Marshall, R., and Christie, R. V.: The visco-elastic properties of the lungs in acute pneumonia, Clin. Sci. 13:403, 1954.

34. Mead, J.: Control of respiratory frequency, J. Appl. Physiol. 15:325, 1960.

35. Comroe, J. H.: The hyperpnea of muscular exercise, Physiol. Rev. 24:31, 1944.

36. Burnam, J. F., Hickam, J. B., and McIntosh, H. D.: The effect of hypocapnia on arterial blood pressure, Circulation 9:89, 1954.

37. Finesinger, J. E.: Effect of pleasant and unpleasant ideas on respiration in psychoneurotic patients, Arch. Neurol. & Psychiat. 42:425, 1939.

38. Finesinger, J. E., and Mazick, S. G.: Respiratory responses of psychoneurotic patients to ideational and sensory stimuli, Am. J. Psychiat. 97:27, 1940.

39. Du Bois, E. F.: Basal Metabolism in Health and Disease, Philadelphia, Lea & Febiger, 1936.

40. Bazett, H.: Physiological responses to heat, Physiol. Rev. 7:531, 1927.

41. Himwich, H. E., and Barr, D. P.: Studies in the physiology of muscular exercise and oxygen relationships in the arterial blood, J. Biol. Chem. 57:363, 1923.

42. Mitchell, J. H., Sproule, B. J., and Chapman, C. B.: Factors influencing respiration during heavy exercise, J. Clin. Invest. 37:1693, 1958.

43. Yamamoto, W. S., and Edwards, M. W., Jr.: Homeostasis of carbon dioxide during intravenous infusion of carbon dioxide, J. Appl. Physiol. 15:807, 1960.

44. Pi Suner, A.: The regulation of the respiratory movements by peripheral chemoreceptors, Physiol. Rev. 27:1, 1947.

45. Fry, D. L., Ebert, R. V., Stead, W. W., and Brown, C. C.: The mechanics of pulmonary ventilation in normal subjects and in patients with emphysema, Am. J. Med. 16:80, 1954.

46. Lukas, D. S.: Pulmonary function in health and disease, M. Clin. North America 39:661, 1955.

47. West, J. R., Baldwin, E. de F., Cournand, A., and Richards, D. W., Jr.: Physiopathologic aspects of chronic emphysema, Am. J. Med. 10:481, 1951.

48. Harvey, R. M., Ferrer, I., Richards, D. W., Jr., and Cournand, A.: Influence of chronic pulmonary disease on the heart and circulation, Am. J. Med. 10:719, 1951.

49. Baldwin, E. de F., Cournand, A., and Richards, D. W., Jr.: Pulmonary insufficiency. II. A study of thirty-nine cases of pulmonary fibrosis, Medicine 28:1, 1949.

50. Austrian, R., et al.: Clinical and physiologic features of some types of pulmonary disease with impairment of alveolar-capillary diffusion. The syndrome of "alveolar-capillary block," Am. J. Med. 11:667, 1951.

51. Lukas, D. S.: Pulmonary function in a group of young patients with bronchial asthma, J. Allergy 22:411, 1951.

52. Herchfus, J. A., Bresnick, E., and Segal, M. S.: Pulmonary function studies in bronchial asthma. I. In the control state, Am. J. Med. 14:23, 1953.

53. Lewis, B. M., Houssay, H. E., Haynes, F. W., and Dexter, L.: The dynamics of both right and left ventricles at rest and during exercise in patients with heart failure, Circulation Res. 1:312, 1953.

54. Lukas, D. S., and Dotter, C. T.: Modifications of the pulmonary circulation in mitral stenosis, Am. J. Med. 12:639, 1952.

55. Araujo, J., and Lukas, D. S.: Interrelationships among pulmonary "capillary" pressure, blood flow and valve size in mitral stenosis. The limited regulatory effects of the pulmonary vascular resistance, J. Clin. Invest. 31:1082, 1952.

56. Brown, C. C., Jr., Fry, D. L., and Ebert, R. V.: The mechanics of pulmonary ventilation in patients with heart disease, Am. J. Med. 17:438, 1954.

57. Perera, G. A., and Berliner, R. W.: The relation of postural hemodilution to paroxysmal dyspnea, J. Clin. Invest. 22:25, 1943.

58. Doyle, J. T., Wilson, J. S., Estes, E. H., and Warren, J. V.: The effect of intravenous infusions of physiologic saline solution on the pulmonary arterial and pulmonary capillary pressure in man, J. Clin. Invest. 30:345, 1951.

59. Sharp, J. T., Griffith, G. T., Bunnell, I. L., and Greene, D. G.: Ventilatory mechanics in pulmonary edema in man, J. Clin. Invest. 37:111, 1958.

60. Sharp, J. T., Bunnell, I. L., Griffith, G. T., and Greene, D. G.: The effects of therapy on pulmonary mechanics in human pulmonary edema, J. Clin. Invest. 40:665, 1961.

61. Brown, H. W., and Plum, F.: The neurologic basis of Cheyne-Stokes respiration, Am. J. Med. 30:849, 1961.

62. Lange, R. L., and Hecht, H. H.: The mechanism of Cheyne-Stokes respiration, J. Clin. Invest. 41:42, 1962.

63. Plum, F., and Swanson, A. G.: Central neurogenic hyperventilation in man, Arch, Neurol. & Psychiat. 81:535, 1959.

64. Karp, H. R., Sieker, H. O., and Heyman, A.: Cerebral circulation and function in Cheyne-Stokes respiration, Am. J. Med. 30:861, 1961.

65. Guyton, A. G., Crowell, J. W., and Moore, J. W.: Basic oscillating mechanism of Cheyne-Stokes breathing, Am. J. Physiol. 187:395, 1956.

66. Brannon, E. S., Merrill, A. J., Warren, J. V., and Stead, E. A.: The cardiac output in patients with chronic anemia as measured by the technique of right atrial catheterization, J. Clin. Invest. 24:332, 1945.

67. Sharpey-Shafer, E. P.: Transfusion and the anemic heart, Lancet 2:296, 1945.

68. Leight, L., Snider, T. H., Clifford, G. O., and Hellems, H. K.: Hemodynamic studies in sickle cell anemia, Circulation 10:653, 1954.

69. Ryan, J. M., and Hickam, J. B.: The alveolar-arterial oxygen pressure gradient in anemia, J. Clin. Invest. 31:188, 1952.

17

Cyanosis

Daniel S. Lukas and David P. Barr

Definition. Cyanosis is the diffuse bluish color that is due to the presence of reduced hemoglobin in increased amounts in the subpapillary venous plexus of the skin. It is not to be confused with the leaden color associated with the presence in the blood of methemoglobin or sulfhemoglobin or with argyria due to deposition of silver after prolonged use of medications containing this metal. Cyanosis is not synonymous with hypoxemia or hypoxia. It does not appear in carbon monoxide poisoning, in which hypoxemia is extreme, in severe anemia, which may be characterized both by hypoxemia and hypoxia, nor in cyanide poisoning, in which there is profound hypoxia without hypoxemia. Thus the presence of cyanosis implies hypoxemia, but the absence of cyanosis does not preclude severe hypoxia.

Pigmentation and thickness of the skin modify the appearance of cyanosis or may hide it completely. The presence in the blood of other pigments, such as methemoglobin or bilirubin, may add to the difficulty of recognition, while dilatation of surface vessels makes the color more obvious. Cyanosis can best be seen and recognized in places where the skin is thick, unpigmented and flushed, favorable sites being the lobes of the ears, the cutaneous surfaces of the lips and the fingernail beds. It is somewhat less apparent in the mucous membranes and in the retina, but these may be important sites for detection of cyanosis in patients with dark skin. The nature of the light under which the subject is examined is of considerable importance in identifying cyanosis. Bright daylight is best. Under certain types of fluorescent light, even normal individuals appear cyanotic.

NORMAL OXYGEN RELATIONSHIPS

The transport of oxygen is almost entirely dependent on the presence of hemoglobin, for the amount of oxygen which is carried in simple solution under normal conditions of breathing is only 0.3 volumes per cent, and is negligible from the standpoint of metabolic requirements. Normal blood contains approximately 15 Gm. of hemoglobin per 100 ml. Since each gram when fully saturated can carry 1.34 ml. of oxygen, this amount of hemoglobin is equivalent to an oxygen capacity of 20 volumes per cent.

The blood in passing through pulmonary capillaries under normal conditions is exposed to about 100 mm. Hg of oxygen tension, but is not more than 95 to 97 per cent saturated.[1] Therefore, arterial blood leaves the lungs with approximately 19 volumes per cent of oxygen. As the blood passes through the peripheral capillaries, oxygen is removed according to the needs of the tissues. By the technic of cardiac catheterization the arteriovenous oxygen difference for the whole body under resting conditions has been found to be 3.6 to 4.5 volumes per cent.[2] The mixed venous blood returning to the lungs still contains approximately 15 volumes per cent which represents an oxyhemoglobin saturation of 75 per cent and an oxygen tension of 40 mm. Hg. The amount of oxygen extracted from each 100 ml. of blood varies with each organ. In the skin this is probably not much more than 5 ml. Therefore its venous blood is 70 per cent saturated. Blood oxygen relationships for the skin may be represented as follows:

	Oxygen Vol. Per Cent	Oxy-hemo-globin Gm. Per Cent	Reduced Hemo-globin Gm. Per Cent
Oxygen capacity.	20	15.00	0.00
Oxygen content arterial blood..	19	14.25	0.75
Oxygen content venous blood...	14	10.50	4.50

The rate at which oxygen unsaturation develops during the passage of blood through the capillary bed is not known and cannot be determined in the individual case. However, for purposes of calculation it is usually assumed that the loss of oxygen is uniform from the arterial to the venous end of the capillary, and that the mean oxygen deficit and the mean concentration of reduced hemoglobin may be designated as one half of the sum of the arterial and the venous values. Expressed in values of reduced hemoglobin, the normal conditions of the preceding example may be represented as follows:

$$\frac{0.75 + 4.50}{2} = 2.62 \text{ Gm. } \% = \text{mean concentration of reduced hemoglobin}$$

This value would correspond to a normal color of the skin; although a considerable amount of reduced hemoglobin is present, cyanosis is not apparent. Lundsgaard[3] found that the mean content of reduced hemoglobin in the capillaries must rise to almost double the normal value, namely, to about 5.0 Gm. or its equivalent of 6.7 volumes per cent of oxygen unsaturation, before cyanosis became perceptible. This state may be attained by an increase in the amount of reduced hemoglobin, either in the arterial or in the venous blood.[4] Such

an increase in reduced hemoglobin may result from either inadequate oxygenation of arterial blood or excessive removal of oxygen from capillary blood, or both factors may be operative. Thus, if the arterial unsaturation is approximately normal (1 volume per cent) and the amount of oxygen removed in the passage of blood through the skin is excessive and amounts to 12 volumes per cent instead of the normal 5 volumes per cent, the venous blood will be 13 volumes per cent unsaturated, and the average deficit of oxygen in the capillary blood will be:

$$\frac{1 + 13}{2} = 7 \text{ volumes } \% = \frac{5.22 \text{ Gm. } \%}{\text{reduced hemoglobin}}$$

On the other hand, if the blood for some reason is incompletely saturated with oxygen during its passage through the pulmonary capillaries so that the arterial blood leaving the lung contains only 15.5 volumes per cent, the deficiency of oxygen in the arterial blood will be 4.5 volumes per cent, and after the normal utilization of oxygen by the skin the unsaturation of the venous blood will be 9.5 volumes per cent. Obviously the oxygen deficit and the concentration of reduced hemoglobin in the capillary blood will be the same as in the previous example and there will be in each

$$\frac{4.5 + 9.5}{2} = 7 \text{ volumes } \% = \frac{5.22 \text{ Gm. } \%}{\text{reduced hemoglobin}}$$

case faint cyanosis in the exposed skin.

The degree of cyanosis is dependent upon the *absolute amount of reduced hemoglobin* and not upon the relative amounts of oxyhemoglobin and reduced hemoglobin. Thus, an extremely anemic individual might have only 3.0 Gm. of hemoglobin in 100 ml. of blood. Under such circumstances, it is obvious that complete unsaturation of all of the hemoglobin and hypoxemia sufficient to threaten life may develop without the clinical appearance of cyanosis. Lesser degrees of anemia may permit the appearance of the blue color, which in times of emergency can unfortunately conceal the pallor. On the other hand, a patient suffering from polycythemia with a hemoglobin concentration of 20 Gm. of hemoglobin per 100 ml. of blood may develop cyanosis with a lesser degree of oxygen unsaturation than would a normal person. In such a patient, hypoxemia might be only moderate even at a time when the cyanosis appears somewhat alarming.

CAUSES OF CYANOSIS

Peripheral cyanosis is due to abnormal reduction of oxyhemoglobin in the systemic capillaries. It may arise either from an increased utilization of oxygen, such as occurs in very strenuous muscular exertion, or from a decreased or retarded blood flow. The relationships of the oxygen consumed by a particular organ or tissue, the blood flow to it and the difference in oxygen content between the arterial blood supplying it and the venous blood draining it, are stated in the Fick principle:

Rate of blood flow to organ =

$$\frac{\text{rate of } O_2 \text{ consumption by organ}}{\left\{ \begin{array}{l} \text{arterial blood } O_2 \text{ content} - O_2 \text{ content of venous blood from organ} \end{array} \right\}}$$

The commonest type of cyanosis is dependent upon a decreased blood flow through the peripheral capillary bed. This necessitates the removal of more than the usual amount of oxygen from each unit of blood during its passage through the tissues. This condition may be produced locally in normal persons by chilling or cold applications or by exposure of the body to low environmental temperatures. Under these circumstances cyanosis is particularly apparent in the nailbeds of the extremities.

Slight blueness of the toe nailbeds is common in anxious individuals. Contraction of the superficial vessels is responsible for this phenomenon and for the pale, cold skin that is also frequently present. In polycythemia, the increased viscosity of the blood may result in slower blood flow through peripheral capillaries, with resultant cyanosis. The symptom may be a striking feature of Raynaud's disease, in which spasmodic contraction of arteries leads to a diminution of arterial blood flow to the tissues, particularly to the fingers. Cyanosis

may occur for analogous reasons in thromboangiitis obliterans or with the endarteritic occlusion of arteriosclerosis. Blood flow in the peripheral capillaries may also be slowed because of obstructed veins, and cyanosis of the affected part may be notable in phlebitis, in thrombosis, and even with varicosities.

Peripheral cyanosis may be a very striking feature of the low output varieties of cardiac failure. The arteriovenous oxygen difference is increased, but at rest is seldom greater than 9 volumes per cent. In the cyanotic areas the arteriovenous oxygen difference, therefore, must be greater than it is for the body as a whole. This implies a disproportionate reduction of blood flow to these areas. During exercise the arteriovenous difference becomes greater than normal, since cardiac output does not increase appropriately or may even fall. Consequently cyanosis is more apparent during exertion. Pulmonary factors may play an additional slight role in the cyanosis of cardiac failure in which pulmonary congestion is a feature. Unless pulmonary edema is present, however, the hypoxemia is usually mild or absent.[5]

Dilatation and prominence of the venules in the skin secondary to a high venous pressure also affect skin color. The relative fullness of the venules is particularly important in those diseases in which the venous pressure is markedly and chronically elevated, such as tricuspid insufficiency.[6] In advanced tricuspid valvular disease jaundice may occur together with cyanosis, producing a curious combination of colors, known as icterocyanosis.

The cardiac output is profoundly lowered in shock and cyanosis is observed frequently.

The peripheral cyanosis in cardiac failure with a very low output or in acute reductions of the cardiac output (as when a ballvalve thrombosis obstructs the orifice of the mitral valve) is characteristically most marked in distal regions such as the hands, the feet and the tip of the nose. Peripheral cyanosis from any cause may be differentiated from central cyanosis due to hypoxemia, as Sir Thomas Lewis suggested,[7] by massaging the cyanotic part or applying heat to it. The ensuing increase in blood flow to the part will abolish peripheral, but not central, cyanosis.

Pulmonary Cyanosis. Hypoxemia, and therefore cyanosis, may occur when the normal state of gas exchange between alveolar air and pulmonary capillary blood is disturbed. Such a disturbance may result from an inadequate alveolar ventilation (as in paralysis of the chest cage, depression of the respiratory center, or laryngeal obstruction), from maldistribution of inspired air and blood among the alveoli with consequent underventilation of many alveoli relative to their blood supply (as in emphysema, asthma or pulmonary edema), from decrease in the diffusion capacity of the alveolar-capillary membrane (as in pulmonary fibrosis, or any condition in which the alveolar septa are infiltrated by inflammatory or neoplastic cells),[8,9] or from blood flowing through the lungs without coming into contact with alveolar air (pulmonary arteriovenous shunts). The hypoxemia of chronic pulmonary disease frequently is exaggerated by exercise, particularly if the diffusion capacity of the alveolar-capillary membrane is restricted severely.

The syndrome of alveolar hypoventilation of sufficient degree to cause hypoxemia, polycythemia and cyanosis with essentially normal function of the lungs may occur when the work of moving the chest bellows is greatly increased, as in advanced kyphoscoliosis or marked obesity.[10] Cyanosis is also seen in patients with impairment of the respiratory muscles due to primary diseases of muscle, a previous attack of poliomyelitis, or other forms of neuritis or neuropathy involving motor nerves. When it is due to primary failure of the respiratory center of obscure origin the clinical picture may be puzzling, since there is no evidence of lung disease, impairment of the chest bellows, or right–left shunt within the heart or the lungs.[11] In this disorder, arterial oxyhemoglobin saturation, which is decreased, and the carbon dioxide tension, which is increased, can both be brought to normal levels by increasing alveolar ventilation either volitionally or by a mechanical ventilator. A cardinal feature of the condition is a markedly decreased or absent ventilatory response to inhalation of carbon dioxide.

Hypoxemia also occurs when the pressure of oxygen in the inspired air is decreased by a reduction in barometric pressure, such as occurs at altitudes above sea level, or by a subnormal concentration of oxygen in air being breathed at sea level.

It is essential to bear in mind that when cyanosis is due to arterial hypoxemia alone it is a sign of a very advanced disturbance in gas exchange. Because the upper segment of the oxyhemoglobin dissociation curve is relatively flat, a fall of alveolar oxygen pressure as large as 35 mm. Hg may occur without great change in arterial oxyhemoglobin saturation. Cyanosis may not be apparent until the saturation has dropped to 85 per cent, and is usually, but not always, discernible at 75 per cent even by well-trained observers.[12] The arterial oxygen tensions at these saturations are 51 and 40 mm. Hg respectively, about one half the normal of 95 mm. The consequent loss of pressure-head that drives oxygen into the tissues may be critically important to previously ischemic areas.

Right–Left Shunts. Cyanosis in congenital heart disease is mainly attributable to contamination of the arterial stream by venous blood. Such a right–left shunt may occur through any of the various defects that may exist between the right and the left sides of the heart or between the great vessels. Whether or not a shunt exists will depend on the relationship between the pressures on either side of the communication. Normally both the systolic and the diastolic pressures on the left side exceed those on the right. In atrial and ventricular septal defects and patent ductus arteriosus, the shunt is mainly from left to right, and cyanosis is absent. If the pressures on the right side are increased greatly, as they may be when pulmonary vascular lesions develop or cardiac failure supervenes, the shunt may become bi-directional or be reversed completely. In pulmonic stenosis, pressures in the right ventricle, and also secondarily in the right atrium, are increased and may give rise to a right–left shunt through a ventricular septal defect, a patent foramen ovale, or an atrial septal defect. Pressure relationships between the atria may be altered transiently by vigorous crying, the Valsalva maneuver, or heavy exertion, and thereby cause partial reversal of a left-to-right interatrial shunt.

Several factors determine the presence or absence and degree of cyanosis in congenital heart disease. Most important is the size of the shunt relative to the systemic blood flow. If the systemic blood flow is normal, one third of it may be composed of venous blood without the appearance of cyanosis, since the arterial oxyhemoglobin saturation would be greater than 85 per cent. This is demonstrated in the following mixture calculation:

Pulmonary factors ordinarily do not play a role in producing the hypoxemia unless cardiac failure with pulmonary congestion develops. The sclerotic and the thrombotic lesions that may occur in the small pulmonary arteries do not interfere appreciably with gas exchange across the alveolar-capillary membrane. Pulmonary arteriovenous fistula, a congenital vascular lesion, may give rise to cyanosis and polycythemia without disturbing cardiac function. In some cases multiple fistulae occur, and the cyanosis may be pronounced.

The anatomic distribution of cyanosis in the various congenital cardiovascular disorders is like that due to arterial hypoxemia

Source of Blood	Amount	Oxygen Content, Vol. Per Cent	Oxyhemoglobin Saturation, Per Cent
Right–left shunt.................	1 part	13.0	65
Pulmonary veins................	2 parts	19.4	97
Total (i.e., arterial).............	3 parts	17.3	86.5

Another factor is the oxyhemoglobin saturation of the venous blood. If the systemic blood flow is less than normal in a case of cyanotic congenital heart disease, the arteriovenous oxygen difference is increased, and the mixed venous blood that is shunted into the arterial circulation is less saturated with oxygen. Under these circumstances a small shunt may produce a significant degree of hypoxemia. During exercise the oxyhemoglobin saturation of mixed venous blood normally falls. This change may be exaggerated in cyanotic congenital heart disease because of an inability to increase cardiac output appropriately. This factor, as well as an increase in the size of the shunt, accounts for the exaggerated anoxemia and cyanosis that develop during exertion. In some patients cyanosis may not be evident except with exertion. Therefore, observation of the patient during some simple form of exercise constitutes an important part of the examination.

Secondary polycythemia occurs frequently and is another factor that is responsible for the very profound degree of cyanosis that is observed in these disorders.

of any cause. However, there are instances in which the distribution is not uniform. Cyanosis of the lower extremities with absence of or a lesser degree of cyanosis in the upper extremities occurs in patent ductus arteriosus when the usual direction of blood flow through the ductus is reversed as a result of severe pulmonary arterial hypertension.[13] Since the ductus is inserted into the aorta distal to the bronchiocephalic arteries, the venous blood is directed mainly into the descending aorta. Occasionally the left hand is more cyanotic than the right because the left subclavian artery, which is almost opposite the ductus, receives some of the shunt. The differential cyanosis between the upper and the lower extremities is often associated with differential clubbing and is of diagnostic importance, and the "machinery" murmur typical of a patent ductus is absent under these circumstances (reversed flow).[13] Reversal of ductus flow also occurs in coarctation of the aorta when a coexisting ductus inserts into the aorta beyond the coarctation.

Normally, a very small quantity of venous blood is shunted into the systemic arterial stream via anastomotic connections between the bronchial and the pulmonary veins, and by drainage of the Thebesian and the anterior cardiac veins into the left heart. This venous admixture does not exceed 1 per cent of the pulmonary blood flow.[14] In some patients with cirrhosis of the liver, venous admixture is increased by the development of anastomoses between the portal, the mediastinal and the pulmonary veins.[15] This venous admixture, although apparently not large, may contribute to the decreased arterial oxyhemoglobin saturation and the consequent cyanosis that occasionally occur in patients with alcoholic cirrhosis.[14]

Abnormalities of Hemoglobin. The binding of oxygen by hemoglobin is influenced by the nature of the amino acid chains in the globin portion of the molecule.[16] Among the score or more abnormal human hemoglobins that have been identified, a few have an altered affinity for oxygen that has been related to the abnormal configuration of the globin. The affinity of hemoglobin M for oxygen appears to be reduced sufficiently to produce cyanosis.[17] This hemoglobin also has a tendency to become oxidized, and a large fraction of it in vivo may exist in the met-hemoglobin form.

A recently characterized hemoglobin was obtained from a 14-year-old boy who was completely normal except for cyanosis which had been present since birth.[18] His hemoglobin showed a striking reduction in its affinity for oxygen; although the arterial blood oxygen tension was normal (100 mm. Hg), the hemoglobin was only 60 per cent saturated with oxygen. Saturation attained a level of 94 per cent during oxygen breathing. Hemoglobin from the patient's mother showed a quantitatively similar decrease in ability to bind oxygen.

A shift of the oxyhemoglobin dissociation curve to the right in sickle cell anemia partially accounts for the low arterial oxygen saturation in some patients with this disease.[19] The shift of the curve is due to abnormalities within the red cell, since solutions of hemoglobin S have a normal dissociation curve.

Hemoglobin H has an affinity for oxygen that is 10 times greater than normal.[20]

RELATION OF CYANOSIS TO HYPERCAPNIA

Hypoxemia and cyanosis are not always accompanied by elevation of the carbon dioxide tension in the arterial blood. However, when hypoxemia is due to an over-all diminution of alveolar ventilation, the tension of carbon dioxide in alveolar air and arterial blood also is increased (see chapter on Dyspnea). Characteristically, in instances of uneven distribution of air and blood among the alveoli, such as may be caused by obstruction of the intrapulmonary airways (emphysema, asthma, pulmonary edema), an increase in carbon dioxide tension and consequent respiratory acidosis occur only when many alveolar areas are underventilated and anoxemia already is advanced. This phenomenon is explained by the fact that other areas of the lung are hyperventilated. Carbon dioxide output from the overventilated alveoli can balance, or even overcompensate for the retention of this gas in the blood of poorly ventilated alveoli because of the steepness of the blood carbon dioxide dissociation curve. On the other hand, the oxyhemoglobin dissociation curve is relatively flat in the usual physiologic range. The additional amount of oxygen that can be bound by the blood in the overventilated alveoli is not sufficient to compensate for the inadequate oxygenation of blood in the underventilated regions.[9]

If the alveolar-capillary membrane is abnormal, hypoxemia may be severe, but because of the much greater diffusibility of carbon dioxide as compared to oxygen, exchange of carbon dioxide is relatively undisturbed unless inadequacy of alveolar ventilation and ventilation/perfusion defects are superimposed.

The blood vessels of the skin are dependent for their normal state of dilatation upon the presence of a normal carbon dioxide tension. Diminution in the pressure of carbon dioxide may result in contraction of these vessels although it causes dilatation of other systemic arterioles. Under such circumstances the skin becomes pallid and pallor so caused, if combined with cyanosis, may give rise to a distinctive gray or helio-trope color, which has been much empha-sized by all who have studied the variations of cyanosis.[21] This shade of cyanosis also is observed frequently in patients with shock and pulmonary edema secondary to myo-cardial infarction.

RATIONALE OF OXYGEN THERAPY

When pure oxygen is breathed the pres-sure of oxygen in the alveolar air and arterial blood is increased six-fold. The amount of oxygen carried in solution con-sequently rises to 1.8 volumes per cent, and an additional 0.6 to 1.0 volume per cent is bound by the hemoglobin, since it becomes almost fully saturated. The net increase in arterial oxygen content is therefore 2.4 to 2.8 volumes per cent.

Amelioration of any type of cyanosis will occur on breathing pure oxygen. In the example of peripheral cyanosis cited above if the arterial blood oxygen content is raised to 22.5 volumes per cent and the amount of oxygen extracted by the tissues contin-ues at 12 volumes per cent, the venous blood will be only 9.5 volumes per cent unsaturated. The average deficit of oxygen in the capillary blood will be 4.25 volumes per cent (3.2 Gm. of reduced hemoglobin) instead of 7 volumes per cent, and cyanosis will disappear. However, oxygen will not abolish cyanosis when the peripheral blood flow is more restricted, and the arterio-venous oxygen difference in the tissue be-ing examined is consequently greater than in this example.

In the case of a right–left shunt, breath-ing of oxygen will also lessen the hy-poxemia and relieve cyanosis by increasing the amount of oxygen in both the pul-monary venous blood and in the systemic venous blood that is being shunted. In the mixture calculation described above, in the section on congenital heart disease, the pul-monary venous oxygen content will increase to 22.5 volumes per cent, the right–left shunt content to 16.05 volumes per cent, and the arterial content to 20.35 volumes per cent. Complete saturation of the ar-terial blood with oxygen, however, will not occur if the shunt is greater than 40 per cent of the systemic blood flow or if the arteriovenous oxygen difference is greater than normal.

The most dramatic relief of anoxemia and cyanosis that is achieved by adminis-tration of oxygen occurs when gas ex-change is impaired by disturbances in pul-monary function. Regardless of whether these disturbances consist of marked over-all deficiency in alveolar ventilation, mal-distribution of air and blood among the alveoli, decrease in oxygen diffusion ca-pacity of the alveolar-capillary membrane, or a combination of these factors (as is so often the case), administration of oxygen will almost always increase the arterial blood oxyhemoglobin saturation to or near normal. Oxygen therapy is therefore of considerable value especially in acute con-ditions like pulmonary edema, pneumonia, chronic pulmonary disease complicated by a respiratory infection and severe asthma. Frequently it may be life-saving.

Some reservations about the use of oxygen should be noted. When alveolar ventilation is decreased seriously by re-spiratory paralysis resulting from polio-myelitis or depression of the respiratory center, oxygen will promptly abolish hy-poxemia and cyanosis but it will not cor-rect the coexisting hypercapnia. The pa-tient may be spared the dangers of anoxia while receiving oxygen but may develop all the serious mental and neurologic con-sequences of a markedly increased blood carbon dioxide tension and respiratory acidosis. Artificial ventilation is the es-sential therapy in these conditions and is the only way to control the concentration of carbon dioxide in the alveolar air and the arterial blood.[8,22]

In chronic pulmonary disease compli-cated by chronic hypoxemia and respira-tory acidosis, as is often the case in emphy-sema, oxygen may produce *undesirable* sequelae. The respiratory centers of such patients are relatively insensitive to car-bon dioxide and increase in blood hydro-gen ion concentration. A greater than nor-mal portion of central neurogenic drive to respiration arises from hypoxic reflexes originating in the oxygen-sensitive aortic and carotid bodies. Elevation of the arterial oxygen tension to normal or above on breathing oxygen abolishes the anoxia-induced impulses, and ventilation may drop precipitously. Pre-existing inadequacy of alveolar ventilation is aggravated thereby. Alveolar and arterial carbon dioxide tensions rise sharply, and the various manifestations of the *carbon dioxide narcosis syndrome* may appear.[8]

If oxygen therapy is required, as it often is when the chronic pulmonary insufficiency is acutely aggravated, it is best given intermittently and with caution. It may be necessary to resort to a mechanical respirator, such as an *intermittent* positive pressure mask, in order to maintain ventilation.[23]

Until recent years the clinical importance of carbon dioxide has been poorly appreciated. In high concentrations this gas produces unconsciousness. In lesser concentration, delirium, stupor and somnolence are common effects. In very high concentrations it can produce death. The exact concentrations at which these phenomena occur is not known. Stupor has been observed in young men breathing 10.4 per cent carbon dioxide for 3 to 4 minutes,[21,24] and patients with pulmonary disease whose arterial carbon dioxide tension rises to the range of 100 mm. Hg frequently become comatose. Normal subjects lose consciousness in 20 to 30 seconds upon breathing a mixture of 30 per cent carbon dioxide and 70 per cent oxygen.[25]

Carbon dioxide is a powerful dilator of the cerebral vessels.[26] The sudden dilatation of these vessels that occurs with increments in arterial carbon dioxide tension causes an abrupt increase in cerebrospinal fluid pressure.[27] This change may be of sufficient degree to produce papilledema.[28] Carbon dioxide directly constricts other systemic vessels and may produce a rise in blood pressure. In high concentrations it may cause cardiac arrhythmias, both auricular and ventricular.[25]

REFERENCES

1. Roughton, F. J. W., Darling, R. C., and Root, W. S.: Factors affecting the determination of oxygen capacity, content and pressure in human arterial blood, Am. J. Physiol. 142:708, 1944.

2. Cournand, A., Riley, R. L., Breed, E. S., Baldwin, E. de F., and Richards, D. W.: Measurements of cardiac output in man; using the technique of catheterization of the right auricle or ventricle, J. Clin. Investigation 24:106, 1945.

3. Lundsgaard, C.: Studies of oxygen in the venous blood, J. Biol. Chem. 33:133, 1918; J. Exper. Med. 27:179, 199, 219, 1918; 30:147, 259, 271, 295, 1919.

4. Lundsgaard, C., and Van Slyke, D. D.: Cyanosis, Medicine 2:1, 1923.

5. Carroll, D., Cohen, J. E., and Riley, R. L.: Pulmonary function in mitral valvular disease: Distribution and diffusion characteristics in resting patients, J. Clin. Invest. 32: 510, 1953.

6. Sepulveda, G., and Lukas, D. S.: The diagnosis of tricuspid insufficiency. Clinical features in 60 cases with associated mitral valve disease, Circulation 11:552, 1955.

7. Lewis, T.: Diseases of the Heart, London, Macmillan, 1933.

8. Lukas, D. S.: Pulmonary function in health and disease, M. Clin. North America 39:661, 1955.

9. Comroe, J. H., Jr., Forster, R. E., II, Du Bois, A. B., Briscoe, W. A.: The lung. Clinical Physiology and Pulmonary Function Tests, Chicago, Yr. Bk. Pub., 1955.

10. Fishman, A. P., Turino, G. M., and Bergofsky, E. H.: The syndrome of alveolar hypoventilation, Am. J. Med. 23:333, 1957.

11. Rodman, T., Resnick, M. E., Berkowitz, R. D., Fenelly, J. F., and Olivia, J.: Alveolar hypoventilation due to involvement of the respiratory center by obscure disease of the central nervous system, Am. J. Med. 32:208, 1962.

12. Comroe, J. H., and Botelho, S.: The unreliability of cyanosis in the recognition of arterial anoxemia, Am. J. Med. Sci. 214:1, 1947.

13. Lukas, D. S., Araujo, J., and Steinberg, I.: The syndrome of patent ductus arteriosus with reversal of flow, Am. J. Med. 17:298, 1954.

14. Fritts, H. W., Jr., Hardewig, A., Rochester, D. F., Durand, J., and Cournand, A.: Estimation of pulmonary arteriovenous shunt-flow using intravenous injections of T-1824 dye Kr,[85] J. Clin. Invest. 39:1841, 1960.

15. Calabresi, P., and Abelmann, W. H.: Porto-caval and porto-pulmonary anastomoses in

Laennec's cirrhosis and in heart failure, J. Clin. Invest. 36:1257, 1957.

16. Wyman, J., and Allen, D. W.: The problem of heme interactions in hemoglobin and the basis of the Bohr effect, J. Polym. Sci. 7:499, 1951.

17. Gerald, P. S., and George, P.: Second spectroscopically abnormal methemoglobin associated with hereditary cyanosis, Science 129: 393, 1959.

18. Reissmann, K. R., Ruth, W. E., and Nomura, T.: A human hemoglobin with lowered oxygen affinity and impaired heme-heme interactions, J. Clin. Invest. 40:1826, 1961.

19. Rodman, T., Close, H. P., Cathcart, R., and Purcell, M. K.: The oxyhemoglobin dissociation curve in the common hemoglobinopathies, Am. J. Med. 27:558, 1959.

20. Benesch, R., Ranney, H. M., and Benesch, R. E.: Some properties of hemoglobin H, Fed. Proc. 20:70, 1961.

21. Haldane, J. S.: Respiration, New Haven, Yale Univ. Press, 1922.

22. Plum, F.: Respiratory failure in neuromuscular disorders. Monographs in Medicine. Series 1:225, Baltimore, Williams & Wilkins, 1952.

23. Cohn, J. E., Carroll, D. G., and Riley, R. L.: Respiratory acidosis in patients with emphysema, Am. J. Med. 17:447, 1954.

24. Dripps, R. D., and Comroe, J. H., Jr.: The respiratory and circulatory response of normal man to inhalation of 7.6 and 10.4 per cent O_2 with a comparison of the maximal ventilation produced by severe muscular exercise, inhalation of CO_2 and maximal voluntary hyperventilation. Am. J. Physiol. 149:43, 1947.

25. MacDonald, F. M., and Simonson, E.: Human electrocardiogram during and after inhalation of 30 per cent carbon dioxide, J. Appl. Physiol. 6:304, 1953.

26. Schieve, J. F., and Wilson, W. P.: The changes in cerebral vascular resistance of man in experimental alkalosis and acidosis. J. Clin. Invest. 32:33, 1953.

27. Davies, C. E., and Mackinnon, J.: Neurological effects of oxygen in chronic cor pulmonale. Lancet 2:883, 1949.

28. Simpson, T.: Papilloedema in emphysema. Brit. M. J. 2:639, 1948.

18

Anorexia, Nausea and Vomiting

JOHN L. HORNER AND STEWART WOLF

Disturbances in the ability to ingest or retain nutriment are among the commonest of symptoms. The significance of anorexia, nausea or vomiting is often minor, indicative of only temporary or mild disorders. Frequently, however, investigation of these manifestations is necessary, especially if they are severe or recurrent or chronic. Many different types of gastrointestinal disease may be responsible for these symptoms, but often the cause lies in quite another body system and is only expressed through the enteric tract.

NERVE SUPPLY TO GASTRO-INTESTINAL TRACT

A consideration of the mechanisms involved in the production of the common symptoms of anorexia, nausea and vomiting requires frequent reference to the peripheral nerve supply to the gastrointestinal tract and its connections with the higher centers of the central nervous system. A brief review of the pathways by which a reciprocal interplay is constantly maintained between the gastrointestinal tract and the nervous system therefore follows.

That the gastrointestinal tract can continue to function with some efficiency after degenerative section of its extrinsic nerve supply has been demonstrated by numerous investigators. It is apparent that there must be intrinsic reflex arcs, and that they must be important in co-ordinating conduction through the intestine, in helping to prevent localized spasm, in transmitting impulses from the mucosa to the longitudinal and the circular muscles and in protecting the bowel from violent extraneous stimuli. This intrinsic reflex function is presumably exercised by the submucosal and myenteric plexuses, which have been shown to contain the essentials of a local reflex mechanism.[1]

The alimentary tract does not, however, in the intact animal or man, function in an autonomous manner, despite the fact that it is possible for it to do so. Under normal circumstances the vagus, the splanchnic and the pelvic nerves play an important role in transmitting impulses between the central nervous system and the viscera.

In attempting to define the functions of different parts of the autonomic nervous system, experiments have yielded somewhat confusing results. This should not be surprising, in view of the profuse synapses in the peripheral ganglia between terminal fibers of the sympathetic and parasympathetic "systems." Thomas, who has been instrumental in attempting to bring our theories of autonomic function into line with physiologic experiments, believes that the time-honored classification into systems has lost much of its significance.[2] He points out that all preganglionic, most parasympathetic postganglionic and some sympathetic postganglionic fibers release acetylcholine at their terminals. This common pharmacologic mechanism justifies designating these fibers as "cholinergic." Most sympathetic postganglionic nerves release arterenol (and perhaps epinephrine) and are "adrenergic." He further argues that even if we adopt the more physiologic concept of adrenergic and cholinergic nerves, rather than the traditional anatomic classification, we do not necessarily find strict antagonism in their function. Thomas therefore suggests that the entire autonomic nervous system be considered as a unit, with the individual fibers, whether sympathetic or parasympathetic, being used by the organism in accord with its needs at the moment.[3]

Abandonment of the traditional classification at this stage of our knowledge would, unfortunately, advance little our understanding of gastrointestinal function. The concept of duality is too convenient for interpreting some facts for which we otherwise have little or no explanation. It seems wise, therefore, with due regard to the defects of the theory, to still consider the *parasympathetic* system as generally increasing the tone and the motility of the alimentary tract, as a result of reinforcement of reflexes mediated through the local nerve plexuses. The *sympathetic* system, although apparently of little significance in regulating ordinary day-to-day activity, is generally inhibitory.[4]

The gastrointestinal parasympathetic efferent fibers arise from cells in the medulla and also from the sacral region of the spinal cord. They typically undergo synapsis with ganglion cells within or adjacent to the viscus they are innervating. This results in each fiber conducting impulses to a small localized area.

The sympathetic efferent nerves arise from cells in the lateral horns of the eighth cervical or the first thoracic to the second or the third lumbar segments of the cord. They pass by way of the white rami communicantes to the paravertebral ganglionic chain, some fibers synapsing there with several postganglionic fibers, some ascending or descending the sympathetic chain before undergoing synapsis, and others passing through to synapse with cells in the prevertebral ganglia. The wide synaptic connection of each preganglionic fiber with many postganglionic fibers insures a diffuse discharge of impulses, not limited to a single organ.

Afferent impulses from the viscera travel to the central nervous system primarily by way of the vagus, the pelvic and the splanchnic nerves. Since the cells of origin for the splanchnic and the pelvic nerves are in the posterior roots of the cord and since the fibers are histologically no different from ordinary somatic sensory fibers, these afferent neurones are technically not part of the sympathetic system. Nevertheless, they serve to complete the visceral reflex arc.

Many viscerovisceral reflexes are routed through the spinal cord without involving higher centers. Others are controlled or modified by medullary and hypothalamic nuclei. The hypothalamus serves as a co-ordinating mechanism for activities involving simultaneous visceral and somatic expression.[3] Still higher in the segmental level the cortex of the cerebrum and the cerebellum serves as the chief connecting station between sensory and motor autonomic and somatic functions. It is through the reflexes mediated at this highest level that mental states exert stimulative or depressive effects on the gastrointestinal tract.

This introduction would be incomplete without reference to the effect of hormones on the alimentary tract. The results of research in this field have made it apparent that these substances will have to be increasingly considered in any physiologic field. At the present time, however, they cannot be considered apart from the autonomic nervous system. It is true that, when injected into the experimental animal, they act without regard to the extrinsic visceral nerve supply, but in normal daily activities their release depends on intact local nerve plexuses or hypothalamic stimulation. In other words, even where the hormone is the final action effector, it is produced at the direction of the autonomic nervous system. Therefore this discussion of the etiology of anorexia, nausea and vomiting will for the most part be in terms of the role of the nervous system.

ANOREXIA

To understand anorexia, the loss of appetite, it would be necessary to understand appetite itself, a subject not yet clearly explained.

Most observers consider appetite to be a state of mind, one that implies an agreeable relationship to food, often to a certain specific food. For example, at one time a person may have an appetite for one article of diet, but not another. Appetite may be present when there is no hunger, or when hunger has been thoroughly satisfied.

Conversely, although satiety usually implies a lack of appetite, it is certainly not the same thing as anorexia.

Appetite can perhaps be best considered as one of the mechanisms available for the regulation of food intake, although eating behavior may or may not correspond appropriately to the presence or the absence of appetite.

A person may eat compulsively in the absence of appetite or hunger, or he may be unable to eat despite a desire and need for food.

Hunger. Since the experiments of Cannon and Washburn it has been known that hunger often is accompanied by strong peristaltic contractions of the stomach.[5] Until recent years it was assumed that these contractions were responsible for the hunger "pangs," as well as reflexly causing the accessory symptoms of weakness, emptiness, irritability, headache and even nausea. Now it can be stated, through the work of several groups of investigators, that the hunger sensations are initiated in the hypothalamus.[6] The hunger pangs are produced by stimuli flowing to the stomach through vagus fibers. They help to make us aware of our need for food, but are not indispensable. After vagotomy, gastric contractions cease, the "pangs" disappear, but the patient still develops sensations of hunger.

Hunger, then, may be defined as a primitive, uncomfortable, unconditioned physiologic state due to privation of food. The mechanism of the production of the hunger sensations is as yet unknown. In some patients hunger, with weakness and headache, is clearly connected with low blood glucose levels. This is true with various types of spontaneous hypoglycemia (functional hypoglycemia following excessive carbohydrate ingestion, Addison's disease, pancreatic islet cell tumors) and in diabetic and nondiabetic patients after insulin injection. Prompt relief follows the oral or intravenous administration or dextrose. That this is a central mechanism was proved when Grossman and coworkers produced definite augmentation of food intake in dogs and man by insulin injection even after complete denervation of the upper gastrointestinal tract.[7]

To account for the association of hunger with relative hypoglycemia it has been suggested that the lateral hypothalamic hunger centers, and the medially placed satiety centers, contain glucoreceptor cells which are sensitive to changes in blood sugar levels.[8] Despite the attractiveness of the theory no proof is as yet available, and a number of facts cast doubt on it. For example, why does eating a hearty meal relieve the symptoms of hunger before the blood sugar begins to rise? Why does putting inert material such as celluflour into the stomach cause temporary satiety?[9] Why does hyperglycemia produced by parenteral glucose administration not depress hunger sensations and food intake?[10] It is apparent that at present there are many more questions than answers about the mechanism of hunger production.

To summarize what we do know about hunger we may quote Grossman, one of the most active investigators in this field. In his words, hunger is a psychic correlative of the bodily processes which regulate nutrient balance. The special hypothalamic areas participating in this control may be affected by oropharyngeal stimulation, gastrointestinal distention, blood levels of nutrients such as glucose, and tissue storage of nutrients.

Appetite. It is apparent that appetite, by the definition previously given, is largely a central phenomenon. There is ample experimental and clinical exidence to support this concept. For example, patients who have had combined sympathetic and parasympathetic denervation of the stomach, small bowel and proximal colon may have the sensation of appetite unaffected.[4] Patients who have had a complete gastrectomy still have a selective desire for foods. Also it has long been known that areas in the parietal and the frontal lobes of the brain may be so involved by disease as to decrease the appetite.

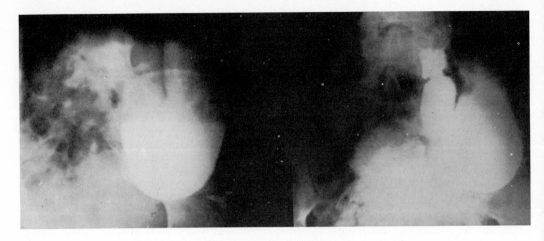

Fig. 102. Hypotonia of the stomach during an attack of nausea.

Before accepting the concept of appetite as purely central, however, it would be well to consider the accompanying visceral manifestations. Many years ago it was observed by Barclay that the appearance of appetite was associated with an increase in gastric tone.[11] By this is meant an approximately equal shortening of all the muscle fibers in the stomach wall, so that the stomach seems smaller and tenser. It has no connotation as to peristalsis, which can take place whether tone is good or poor, but is restricted by excessive tone. Wolf and Wolff demonstrated, in their gastrostomy subject, that the thought of good food was associated with accelerated acid secretion, together with hyperemia and hypermotility of the stomach.[12] However, they were able to show that these changes were the result, rather than the cause, of appetite.

Anorexia is usually associated with hypofunction of the stomach, manifested by pallor of the mucosa, hypoacidity, and hypomotility. Anorexia may occur, however, with gastric hyperfunction as in the case of peptic ulcer, especially in the presence of pain. Anorexia is commonly a stage which precedes nausea and then vomiting. However, any of the three disorders may appear in the absence of the others. Anorexia may be induced by excessive eating, especially of fat or sugar, by odors, and sights of various sorts. In some, smoking and drinking curb the appetite. They whet the appetite of others.

A common denominator seems to be that central effects producing loss of appetite cause hypoactivity and hypotonicity of the stomach, whereas primary visceral states associated with gastric inactivity cause anorexia.

The central and the visceral manifestations may be precipitated by thoughts or odors, tastes, sights or sounds which are unpleasant ("disgusting," literally taking taste or appetite away). Often, however, the central stimulus need only be "exciting," primarily adrenergic in effect, as a rule), and anorexia results.

The association of appetite with olfactory acuity has been the subject of some study. One group found that the keenness of the sense of smell exhibited diurnal variations closely related to habitual hours of eating. A simple sugar solution was capable of producing a decrease in olfactory acuity, and of bringing about a conversion of the sensation of appetite into one of satiety, but these effects occurred only if the subjects were permitted both to taste and to ingest the carbohydrate.[13] These observations have not been confirmed by others.[14]

In summary, appetite may be considered as a mental state characterized by a desire to eat certain foods, with which there are associated visceral changes. As with any other learned sensation it is reasonable to assume that appetite may be affected by a number of factors. Of particular importance are the emotional state, chemical and vascular variations and impulses transmitted to the midbrain from the viscera and the other organs. Visceral stimuli are, of course, carried to the central nervous system through the vagus, the pelvic and the sympathetic nerves. In later discussion it will be convenient to consider as reflex or visceral causes of anorexia those agents which stimulate the appetite adversely by stimulation of the autonomic visceral nerves.

NAUSEA

It is only a step from anorexia (lack of desire for food) to nausea (a feeling of revulsion for food). Is the physiologic mechanism the same, differing only in degree? We know that many drugs which in small doses cause loss of appetite will, in larger doses, cause the stomach to rebel actively. Some patients who complain of anorexia, whatever the etiology, will become nauseated when food is brought into their pres-

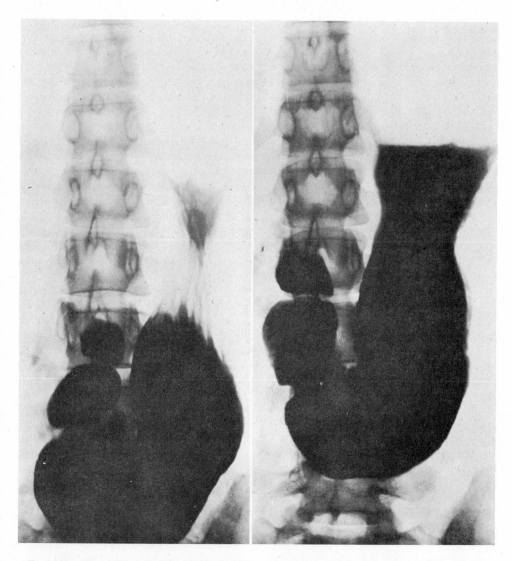

FIG. 103. The effect of abdominal muscle contraction on the appearance of gastric tone. (*Left*) Apparent hypotonicity with relaxed abdominal muscles. (*Right*) Normal appearance in same patient with contraction of abdominal muscles.

ence. With both sensations, changes in the tonicity and the activity of the stomach and the small bowel can be observed and recorded. With nausea these changes are more readily apparent.

Nausea is usually associated with other symptoms, such as salivation, sweating, and tachycardia, followed by bradycardia—all indications of imbalance of the autonomic nervous system.

Nausea is an intensely unpleasant sensation referred to the "back of the throat" or the "pit of the stomach." The patient may say just that he "feels sick" or is "sick at the stomach." When only mild, it may be described as a sinking sensation in the epigastrium.

Nausea is generally considered to be a sensory experience mediated by peripheral nerves which are located in the epigastrium and travel in either the splanchnic or vagal pathways. It should be noted, however, that nausea has been felt by subjects who have had both bilateral thoraco-lumbar splanchnicectomy and vagotomy. Nausea is a parodoxical sensation, difficult for the subject to describe and usually described only vaguely, yet very real and often severe.

Most people localize nausea in the epigastrium, but not very precisely. It is not exactly painful but does at times resemble a cramp or pulling sensation. The peripheral mechanism responsible for nausea has not been discovered as yet but there has been a good deal of study of the associated changes in the stomach and duodenum.

The stomach during nausea becomes inactive in terms of acid secretion and contractions. The hypotonic walls hang loosely, as those of a bag. The walls of the duodenum, in contrast, usually undergo an increase in contractile state so that a reversal of the usual pressure gradient occurs, with regurgitation of duodenal contents backward into the stomach. The hypotonic stomach characteristic of nausea is illustrated in Figure 102. Barclay noted that the lower border of the stomach descended as much as 3 inches in response to nauseous odors. He did not explain the mechanism behind this action, but it is apparent from Figure 103 that it could be due in part to relaxation of the abdominal muscles. In fearful soldiers the stomach relaxed just prior to the onset of nausea and peristalsis ceased.[15] One learns to anticipate vomiting in patients undergoing gastric fluoroscopy when there is a sudden loss of tonicity, with a drop in the lower border of the stomach. Since the drop would cause a pull on the mesenteric and the peritoneal attachments, it is of interest that nausea has been produced during abdominal operations under local anesthesia by pulling on the mesentery.

There are many observations on record of nausea caused by balloon distention of the lower end of the esophagus, the stomach and particularly the duodenum. Wolf and Wolff discovered also, in their gastrostomy subject, that nausea occurred consistently, accompanied by pain of moderate intensity and with vigorous peristaltic contractions, when pressure was applied to the stomach wall with a blunt glass rod.[16]

Often the question is raised whether reverse peristalsis in the small bowel has anything to do with nausea. Oppenheimer and Mann have studied the intestinal activity in dogs which precedes the act of vomiting.[17] This period may coincide with the sensation of nausea in man. They found at times considerable activity in exteriorized jejunal and ileal loops, some of it antiperistaltic. Another group demonstrated, in man, that periods of transitory duodenal contraction characteristically, but not invariably, accompanied nausea. They conclude that duodenal contraction is not essential to the sensation of nausea, and probably is produced at the direction of the central nervous system, since Dramamine, a centrally acting agent, eliminated duodenal spasm as well as nausea following vestibular stimulation.[18] On the other hand Wolf suggested that the duodenum could be the site of the peripheral sensation of nausea, on the basis of balloon studies in soldiers which demonstrated an increase in the duration and the amplitude of contractions at the time nausea was experienced.[15]

In regard to the depression of gastric secretion that uniformly follows the onset of nausea, whether spontaneous or induced, work in Ivy's laboratory demonstrated that this phenomenon must be vascular or hormonal in nature.[19] Abdominal splanchnicectomy and lumbar sympathectomy do not abolish the effect.

The evidence which has been cited shows that the visceral components of nausea are easily demonstrated. Nevertheless nausea, like anorexia, is largely of central origin, with the sensation being elicited by stimuli brought to the hypothalamic nuclei through the blood stream, by direct pressure and through strong stimuli carried over cranial, spinal and autonomic nerves. Thus anorexia may be due to a few synaptic connections through the emetic or other hypothalamic nuclei; nausea, to a greater number of such connections.

Gastric Hypofunction

While nausea and vomiting are characteristically associated with a decrease in mucosal blood flow, acid secretion, and motor activity, the presence of such gastric hypofunction does not necessarily imply the presence of nausea. Most commonly, the full or bloated sensations of "indigestion" are felt when there is a lack of contractile activity in the stomach and a failure of the contents to move on to the duodenum. Belching of air may occur in an attempt to relieve the feeling of pressure. If the normal, brisk, propulsive movements fail to occur in the stomach and the upper portion of the small intestine, the partially digested food does not become thoroughly mixed with the digestive juices and is not uniformly exposed to the membranous lining of the intestine, where absorption occurs. Gas is formed in the desultory digestive processes so that the lax wall of the stomach and duodenum are distended, further aggravating the sensation of fullness, tightness, or indigestion. Aerophagia plus gas formation produces a sensation of bloating and the affected person becomes demonstrably distended. Actual pain may result when such distention becomes very pronounced. The bloated sensation often seems to merge imperceptibly into the sensation of nausea.

VOMITING

Vomiting may be defined as the sudden, forceful ejection of the stomach contents through the mouth. It is a frequent consequence of nausea, since a stimulus that will produce a "sick feeling" will usually in greater strength cause attempted emptying of the stomach.

The existence of a vomiting center in the medulla oblongata has been accepted by most physiologists. Its precise location is perhaps in some doubt. Destruction of a tiny area in the dorsal portion of the lateral reticular formation in dogs and cats prevents vomiting, while local application of minute amounts of apomorphine and certain other chemicals induces it. However, Borison and Wang have demonstrated a "chemoreceptor zone" adjacent to the vomiting center.[20] They believe the emetic center is activated directly by afferent impulses arising in the gastrointestinal tract, whereas the chemoreceptor trigger zone appears to be the site of emetic action for many circulating drugs. The latter zone is unable to act independently, and therefore must be a way station transmitting stimuli to an intact emetic center. Borison emphasizes that these findings are based on animal experimentation and hence cannot be applied directly to the vomiting mechanism in the human.[21] However, it would certainly seem that their studies on emetic action of drugs should be of some value in their clinical application.

If the original impulse arises in the gastrointestinal tract the afferent fibers involved in the emetic reflex are principally those in the vagus and the splanchnic nerves. Many other nerve tracts may carry the afferent impulse, for example: vestibular, glossopharyngeal, optic and olfactory nerves. The efferent fibers are found in the vagi and the splanchnic nerves also, but equally important are the phrenics, the spinal nerves to the abdominal muscles, and the cranial nerves to the muscles of the pharynx, the palate and the epiglottis.

The vomiting center in the medulla oblongata lies in close relation to, but is quite distinct from, the respiratory centers. It is one of a number of visceral centers which are situated close together anatomically, and which likewise have coordinated physiological actions: salivatory nuclei, defecation and vasomotor centers, vestibular nuclei, etc.

INDUCTION OF VOMITING

The complex group of reflexes resulting in the physical response called vomiting results from excitation of the vomiting center by (1) impulses arising in the stomach, other parts of the gastrointestinal tract or elsewhere in the body, (2) impulses received from cerebral centers, or (3) chemical materials carried to it by the blood.

THE ACT OF VOMITING

Nausea is usually part of the complex series of phenomena preceding and accompanying emesis. There may be a number of vasomotor and autonomic manifestations, especially salivation and sweating. The affected person may become weak and feel faint, become pale, and experience vertigo, headache, or tachycardia. Breathing becomes rapid and irregular, the blood pressure falls and retching may occur, consisting of spasmodic contraction of the expiratory muscles of the chest, descent and sudden spasm of the diaphragm, with simultaneous sudden contraction of the abdominal muscles. Such retching (unproductive vomiting movements) may be brief or repeated for some time before actual emesis results. During the act of vomiting the blood pressure may oscillate greatly, the heart rate may become quite slow, and respiration is halted.

The sequence of events when emesis occurs has been observed many times in animals and man. First of these is a relaxation of the upper half of the stomach and the esophageal cardia. This is followed by one or more deep peristaltic contractions passing from the mid-portion of the stomach to the incisura angularis, apparently fading out at this level. A strong contraction at the incisura then forms and persists, dividing the stomach and preventing its contents from passing into the gastric antrum and the duodenum. Following this there is a sudden vigorous contraction of the dia-

phragmatic and the abdominal muscles, causing increased intra-abdominal pressure. This pressure, transmitted to the flaccid main portion of the stomach, causes the orad movement of the gastric contents. At the same time the glottis is closed; respiration ceases; the larynx and the hyoid bones are drawn and held forward, and the soft palate is elevated against the nasopharynx.

It will be noted that reverse peristalsis in the stomach has no part in the mechanism of vomiting. Apparently, in man at least, it rarely has been observed. It is further remarkable that stomach activity is not decidedly important in this entire sequence, except as it prevents the caudad movement of its contents. Reverse peristalsis in the small bowel probably does occur, and results in the passage of some of the intestinal content into the stomach.[18] Hence the presence of bile in the vomitus after repeated retching. But it is not a factor in the actual vomiting act, as Gregory has shown.[22] Denervation of the mesenteric pedicles to the upper small bowel loops will abolish reverse peristalsis, but vomiting can be produced as before.

The ease with which some persons vomit must depend to some extent on the state of relaxation at the esophageal cardia. Obviously, if the cardia becomes contracted rather than relaxed, retching may occur, but vomiting, as it has been defined, cannot.

CAUSES OF ANOREXIA, NAUSEA AND VOMITING

In the past it has been customary to divide the various diseases, the conditions and the drugs that may induce anorexia, nausea and vomiting into central and reflex groups. Paradoxically, with increasing knowledge of the mechanisms involved, it has become increasingly difficult to "pigeonhole" the various causes, and there seems little point in perpetuating a distinction which has lost its usefulness. We will not attempt central and reflex classification. With some causes there is insufficient evidence at hand to warrant arbitrary classification of any kind. Nevertheless, because some organization into groups helps to clarify thinking, the following headings will be used in the discussion which is to follow: cerebromedullary, toxic, visceral, deficiencies and motion sickness.

CEREBROMEDULLARY

Stress, Fear, Depression. Emotional and psychic reactions to life situations often cause anorexia, nausea or vomiting.[26] The situation is frequently not an unpleasant one but simply exciting, stressful, adrenergic, preparing for a party, an athletic contest, a speech, etc. More often the situation is associated with fear or depression, frustration and a tendency to withdrawal.[15] The stomach studied in such circumstances is pale and inactive. In many instances the patient may be apparently unaware or only partially aware of the possibility that his emotional and psychic responses may be causing his recurrent or chronic anorexia, his frequent feelings of fullness, and occasional nausea and vomiting. Such reactions were often encountered among soldiers overseas during World War II in the horrifying circumstances of the war in the jungle against the Japanese. One patient observed in New Guinea during the war years is particularly characteristic of this disorder. A 27-year-old infantryman complained mainly of insomnia, loss of appetite, nausea, vomiting, and weight loss. He appeared dejected, inactive, spoke very little, and was considerably slowed mentally. In the past he had always been unduly timid and dependent on his mother. Four years earlier, when his father had met accidental death, he had become depressed and fearful and had morning vomiting for weeks. Early in the war he had joined the Merchant Marine, but had had to give it up because of seasickness. His present episode of incapacity had been associated with inability to face the fact that he was involved in the war in New Guinea. As he expressed it "The jungle gets me down."

In studies on others it was observed that situations which induced feelings of disgust were commonly accompanied by nausea, as were despondency and feelings of dejection from whatever cause. The common denominator appeared to be an attitude of defeat or of being overwhelmed, accompanied by a desire to reject or eject the offending situation. Among soldiers overseas, those who had the most difficulty with nausea in the combat zone were those who, earlier in life, had been unduly dependent and passive, showing indecisiveness and failure to take aggressive action. The pattern of gastric underfunctioning was extremely common, however, and occurred during the war in many individuals without neurotic backgrounds. This is doubtless because of the intensity of the situational stimuli which more or less naturally gave rise to feelings of dejection and the desire to withdraw.

Thus, while anorexia, nausea, and vomiting may be indicative of structural disease and disorders of various sorts, the symptoms probably occur more commonly as manifestations of a troubled spirit, reflecting fear, sadness, or discouragement. Indeed, these symptoms may be the only manifestations, the patient having repressed other responses to the troublesome situation and his feelings about it.

The visceral changes are secondary to hypothalamic stimulation. Whether the latter acts through release of hormones resulting in adrenalin secretion, or directly through the sympathetic nerves to the stomach, is not known. In animals it has been shown that stress situations involving fear can cause gastric mucosal vasodilatation even to the point of hemorrhage. It has been theorized that this is due to histaminemia and heparinemia as a result of degranulation of mast cells.[23] If this could be demonstrated in man, it would be apparent that nausea would then result from the nerve reflexes originating within the stomach. This would then become a visceral rather than a cerebromedullary cause.

Neuroses and Psychoses. As might be expected from the importance of the psychic element in appetite, frequent sources of anorexia are the neuroses. From early infancy the satisfaction of hunger and appetite is inseparably linked with the striving for security and the desire for love. When these emotions are repressed in later life, as they frequently must be, there may result a tension, an unconscious feeling of guilt, that results in a refusal to enjoy eating. If the neurosis is more deeply ingrained, there may be nausea and even vomiting of severe degree. Psychoanalysis in such cases interprets the organic symptoms as expressing the need of the patient to "give back what he receives."

Recent experiments would suggest that in major psychoses there is a depression of gastrointestinal function concomitant with the depression of mental reactions.[24] When the feelings of anxiety, fear and guilt have been relieved by prefrontal lobotomy, the alimentary tract tends to resume normal function. It seems apparent that the gastrointestinal changes are secondary to changes in the hypothalamic nuclei induced by cerebral repression.

The most dramatic form of anorexia of psychoneurotic origin is known as anorexia nervosa. Except for its great severity, with occasional fatal results, it is believed by most psychiatrists to be little different from any other neurotic loss of appetite.[25] It usually occurs in neurotic young women and is accompanied by severe weight loss, amenorrhea and low basal metabolic rate. Differentiation from pituitary hypofunction of the cachectic type (Simmonds' disease) may be difficult, since severe functional hypopituitarism is present in prolonged starvation states.

Shock. Both primary (neurogenic or psychogenic) shock and secondary shock (resulting from trauma, hemorrhage, vascular accidents, toxins, etc.) are apt to be accompanied by anorexia, nausea and vomiting. There is widespread peripheral capillary dilatation, reduction in cardiac output, slowing of peripheral blood flow and a fall in blood pressure. Nausea and vomiting may occur because of reduced blood supply to the cerebromedullary center. Vasoconstriction of the splanchnic areas occurs in shock and may play a role in causing anorexia, nausea or vomiting.

Pain. Sudden severe pain or frequently recurring or chronic pain often is the cause of anorexia, nausea or vomiting. Certain types of pain are particularly known to cause these symptoms, probably because of their high intensity. Two of these are migraine, and visceral pain such as that following trauma to the testes. Vomiting may occur because of central nervous connections and effects upon the vomiting center

or because of shock effects produced by the pain.

Hypoxemia. Reduction of the oxygen supply to the vomiting center through reduction of the oxygen content of the inspired air lowers its threshold and may cause anorexia, nausea or vomiting (aviation, mountain climbing). Limitation of the blood supply to the vomiting center has a similar effect and may result from anemia, hemorrhage, vascular occlusion or increased intracranial pressure.

Hot Weather. The loss of appetite experienced by many persons during hot weather is difficult to explain, although it obviously is the means by which the body adjusts to a lessened need for energy output. Normal men doing hard work at 120° F. do not experience anorexia or any signs of decreased gastrointestinal activity except in actual heat exhaustion.[27] These observations are consistent with the fact that farmers working in hot fields will eat a hearty midday meal. It seems likely that the ordinary mild anorexia of summertime is psychic in origin, possibly induced by bodily discomfort. As more and more of us live, work and eat in air-conditioned comfort, the less noticeable will be the seasonal change in eating habits.

An increase in intracranial pressure is frequently associated with emesis, with or without preceding nausea, often with preceding anorexia. This type of vomiting is often called "projectile," since the ejection of the stomach contents is usually more forceful than in other types, perhaps because of the suddenness of the impulse. Examples of lesions causing increased intracranial pressure and vomiting are concussion of the brain, cerebral tumor and abscess, hydrocephalus, meningitis, lateral sinus thrombosis and cerebral hemorrhage. Migraine might also be included in this list. The increased sensitiveness of the emesis center associated with intracranial hypertension is probably due to interference with the blood supply to the center. Evidence for this may be found in the vomiting which always accompanies the experimental ligation of the carotid arteries in animals. Then, too, it is well known that

Plate 3

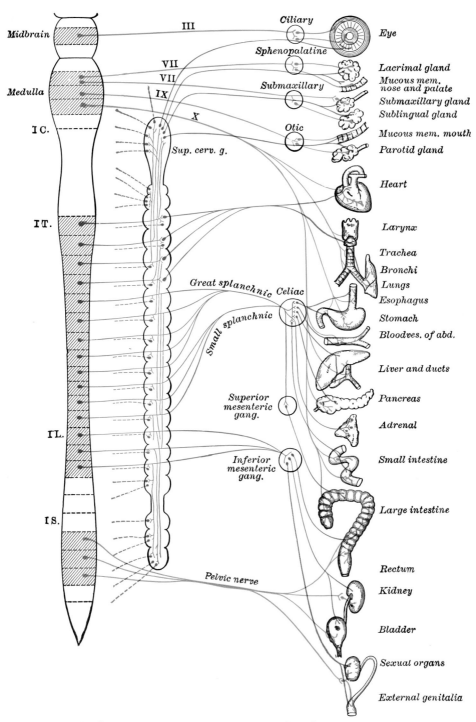

Diagram of efferent autonomic nervous system. (*Blue*) Cranial and sacral outflow, parasympathetic. (*Red*) Thoracolumbar, sympathetic. (*Dotted red line*) Postganglionic fibers to spinal and cranial nerves to supply vasomotors to head, trunk and limbs, motor fibers to smooth muscles of skin and fibers to sweat glands. (Modified after Gottlieb. Gray: Anatomy of the Human Body, ed. 24, Philadelphia, Lea & Febiger)

severe anemia increases the likelihood of vomiting.

Oral sepsis and badly fitting dentures are common causes of anorexia, due to discomfort or bad taste connected with eating. As has been pointed out, appetite is a pleasurable mental state. If a person is deprived of the pleasure of eating he will not eat as much. There is no reliable evidence that these disorders of dentition result in a chronic gastritis.

Carminatives, which have been used for centuries to improve appetite, have no consistent effect on secretion or motility of the stomach or small bowel. Possibly foods taste better by contrast with the bitterness of such carminatives as gentian, or iron, quinine and strychnine. Possibly the effect is purely one of suggestion, and a conditioned reflex is set up. Highly seasoned appetizers, hot soups and the like might be expected to stimulate some increase in gastric tone and secretion through their effect on the sensory nerve endings in the mouth, but this could not be demonstrated experimentally. The use of spices appears to be conditioned more by the habits of the individual than by the taste of any particular spice.[28] The increase in appetite that frequently follows the ingestion of moderate quantities of alcoholic beverages is largely a central effect, due to improvement of mood and blocking of inhibitory impulses. Another factor increasing appetite *after* alcohol ingestion is probably the increased gastric secretion of hydrochloric acid causing localized gastric consciousness. The effect of alcohol on the stomach itself is, according to Beazell and Ivy, actually one of inhibition of hunger contractions.[29]

Toxic

Drugs may bring about anorexia, or nausea and vomiting, in one of two ways. Many of them have direct action on the cerebrum, the hypothalamus or the brain stem, and produce gastrointestinal symptoms only after absorption into the circulation, or after parenteral injection. Others have an irritant effect on the gastric or small bowel mucosa, with emesis center stimulation mediated through vagal or sympathetic nerve fibers. A few have both modes of action. As previously described, Borison and Wang make a distinction, on the basis of animal experiments, between the vomiting center itself and a nearby "chemoreceptor zone." The latter appears to be necessary for the emetogenic action of many circulating drugs, although it cannot act independently of an intact vomiting center.[20]

Mercury bichloride, ammonium chloride, copper sulfate, ipecac and aminophylline are examples of drugs which cause mucosal irritation in almost all persons, although some are much more susceptible than others.[47] These, and many other drugs, do not affect the appetite or cause nausea until they enter the duodenum, and are hence not gastric irritants, as formerly thought. Wolf and Wolff demonstrated this fact in their gastrostomy subject. However, salicylates have a topical irritant action, sometimes with superficial or deep capillary thrombosis and gastric mucosal necrosis.[30] Despite this fact, they may in large doses exert most of their unfavorable effect through the higher nerve centers, since intravenous therapy may produce the same symptoms of nausea and vomiting. Copper sulfate and ipecac, too, have central effects in addition to peripheral irritation. After absorption they have a direct action on the medullary chemoreceptor trigger zone, as shown by Wang and Borison.[20] Many of the drugs in common use today will occasionally cause anorexia or nausea due to peripheral irritation; the mycins are classic examples. This is a matter of individual tolerance, as it is with certain foodstuffs such as onions.

Irritation of the mucosa by amines is probably the mode of action of "spoiled" food. With regard to ingesta contaminated by bacteria, notably staphylococci, it is believed that nausea and vomiting are produced through the medium of toxins acting locally or, after absorption, centrally. The central effects of the enterotoxin have been proved experimentally, whereas the peripheral irritation rests more on clinical observation.[31] Acute gastric mucosal changes have been demonstrated gastroscopically as long as 3 to 4 weeks after a brief attack of food poisoning.[32] Likewise acute gastritis is blamed for the upsets occurring after the unwise ingestion of heavily seasoned food mixtures. Alcohol may cause acute gastritis if ingested in concentrated form or in large quantity. More often nausea and vomiting from alcohol is probably central in origin, since it can be demonstrated by intravenous injection that the action is similar to that of other anesthetics —irritation of hypothalamic nuclei.

Almost all drugs which give rise to nausea and vomiting when administered parenterally do so through direct action on the brain stem or the hypothalamus. The site of action of the majority of them is the vomiting center or the chemoreceptor trigger zone of Borison and Wang. This has been proved in many cases by the emetogenic action of minute amounts of the drug applied directly to the vomiting center of experimental animals. The classic example is apomorphine. Others are morphine, emetine, histamine and epinephrine. Because nicotine has a similar action, tobacco smoking, before tolerance is acquired, may initiate anorexia, nausea and emesis. The improvement in appetite when the use of tobacco is discontinued is a well known phenomenon, but other factors may be involved.

Amphetamine is widely and successfully used today for its ability to help obese patients lose weight by causing anorexia. This drug is among the central stimulants, but it acts upon the brain to reduce appetite. Its action is not affected by complete extrinsic denervation of the stomach and the intestine.[33] By improving mood it also has psychological benefit for those who eat excessively because of a neurosis.

For many years, following the investigations of Hatcher and Weiss, it was considered that digitalis exerted an emetic action through the stimulation of the vagal and sympathetic terminals in the overdigitalized heart.[34] They found that sectioning of the cardiac nerves in the cat abolished this emetic action. Many others since have challenged this opinion. In particular, Dresbach found that glycoside emesis could still be produced after cardiac deafferentation, abdominal vagotomy and complete

visceral deafferentation. These and other studies have demonstrated that digitalis definitely has a central action, placed by Borison and Wang in the medullary chemoreceptor zone.[35] They state, however, that their work proves the existence of peripheral receptors which lie outside of the gastrointestinal tract, and that it is these receptors which largely initiate the vomiting caused by orally administered digitalis. At the present time, therefore, it can be stated that the nausea and the vomiting accompanying excessive doses of the cardiac glycosides is definitely not due to gastrointestinal irritation, but there is not complete agreement about the role of other peripheral and central receptors.

The gastrointestinal effects and the central nervous system responses resulting from the oral intake of a concentrated toxic chemical substance (a poison) are protective in nature. The local enteric effects limit absorption and may result in emesis with ejection of the toxin. Even very small amounts of the toxin which may be absorbed and reach the chemoceptor trigger zone through the blood stream promote emesis.

A prototype for the sequence anorexia, nausea, and vomiting is provided by the chain of events which follows the ingestion of poison. Here, the series of reactions is highly appropriate and protective. Within a very few minutes after a poison such as ipecac or copper sulfate is swallowed, relaxation of the stomach wall occurs, with an accompanying marked slowing of gastric emptying or no emptying at all. The lining membrane of the stomach becomes pale and flat and the secretion of hydrochloric acid and other components of the gastric juice is greatly reduced. The welfare of the person is served by this type of reaction, since the lack of stomach activity reduces the likelihood of assimilation of the poison and the associated pale membrane and underactivity of the glands substantially reduce the likelihood of digestive activity and absorption within the stomach. Finally, the failure of the stomach to pass its contents on to the duodenum reduces the chance of absorption of the noxious material. When nausea and vomiting ultimately occur the body is able to rid itself of the ingested poison.

Acute febrile diseases, whatever the type of infection, often are heralded by loss of appetite; in children, particularly, nausea and vomiting are common. That this effect is not due primarily to fever itself is indicated by the fact that the anorexia may precede by many hours the rise in temperature. Further, artificial mechanical hyperthermia is entirely compatible with a good appetite. Therefore, it seems likely that the autonomic centers are affected by the toxicity that also produces headache, malaise and a feeling of general weakness. Whether the effect is produced by changes in blood volume, vasconstriction or changes in circulating hormones is not known. Chronic infections, e.g. pulmonary tuberculosis, brucellosis and empyema, presumably affect the appetite in much the same manner. Here, however, the effect of long-continued inadequate vitamin intake and poor absorption of vitamins and minerals must also be taken into consideration.

Some systemic diseases are attended by nausea and vomiting. Toxins, in the form of abnormal metabolites, are probably responsible in uremia and severe liver disease. The nature of the toxin is not as yet known in either of these diseases. Certainly in uremia it is not urea, uric acid or other known products of protein metabolism that are at fault, since these may be greatly elevated in the blood stream without concurrent nausea. Both in uremia and diabetic acidosis vomiting appears usually with the advent of acidosis; usually blood potassium is elevated and it is known experimentally that this can cause emesis. In Addison's disease nausea and vomiting are common; again changes in blood and tissue levels of electrolytes occur. Whether they then act as toxins on the emesis center cannot be stated. Obviously the lack of adrenocortical hormones themselves may be of much more fundamental importance, but the effect of such a lack on the gastrointestinal tract has not been well demonstrated. In hyperthyroidism, particularly in the crisis of thyrotoxicosis, there is marked irritability of the entire central nervous system, in which the emesis center presumably

shares. In diabetic patients, nausea and vomiting may result from gastroparesis as a result of stress.[36] This is probably due to an enteric peripheral neuropathy, similar to the neuropathy producing diarrhea.

VISCERAL

Allergy has been described as a cause of apparent poor appetite in children. They actually may have some degree of pain and nausea after eating foods to which they are sensitive and they translate these sensations into an expression of dislike for such foods. Acute intestinal allergy and Henoch's purpura produce spasm of the intestinal musculature, hyperemia and edema of the bowel wall, exudation, and peritoneal urticaria and hemorrhage. Although pain may be the most prominent symptom, nausea and vomiting are usually present. Irritative impulses arising in the wall of the bowel and the peritoneum reflexly give rise to the emesis and its premonitory symptom.

Obstruction to the passage of food and food residue anywhere in the gastrointestinal tract will eventually produce emesis. It is logical that the higher the obstruction the quicker the onset of vomiting. In pyloric obstruction, whether from ulcer or carcinoma, the stomach is able to compensate for a time by gradual stretching of the muscle fibers, without great increase in intragastric pressure. Tone is usually lost within a short time. As the dilatation increases the limit of elasticity is reached and the pressure rises. This is in itself a stimulus to nausea and vomiting, and makes regurgitation through the cardia easier. In hypertrophic pyloric stenosis of infancy the mechanism is presumably the same, i.e., rising intragastric pressure. In addition much of the gastric residue is simply regurgitated from the overfilled stomach, an action that takes place much more readily than it does in adults.

Intestinal obstruction may be caused by tumors, benign or malignant, cicatricial adhesions, volvulus, infections, etc. The violence of the symptoms will depend on whether the obstruction is high or low in the bowel, acute or chronic, partial or complete. If acute, the intestine orad to the blocked point has no chance to accommodate itself to the sudden increased pressure. If chronic, and hence incomplete, the bowel may dilate for some time, as the stomach does in gradually developing pyloric obstruction. It will hypertrophy and keep some of the chyme passing through the partially blocked lumen. In acute ileus there may be no actual mechanical obstructions. It is well recognized that functional intestinal obstruction can occur with bruising or disease of the intestinal wall, without narrowing of the lumen. According to the gradient theory of Alvarez the level of irritability of the bowel is raised at the point of trauma or disease, reversing the normal downward gradient for some distance above the irritated segment. When peristaltic waves reach the area of the reversed gradient they can no longer continue downward and gradually fade out. A localized distention then occurs. The generalized ileus which may eventually occur, with mechanical or functional obstruction, is a result of inhibition of the entire small bowel by the localized distention. The reflex is mediated by the sympathetic nerves, or experimentally even by the intrinsic pathways. The longer the section of bowel being distended, the lower the pressure that is required to elicit the reflex.[37] Distention, with increased intraluminal tension, is also the cause of the nausea and the vomiting accompanying the ileus.[38] Again the agent is the sympathetic nervous system, as shown by the fact that splanchnicotomy and excision of the lumbar chain will prevent emesis in intestinal obstruction or with simple distention. Experimentally, anorexia remains, unless the vagi are also cut.

In the ileus so often complicating the course of peritonitis, peritoneovisceral reflexes are responsible. It is possible to abolish the intestinal inhibition accompanying chemical (iodine) peritonitis by spinal anesthesia, which blocks inhibitory splanchnic impulses.[39]

Constipation. In many persons constipation will produce not only anorexia but also nausea, which disappears promptly with evacuation of the rectum. These symptoms, along with headache, mental depression and giddiness, are not, as was formerly thought, due to "auto-intoxication." This theory is disproved by the rapidity with which the symptoms disappear after evacuation of the rectum, by failure to find toxins in the blood and by reproduction of the symptoms when an inert material such as cotton is stuffed into the rectum.[40] Actually, the nausea is the result of viscerovisceral reflexes, similar to those seen in more severe form in intestinal obstruction. "Biliousness," another term used to describe this syndrome, would suggest that a "sluggish liver" rather than constipation is at fault. Calomel usually will give relief from biliousness, but is it through its laxative rather than its supposed choleretic action.

Diseases of the stomach frequently are heralded first by the appearance of anorexia. In linitis plastica the appetite invariably is decreased, as might be expected from the diffuse involvement of the musculature and the nerve terminals. In other types of gastric carcinoma anorexia may be an early or a late symptom. Although victims of peptic ulcer may have a lowered food intake it is the fear of pain following the meal rather than a poor appetite that is responsible. Usually, however, the appetite is excellent and the caloric intake entirely adequate. A direct effect on the gastric tonus may be the mechanism of production of anorexia in acute and chronic gastritis. In the latter condition, however, neurotic factors may be partly responsible, since in many cases chronic gastritis is associated with a psychic disturbance.

Acute inflammatory diseases of the abdominal and pelvic organs cause nausea, and frequently vomiting as well, primarily through viscerovisceral reflexes. Particularly common offenders are acute appendicitis, salpingitis, cholecystitis, hepatitis and pancreatitis. In all cases the physiologic mechanism is essentially the same. Stimuli pass through the vagus and the splanchnic afferent fibers to the medullary vomiting centers, where synaptic connections are made with efferent vagal, splanchnic and spinal nerves to the pharynx, the esophagus, the cardia, the stomach, the abdominal muscles and the diaphragm. Viscerovisceral reflexes are also responsible for the nausea and the vomiting of gall-stone and kidney stone colic. As previously noted, with peritonitis there are peritoneovisceral reflexes which produce ileus. These same reflexes initiate vomiting. Many patients with acute hepatitis have been observed gastroscopically with the thought that gastric mucosal changes might account for the usual occurrence of nausea. Some patients show a superficial form of gastritis, but the changes are not consistent enough to cause anorexia or emesis.[41]

The nausea and vomiting of pregnancy continues to pose questions which cannot yet be answered with finality. Many theories of its etiology have been considered; none have met widespread acceptance.[42] According to one viewpoint the important factors are carbohydrate starvation, decreased liver glycogen reserve and dehydration with ketosis. According to another, avitaminosis B, particularly a lack of pyridoxine, is responsible. Various endocrine factors associated with pregnancy have been incriminated by other authors, among them low estrogen levels, adrenocortical failure, allergy to the corpus luteum hormone, and some substance produced by the growing chorion. Many obstetricians today believe that neurotic influences are the most important, since the nausea and vomiting of pregnancy occurs so frequently in the tense, emotionally high-strung patient. However, this may simply mean that the vomiting center is more sensitively "triggered" in these persons, and not that there is always a protest against pregnancy on the part of the subconscious mind. The preceding discussion, of course, applies only to the disturbances of early pregnancy, not to those occurring later in the pre-eclamptic and eclamptic states. Among the maze of possible causes mentioned it is impossible to pick only one that is supported by overwhelming evidence. Indeed, it is possible that many or all of them may, at different times and in different persons, be active.

Disease of the heart may cause gastrointestinal disturbances of considerable severity. In acute and chronic congestive failure it is most often edema of the liver and the intestine that produces nausea and vomiting, although impulses arising in a dilated heart muscle may be contributory in the acute variety. Certainly in acute coronary spasm or occlusion the afferent limb of the vomiting reflex must traverse fibers originating in the ischemic cardiac muscle. In congestive failure, however, changes in blood and tissue electrolytes, particularly potassium, must be considered. Some of these changes are induced by the physician, and account for the profound anorexia following overvigorous diuretic measures. Then too, it is important to distinguish anorexia and nausea of heart failure from that as a result of digitalis toxicity.

Other Visceral Diseases. With chronic renal disease anorexia is often a severe and disturbing symptom. It may be due to reflex changes in gastric tonus resulting from impulses arising in the diseased kidneys themselves. However, many other factors may be wholly or partly responsible, among them the toxicity and the acidosis associated with nitrogen retention, edema of the gastrointestinal mucosa, nutritional deficiency, drugs such as ammonium chloride which cause irritation of the intestinal mucosa and psychological disturbance attendant on an unpalatable salt-poor diet. The visceroviseral reflexes here involved are readily understandable if it is recalled that the urinary tract has a common autonomic nerve supply with the gastrointestinal tract.

Cirrhosis of the liver commonly causes loss of appetite. Among the etiologic factors may be nutritional deficiencies, visceroviseral reflexes, the direct effect of circulating toxins due to failure of the detoxifying function of the liver and to chronic gastritis.[46]

In pulmonary disease, particularly tuberculosis and bronchiectasis, nausea and vomiting often occur following a paroxysm of coughing. The cough, especially when productive of offensive sputum, causes gagging by direct stimulation of the pharynx. Again, as with any chronic disease, nutritional defects may be an additional factor.

DEFICIENCIES

Severe avitaminosis invariably causes anorexia. The evidence at the present time indicates that the vitamins of the B group are primarily responsible. Williams and co-workers showed that subjects fed diets adequate in every known respect except in regard to thiamine develop a loss of appetite very early.[43] Concomitant with the appearance of anorexia there was found a lowered gastric acidity to a test meal and impairment of gastrointestinal motility by roentgenographic examination after a barium meal. Function became normal after thiamine therapy. The longer the period of deprivation, the slower was the return of appetite to normal. Other vitamin B fractions may be important. Vitamin B_{12} produces a remarkable increase in appetite (even when given orally) to children who are malnourished or who are recovering from simple growth failure.[44] Lack of any of these and other factors that are necessary for optimum nutrition interferes with muscle and nerve cell metabolism and hence causes lowered gastric and intestinal muscle tonus. Nutrional influences upon cerebral centers is not so well known, but obviously may be of even more importance in influencing the sensation of appetite.

Fasting and Starvation. The effect of fasting and starvation on appetite is known to be deleterious after several days, but the resulting lack of interest in food depends on a number of factors, some of which have been discussed already. It is an interesting fact that anorexia may appear at a time when the stomach is still hypertonic, indicating that psychic and organocerebral depression may be of most importance. Complete lack of food and water quickly leads to loss of chloride and sodium and rise in the blood potassium level. If water is available but no food, hydration may be maintained for some time, and the chemical balance is not disturbed quickly. It is a seeming paradox that animals deprived of one important factor in metabolism, such as chloride, will die sooner than when starved completely.

Endocrine Disorders. Allusion has already been made to endocrine deficiencies. Hypothyroidism usually causes anorexia. There is a generalized slowing of the metabolic processes, with impaired gastrointestinal motility and tone. Presumably the hypothalamic nuclei are involved as well. In Addison's disease profound anorexia, nausea and vomiting are common. Little is known about the effect on the alimentary tissues of lack of adrenocortical hormones. It seems likely that the symptoms are related more to biochemical changes and the attendant disturbance of function in the hypothalamic nuclei. Potassium retention has been shown to have an adverse effect on food intake.

MOTION SICKNESS

Motion sickness is a term used to designate inclusively seasickness, airsickness, trainsickness, etc., all having a common physiopathologic background involving numerous etiologic factors. The symptoms, in the order of their appearance, are anorexia, apathy, salivation, sweating, nausea, headache and vomiting. Both motion sickness and caloric stimulation of the labyrinth are associated with decreased gastric tone, peristalsis and secretion. Hence there is little doubt of the importance of labyrinthine impulses in the causation of this syndrome. The exact site in the labyrinth has been determined to be the utricular macula, and the type of motion a linear acceleration.[45] The changes in tone and motility of the gastrointestinal tract are obviously secondary ones, since the impulses transmitted over the vestibular nerve would go first to the midbrain and the hypothalamus. Nevertheless, gastrointestinal factors are of primary etiologic importance in jolting or in rapid elevator acceleration or deceleration, where pull on the mesentery occurs.

Other sources of stimuli which, in addition to the labyrinth and the gastrointestinal tract, may at times play a role in the causation of motion sickness are psychic, olfactory, visual and proprioceptive nerve endings. For example, a sailor in rough seas may be fairly comfortable when he is lying in his bunk. When he comes on deck and watches the rolling waves he may become ill. The summation of labyrinthine, optic and proprioceptive stimuli may result in vomiting, when motion-induced impulses from the labyrinth alone do not.

The vestibular nerve is the afferent limb of the reflex which causes the nausea and vomiting accompanying the vertigo of Ménière's disease, and that following the "fenestration" operation. Other disorders involving the vestibulocerebellar pathways, including otitis media, act similarly.

SUMMARY

Appetite is a conditioned reflex, a state of anticipation, stimulated by the smell, the sight or even the memory of agreeable food. Hunger is a primitive, unconditioned physiologic state due to privation of food. As commonly used, the term anorexia indicates lack of both appetite and hunger. Of importance in its causation are the emotional state, chemical and vascular changes from the norm and impulses transmitted to the brain from the viscera and other organs.

It is only a step from anorexia (lack of desire for food) to nausea (a feeling of revulsion for food). Likewise, nausea thus is considered to be largely of central origin. It may or may not result in its logical consequence, vomiting.

The vomiting center in the medulla receives impulses from the viscera, from the higher centers in the nervous system, and from the chemoreceptor trigger zone (CTZ) located nearby. Centrally-acting emetic drugs, formerly thought to stimulate the vomiting center directly, apparently excite the CTZ or forebrain or hypothalamus, which then transmit impulses to the medullary vomiting center.

As might be expected from the importance of the psychic element in appetite, the most frequent sources of anorexia and nausea are the neuroses. Pain, fright and grief, offensive smells, tastes and sights are associated with reflex inhibition of the stomach mediated through the higher nerve centers. The increased sensitiveness of the emesis center associated with concussion, brain tumor, brain abscess and cerebral hemorrhage is probably due to interference with the blood supply to the center.

Drugs may bring about anorexia, or nausea and vomiting, in one of two ways. Many of them (mercury, copper sulfate and aminophylline) cause gastric or intestinal mucosal irritation, with stimulation of the emesis center by vagal or sympathetic nerve fibers. Others (apomorphine, nicotine, alcohol and amphetamine) act directly on the brain centers after absorption into the circulation. Still others (digitalis and staphylococcus toxin) have more than one mode of action.

Acute febrile diseases affect food intake adversely by general "toxicity." Presumably toxins are responsible also in uremia and in severe liver disease. In other chronic diseases nutritional factors are often important.

In the case of "visceral" causes of anorexia, nausea and vomiting, stimuli arising in the inflamed or diseased viscus are transmitted centrally over the vagus or sympathetic nerves. Food allergy, intestinal obstruction, constipation, intestinal neoplasms, appendicitis and cholecystitis are examples of abdominal visceral disorders which may sharply limit food intake. In cardiac decompensation, edema of the liver and dilatation of the heart chambers may be contributory.

Nutritional and endocrine deficiencies interfere with muscle and nerve cell metabolism, peripheral as well as central, and hence reduce appetite. The results of total starvation experiments involve so many different factors that it is difficult to state why anorexia occurs within a few days. Presumably it is related to the general slowing down of metabolic processes which is designed to conserve the bodily reserves.

Motion sickness is produced primarily by the effect of linear accelerations on the labyrinth. However, other contributing stimuli may be optic, olfactory and gastrointestinal.

REFERENCES

1. Kuntz, A.: On the occurrence of reflex arcs in myenteric and submucous plexuses, Anat. Rec. 24:193-210, 1922.
2. Thomas, J. E.: The autonomic nervous system in gastrointestinal disease, J.A.M.A. 157:209-212, 1955.
3. ———: Recent advances in gastrointestinal physiology, Gastroenterology 12:545-555, 1949.

4. Bingham, J. R., Ingelfinger, F. J., and Smithwick, R. H.: The effects of sympathectomy on the motility of the human gastrointestinal and biliary tracts, Gastroenterology 15: 6-17, 1950.

5. Cannon, W. B., and Washburn, A. L.: An explanation of hunger, Am. J. Physiol. 29: 441-454, 1912.

6. Grossman, M. I., and Stein, I. F., Jr.: Vagotomy and the hunger-producing action of insulin in man, J. Appl. Physiol. 1:263-269, 1948; Anand, B. K., and Brobeck, J. R.: Localization of "feeding center" in hypothalamus of rat, Yale J. Biol. and Med. 24: 141, 1951.

7. Grossman, M. I., Cummins, G. M., and Ivy, A. C.: The effect of insulin on food intake after vagotomy and sympathectomy, Am. J. Physiol. 149:100-104, 1947.

8. Mayer, J.: Genetic, traumatic and environmental factors in the etiology of obesity, Physiol. Rev. 33:472-508, 1953.

9. Share, I., Martyniuk, E., and Grossman, M. I.: Effect of prolonged intragastric feeding on oral food intake in dogs, Am. J. Physiol. 169:229, 1952.

10. Grossman, M. I.: Integration of current views on the regulation of hunger and appetite, Army Medical Nutrition Laboratory Report 145, (Dec.) 1954.

11. Barclay, A. E.: The Digestive Tract, New York, Macmillan, 1936, p. 85.

12. Wolf, S., and Wolff, H. G.: Human Gastric Function, London, Oxford, 1943, p. 111.

13. Goetzl, F. R., Goldschmidt, M., Wheeler, P., and Stone, F.: Influence of sugar upon olfactory acuity and upon the sensation complex of appetite and satiety, Gastroenterology 12:252-256, 1949.

14. Janowitz, H. D., and Grossman, M. I.: Gusto-olfactory thresholds in relation to appetite and hunger sensations, J. Appl. Physiol. 2:217-222, 1949.

15. Wolf, S.: Observations on the occurrence of nausea among combat soldiers, Gastroenterology 8:15-18, 1947.

16. Wolf, S., and Wolff, H. G.: Human Gastric Function, London, Oxford, 1943, p. 146.

17. Oppenheimer, M. J., and Mann, F. C.: Role of small intestine during emesis, Am. J. Dig. Dis. 8:86-89, 1941.

18. Abbott, F. K., Mack, M., and Wolf, S.: The relation of sustained duodenal contraction to nausea and vomiting, Gastroenterology 20:238-248, 1952.

19. Grossman, M. I., Woolley, J. R., Dutton, D. F., and Ivy, A. C.: The effect of nausea on gastric secretion, Gastroenterology 4:347-351, 1945.

20. Borison, H. L., and Wang, S. C.: Physiology and pharmacology of vomiting, Pharmacol. Rev. 5:193-230, 1953.

21. Borison, H. L.: Personal communication.

22. Gregory, R. A.: Changes in intestinal tone and motility associated with nausea and vomiting, J. Physiol. 105:58-66, 1946.

23. Räsänen, T.: A mucosal bleeding mechanism in the upper part of the gastrointestinal tract, Gastroenterology 44:168-177, 1963.

24. Reed, J. A.: A study of gastric acids in prefrontal lobotomy, Gastroenterology 10:118-119, 1948.

25. Bliss, E. L.: Anorexia nervosa: psychogenic malnutrition, South. Med. Journ. 56:529-533, 1963.

26. Wolf, S., and Wolff, H. G.: Human Gastric Function, London, Oxford, 1943.

27. Henschel, A., Taylor, H. L., and Keys, A.: The gastric emptying time of man at high and normal environmental temperatures, Am. J. Physiol. 141:205-208, 1944.

28. Sanchez-Palomera, E.: Action of spices on acid gastric secretion, on appetite and on caloric intake, Gastroenterology 18:254-268, 1951.

29. Beazell, J. M., and Ivy, A. C.: The influence of alcohol on the digestive tract, Quart. J. Stud. on Alcohol 1:45-73, 1940-1941.

30. Roth, J. L. A., Valdes-Dapena, A., Pieses, P., and Buchman, E.: Topical action of salicylates in gastrointestinal erosion and hemorrhage, Gastroent. 44:146-158, 1963.

31. Bayliss, M.: Mechanism of vomiting produced by Staphylococcus enterotoxin, J. Exper. Med. 72:669-684, 1940.

32. Schwartz, I. R.: A gastroscopic study following an outbreak of food poisoning, Gastroenterology 6:105-108, 1946.

33. Harris, S. C., Ivy, A. C., and Searle, L. M.: The mechanism of amphetamine-induced weight loss, J.A.M.A. 134:1468-1475, 1947.

34. Hatcher, R. A., and Weiss, S.: Reflex vomiting from the heart, J.A.M.A. 89:429-432, 1927.

35. Borison, H. L., and Wang, S. C.: Locus of the central emetic action of the cardiac glycosides, Proc. Soc. Exper. Biol. & Med. 76: 335-338, 1951.

36. Howland, W. J., and Drinkard, R. V.: Acute diabetic gastric atony, J.A.M.A. 185:214-216, 1963.

37. Youmans, W. B.: The intestino-intestinal inhibitory reflex, Gastroenterology 3:114-118, 1944.

38. Herrin, R. C., and Meek, W. J.: Afferent nerves excited by intestinal distention, Am. J. Physiol. 144: 720-723, 1945.

39. Walton, F. E., Moore, R. M., and Graham, E. A.: The nerve pathways in the vomiting of peritonitis, Arch. Surg. 22:829-837, 1931.

40. Alvarez, W. C.: Intestinal autointoxication, Physiol. Rev. 4:352-393, 1924.

41. Bank, J., and Dixon, C. H.: Gastroscopy in acute and chronic hepatitis, J.A.M.A. 131: 107-108, 1946.

42. Hall, M. B.: Nausea and vomiting in pregnancy, Am. J. Med. Sc. 205:869-875, 1943.

43. Williams, R. D., Mason, H. L., Wilder, R. M., and Smith, B. F.: Observations on induced thiamin deficiency in man, Arch. Int. Med. 66:785-789, 1940.

44. Wetzel, N. C., Fargo, W. C., Smith, I. H., and Helikson, J.: Growth failure in school children as associated with vitamin B_{12} deficiency—response to oral therapy, Science 110:651-653, 1949.

45. Shaw, C. C.: A common dynamic factor in motion sickness, Mil. Surgeon 114:347-350, 1954.

46. Dagradi, A. E., Olson, D., and Stempien, S.: The gastric mucosa in liver cirrhosis, Gastroenterology 31:74-78, 1956.

47. Wolf, S.: Studies on nausea. Effects of ipecac and other emetics on the human stomach and duodenum, Gastroenterology 12:212, 1949.

48. Wolf, S.: The relation of gastric function to nausea in man, J. Clin. Invest. 22:887, 1943.

19

Constipation and Diarrhea

JOHN L. HORNER

It is important at the outset of this discussion to define in what sense the terms constipation and diarrhea will be used, since the patient's statements of these complaints often cannot be taken at face value. This is particularly true with regard to constipation, for lay persons vary widely in their concept of what constitutes normal bowel action. Does the patient mean that he does not have a bowel action every day; that the stool is too hard, or too small; or that he never has a feeling of complete evacuation? The details may reveal that he needs reassurance rather than a laxative. Before attempting a precise definition, therefore, it is necessary to discuss the normal physiology concerned with the formation of feces.

Within a few minutes after food enters the stomach some of it passes into the duodenum. The rate of gastric emptying depends upon a number of factors, among them the quantity and the quality of the food, the emotional state of the individual, his nutritional status and the time interval since the previous food intake. On the average, after an ordinary mixed meal, the stomach is empty in 3 to 4 hours. With a meal containing much fat there may be a a delay of 6 hours or more.

In the small intestine the rate of transmission of chyme is relatively rapid in the duodenum and jejunum, slowing considerably in the ileum, particularly in the distal 12 to 14 inches. A mixed meal will begin to pass through the ileocolic sphincter in from 2 to 3 hours after it is consumed and will have completed its passage into the cecum in from 6 to 9 hours. The consistency of the food mass remains semiliquid throughout the small gut. A great deal of the water content is absorbed, but the fluid is partially replaced by the addition of pancreatic juice, bile and succus entericus.

Stool which enters the cecum in a semiliquid state is ejected from the rectum as a soft, formed, plastic mass. Most of this transformation takes place in the cecum and the ascending colon, since there is some molding of the fecal material by the time it has reached the proximal transverse colon. This does not involve as much change in water content as might be imagined, since liquid stool may contain as little as 10 per cent more water than the hardest scyballum. The mucosa of the proximal colon thus contains an efficient mechanism for absorbing water. It apparently can also absorb some products of bacterial decomposition and can excrete certain substances, particularly potassium and heavy metals. In the cecum there is considerable mixing of the residue from one meal with that of previous meals.

Understanding of normal intestinal and colonic motility has been obscured by the variety of results obtained by different methods of study. Much has been learned from fluoroscopic observation of a barium suspension and from placing of liquid- or air-filled balloons in the intestine, but these two methods introduce factors which are certainly not physiologic in the gastrointestinal tract. Two recent methods of study, (1) the swallowing of a radiotelemetering capsule,[1] and (2) the use of water-filled polyethylene tubes,[2] produce much less interference with normal gastrointestinal function. When one puts the results of all these studies together it seems likely that food residue passes down the intestine primarily because there is a progressive decrease in the frequency and intensity of the muscle contractions from duodenum to rectum, with mass peristalsis playing a secondary role. The time involved in this passage depends somewhat on intestinal tone, since increased tone reduces propulsive motility.

Recent years have brought renewed interest in the factors controlling normal intestinal motility, particularly with regard to the role of the autonomic nervous system and various hormones and enzymes. It has long been known that the gastrointestinal tract *can* continue to function effectively after degenerative section of its extrinsic nerve supply, yet it probably is not autonomous in the intact animal or man. Under normal conditions the vagus, the splanchnic and the pelvic nerves may play a significant role in transmitting impulses between the central nervous system and the viscera. These connections are shown in Plate 3. The parasympathetic efferent supply of the small bowel and the proximal third of the colon is supplied via the vagus and that of the remainder of the colon via the lower sacral segments of the spinal cord, through the pelvic nerves. The splanchnic nerves supply the sympathetic innervation. The afferent autonomic nerve distribution is also through the vagus, the splanchnic and the pelvic nerves. (p. 352)

Of the several types of muscular activity encountered in the small intestine, the segmenting and pendular movements (movements of mixing and churning) are inherent in the muscle itself. The peristaltic contractions are accomplished through local myenteric reflexes,[3] but it is usually considered that they may be augmented by vagus and pelvic efferent impulses and inhibited by splanchnic efferent impulses. Augmentation and inhibition effects are likewise exerted by these nerves on the tone of the intestine. The sympathetic fibers are believed to exert a continuous inhibitory effect, whereas the vagal impulses are intermittent.

Similarly, in the colon the chief effect of sympathetic activity is inhibition, although this may not be apparent in post-sympathectomy patients except under conditions of stress. Hence the tone and the peristaltic activity of the small bowel and colon may be profoundly affected by impulses received through their extrinsic nerves—impulses that may originate in the higher nerve centers or in the cord as part of a reflex arc.

Of course the influence of the nervous system cannot be considered without also taking into account the chemicals which are released when these nerves are stimulated. Acetylcholine is produced at the terminals of the parasympathetic postganglionic fibers and thus increases tone and activity of the intestine. It is also a factor in transmission of all preganglionic and some sympathetic postganglionic impulses.[4] Most sympathetic postganglionic nerves release norepinephrine (and perhaps epinephrine) and are therefore termed "adrenergic." Much recent work suggests that serotonin (5-hydroxytryptamine), found in large quantities in the intestinal tract, alters intestinal motility in the direction of increased activity. The release of serotonin is probably not controlled by extrinsic nerves,[5] since its site of action is distal to the ganglionic synapse. Its release may possibly be controlled by neural elements within the intestinal wall.[6] At present the available evidence indicates that serotonin helps to regulate peristaltic activity by mediating pressure reception in the mucosa. Other chemicals may be important in normal intestinal motor function—certainly potassium plays a role in the functioning of nerve and muscle cells within the gut wall.

With this brief description of the normal physiologic processes in mind, it is now possible to attempt a definition of terms.

Constipation may be considered as simply undue delay in the evacuation of feces. This

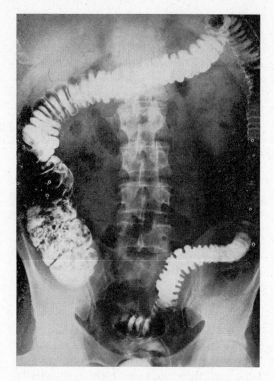

FIG. 104. Often this type of hypertonic or "spastic" colon is associated with constipation, due to failure of normal transit in the descending colon.

usually results in the passage of hard dry stools, or no stool at all for an inordinate number of days. The evacuation of hard stools is accomplished only with some difficulty involving excessive use of the voluntary muscles. The definition here given does not imply that there need normally be a bowel movement every 24 hours. There are healthy persons who pass a well-formed stool of normal consistency once every two or even three or more days. They are not constipated. The definition does not imply that the constipated stool is small, though it may be if it contains less water and fiber. Neither does it imply that there need be a feeling of gratification, of complete evacuation, after defecation, though this normally occurs. A feeling of incomplete evacuation may be due to local conditions in the rectum or, more frequently, to psychic factors.

Diarrhea, as the opposite of constipation,

means undue precipitation in the passage of the feces, with resultant discharge of loose stools. It may, or may not, be accompanied by abdominal cramping or tenesmus. The number of stools does not enter into the definition of diarrhea, although commonly the frequency of the bowel movements is increased. In regard to both of these definitions it has been suggested that the disorder must be habitual before it can be considered either constipation or diarrhea. This technicality can be disposed of if the modifying adjectives, acute and chronic, are used.

CAUSES OF CONSTIPATION

By definition, any factor that delays evacuation of the feces is a cause of constipation. For purposes of logical discussion some classification of such factors is obviously desirable, and, since the viewpoint of this presentation is physiologic, a classification based on physiologic causes will be attempted. We are not interested here in a differential diagnosis. We are interested in "why". Therefore the following headings will be used: *central,* indicating that the underlying cause is in the central nervous system; *reflex,* the disturbance being secondary to visceral disease or malfunction; and *mechanical,* suggesting a breakdown in the anatomic factors necessary for normal healthy defecation. As with any physiologic classification based on imperfect knowledge, some overlapping will occur, and an etiologic factor, if completely elucidated, might account for disturbances under several of these functional headings. From time to time attention will be called to such difficulties.

CENTRAL CONSTIPATION

Lack of Regularity. Although the number of causes that can be listed under this heading is small, the number of patients suffering from these causes is disproportionately large. When stool enters the rectum in sufficient quantity to stimulate the pressure receptors, the patient is aware of the need to defecate but is able to overcome the need by voluntary contraction of the external sphincter and associated muscles. The rectum then adjusts itself to the increased tension and ceases to send out afferent impulses, or the rectum may actually return stool into the sigmoid. If this is done habitually, the reflex ceases to function. The difficulty may stem from lack of childhood training, or more often from failure of adults to allow sufficient time because of the pressures of business, family responsibilities or overcrowded toilet facilities.

Constipation of this type might be considered in the reflex category, since it is the defecation reflex that fails eventually; but the primary disorganization is central, since the reflex (unlike that of undomesticated animals) is a conditioned one—conditioned to time and to type of activity. The constipation that many persons experience when traveling is often ascribed to the "change in water." Actually, in most cases, it is the conditioned reflex which temporarily breaks down.

Excessive Tone. Another large group of constipated persons suffers from excessive tone of the circular muscle of the intestines, particularly of the distal colon, induced by an imbalance of the autonomic nervous system. Experimentally, markedly increased contraction of the colon has been observed with a wide variety of stressful situations, such as exposure to cold, pain, compression of the head and discussion of troublesome life situations.[7] Further, patients with spastic colons overreact to prostigmine. Since it is well known that excessive tone (spasm) interferes with propulsive motility, it is easy to understand why these patients have difficulty with constipation, and why the stool produced is usually small in character and segmented. This is a central type of constipation, since it must be presumed that cortical and subcortical impulses travel to parasympathetic centers, with resultant activation of sacral, and possibly vagal, fibers supplying the colon. (Fig. 104)

Psychogenic. Constipation may result from certain types of acute emotional disturbances (grief, anger, abject fear) which produce increased epinephrine production with inhibition of peristalsis.[8] Paranoid psychoses are often accompanied by constipation. Such patients often exhibit marked chronic fear and anger.

Acute infectious diseases may be associated with absent or difficult defecation. This may be central effect from toxemia, but a breakdown in the conditioned reflex, as well as a lack of food and fluid, may be a contributory factor. The specific action of some toxins on the gastrointestinal tract will be considered later.

Traumatic lesions and organic diseases of the nervous system, such as tabes dorsalis, multiple sclerosis, brain and cord tumors, meningitis and the like, may produce constipation. Stimuli from the higher nerve centers may directly influence bowel activity. Such influences are evident from both clinical and experimental studies. Cord involvement is, however, more likely to upset gastrointestinal motility than are diseases of the brain, possibly because the effect may be on only one set of autonomic nerves, leaving the "opposing" set in control. For example, tabes dorsalis may activate parasympathetic nerve fibers and produce severe hypertonus, which interferes with peristaltic activity. Traumatic lesions may destroy efferent nerves concerned with the defecation reflex. When the spinal cord is unable to recognize the presence of stool in the rectum there is no stimulus to start the reflex. At the higher level, again, many patients with strokes are unable to recognize the pressure produced by rectal stool accumulation. These patients are usually constipated at first, and are then likely to have involuntary liquid stools as the spinal cord takes over the reflex.

Drugs. A few drugs, given orally or parenterally, delay the passage of intestinal contents. *Morphine* and, to a lesser extent, *codeine,* increase the tone of the small intestine and the colon, decreasing propulsive motility. In the small intestine this is followed by atony in about 1 hour. The colon becomes atonic in 3 or 4 hours. Efforts to block the effect of morphine by various means have shown that its spasmogenic action is mediated through postganglionic fibers of the extrinsic intestinal nerves, but whether by stimulation of the cholinergic fibers or by blocking the adrenergic inhibitory supply is not known. The latter is suggested by recent in vitro experiments.[9]

Atropine decreases motility by paralyzing parasympathetic nerve terminals. So do the synthetic parasympathetic drugs, such as elorine,[10] probanthine, etc. Tetraethylammonium chloride, which paralyzes both parasympathetic and sympathetic nerve terminals, produces almost complete inertness of the bowel as does dibutoline, which, like atropine, is parasympatholytic, but also has a direct inhibitory action on nonstriated muscle.

REFLEX CONSTIPATION

In this classification are included many conditions and diseases related to each other only by their reflex inhibition or failure to support integrated bowel motility and defecation.

Lack of sufficient bulky foods in the ingesta may cause deficient reflex activity. It is commonly thought that bulk is directly proportional to the fiber content of foods, but this is not necessarily true.[11] Some fiber-containing foods (such as fruit) are digested to a considerable extent, whereas others (such as bran) remain completely undigested. Furthermore, there are several factors other than bulk which are responsible for the laxative action of these foods. These are organic acids produced by bacterial decomposition, increased bacterial residue, moisture content and the highly dispersed gases which are liberated. Certain fruits have laxative properties due to unique chemical constituents. In prunes this is di-hydroxyphenyl isalin. Because of these variables it is not always possible to predict what the effect of ingestion of fiber-containing foods on bowel motility will be in a given individual, but the great majority of persons will be constipated on a diet rich in concentrated sweets, pastries and protein foods, because there will not be adequate enteric stimuli to peristalsis.

Excessive use of laxatives may lead to constipation by overstimulating the bowel and "wearing out" the effect; therefore most habitually constipated persons have to abandon a favorite laxative after a time for another with a slightly different mode of action. The sensitive nerve terminals in the intestinal mucosa presumably become fatigued or perhaps even damaged. However, the fact often unrealized by the patient is that the bowel cannot be expected to resume activity after purgation until enough residue from food ingestion has accumulated to stimulate peristalsis.

Heart Failure. In the constipation so frequently accompanying congestive heart failure many factors are involved. The patient is often poorly nourished, the diet is inadequate in bulk, and there is lack of physical activity as in any chronic illness. In addition there is hypoxia. With lowered oxygen pressures, there is depression of motor activity of the colon due to hypoxic stimulation of the sympathetic nervous system, and probably also to a direct inhibition of local metabolic processes.

Peptic ulcer recurrences are often associated with constipation. Pyloric obstruction may obviate normal intestinal peristaltic initiation, ulcer medications inhibit peristalsis and dietary restrictions may fail to provide sufficient bulk.

Inflammation of the abdominal and pelvic viscera is frequently a cause of constipation through a viscerovisceral reflex mechanism. Peritonitis is a particularly powerful stimulant of the sympathetic inhibitory nerves, with the production of the classic *paralytic ileus,* but appendicitis, salpingitis and cholecystitis may have a similar effect. In patients with cholecystitis and cholelithiasis there is the additional factor of failure of excretion of concentrated bile which has somewhat of a cathartic action. In all of these illnesses enforced bed rest and diet limitations may discourage bowel activity.

Intrinsic lesions of the ileum and colon, even though not mechanically obstructing, may cause constipation through viscerovisceral reflex inhibition. Even a very localized distention may reflexly inhibit the entire small bowel. In many patients there is the additional mechanical factor of the difficulty of forcing an already formed stool through a narrow lumen, such as occurs in *annular carcinoma* and *diverticulitis.* With *hemorrhoids, cryptitis, anal fissure* and *perirectal abscess* it is often found that stool does not even enter the rectum because of inhibition of sigmoid function. Further, because of the natural reluctance of the patient to experience pain, he does not attempt to force hard stool which has entered the ampulla through the spastic anus. The spasm is, of course, a very local reflex action in which the external nerve supply is not involved.

Extra-alimentary tumors, such as fibroids of the uterus, large ovarian cysts, hypernephromata and gravid uteri may produce constipation by the mechanical effect of narrowing the bowel lumen by compression, or through viscerovisceral reflexes. Acute renal diseases, such as glomerulonephritis, renal lithiasis and hydronephrosis, may cause reflex ileus through stimulation of the nerve supply in the distended or inflamed kidney capsule.

MECHANICAL CONSTIPATION

The bowel may be unable to move the chyme or stool distally in the usual length of time because of weakness of the bowel muscles, weakness of the voluntary muscles of defecation, an abnormal physical state of the bowel content or mechanical obstruction of the lumen of the bowel. In these situations, there may be no abnormal reflex activity and no disturbing impulses directly from the central nervous system.

Weakness of the intestinal muscles occurs in cachexia from any cause, in congenital hypoplasia or atony of the bowel, and particularly in senile hypoplasia. Hypothyroidism leads to slowed function, tissue edema and eventually atrophy of the muscles of the intestine as elsewhere. Deficiency of specific factors may be at fault; well known is the sluggish intestinal motility found with thiamin deficiency and lack of adequate amounts of niacin. These members of the vitamin B group are needed in the synthesis of coenzymes required in muscle and nerve cell metabolism. However, severe niacin lack causes diarrhea, through a mechanism to be explained later. Lowered serum calcium leads to impaired gut motility. Potassium, too, plays a role in normal functioning of nerve and muscle cells within the intestinal wall, and a decreased potassium concentration may lead to intestinal paralysis.[12]

The constipating action of lead is probably due to spasm of the smooth muscle caused by direct irritation. However, there may be additional damage to the intrinsic and extrinsic nerves. Iron is commonly thought to cause constipation by producing muscle spasm. A recent study utilizing the double blind technic throws doubt on the idea that there is any actual intestinal intolerance to iron.[13]

Weakness of the voluntary muscles occurs with cachexia, obesity, emphysema, pregnancy and ascites. Because of the important role of the abdominal, the pelvic and the diaphragmatic muscles in initiating and completing defecation in man, diseases affecting the strength of these muscles will obviously make evacuation difficult. This is seen most conspicuously in the stretching and thinning of muscle tissue associated with severe rectocoele. An additional mechanical factor here involved is the angulation of the ampulla, causing the propulsive force to be directed against the perineum rather than toward the anus.

Dehydration is a cause of constipation only when it is extreme, as a result of prolonged vomiting, diabetic acidosis and the like. Seldom can bowel function be improved in the normal individual by forcing fluids, since the ileum and the colon are perfectly capable of absorbing the additional water.[11] The length of the colon may, in some persons, favor constipation because of the opportunity for excessive absorption; theoretically, at least, marked redundancy of the distal segments of the bowel should result in hard dry stools which would be passed with difficulty. This has nothing to do with the long-discredited "ptosis" of the bowel. It is now recognized that the position of the intestine in the abdominal cavity has little to do with its function, and that the transverse colon in the upright person is normally in the pelvis, and not, as was originally thought, in the hypochondrium.

Megacolon. In Hirschsprung's disease a section of rectum including the internal anal sphincter is congenitally without myenteric or submucosal plexuses.[14] Blockage occurs because peristalsis cannot pass through this section. Further, this segment is narrowed because smooth muscle contracts when separated from the nearest ganglion cell.

Mechanical obstruction, of such a degree that even strong intestinal and abdominal muscles cannot force the intestinal content through it, is usually acute. A gradually developing stenosis is more likely to produce constipation through reflex inhibition. Common causes of acute obstruction are strangulated hernia, intussusception and volvulus.

CAUSES OF DIARRHEA

By definition, any factor that hastens evacuation of the feces may be a cause of diarrhea. However, hypermotility in the small bowel and the proximal colon can be compensated for by slightly longer retention and dehydration in the distal colon. Furthermore, hypermotility in the distal colon may result in little abnormality if the stool is already of normal consistency. It is helpful to recall in this regard that a liquid stool contains only about 10 per cent more water than the hardest scyballum, so that addition or removal of relatively small amounts of fluid can alter physical characteristics of excreta tremendously.

As with constipation, so with diarrhea, many classifications have been suggested. None is completely satisfactory because it is impossible to include all of the many factors involved, such as the etiology, the pathology, the chemistry, the clinical picture and the characteristics of the excreta. Since the present discussion is based on physiologic rather than specific causation, the previously employed and admittedly imperfect designations of central, reflex and mechanical will be used.

CENTRAL DIARRHEA

Diarrhea resulting from direct irritation or stimulation of the central and autonomic nervous systems may be classified as central. In diarrheas of this type reflex stimuli from the intestine or other organs are not of etiologic significance.

Neuroses. In most patients with chronic diarrhea the passage of loose stools is simply the most obvious expression of a psychoneurotic condition or a reaction to unusual stress in a stable individual. Studies of intestinal motility have amply demonstrated that emotionally charged interviews do cause changes in the number and amplitude of contraction waves,[2] and further, that patients with the irritable colon syndrome overreact to parasympathicomimetic drugs such as prostigmine. Although the actual mechanism for the production of diarrhea in some of these patients has yet to be clearly demonstrated, it is logical to assume that the parasympathetic centers in the brain stem, under the influence of an emotional disturbance, produce a periodic hyperactivity of the intestinal tract, particularly of the small bowel and the right colon supplied by the vagus nerve.

Why do certain strong emotions tend to be associated with diarrhea, whereas others cause constipation? As we have seen in a previous section, hostile feelings, anger and abject fear result in increased epinephrine production with inhibition of peristalsis, thus teleologically preparing the individual for conflict or flight. On the other hand, anxiety, guilt, and dependence have been shown in a classical study to be characteristic of patients with "mucous colitis."[15] In psychoanalytic terms, the patient compensates for inadequacy and passivity by overactivity in symbolic form.

Ulcerative Colitis. The etiology of this disease is still obscure, and it is discussed here because many physicians have long believed it to be, in some way, an emotional illness. Innumerable recent studies have thrown grave doubt on this hypothesis and have even suggested that there may not be one cause but several. The psychiatric components are now relegated by most investigators to a contributory role. Nevertheless, certain consistent patterns of behavior are found quite commonly in these patients—notably obsessive-compulsive neatness, rigid attitudes toward morality and extreme dependence upon a parent or parental figure.[16] In what way these patterns fit into the initiation or maintenance of the clinical picture of ulcerative colitis has not been demonstrated. Certain it is that the patient suffering from this illness responds in greater degree to an emotionally charged interview than does the normal individual. Perhaps, when the colon is inflamed, the nerve endings react excessively to impulses which would cause little or no change in the same subject if his colon were healthy.[2]

The idea that this disease, and also regional enteritis, are due to an autoimmune mechanism has long been championed by a few people, but only in the past few years have studies been reported which offer scientific support for the presence of specific antibodies in ulcerative colitis patients which do not appear in normal controls.[17] There is no agreement, however, about the nature of the offending antigen. There is some agreement that the colonic mucosa of these patients contains increased numbers of mast cells, which are important in antigen-antibody

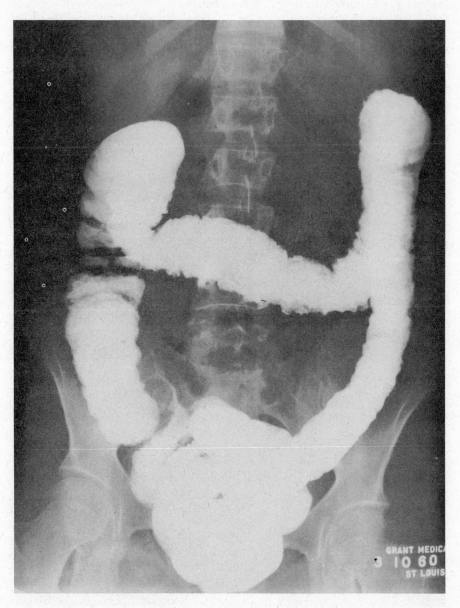

FIG. 105. The colon in acute ulcerative colitis, with barium clearly outlining many of the ulcers. Admixture of mucus, pus and blood to the mushy fecal content results in a characteristic type of diarrhea.

reactions, but it is not clear whether this should be considered cause or effect.[18]

Whatever the pathogenesis of ulcerative colitis, it is quite apparent why diarrhea occurs. Hyperactivity of the colon can easily be demonstrated by clinical observation and by roentgenologic and manometric studies. Once the disease is established, impulses from the inflamed mucosa stimulate propulsive motility by reflex parasympathetic activity. Further contributing to the diarrheal nature of the stool is the addition to it of mucus, pus and blood.

Diabetes. Diabetic diarrhea is a long-recognized but puzzling phenomenon. Except in those cases in which there is steatorrhea due to failure of exocrine pancreatic secretion, no anatomic lesion can be found at autopsy or on peroral biopsy, but autonomic neuropathy is inferred since evidence of other peripheral and autonomic neuropathies may often be present.[19] This would then be a "central" diarrhea.

One of the puzzling features of this diarrhea is its tendency to occur at night. This might be due to removal of central inhibi-

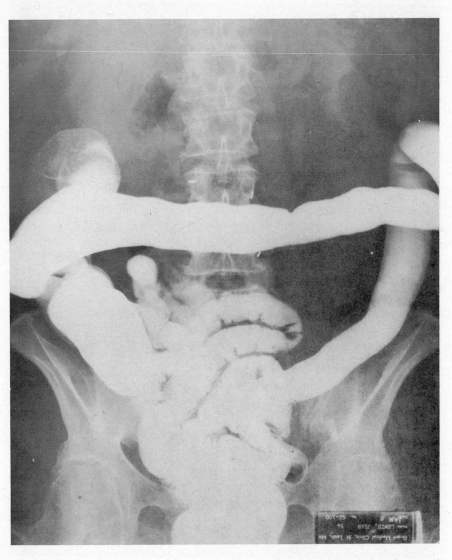

Fig. 106. In the patient with chronic ulcerative colitis the tubular shortened colon discharges the fecal content in the same mushy state in which it is received from the ileum. Because of extensive damage to the mucosal cells very little water can be absorbed.

tory influences cut off during sleep. Or, as recently suggested, bacteria may migrate proximally during sleep because of the sphincter laxity accompanying autonomic imbalance. In one patient significant numbers of bacteria were cultured from the stomach.[20] In this patient, and in many others, oral antibiotic therapy has induced clinical remission.

Infectious diseases. Diarrhea may be an initial manifestation of certain infectious diseases which produce the picture of *general toxemia.* In relatively mild infections, such as the epidemic diseases of childhood, the pathogenesis is not known, but it may be postulated that the autonomic nerve centers are involved during the period of systemic invasion. Certainly irritability and headache give evidence that there is cerebral irritation.

With more serious infections, in which a state approximating shock may occur, experiments utilizing the intravenous injection of Shiga toxin have shown what may occur. Along with a rise in the hematocrit and the specific gravity of the blood, there is a compensatory vasoconstriction in the intestinal mucosa. The lesions which occur in the gastrointestinal tract are, therefore, the result of *ischemia,* and can be prevented by drugs which block nerve impulse transmission at the sympathetic ganglia.[21]

Pseudomembranous enterocolitis may involve a mechanism similar to that just described. Clinicians have long speculated about the nature of the colitis, sometimes hemorrhagic, which occurs in such a wide variety of conditions as congestive heart failure, severe anemia, traumatic shock, inflammatory pulmonary conditions, myocardial infarction and after surgical procedures. It now seems clear that the common factor in all these situations is a *mesenteric vascular insufficiency* leading to focal areas of necrosis of the bowel mucosa. These areas coalesce and deepen with the eventual formation of the characteristic pseudomembrane.[22] Thus it seems that the mesenteric circulation plays a very important part in maintaining homeostasis by shunting blood to more vital centers. The original pathogenesis of the intestinal abnormality is central; later, of course, the reflex component (from the ulcerated intestine) is predominant.

Drugs. Certain drugs, administered parenterally, induce intestinal hypermotility by their action on the autonomic nervous system. Acetylcholine closely imitates the effects of parasympathetic activity. Pilocarpine and muscarine cause contraction of the smooth muscle of the alimentary tract by direct action on the parasympathetic effector cells. Neostigmine and mecholyl inhibit the destructive action of cholinesterase on acetylcholine and therefore produce intestinal overactivity. It is notable that in moderate doses these drugs stimulate only the proximal colon, but in larger doses both proximal and distal segments are affected, suggesting that the left colon contains more cholinesterase.[23] Urecholine, which is unaffected by cholinesterase, is an intestinal stimulant.

Serotinin or 5-hydroxytryptamine, relatively unknown a few years ago, has been the subject of intensive study to determine its normal site of action in the gastrointestinal tract ever since its role in the symptomatology of the carcinoid syndrome was first discovered. Diarrhea is a prominent feature in this syndrome. Experimentally, serotonin, either applied directly to the mucosa or injected intravenously, stimulates peristalsis. Its prescursor, 5-hydroxytryptophan, is an even more potent peristaltic stimulant. Serotonin does not act via cholinergic pathways, but does appear to act as a modulator of the cholinergic system by reducing the threshold of the pressoreceptors in the gut wall.[24]

Some drugs used in the treatment of hypertension may cause diarrhea. For example, guanethidine exerts a selective inhibitory effect on the sympathetic nervous system at the junction of nerves and arterioles.[25] Parasympathetic action remains unopposed. Reserpine may induce intestinal overactivity because of its effect on serotonin release.

REFLEX DIARRHEA

This comprises a large group, as it includes not only disorders in which the irritating impulses arise in organs outside the alimentary tract, but also those in which the irritation involves the intestinal mucosa itself. In this latter group, the irritation may be mechanical, but the increased propulsion is reflex, mediated through myenteric reflex arcs, as well as through reflexes involving the extrinsic nerves.

Pancreatic disease. In recent years many reports have described the clinical picture in patients with noninsulin-secreting islet cell tumors of the pancreas or, occasionally, with islet-cell hyperplasia. Many of these patients suffer from a watery diarrhea so profuse that severe hypokalemia occurs.[26] In some of them steatorrhea is prominent. In others intractable peptic ulcer has oc-

curred (Zollinger-Ellison syndrome). Several authors believe that the involvement of the pancreas is only part of a polyendocrine adenomatosis, in which the pituitary, the parathyroid and the adrenal glands also participate.

Diarrhea in patients with this syndrome is due to the tremendous load of *acid gastric juice* presented to the small intestine, perhaps combined with inhibition of the resorptive capacity of the ileum and cecum by a humoral substance elaborated by the tumor. At the low pH of 1.8 lipase and trypsin are inactivated and emulsifica-

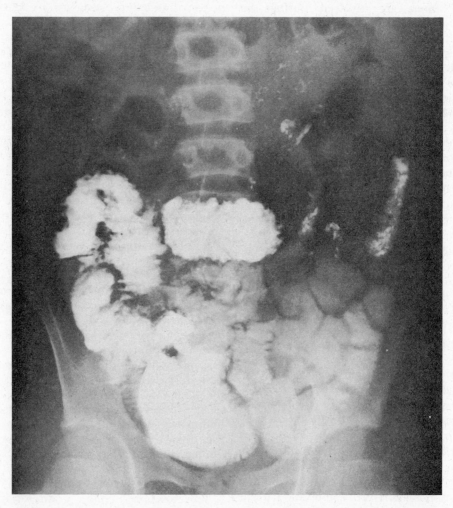

Fig. 107. The characteristic roentgenologic picture in the malabsorption states. Dilated loops of small bowel are divided into sausage-shaped segments. Fluid and fat are not absorbed adequately by the flattened shortened villi, and a bulky foamy stool results.

tion and digestion of fat are inhibited with resultant steatorrhea. This mechanism has been demonstrated by showing that aspiration of all gastric secretion results in cessation of the diarrhea and the loss of fat.[27] Furthermore, neutralization of the gastric aspirate and returning it to the duodenum permits almost normal fat absorption. Removal of the pancreatic adenoma halts the tremendous gastric secretion and the diarrhea ceases.

Deficiency of the sugar-splitting enzymes, lactase, maltase and invertase, may occur and be accompanied by excessive lactic acid in the stools. These syndromes have been demonstrated primarily in infants.

Deficiency of pancreatic juice occurs in chronic pancreatitis and with obstruction of the pancreatic ducts by cancer or calculi. The stools are bulky because of the lack of digestion and absorption of fat and, to a lesser extent, of protein. Increased *bulk* is itself a stimulus to rapid motility through the bowel. In addition, the presence of large amounts of unsplit *fat* in the chyme is irritating to the mucosa. Nerve terminals in the mucosa and the wall of the bowel initiate the myenteric reflexes.

Malabsorption syndromes, including sprue, nontropical sprue and celiac disease are somewhat better understood in recent years largely because of the relative ease with which biopsies of the small bowel can now be obtained. Familiar now are the short, blunt villi and lengthened dilated crypts in the mucosa of these patients, and the fact that the rates of mucosal cell loss and cell renewal are significantly increased. Nevertheless the cause of these anatomic changes is still obscure. There is evidence that tropical sprue, nontropical sprue and celiac disease are all manifestations of a complex metabolic disorder, genetically transmitted, with disturbed enzymatic pathways.[28] As a result, there is defective intestinal absorption of many factors. There is defective metabolism of electrolytes, water, protein, lipids and vitamins, not only because of decreased mucosal surface but also because of deficiency in the chemical organization of absorptive cells, especially in relation to active transport. There is difficulty in

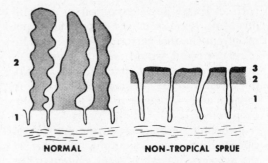

NORMAL   **NON-TROPICAL SPRUE**

Fig. 108. Epithelial zonation in the human jejunum. The zonation of the normal and abnormal intestinal epitheliums is derived from histochemical characteristics. Zone 1 comprises the crypts, and this germinal region is more extensive in nontropical sprue. Zone 2 represents the villous epithelium; in sprue this area is considerably smaller. Zones 1 and 2 in sprue are identical histochemically to zones 1 and 2, respectively, of the normal intestine. Zone 3 is the location of the peculiar surface epithelium of sprue, and it shows striking deviations from the normal absorptive epithelium. (Padykula, Gastroenterology 40:738)

handling residues of wheat gluten, as evidenced by the frequency with which clinical remissions occur on a gluten-free diet. Yet gluten may be only one of several triggering mechanisms. The stress of tropical climates, malnutrition and psychological upsets may be others.

The question of cause and effect with regard to the relation of malabsorption to the small intestinal mucosal abnormalities is raised by experiments involving induced niacin deficiency. Diarrhea regularly occurs in this situation due to decreases in the absorption of water, sodium and potassium.[29] Of most interest, however, is that during niacin deficiency the epithelial lining of the duodenal and the ileal loops changes from the normal regular columnar type to a disordered cuboidal type, and there is clubbing of the villi as in nontropical sprue.

Short-term neomycin administration is also capable of producing malabsorptive defects resembling those observed in idiopathic steatorrhea.[30] Diarrhea occurs along with increased fecal excretion of fat and nitrogen. Because of the known action of neomycin on the bacterial flora of the intestinal tract it would seem reasonable to ascribe the effects observed to this action, but actually they are more likely due to inflammatory changes in the jejunal mucosal cells.

Although the etiology of the malabsorption syndrome remains unsolved reasons for the resultant diarrhea seem evident. The large quantity of unabsorbed, unsplit fat creates bulk and mucosal irritation just as in the steatorrhea of pancreatic disease. Apparently there is also an increase in the bacterial flora of the small bowel, causing an increase in intestinal motility, perhaps through an elevated 5 hydroxy-indole-acetic acid and indole-3-acetic acid production and excretion.[31]

Secondary malabsorption syndromes occur with many anomalies or diseases which lead to impaired or incomplete digestion and absorption from the small bowel. The list of these diseases is extensive and includes regional enteritis, amyloidosis, scleroderma, radiation enteritis, intestinal lipodystrophy, lymphoma, jejunal diverticulosis, internal fistulas, the blind loop syndrome and others. It is apparent that a number of factors may be involved in the diarrhea which is associated with these disorders, but basically the stimuli are the same—an increase in fecal bulk due to undigested residue, and an increase in small intestinal bacterial content. Of particular interest are the patients with small-intestinal diverticulosis, who have been intensively studied. Here a heavy growth of endodiverticular bacteria may produce chronic inflammation and edema and therefore rapid intestinal transit and decreased absorption of fat. Bacterial-induced conversion of conjugated bile salts to toxic unconjugated salts may interfere further with fat absorption. And lastly, the microorganisms may utilize the nutrients in the chyme, such as vitamin B_{12}, at the expense of the patients' nutritional status. It is this last factor which accounts for the anemia so commonly found in a number of the secondary malabsorption states.

Food poisoning, if the term is used to indicate the ingestion of spoiled food, results in the irritation of the intestinal mucosa by decomposition products or toxins. The irritation is mechanical, and the diarrhea is reflexly induced through the myenteric pathways. On the other hand, the intake of contaminated food, containing large numbers of bacteria such as staphylococci, causes a true inflammation of the mucosa, a bacterial enteritis. There may also be a marked central effect from absorption of toxins.

Dietary indiscretions may result in the passage of loose stools due to irritation of the mucosa by coarse foods, seasonings, excess alcohol, etc.

Allergy to a certain food is not an uncommon cause of transient or even of chronic diarrhea. The sensitized mucosa becomes hyperemic and edematous and pours out mucus, and there is increased peristalsis stimulated by irritation of the mucosal nerve endings. As mentioned previously, ulcerative colitis is considered by some to involve an autoimmune mechanism.

Infections. All of these diarrheas due to food poisoning, contaminated foods, dietary indiscretions and allergy are usually acute and brief. More chronic effects may result from the multiplication of other bacteria and parasites, such as the Shigella and Salmonella bacilli, *Endamoeba histolytica, Vibrio cholerae, Leishmania donovani, Strongyloides stercoralis,* etc. Further discussion of these important, common, and serious causes will not be undertaken, since the mechanism of the production of diarrhea is the same in all cases—stimulation of nerve terminals in the mucosa and the walls of the intestine by inflammation, edema and ulceration, with hyperactivity of the small or the large intestine produced through myenteric and extrinsic reflexes.

Staphylococci have been cultured from the stool in some patients with pseudomembranous enterocolitis and have therefore often been thought to be the cause of this condition. Previous discussion has brought out the fact that mesenteric vascular insufficiency is the usual basic cause, with toxin-producing staphylococci sometimes playing a secondary role. There is, however, a true staphylococcic enteritis, separate from the pseudomembranous type, which may occur after antibiotics have eliminated most of the usual intestinal flora.

Turista, an explosive diarrhea which affects a large proportion of international travelers, has long been the subject of speculation. The cause is unknown, but recent studies have suggested that qualitative or quantiative alterations in the colonic bacterial population may be involved.[33]

"Intestinal flu" is a very common epidemic dysentery. Many types of enteroviruses, including Echo and Coxsackie viruses, have been established as capable of causing this sudden, usually brief illness.

Intestinal tuberculosis, regional ileitis, diverticulitis, or carcinoma of the bowel may induce marked irritability of involved segments of intestine and hurry the intestinal contents distally. The effect of a neoplasm, benign or malignant, depends on its location and type, and perhaps on other less well understood factors. If it is in the small intestine or the proximal colon, the tumor may cause diarrhea because of the still liquid consistency of the stool in these segments. Obviously, an ulcerative type of neoplasm will produce more local irritation than a scirrhous type. Although malignancies of the distal colon are more often associated with constipation than diarrhea, lesions of the rectum frequently cause diarrhea, perhaps because of stimulation of the defecation reflex with resultant increased motility proximally. One should remember also that the rectal ampulla has many times the diameter of the colon, so that feces can more readily bypass a tumor in this area. For the same reasons fecal impaction is frequently followed by the passage of liquid stools through or around the hard impacted stool. With villous adenomata of the rectum and lower bowel, dirrhea occurs because of excretion of large quantities of fluid and mucus by the tumor itself.[34]

Cathartics are variously classified. Most of them produce loose stools through mucosal irritation. The group of emodin or anthracene cathartics, which includes cas-

cara, senna, rhubarb and aloe, acts by direct irritation and stimulation of the colon after passage through the small bowel. Hence, there is a lag of several hours before the effect is evident. Bisacodyl and phenolphthalein have a similar action, but phenolphthalein has an additional stimulant effect on the motor nerves of the colon. The resinous cathartics (e.g., colocynth) and certain oils (e.g., castor oil) have an irritant action on the mucosa of the small bowel. Calomel purges because of the irritation produced by the mercuric ion liberated in the bowel, not because of any flushing action on the liver.

The saline cathartics, such as magnesium sulfate and magnesium citrate, are hygroscopic agents. They retain the water ingested with them in the bowel and even increase the water bulk by osmotic pressure. The fluid bulk distends and stimulates the intestine to great activity by stretching the nerve terminals in the mucosa and circular muscle. A somewhat similar action is obtained by the use of indigestible celluloses and hemicelluloses, such as are contained in agar and psyllium seed. With these substances, however, an important added factor may be their breakdown by intestinal bacteria into irritating organic acids. This is not true of methylcellulose, which passes through the alimentary tract unchanged. Mineral oil has to some extent a bulk-producing action and also acts as a lubricant. Water retention results from the ingestion of certain detergents such as dioctyl sodium sulfosuccinate.

Many poisons, ingested accidentally or with suicidal intent, have a purging action. Of these, perhaps the commonest is mercury, in the form of mercury bichloride. Mercury is a protoplasmic poison, producing violent local irritation and ulceration. When given parenterally in the form of a complex salt as a diuretic it may be deposited in the intestinal wall in sufficient concentration to cause injury to the cells, with resultant diarrhea. *Arsenic* also may stimulate peristalsis when ingested or given parenterally, but in a different manner. It produces capillary dilatation and hyperemia, with exudation of plasma. Such irritation is enough to cause diarrhea. With larger doses, blisters may form and rupture. Plasma then escapes into the bowel in large quantities, along with mucus, mucosal shreds and blood, giving rise to a more violent dysentery. *Alcohol* in high concentration or in large amounts induces hyperemia and edema of the small bowel, with irritation of the nerve terminals. It is also possible that cerebral and brain stem irritation may be responsible for some of the bowel overactivity due to alcohol.

MECHANICAL DIARRHEA

There are a very few conditions that increase the activity of the bowel other than through stimulation of the autonomic nervous system or the myenteric nerve reflexes. However, it is possible that certain disorders which are associated with increased neuromuscular excitability may cause the gut to be more active and to respond more readily to reflex impulses of all kinds. They could, of course, be placed in the reflex group, since reflexes that would usually result in normal intestinal motility could in these conditions be overactive, producing excessively rapid food transport. Such diseases could also be classified as central, since they probably affect the nerve terminals directly. They are here termed mechanical primarily to contrast them with the opposite factors inducing constipation.

Thyrotoxicosis is an instance of an abnormal condition leading at times to overwhelming excitation of the nervous system. The high metabolic rate with greater food intake (and thus greater residue) plus autonomic hyperactivity usually causes frequent, and sometimes loose, stools.

Parathyroid deficiency is accompanied by a reduction in the concentration of ionized calcium in the body fluids and tissues, which in turn increases neuromuscular excitability. The bowel may be hyperirritable and diarrhea may result.

In uremia diarrhea may be severe. The failing kidney is unable to excrete phosphate, a compensatory reduction in ionized calcium occurs, and hyperexcitability of the neuromuscular mechanism follows.

SUMMARY

Constipation and diarrhea are best understood as abnormal variants of intestinal motility and function. Normally an ordinary mixed meal has passed completely into the colon in about 6 hours, entering the cecum as a thin mush. Water is absorbed as the stool passes through the colon. If the passage is slow, more of the water content is absorbed and the resultant stool is hard and dry. If the passage is rapid a fluid or soft stool results.

Peristaltic contractions in the small bowel and colon are accomplished through local myenteric reflexes, but it is usually considered that they are augmented by vagus efferent impulses and inhibited by splanchnic efferent impulses. These impulses may originate in the higher nerve centers or in the cord as part of a reflex arc.

Constipation may be defined as undue delay in the evacuation of feces. Such delay may result in the passage of hard dry stools, or no stool at all. Diarrhea indicates excessive speed in the transport of feces with resultant passage of loose stools. These conditions may occur because of central nervous system overactivity or inhibition, reflex influence on motility from factors arising within the intestine or in other organs, and, finally, from mechanical factors.

A central constipation or diarrhea is one induced by direct stimulation or inhibition of the autonomic nerves. The impulse may arise in the brain, the hypothalamus, the medulla, the cord or the peripheral nerve endings. Examples of constipation on this basis are failure of the conditioned defecation reflex due to lack of regularity or prolonged bed rest, stressful situations, emotional disturbances, organic diseases or traumatic lesions of the central nervous system, and certain drugs, such as morphine. Central disorders causing diarrhea include certain types of neuroses, poorly controlled diabetes, infectious diseases involving toxemia and some parenterally administered drugs such as prostigmine.

Most of the disorders that disturb the motility of the bowel do so in a reflex manner. The impulse may originate in the mucosa or the wall of the intestine and the rectum, in other abdominal viscera, in the kidney, etc. For example, intrinsic bowel lesions may stimulate inhibitory action of the sympathetic nerves and produce constipation. Other types of mucosal irritation, such as that produced by ulcerative colitis, food poisoning and cathartics will cause diarrhea because of marked stimulation of local myenteric reflex arcs or parasympathetic autonomic nerves.

Mechanical constipation may occur if there is weakness of the voluntary muscles used in defecation or weakness of the intestinal muscles, and also in acute obstruction when the lumen is completely blocked. Diarrhea may result from increased neuromuscular excitability, such as is found with thyrotoxicosis, parathyroid deficiency and uremia.

REFERENCES

1. Horowitz, L., and Farrar, J. T.: Intraluminal small intestinal pressures in normal patients and in patients with functional gastrointestinal disorders, Gastroenterology 42:455-464, 1962.
2. Chaudhary, N. A., and Truelove, S. C.: Human colonic motility: a comparative study of normal subjects, patients with ulcerative colitis, and patients with the irritable colon syndrome, Gastroenterology 40: 1-36, 1961.
3. Bülbring, E., Lin, R. C. Y., and Schofield, G.: An investigation of the peristaltic reflex in relation to anatomic observations, Quart. J. Exper. Physiol. 43:26-35, 1958.
4. Thomas, J. E.: The autonomic nervous system in gastrointestinal disease, J.A.M.A. 157:209-212, 1955.
5. Lee, C. Y.: The effect of stimulation of extrinsic nerves on peristalsis and on the release of 5-hydroxytryptamine in the large intestine of the guinea-pig and of the rabbit, J. Physiol. 152:405, 1960.
6. Haverback, B. J., and Davidson, J. D.: Serotonin and the gastrointestinal tract, Gastroenterology 35:570-578, 1958.
7. Almy, T. P., Hinkle, L. E., Jr., Berle, B., and Kern, F., Jr.: Alteration in colonic function in man under stress, Gastroenterology 12: 437-444, 1949.
8. Grace, W. J., Wolf, S., and Wolff, H. G.: Life situations, emotions and colonic function, Gastroenterology 14:93-108, 1950.
9. Daniel, E. E., Sutherland, W. H., and Bogoch, A.: Effects of morphine and other drugs on motility of the terminal ileum, Gastroenterology 36:510-523, 1959.
10. Fink, S., and Friedman, G.: The differential effect of drugs on the proximal and distal colon, Am. J. Med. 28:535-540, 1960.
11. Kramer, P., Kearney, M. M., and Ingelfinger, F. J.: The effect of specific foods and water loading on the ileal excreta of ileosteomized human subjects, Gastroenterology 42:535-546, 1962.
12. Spencer, R. P.: Potassium metabolism and gastrointestinal function: a review, Am. J. Dig. Dis. 4:145-158, 1959.
13. Kerr, D. N. S., and Davidson, S.: Gastrointestinal intolerance to oral iron preparations, Lancet 2:489-492, 1958.
14. Fisher, J. H., and Swenson, O.: Aganglionic lesions of the colon, Am. J. Surg. 99:134-136, 1960.
15. White, V. W., Cobb, S., and Jones, C. M.: Mucous Colitis, Psychosom. Med., Monograph 1, 1939.
16. Engel, G. L.: Studies of ulcerative colitis, Am. J. Med. 19:231, 1955.
17. Thayer, W. R., Calabresi, P., and Spiro, H. M.: Further observations on the antinuclear globulin in ulcerative colitis and regional ileitis, Gastroenterology 40:695-699, 1961.
18. Almy, T. P.: Ulcerative colitis, Gastroenterology 41:391-400, 1961.
19. Bridwell, T., Whitehouse, F. W.: Peroral jejunal biopsy in a patient with diabetic diarrhea, Diabetes 10:58-59, 1961.
20. Finlay, J. M., and Sumi, S. M.: On the pathogenesis of diabetic steatorrhea, Ann. Int. Med. 55:994-997, 1961.
21. Penner, A.: The pathogenesis of experimental dysentery intoxication: Further studies in the inhibition of the lesions, Gastroenterology 19:855-861, 1951.
22. Birnbaum, D., Lanfer, A., and Freund, M.: Pseudomembranous enterocolitis, Gastroenterology 41:345-352, 1961; Corday, E., and Williams, J. H.: Effect of shock and vasopressor drugs on regional circulation of brain, heart, kidney and liver, Am. J. Med. Sc. 29:228-241, 1960.
23. Fink, S., and Friedman, G.: The differential effect of drugs on the proximal and distal colon, Am. J. Med. 28:535-540, 1960.
24. Sleisenger, M. H., Law, D. H., Smith, F. W., Pert, J. H., and Lewis, C. M.: Studies of colon contractility in dogs. 1. Description of method and effect of parasympathomimetic agents and serotonin, J. Clin. Invest. 38:2199-2130, 1959.

25. Klapper, M. S., and Richard, L.: Guanethidine in hypertension, South. Med. J. 55: 75-80, 1962.

26. Morrison, A. B., Rawson, A. J., and Fitts, W. T., Jr.: The syndrome of refractory watery diarrhea and hypokalemia in patients with a noninsulin-secreting islet cell tumor, Am. J. Med. 32:119-127, 1962.

27. Haubrich, W. S., O'Neil, F. S., and Block, M. A.: Observations on steatorrhea associated with gastric hypersecretion and pancreatic islet cell neoplasm, Ann. Int. Med. 56:302-307, 1962.

28. Padykula, H. A., Strauss, E. W., Ladman, A. V., and Gardner, F. H.: A morphologic and histochemical analysis of the human jejunal epithelium in non-tropical sprue, Gastroenterology 40:735-765, 1961; Frazer, A. C.: Pathogenetic concepts of the malabsorption syndrome, Gastroenterology 38:389-398, 1960; di Sant' Agnese, P. A., and Jones, W. O.: The celiac syndrome (malabsorption) in pediatrics, J.A.M.A. 180:308-316, 1962.

29. Nelson, R. A., Code, C. F., and Brown, A.

L.: Sorption of water and electrolytes, and mucosal structure, in niacin deficiency, Gastroenterology 42:26-35, 1962.

30. Jacobson, E. D., Chodos, R. B., and Faloon, W. W.: An experimental malabsorption syndrome, Am. J. Med. 28:524-533, 1960.

31. Haverback, B. J., Dyce, B., and Thomas, H. V.: Indole metabolism in the malabsorption syndrome, New England J. Med. 262:754-757, 1960.

32. Schiffer, L. M., Faloon, W. W., Chodos, R. B., and Lozner, E. L.: Malabsorption syndrome associated with intestinal diverticulosis, Gastroenterology 42:63-68, 1962; Johnson, P. M., Wysor, W. G., Jr.: Mimetic aspects of small intestinal diverticulosis, Arch. Int. Med. 108:370-375, 1961.

33. Kean, B. H., Schaffner, W., Brennan, A. B., and Waters, S. R.: The diarrhea of travelers, J.A.M.A. 180:367-371, 1962.

34. Rabinowitz, P., Farber, M., and Friedman, I. S.: A depletion syndrome in villous adenoma of the rectum, Arch. Int. Med. 109: 265-269, 1962.

20

Hematemesis and Melena

Leon Schiff

GENERAL CONSIDERATIONS

Definitions. *Hematemesis* is the vomiting of blood, whether fresh and red or digested and black.

Melena by derivation means black and is usually used to describe the passage of black "tarry" stools, with the coal-black, clotted, gummy appearance of tar. However, melena is used clinically in a wider sense to describe the passage of blood in the stools, whether the color is visibly altered or not and whether the color is light, reddish or (as is more common) dark brown or blackish.

Pathogenesis. Bleeding in the gastrointestinal tract may result from:

1. Disease of, or trauma to, tissue, with secondary erosion or rupture of blood vessels

2. Primary disorders affecting the walls of the blood vessels (increased capillary fragility, varices, aneurysm, arteriosclerosis, etc.)

3. Disturbance of the blood-clotting mechanism.

In general, any of the disorders discussed in the chapter on Pathologic Bleeding may result in the presence of some blood in the gastrointestinal tract, but only when fairly large amounts are present does hematemesis occur or does melena become obvious.

Source of Hemorrhage

The vomiting of large amounts of blood or the passage of tarry stools are symptoms that usually appear with dramatic suddenness. They may supervene in patients with pre-existing digestive disturbances or may, of themselves, prove the harbingers of disease. Their occurrence may clarify the significance of existing symptoms or may constitute the sole evidence of disease. It is well known that they occur most commonly in a number of disorders, which will be considered separately. The occurrence of hematemesis indicates a bleeding point proximal to the ligament of Treitz. The appearance of the vomitus, whether resembling coffee-grounds or bright-red and obviously bloody, has proved of little diagnostic value.

Melena Without Hematemesis. While it is generally true that the occurrence of melena (tarry stools) without hematemesis indicates a lesion distal to the pylorus, usually a duodenal ulcer, this is not invariably so. We have seen melena without hematemesis in cases of ruptured esophageal varix associated with hepatic cirrhosis and in cases of gastric cancer. Ratnoff and Patek[1] noted 9 instances of melena without hematemesis in 386 cases of hepatic cirrhosis. Benedict[2] reported melena alone in 5 of 20 cases of hemorrhage from gastritis. Jones[3] observed melena only in 6 fatal cases of bleeding gastric ulcer. A common feature of these 6 cases was their extremely poor general condition, and it was suggested that the patients may have been too weak to vomit.

Color of Stools. While the presence of bright blood in the stools usually indicates a bleeding point low in the intestine, this is not an infallible sign. In the presence of hypermotility, the blood may be swept through the intestinal tract so rapidly as to appear unaltered in the feces. The presence of bright blood in the stools has been noted in 3 individuals 4 to 17 hours after they were given 1,000 ml. of citrated human blood intragastrically; none of them passed a tarry stool.[4] Tarry stools are said to occur when blood is introduced in the cecum, particularly in the presence of delayed colonic motility.[5] The author has seen truly tarry stools in hemorrhage arising just distal to the ileocecal valve; but not when bleeding took place beyond this area. According to Hilsman,[5] the color of the stools (whether bright red, dark red, brown or tarry) depends more on the time the blood remains in the intestine than on the level at which the bleeding occurs.

CHARACTERISTICS OF MELENA

Amount of Blood Necessary. Daniel and Egan[6] reported the occurrence of tarry stools after the oral administration of from 50 to 80 ml. of fresh human blood. The writer and his associates have reported the occurrence of tarry stools after the oral administration of 100 ml. of citrated human "bank" blood. These observations indicate that the passage of a tarry stool does not necessarily indicate severe blood loss.

Duration of Tarry Stools. Tarry stools may be passed for from 3 to 5 days following the intragastric administration of 1,000 to 2,000 ml. of citrated human blood to human subjects.[4] This indicates that the passage of a tarry stool is no proof that

hemorrhage is continuing. The number of tarry or bloody stools that follow the intragastric administration of blood is not necessarily related to the quantity of blood introduced.

Duration of Occult Blood. Hesser[7] has pointed out that occult blood is usually present in the stools for from 2 to 3 weeks following hematemesis or melena in patients with bleeding peptic ulcer. We have been able to confirm this experimentally, upon oral or intragastric administration of citrated human blood. The persistence of a positive test for occult blood is, therefore, not necessarily an indication that hemorrhage is continuing.

SEVERITY OF HEMORRHAGE

It is difficult to estimate the amount of blood lost through that appearing in the vomitus: first, because of the admixture of gastric contents; second, because only part of the effused blood is vomited. One not infrequently hears a patient proclaim that he has vomited a gallon or two of blood! As Cullinan and Price[8] have well put it, the amount of blood vomited varies with the patient's imagination.

It may be difficult to estimate the severity of the bleeding when the patient is first seen clinically, for, as Black[9] has stated, the rate of blood loss may influence the patient's appearance. Thus, "the rapid loss of a small amount of blood may produce as much appearance of circulatory failure" as the gradual loss of a larger quantity. The pulse rate may be misleading for, as Wallace and Sharpey-Schafer[10] have shown, the heart rate may be slowed, increased or unchanged after the rapid removal of up to 1,150 ml. of blood in control subjects. We have been impressed with the frequency of a normal pulse rate in the presence of a rather marked fall in blood pressure soon after massive hematemesis or melena. The hemoglobin percentage may prove unreliable shortly after hemorrhage, as the lowest values are usually obtained from 6 to 48 hours later[9] as a result of dilution of the blood by tissue fluids. Wallace and Sharpey-Schafer[10] obtained maximum blood dilution (and lowest hemoglobin percentage) from 3 to 90 hours after the rapid removal of up to 1,150 ml. of blood in control subjects. They found the time of maximal dilution to vary in the same individual on different occasions.

Ebert, Stead and Gibson[11] removed 760 to 1,220 ml. of blood from six normal subjects in 6 to 13 minutes. They found a sharp drop in plasma volume immediately after hemorrhage, after which the plasma volume was gradually increased, until at the end of three to four days it was greater than the original plasma volume by an amount approximately equal to the volume of red cells removed. After the first two hours the change in plasma volume was much more accurately reflected by the hematocrit value than by the protein concentration. "If the difference between the original hematocrit reading and that made 72 hours after venesection is taken as 100 per cent, it is found that 14 to 36 per cent of this drop occurred in two hours, 36 to 50 per cent in eight hours, and 63 to 77 per cent in twenty-four hours."

Estimations of blood volume might theoretically be helpful in determining the severity of blood loss, but a simple method of measuring circulating blood volume is not available. Furthermore, by the time such a procedure can be carried out clinically, usually sufficient plasma dilution will have occurred so as to obviate the determination of the original blood volume.

Howarth and Sharpey-Schafer[12] describe three low-blood-pressure phases after hemorrhage. The first phase is that of sudden vasovagal reaction with bradycardia and muscle vasodilatation which develops suddenly during or after bleeding. The second phase is associated with increased heart rate, low right-auricular pressure and low cardiac output. Large transfusions raise right-auricular pressure, cardiac output and blood pressure. The third phase "takes time to develop and persists over long periods. Severe anemia may be a causal factor in this phase. Right auricular pressure and cardiac output are increased. Large transfusions may be dangerous from overloading." The writer has seen instances of pulmonary edema following blood transfusions in patients with severe gastrodu-

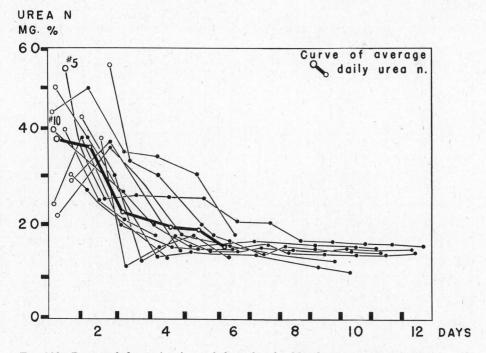

Fig. 109. Repeated determinations of the value for blood urea nitrogen in 12 cases of single hemorrhage followed by recovery. (Arch. Int. Med. 64:1239-1251)

odenal hemorrhage, who were probably in phase 3 of Howarth and Sharpey-Schafer, and in whom the cardiac output probably fell as the result of the transfusion (instead of increasing as it would normally, according to Sharpey-Schafer[13]).

AZOTEMIA

The frequent occurrence of azotemia following hematemesis and melena has been confirmed by numerous observers, since it was first pointed out by Sanguinetti,[14] in 1933, in cases of bleeding gastric and duodenal ulcer. The writer and his associates[15] reported an elevation of the blood urea nitrogen to 30 mg. per cent or more in about two-thirds, and elevation of 50 mg. per cent or more in one-fifth of 135 cases of hematemesis or melena due to various causes. Following a single nonfatal hemorrhage, the blood urea nitrogen may increase within a few hours, usually reaches a maximum within 24 hours and drops sharply to normal by the third day.[16]

The rate of subsidence of the azotemia can be increased by slow-drip blood transfusion but not be infusion of plasma in comparable amount.[17] In cases in which there is a second (nonfatal) hemorrhage, there is a secondary increase within 24 hours with a drop to normal by the third day. In cases in which repeated hemorrhages occur and ultimately prove fatal, there is an increasingly or persistently high level of the urea nitrogen in the blood. The kidneys have generally been found normal at autopsy.

The mechanism of the azotemia is not the same as that associated with high intestinal obstruction as it occurs in the absence of any vomiting, that is, in the presence of melena alone, and is associated with a normal or increased blood chloride concentration and a normal carbon dioxide combining power of the blood.

Other things being equal, the degree of azotemia is determined by the amount of blood entering the intestinal tract in a

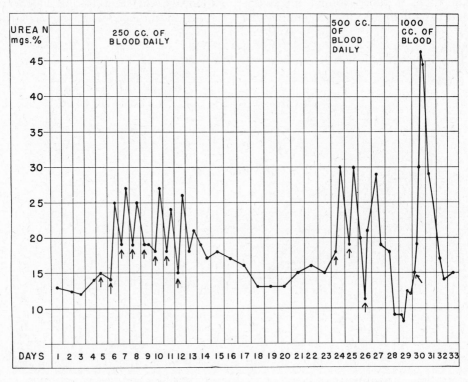

Fig. 110. Blood urea nitrogen following intragastric administration of varying quantities of citrated blood in one patient. (Am. J. Digest. Dis. 6:597-602)

given period of time. The time factor is important, for it has been shown that if a given quantity of blood is introduced into the gastrointestinal tract over a period of days, the maximum elevation of the blood urea nitrogen obtained on any single day may be much less than if a fraction of the blood is given quickly. (Thus, the administration of 250 ml. of citrated human blood daily to a control subject for 8 days yielded a maximum blood urea nitrogen value of 26 mg. per cent; while giving 1,000 ml. of blood intragastrically during a half hour yielded a maximum elevation of 47 mg. per cent.[18]) The time element may explain the disparity between the degree of anemia and the level of the blood urea nitrogen in some patients with hematemesis. Thus, if a patient loses 2,000 ml. of blood over a period of 8 days, one might not expect the same degree of elevation of the blood urea nitrogen that would follow the sudden loss of this quantity of blood, although comparable degrees of anemia might develop.

The azotemia occurs irrespective of the cause of hemorrhage into the upper digestive tract. It does not appear in hemorrhage from the colon, a fact that may prove of value in differential diagnosis. It does not follow the sudden withdrawal of up to 1,150 ml. of blood in control subjects except in the presence of renal impairment.[10]

The factors that may influence the azotemia include *dehydration, shock, impairment of renal function, increased catabolism of tissue protein,* and *absorption of products of decomposition of the blood liberated into the intestinal tract.* Observations on both man and animals indicate the importance of the digestion and the absorption of the blood liberated into the intestinal tract in the production of the azotemia.[18,19,20,21,22] Black,[9] though admitting the role of the blood in the intestinal tract, nevertheless believes that functional renal failure, resulting from a fall in the pressure and the amount of the blood supplied to the kidneys, plays an important role at the time the blood urea nitrogen is rising. He believes that the rise of the blood urea that follows the giving of large amounts of blood by mouth is smaller and slower in onset than the azotemia of severe hematemesis. The observations of Gregory *et al.*[22] in experimental animals indicate that the azotemia may be due to decreased renal function caused by low blood pressure and dehydration or to absorption of digested blood protein. They found the rise in the blood urea nitrogen that fol-

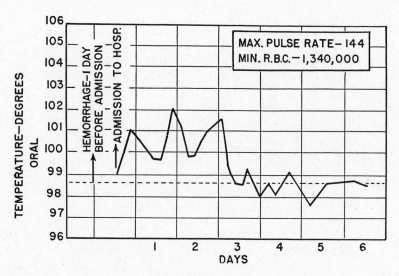

Fig. 111. Temperature curve following hemorrhage in case of J. P. (bleeding gastric ulcer).

lowed maintenance of a low blood pressure through bleeding to be slower and more sustained than that which followed the giving of blood by stomach tube.

Although we admit that functional renal failure may occur in many instances, particularly in the presence of shock, we believe that it is not essential to the genesis of the azotemia. This is substantiated by the production of azotemia through the intragastric administration of blood to individuals without obvious renal disease (producing in some instances a curve almost exactly the same as that which followed hematemesis in the same subject), by the demonstration that the introduction of such blood does not cause impairment of renal function, and by the demonstration of normal renal function in the presence of azotemia.[23]

We thoroughly endorse Black's statement that "the level to which the blood urea nitrogen rises is of value in judging the severity of gastroduodenal hemorrhage and repeated estimation a good measure of progress." In a series of 135 cases, the writer and his associates[15] reported a maximum blood urea nitrogen of less than 30 mg. per cent to be a favorable prognostic sign in patients with hematemesis due to peptic ulcer, hepatic cirrhosis, or undetermined cause. Exceptions noted were two cases of ruptured aortic aneurysm and one of perforated peptic ulcer. (Subsequent observations include a fatal case of bleeding peptic ulcer without significant elevation of the blood urea nitrogen in which death was due to pneumonia.) The presence of a maximum blood urea nitrogen content of 50 mg. per cent or more was followed by a fatal outcome in one third of the cases, while an elevation of 70 mg. per cent or more was accompanied by a fatal outcome in about two thirds of the cases. In interpreting azotemia in a given case, one should keep in mind that the blood urea nitrogen level may be affected by such complicating factors as starvation, dehydration, alkalosis, or pre-existing renal disease. In our experience a blood urea nitrogen content of over 100 mg. per cent has been found to indicate pre-existing kidney disease. Evidently the functional renal failure and the amount of blood entering the intestinal tract are clinically not sufficient to produce a degree of azotemia above this level.

Fever

Fever occurs in the majority of patients with hematemesis and melena irrespective of the cause of hemorrhage (Figs. 111-114). It usually appears within 24 hours, lasts from a few days to a week or slightly

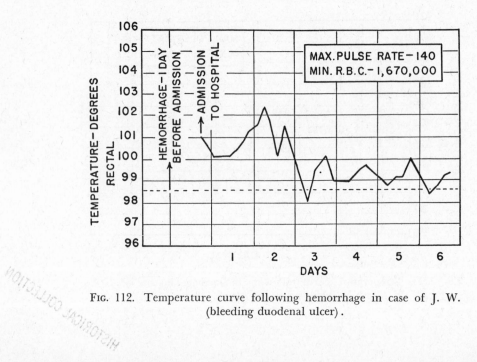

Fig. 112. Temperature curve following hemorrhage in case of J. W. (bleeding duodenal ulcer).

longer and may reach a maximum of 103°. It more frequently follows massive or moderately severe than mild hemorrhage.

The cause of the fever is not known. According to Dill and Isenhour,[24] numerous factors have been invoked, including absorption of blood decomposition products, reduction in blood volume, anemia, associated gastritis, or increased lability of the heat-regulating center as a result of asthenia or shock. The absorption of blood decomposition products has been considered the most likely cause by a number of European observers. Black[9] suggests that the fever may possibly be related to the endogenous breakdown of the body protein which may occur after hemorrhage. However, the experimental observations of Dill and Isenhour, both in man and animals, and our own observations in man[25] indicate that the intragastric administration of large quantities of citrated blood is not followed by any significant elevation of temperature. Incidentally, no change in the white-blood-cell count followed the administration of such blood.

Factors Influencing Hemorrhage in General

Vitamin-C Deficiency. A number of observers have focused attention on the low plasma vitamin-C level in patients with peptic ulcer, particularly those with hematemesis. Though the vitamin-C deficiency has been attributed to the restricted ulcer diet, the relationship of scorbutic states to hemorrhage has been emphasized. Studies reported from the Gastric Research Laboratory of the Cincinnati General Hospital[26] have shown that the plasma vitamin-C content may be normal in patients with hematemesis or melena due to peptic ulcer or undetermined cause. The average plasma vitamin-C level of patients with bleeding peptic ulcers, though reduced, may be higher than that of patients with peptic ulcers without hemorrhage. Furthermore, the low plasma vitamin-C level seen in patients with bleeding peptic ulcers or hematemesis of undetermined cause usually persists after cessation of hemorrhage.

Prothrombin Content of Blood. Frank[27] reported a decrease in the prothrombin content of the blood in patients with peptic ulcer and hemorrhage. Our own studies failed to reveal any significant prolongation of prothrombin time (method of Quick[28]) or reduction of prothrombin content of the blood (method of Smith and associates[29]) in patients with hematemesis or melena due to peptic ulcer or undetermined cause. Recently, however, significant variations from the normal have been reported in prothrombin concentrations of the blood of patients with massive gastrointestinal hemorrhage.[30] Significant

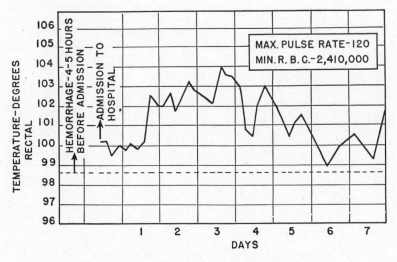

Fig. 113. Temperature curve following hemorrhage in case of L. G. (gastric carcinoma).

changes also were observed in the platelet count during and after gastrointestinal bleeding in patients with and without liver disease.[31] Abnormalities in other clotting factors have been reported also following massive gastrointestinal hemorrhage.[30]

ETIOLOGY

Vomiting of blood or the passage of tarry stools may be due to a variety of disorders. The most common of these is bleeding peptic ulcer. Alsted[32] has pointed out that reports on the etiology of gastrointestinal hemorrhage coming from various clinics seem to fall into two groups. In the first, the cause of the hemorrhage was almost always determined, with peptic ulcer comprising about three-fourths of the cases; in the second, the cause of the hemorrhage was undetermined in from one-fourth to one-half of the cases. He indicates that the patients in the first group were admitted to institutions treating selected chronically ill patients while those of the second group entered municipal hospitals dealing largely with acutely ill patients.

In our own experience with 640 cases of hematemesis and melena admitted to the Cincinnati General Hospital over a ten-year period, peptic ulcer comprised 339, or 52.9 per cent of the causes; the cause was undetermined in 132, or 20.6 per cent; hepatic cirrhosis was present in

80, or 12.5 per cent; gastric carcinoma in 15, or 2.3 per cent; hiatal hernia in 14, or 2.1 per cent; gastritis with mucosal erosions in 7, or 1.1 per cent; aortic aneurysm rupturing into the esophagus in 5, or 0.8 per cent; and miscellaneous causes were found in 48, or 7.5 per cent (Fig. 115).

The etiologic factors in other series of cases[33,34] are listed in Tables 18 and 19. In Palmer's series the diagnoses were based on the author's "vigorous diagnostic approach" which consists of ice water lavage of the stomach as soon as the history and physical examination have been completed, followed by immediate esophagogastroscopic and contrast roentgenologic examinations. Using this type of approach, Palmer reports a diagnostic accuracy of 87.1 per cent in 650 patients as compared with an accuracy of 34.9 per cent obtained in 212 patients using the classical approach. The advantage of Palmer's method lies in the greater frequency with which bleeding can be traced, as contrasted with the mere demonstration of a lesion capable of explaining bleeding.

HISTORY AND PHYSICAL EXAMINATION

Inquiry should be made regarding bleeding tendencies during childhood and early adulthood which, if present, should suggest a blood dyscrasia. A family history of

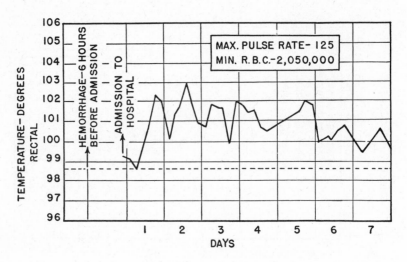

Fig. 114. Temperature curve following hemorrhage in case of F. W. (hepatic cirrhosis with ruptured esophageal varix).

gastrointestinal bleeding is suggestive of hemophilia or Osler-Rendu-Weber disease. Questioning should be directed toward eliciting a history of ingestion of drugs capable of inducing gastrointestinal bleeding, such as steroids, aspirin, butazolidin and rauwolfia alkaloids. A history of alcoholism should favor erosive gastritis or bleeding esophageal varices. The passage of possibly tarry stools should be checked by inquiry regarding concomitant faintness or weakness, ingestion of iron and bismuth compounds and the eating of licorice candy or foods which may discolor the stools. The typical peptic ulcer syndrome may frequently be absent prior to ulcer bleeding.

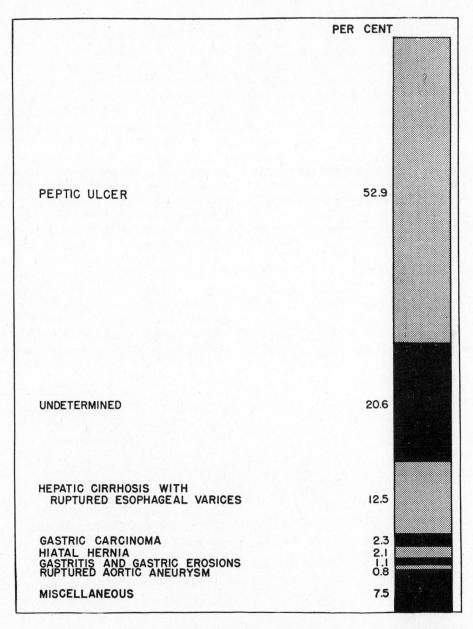

PER CENT

PEPTIC ULCER — 52.9

UNDETERMINED — 20.6

HEPATIC CIRRHOSIS WITH
 RUPTURED ESOPHAGEAL VARICES — 12.5

GASTRIC CARCINOMA — 2.3
HIATAL HERNIA — 2.1
GASTRITIS AND GASTRIC EROSIONS — 1.1
RUPTURED AORTIC ANEURYSM — 0.8

MISCELLANEOUS — 7.5

FIG. 115. Etiology of hematemesis and melena in 640 cases admitted to the Cincinnati General Hospital over a 10-year period.

TABLE 18.

ETIOLOGY OF UPPER GASTROINTESTINAL BLEEDING IN 5,192 CASES—12 AUTHORS—YEARS 1950-57*

	PEPTIC ULCER	ESOPHAGEAL VARICES	GASTRITIS	GASTRIC CANCER	HIATUS HERNIA	OTHER	UNDETER- MINDED
Average	65%	9%	11%†	1%	2%	2%	10%

* Data from Gray, S. J., *et al.:* Med. Clin. N. Am. 41:1327.
†Acute ulceration gastroscopically not seen by x-ray.

Prominent heartburn and epigastric or low substernal discomfort or pain, particularly in the recumbent position and brought on by large meals or by stooping over as in lacing one's shoes, should suggest the presence of a hiatal hernia.

The examination of a patient with massive hematemesis or melena must of necessity be cursory. Attention should be concentrated on pulse rate, blood pressure and

TABLE 19. THE BLEEDING LESIONS— 650 VDA PATIENTS*

	NO. OF PATIENTS	PER CENT OF TOTAL
Esophagus, varices.......	111	17.1
erosive esophagitis.....	62	9.5
ulcer...............	8	1.2
adenoma............	1	
Stomach, erosive gastritis.	98	15.1
ulcer...............	67	10.3
Mallory-Weiss syndrome	23	3.5
Osler-Rendu-Weber disease............	8	1.2
varices..............	5	
leiomyoma...........	3	
sarcoma.............	2	
gastric leukemia.......	2	
gastric and duodenal ulcer.............	2	
mucosal prolapse into esophagus.........	1	
sarcoidosis..........	1	
adenoma............	1	
Duodenum, ulcer.......	165	25.3
leiomyoma..........	2	
ulcer and varices......	1	
rupture aortic aneurysm	1	
Jejunum, stomal ulcer....	16	2.5
adenoma at stoma.....	1	
Liver, post-traumatic.....	2	
Undetermined.........	67	10.3

* Palmer, E. D.: Diagnosis of Upper Gastrointestinal Hemorrhage, Thomas, Springfield, 1961.

general appearance. Icterus, if present, should direct attention to disease of the liver, as should the presence of vascular spiders on the face, neck, upper trunk or upper limbs. Search should be made on the skin of the face, the lips, the mucocutaneous junction and the mucous surfaces of the mouth for the brownish, frecklelike melanin spots of the Peutz-Jeghers Syndrome. The telangiectasia of the Osler-Rendu-Weber Syndrome are usually reddish (occasionally purplish) and are commonest on the lips, the tongue, the ears, the fingers and the toes, and frequently can be demonstrated to pulsate (Fig. 116). Also to be looked for are the skin changes characteristic of pseudoxanthoma elasticum: the yellowish discoloration and the lax, redundant and relatively inelastic quality with thickening and a grooved appearance of "coarse Moroccan leather."[35,36] According to McKusick, the regions prone to be involved are the face, the neck, the axillary folds, the cubital areas, the inguinal folds and the periumbilical area[36] (Fig. 117). Examination of the ocular fundi may furnish evidence of arteriosclerosis and the angioid streaks of pseudoxanthoma elasticum.[37] These streaks are brownish or gray, are four or five times wider than veins and resemble vessels (Fig. 118). A smooth or red tongue may indicate the presence of achlorhydria or nutritional deficiency, which in turn should direct attention to the possibility of gastric carcinoma or hepatic cirrhosis. The left supraclavicular space should be felt for the presence of "sentinel glands." The time-honored practice of palpating the abdomen gently and briefly in cases of upper digestive tract hemorrhage for fear of reinducing bleeding by the usual form of palpation is probably

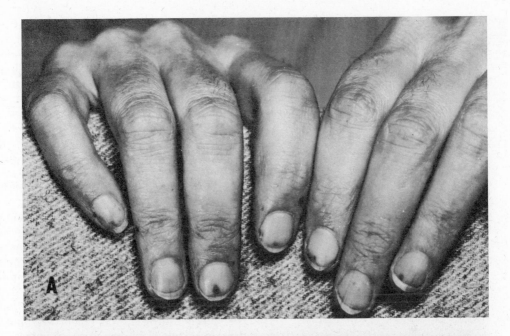

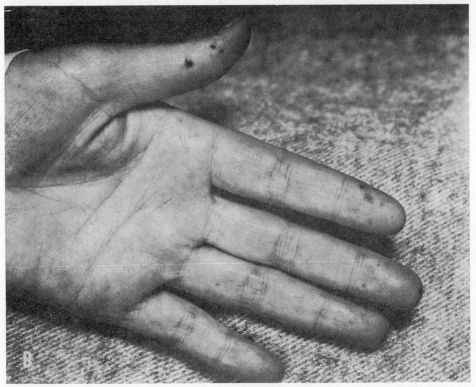

FIG. 116. Osler's disease. Telangiectatic lesions with characteristic punctate areas on the palmar surface of the fingers and the typical diffuse, sometimes linear spots under the nails. These ordinarily do not have very sharply defined margins. (Bean, W. B.: Vascular Spiders and Related Lesions of the Skin, Springfield, Ill., Thomas)

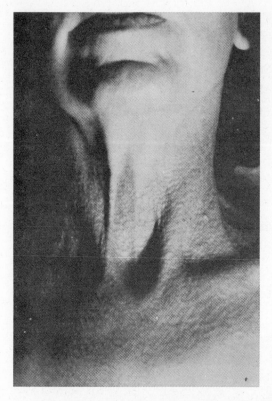

FIG. 117. Pseudoxanthoma elasticum, revealing the leathery, ridged, yellowish skin of the anterior portion of the neck. (Bean, W. B.: Vascular Spiders and Related Lesions of the Skin, Springfield, Ill., Thomas)

no longer tenable. It is indeed difficult to picture dislodgement of a clot from an esophageal varix by pressing on the abdomen. Hemostasis in the capillary bleeding of erosive gastritis and esophagitis is said to be accomplished by the prevention of filling of the injured capillaries through the opening of arteriovenous shunts of the mucosal vascular system rather than by clot formation.[34] Furthermore, the importance of surface clotting in the hemostasis of bleeding peptic ulcer has been seriously questioned.[34]

A palpable liver of increased consistency should strongly suggest the presence of hepatic cirrhosis, as should the presence of ascites or distended veins over the chest and the abdomen. Splenomegaly should indicate hepatic cirrhosis or Banti's syndrome; but it should be remembered that the spleen contracts after hemorrhage, and thus for a time it may not be palpable. It is needless to add that the presence of an abdominal tumor should suggest carcinoma. Search for the characteristic continuous murmur of splenic arteriovenous fistula should be made over the lower left posterolateral ribs in young patients with suspected portal hypertension and hypersplenism in the absence of hepatomegaly and abnormal liver function tests.[38] Palpation of the radial pulse may furnish

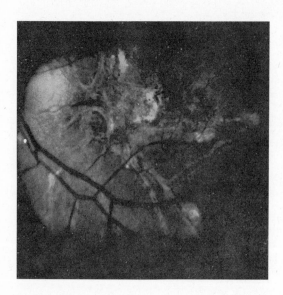

FIG. 118. Angioid streaks and proliferative changes in fundus oculi. (McKusick, V. A.: Heritable Disorders of Connective Tissue, ed. 2, St. Louis, Mosby)

evidence of arteriosclerosis, which may prove of importance in prognosis and in the choice of emergency surgical therapy for bleeding peptic ulcer.

X-RAY EXAMINATION

The great value of x-ray examination in furnishing direct evidence of peptic ulcer or gastric cancer need only be mentioned in passing. Unfortunately, the roentgenogram has proved to be of little value in the diagnosis of gastritis.[39] In Benedict's series of 42 cases of gastritis with hemorrhage,[2] roentgenologic examination suggested the presence of gastritis in 9 instances. Gastric erosions are rarely demonstrated roentgeno-

logically. Roentgen examination may prove of particular value in the diagnosis of esophageal varices (Fig. 119). Sometimes the roentgen demonstration of such varices may furnish the sole anatomic evidence of hepatic cirrhosis.[40]

In an excellent discussion of the subject, Schatzki[40] points out that the principle of roentgen visualization of esophageal varices rests on the fact that the dilated veins bulge into the lumen of the esophagus and produce an "uneven wormlike surface." Large varices may be detected fluoroscopically, whereas small ones may be visible only on a roentgenogram. Occasionally varices may be seen in the cardiac end of

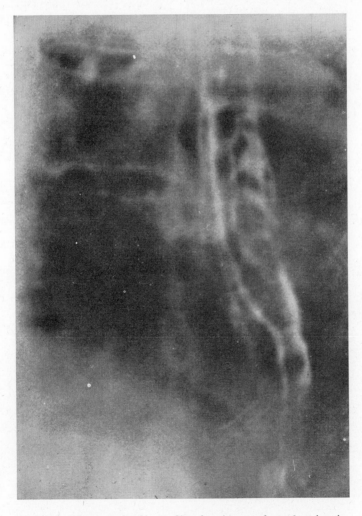

FIG. 119. Photograph of x-ray film showing esophageal varices in a case of hepatic cirrhosis (patient R. R.).

the stomach and be mistaken for the enlarged folds of a localized hypertrophic gastritis or even for tumor[41] (Fig. 120). He advises that the examination be made with the patient in the horizontal position, as varices become smaller in the erect position. He uses a suspension of equal parts of barium and water and advises coating the inner surface of the esophagus with only a thin layer of barium, as filling the organ with a large amount of the opaque medium will obliterate the protruding vessels. Films should be taken in several projections after slight inspiration, since during this phase the lower end of the esophagus is stretched slightly, thus avoiding misinterpreting of tortuous folds in a slack esophagus. Nelson[42] recommends the admixture of carboxymethylcellulose (0.25 to 0.75 per cent) to increase the adherence of the barium to the esophageal and gastric mucosa, or the administration of atropine, 0.5 to 1.0 mg., subcutaneously 30 minutes before the examination. He stresses the value of the Valsalva maneuver in demonstrating varices and states that the Müller maneuver may occasionally show varices when all other methods have failed. Barium studies of the esophagus are much less reliable than either esophagoscopy or splenoportography for the demonstration of esophageal varices.[43] It has been estimated that the radiologist is only able to visualize varices in about 30 to 50 per cent of the cases.[42] Even when special techniques are employed, only 70 per cent are said to be demonstrated.[43]

It has been customary to defer roentgenologic examination of the upper digestive tract in patients with hematemesis or melena until two or three weeks after the hemorrhage. The reason for this delay has been the fear of reinducing hemorrhage through the manipulation of the abdomen. The disadvantage of deferring the examination has been twofold: (1) an ulcer may heal within one to three weeks after hemorrhage (Benedict,[2] Hampton,[44] Jones[3] and Schiff[45]) and thus escape detection, and (2) it withholds the means of establishing promptly the diagnosis of peptic ulcer in patients past 50 years of age with massive hemorrhage, in whom immediate surgery may be contemplated.

Hampton[44] devised a technic for the roentgenologic demonstration of bleeding duodenal ulcers in which neither abdominal palpation nor compression is used, in order to obviate the danger of reinducing hemorrhage. The patient is taken to the x-ray room in his bed and is transferred to the horizontal roentgenoscopic table by means of a sheet. Four ounces of the following mixture are taken through a drinking tube:

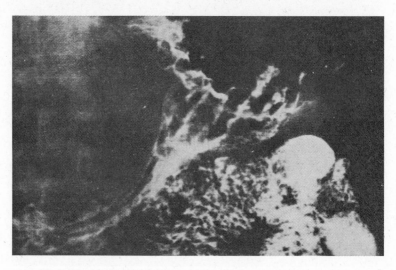

FIG. 120. Film showing a lobulated mass at the esophagogastric junction. (Karr, S., and Wohl, G. T.: New England J. Med. 263:667)

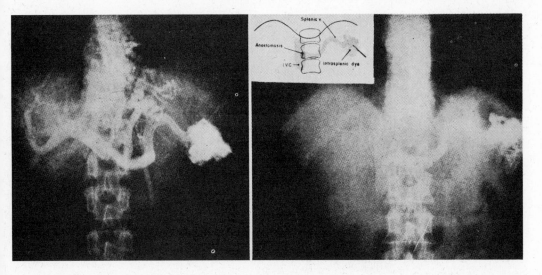

Fig. 121. Splenoportogram in Laennec's cirrhosis with bleeding varices. (*Left*) Preoperative study. The coronary and short gastric veins are dilated and there are gastric and esophageal varices. There is backflow into the inferior mesenteric vein. The portal radicles in the liver are attenuated. Intrasplenic pressure 28.5 cm. (*Right*) Repeat study two months after portacaval shunt. The anastomosis is patent and there is no collateral filling. Splenic pressure, 16 cm. (Ann. Int. Med. 52:782)

Plain barium sulfate.......... 4 oz. (volume)
Water .... 3 oz. (volume)
Plain Petrogalar .... 1 teaspoonful

The mixture should be freshly prepared and have the consistency of cream.

After the patient has ingested the barium as he lies upon his back, he is rotated toward his right side and allowed to remain in this position under roentgenoscopic observation until the first part of the duodenum has filled and emptied two or three times. Then when the duodenum is completely filled, he is promptly returned to the face-up position and rotated more to the left side until the pyloric valve and first portion of the duodenum are seen in profile. Roentgenograms are taken with the roentgenoscopic tube immediately, while the duodenum is still filled.

Since compression or palpation is not used because of the traditional fear of starting further hemorrhage, some method must be used which would permit visualization of the inner relief of the posterior wall of the duodenum. This is done by taking films after the duodenum has emptied. Thick barium will adhere to the duodenal mucosa and by the force of gravity will remain in such ulcer craters as are present.

The double contrast examination is then done. There is usually a gas bubble present in the stomach, but if this is not the case the patient should be instructed to swallow four to five times. Gas in the stomach will, of course, pass upward when the patient is on the left side and this gas can be seen to pass through the pyloric valve. It is during the time that the fundus gas bubble is in the antrum, the pyloric valve and the duodenum that films are taken for double contrast examination.

At the Cincinnati General Hospital, the Hampton technic has been carried out since 1938 in many patients with severe hematemesis and melena within a few hours or a day or so after admission to the hospital. The procedure has proved to be quite safe and of great value in establishing an early diagnosis in cases of severe gastroduodenal hemorrhage. In a series of unselected cases[46] examined by this method during a 1-year period, a diagnostic accuracy of 86 per cent was obtained. Early radiologic examination of the upper digestive tract has recently been carried out

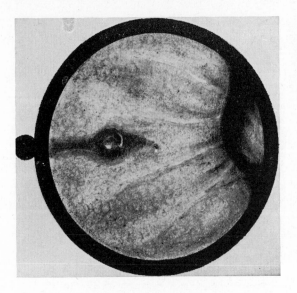

FIG. 122. Photograph of drawing of a bleeding mucosal erosion seen at gastroscopy. There was associated hypertrophic gastritis as evidenced by the polygonal pattern of the near-by mucosa.

with a portable x-ray apparatus.[47] Four ounces of barium suspension are drunk as rapidly as possible by the patient who is then turned into the right lateral position with the film cassette and grid beneath him. An exposure is made in this position, followed in quick succession by right anterior oblique, right posterior oblique, and anteroposterior projections.

Esophageal varices may also be demonstrated by means of percutaneous splenoportal venography (Fig. 121).

ESOPHAGOSCOPY AND GASTROSCOPY

The mere demonstration of esophageal varices by x-ray examination or endoscopy prior to an episode of bleeding is no proof that they are the actual source of hemorrhage. The purpose of performing esophagoscopy in the presence of upper gastrointestinal hemorrhage is not only to determine the presence (or absence) of esophageal varices, but to see if they are bleeding. The hazard incurred by the pro-

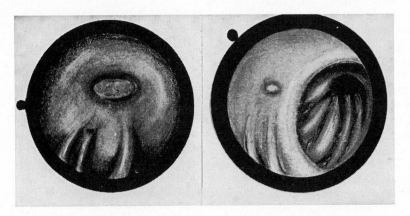

FIG. 123. (Left) Photograph of drawing of superficial gastric ulcer made at gastroscopy 3 days after massive hematemesis. (Right) Gastroscopic findings after 15 days on Meulengracht Diet. Note marked reduction in size of ulcer.

Fig. 124. Photograph of drawing made at gastroscopy of a large benign gastric ulcer containing several large clots (patient C. F.). There was no antecedent history of hematemesis or melena. The lesion disappeared following medical therapy.

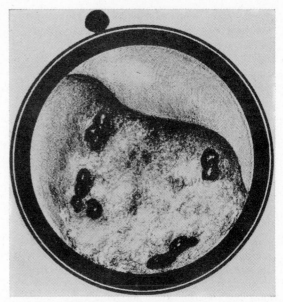

cedure has probably been exaggerated. In the hands of the particularly interested and experienced esophagoscopist it is said to be minimal.[34,48] As Smith[48] has indicated, "esophagoscopy in the presence of actively bleeding esophageal varices is not for the occasional endoscopist."

In addition to being prerequisite in the clinical diagnosis of gastritis, gastroscopy is particularly valuable in revealing erosions or small superficial or acute ulcers that usually are not demonstrable on roentgen examination (Figs. 122 and 123). In some cases of gastritis, there may be oozing from the mucosa without definite erosion (Benedict,[49] Schindler[50]), and in others fresh or old blood may be seen without demonstrable erosion (Benedict[49]). Schindler[51] believes that hemorrhagic erosions may occur in the absence of demonstrable gastritis and our experience would confirm this view. The erosions are small, usually less than 5 mm. in diameter, and deep. They may be reddish, grayish-red or brownish-red in color. Occasionally a gastric ulcer containing clots may be seen without an antecedent or subsequent history of hemorrhage (Fig. 124).

Mucosal hemorrhages may not necessarily be significant since they may be present in the normal stomach. Ruffin and Brown[52] believe that they may result from the suc-

tion employed prior to introduction of the gastroscope. In this connection, the important observations of Wolf and Wolff[53] made in their experimental subject must be kept in mind, namely, that acceleration of acid production and motor activity were always accompanied by hyperemia and engorgement of the mucosa. When vascular engorgement was prolonged, the rugae became intensely red, thick and turgid, presenting the picture of what has been called hypertrophic gastritis. In this state the mucosa was unusually fragile, hemorrhages and small erosions resulting from the most minor traumata.

Since it is known that erosions may heal within a few days and that peptic ulcers may heal within two weeks, it is most desirable to perform gastroscopy within two or three days after hemorrhage. Jones[3] performed successful gastroscopy mainly between the third and tenth day following hemorrhage in 116 out of 217 cases without radiologic proof of peptic ulcer (the so-called acute lesion group). A gastric ulcer was found in 65 of these cases, and valuable diagnostic information was obtained in 31 additional instances.

BLEEDING PEPTIC ULCER

Hemorrhage in patients with peptic ulcer is generally due to erosion of an artery lying at the base of the ulcer. Ulcers on the posterior wall of the superior portion of the duodenum are unusually prone to bleed. In some cases the stomach itself may be eroded as the result of an associated gastritis (Benedict,[2] Alsted[32]). Chronic gastric ulcers are apt to bleed more severely than duodenal ulcers, due probably to erosion of larger-sized arteries, i.e., the main trunks of the right or the left gastric arteries as compared with branches of the gastroduodenal or pancreaticoduodenal arteries.[54]

In discussing cases of bleeding peptic ulcer, Jones[3] states:

At necropsy it was usual to find one large open vessel in the floor of the ulcer, and it was remarkable that death had occurred usually not quickly but after several recurrent bleedings in the course of as many days. Bleeding with acute collapse must have occurred from the large exposed vessel, not once but perhaps six times. It would seem probable that in most cases bleeding from such a large vessel could have occurred for only a short period, perhaps 10 to 15 minutes, and then ceased. At operation the vessel usually did not begin to spurt until it was manipulated.

If the loss of blood is severe, there is a prompt fall in blood pressure which in itself, if not too great, is advantageous since it helps curtail further bleeding. Clotting of the blood serves to close the opening in the blood vessel. Effectual sealing of the vascular wall is furthered by the retraction of the open end of the artery. Only after a few days does the clot begin to harden. It is apparent that if the eroded artery is sclerotic it may not be able to retract sufficiently to prevent further bleeding, which may prove fatal.

It is generally agreed that during hunger the stomach exhibits active contractions, and it is conceivable that such contractions may dislodge the clot. The administration of food has a quieting effect on these hunger contractions (Christensen[55]). This fact, among others, led Meulengracht[56] to begin the immediate feeding of patients suffering from bleeding peptic ulcer. Most reports, including our own,[57] indicate that immediate feeding has resulted in a substantial reduction in mortality and a shortening of hospital stay. According to Crohn[58] and Hurst[59] the frequency of hemorrhage in

peptic ulcer is probably about 10 per cent if patients not admitted to the hospital as well as hospital patients are included.

The relative frequency of hematemesis versus melena varies in different statistics. In hospital cases, hematemesis accompanied by melena occurs more frequently than melena alone. This may be explained by the fact that melena may be unnoticed or disregarded by the ambulatory patient, whereas hematemesis is more apt to cause him to seek hospital care.

Hemorrhage is an indication of activity of the ulcerative process. It is said to occur rarely in patients under strict treatment. In most cases ulcerlike symptoms precede hemorrhage for varying periods of time, usually for many years. In some cases, however, there are no antecedent symptoms, or symptoms have been present for only a few days or weeks.

Disappearance of pain for weeks or longer following hemorrhage has been pointed out by Hurst[59] and has been quite striking in our experience. The cause of this phenomenon is not clear. In some instances it has been found to be associated with actual healing of the ulcer. It is possible that the lack of gastric tone occurring as a result of the anemia may play a role (Carlson[60]). Bonney and Pickering[61] suggest that the blood in the crater may increase the thickness of the protective layer of slough which may cover the pain nerve endings and hinder their excitation by the hydrochloric acid. Another explanation of the initial loss of pain may be the neutralizing effect of the blood in the stomach on the gastric acidity.[62]

The symptoms of bleeding peptic ulcer depend upon the severity of the hemorrhage. In mild cases there may be little more than hematemesis or melena. In more severe hemorrhage there may be weakness, dizziness, faintness, excessive perspiration, thirst, or actual syncope and shock. Headache may be quite severe and in several of our patients was relieved by inhalation of oxygen or by a blood transfusion. Hematemesis may precede or follow the passage of loose tarry stools. Syncope not infrequently takes place in the bathroom and may be due to a fall in blood pressure upon assumption of the erect position. In this connection, Wallace and Sharpey-Schafer[10] reported syncope following assumption of the erect position as long as 5 or 6 hours after venesection in some of their control subjects. They found that the rapid removal of from 900 to 1,150 ml. of blood resulted in an exaggerated "postural response" in every instance immediately after removal of the blood.

In one patient with duodenal ulcer and a rather severe hemorrhage manifesting itself by melena, the first complaint was marked shortness of breath which she experienced after climbing two flights of stairs on her way to dinner. Earlier in the day she fainted at the hairdresser's and felt faint on two other occasions. She had passed a tarry stool the day before the attack of dyspnea but recalled this only after passing several more tarry stools the following day. Another patient felt a little weak and sweated a little after a round of golf on a cool October day. He was driven home by a friend. Before entering his home, he sat on the porch but grew weaker and became frightened. He called his family physician, who advised a suppository. He noticed that his stool was black but he

went to bed without notifying anyone. He passed three black stools during the night and the following morning fainted in the bathroom. Another patient, not included in this study, became a little faint and sweated as he was dictating a letter to his stenographer. That night he passed a tarry stool and was brought to a hospital.

Although coronary thrombosis has been precipitated by gastroduodenal hemorrhage,[3,63,64,65,66] electrocardiographic changes may occur after acute gastrointestinal hemorrhage without subsequent evidence of coronary artery disease. Rasmussen and Foss[67] reported flattening, isoelectric or negative T-waves, and lowering of the S-T interval in about half the cases. They were unable to correlate the changes with anemia or fall in blood pressure, but did find some relationship to azotemia. Like Scherf and associates,[68] they attribute the changes to myocardial anoxemia secondary to coronary spasm associated with the generalized vasoconstriction following hemorrhage. On the other hand, Master and his associates[69] stress the degree of shock, drop in blood pressure, tachycardia and decrease in hemoglobin level as factors responsible for precipitating these changes, which they inter-

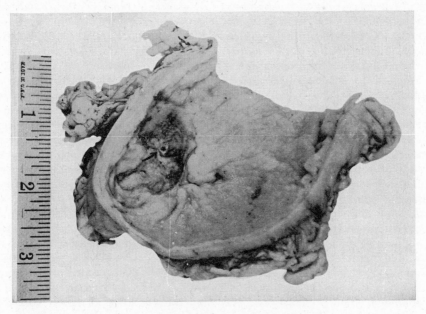

Fig. 125. Photograph of specimen of stomach showing malignant gastric ulcer with a gaping sclerotic artery in its base (patient J. S.) .

pret as evidence of acute coronary insufficiency. They regard the decreased blood volume resulting from hemorrhage as the major mechanism.

Association of acute emotional distress with gastroduodenal hemorrhage is frequent.[3,70,71] The engorging effect on the gastric mucosa of sustained resentment, frustration and anxiety may play an important role in the genesis of the ulceration.[53] The additional factors of missed meals, extra smoking and drinking have been suggested as possibly causing sudden extension of the ulceration.[3]

CARCINOMA OF THE STOMACH

Bleeding in cases of gastric carcinoma is usually due to ulceration of the stomach or necrosis and sloughing of papillary growths. "Because of the small vessels involved, the bleeding is usually in the form of oozing or seepage."[72] However, if there is erosion of a medium-sized or large vessel, massive hemorrhage may result as occurred in the case shown in Figure 125. In one patient with a large carcinomatous ulcer, fifteen small vessels were seen projecting from the base of the lesion at autopsy. Three of them were capped with thrombi.

Massive hemorrhage may be the initial symptom in patients with gastric carcinoma and is probably not as rare as is generally supposed. It was the presenting symptom in 10 such patients seen at the Cincinnati General Hospital, taking the guise of hematemesis followed by melena in 8 and of melena alone in 2. Massive hemorrhage in gastric carcinoma may occur in the absence of any demonstrable lesion either by physical or x-ray examinations.[73,74] Temporary improvement may occur in patients with gastric cancer and may suggest the presence of a benign rather than a malignant ulcer. If the disease is sufficiently advanced, physical examination may reveal the presence of enlarged supraclavicular glands on the left, an abdominal mass, an enlarged nodular liver or a "Blumer's shelf."

X-ray and gastroscopic examinations are of recognized value in the diagnosis of gastric carcinoma. The presence of a persistent posthistamine achlorhydria in a patient with hematemesis and melena should exclude the possibility of peptic ulcer and should lead to a suspicion of gastric cancer.

Exfoliative cytology as applied to gastric aspirates has proved of diagnostic value in areas where it is properly performed. Determination of the lactic dehydrogenase activity of gastric juice may also prove helpful in diagnosis.[75].

BLEEDING ESOPHAGEAL VARICES

Hematemesis in patients with hepatic cirrhosis is usually due to a ruptured varix in the lower end of the esophagus. Rupture may occur spontaneously, or may follow excessive physical activity, uncontrolled vomiting and coughing.[76] Esophageal varices develop because of obstruction to the return of the portal blood to the systemic venous system. The site of the portal block may be either in the liver (the intrahepatic type secondary to portal cirrhosis), or in the portal vein itself (the extrahepatic type as seen in Banti's syndrome).[77,78] According to Whipple, the most easily established collaterals are those between the gastric, the lienogastric and the esophageal veins, carrying a large part of this shunted blood to the superior vena cava through the azygos route.

Bleeding varices may occur in the absence of either intrahepatic or extrahepatic obstruction of the portal vein.[79,80] To explain this occurrence, Tisdale postulates functional or structural alterations of the vessels of the gastrointestinal tract, the spleen and the liver as permitting increased flow of blood into the portal vein with a resultant rise in pressure. On the basis of a similar mechanism, portal hypertension may result from splenic arteriovenous fistulas. Aneurysm of the hepatic artery may produce portal hypertension and bleeding esophageal varices by compression of the portal vein or by direct communication with the portal vein in the nature of an arteriovenous shunt.[81] Bleeding varices have also been noted in obstruction of the superior vena cava from idiopathic mediastinal fibrosis.[82,83] Their occurrence in young individuals without demonstrable liver disease or abnormalities of liver function tests should suggest the possibility of polycystic liver.[84,85] Opinion differs as to the relative importance of the increase in portal venous pressure and the presence of peptic esophagitis in the causation of variceal rupture.[86,87,88]

Whipple believes that the esophageal veins are prone to thinning, dilatation and varix formation because of a combination of portal hypertension and meager support by the tissues and organs in the mediastinum. He also points out that the varices are subject to trauma because of the frequent contractions of the esophagus, and the pressure and passage of boluses of ingested food. Wangensteen[87] has suggested that rupture of esophageal varices may be due to peptic ulceration of the esophageal mucosa over them because of the reflux of acid contents into the esophagus. Another possible cause of esophageal bleeding which has been postulated is based on the assumption that intravariceal pressure is sufficient to cause necrosis of the thin-walled vessel and overlying attenuated mucosa.[89] In some instances the source of the blood may be an erosive gastritis, a gastric varix, or a coexisting peptic ulcer.[90]

Ratnoff and Patek[1] reported nine instances of melena without hematemesis in a series of 386 cases of Laennec's cirrhosis. They also pointed out the frequency of other hemorrhagic phenomena such as epistaxis, purpura, and bleeding from the gums. Morlock and Hall[91] have emphasized the occurrence of *thrombopenia* which they believe may increase the bleeding hazard.

Hematemesis occurs in about one-fourth of patients with hepatic cirrhosis, the initial bout being fatal in about one-third of the cases in whom it occurs.[1] It may be the first manifestation of disease in about 10 per cent of cases and was the only symptom in 10 of Preble's 60 fatal cases of hematemesis.[92] While frequently fatal, hematemesis sometimes recurs over long periods of time. In one of our patients who subsequently came to autopsy, it recurred during a 10-year period. In some instances it may be followed by a decline in serum protein and development of ascites.[1] Hematemesis is frequently a forerunner of hepatic coma. The presence of blood in the intestinal tract may produce an elevation of the blood ammonia concentration.[93]

White and Chalmers[94] have emphasized the uniform presence of abnormal bromsulphalein excretion in cases of hepatic cirrhosis with hematemesis, particularly during shock. While they encountered abnormal dye retention in occasional cases of bleeding peptic ulcer, "at the time of shock or soon after," they believe that a normal bromsulphalein test soon after a severe hemorrhage practically rules out bleeding esophageal varices associated with hepatic cirrhosis. The bromsulphalein excretion test and determination of blood ammonia concentration, when considered together, have been reported to be very useful in differentiating bleeding esophageal varices from bleeding peptic ulcer.[95,96,97,98] These tests have not proved as helpful as expected in patients with upper digestive tract hemorrhage associated with portal hypertension and known liver disease because abnormal bromsulphalein retention and elevated blood ammonia levels are apt to occur regardless of the source of bleeding.

Gastrointestinal symptoms such as anorexia, morning nausea, vomiting, flatulence and not infrequently diarrhea may precede the attacks of hematemesis. Of value in establishing a diagnosis of hepatic cirrhosis are a history of chronic alcoholism, a diet deficient in meat and dairy products,[1] the presence of icterus, ascites, vascular spiders on the skin of the face, the neck, the upper chest and the upper extremities, distended veins on the abdomen and the chest, a firm, palpable liver and a palpable spleen. Laboratory tests suggesting cirrhosis include a positive cephalin flocculation test, increased thymol or zinc sulfate turbidity, retention of bromsulphalein, reduction of serum albumin content and elevation of gamma globulin. Needle biopsy of the liver is extremely helpful in diagnosis, but is best carried out following recovery from hemorrhage. The demonstration of esophageal varices by roentgenologic examination, esophagoscopy or portal venography[99] may clinch the diagnosis if congestive splenomegaly due to extrahepatic portal block or hepatoma can be excluded.

Merigan and associates[100] found that patients with cirrhosis who underwent acute hepatic decompensation were more apt to be bleeding from esophageal varices, and were less apt to be bleeding from sites other than varices, than those who bled without hepatic decompensation. Bleeding in patients who have had a recent portacaval shunt may not necessarily indicate recurrence of esophageal varices, but rather prove to be due to a peptic ulcer developing following the shunt.[101,102] In dogs, the secretion of hydrochloric acid from a Heidenhain pouch has been shown to increase greatly after portacaval transposition. This may be due to the increased effect of a humoral secretagogue which originates in the abdominal viscera and is normally inactivated by the liver.

Panke and associates[103] have stressed the value of determining the intrasplenic pulp pressure, a measure of the portal venous pressure, in patients with upper digestive tract hemorrhage. In a series of 130 patients they found bleeding esophagogastric varices never to be associated with a splenic pulp pressure below 250 mm. of water. Contrariwise, bleeding from other lesions was never associated with pressures above 290 mm. of water. Variceal bleeding was associated with high splenic pulp pressures regardless of the presence of shock. They reported a 90 per cent accuracy in determining the presence or absence of varices.

GASTRITIS AND ESOPHAGITIS

Gastritis has long been recognized as a cause of varying degrees of hemorrhage, particularly by European observers. This relationship has been stressed, among others, by Faber,[104] Moutier,[105] Henning,[106] and Benedict.[2] In a series of 42 cases of hemorrhage from gastritis, Benedict reported a mild degree of hemorrhage in 7, a moderate degree in 14 and a severe degree in 21. The bleeding occurring in chronic gastritis usually takes place from erosions in the mucous membrane (Figs. 126 and 127), which most commonly occur on the crests of the folds. In some cases there may be oozing from the mucosa without definite erosion (Benedict,[2] Schindler[50]). Schindler believes that most of the profuse hemorrhages in gastritis occur in the chronic hypertrophic form from an ulceration eroding a small blood vessel.

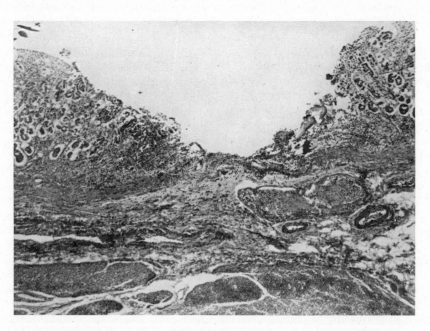

Fig. 126. Photomicrograph of a gastric mucosal erosion which produced fatal hemorrhage. × 30. A blood clot covers the erosion. (Dr. Ralph Fuller)

Fig. 127. Biopsy at edge of erosion in case of erosive esophagitis. The hemorrhage stopped about half an hour before the specimen was taken. No clot has formed on the erosion's surface, in the mucosa's capillaries, or in the other vessels. (Palmer, E. D.: Diagnosis of Upper Gastrointestinal Hemorrhage, Springfield, Ill., Thomas)

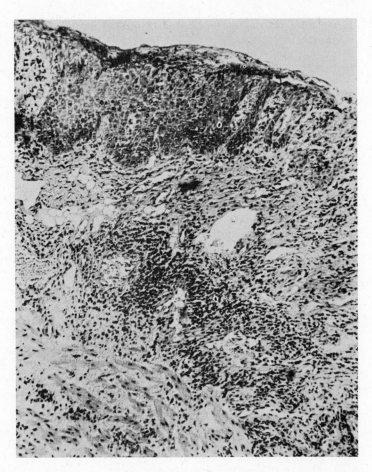

Among the 42 cases reported by Benedict, the gastritis was superficial in 13, hypertrophic in 12, atrophic in 2, "postoperative" in 5, and mixed in 10. This author stresses excessive use of alcohol as the most important etiologic factor in massive bleeding from gastritis. According to Palmer ingestion of large amounts of alcohol during a brief period produces an acute gastritis with frequently demonstrable erosions with return of the gastroscopic appearance to normal soon after avoidance of alcohol.[107]

Benedict[49] believes that gastritis may reasonably be assumed to be the cause of hematemesis if no other pathologic changes have been found and there is gastroscopic evidence of severe gastritis. While we realize that this view may be correct, we have been hesitant to follow it in the absence of demonstrable erosions. In this connection it must be realized that one is particularly apt to be in error if the gastroscopic examination is made, as is customary, two or three weeks after the hemorrhage, since erosions may heal within a few days.

The relatively high incidence of subacute erosive esophagitis and acute erosive gastritis as a cause of upper digestive tract hemorrhage in Palmer's series of cases is testimony to the diagnostic value of early endoscopy, particularly in cases where roentgenographic examination is apt to prove negative. Palmer recommends a swallow of 10 per cent fluorescin several minutes before the procedure to improve the visualization of both esophageal and gastric erosions, particularly following ice-water lavage.

HIATAL HERNIA

Bleeding in cases of hiatal hernia may be due to congestion of the blood vessels in

TABLE 20. CAUSES OF HEMATEMESIS AND MELENA IN MISCELLANEOUS GROUP OF 43 PATIENTS OVER A 10-YEAR PERIOD

CAUSE OF HEMORRHAGE	NUMBER OF PATIENTS
Acute esophagitis with pancreatic necrosis	1
Banti's syndrome (extrahepatic block)	2
Benign tumor of the stomach	1
Blood dyscrasia	8
Carcinoma of the esophagus	3
Chronic relapsing pancreatitis	1
Cirrhosis with esophageal diverticulum	1
Cholecystoduodenal fistula	1
Curling's ulcer	1
Erosive esophagitis and/or erosive gastritis associated with liver disease	8
Erosion of the aorta due to periaortitis	1
Gastric varices	1
Lymphosarcoma of the stomach	1
Malignancy eroding the gastrointestinal tract	3
Mesenteric thrombosis	5
Prolapsed gastric mucosa	1
Ulcerative esophagitis	3
Ulcerated heterotopic gastric tissue	1

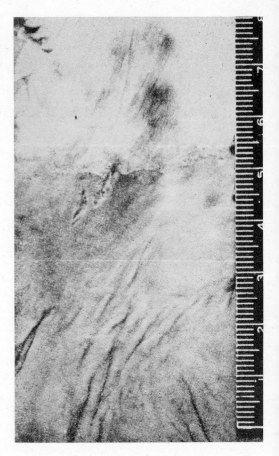

FIG. 128. Specimen showing two small 1 cm. lacerations just inferior to the gastroesophageal junction. (Decker, J. P. *et. al.*: New England J. Med. 249:957)

the herniated portion of the stomach, gastritis or ulceration.[108] There may be ulceration of the esophagogastric junction or there may be a gastric ulcer adjacent to the neck of the sac where it passes through the diaphragm. The symptoms of hiatal hernia have been well described.[109,110,111] At the time of admission it may be difficult to prove the hiatal hernia as the cause of the bleeding. Esophagoscopy and gastroscopy may prove helpful. In some instances presumptive proof may be based on the lack of recurrence of bleeding following repair of the hernia.

HEMATEMESIS AND MELENA DUE TO MISCELLANEOUS CAUSES

Miscellaneous causes of hematemesis and melena found in 43 patients (48 cases) of a series of 640 cases seen at the Cincinnati General Hospital are listed in Table 20. Other causes include hemorrhage from localized arteriosclerosis of gastric vessels,[112] hereditary telangiectasia,[113,114,115] tumors of the small intestine,[116] rupture of aneurysm of the hepatic artery[117] or splenic artery,[118] aortic stenosis,[119] pseudoxanthoma elasticum,[35,36,37] ruptured aortic aneurysm, periarteritis nodosa,[120] jejunal diverticulosis,[121] multiple hemangiomas of the jejunum[122] and gastric carcinoid.[123] Bleeding may also arise from Meckel's diverticulum or diverticulitis of the colon.

Hematemesis and melena have been ascribed to aspirin ingestion.[124-136] Slight to intense hyperemia and even submucous hemorrhage have been reported on gastroscopic examination made in patients following the ingestion of three crushed aspirin tablets.[125] Acute gastric erosions attributed to salicylates have been described at gastroscopy[126,128] and laparotomy.[134] The mechanism may possibly be related to the hypoprothrombinemic action of salicylic acid.[137,138] Muir and Cossar gave aspirin shortly before partial gastrectomy and found less reaction in the resected specimens when soluble aspirin was given as contrasted with ordinary aspirin. In one case, a half aspirin tablet was found imbedded in the mucosa of the greater curvature, lying beneath overlapping edematous and congested rugae.[139] According to Winkelman and Summerskill,[130] factors involved in mucosal damage and resistance seem more important than hydrochloric acid secretion in relation to gastrointestinal bleeding following consumption of aspirin. They could establish no relationship between massive gastrointestinal bleeding, subjective intolerance to salicylate compounds and hydrochloric acid secretion in response to administration of salicylates. They found blood to be present in specimens of gastric juice much more frequently after standard or soluble aspirin tablets were ingested than after oral or intravenous administration of sodium salicylate.

Hemorrhage from gastroesophageal lacerations at the cardiac orifice of the stomach—the so-called Mallory-Weiss syndrome[140,141]—is an uncommon cause of massive bleeding (Fig. 128). It occurs in alcoholics and is usually preceded by violent or protracted retching and vomiting. It may occur in the absence of alcoholism, as in the vomiting of pregnancy or even obstructing ulcer.[34] There may be one laceration[34] or two to four as originally described. Mallory and Weiss[140] reported the lesions to be characteristically arranged around the circumference of the cardiac opening, along the longitudinal axis of the esophagus. In their report, the size of the lesions varied from 3 to 20 mm. in length and from 2 to 3 mm. in width. According to Palmer, the laceration is found at gastroscopy to be a straight cleft running roughly parallel to the esophageal axis. The cleft is usually an estimated centimeter in length and rarely may extend for as many as 4 centimeters. A characteristic feature of the laceration is rather steep elevation of its edges, with fairly wide gaping. The cleft is always filled with clot and it is presumed that the

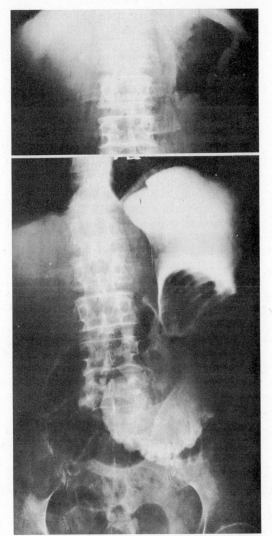

FIG. 129. (*Top*) A lobulated mass is shown projecting into the lumen of the distal stomach. (*Bottom*) Following a barium swallow the mass in the stomach shows valvulae conniventes on its surface. There is obstruction of the duodenum and proximal jejunum secondary to the intussusception.

ridge-like elevation is due to bleeding beneath the laceration's edges. Mallory and Weiss considered the pressure changes in the stomach during the disturbed mechanism of vomiting together with regurgitation of the gastric juice and the corrosive effect of alcohol to be responsible for the lesions described in their cases.

Heuer[142] reported a case in which the pathologist failed to find any erosion of the mucosa of the stomach or duodenum, but, on injecting the gastric artery with saline from a pressure bottle, he was able to observe a jet of fluid from the mucosal lining. Serial sections of the area showed a small ruptured aneurysm concealed by overlying, mucosal folds. It appears quite plausible that this type of lesion may be the underlying cause of hemorrhage in some otherwise unexplained cases.

Retrograde jejunogastric intussusception occurs more often in women than in men, is much more frequent after gastroenterostomy than after gastric resection and may occur as long as 18 years after operation with an average interval of 6 years[143] (Fig. 129). In the majority of cases, vomiting of food and bile precedes hematemesis. A mass may be palpable above and to the left of the umbilicus in more than half the cases. The x-ray finding within the lumen of the stomach of a partially moving filling defect simulating the normal pattern of small intestinal folds (Kerckring folds or valvulae conniventes) is characteristic.

Fistulization between the intestinal tract and an abdominal aortic prothesis is a common cause of late graft failure and usually occurs at suture lines which are contiguous with bowel loops.[144] "Any massive gastrointestinal hemorrhage after an abdominal aortic operation should be considered of aortic origin until proved otherwise."[144]

Massive gastrointestinal bleeding may result from hemorrhage into the bile ducts.[145-149] Hemobilia, as this condition has been called, is most commonly due to aneurysm of the hepatic artery or liver trauma. Sparkman[146,147] stressed the triad of abdominal injury, gastrointestinal hemorrhage and biliary colic as highly suggestive of traumatic hemobilia. The pain is characteristic of biliary colic and the patient, having previously experienced such pain before bleeding, may rightly warn the physician that he is about to bleed again. Transient jaundice is a common accompaniment. An intrahepatic cavity that periodically empties its contents into the biliary tract is the basis of the syndrome. According to Schatski,[149] scintillating scanning of the liver may reveal the hepatic cavity acting as the source of the bleeding. In a recent case report the bleeding originated in an hepatic abscess.[150]

Pseudoxanthoma elasticum should be recognized by the characteristic skin changes and the angioid streaks in the retina. Superficial ulceration has been observed at gastroscopy and in the resected stomach. In some cases gastroscopy soon after hematemesis has been negative.[151] The bleeding point may be in the duodenum or there may be multiple bleeding points in other parts of the intestine.

SUMMARY

Bleeding into the gastrointestinal tract may be brought to the attention of the patient and the physician through vomiting of blood (hematemesis) or through the detection of blood in the stools (melena).

Pathogenic mechanisms include (1) conditions involving the tissues of the walls of the gastrointestinal tract, (2) disorders of blood vessel walls, and (3) disturbances of blood clotting.

The commonest clinical causes are peptic ulcer, esophageal varices associated with hepatic cirrhosis, gastric cancer, hiatus hernia, gastritis and esophagitis. Examination by roentgenography and by gastroscopy and esophagoscopy is of great assistance in the differential diagnosis of the more usual causes of gastrointestinal bleeding.

Among the less frequent causes are blood dyscrasias, the Mallory-Weiss Syndrome, mesenteric thrombosis, gastrointestinal neoplasms other than gastric carcinoma, diverticula of the alimentary tract, pseudoxanthoma elasticum and a few rare miscellaneous conditions.

Bleeding into the gastrointestinal tract is of serious import, whether acute and dramatic or chronic and obscure. Discovery of the cause should be as prompt as possible so that proper therapy can be used to prevent death, various complications or chronic disability.

REFERENCES

1. Ratnoff, O. D., and Patek, A. J., Jr.: The natural history of Laennec's cirrhosis of the liver; an analysis of 386 cases, Medicine 21: 207, 1942.

2. Benedict, E. B.: Hemorrhage from gastritis; a report based on pathological, clinical, roentgenological and gastroscopic findings, Am. J. Roentgenol. 47:254, 1942.

3. Jones, F. Avery: Haematemesis and melaena with special reference to bleeding peptic ulcer, Brit. M. J. 2:441; 477, 1947.

4. Schiff, L., Stevens, R. J., Shapiro, N., and Goodman, S.: Observations on the oral administration of citrated blood in man; II, The effect on the stools, Am. J. M. Sc. 203: 409, 1942.

5. Hilsman, J. H.: The color of blood-containing feces following instillation of citrated blood at various levels of the small intestine, Gastroenterology 15:131, 1950.

6. Daniel, W. A., Jr., and Egan, S.: Quantity of blood required to produce a tarry stool, J.A.M.A. 113:2232, 1939.

7. Hesser, S.: Über die Dauer von Magengeschwürblutungen, Acta med. Scandinav., supp. 59, p. 367, 1934.

8. Cullinan, E. R., and Price, R. K.: Haematemesis following peptic ulceration; prognosis and treatment, St. Barth. Hosp. Rep. 65:185, 1932.

9. Black, D. A. K.: Critical review; azotaemia in gastro-duodenal haemorrhage, Quart. J. Med. 11:77, 1942.

10. Wallace, J., and Sharpey-Schafer, E. P.: Blood changes following controlled haemorrhage in man, Lancet 2:393, 1941.

11. Ebert, R. V., Stead, E. A., Jr., and Gibson, J. G., II: Response of normal subjects to acute blood loss, with special reference to the mechanism of restoration of blood volume, Arch. Int. Med. 68:578, 1941.

12. Howarth, S., and Sharpey-Schafer, E. P.: Low blood-pressure phases following haemorrhage, Lancet 1:18, 1947.

13. Sharpey-Schafer, E. P.: Transfusion and the anaemic heart, Lancet 2:296, 1945.

14. Sanguinetti, L. V.: Curvas azohemicas en las hemorragias retenidas del tubs digestiva, Arch. argent. de enferm. d. ap. digest. y de la nutrición 9:68, 1933.

15. Schiff, L., Stevens, R. J., and Moss, H. K.: The prognostic significance of the blood urea nitrogen following hematemesis or melena, Am. J. Digest. Dis. 9:110, 1942.

16. Schiff, L., and Stevens, R. J.: Elevation of urea nitrogen content of the blood following hematemesis or melena, Arch. Int. Med. 64:1239, 1939.

17. Black, D. A. K., and Smith, A. F.: Blood and plasma transfusion in alimentary haemorrhage, Brit. M. J. 1:187, 1941.

18. Schiff, L., Stevens, R. J., Goodman, S., Garber, E., and Lublin, A.: Observations on the oral administration of citrated blood in man; I, The effects on the blood urea nitrogen, Am. J. Digest. Dis. 6:597, 1939.

19. Kaump, D. H., and Parsons, J. C.: Extrarenal azotemia in gastro-intestinal hemorrhage; II, Experimental observations, Am. J. Digest. Dis. 7:191, 1940.

20. Chunn, C. F., and Harkins, H. N.: Experimental studies on alimentary azotemia; I, Role of blood absorption from the gastrointestinal tract, Surgery 9:695, 1941.

21. ———: Alimentary azotemia due to whole blood absorption from the gastrointestinal tract, Proc. Soc. Exper. Biol. & Med. 45:569, 1940.

22. Gregory, R., Ewing, P. L., and Levine, H.: Azotemia associated with gastrointestinal hemorrhage; an experimental etiologic study, Arch. Int. Med. 75:381, 1945.

23. Stevens, R. J., Schiff, L., Lublin, A., and Garber, E. S.: Renal function and the azotemia following hematemesis, J. Clin. Investigation 19:233, 1940.

24. Dill, L. V., and Isenhour, C. E.: Observations on the incidence and cause of fever in patients with bleeding peptic ulcers, Am. J. Digest. Dis. 5:779, 1939.

25. Schiff, L., Shapiro, N., and Stevens, R. J.: Observations on oral administration of citrated blood in man; III. The effect on temperature and the white blood cell count, Am. J. M. Sc. 207:465, 1944.

26. Moss, H. K., Schiff, L., Stevens, R. J., and Rich, M. L.: The blood in cases of hematemesis and melena with reference to factors influencing hemorrhage, Am. J. Digest. Dis. 7:490, 1940.

27. Frank, L. W., in discussion on La Due, J. S.: The treatment of massive hemorrhage due to peptic ulcer, J.A.M.A. 113:373, 1939.

28. Quick, A. J.: The nature of the bleeding in jaundice, J.A.M.A. 110:1658, 1938.

29. Smith, H. P., Warner, E. D., and Brinkhous, K. M.: Prothrombin deficiency and the bleeding tendency in liver injury

(chloroform intoxication), J. Exper. Med. 66:801, 1937.

30. Chalmers, T. C., Bigelow, F. S., and Desforges, J. F.: The effects of massive gastrointestinal hemorrhage on hemostasis; II, Coagulation factors, J. Lab. & Clin. Med. 43:511, 1954.

31. Desforges, J. F., Bigelow, F. S., and Chalmers, T. C.: The effects of massive gastrointestinal hemorrhage on hemostasis; I, The blood platelets, J. Lab. & Clin. Med. 43:501, 1954.

32. Alsted, G.: Changing Incidence of Peptic Ulcer, Copenhagen, E. Munksgaard, 1939.

33. Gray, S. J., Olson, T. E., Manrique, J.: Hematemesis and melena, Med. Clin. N. Am. 41:1327, 1957.

34. Palmer, E. D.: Diagnosis of Upper Gastrointestinal Hemorrhage, Pub. 443, Am. Lect. Series, Springfield, Ill., Thomas, 1961.

35. Strandberg, J.: Pseudoxanthoma elasticum, Zbl. Haut Geschlechtskr. 31:689, 1929.

36. McKusick, V. A.: Heritable Disorders of Connective Tissue, ed. 2, St. Louis, Mosby, 1960.

37. Grönblad, E.: Angioid streaks—pseudoxanthoma elasticum: verläufige mitheilung, Acta Ophth. 7:329, 1929.

38. Murray, M. J., Thal, A. P., and Greenspan, R.: Splenic arteriovenous fistulas as a cause of portal hypertension, Am. J. Med. 29:849, 1960.

39. Ansprenger, A., and Kirklin, B. R.: The roentgenologic aspects of chronic gastritis; a critical analysis, Am. J. Roentgenol. 38:533, 1937.

40. Schatzki, R.: Roentgen demonstration of esophageal varices; its clinical importance, Arch. Surg. 41:1084, 1940.

41. Karrs, S., and Wohl, G. T.: Clinical importance of gastric varices, New England J. Med. 263:665, 1960.

42. Nelson, S. W.: The roentgenologic diagnosis of esophageal varices, Am. J. Roentgenol. 77:599, 1957.

43. Leevy, C. M., Cherrick, G. R. and Davidson, C. S.: Medical progress. Portal Hypertension, New England J. Med. 262:397-403, 451-456, 1960.

44. Hampton, A. O.: A safe method for the roentgen demonstration of bleeding duodenal ulcers, Am. J. Roentgenol. 38:565, 1937.

45. Schiff, L.: Unpublished observation.

46. Knowles, H. C., Felson, B., Shapiro, N., and Schiff, L.: Emergency diagnosis of upper digestive tract bleeding by roentgen examination without palpation ("Hampton Technic"), Radiology, 58:536, 1952.

47. Chandler, G. N., Cameron, A. D., Nunn, A. H., and Street, D. F.: Early investigations of haemetemesis, Gut, 1:6, 1960.

48. Smith, H. W.: Esophagoscopy during active upper gastrointestinal hemorrhage, Conn. Med. 23:519, 1959.

49. Benedict, E. G.: Personal communication.

50. Schindler, R., in discussion on Benedict, E. B.: Hemorrhage from gastritis; a gastroscopic study, Am. J. Digest. Dis. 4:657, 1937.

51. Schindler, R.: Gastroscopy, The Endoscopic Study of Gastric Pathology, ed. 2, p. 223, Chicago, Univ. of Chicago Press, 1950.

52. Ruffin, J. M., and Brown, I. W., Jr.: The significance of hemorrhagic or pigment spots as observed by gastroscopy, Am. J. Digest. Dis. 10:60, 1943.

53. Wolf, S., and Wolff, H. G.: Human Gastric Function, ed. 2, p. 149, New York, Oxford, 1947.

54. Shapiro, N., and Schiff, L.: Ten years' experience with bleeding peptic ulcer with emphasis on 45 fatal cases, Surgery 31:327, 1952.

55. Christensen, O., cited by Meulengracht, E.: Behandlung von Hämatemesis und Meläna mit uneingeschränkter Kost, Wien. klin. Wschr. 49:1481, 1936.

56. Meulengracht, E.: Treatment of haematemesis and melaena with food; the mortality, Lancet 2:1220, 1935.

57. Schiff, L.: The Meulengracht diet in treatment of bleeding peptic ulcer, J. Am. Dietet. A. 18:298, 1942.

58. Crohn, B. B.: Affections of the Stomach, Philadelphia, Saunders, 1927.

59. Hurst, A. F., and Stewart, M. J.: Gastric and Duodenal Ulcer, London, Oxford, 1929.

60. Carlson, A. J.: Personal communication.

61. Bonney, G. L. W., and Pickering, G. W.: Observations on mechanism of pain in ulcer of stomach and duodenum; nature of the stimulus, Clin. Sc. 6:63, 1946.

62. Van Liere, E. J., Sleeth, C. K., and Northup, D.: Effect of acute hemorrhage on emptying time of the stomach, Am. J. Physiol. 117:226, 1936.

63. McLaughlin, C. W., Baker, C. P., and Sharpe, J. C.: Bleeding duodenal ulcer complicated by myocardial infarction, Nebraska M. J. 25:266, 1940.

64. Blumgart, H. L., Schlesinger, M. J., and Zoll, P. M.: Multiple fresh coronary occlu-

sions in patients with antecedent shock, Arch. Int. Med. 68:181, 1941.

65. McKinlay, C. A.: Coronary insufficiency precipitated by hemorrhage from duodenal ulcer, Journal Lancet 63:31, 1943.

66. Kinney, T. D., and Mallory, G. K.: Cardiac failure associated with acute anemia, New England J. Med. 232:215, 1945.

67. Rasmussen, H., and Foss, M.: The electro-cardiogram of acute hemorrhage from stomach and intestines, Acta med. Scandinav. 111:420, 1942.

68. Scherf, D., Reinstein, H., and Klotz, S. D.: Electrocardiographic changes following hematemesis in peptic ulcer, Rev. Gastroenterol. 8:343, 1941.

69. Master, A. M., Dack, S., Grishman, A., Field, L. E., and Horn, H.: Acute coronary insufficiency: an entity; shock, hemorrhage and pulmonary embolism as factors in its production, J. Mt. Sinai Hosp. 14:8, 1947.

70. Davies, D. T., and Wilson, A. T. M.: Personal and clinical history in haematemesis and perforation, Lancet 2:723, 1939.

71. Gainsborough, H., and Slater, E.: A study of peptic ulcer, Brit. M. J. 2:253, 1946.

72. Rivers, A. B.: Hemorrhage from the stomach and duodenum, in Eusterman, G. B., and Balfour, D. C.: The Stomach and Duodenum, p. 759, Philadelphia, Saunders, 1935.

73. Palmer, W. L.: Peptic ulcer, in Portis, S. A.: Diseases of the Digestive System, ed. 2, p. 208, Philadelphia, Lea & Febiger, 1944.

74. Schiff, L.: Unpublished observation.

75. Smyrniotis, F., Schenker, S., O'Donnell, J., and Schiff, L.: Lactic dehydrogenase activity in gastric juice for the diagnosis of gastric cancer, Am. J. Digest. Dis. 7:712, 1962.

76. Snell, A. M., and Butt, H. R.: Chronic atrophy of the liver, in Barr, D. P.: Modern Medical Therapy in General Practice, p. 2,386, Baltimore, Williams & Wilkins, 1940.

77. Linton, R. R.: The surgical treatment of bleeding esophageal varices by portal systemic venous shunts, with a report of 34 cases, Ann. Int. Med. 31:794, 1949.

78. Whipple, A. O.: Portal Bed Block and Portal Hypertension in Advances in Surgery, vol. 2, p. 155, New York, Interscience, 1949.

79. Garrett, N., Jr., and Gall, E. A.: Esophageal varices without hepatic cirrhosis, Arch. Path. 55:196, 1953.

80. Tisdale, W. A., Klatskin, G., and Glenn, W. W. L.: Portal hypertension and bleed-ing esophageal varices. Their occurrence in the absence of both intrahepatic and extra-hepatic obstruction of the portal vein, New England J. Med. 261:209, 1959.

81. Liebowitz, H. R.: Bleeding Esophageal Varices, Portal Hypertension, Springfield, Ill., Thomas, 1959.

82. Snodgrass, R. W., and Mellinkoff, S. M.: Bleeding varices in the upper esophagus due to obstruction of the superior vena cava, Gastroenterology 41:505, 1961.

83. Felson, B., Zeid, S., and Schiff, L.: Unpublished observations.

84. Campbell, G. S., Bick, H. D., Paulsen, E. P., Lober, P. H., Watson, C. J., and Varco, R. L.: Bleeding esophageal varices with polycystic liver, New England J. Med. 259:904, 1958.

85. Sedacca, C. M., Perrin, E., Martin, L., and Schiff, L.: Polycystic liver: An unusual cause of bleeding esophageal varices, Gastroenterology 40:128, 1961.

86. Liebowitz, H. R.: Pathogenesis of esophageal varix rupture, J.A.M.A. 175:874, 1961.

87. Wangensteen, O. H.: The ulcer problem (Listerian oration), Canad. M. A. J. 53:309, 1945.

88. Chiles, N. H., Baggenstoss, A. H., Butt, H. R., and Olsen, A. M.: Esophageal varices: Comparative incidence of ulceration and spontaneous rupture as a cause of fatal hemorrhage, Gastroenterology 25:565, 1953.

89. Child, C. G., III, and Donovan, A. J.: Surgical treatment of portal hypertension, Am. J. Digest. Dis. 3:114, 1958.

90. Rolleston, H. D., and McNee, J. W.: Diseases of the Liver, Gall-Bladder and Bile Ducts, ed. 3, New York, Macmillan, 1929.

91. Morlock, C. G., and Hall, B. E.: Association of cirrhosis, thrombopenia and hemorrhagic tendency, Arch. Int. Med. 72:69, 1943.

92. Preble, R. B.: Conclusions based on sixty cases of fatal gastro-intestinal hemorrhage due to cirrhosis of the liver, Am. J. M. Sc. 119:263, 1900.

93. Young, P. C., Burnside, C. R., Knowles, H. C., Jr., and Schiff, L.: The effect of the intragastric administration of whole blood on the blood ammonia, blood urea nitrogen and non-protein nitrogen in patients with liver disease, J. Clin. Invest. 35:747, 1956.

94. White, F. W., and Chalmers, T. C.: The problem of gross hematemesis in a general hospital, Tr. A. Am. Physicians, 61:253, 1948.

95. Zamcheck, N., Chalmers, T. C., White, F.

W., and Davidson, C. S.: The bromsulpha-lein test in the early diagnosis of liver disease in gross upper gastrointestinal hemorrhage, Gastroenterology 14:343, 1950.

96. Stahl, J., and Bockel, R.: L'ammoniémie dans le diagnostic de hémorrhagies digestives, Strasbourg med. 7:389, 1956.

97. McDermott, W. V., Jr.: A simple discriminatory test for upper gastrointestinal hemorrhage, New England J. Med. 257:1161, 1957.

98. Belkin, G. A., and Conn, H. O.: Blood ammonia concentration and bromsulfalein retention in upper gastrointestinal hemorrhage, New England J. Med. 260:530, 1959.

99. Atkinson, M., Barnett, E., Sherlock, S., and Steiner, R. E.: The clinical investigation of the portal circulation, with special reference to portal venography, Quart. J. Med. 24:77, 1955.

100. Merigan, T. C., Jr., Hollister, R. M., Gryska, P. F., Starkey, G. W. B., and Davidson, C. S.: Gastrointestinal bleeding with cirrhosis, New England J. Med. 263:579, 1960.

101. Clarke, J. S., Ozeran, R. S., Hart, J. C., Cruze, K., and Crevling, V.: Peptic ulcer following portacaval shunt, Ann. Surg. 148:551, 1958.

102. Dubuque, T. J., Jr., Mulligan, L. V., and Neville, E. C.: Gastric secretion and peptic ulceration in the dog with portal obstruction and portacaval anastomosis, Surg. Forum: Clin. Cong. Am. Coll. Surgeons 8:208, 1957.

103. Panke, W. F., Moreno, A. H., and Rousselot, L. M.: The diagnostic study of the portal venous system, Med. Clin. N. Am. 44:727, 1960.

104. Faber, K.: Gastritis and Its Consequences, London, Oxford, 1935.

105. Moutier, F.: Traité de gastroscopie et de pathologie endoscopique de l'estomac, Paris, Masson, 1935.

106. Henning, N.: Die Entzündung des Magens, Leipzig, Barth, 1934.

107. Palmer, E. D.: Gastritis: a revaluation, Medicine 33:199, 1954.

108. Sahler, O. D., and Hampton, A. O.: Bleeding in hiatus hernia, Am. J. Roentgenol. 49:433, 1943.

109. Jones, C. M.: Hiatus esophageal hernia; with special reference to a comparison of its symptoms with those of angina pectoris, New England J. Med. 225:963, 1941.

110. Harrington, S. W.: Diagnosis and treatment of various types of diaphragmatic hernia, Am. J. Surg. 50:377, 1940.

111. Olsen, A. M., and Harrington, S. W.: Esophageal hiatal hernias of the short esophagus type; etiologic and therapeutic considerations, J. Thoracic Surg. 17:189, 1948.

112. Frank, W.: Hematemesis associated with gastric arteriosclerosis; review of literature with case report, Gastroenterology 7:231, 1946.

113. Griggs, D. E., and Baker, M. Q.: Hereditary hemorrhagic telangiectasia with gastrointestinal bleeding, Amer. J. Digest. Dis. 8:344, 1941.

114. Kushlan, S. D.: Gastro-intestinal bleeding in hereditary hemorrhagic telangiectasia; historical review and case report with gastroscopic findings and rutin therapy, Gastroenterology 7:199, 1946.

115. Bean, W. B.: Enteric bleeding in rare conditions with diagnostic lesions of the skin and mucous membrane, Trans. Am. Clin. Climat. Ass. 69:72, 1957.

116. Segal, H. L., Scott, W. J. M., and Watson, J. S.: Lesions of small intestine producing massive hemorrhage, with symptoms simulating peptic ulcer, J.A.M.A. 129:116, 1945.

117. Gordon-Taylor, G.: Rare causes of severe gastro-intestinal haemorrhage, with note on aneurysm of hepatic artery, Brit. Med. J. 1:504, 1943.

118. Murphy, B.: Aneurysm of splenic artery; death from haematemesis, Lancet 1:704, 1942.

119. Williams, R. C., Jr.: Aortic stenosis and unexplained gastrointestinal bleeding, Arch. Int. Med. 108:859, 1961.

120. Lee, H. C., and Kay, S.: Primary polyarteritis nodosa of the stomach and small intestine as a cause of gastro-intestinal hemorrhage, Ann. Surg. 147:714, 1958.

121. Denkewalter, F. R., Molnar, W., and Horava, A. P.: Massive gastro-intestinal hemorrhage in jejunal diverticulosis, Ann. Surg. 148:862, 1958.

122. Evans, A. L., Cofer, O. S., and Gregory, H. H.: Multiple hemangiomas of the jejunum as a cause of massive gastrointestinal bleeding, J. Med. Ass. Georgia 47:600, 1958.

123. Schoenfeld, R., Cahan, J., and Dyer, R.: Gastric carcinoid tumor—An unusual cause of hematemesis, Arch. Int. Med. 104:649, 1959.

124. Aspirin poisoning, symposium section, Internat. Med. Digest 56:54, 1950.

125. Douthwaite, A. H.: Some recent advances in medical diagnosis and treatment, Brit. M. J. 1:1143, 1938.

126. Douthwaite, A. H., and Lintott, G. A. M.: Gastroscopic observation of the effect of aspirin and certain other substances on the stomach, Lancet 2:1222, 1938.

127. Hurst, A. F.: Aspirin and gastric hemorrhage, Brit. M. J. 1:768, 1943.

128. Hurst, A. F., and Lintott, G. A. M.: Aspirin as a cause of haematemesis; a clinical and gastroscopic study, Guy's Hosp. Rep. 89: 173, 1939.

129. Crismer, R.: Gastric hemorrhage provoked by acetylsalicylic acid, Acta clin. belg. 2:193, 1947.

130. Winkelman, E. I., and Summerskill, W. H. J.: Gastric secretion in relation to gastrointestinal bleeding from salicylate compounds, Gastroenterology 40:56, 1961.

131. Allibone, A., and Flint, F. J.: Gastrointestinal haemorrhage and salicylates, Lancet 2:1121, 1958.

132. Kelly, J. J., Jr.: Salicylate ingestion: A frequent cause of gastric hemorrhage, Am. J. Med. Sci. 232:119, 1956.

133. Lange, H. F.: Salicylates and gastric hemorrhage. II. Manifest bleeding, Gastroenterology 33:778, 1957.

134. Muir, A., and Cossar, I. A.: Aspirin and gastric haemorrhage, Lancet 1:539, 1959.

135. Waterson, A. P.: Aspirin and gastric haemorrhage, Brit. Med. J. 2:1531, 1955.

136. Pierson, R. N., Jr., Holt, P. R., Watson, R. M., and Keating, R. P.: Aspirin and gastrointestinal bleeding. Chromate[51] blood loss studies, Am. J. Med. 31:259, 1961.

137. Shapiro, S., Redish, M. H., and Campbell, H. A.: Studies on prothrombin, IV. The prothrombinopenic effect of salicylate in man. Proc. Soc. Exper. Biol. & Med. 53:251, 1943.

138. Meyer, O. O., and Howard, B.: Production of hypoprothrombinemia and hypocoagulability of the blood with salicylates, Proc. Soc. Exper. Biol. & Med. 53:234, 1943.

139. Muir, A., and Cossar, I. A.: Aspirin and ulcer, Brit. M. J. 2:7, 1955.

140. Mallory, G. K., and Weiss, S.: Hemorrhages from lacerations of the cardiac orifice of the stomach due to vomiting, Am. J. Med. Sci. 178:506, 1929.

141. Decker, J. P., Zamcheck, N., and Mallory, G. K.: Mallory-Weiss syndrome. Hemorrhage from gastroesophageal lacerations at the cardiac orifice of the stomach, New England J. Med. 249:957, 1953.

142. Heuer, G. J.: The surgical aspects of hemorrhage from peptic ulcer, New England J. Med. 235:777, 1946.

143. Foster, D. G.: Retrograde jejunogastric intussusception—a rare cause of hematemesis. Review of the literature and report of two cases, Arch. Surg. 73:1009, 1956.

144. Cordell, A. R., Wright, R. H., and Johnston, F. R.: Gastrointestinal hemorrhage after abdominal aortic operations, Surg. 48:997, 1960.

145. Sandblom, P.: Hemorrhage into the biliary tract following trauma: "Traumatic hemobilia," Surg. 24:571, 1948.

146. Sparkman, R. S.: Massive hemobilia following traumatic rupture of liver: Report of a case and review of the literature, Ann. Surg. 138:899, 1953.

147. Sparkman, R. S., and Fogelman, M. J.: Wounds of the liver: Review of 100 cases, Ann. Surg. 139:690, 1954.

148. Ferguson, L. K., and Nusbaum, M.: Idiopathic massive hemobilia, Am. J. Surg. 102:109, 1961

149. Schatzki, S. C.: Hemobilia, Radiology 77: 717, 1961.

150. Karam, J. H., and Jacobs, T.: Hemobilia: Report of a case of massive gastrointestinal bleeding originating from a hepatic abscess, Ann. Int. Med. 54:319, 1961.

151. Stokes, J. F., and Jones, F. A., *in discussion of* Edwards, H.: Haematemesis due to pseudoxanthoma elasticum, Gastroenterologia 89:345, 1958.

21

Jaundice

LEON SCHIFF

Jaundice, or icterus, is the condition recognized clinically by a yellowish discoloration of the plasma, the skin and the mucous membranes caused by staining by bile pigment. It may be the first and sometimes the sole manifestation of disease. It is detected best in the peripheral portions of the ocular conjunctivae and can be observed also in the mucous membrane of the hard palate or in the lips when compressed with a glass slide. It may be overlooked in poor or artificial light. Attention may be first directed to it by a laboratory report of "serum icteric."

BILIRUBIN METABOLISM

It is now generally accepted that the formation of bilirubin from hemoglobin occurs mainly in the cells of the reticuloendothelial system. Studies with erythrocytes labeled with Cr^{51} and Fe^{59} have shown that the principal sites of hemoglobin catabolism are the bone marrow, the spleen and the liver, while the kidneys, the lungs and the intestines play a minor role.[1,2]

In the normal individual, 1/120 of the total circulating erythrocytes are destroyed daily. In the adult this represents 7.5 Gm. of hemoglobin. The released hemoglobin is broken down into heme and globin; the latter being further catabolized into its constituent amino acids, which are reutilized. The heme is broken down into inorganic iron and protoporphyrin; the protoporphyrin being further catabolized into bilirubin. The daily breakdown of hemoglobin (7.5 Gm.) should result in the formation of 300 mg. of bilirubin. The bilirubin is liberated into the circulation and is bound mainly to plasma albumin and to a slight extent to alpha-1-globulin.[3,4]

In its passage through the liver cell, unconjugated ("indirect-reacting") bilirubin is converted into a water-soluble ("direct-reacting") conjugated form, which is then excreted into the bile.[5,8] Uridine diphosphate glucuronic acid (UDPGA) acts as the glucuronyl donor for the conjugation of bilirubin; the conjugating enzyme, glucuronyl transferase, being located in the microsomes of the liver cells. The series of enzymic reactions involved in the synthesis of bilirubin glucuronide is given in Figure 130. An enzymic system capable of conjugating bilirubin as the sulphate has also been demonstrated in the liver; "active sulfate" (adenosine-3-phosphate-5-phosphosulfate) is the sulfate donor in this reaction.[9]

The normal values given for plasma bilirubin depend on the analytic technics employed, but in general they range from 0 to 1.3 mg./100 ml. with a mean value of approximately 0.5 mg./100 ml. The amount of conjugated bilirubin in plasma as determined by the Malloy and Evelyn technic is usually less than 0.3 mg./100 ml. This figure indicates, in part, the fraction of unconjugated bilirubin that couples in the absence of alcohol. The amount of conjugated bilirubin in normal plasma, if it exists, is therefore very small.

The over-all metabolism of bilirubin by the liver cell involves three processes: (1) transport of bilirubin from the plasma to the liver (uptake), (2) conjugation of bilirubin primarily with glucuronic acid, and (3) excretion of the water-soluble conjugate into the biliary system (Fig. 131). It is not known whether bilirubin enters the hepatic cell bound to plasma proteins or in a free state, and little is known about the excretion mechanism. Jaundice can result from interference with any of the three processes involved in the metabolism of bilirubin by the liver cell.

In normal subjects, bilirubin is rarely excreted in the urine. In fresh specimens of icteric urine only the conjugated pigments can be detected. There is a poor correlation between the concentration of conjugated bilirubin in the plasma and that in the urine, particularly in viral hepatitis in which, at the onset of the disease, bilirubin may appear in the urine with serum levels of 2 to 3 mg./100 ml., but during convalescence it often fails to appear with levels of 6 to 8 mg./100 ml.[10] It has generally been accepted that the pigments are excreted by the renal tubules.[11] However, little is known of the underlying mechanisms, since purified pigments are not available for the necessary investigations.

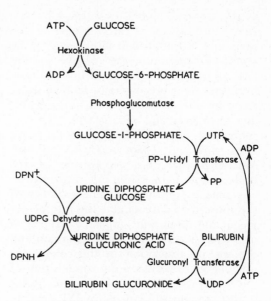

Fig. 130. A possible mechanism for the conjugation of bilirubin with glucuronic acid. (Billing, B. H., and Lathe, G. H.: Am. J. Med. 24:111)

After it enters the small intestine, the bilirubin is reduced to urobilinogens (Fig. 132), which are partially reabsorbed and re-excreted into the intestine (Fig. 133). It is now generally accepted that the urobilinoid pigments are formed from conjugated bilirubin in the intestine by the bacterial flora. The presence of conjugated, rather than free, bilirubin appears to be necessary,[12] and although the individual enzyme systems have not been isolated, in-vitro studies have shown that fecal bacteria, such

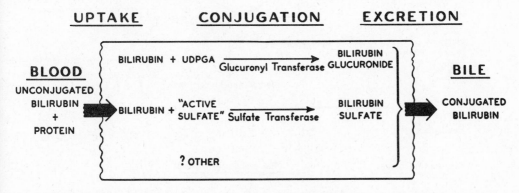

Fig. 131. Schematic representation of the metabolism of bilirubin by the liver cell. (Arias, I. M.: Med. Clin. N. Am. 44:610)

as the Clostridium-like organism G62 and *E. coli,* are capable of carrying out the conversion of bilirubin to urobilinogen.[13,14] Attempts to determine the relative proportions of urobilin IX_a, stercobilin and d-urobilin and their precursors in fecal urobilin have, for the most part, been unsuccessful due to difficult and unsatisfactory analytic procedures, and conflicting results have been obtained. More recently Watson[15] concluded that the composition of the urobilin group in urine, bile and feces at any time is controlled by the mobility of the intestinal contents and the rate of filling of the colon, and appeared to depend on the efficiency of bacterial reduction and the site of absorption in the colon. He was unable to correlate the composition of the fecal urobilin with the state of health or disease; and while urobilin IX_a predominated in some subjects, stercobilin was the dominant pigment in others. The administration of broad-spectrum antibiotics resulted in d-urobilin becoming the dominant pigment in feces, bile and urine. However, this pigment was found in appreciable quantities in some subjects who had never received antibiotic therapy and may be normally present in all subjects in small amounts, which are not detected by our present technics.

McMaster and Elman[16] postulated, as the result of experiments with dogs, that urobilinogen was normally reabsorbed from the intestine and re-excreted by the liver, and that in the presence of liver damage re-excretion was impossible, so that the pigment passes instead to the kidney and is excreted in the urine. The form in which reabsorbed stercobilinogen is normally excreted in the bile is unknown, for it is only in the presence of infection that appreciable amounts of urobilinoids and bile pigments, other than bilirubin, can be detected.

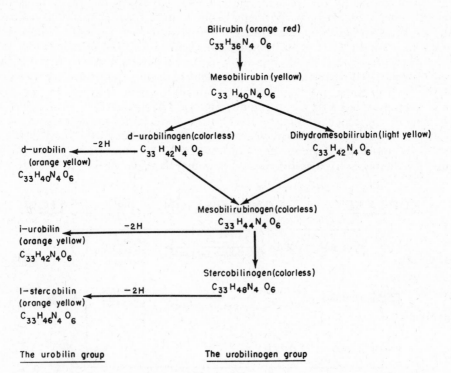

FIG. 132. The bacterial reduction of bilirubin by the human intestinal flora. (Watson, C. J., Lowry, P., Collins, S., Graham, A. and Ziegler, N. R.: Tr. A. Am. Physicians 67:242)

CLASSIFICATION AND MECHANISMS

The fact that various classifications of jaundice have been proposed would indicate the lack of an ideal one. With advances in knowledge of cellular structure, increasing interest in cellular physiology and the discovery of the conjugation of bilirubin, more attention is being focused on the liver cell itself in the pathogenesis of icterus.

McNee's classification[17] into (1) obstructive hepatic, (2) toxic and infective hepatic and (3) hemolytic types has maintained its clinical usefulness. Watson's[18] division of regurgitation jaundice into the cancerous, calculous and parenchymal types, based largely on the extent of biliary obstruction, has been of further help in clinical practice. Watson considers biliary obstruction to be complete when the daily fecal excretion of urobilinogen is less than 5 mg. (normal range is 40 to 280 mg.). Factors which diminish urobilinogen production in the intestine, such as diarrhea and ingestion of antibiotics, must of course be excluded.

TABLE 21.   CLASSIFICATION OF JAUNDICE

1. Hemolytic
2. Hepatocellular
   A. Without features of biliary obstruction
   B. With features of biliary obstruction
      (Cholestatic Jaundice)
   C. Congenital
3. Obstructive

Watson found complete biliary obstruction in 92 per cent of his cancerous cases in contrast with only 3.5 per cent of the parenchymal and 11.5 per cent of the calculous groups.

The author prefers the classification of jaundice shown in Table 21. The hepatocellular type comprises the various forms of hepatitis and hepatic cirrhosis and includes the intrahepatic cholestatic forms of hepatitis (which are chiefly of viral or drug origin) and the hereditary hyperbilirubinemias. The obstructive form includes biliary obstruction due to neoplasm, gallstones, stricture, cholangitis or contiguous inflammatory processes or cysts.

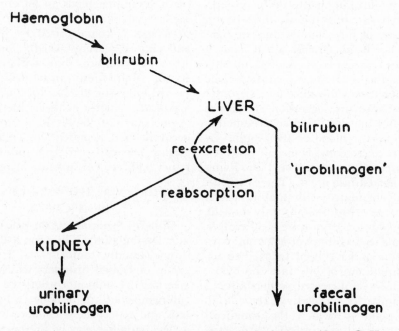

FIG. 133. Fate of bilirubin after excretion into the gut. (Gray, C. H.: The Bile Pigments, London, Methuen)

HEMOLYTIC JAUNDICE

In hemolytic disease there is an increased production of bilirubin, most of which is excreted by the liver. Therefore, an elevated fecal urobilinogen excretion occurs, and excessive amounts of urobilinogen may appear in the urine. Unconjugated bilirubin is the main pigment found in the serum of these patients. Therefore, bilirubinuria is not usually observed. However, small amounts of conjugated bilirubin may be detected, but these will not exceed 15 per cent of the total serum bilirubin concentration unless there is considerable hepatocellular damage present, which will interfere with the normal excretion of conjugated bilirubin.[19]

OBSTRUCTIVE AND HEPATOCELLULAR JAUNDICE

Controversy still exists regarding the mechanisms of the development of jaundice. It has generally been accepted that obstructive jaundice is caused by hydrostatic dilatation and rupture of the bile capillaries with leakage of bilirubin back from the biliary system into the lymphatics of the liver and thence to the blood stream. Gonzalez-Oddone[20] observed the prompt appearance of bilirubin (mainly of the prompt-reacting type) in the thoracic duct lymph after ligature of the common duct in dogs. On the other hand, Grafflin and Chaney[21] studied the excretion of fluorescent substances by the liver after ligature of the common duct in white mice and were unable to visualize any suggestion of rupture or leakage of the dye ("and so presumably of bile") into the blood or the lymph. By fluorescence microscopy, Hanzon[22] observed the movement of uranin injected into living rats with ligated bile ducts. The canaliculi became much dilated with uranin, which was then observed to flow abruptly into the blood. In addition to rupture of bile capillaries secondary to biliary obstruction, various mechanisms have been invoked to explain regurgitation of bile into the blood. These include (1) increased permeability of the bile capillaries, especially at the ampullae (the point at which the canaliculi emerge from the liver cords),[23] (2) necrosis of liver cells,[24] (3) swelling of the parenchymal cells of the liver with obstruction of the bile canaliculi,[25] (4) swelling of the liver cords, edema of the spaces of Disse and fibrosis of the portal areas,[26] (5) obstruction of the intralobular canaliculi by bile thrombi,[27,28] and (6) compression or rupture of the canals of Hering in the region of the periportal fields as a result of exudative processes.[29] With the use of the electron microscope Popper and Schaffner[30] have more recently pointed out dilatation of the bile canaliculi with diminution and distortion of the microvilli, and rupture of the canaliculus into the surrounding tissue space both in intrahepatic cholestasis and extrahepatic obstructive jaundice. Decrease in the microvilli and dilatation of the canaliculi may interfere with the normal hydration of bile, thus favoring cholestasis.

Where the injured liver cells appear to be histologically normal, particularly in instances of hepatocellular jaundice, the studies of Hanzon[22] suggest an impairment of the unidirectional transport mechanism of the hepatic cell affecting its permeability and thereby permitting regurgitation of the bile through the cell from the canaliculi.

Cholestatic jaundice has proved to be the main stumbling block to an entirely satisfactory classification of jaundice. This type of icterus is characterized by biochemical and clinical features usually found in obstructive jaundice, but without demonstrable obstruction. It occurs most commonly following the use of such drugs as arsenicals, chlorpromazine, methyl testosterone and norethandralone but may also occur in viral hepatitis[31] (so-called cholangiolitic hepatitis). It may appear in pregnancy and recur in subsequent pregnancies.

HEREDITARY HYPERBILIRUBINEMIAS (IN THE ADULT)

Gilbert's Syndrome (Constitutional Hepatic Dysfunction). The term Gilbert's syndrome usually comprises a heterogenous group of benign disorders which are characterized by mild unconjugated hyperbilirubinemia not attributable to overt hemolysis and is seen most commonly in young males. Jaundice may be present from birth or may be noted first in adult life and persists into old age but tends to lessen with age. The icterus fluctuates in degree and may be increased by fatigue, emotional tension, excessive intake of alcohol or intercurrent infection. Neither hepatomegaly nor splenomegaly is present. Hepatic function is usually normal, except for an impaired bilirubin tolerance, and the liver is usually normal on histologic examination, although fatty infiltration of the liver has been reported.

The majority of patients have an unconjugated bilirubinemia of 1 to 4 mg./100 ml. It has been postulated that a defect in the uptake of bilirubin by the liver cell is responsible for the jaundice in these patients. Analysis of plasma bilirubin disappearance curves, following an injection of bilirubin, tends to substantiate this hypothesis.[32]

Patients with hyperbilirubinemia greater than 5 mg./100 ml. are rare, and it seems likely that in these subjects there may be a defect in glucuronide formation such as is seen in infants with the Crigler-Najjar syndrome but to a varying extent.[33] Fecal urobilinogen excretion is usually decreased. The administration of ACTH or prednisolone does not appear to affect the degree of jaundice in these patients.[34]

Chronic Idiopathic Jaundice (Dubin-Johnson Syndrome). This disorder, which was first described independently by two groups of workers, Dubin and Johnson[35] and Sprinz and Nelson,[36] is a chronic or intermittent form of jaundice with both free and conjugated bilirubin in the plasma. It is characterized by the presence of large amounts of a yellow-brown lipofuscinlike pigment in the liver cells. It has been proposed that the pigment is melanin,[37-39] but this has not been generally accepted.

As in Gilbert's syndrome, this disorder manifests itself as a form of chronic or intermittent jaundice most commonly seen in young people and frequently familial in occurrence. According to Dubin[35] most patients complain of abdominal pain in the region of the liver, and the liver is palpable and tender in about one half of the cases. A striking feature is the failure of the gallbladder, although normal, to visualize on oral cholecystography. The liver is normal except for the pigment in its cells, which may be so abundant as to discolor it green, slate blue, or black. This gross discoloration may be detected in a needle biopsy specimen.

Jaundice may be precipitated or aggravated by many factors, including pregnancy, surgical operations, severe physical strain, alcoholism and infectious diseases.[35] The icterus may be mistaken for the obstructive variety because of abdominal pain, dark urine, pale stools, increase in direct-reacting bilirubin, and a nonvisualizing gallbladder. Prognosis is excellent, as indicated by the long duration of the disease and the absence of progressive hepatic damage in cases of long standing.[35]

Except for the presence of pigment, the hepatic cells appear to be histologically normal. Such tests of liver function as serum proteins, transaminases, bile acids, alkaline phosphatase and flocculation tests are usually within normal limits but may be raised slightly. On the other hand, all patients show a marked retention of such dyes as bromsulphalein,[35,40] rose bengal,[41] indocyanine green,[42] and methylene blue[43] which appears to be due to a defect in the hepatic cells. During the first 30 minutes after the injection the dye is cleared from the plasma at a rate similar to or slightly reduced from that seen in the normal subject. The level of the dye in the plasma then rises again and remains elevated for many hours, so that it can still be detected after 48 to 72 hours (Fig. 134). With bromsulphalein the proportion of dye conjugated with glutathione in the plasma gradually rises, and an appreciable amount of the injected dye can be recovered from the urine.

Measurements of serum bilirubin show elevation of both the conjugated (direct) and the total levels. These levels tend to fluctuate under the influence of the factors mentioned above and range from normal to 19 mg./100 ml. of plasma. Approximately 60 per cent of the cases have total bile pigment concentrations under 6 mg./100 ml. of plasma.

Familial Nonhemolytic Jaundice With Conjugated Bilirubin in the Serum and

Normal Liver Histology. Although this disorder was described by Rotor and associates in 1948,[44] it is only within the past 3 or 4 years that interest in familial non-hemolytic jaundice with conjugated bilirubin in the serum has been renewed.[45-52]

The disease appears to be familial in occurrence, with both sexes probably equally represented, and is characterized by a chronic, relatively mild jaundice, fluctuating in degree. As in Gilbert's syndrome, the icterus may increase with fatigue, emotional upsets, or respiratory infections.[48] In one patient the icterus was said to diminish during each of 3 pregnancies,[48] in direct contrast with behavior of cases of the Dubin-Johnson syndrome.[35] In one of Rotor's cases, ingestion of fatty foods was said to deepen the jaundice. Abdominal pain is usually absent, and the liver and the spleen are not enlarged.

The disorder is chronic, not incapacitating, requires no treatment and appears to be compatible with a normal life. In contrast with the Dubin-Johnson syndrome, the oral cholecystogram is normal, and no pigment is present in the liver cells. However, the bile ducts may fail to visualize roentgenologically following the intravenous injection of iodipamide,[47,50] although shown to be patent and otherwise normal at peritoneoscopy and laparotomy.[51,52] Davis and Young have observed coincidental gallbladder calculi. The liver biopsy specimen is essentially normal on light microscopy and fluorescence microscopy and probably so on electron microscopy.[47] In the case studied by Arias[49] the pericanalicular lysosomes appeared to be increased in numbers and in dispersion throughout the cell as examined with the electron microscope.

Information based on the few cases studied would indicate that the cephalin flocculation test is sometimes abnormal, but the thymol turbidity, zinc sulfate turbidity, total lipids, serum proteins and serum transaminases are within normal limits. The serum alkaline phosphatase activities may tend toward the low side of normal; the level of the serum trihydroxy and dihydroxy bile acids may be within normal range.

There is abnormal retention of bromsulphalein in the plasma, and the appearance

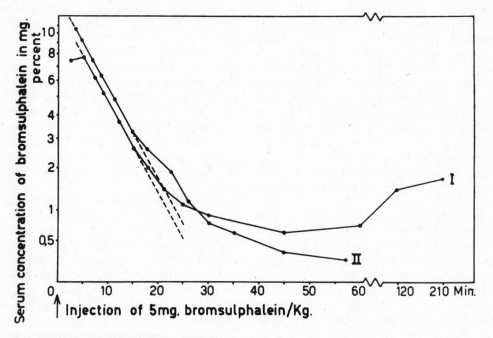

Fig. 134. Bromsulphalein disappearance curve. (I) Case III, (II) Normal, subject. (Mandema, E., de Fraiture, W. H., Nieweg, H. O., and Arends, A.: Am. J. Med., 27:47)

of the dye in the bile following intravenous injection may be somewhat delayed. The retained bromsulphalein has been found to be almost entirely in the unconjugated form[47,50] at 45 minutes after injection of the dye, but at 100 minutes Arias has found most of the dye in the serum to be conjugated. He found the hepatic storage of bromsulphalein to be normal and the hepatic Tm (transport maximum) for bromsulphalein to be markedly reduced.

The serum bilirubin levels fluctuate and are usually less than 10 mg. per cent, with the free and conjugated pigments present in about equal proportions. Bile pigments can be detected in the urine, provided that the level of conjugated pigments is sufficiently high. Abnormal amounts of urinary urobilinogen are usually not present, although they have been reported. The fecal urobilinogen is not increased.

CLINICAL APPROACH

The clinician usually has little difficulty in distinguishing hemolytic from hepatocellular and obstructive jaundice. His usual task is to differentiate jaundice due to primary liver disease from that due to obstruction of the extrahepatic bile ducts. In the differentiation of the various forms of jaundice, he has available four methods of approach, short of surgical intervention or peritoneoscopy: (1) the history and the physical examination, (2) laboratory tests, including the so-called liver function tests, (3) x-ray examination and (4) needle biopsy of the liver in selected cases.

HISTORY

Family History. The familial occurrence of icterus should suggest the possibilities of congenital hemolytic jaundice, Gilbert's syndrome, the Dubin-Johnson syndrome and the familial nonhemolytic jaundice with conjugated bilirubin in the serum.

Occupation. The increased likelihood of hepatic cirrhosis in bartenders and brewery workers and the predisposition to Weil's disease among workers in rat-infested premises are well known.

Recent contact with a jaundiced individual should suggest the possibility of infectious hepatitis.

The ingestion or the administration of or exposure to hepatotoxic drugs, particularly arsenicals, carbon tetrachloride, phosphorus, thorazine, methyl testosterone, norethandralone, and mono-amine-oxidase inhibitors should suggest the possibility of a toxic or drug hepatitis.

Needle puncture or transfusion from 6 weeks to 6 months prior to the onset of jaundice should lead to suspicion of homologous serum hepatitis.

A history of a recent gallbladder operation should lead to suspicion of a residual common duct stone or stricture as the cause of icterus, but careful inquiry should be made as to the transfusion of blood or plasma at the time of surgery in order to exclude homologous serum hepatitis.[53]

History of Resection of a Malignant Tumor. If the interval between resection of the tumor and the appearance of icterus is more than 3 or 4 years, an unrelated cause of the icterus should be considered. Metastatic tumor of the liver is more apt to appear within 2 or 3 years.[54]

While **chills and fever** in a jaundiced patient are usually indicative of cholangitis, it is well to remember that they may be prominent during the preicteric phase of infectious hepatitis and may occur in thorazine jaundice.

Pruritus. As George Budd pointed out over 100 years ago, pruritus is most pronounced in cases of occlusion of the common bile duct, particularly by tumor. Itching is often prominent in patients with biliary cirrhosis and occasionally occurs in viral hepatitis, and in nutritional cirrhosis.

Abdominal pain is usually inconspicuous in patients with viral hepatitis or hepatic cirrhosis. In cases of *common duct stone* the pain is generaly colicky and is accompanied by nausea and vomiting and usually requires an opiate for relief.

It is well recognized that pain occurs in most cases of *pancreatic carcinoma*. While the nature of the pain is not pathognomonic, it is usually located in the epigastrium, is often described as boring in nature and frequently radiates to the back. As pointed out by Chauffard,[55] it is worse when the patient lies on his back and is lessened by turning on one side and drawing up the knees, by changing to the prone position, or by sitting up and bending forward. It is frequently so severe as to require an opiate. An atypical pain pattern may be produced by *peritoneal tumor implants.*

Abdominal pain is usually prominent in cases of *malignant tumor of the liver,* primary more than metastatic. It is usually localized to the right hypochondrium and may be dull or sharp and intermittent in character. It may radiate to the right infrascapular area or right flank and may be increased by deep breathing, coughing, exertion or changes in posture. It is presumably due to invasion or stretching of the liver capsule by the neoplasm.

Physical Examination

Age and Sex. The age and the sex of the patient are of diagnostic help. Infectious hepatitis is seen most commonly in young adults, while common duct stone and neoplastic jaundice usually occur in middle-aged or older individuals. Weil's disease, at least in this country, is said to be rare in females and in children.[56] Portal cirrhosis, hepatoma, pancreatic cancer and primary hemochromatosis predominate in the male, while common duct stone, primary biliary cirrhosis and carcinoma of the gallbladder are more prevalent in the female.

Vascular Spiders.[57] These structures should be looked for carefully with the aid of a good light. Inspection with a hand lens may be necessary to distinguish them from small papular lesions. They may pulsate and can be obliterated by pressing on their central point with the end of a pencil. They usually indicate the presence of hepatic cirrhosis.

Breath. A peculiar sickly sweetish breath (hepatic foetor) is characteristic of severe hepatic disease with necrosis.[58] According to Hoffbauer,[59] hepatic foetor is sometimes detected on the breath of patients with well-compensated hepatic cirrhosis, or it may follow the therapeutic use of large quantities of pure methionine. Methyl mercaptan has been isolated from the urine of patients with hepatic foetor,[60] and this, coupled with a high plasma level of methionine, suggests that the mercaptan arises by

hydrolytic or reductive fission of the sulfur-carbon bond in methionine.

Cervical lymphadenopathy should suggest the presence of viral hepatitis or infectious mononucleosis.

Prominent superficial abdominal veins are observed most often in patients with hepatic cirrhosis but may occur in the presence of peritoneal tumor implants, obstruction of the portal vein by tumor or in cases of inferior caval obstruction. In portal hypertension the blood flow in the abdominal veins is radially away from the umbilicus, whereas in inferior caval obstruction it is always upward over the abdominal wall.[61]

Liver. The normal liver is soft, smooth and frequently tender. It has a sharp edge which may not be palpable or may be felt 1 to 2 fingerbreadths below the right costal margin. While a reliable method for estimating liver size is not available, it is safe to assume that a liver which extends 3 fingerbreadths or more below the right costal margin is probably enlarged (and hence the seat of disease) provided that one may exclude downward displacement by right pleural cavity fluid or marked pulmonary emphysema, and that the body habitus is not hyposthenic. Variations in the shape and the position of the liver appear to accompany body types. In a stocky person, the liver may often extend to the left lateral abdominal wall with its lower edge lying relatively high; it may not be palpable beneath the costal margin. In a lanky individual, the normal liver, including the left lobe, may lie entirely in the right abdomen and may extend 5 fingerbreadths below the costal margin.[62]

A liver which is unduly firm is apt to be diseased, as is one with a blunted edge or an irregular contour. An irregular, firm, nodular liver is most commonly indicative of intrahepatic malignant neoplasm. However, the large regenerating nodules of postnecrotic cirrhosis may produce an irregularity of contour which may closely simulate that produced by tumor. The same may hold true in the fatty or cystic liver.

The liver may not extend below the right costal margin in cases of hepatitis or cirrhosis. It is usually found from 1 to 2 (or

2 to 3) fingerbreadths below the right costal margin in viral hepatitis and is frequently tender in this disease. A very large liver (one extending 4 to 5 fingerbreadths or more below the right costal margin) is usually indictive of fatty vacuolization, cirrhosis, tumor, amyloidosis or congestive failure, and is most unusual in viral hepatitis (Fig. 135). Enlargement of the left lobe of the liver should suggest hepatic syphilis but may be caused by primary or metastatic tumor or by abscess.

The absence of a palpable liver in a patient who has had jaundice for 2 to 3 weeks or more would tend to exclude neoplastic obstruction of the bile ducts, since sufficient bile stasis should result, by this time, to produce detectable hepatic enlargement.[63]

Gallbladder. The presence of a smooth, nontender, distended gallbladder in a jaundiced patient is almost always indicative of neoplastic obstruction of the common bile duct in accordance with Courvoisier's law. It is found much more frequently at operation or necropsy than it is on physical examination; a discrepancy accounted for by the overlying right lobe of the liver or, less frequently, by a thick abdominal wall. Painless distention of the gallbladder may be encountered in patients who have been vomiting and not ingesting fats.[64]

Spleen. In the absence of hemolytic jaundice a palpable spleen is usually indicative of hepatocellular jaundice. The spleen is palpable in about one half of patients with hepatic cirrhosis, in about 10 to 15 per cent of patients with viral hepatitis and about 20 per cent of cases of hepatic neoplasm.[65] It is well to bear in mind that in obstructive jaundice of long standing, splenomegaly may be a manifestation of obstructive cirrhosis. In cancer of the body and the tail of the pancreas splenic enlargement may result from encroachment of the tumor on the splenic vein.[66] Splenomegaly is also encountered occasionally in periampullary tumor.

Ascites. The presence of ascites in a jaundiced patient is usually indicative of hepatic cirrhosis but may also be observed in massive hepatic necrosis or very severe hepatitis, in subacute hepatic necrosis, in the presence of peritoneal tumor implants or following invasion of the portal vein by tumor.

Palmar Erythema. Patek[67] and Perera[68] have pointed out the frequency of a symmetric erythema—so-called palmar erythema—involving the eminences of the

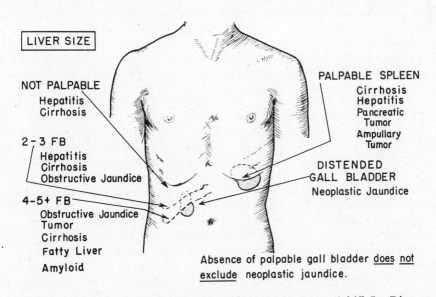

FIG. 135. Abdominal findings in various forms of jaundice. (Schiff, L.: Diseases of the Liver, ed. 2, Philadelphia, Lippincott)

palms and the digits of the hands in patients with hepatic cirrhosis.

"Routine" Tests

Blood Count. According to Havens[69] the white cell count is usually reduced during the preicteric and normal during the icteric phase of infectious hepatitis, although Jones and Minot[70] reported leukocytosis within the first few days of the disease. The chief value of a white cell count in a patient with jaundice is in helping to distinguish uncomplicated viral hepatitis in which there is usually no leukocytosis from conditions in which leukocytosis is found frequently, such as toxic hepatitis, amebic hepatitis, metastatic hepatic neoplasm, common duct stone (with cholangitis) and Weil's disease. The presence of eosinophilia should suggest toxic hepatitis.

Blood Urea Nitrogen. Elevation of the blood urea nitrogen in a patient with jaundice should suggest the possibility of Weil's disease or exposure to a hepatotoxic agent which is also injurious to the kidney, such, for example, as carbon tetrachloride.

Urine Analysis. The presence of albuminuria should suggest the possibility of Weil's disease, although it may occur in the preicteric and the early icteric phases of viral hepatitis. Since jaundice may occur in amyloidosis, the simultaneous occurrence of marked albuminuria should also arouse suspicion of this disorder.

Stool Examination. Strongly positive tests for occult blood in the stools should arouse suspicion of an ulcerating periampullary lesion or a pancreatic cancer eroding the stomach or the duodenum.

Serum Lipids. Increase in serum lipids should suggest biliary cirrhosis, fatty liver or Zieve's syndrome.[71]

Liver Profile

The writer and his associates have employed the following profile in the differential diagnosis of jaundice: (1) serum bilirubin (method of Malloy and Evelyn as modified by Ducci and Watson); upper limit for 1-minute bilirubin, 0.25 mg. per cent, and for total bilirubin, 1.50 mg. per cent,[72,73] (2) cephalin-cholesterol flocculation (method of Hanger:[74] 1 to 2+ in 24 hours considered normal); (3) thymol turbidity (Shank and Hoagland's modification[75] of Maclagan's method,[76]) with normal range of 0 to 5 units; (4) zinc sulfate turbidity (method of Kunkel[77]) with normal values of 12 units or less; (5) thymol flocculation (Neefe), 1+ flocculation considered normal;[78] (6) serum alkaline phosphatase (Bodansky method[79]), with normal for adults 0 to 4 units per 100 ml.; (7) serum glutamic oxaloacetic[80] (SGOT) and serum glutamic pyruvic transaminase[81] (SGPT), normal range 4 to 40 units; (8) 5-nucleotidase,[82] normal value 0.3 to 3.2 units per 100 ml.

In *hepatocellular jaundice* there usually are a positive cephalin-cholesterol flocculation, increased thymol and zinc turbidity, positive thymol flocculation, and little or no increase in the serum alkaline phosphatase (less than 10 Bodansky units per 100 ml. or 30 to 35 King-Armstrong units). By contrast, we note that the usual findings in cases of *obstructive jaundice* are a negative cephalin-cholesterol flocculation, normal thymol and normal or decreased zinc turbidity, negative (or 1+) thymol flocculation and increase in the serum alkaline phosphatase of more than 10 Bodansky units per 100 ml. (or more than 30 to 35 King-Armstrong units).

While obstructive jaundice is virtually always accompanied by an increase in the serum alkaline phosphatase, this increase may be of moderate degree, less than 10 Bodansky units per 100 ml., even in cases of biliary obstruction due to neoplasm.[83] A steadily rising concentration of both serum alkaline phosphatase and serum bilirubin, coupled with a negative cephalin flocculation test, constitute a most reliable index of obstructive jaundice.[84] One may exclude increases in the enzyme concentration attributable to bone disease by determining the concentration of serum 5-nucleotidase, which is not influenced by osseous factors.[82] On the other hand, the serum 5-nucleotidase may rarely be increased in the face of a normal serum-alkaline phosphatase concentration.

Determination of the serum glutamic oxaloacetic (SGOT) and serum glutamic pyruvic (SGPT) transaminase levels may be of value in the distinction between hepatocellular and obstructive jaundice. In obstructive jaundice the concentration of these enzymes is usually not greater than 300 units, whereas in the very early stages of hepatitis, an increase of 1,000 or more units is frequent. However, we have seen a patient with obstructive jaundice due to carcinoma of the head of the pancreas in whom the serum transaminase (SGPT) was reported to be 750 units, and a case of carcinoma of the ampulla of Vater with a value of approximately 600 units. The diagnostic value of these enzyme determinations decreases with increase in the duration of jaundice. The most marked increases occur in the very early stages of hepatitis. Thus, in patients first seen 2 or 3 weeks after the onset of symptoms, the enzyme concentration may have fallen to the levels ordinarily observed in obstructive jaundice.[83]

It is well recognized that most of the individual laboratory tests constituting the so-called liver profile are not specific liver function tests and hence may be positive in the absence of liver disease. The importance of the clinical examination in the interpretation of the results of these liver function tests becomes evident. As Himsworth[25] has stated so well, "There is yet no test which approaches in value a careful clinical assessment of the patient and none which can be interpreted without it." This is well exemplified by increases in the serum alkaline phosphatase which occur in the presence of osseous lesions such as Paget's disease and hyperparathyroidism and by positive cephalin flocculation tests observed in infectious mononucleosis, hemolytic jaundice, disseminated lupus erythematosus, pernicious anemia, acute leukemia, chronic malaria, and diffuse diseases of the reticuloendothelial system.[84]

PROTHROMBIN RESPONSE TO VITAMIN K[85-87]

Four of the clotting factors in plasma appear to be synthesized exclusively in the liver, namely, prothrombin, Factor VII (pro-SPCA or proconvertin), Factor X (Stuart-Power factor) and Christmas factor (plasma thromboplastin component). Their formation depends on the normal absorption of vitamin K from the intestine and the functional integrity of the liver cells. Three of these factors (prothrombin, Factor VII and Factor X) influence the one-stage prothrombin time. Thus a long prothrombin time may be due to the exclusion of bile from the intestine and/or severe liver injury. If the prothrombin time of the blood of an icteric patient is markedly prolonged (that is, if the "prothrombic activity" is under 40 per cent of normal) and becomes normal within 24 hours after parenteral administration of vitamin K, it is probable that liver cell function is reasonably good and that the jaundice is due to extrahepatic obstruction. The failure of the prothrombin time to shorten under these circumstances would indicate the presence of parenchymal liver disease. An adequate amount of vitamin K is provided by 10 mg. of menadione sodium bisulphite (Hykinone) given subcutaneously. In order to exclude intrinsic errors in the test itself, it is best to determine the blood prothrombin time on two separate days both before and after the administration of the vitamin K. A recent case of common duct stones presented itself with purpura and a marked hypoprothrombinemia which responded to vitamin K administration. No other clinical features of common duct stone were present.

RESPONSE TO STEROIDS

The response of the serum-bilirubin to steroid therapy may prove to be very helpful in the differential diagnosis of jaundice in spite of earlier conflicting reports.[88-92] A period of 4 or 5 days is usually chosen during which ACTH or corticosteroids are given and the affects on the serum bilirubin concentration observed. The ACTH is usually administered intramuscularly in doses of 60 to 120 units per day; while the corticosteroids are given in the form of 30 to 60 mg. of prednisone daily. A drop in serum bilirubin concentration of 40 to 50 per cent or more is strongly indicative of hepatitis; the drop is rapid in the first 24 to 48 hours and is followed by a slower fall. In obstructive jaundice (and cirrhosis) the drop is less marked, and when treatment is

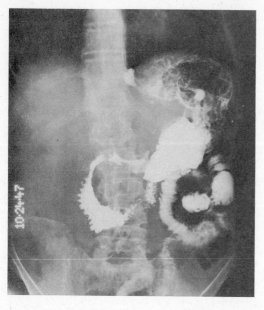

Fig. 136. P. M. Carcinoma of the head of the pancreas, producing extrinsic pressure on bulb and smoothing of inner border of duodenum. (Schiff, L.: Clinical Approach to Jaundice, Springfield, Ill., Thomas)

discontinued the value promptly returns to pretreatment levels.

The mechanism of the resulting decrease in serum bilirubin is not known. It is not that of increased biliary excretion, increased renal clearance of bile pigments or decrease in the rate of red cell breakdown. An additional metabolic pathway for bilirubin has been suggested,[92] as has inhibition of hepatic bilirubinogenesis.[93]

DUODENAL DRAINAGE

Duodenal drainage may be helpful in the differential diagnosis of jaundice by

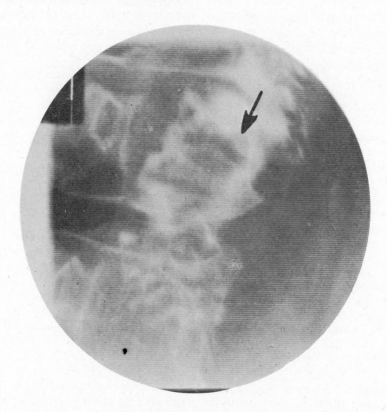

Fig. 137. (R.R. 32331). Carcinoma of the ampulla of Vater. Spot film showing defect in descending duodenum. (Schiff, L.: Clinical Approach to Jaundice, Springfield, Ill., Thomas)

furnishing material for clinical, microscopic and cytologic examinations.[94]

ROENTGEN EXAMINATION

X-ray examination has been of limited value in the differential diagnosis of jaundice, due largely to four factors: (1) inability to furnish direct evidence of hepatitis, (2) inadequacies of present-day technics in the demonstration of tumors producing jaundice, (3) limitations of cholecystography and intravenous cholangiography, and (4) lack of proof that gallstones are the cause of jaundice by their mere demonstration.

X-ray changes caused by tumors producing icterus depend largely on pressure or displacement effects upon contiguous structures resulting from expansion of the neoplasm and may not be present during the early stages of tumor growth. A carcinoma of the head of the pancreas producing jaundice may not be large enough to bulge appreciably on the surface of the gland and therefore may escape detection on roentgen examination.

Cholecystography has been of little diagnostic value in cases of hepatocellular or obstructive jaundice, since the gallbladder may fail to visualize because of the liver's impaired ability to excrete the dye.

Despite its limitations, the roentgen examination may be helpful in the diagnosis of the cause of jaundice. A plain film may reveal enlargement of the liver and the spleen, a stone in the common bile duct, a ground-glass appearance suggestive of ascites, or an elevated right diaphragm indicative of hepatic tumor or abscess. Esophageal varices may be visualized in cases of hepatic cirrhosis or hepatoma. By revealing the presence of a primary neoplasm in the alimentary canal or other body system, the roentgen examination may help to confirm the diagnosis of a metastatic hepatic tumor; or, by failing to reveal a

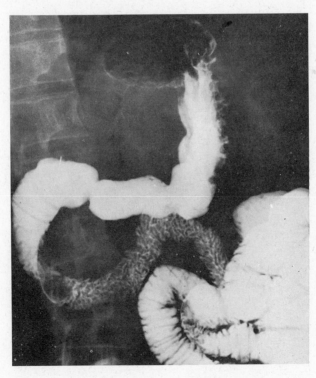

Fig. 138. (E.T. 158725). Defect in descending duodenum.

primary site elsewhere, it may strengthen the clinical impression of hepatoma. It may furnish evidence of an enlarged liver by demonstrating displacement of the stomach posteriorly and/or to the left, or displacement of the hepatic flexure of the colon downward.

A pancreatic tumor may produce anterior displacement of the duodenal loop, downward displacement of the duodenal-jejunal juncture, compression or invasion of the duodenum or the stomach or widening of the duodenal loop (Fig. 136). Periampullary tumor may produce a filling defect in the descending duodenum (Figs. 137 and 138) or Forstberg's reversed-3 sign (Fig. 139).

By demonstrating calcification in the pancreas the roentgen examination may lead to the diagnosis of relapsing pancreatitis as a cause of icterus.

Intravenous cholangiography may be em-ployed successfully when the serum bilirubin has dropped to 3 mg. per cent or less (Fig. 140) or when bromsulphalein retention is less than 15 to 30 per cent.[95,98] The common duct is demonstrated best within the first hour. It is well to remember that the normal common bile duct measures up to 10 mm. in diameter on the roentgenogram and that following cholecystectomy the common duct may dilate up to 16 mm. in diameter. More marked dilatation or persistent opacification on 2- or 3-hour films is indicative of obstructive disease.

Oral cholangiography may be accomplished by repeating the dose of iopanoic acid (Telepaque), giving it on the evening before and again on the morning of the x-ray examination[97] or by administering iopanoic acid in doses of 1.0 Gm. (2 tablets) after each meal for a 4-day period with the patient on a relatively fat-free diet.[98,99] On the morning of the 5th day, roentgenograms

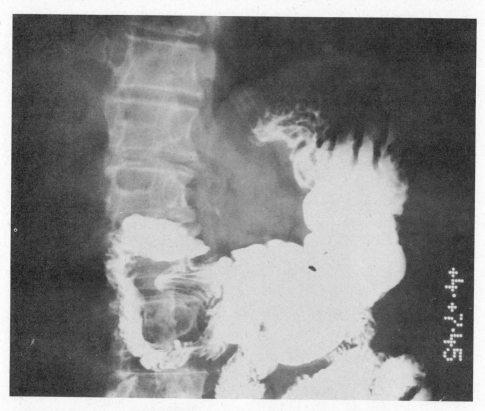

Fig. 139. (W.B. 539). Reversed-3 sign in the descending portion of the duodenum with clinical evidence suggestive of carcinoma of the ampulla of Vater. (Schiff, L.: Differential Diagnosis of Jaundice, Chicago, Year Book)

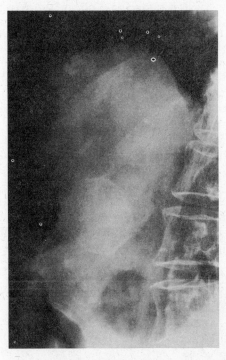 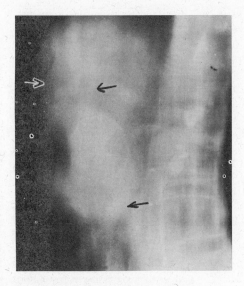

Fig. 140. (*Left*) Large calculus demonstrated by 4-day dye (Telepaque) test not previously revealed on plain film or after attempt at intravenous cholangiography. (*Right*) Calculus shown in common bile duct following intravenous cholangiograph performed immediately after demonstration by 4-day technique. Upper arrows indicate degree of dilatation of common bile duct. Lower arrow indicates narrowing of duct distal to the calculus.

are taken with the patient fasting. By this technic, opacification of radiolucent biliary calculi may result from deposition of the Telepaque on the surface of the stones (Fig. 140 Left).

Percutaneous transhepatic cholangiography[100-103] is being used increasingly for demonstrating the presence of obstructive jaundice and indicating the site and nature of the obstructing lesion, with reports indicating that the risk from this procedure may have been exaggerated. One particular advantage is that it may be used when intravenous cholangiography is contraindicated, i.e., when the serum bilirubin is over 3 mg. per cent. It is the best means presently available for distinguishing intrahepatic cholestasis from extrahepatic obstructive jaundice (Figs. 141 and 142). The technic has recently been modified by introducing the contrast material into the liver through a polyethylene catheter drawn over a short

beveled needle 12 cm. in length and of 1 mm. bore; the catheter being left in situ after the cholangiogram is obtained, thus permitting biliary drainage and decreasing the risk of bile periotonitis.[103] In cases of hepatitis the bile passages are not dilated and hence cannot be entered by the needle, and a cholangiogram will not be obtained.

According to Atkinson *et al.*, the incidence of leakage of bile from the puncture wound in the liver is 5 per cent. Santos *et al.* reported 1 instance of bile peritonitis and 2 instances of shock in 46 cases in which the procedure was carried out. If a bile duct is punctured and a diagnostic cholangiogram is obtained, surgery is usually undertaken within 24 hours. Failure to puncture a dilated duct in patients with obstructive jaundice is considered to afford strong presumptive evidence of an intrahepatic cause for the jaundice.[103] Further experience is required to assess both the risk of the method and its true value.

The importance of operative and postoperative cholangiography in the detection of stones in the common and the intrahepatic ducts is well known (Figs. 143 and 144). It has been estimated that common duct calculi may be overlooked by ordinary methods in between 10 and 30 per cent of operated cases. The necessity for meticulous technic and intimate teamwork on the part of the anesthetist, the roentgenologist and the surgeon has been stressed. For details the reader is referred to the monographs of Mirizzi,[104,105] Norman,[106] Partington and Sachs[107] and to the studies of Isaacs and Daves.[108]

NEEDLE BIOPSY OF THE LIVER

The use of needle biopsy of the liver should be confined to selected, unsolved cases of jaundice for many reasons: (1) the diagnosis of the cause of jaundice can be made in 85 to 90 per cent of cases on the basis of the clinical examination and the results of laboratory tests;[26,83,109] (2) the diagnostic use of steroids has decreased the need for needle biopsy in the jaundiced patient, particularly when marked lessening of the icterus results, and the steroids are then continued therapeutically; (3) marked increases of the serum glutamic transaminases (of an order of 1,000 units or more) justify deferment of the biopsy because of

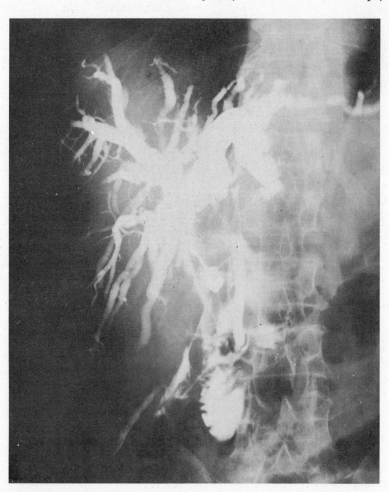

Fig. 141. W.G. Biliary tract dilatation due to carcinoma of bile ducts as shown on transhepatic cholangiogram. (Schiff, L.: Diseases of the Liver, ed. 2, Philadelphia, Lippincott)

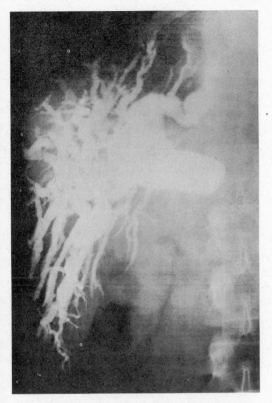

FIG. 142. B.K. Transhepatic cholangiogram showing biliary tract dilatation associated with carcinoma of head of pancreas. (Schiff, L.: Diseases of the Liver, ed. 2, Philadelphia, Lippincott)

the likelihood of hepatitis; (4) there is the added danger of hemorrhage and, in cases of obstructive jaundice, bile peritonitis.[110] Nevertheless, in carefully selected patients who are observed closely after the procedure and treated promptly when indications arise, the danger is slight. The overall risk of needle biopsy of the liver includes a mortality of 0.1 per cent and a complication rate of 0.32 per cent according to the reviews of Terry[111] and Zamcheck and Klausenstock.[112]

Actually, the procedure probably will *be indicated* in less than 10 per cent of cases of jaundice, and includes the following situations:

When Difficulty Exists in Distinguishing Medical from Surgical Cases. Needless surgery may be averted by demonstrating the presence of hepatitis (Figs. 145 and 146); conversely, surgical therapy may be expedited in cases of obstructive jaundice (Figs. 147 and 148).

It should be emphasized that the biopsy specimen is almost of no help in determining the cause of extrahepatic obstruction; hence, needle biopsy of the liver should not be performed when the jaundice is obviously due to extrahepatic obstruction! Instead, surgery should be carried out.

The Presence of an Obscure Systemic Disorder. Unsuspected granulomatous disease may be revealed in the biopsy specimen.

Suspicion of Metastatic Neoplasm of the Liver. In over 100 cases of proved neoplasm of the liver the specimens obtained by needle biopsy were positive for tumor in 74 per cent; and, interestingly enough, the positive incidence was as high with the transthoracic as with the transabdominal approach.[113] In an experience which now covers the procurement of needle specimens in about 200 cases of malignant neoplasms

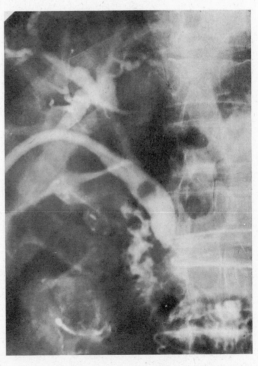

FIG. 143. W.J. Operative cholangiogram showing common duct stone. (Schiff, L.: Clinical Approach to Jaundice, Springfield, Ill., Thomas)

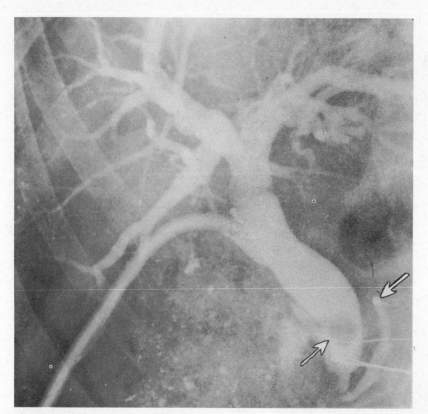

Fig. 144. W.J. Note shift of stone on comparing with Fig. 143. Upper arrow points to pancreatic duct. (Schiff, L.: Clinical Approach to Jaundice, Springfield, Ill., Thomas)

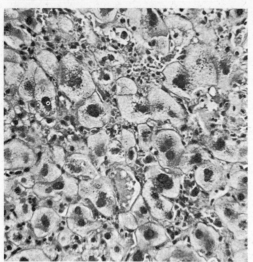

Fig. 145. Acute viral hepatitis. A high-power view, demonstrating swollen parenchymal elements ("balloon cells") with ground-glass cytoplasm and amitotic nuclear division. Focal inflammatory aggregates are evident, but the liver cells exhibit no fatty vacuolization. (Schiff, L.: Diseases of the Liver, ed. 2, Philadelphia, Lippincott)

Fig. 146. Infectious (viral) hepatitis. A portal area is the seat of marked infiltration with lymphocytes and monocytes but shows no other significant alteration. Hepatic cells are swollen, pale staining, granular and often multinucleated. Near the upper center of the photograph may be seen a single cell which has become shrunken, rounded, hyperchromatic and separated from its neighbors. (Weisbrod, F. G., Schiff, L., Gall, E. A., Cleveland, F. P., and Berman, J. R.: Gastroenter. 14:56)

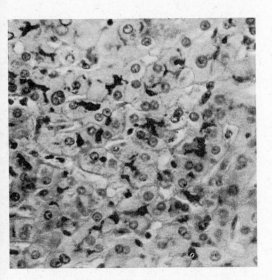

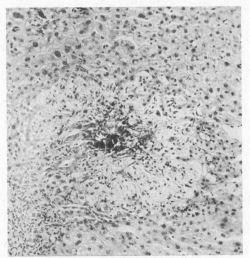

Fig. 147. Obstructive bile stasis, carcinoma of the head of the pancreas. Intercellular bile capillaries are brought into prominence by dark-staining inspissated plugs of static bile. Liver cells are essentially normal in appearance and exhibit none of the features observed in viral hepatitis. (Schiff, L.: Diseases of the Liver, ed. 2, Philadelphia, Lippincott)

Fig. 148. Obstructive bile stasis. A bile lake pathognomonic of extrahepatic biliary obstruction. Characteristic are a central pool of extravasated bile surrounded by a radial zone of degenerated parenchyma exhibiting a peculiar feathery reticulated appearance. (Taken from Weisbrod, F. G., Schiff, L., Gall, E. A., Cleveland, F. P., Berman, J. R.: Gastroenterol. 14:56)

of the liver, the high percentage of positive yields remains unaltered, and the risk of procedure has not been increased by the presence of neoplasm. This has also been the experience of Fenster and Klatskin.[65] Whether or not preliminary photo-scans of the liver to help determine the proper or most promising site of needle biopsy will increase the positive yields in the needle specimens awaits further study.

Hepatomegaly of Undetermined Cause. A fatty liver may be discovered in a patient thought to have cirrhosis, neoplasm or hepatitis. Histologic changes of obstructive jaundice may be found in patients with suspected hepatitis, and vice versa.

CONCLUSION

As was so well stated more than a century ago,

Jaundice is rather a symptom of disease than a disease itself, and may arise from various causes which it is very important that we should be acquainted with; because knowledge of the cause, or of the circumstances under which the jaundice arose in any particular case, often gives us an insight into its real nature, which we could scarcely obtain from considering the symptoms merely.*

Excluding the hemolytic and hereditary varieties, most cases of jaundice comprise the various forms of hepatitis and cirrhosis or obstructive types due to gall stones or neoplasms. In the interpretation of the significance of jaundice, even in the present-day laboratory age the physician will derive greatest help from the clinical approach. Nevertheless, he should be wary lest certain diagnostic clues prove misleading. These pertain particularly to the age of the patient and a history of alcoholism, which, while favoring certain causes of jaundice do not of themselves exclude others. Similarly, the physician should bear in mind that *exposure* to an hepatotoxic agent does not necessarily establish a causal relationship, since there is at present no specific means of proving such a relationship in the form of a reliable skin test or

*George Budd, On Diseases of the Liver, 1846.

by the demonstration of specific circulating antibodies. He should also realize that obstructive jaundice due to neoplasm, particularly that arising in the bile ducts, may sometimes endure for several years and may even escape detection at laparotomy. Since jaundice is rarely, if ever, a surgical emergency, biding one's time may prove of help in diagnosis as the result of variations in the intensity of the icterus or its actual disappearance.

In the past few decades, aids in the diagnosis of the cause of jaundice have been provided through the introduction of new biochemical tests, advances in roentgenologic technics and the procurement of needle specimens of the liver. As time passes, additional advances will be forthcoming, but as those of the past, all will undoubtedly have their limitations, some their risks, and none will replace the clinical examination of the patient. It is hoped that these advances will soon include isolation of the hepatitis virus or viruses and the development of serologic tests for hepatitis and that they will thus better enable the clinician to meet the challenge posed by the appearance of jaundice.

REFERENCES

1. von Ehrenstein, G., and Lockner, D.: Physiologischer erythrozytenabbau, Acta Haemat. 22:129, 1959.
2. Hughes-Jones, N. C., and Cheney, B.: The use of Cr^{51} and Fe^{59} as red cell labels to determine the fate of normal erythrocytes in the rat, Clin. Sci., 20:323, 1961.
3. Gray, C. H., and Kekwick, R. A.: Bilirubin-serum protein complexes and the van den Bergh reaction, Nature 161:274, 1948.
4. Martin, N. H.: Bilirubin serum complexes, Biochem. J., vol. 42, Proc. XV, 1948.
5. Billing, B. H.: The Role of Conjugation in the Excretion of Bilirubin, Elsevier Monograph, Amsterdam, 1961.
6. Billing, B. H., Cole, P. G., and Lathe, G. H.: The excretion of bilirubin as a diglucuronide giving the direct van den Bergh reaction, Biochem. J. 65:774, 1957.
7. Schmid, R.: The identification of "direct-reacting" bilirubin as bilirubin glucuronide, J. Biol. Chem. 229:881, 1957.
8. Talafant, E.: Properties and composition of the bile pigment giving a direct diazo reaction, Nature 178:312, 1956.
9. Isselbacher, K. J., and McCarthy, E. A.: Studies on bilirubin sulfate and other non-glucuronide conjugates of bilirubin, J. Clin. Invest. 38:645, 1959.
10. Nosslin, B.: The direct diazo-reaction of bile pigments in serum. Scand. J. Clin. Lab. Invest. vol. 12, Supp. 49, 1960.
11. Nizet, E., and Barac, G.: Localization intra-rénale de la bilirubine chez le chien ictérique, C. R. Soc. Biol. 146:1282, 1952.
12. Watson, C. J., Campbell, M., and Lowry, P. T.: Preferential reduction of conjugated bilirubin to urobilinogen by normal fecal flora, Proc. Soc. Exp. Biol. Med. 98:707, 1958.
13. Gustafsson, B. E., and Lanke, L. S.: Bilirubin and urobilins in germfree, ex-germ-free and conventional rats, J. Exp. Med. 112:975, 1960.
14. Matsui, K.: Studies on the reduction products of bilirubin in the small intestine, Igaku Kenkyu 29:1086, 1959.
15. Watson, C. J.: Composition of the urobilin group in urine, bile, and feces and the significance of variations in health and disease, J. Lab. Clin. Med. 54:1, 1959.
16. McMaster, P. D., and Elman, R.: Urobilin physiology and pathology, Ann. Int. Med. 1:68, 1927.
17. McNee, J. W.: Jaundice: a review of recent work, Quart. J. Med. 16:390, 1922-23.
18. Watson, C. J.: Regurgitation jaundice: clinical differentiation of the common forms, with particular reference to the degree of biliary obstruction, J.A.M.A. 114:2427, 1940.
19. Tisdale, W. A., Klatskin, G., and Kinsella, E. D.: The significance of the direct-reacting fraction of serum bilirubin in hemolytic jaundice, Am. J. Med. 26:214, 1959.
20. Gonzales-Oddone, M. V.: Bilirubin, bromsulfalein, bile acids, alkaline phosphatase and cholesterol of thoracic duct lymph in experimental regurgitation jaundice, Proc. Soc. Exp. Bio. Med. 63:144, 1946.
21. Grafflin, A. L., and Chaney, V. E., Jr.: Studies of extrahepatic biliary obstruction in the white mouse by flourescence microscopy, Bull. Johns Hopkins Hosp. 93:107, 1953.
22. Hanzon, V.: Liver cell secretion under normal and pathologic conditions studied by fluorescence microscopy on living rats, Acta Physiol. Scand. (supp. 101) 28:1 1952.
23. Watson, C. J.: The bile pigments, New England J. Med. 227:705, 1942.

24. Rich, A. R.: The pathogenesis of the forms of jaundice, Bull. Johns Hopkins Hosp. 47:338, 1930.

25. Himsworth, H. P.: Lectures on the Liver and Its Diseases, ed. 2, Cambridge, Mass., Harvard, 1950.

26. Watson, C. J.: An approach to the distinction of medical and surgical jaundice, Minn. Med. 32:973, 1949.

27. Eppinger, H.: Die Leberkrankheiten: Allgemeine und Spezielle Pathologie und Therapie der Leber, Vienna, Springer, 1937.

28. Lucke, B.: The pathology of fatal epidemic hepatitis, Am. J. Path. 20:471, 1944.

29. Steigmann, F., and Popper, H.: Intrahepatic obstructive jaundice, Gastroenterology 1:645, 1943.

30. Popper, H., and Schaffner, F.: Response of the liver to injury, in Popper and Schaffner (eds.): Progress in Liver Disease, p. 86, New York, Grune & Stratton, 1961.

31. Watson, C. J., and Hoffbauer, F. W.: The problem of prolonged hepatitis with particular reference to the cholangiolitic type and to the development of cholangiolitic cirrhosis of the liver, Ann. Int. Med. 25: 195, 1946.

32. Billing, B. H., and Williams, R. S.: Unpublished data.

33. Arias, I. M.: Panel: Bilirubin metabolism, Gastroenterology 36:166, 1959.

34. McMahon, F. G.: Effect of prednisolone, physical activity, fat intake and choleretic agents on the serum bilirubin level in a case of constitutional hepatic dysfunction (Gilbert's disease), Gastroenterology 32: 325, 1957.

35. Dubin, I. N.: Chronic idiopathic jaundice: a review of 50 cases, Am. J. Med. 24:268, 1958.

36. Sprinz, H., and Nelson, R. S.: Persistent nonhemolytic hyperbilirubinemia associated with lipochrome-like pigment in liver cells: Report of four cases, Ann. Int. Med. 41:952, 1954.

37. Bynum, W. T.: Mavero-hepatic icterus (black liver jaundice), Gastroenterology 33:97, 1957.

38. Caroli, J.: Int. Ass. Study Liver Dis., 1st Mtg., London, Apr. 1960, Lancet 1:1066, 1960.

39. Wegmann, R., Weinmann, S., and Rangier, M.: Infra-red spectrography of the black pigment extracted from the spleen. Rev. Med. Mal. Foie, 35:95, 1960.

40. Mandema, E., de Fraiture, W. H., Nieweg, H. O., and Arends, A.: Familial chronic idiopathic jaundice (Dubin-Sprinz disease) with a note on bromsulphalein metabolism in this disease, Am. J. Med. 28:42, 1960.

41. Wolf, R. L., Pizette, M., Richman, A., Dreiling, D. A., Jacobs, W., Fernandez, O., and Popper, H.: Chronic idiopathic jaundice; a study of 2 afflicted families, Am. J. Med. 28:32, 1960.

42. Shaldon, S., and Caeser, J. J.: Personal communication.

43. Calderon, A., and Goldgraber, M. B.: Chronic idiopathic jaundice: a case report, Gastroenterology 40:244, 1961.

44. Rotor, A. B., Manahan, L., and Florentin, A.: Familial non-hemolytic jaundice with direct van den Bergh reaction, Acta Med. Philipp. 5:37, 1948.

45. Stransky, E.: Uber kongenitalen, familiären, nichthämolytischen icterus, Ann. Pediat. 175:301, 1950.

46. Dagnini, G., and Moreschi, E.: Ittero famigliare epatogeno a bilirubina diretta, Recenti Progr. Med. 23:47, 1957.

47. Schiff, L., Billing, B. H., and Oikawa, Y.: Familial nonhemolytic jaundice with conjugated bilirubin in the serum; a case study, New England J. Med. 260:1315, 1959.

48. Haverback, B. J., and Wirtschafter, S. K.: Familial non-hemolytic jaundice with normal liver histology and conjugated bilirubin, New England J. Med. 262:113, 1960.

49. Arias, I. M.: Studies of chronic familial non-hemolytic jaundice with conjugated bilirubin in the serum with and without an unidentified pigment in the liver cells, Am. J. Med. 31:510, 1961.

50. Peck, O. C., Rey, D. F., and Snell, A.: Familial jaundice with free and conjugated bilirubin in the serum and without liver pigmentation, Gastroenterology 39: 625, 1960.

51. Davis, W. D., and Young, P. C.: An unusual type of hyperbilirubinemia with bromsulfalein retention and microscopically normal liver, Gastroenterology 37:206, 1959.

52. Charbonnier, A.: Personal communication.

53. Schiff, L.: Homologous serum hepatitis: clinical implications, New Orleans M. S. J. 99:611, 1947.

54. ———: Diagnostic significance of the time interval between resection of a malignant tumor and the appearance of jaundice, Am. J. Dig. Dis. 5:573, 1960.

55. Chauffard, M. A.: Le cancer du corps de pancréas, Bull. Acad. Med. 60:242, 1908.

56. Ashe, W. F., Pratt-Thomas, H. R., and Kumpe, C. W.: Weil's disease: a complete review of American literature and abstract of the world literature; 7 case reports, Medicine 20:145, 1941.

57. Bean, W. B.: The cutaneous arterial spider: a survey, Medicine 24:243, 1945.

58. Watson, C. J.: The prognosis and treatment of hepatic insufficiency, Ann. Int. Med. 31:405, 1949.

59. Hoffbauer, F. W.: Bedside diagnosis of jaundice, Northwest Med. 48:757, 1949.

60. Challenger, F., and Walshe, J. M.: Foetor hepaticus, Lancet 1:1239, 1955.

61. Sherlock, S.: Cirrhosis of the liver, Postgrad. M. J. 26:472, 1950.

62. Fleischner, F. G., and Sayegh, V.: Assessment of the size of the liver; roentgenologic considerations, New England J. Med. 259:271, 1958.

63. Schiff, L.: Absence of a palpable liver: a sign of value in excluding obstructive jaundice due to pancreatic cancer, Gastroenterology 32:1143, 1957.

64. Jones, C. M.: Personal communication.

65. Fenster, L. F., and Klatskin, G.: Manifestations of metastatic tumors of the liver: a study of 81 patients subjected to needle biopsy, Ann. Med. 31:238, 1961.

66. Duff, G. L.: The clinical and pathological features of carcinoma of the body and tail of the pancreas, Bull. Johns Hopkins Hosp. 65:69, 1939.

67. Patek, A. J., Jr.: *Quoted by* Perera: J.A.M.A. 119:1417, 1942.

68. Perera, G. A.: A note on palmar erythema (so-called liver palms), J.A.M.A. 119:1417, 1942.

69. Havens, W. P., Jr.: Infectious hepatitis, Medicine 27:279, 1948.

70. Jones, C. M., and Minot, G. R.: Infectious (catarrhal) jaundice, an attempt to establish a clinical entity; observations on excretion and retention of bile pigments and on blood, Boston M. & S. J. 189:531, 1923.

71. Zieve, L.: Jaundice, hyperlipemia and hemolytic anemia: a heretofore unrecognized syndrome associated with alcoholic fatty liver and cirrhosis, Ann. Int. Med. 48:471, 1958.

72. Zieve, L., Hill, E., Hanson, M. C. L., Falcone, A. B., and Watson, C. J.: The serum bilirubin, Bull. U. Minn. Hosp. 22:14, 1951.

73. ———: Normal and abnormal variations and clinical significance of the one-minute and total serum bilirubin determinations, J. Lab. Clin. Med. 38:446, 1951.

74. Hanger, F. M.: Serological differentiation of obstructive from hepatogenous jaundice by flocculation of cephalin-cholesterol emulsions, J. Clin. Invest. 18:261, 1939.

75. Shank, R. E., and Hoagland, C. L.: A modified method for the quantitative determination of the thymol turbidity reaction of serum, J. Biol. Chem. 162:133, 1946.

76. Maclagan, N. F.: Thymol turbidity test; a new indicator of liver dysfunction, Nature 154:670, 1944; The thymol turbidity test as an indicator of liver dysfunction, Brit. J. Exp. Path. 25:234, 1944.

77. Kunkel, H. G.: Estimation of alterations of serum gamma globulin by a turbidimetric technique, Proc. Soc. Exp. Biol. Med. 66:217, 1947.

78. Neefe, J. R., Gambescia, J. M., Gardner, H. T., and Knowlton, M.: Symposium on viral hepatitis; comparison of the thymol, cephalin-cholesterol flocculation and colloidal red tests in acute viral hepatitis, Am. J. Med. 8:600, 1950.

79. Bodansky, A.: Phosphatase studies: II. determination of serum phosphatase; factors influencing the accuracy of the determination, J. Biol. Chem. 101:93, 1933.

80. Cabaud, P., Leeper, R., and Wroblewski, F.: Colorimetric measurement of serum glutamic oxaloacetic transaminase, Am. J. Clin. Path. 26:1101, 1956.

81. Wroblewski, F., and Cabaud, P.: Colorimetric measurement of serum glutamic pyruvic transaminase, Am. J. Clin. Path. 27:235, 1957.

82. Young, I. I.: Serum 5-nucleotidase: characterization and evaluation in disease states, Ann. N.Y. Acad. Sci. 75:357, 1958.

83. Schenker, S., Balint, J., and Schiff, L.: Differential diagnosis of jaundice: a prospective study of 61 proved cases, Am. J. Dig. Dis. 7:449, 1962.

84. Hanger, F. M.: The meaning of liver function tests, Am. J. Med. 16:565, 1954.

85. Giansiracusa, J. E., and Althausen, T. L.: Diagnostic management of patients with jaundice, J.A.M.A. 134:589, 1947.

86. Lord, J. W., Jr., and Andrus, W. DeW.: Differentiation of intrahepatic and extrahepatic jaundice: response of the plasma prothrombin to intramuscular injection of menadione (2 methyl-1, 4-naphthoquinone) as a diagnostic aid, Arch. Int. Med. 68:199, 1941.

87. Turner, R. H.: *Quoted by* Schiff, L.: Differential Diagnosis of Jaundice, p. 250, Chicago, Year Book Pub., 1946.

88. Chalmers, T. C., Gill, R. J., Jernigan, T. P., Svec, F. A., Jordan, R. S., Waldstein, S. S., and Knowlton, M.: Evaluation of a 4-day ACTH test in the differential diagnosis of jaundice, Gastroenterology 30:894, 1956.

89. Ingelfinger, F.: Differential diagnosis of jaundice, DM, Nov. 1958, Chicago, Year Book Pub.

90. Solem, J. H.: The value of ACTH administration in the differential diagnosis of jaundice, Gastroenterologia 87:23, 1957.

91. Summerskill, W. H. J., Clowdus, B. F., Bollman, J. L., and Fleisher, G. A.: Clinical and experimental studies on the effect of corticotropin and steroid drugs on bilirubinemia, Am. J. M. Sc. 241:555, 1961.

92. Williams, R., and Billing, B. H.: Action of steroid therapy in jaundice, Lancet 2:392, 1961.

93. Katz, R., Ducci, H., and Alessandri, H.: Influence of cortisone and prednisolone on hyperbilirubinemia, J. Clin. Invest. 36: 1370, 1957.

94. Schiff, L. (ed.): Diseases of the Liver, ed. 2, Philadelphia, J. B. Lippincott, 1963.

95. Berk, J. E., and Feigelson, H. H.: Current status of intravenous cholecystography and cholangiography, Southern Med. J. 50:421, 1957.

96. Johnson, G., Jr., Pearce, C., and Glenn, F.: Intravenous cholangiography in biliary tract disease, Ann. Surg. 152:91, 1960.

97. Twiss, J. R., and Gillette, L.: Oral cholangiography; a method of visualizing the "nonvisualized" gallbladder, J.A.M.A. 169: 1275, 1959.

98. Salzman, E., and Warden, M. R.: Telepaque opacification of radiolucent biliary calculi; the "rim sign," Radiology 71:85, 1958.

99. Watkins, D. H., and Salzman, E.: Opacifying gallstones, Arch. Surg. 80:986, 1960.

100. Atkinson, M., Happey, M. G., and Smiddy, F. G.: Percutaneous transhepatic cholangiography, Gut 1:357, 1960.

101. Kaplan, A. A., Traitz, J. J., Mitchell, S. D., and Block, A. L.: Percutaneous transhepatic cholangiography, Ann. Int. Med. 54:856, 1961.

102. Santos, M., Figueroa, L., and Lopez, O.: Percutaneous transhepatic cholangiography in the diagnosis of posthepatic jaundice, Surgery 48:295, 1960.

103. Shaldon, S., Barber, K. M., and Young, W. B.: Percutaneous transhepatic cholangiography, a modified technique, Gastroenterology 42:371, 1962.

104. Mirizzi, P. L.: Fisiopathologia del Hepato-Coledaco: Colangio-grafia operatoria, vol. 26, Buenos Aires, Ateneo, 1939.

105. ———: La cholangiographie operatoire. Quinze annes d'experience, Lyon chir. 43: 385, 1948.

106. Norman, O.: Studies on the hepatic ducts in cholangiography, Acta Radiol., Supp. 84, pp. 1-81, 1951.

107. Partington, P. F., and Sachs, M. D.: Cholangiography, in Carter, B. N. (ed.): Monographs on Surgery, p. 75, New York, Nelson, 1951.

108. Isaacs, J. P., and Daves, M. L.: Technique and evaluation of operative cholangiography, Surg., Gynec. & Obst. 111:103, 1960.

109. Hanger, F. M.: Diagnostic problems of jaundice, Arch. Int. Med. 86:169, 1950.

110. Gallison, D. T., Jr., and Skinner, D.: Bile peritonitis complicating needle biopsy of the liver, New England J. Med., 243:47, 1950.

111. Terry, R.: Risks of needle biopsy of the liver, Brit. M. J. 1:1102, 1952.

112. Zamcheck, N., and Klausenstock, O.: The risk of needle biopsy, New England J. Med. 249:1062, 1953.

113. Ward, J., Schiff, L., Young, P., and Gall, E. A.: Needle biopsy of the liver: IX. Further experiences with malignant neoplasm, Gastroenterology 27:300, 1954.

22

Fever

ELISHA ATKINS*

Definition. Fever is an elevation of body temperature due to disease.

Proper evaluation of the significance of fever requires some knowledge of the mechanisms of temperature control and of the various ways in which that control may be disturbed. In this chapter, after outlining the principal factors concerned with maintenance of a steady body temperature, we shall consider the kinds of conditions in which fever occurs. In some instances the probable mechanism of the temperature elevation will be suggested; more often, however, the actual pathogenesis of this important manifestation of disease will be listed only as a subject for hypothesis.

REGULATION OF BODY TEMPERATURE

In order to maintain a relatively constant body temperature, a fine balance between heat loss and heat production must be maintained, so that a slight increase or decrease of one is promptly compensated by a similar increase or decrease of the other. Maintenance of body temperature within the normal range is accomplished through the agency of a number of physiologic processes, involving both chemical and physical transfer of heat energy. The op-

eration of these mechanisms is integrated by the central nervous system.

SOURCES OF BODY HEAT

Small, and usually inconsequential quantities of heat may be derived from external sources: by radiation from the sun or a heating fixture, or by conduction from an electric heating pad or hot water bottle.

The principal source of heat is combustion of food within the body. The contribution of various organ systems to the total heat production varies greatly according to circumstances. During rest the proportions are approximately as follows: respiration and circulation one-tenth, brain and muscle metabolism, each two-tenths, abdominal viscera (mainly the liver) one half. During physical work much additional heat is generated in the muscles.[1]

Heat production in the muscular system is of special importance in temperature regulation because it is adapted to maintaining uniform body temperature, being readily increased or decreased according to need.

HEAT ELIMINATION

Three forms of heat elimination are of importance: radiation, vaporization and convection. In addition to these, a small amount of heat is lost by conduction to cooler objects and by the warming of ingested food.

Radiation is the process by which en-

* The author is grateful to Dr. P. B. Beeson who has generously allowed the encorporation of major sections of his text from the previous edition of this chapter.

ergy is transferred from warmer objects to cooler ones by means of electromagnetic waves. Under ordinary conditions about 60 per cent of the body heat is eliminated in this way.

Vaporization of water from the surface of the body takes place constantly, even in the absence of sweating, just as water gradually leaves any moist object that is exposed to the air. Evaporation also occurs in the respiratory passages. Since heat is required for the conversion of a liquid to a vapor, the process cools the body. Under ordinary circumstances vaporization accounts for about 20 to 27 per cent of the total loss of body heat. By pouring out sweat, the amount of heat lost by vaporization can be greatly increased.

Convection is the process by which heat is lost to the air circulating over the body surface and the respiratory passages. This source of heat elimination usually accounts for 12 to 15 per cent of the total heat loss.

In a warm environment the proportionate heat loss by the different mechanisms is altered markedly; radiation and convection become ineffective, so that at external temperatures of 95.0° F. or higher vaporization has to bear the entire burden.

BALANCING OF HEAT PRODUCTION AND ELIMINATION

Under conditions that enhance heat loss, for example on changing to a colder environment, there must be instituted countermeasures to decrease heat elimination and to increase heat production. Heat loss is curtailed by a diminished flow of blood to the skin and the subcutaneous tissues. Greater heat production is brought about by an increase in the activity of the skeletal muscles.

One may increase activity voluntarily, or there may be an involuntary acceleration of muscle activity in response to stimuli from the cerebral temperature-control centers. Burton and Bronk studied the latter phenomenon in the cat.[2] They found that when an animal was chilled there was first merely an increased number of action currents in the muscles. If a moderate increase did not suffice to prevent a further fall in temperature, the number of contractions continued to increase, finally becoming synchronized into gross shivering.

In the event of a positive heat balance, the mechanisms for increased dissipation of heat are activated. More blood is supplied to the skin and the subcutaneous tissues, permitting greater heat loss by radiation, vaporization and convection. The cutaneous tissues of the hands are particularly adapted to this function. Observations on the circulation in the fingers at different environmental temperatures have shown that as the surrounding temperature changes from one extreme to another, the volume of the circulation in these tissues can be altered approximately a hundredfold.[3] There is apparently a continuous ebb and flow in the circulation of the hands, as though the heat-dissipating mechanism were being turned on and off like a mechanical thermostat. In addition to a greater blood flow to the surface of the body, increased heat loss by vaporization may be facilitated by sweating. In a resting subject visible sweating usually appears when the environmental temperature reaches 88° F.

NERVOUS REGULATION

The essential role of the hypothalamus in the regulation of body temperature has been confirmed many times since the original experiments of Barbour in 1912[4] and Isenschmid and Schnitzler in 1914.[5] Evidence from ablation experiments has clearly indicated that neither the cortex nor the thalamus is required for thermoregulation. After removal of the hypothalamus, however, animals are unable to maintain a stable body temperature, and exhibit wide swings in response to alterations in the environmental temperature. The exact manner in which the hypothalamus receives and transmits information necessary to regulate temperature within the narrow limits prescribed by health remains uncertain. When areas within the hypothalamus are subjected to either electrical or thermal stimuli, integrated responses involving either heat loss or heat production may be obtained. Similarly, lesions placed in various areas of the hypothalamus may result in selective loss of ability to maintain body temperature in either a warm or a cold environment. On the basis of experiments of this kind, it has been postulated that there are two anatomically distinct "centers" in the hypothalamus: an anterior part lying largely in the preoptic area which initiates responses leading to the dissipation of body heat (vasodilation, sweating and in animals, panting) and a posterior section that brings into play mechanisms which both generate and conserve body heat (vasoconstriction and shivering).[6,7] These two areas have abundant neural connections and there is evidence that activity of one generally inhibits that of the other. Histologic technics however, have failed to reveal specialized cells in the hypothalamus, and its important location as a "cross-roads" structure in the brain has raised doubts whether it is a center in the classical sense of initiating its own impulses for thermoregulation or whether it acts as a receptor organ, transducing a continual chain of afferent stimuli into impulses along appropriate efferent tracts for maintenance of body temperature.[8]

Recent studies by Benzinger and associates have contributed valuable data in regard to the operation of the thermoregulatory center.[9] They have established that the temperature of a number of structures in the cranium, such as the walls of the ethmoid sinus, the nasopharynx and the eardrum, more accurately reflect small changes in body heat and hence presumably changes in hypothalamic temperature than do either oral or rectal temperatures. By means of cranial thermometry and refined technics of gradient calorimetry for measuring small changes in heat loss and production, Benzinger has shown that under the conditions of his experiments the body has a thermostatic setpoint tenaciously maintained at 37.0° to 37.2° C. Small induced changes in cranial internal temperature above this level were rapidly followed by comparable increases in heat loss as measured by both rate of sweating and vasodilation. On the other hand, wide fluctuations in skin temperature above 33° C., the threshold for warm perception, did not effect evaporative heat loss, suggesting that this response is controlled by a central thermodetector sensitive only to changes in temperature of the blood which exceed the physiologic setpoint.

Thermoregulation at internal temperatures below the setpoint appears to have a different basis. In this situation, heat production is greatly augmented when skin temperatures are below 33° C., the threshold of cold perception. In contrast to the unique role played by cranial temperature in initiating heat-loss responses, Benzinger found that lowering cranial temperatures 0.5° C. or more in man did not affect heat production provided that skin temperatures were held above 33° C. However, when skin temperatures fell below this level, the resulting stimulation of peripheral cold receptors elevated heat production to values which became maximal at skin temperatures of 20° C. In addition, the amount of heat generated at any single skin temperature within this range of cold perception varied directly with the fall in internal temperature below the setpoint. From these data, Benzinger has inferred that the hypothalamus has a heat receptor only, and that at lowered internal temperatures stimuli from the skin, traveling to a separate area in the hypothalamus, reflexly increase heat production, a process which is progressively inhibited by the action of the central thermodetector as body temperature rises to the setpoint.

Despite the elegance of this work, there are both old and recent experiments that cast doubt on Benzinger's conclusion that the stimulus for metabolic heat production, unlike that for heat loss, is virtually entirely peripheral. Sherrington was able to evoke vigorous shivering in the foreparts of dogs with falling core temperatures induced by cooling hind extremities from which all afferent nervous stimuli to the brain were excluded by spinal cord transection. Since these responses occurred at environmental temperatures well above the threshold for peripheral cold stimulation, Sherrington was led to conclude that shivering probably results from direct cooling of a central thermosensitive mechanism.[10]

Similarly, changes in cutaneous vasoactivity induced in one limb by placing another in cold water have been shown to depend in some instances upon change in the temperature of blood reaching a central thermodetector. When an arm is immersed in cold water with its circulation occluded, there is an initial transient vasoconstriction in the opposite arm, followed by a second, prolonged vasoconstriction after circulation from the cold limb is released. Such experiments indicate that the vascular response to cold contains two elements: a reflex arising from receptors in the skin and a second response due to cooling of a central structure. Similar mechanisms control vasodilatory responses to warming although, in agreement with Benzinger's work, increased temperature of the blood appears to be the predominant one. The amount of heat which must be transferred to produce vasodilatation or vasoconstriction indicates that the central thermoregulator responds to changes of less than 0.2° C.[11]

In assessing the role of the various factors which modify vascular tone, as well as the other mechanisms of thermoregulation, it should be stressed that many stimuli may be nonspecific (cf. the characteristic vasoconstrictor response to noxious stimuli) and hence attempts must be made to distinguish between those stimuli which merely affect and those which presumably regulate body temperature.

Recently, Hardy and his associates have adduced further evidence for the role of a thermosensitive central receptor in regulating against cold.[12] Co-ordinated responses for heat conservation, including both vasoconstriction and shivering, were evoked in unanaesthetized dogs during brief periods of hypothalamic cooling resulting in a fall of central temperature of only 1.5° C. It seems probable from the evidence to date that there are central thermodetectors for both warm and cold stimuli in or near hypothalamic structures[12a] and that the responses evoked by changes in hypothalamic temperature may be significantly modified by peripheral stimuli arising from receptors in a number of sites, including the skin and respiratory tract as well as by stimuli contributed by other areas within the cord or elsewhere in the brain. It has been suggested that the combined stimuli from all these receptors throughout the body constitute the temperature which is regulated via the hypothalamus.[13]

The inter-relationships between peripheral and central factors in control of body temperature are undoubtedly exceedingly complex, with a number of feedback mechanisms operative. This can be simply illustrated in the case of shivering. During shivering, skin temperature rises, thus reducing the peripheral drive for this response. However, with the vasodilation which follows the local rise in temperature there is a loss of body heat leading to a further fall in core temperature. This, in turn, reinstitutes a fresh bout of shivering.

Environmental temperature is an important factor determining the relative contribution of the various thermoregulatory mechanisms. In this regard, three zones of environmental temperature have been defined, each with its distinctive effect on thermoregulation: (1) a neutral zone of vasomotor control; (2) a hot zone with both evaporative and vasomotor control; and (3) a cold zone with control of metabolic rate. In the cold and the neutral zones, thermoregulation appears to be largely under control of peripheral receptors, whereas as previously noted by Benzinger, central detectors in the hypothalamus are responsible for regulation in the hot zone and also during exercise when there is need to dissipate excess heat produced in the body.

It should be noted that prolonged direct thermal stimulation of the hypothalamus has a limited effectiveness in modifying body temperature. Modest elevations of 0.5° to 1.0° C and only slightly greater falls (1.0 to 2.5 C.) may be induced by such means, indicating the existence of other thermal inputs as well as the limitations which may be imposed by peripheral stimuli on changes initiated by direct central stimulation. By continuous electrical stimulation of areas adjacent to the hypothalamus it has been possible to drive temperatures down 9.0° C. but only up 0.5° C., a result which again emphasizes that both the main function and capacity of the central structures controlling thermoregulation appear to be directed towards protecting the body against overheating.[13]

The febrile response to bacterial pyrogens is also mediated through areas in the central nervous system. Although neither the cortex nor the thalamus appears to be necessary, there has been conflicting evidence on the role of the hypothalamus in producing this response. In studies by Chambers *et al.,* animals with massive hypothalamic lesions developed fevers when given pyrogens, but decerebrate animals with intact mid-brains and those with transections of the upper cervical cord were unresponsive.[14] However, mid-brain preparations have difficulty conserving heat and although cervical section would appear to interrupt the efferent tracts (sympathetic and extrapyramidal) involved in heat conservation and production, other workers have obtained fevers in similarly prepared animals given pyrogen.[15,16] Two recent careful studies on animals with serial truncations of the brain stem indicate, however, that the ability to develop pyrogen fever requires the functional integrity of the hypothalamic mechanisms which enable an animal to regulate against cold.[17,17a] As will be discussed subsequently, the febrile response to bacterial pyrogen appears to be mediated in most instances by a pyrogen released from host tissues rather than due to a direct pharmacological action of the bacterial endotoxin upon the nervous centers.

There is some evidence, both clinical and experimental, that the thermoregulatory set-point is elevated during fever.[18,19] Direct heating of the hypothalamus may either abort or modify the febrile response to pyrogens, presumably by supplying locally the increase in temperature called for by the action of the pyrogen in resetting the body's thermostat.[20] However, the data may also be interpreted in terms of the opposing effects of the pyrogen and local heat on separate centers in the hypothalamus controlling heat production and loss respectively. The present lack of knowledge as to the manner in which pyrogenic stimuli act upon the thermoregulatory center to cause fever is only part of our ignorance of the cellular mechanisms involved in physiologic temperature regulation.

The actual rise in temperature induced by bacterial pyrogens is brought about in most animals largely by decreased heat loss (through peripheral vasoconstriction).[21,21a] Abolition of muscular activity through curarization does not abolish the temperature response. In man, however, increased heat production (evidenced by frank chills) plays a major role in producing fever with these agents.[22]

In general, the phenomena associated with mechanisms for raising the body temperature are adrenergic (sympathetic), whereas depression of temperature is associated with cholinergic (parasympathetic) mechanisms. When the temperature is rising rapidly adrenergic activity is evidenced by cutaneous vasoconstriction, dilated pupils and erection of hair; during a rapid fall in temperature cholinergic activity is manifested by constricted pupils and cutaneous vasodilatation. Sympatheticotonic drugs, such as ephedrine or epinephrine, in large doses will cause a rise in body temperature.

BODY TEMPERATURE IN HEALTH
ORAL TEMPERATURE

There are available several studies of oral temperatures of groups of healthy individuals. The findings have shown some differences and the conditions under which readings were made were not identical, e.g., some "morning" temperatures were taken before getting out of bed whereas others were taken in the mid-morning after breakfast and activity, etc. The mean value for oral temperature in several of these studies was 98.34° F.; standard deviations have been of the order of 0.47 to 0.50° F.[23] In one attempt to apply statistical methods to such data, taking 98.6° F. as the mean normal oral temperature, and 0.47° F. as the standard deviation, it was concluded that the theoretical distribution of oral temperatures in normal people should extend from 97.0 to 100.4°F.[24]

RECTAL TEMPERATURE

Temperature within the rectum is usually somewhat higher than that of the oral cavity, the average difference being about 0.7° F. However, it must be emphasized that there are comparatively wide variations from person to person, and it is not unusual to encounter a healthy person who exhibits a higher oral than rectal temperature. The rectal temperature is somewhat less variable, and generally has been assumed to be a more accurate and reliable index of internal body or "blood" temperature. From a clinical standpoint rectal temperature determinations are certainly preferable in the case of children or other individuals who cannot keep the mouth closed during the taking of the reading. Furthermore oral temperature may be disturbed grossly immediately after ingestion of hot or cold liquids. Despite these obvious defects of the oral measurement and the traditional respect for rectal measurements, it is interesting to note the findings of Gerbrandy et al.[25] These workers found that oral temperature fluctuates more accurately in response to alterations in body heat balance than does rectal temperature. Therefore, it appears that the cerebral thermoregulatory centers are subject to temperature fluctuations very similar to those in the mouth, whereas rectal temperature fluctuates somewhat independently of body heat balance, and of cerebral regulatory mechanisms.

Temperature of Other Areas

It must be emphasized that oral and rectal temperatures are only spot temperatures which differ significantly from those of other body areas. Such expressions as "blood temperature" or "body temperature" are misleading, since there may be great differences in the warmth of various tissues. With the aid of small thermocouples which can be introduced into various localities, in needles or in venous catheters, observations of the temperature in a variety of locations have been made. In subjects at rest the liver and the brain seem to be the warmest organs in the body. The temperature in the rectum is about equal to that of blood in veins draining the liver and the lungs, and is higher than that of mixed venous blood in the right atrium or of blood in the femoral artery.[26,27] This suggests the possibility that appreciable heat production takes place in the bowel. Suppression of fecal flora by an antibacterial drug did not alter rectal temperatures of test subjects, hence it may be assumed that bacterial metabolism is not responsible for rectal warmth.[28]

Tissues at a distance from the body core are considerably cooler. For example the skin of the hands and the feet is usually 5° to 20° F. below oral temperature. Deeper tissues in distal parts of the extremities are likewise far below "blood heat;" e.g., the temperature of the calf muscles has been found to be as low as 92° F.,[29] and in knee joints 88.6° F.[30] In bone marrow readings have been as much as 7° F. below rectal temperature.[31]

The studies of Bazett and his associates[32] on temperature gradients along the courses of peripheral arteries and veins are of great interest. With the subject in a cold environment it was found that striking cooling occurs in blood passing down the artery of an extremity; differences of as much as 15° F. being recorded between thermocouples in the brachial and the radial arteries. These were found to be associated with corresponding warming of the blood passing out of the extremity in veins accompanying the arteries. The assumption is, then, that in a cold environment heat is transferred from arterial blood to returning venous blood along the course of an extremity, in such a manner as to conserve body heat and to permit the temperature (of hands or feet) to fall far below that of the body core. As Bazett points out, under these conditions physiologic processes in the cold tissues are proceeding under very different circumstances from those at "normal" body temperature: highly significant differences would obtain as regards blood viscosity, pH, electrolyte and gas dissociations, etc.

Diurnal Variation

There is a daily rhythmic change in body temperature, the differences amounting to between 2° and 3° F. The highest point usually is reached between 8 and 11 P.M., and the lowest during sleep between 4 and 6 A.M.[33] This variation does not depend on the environmental temperature and it is not abolished by confinement to bed or by fasting. Nevertheless, the usual explanation is that the higher temperatures are the result of the effects of muscular activity and the digestion of food, while the lowest temperature occurs at the time when these activities are at a minimum. It has been found that in persons accustomed to nocturnal employment (nurses, watchmen, etc.) the pattern of diurnal temperature variation may be inverted from the normal just described.[34] This alteration in temperature rhythm is not uniform in all people; some readily adapt to a new routine, whereas others retain the former cycle for many weeks.

Finally we should note that occasional normal individuals exhibit higher morning than evening temperatures, and that others show a rapid morning rise, then a plateau until after going to sleep at night.

BODY TEMPERATURE IN CHILDREN

In infancy the regulation of body temperature is imperfect, and marked variations occur, depending on changes in environment. Because of this, babies must be protected against excessive cold or warmth. The normal diurnal temperature rhythm becomes established some time during the second year of life, usually about the time the child begins to walk. Some lability of temperature regulation persists until about the time of puberty. Van der Bogert and Moravec studied the temperatures in more than 700 healthy children and noted oral temperatures higher than 98.6° F. at some time in 43 per cent of the children aged 7 and 8, while in the group between 13 and 15 years of age only 8 per cent ever had temperatures higher than 98.6° F.[35] The effect of exercise on body temperature is particularly marked in children; it is not uncommon for them to have temperatures of 100° F. after ordinary play, such as baseball. This fact should be kept in mind in estimating the significance of fever in children.

BODY TEMPERATURE IN OLD PEOPLE

The average body temperature is somewhat lower in the aged and is more likely to be low in cold weather. Furthermore, the diurnal temperature variation may be opposite to the normal.

PHYSIOLOGIC FACTORS AFFECTING BODY TEMPERATURE

Exercise. Muscular activity may cause a considerable elevation in body temperature. Women in the second stage of labor will often register 0.5° to 1.0° F. of fever. Soldiers who have been marching with heavy packs have been found to have rectal temperatures as high as 102.5° F., and after very strenuous exercise in trained athletes the rectal temperature has been observed to reach 106° F.[1] When the exercise is over there is always a quick fall to normal, usually within 30 minutes.

One interesting example of temperature elevation due to exercise is "chewing-gum fever." It has been found that vigorous chewing of gum for a few minutes can raise the mouth temperature by as much as 1.0° F.[36] Presumably this is due to local heat production in the muscles of mastication. Knowledge of this effect of gum-chewing may be useful in explaining an otherwise puzzling fever.

Digestion of Food. Some workers have recorded rise of body temperature of 0.2 to 0.5° F. in experimental subjects after ingestion of a meal.[37] The elevation began in 20 to 30 minutes and reached its peak within 90 minutes. These findings could not be substantiated in the later studies of Mellette et al.[33]

Warm Environment. The average temperature becomes measurably higher in persons who move from temperate to tropical climates. Temporary change to a warm environment may also raise the temperature level slightly. In one experiment it was found that the rectal temperatures of a group of normal subjects rose from an average of 98.06° F. to 99.32°F. when the room temperature was raised from 68.0° to 86.0° F.[38] It is a common experience in hospitals to find that on very hot days many patients who have no other cause for fever register oral temperatures of 99.0° F. or more.

Cold Environment. Exposure to cold causes only a slight reduction in the body temperature of a normal adult, but induces a somewhat greater change in an infant or in an old person.

Menstrual Cycle. There is a rhythmic variation in body temperature associated with the menstrual cycle. Immediately before the onset of menstruation the temperature falls 0.5° to 0.75° F. below its previous level. This relatively low temperature is maintained until the time of ovulation, which is usually about the thirteenth or the fourteenth day of the cycle. Then there is a rise of 0.5° to 0.75° F., which is maintained until just before the next menstrual period. Such variations may be exaggerated in women who have fever from another cause, such as pulmonary tuberculosis. Amenorrheic women have no cyclic temperature change, and in them it has been reported that estrogen therapy depresses body temperature whereas progesterone provokes a rise. Therefore it has been assumed that endogenous estrogens and progesterone are responsible for the biphasic basal temperature of the menstrual cycle. However, certain clinical observations indicate that body temperature change does not always coincide with any narrow phase of the ovarian follicle cycle.[39]

Pregnancy. Early in pregnancy there is a slight rise in average temperature. About the fourth month of gestation a gradual fall begins, and this continues until parturition, when there is a quick return to the normal level.[40]

LIMITS OF BODY TEMPERATURE COMPATIBLE WITH LIFE

Low Temperatures

Formerly it was believed that life would cease if the body temperature fell below about 90.0° F. Fay and others[41] have shown, however, that by administering sedatives and then applying cold, the body temperature can be reduced to 75.0° to 80.0° F. and maintained there for days without evident harm. An extreme example of hypothermia is reported by Laufman.[42] The subject, under influence of alcohol, lay unconscious for many hours out of doors in cold weather. When brought to a hospital the rectal temperature, obtained 90 minutes after warming had begun, was 64.4° F. It was calculated that on admission the rectal temperature must have been in the vicinity of 61° F. This is the lowest recorded internal body temperature in a patient who survived.

Profound hypothermia with a fall in rectal temperature to 87.8° F. has been reported in a patient with disseminated lupus erythematosus treated with cortisone.[43] There were signs of active heat loss with sweating and vasodilatation despite the low temperature, which was felt to be caused by the action of steroid on the thermoregulatory center. ACTH and cortisone also have a marked antipyretic effect in many febrile states, presumably due, like that of other antipyretics, to a direct action on the hypothalamus. Certain of these drugs affect normal body temperature as well and several (such as chlorpromazine) have been used, in conjunction with physical methods, to induce hypothermia in surgery.[44]

High Temperatures

In the medical literature there are reports of fantastic fevers, 130° F. or even 150.0° F. These are undoubtedly the results of fraud or error on the part of either the patients or the physicians. Experiments in animals and acceptable observations in human beings indicate that living tissues are irreversibly damaged at temperatures above the region of 115.00° F. Richet placed the upper possible limit at 114.8° F. (46.0° C.), and this has been endorsed by Mac-Neal[45] after a careful study of the evidence. There are a number of acceptable reports of temperatures as high as 112.0° or 113.0° F. with recovery. In a case of staphylococcal septicemia the fever ranged between 104.0° F. and 112.0° F. continuously for three months.[46]

As has been pointed out by DuBois,[47] there is a sort of temperature "ceiling" in most febrile disease, at about 105° or 106° F. It would appear that the body's thermostat can rarely be disturbed sufficiently to permit an elevation beyond this level. Of special interest is DuBois' analysis of actual temperature readings in 357 patients with febrile diseases. Although the level seldom exceeded 106° F., readings in the range of 104° to 105° F. were obtained more frequently than 103° to 104° F., and twice as frequently as the 102° to 103° F. range. This seems to point to a "secondary thermostat setting" of thermoregulation, operating best in the range of 104° to 105° F.

FEVER: TYPES AND TERMINOLOGY

Fever is an elevation of the body temperature due to disease. It is, of course, only a symptom and, as is discussed subsequently, occurs in a wide variety of pathologic conditions.

Pyrexia is a term usually considered synonymous with fever, although some writers have used it to indicate elevations not due to infection.

Hyperpyrexia and **hyperthermia** usually refer to high fever, 105.0° F. or more.

Habitual hyperthermia has been used to designate a condition in which the average temperature is slightly above the accepted "normal" limit.

An intermittent or quotidian fever is one in which the temperature falls to normal and rises again each day.

In a remittent fever there is a marked variation in the temperature level each day, but the low point is still above the normal line.

A relapsing fever is one in which short febrile periods are interspersed by periods of one or more days of normal temperature. Figure 149 illustrates this in a case of rat-bite fever.

A hectic or septic fever is an intermittent fever in which the daily oscillations are very large; it is often associated with chills and sweating.

PATHOGENESIS OF FEVER

A satisfactory explanation of the genesis of fever must encompass two facts: (1) Fever is a manifestation of many kinds of disease processes, not only infectious diseases, but also injuries, neoplastic diseases, vascular accidents, metabolic disorders, etc. The only obvious common factor in them is tissue injury. (2) Fever occurs in disease of any tissue in the body.

Several theories of the mechanism of the production of fever have been proposed. One is that an abnormal distribution of body water, with hemoconcentration, causes a rise of body temperature by interfering with the transfer and the dissipation of heat. Clinical observations do not substantiate this hypothesis. While it is true that some hemoconcentration usually occurs when the temperature is rising, it is probably only a concomitant process. Certainly there is no constant pattern of temperature variation associated with rapid change in fluid and electrolyte balance. Some workers have sought to explain fever as the result of overfunction of the adrenals and the thyroid, because of histologic evidence of intense activity in these glands following induction of fever in animals.[48] Against this are the facts that fever occurs in animals whose adrenals and thyroid have been destroyed, and that similarly patients with Addison's disease or myxedema may have high fever. Therefore, an endocrine mechanism does not appear capable of explaining all the observed phenomena.

Clinical observation of febrile disorders

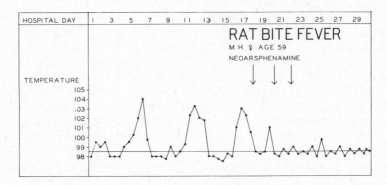

Fig. 149. Rat-bite fever, due to infection with *Spirillum minus*. An example of a relapsing fever. Short febrile periods are separated by two or three days of normal temperature.

suggests strongly that cerebral thermo-regulation is faulty.[49] It may be supposed then that disturbance of the cerebral centers is caused by the action of some product or products of tissue injury.

Most experimental work on the pathogenesis of fever has been carried out with bacterial pyrogens. These substances, also known as endotoxins, are complex lipopolysaccharides of high molecular weight (approximately 1×10^6) which form part of the cell wall of Gram-negative bacteria and, in conjunction with protein, comprise the somatic 'O' antigen. Because of their ubiquity and ability to withstand autoclaving as well as to pass through filters, endotoxins readily contaminate biologic materials and are very difficult to remove from them. Endotoxins are extremely potent pharmacologic agents. In minute amounts they produce a wide variety of reactions in both animals and man, including fever, leukopenia, alterations in blood coagulation and, with large doses, shock and death.[50] Given intravenously, as little as 0.002 gamma/Kg. of purified material regularly produces a pyrogenic response in man.[51]

Two features of the febrile response caused by endotoxins seem relevant to their probable mechanism of action. First, after intravenous inoculation there is a variable latent period (from 15 to 30 minutes in rabbits and up to an hour or more in man) before the onset of fever. Second, during this period, circulating granulocytes virtually disappear from the blood stream due to their adherence to the walls of blood vessels throughout the body. These features of endotoxin-induced fever have given rise to the belief that endotoxins do not act directly on the thermoregulatory center of the brain, but release an intermediary pyrogen from a tissue source within the body, presumably the granulocyte. A considerable body of evidence in support of this view has been accumulated in the past ten years.[52]

A material with pyrogenic properties has been recovered from saline extracts of rabbit granulocytes.[53] This material appears to be a protein and is clearly different from endotoxin. Originally, polymorphonuclear leukocytes were thought to be the only source of this substance; however, a more recent study indicates that extracts of many other normal tissues are similarly pyrogenic.[53a]

A substance known as endogenous pyrogen (EP) with biological properties similar to leukocyte pyrogen appears in the blood of a number of animals,[54] including humans,[55] given endotoxin intravenously. The febrile response corresponds well with the amount of this material in the circulation. Conversely, when circulating granulocytes are virtually abolished by nitrogen mustard, animals do not develop fever to ordinary doses of endotoxin, presumably because such animals cannot release EP.[56] However, these leukopenic animals respond normally when injected with EP. In vitro studies in animals and man have confirmed that both blood and exudate leukocytes release an EP upon addition of endotoxin.

There is evidence that EP plays a role in fevers produced by a number of agents other than the endotoxins of Gram-negative bacteria. Pyrogenic substances which resemble endotoxin-induced EP in their biologic effects are present in a number of human pathologic fluids[56a] and also in the circulation of animals inoculated intravenously with myxoviruses as well as with a variety of Gram-positive bacteria and pathogenic fungi or their soluble products.[56b] Similarly, fevers resulting from the reaction of antigen with antibody in specifically sensitized hosts, appear to be caused by a circulating endogenous pyrogen, though its cellular source remains uncertain.[52] In man, buffy coat incompatibilities[56c] and certain immune hemolytic reactions[56d] are associated with marked leukopenias and fevers resembling those produced by endotoxins. Finally, in studies of fever accompanying peritoneal infections with pneumococci, it has been shown that pyrogen is rapidly liberated by cells in the inflammatory exudate and subsequently reaches the blood by way of the thoracic duct lymph.[57,58]

In all these experimental situations it seems clear that an intermediary pyrogen, liberated from tissues of the host, plays a major role in producing the febrile response. Furthermore, when the brain is perfused directly with this substance, accelerated and augmented fevers are obtained, suggesting that EP has a direct and immediate action on the thermoregulatory centers of the brain.[59]

Recent studies by Wood and his colleagues[60,60a] and Fessler et al.[61] have provided information of great interest on the factors that modify release of pyrogen from granulocytes. The production of this material by granulocytes appears to be an active metabolic process, dependent on temperature and on intact cellular structure, and may be blocked by certain enzyme inhibitors. The composition of the medium is important in determining the amount of pyrogen released. Ions such as K^+ and Ca^{++} prevent its release, presumably by maintaining certain functions of the cell membrane. On the other hand, the inhibiting effects of these ions may be circumvented by a variety of conditions, including phagocytosis, and the addition of endotoxins or agents in inflammatory exudates, all of which have been found to activate granulocytes to produce pyrogen in vitro.

These studies indicate the subtle balance which probably exists between various activators and inhibitors in the body. When the balance is disturbed by certain influences there is production and release of EP which, in turn, causes fever.

Unsolved Questions. It is apparent from this discussion that many questions concerning the pathogenesis of fever remain unanswered. Is there more than one type of endogenous pyrogen? Is the granulocyte the only source of EP? Do cells such as the monocyte and lymphocyte release pyrogenic substances in allergic conditions where they appear to be the sensitive cells? Although EP seems to be the chief factor in producing fever of microbial origin, nothing is known about the cause of fever in malignant tumors, lymphomas, collagen diseases, or certain metabolic diseases such as gout and porphyria. In some of these conditions, factors known to contribute to fever in various infectious diseases, such as inflammation and hypersensitivity, may play a role.

Also, little is known of the specific mechanisms by which EP is activated or of its fate in the body. No attempt has yet been made to determine if this substance has other physiologic properties. Whether EP plays any part in conferring nonspecific resistance to various microbes or their products is unknown, although it seems unlikely that the temperature-elevating effect of EP serves any directly useful role in combating infection.

Finally, the mechanism by which EP stimulates the hypothalamus to produce an increase in body temperature is unknown.

METABOLISM IN FEVER

The basal metabolism is elevated in fever, in proportion to the height of the temperature—roughly 7 per cent for each degree F. In other words, the effect of fever on the metabolic rate follows the principle of van't Hoff: that the velocity of chemical reactions is proportional to the temperature at which they occur. At a temperature of 105.0°F. the basal metabolism is approximately 50 per cent above normal.

The biochemical disturbances that have been noted in fever are not very distinctive. During the first week or two of a febrile disease, there is always some destruction of body protein, evidenced by negative nitrogen balance. Fever is often accompanied by mild to severe dehydration. The biochemical disturbances characteristic of dehydration may become evident: passage of Na and Cl into cells; loss of K, P and N from cells; and loss of cell water as well as of extracellular (plasma and interstitial) water (Chap. 30). Achlorhydria is usually present in persons with high fever, but gastric secretion of acid is resumed when the temperature falls. Mild acidosis is common during infectious fevers.

As stated, the endocrine, metabolic and biochemical evidences of fever are not distinctive but appear to be shared by many conditions associated with stress. In general, fever and the disorders which cause fever also stimulate the hypothalamic-pituitary-adrenocortical system. Thus, adrenocortical hyperactivity is not part of the mechanism which produces fever; it is an important part of the *response* to fever.

COMPLICATIONS OF FEVER

Herpes Simplex. Herpetic lesions about the mouth occur so frequently in certain febrile diseases that they are described in textbooks as manifestations of those diseases. Meningococcal meningitis and pneumococcal pneumonia are particularly likely to be so complicated, while, peculiarly, typhoid fever, typhus fever and primary atypical pneumonia are only rarely accompanied by herpes. Actually, "fever blisters" are due to a separate infection, by the virus of herpes simplex, which apparently is activated by the rise in body temperature. The purest example of the association with fever is found in persons who are given artificial fever therapy; in them the incidence of labial herpes may be as high as 46 per cent.[62] The lesions appear 30 to 48 hours after a treatment.

Albuminuria. Albumin is frequently present in the urine of patients with fever. In many cases this is certainly due to a direct effect of the disease on the kidneys; consequently, there has been some controversy as to whether or not fever alone may cause albuminuria. Welty, however, by studying a group of patients being treated with fever in the Kettering Hypertherm, found that albuminuria occurred solely from the artifically induced rise in body temperature. He reported "true febrile albuminuria" in more than three fourths of his patients.[63]

Chills. In a chill, or rigor, the subject suddenly begins to feel cold. His skin becomes pale, cyanotic and covered with "goose-flesh." Even though covered by several blankets and warmed by hot water bottles, he cannot get warm. His whole body shivers and his teeth chatter—so that the bed shakes and he speaks with difficulty. This state continues for from 10 to 40 minutes, then he gradually feels less cold, his skin becomes pink and warm and there may be sweating. During the "cold" phase there is a rapid rise in body temperature, of from 2° to 7°F. Depending on the underlying process there may or may not be a rapid return of temperature toward normal. The temperature rise is due to a great increase in heat production; the heat elimination remains about normal.[64] The commonest cause of a chill is the introduction of some foreign substance into the blood stream—either living infectious agents or their products, bacterial pyrogens. However, chills can occur in the absence of extraneous substances. For example, they may be experienced by patients with lymphoma or hypernephroma.

When the time at which the chill-producing substance enters the circulation is known, as when typhoid vaccine is injected intravenously, there is always a lapse of approximately one hour before the onset of the chill. Similarly a period of time elapses between instrumentation of infected tissues and subsequent chills. Very probably the lag period is the time necessary for tissue injury to occur, deranged function of the thermoregulatory centers being secondary to this injury. This time relationship is not widely appreciated, since it is commonly believed that the taking of blood cultures should be postponed until "the height of the chill." Actually, the "ideal" time would be about one hour before the chill. Since this is not predictable, the best practice is to take a series of blood cultures, at 30- or 60-minute intervals.

Perera noted that sympathectomized limbs participate in the tremor of a chill but that they do not exhibit the vasoconstriction present in other parts of the body.[65] He found also that in persons with hemiplegia the paralyzed limbs exhibit tremor during chills, and he concludes from this that the efferent tract from the "chill center" is by way of an extrapyramidal pathway in the spinal cord and the motor nerves.

During a chill the rectal temperature rises steadily, while the skin usually remains cool. Microscopic study of the circulation in the capillaries in the nailfolds at this time reveals that the flow of blood almost ceases.[66] This results in more nearly complete removal of oxygen from the blood and is the reason for the characteristic cyanosis. Other observations on the circulatory changes during chill and fever have been reviewed by Altschule and Freedberg.[67]

A sharp drop in the blood leukocyte count occurs during and shortly after a chill; therefore, a leukopenia immediately after a chill may have no diagnostic significance in relation to the primary disease.

In some infectious diseases it is common

to have a series of chills. These include brucellosis, typhus fever, malaria, many acute viral diseases such as influenza, and such pyogenic infections as pyelonephritis, acute osteomyelitis and postpartum infection. In pneumococcal pneumonia, on the other hand, it is unusual to have more than the one chill which occurs at the onset, because the fever is sustained thereafter. However, if an antipyretic drug is given to a patient with pneumonia, his temperature will fall and then may rise again, with a chill.

Sweating. Sweating is the counterpart of the chill. Its facilitates heat loss and tends to produce a rapid fall in temperature. It is usually combined with a rich circulation to the skin, which permits rapid dissipation of heat by vaporization. Sweating is particularly common in diseases associated with intermittent fever, such as tuberculosis, acute brucellosis, or rheumatic fever. In contrast, it does not occur during the febrile period of pneumonia, unless the patient is given an antipyretic drug. When a patient complains of "night sweats" we may suspect that he has an intermittent fever, although it is true that some persons, particularly when convalescing from prolonged illnesses, may have night sweats without fever.

Convulsions. Convulsions may occur at the onset of infectious diseases. This phenomenon is limited to children and in them it appears to be dependent largely on the rapidity with which the temperature rises. Wegman experimented with kittens and noted that they frequently had convulsions if subjected to rapid rise in body temperature; adult cats under the same conditions seldom had convulsions.[68]

The question which is not yet settled is whether febrile convulsions are essentially benign or whether they indicate some abnormality in the central nervous system. Some follow-up studies have provided evidence that children who have suffered febrile convulsions are liable to nonfebrile seizures later, or to exhibit signs of cerebral damage suggestive of conditions such as birth trauma or encephalitis.[69,70]

Delirium. Fever and delirium are often associated. In general it may be said that delirium seldom is present when the fever is less than 104.0° F., although in exceptional instances and in elderly patients it may accompany only a moderate elevation of the temperature. The reason is that delirium depends on several factors: not only the degree of the fever, but also on the temperament of the patient, his previous health, drugs he has received and the nature of his underlying disease.

SPURIOUS FEVER

MacNeal has described some of the ways in which high temperature has been faked by patients.[45] The commonest method is to heat the thermometer with a hot water bottle or other source of heat. This is especially easy if the patient has previously obtained a spare thermometer to substitute for the one given him. Another trick is to hold the bulb of the thermometer tightly between the fingers and rub it against the bedclothes. Skilled malingerers can raise the reading by tapping the bulb end of the thermometer, jarring the mercury upward. In addition to these methods it is said that some individuals are able to warm the thermometer simply by friction with the tongue or anal sphincter. We have already noted that vigorous chewing motion can raise the mouth temperature by as much as 1.0° F. To detect trickery, it is recommended that simultaneous temperatures be taken in the axilla, the rectum and the mouth, with a different observer holding each thermometer in place.

Useful clues in the detection of this state have been summarized by Petersdorf and Bennett and include failure of the temperature curve to follow normal diurnal variation and the absence of correlation of the fever pattern with pulse rate or sweats.[71]

EFFECTS OF FEVER

It is often said that fever assists the host in combating infection. There is no question of the value of fever in neurosyphilis and in certain other types of infection, such as those due to the gonococcus. Moreover, some bacteria and spirilla suffer attenuation of virulence at febrile temperatures. It has been observed too, that failure to develop fever in the presence of a severe

Fig. 150. The typical temperature course in a case of murine typhus fever. There is a remittent fever for about 10 days, then a fall by lysis, usually reaching normal between the 14th and 18th days of illness.

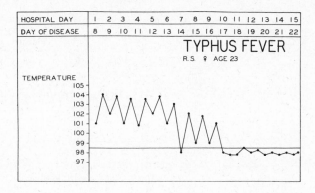

infection usually signifies a grave prognosis. On the other hand, it is probable that in infections the actual presence of fever has little bearing on the outcome, since most organisms do not induce changes in body temperature which would destroy them.[72] The fever that accompanies noninfectious conditions does not appear to serve any useful purpose and may at times be harmful. In malignant disease, for example, high temperature only accelerates weight loss and causes malaise. Likewise, fever that follows myocardial infarction increases the metabolic rate, thereby placing an extra load on the weakened myocardium. The hyperpyrexia of heat stroke may cause death.

CLINICAL CAUSES OF FEVER
INFECTIONS

Infections are certainly the most frequent causes of fever. In general it may be said that any known infection may cause fever; to list a large number of infectious diseases would serve no purpose here. Instead, a few instances will be cited wherein certain infections cause fevers that are particularly characteristic. These are less commonly observed now than formerly, because effective chemotherapy alters their natural courses.

In typhoid and paratyphoid fevers there is a classical temperature course; it consists of a "staircase" rise for several days, a plateau of remittent fever for one to three weeks, then a steplike return to normal temperature.

Typhus fever produces a fairly uniform temperature curve. After a sudden elevation there is a sustained high fever for nine or ten days, then a fall by lysis, returning to normal about the fourteenth to the eighteenth day of disease. An example of this is shown in Figure 150.

Gonococcal endocarditis may have a unique fever: two steeplelike rises and falls in each 24-hour period—double quotidian.[73] This is also described as a feature of kala-azar. It may occasionally be present in other severe infections. We have seen a double quotidian fever in miliary tuberculosis.

In dengue a "saddle-back" temperature curve is typical. By this is meant a fever that rises rapidly, declines somewhat during the succeeding two or three days, then rises again to a peak on about the sixth day, after which it subsides quickly.

Localized collections of pus as in subdiaphragmatic abscess or osteomyelitis, frequently lead to a hectic type of fever, associated with chills and sweating. This may also be seen in patients with pyelonephritis, ascending cholangitis (Charcot's biliary fever) and thrombophlebitis.

Diseases that cause relapsing fevers are not very frequent in the United States. The following diagnostic possibilities should receive special consideration: (1) malaria; (2) rat-bite fever, caused by either *Spirillum minus* or *Streptobacillus moniliformis* (Fig. 149); (3) relapsing fever, caused by *Spirillum recurrentis;* and (4) chronic meningococcemia.

DISEASES OF THE CENTRAL NERVOUS SYSTEM

Head Injury. Fever is nearly always present after head injury, and the height

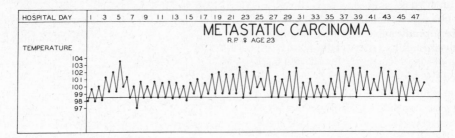

Fig. 151. Temperature chart of a young woman with fever due to carcinoma of the pancreas with metastasis to the liver.

of the temperature may be of some value in estimating prognosis. In slight concussions there is a rise to 101° F. or less, whereas in more serious cases the fever is often higher, and in the most severe injuries there may be a rapid ascent to a hyperthermic level before death. Erickson states that following middle meningeal hemorrhage, a person may be more or less poikilothermic, his body temperature fluctuating markedly with changes in the environmental temperature.[74]

Cerebral Vascular Accident. Hemorrhage or thrombosis in the vessels of the brain is usually attended by a moderate fever—100° to 102° F. In large hemorrhages very high fever may develop just before death.

Neurogenic Hyperthermia. Following surgical operations in the region of the pituitary fossa and the third ventricle, a serious hyperthermia sometimes occurs. The rectal temperature rises steadily during the first few hours after operation. The skin of the extremities is cold, while that of the trunk is relatively warm. There is complete absence of sweating. Energetic treatment of the fever is indicated: application of ice bags, alcohol rubs, cold air fan, etc.[74]

Degenerative Disease. Disturbances in temperature regulation are occasionally noted after recovery from encephalitis. Children who have sustained cerebral trauma in a birth injury often have faulty temperature regulation. Approximately 50 per cent of cases of multiple sclerosis have a low fever at some time.[75]

Spinal Cord Injury. Holmes made a study of the effects of spinal cord injuries and observed that injury to the cervical cord was frequently followed by severe disturbance of temperature regulation. Injury to the lower cervical cord usually resulted in very low body temperature, while patients with upper cervical cord injury often had high, irregular fevers.[76] The cause of this temperature disturbance probably is the interruption of the tracts leading to and from the hypothalamus.

Neoplasms

Malignant growths frequently cause fever. Sometimes, for example in carcinoma of a bronchus, this fever may be the result of an associated infection; but often the tumor alone appears to be responsible. Hypernephroma is notorious in this respect; it may even cause a hectic fever with chills and sweats. Primary or metastatic carcinoma in the liver is also frequently attended by fever. Figure 151 shows the temperature chart of a patient with primary carcinoma of the pancreas, with metastases to the liver. Harsha has reviewed the literature on fever in malignant disease, and reports a case in which there was dramatic cessation of a hectic fever after removal of a retroperitoneal malignant tumor.[77] Similar defervéscence has followed extirpation of mesotheliomata of the pleura.[78] The cause of the fever in malignancy is thought to be the liberation of products from the tissue destroyed by the invading neoplasm but there is, in fact, a poor correlation between the degree of fever and the extent of tissue necrosis. Infection and obstruction are a more frequent cause of fever in malignancy than the disease itself.[79] The fever of malignancy presents no characteristic features, although low grade or regularly recurrent fevers seem more common in tumors not associated with infection.[80]

Lymphoma. Fever is an almost constant accompaniment of this group of neoplastic diseases and is often the first symptom. Consequently, such conditions as Hodgkin's disease, lymphosarcoma and leukemia must always be considered in investigating cases of obscure fever. A few persons with Hodgkin's disease exhibit a peculiar relapsing fever, in which periods of from 7 to 10 days of normal temperature alternate with equal periods of fever. This is called the Pel-Ebstein fever. An example is shown in Figure 152.

BLOOD DISEASES

Acute leukemia is always a febrile disease,[80a] as is also any acute hemolytic anemia. Hemorrhagic disorders, such as thrombocytopenic purpura, hemophilia and scurvy, also cause fever if there is hemorrhage into the tissues. Severe anemia from chronic blood loss is not a cause of fever. Chronic aplastic anemia, chronic lymphocytic leukemia (in the absence of infection) and myelofibrosis are rarely febrile diseases, but high fevers are often present in acute agranulocytosis.

EMBOLISM AND THROMBOSIS

Embolism or aseptic thrombosis in a large artery or vein is often associated with fever. This probably depends on the occurrence of tissue necrosis (and attendant inflammation) due to interference with the nutrition of the part supplied by the vessel. In myocardial infarction, for example, low fever is expected during the first few days, and elevations as high as 103° to 104° F. are sometimes seen.

HEAT STROKE

Heat stroke is a serious condition characterized by high fever, coma and absence of sweating. It should not be confused with heat cramp or heat exhaustion, neither of which causes a change in body temperature. Heat stroke is induced by prolonged high environmental temperature; it occurs most commonly in old people, or in those who have been consuming alcohol. Apparently the fault here is failure of the cerebral centers of heat regulation. The onset of symptoms is usually sudden, with loss of consciousness. The affected person ceases to sweat just prior to his collapse. Ferris and his associates carried out an excellent study on 44 patients with heat stroke during a single period of hot weather.[81] The body temperatures of their patients ranged from 104° to 112° F. Absence of sweating was noted in all of them. Biochemical studies revealed normal bloood chlorides, but there was some acidosis and hemoconcentration. The reason for the sudden cessation of sweating could not be ascertained. Seventeen of the 44 patients died. It was concluded that energetic measures must be employed in an effort to reduce the body temperature quickly; the procedures recommended were ice-water tubbing combined with massage.

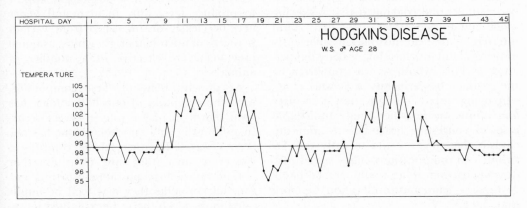

FIG. 152. An example of the Pel-Ebstein type of fever, in a case of Hodgkin's disease.

DISTURBANCES IN FLUID BALANCE

Dehydration is commonly held to be responsible for fever. However, there is little evidence that this is true in adults and the best clinical practice is to search for some other cause.

There can be little doubt that infants during the first few days of life can have temperature elevation due to lack of water—the so-called dehydration or inanition fever. Administration of adequate fluid is followed by prompt cessation of the fever. The mechanism of this is obscure.

Fever may be observed in severe diabetic acidosis, and some persons have ascribed this to dehydration. Himwich produced acidosis and high fever in depancreatized dogs by withholding water and insulin; then by giving fluids he found that the temperature returned to normal. Insulin alone did not have this effect.[82] However, the temperature is frequently normal or subnormal in diabetic acidosis; consequently the presence of fever should stimulate a search for some other disease process.

HEART FAILURE

Fever is almost invariably present in patients with congestive heart failure, but often there is some complication present which could cause it, such as bronchopneumonia, pulmonary infarction, rheumatic fever, myocardial infarction or thrombophlebitis. Nevertheless, there are many instances in which no such complication is obvious and where fever appears with failure and disappears when compensation is regained. Steele studied this problem experimentally and concluded that a slowing blood flow to the surface of the body could interfere with heat dissipation sufficiently to bring about an elevation of body temperature.[83] This hypothesis was supported by the results of experiments of Stewart *et al.*, employing rapid digitalization.[84] Kinsey and White, on the other hand, studied 200 cases of congestive heart failure and concluded that fever could usually be attributed to complications. They stated that decompensation alone would not be likely to cause a temperature elevation of more than 1.0 F.[85]

THYROID DISEASE

It is common to find a slight temperature elevation—99.5° to 100.5° F.—in persons who have thyrotoxicosis. This is probably due to the excessive heat production which accompanies the increased metabolism. In a thyroid crisis, which may appear spontaneously or may occur immediately after surgery of the thyroid (occasionally also after other surgical procedures), there is a rapid rise in body temperature to 104° F. or higher, accompanied by tachycardia, thready pulse, restlessness, sometimes mania, and eventually stupor.

STEROID FEVER

Recent studies have shown that a number of steroid metabolites of the pregnane and etiocholane type, when given by either intravenous or intramuscular routes,[86] produce marked pyrogenic responses in man, associated with leucocytosis, headache, myalgia and arthralgia. One of these hormones, the urinary ketosteroid, etiocholanolone, has been detected in the blood during febrile episodes in *periodic disease,* a benign cyclic disease of previously undetermined etiology.[87] At present, the mechanism by which these agents cause fever is unknown but appears to be highly specific since minor structural modifications of the molecule abolish its pyrogenic properties. Since there is a prolonged delay before the onset of fever, it seems doubtful that these agents act directly on the thermoregulatory center, but no intermediary pyrogens have been detected in the circulation during the febrile response. These substances appear to produce fever only in man and hence may be clearly distinguished from various pyrogens of microbial origin which, as noted previously, are effective in a number of animals.

At present, none of these compounds, with the exception of etiocholanolone, has been shown to play a role in fevers occurring clinically, and etiocholanolone has not been detected in other febrile conditions. However, since they are transformation products of endogenous adrenocortical and gonadal hormones they may well be implicated in certain hitherto unexplained fevers associated with various hepatic and endocrine disorders.

In familial Mediterranean fever, a disease which clinically resembles periodic disease but appears to be almost entirely restricted to Jews and Armenians, and is often associated with amyloidosis, no abnormal steroids have been detected.

Liver Diseases

Various diseases of the liver are prone to produce fever. Liver abscess, amebic or bacterial, may cause a hectic type of fever. The frequency of temperature elevation in neoplastic disease of the liver has already been mentioned. McCrae and Caven noted fever in 80 per cent of their cases of syphilis of the liver.[88] About half of all patients with cirrhosis of the liver have temperature elevations which are typically moderate and prolonged in uncomplicated cases.[88a]

Tissue Trauma

Crushing injuries and fractures of large bones are usually followed by some rise in body temperature. Also, a moderate elevation is to be expected during the first day or two after an extensive surgical procedure. The inflammation resulting from release of products of damaged tissue is probably the cause of these fevers.

Peptic Ulcer

European physicians have reported fever in from 8 to 25 per cent of patients with uncomplicated peptic ulcer.[89] The elevation seldom exceeds 100.5° F. Dill and Isenhour in this country investigated the subject.[90] They found fever in 46 per cent of a group of patients with uncomplicated peptic ulcer, but the significance of the finding was somewhat clouded by the fact that the same criteria for fever were satisfied in 37 per cent of their control group—persons with digestive symptoms but without demonstrable organic lesions. Upon the available evidence, the statement that uncomplicated peptic ulcer is a cause of fever is still open to question.

Massive hemorrhage from a peptic ulcer results in fever in at least 80 per cent of cases. Attempts to produce this type of fever in normal subjects by the introduction of large quantities of blood into the intestinal tract were unsuccessful.[91] One could speculate that the fever in bleeding ulcer is due to increased heat produced by the specific dynamic action of a large quantity of protein absorbed from the intestinal tract in a subject whose means of heat dissipation is handicapped by the circulatory embarrassment of blood loss. One factor which perhaps is not appreciated sufficiently in evaluating fever after gastrointestinal hemorrhage is the effect of blood transfusions which these patients receive. The findings of Selesnick and White indicate that the fever of gastrointestinal hemorrhage rarely exceeds 100° F. except after transfusion.[92]

Abnormalities of the Skin

Persons who have congenital absence of the sweat glands or other generalized skin disease may be seriously handicapped in hot weather, when vaporization is the principal means of heat loss. Under such conditions they may develop fever. Woodyatt reported this in the case of a woman with extensive ichthyosis. In the winter she was able to work normally, but in summer she would develop fever and symptoms resembling those of effort syndrome.[93]

Serum Sickness and Allergy

Serum sickness, with fever arthralgia and urticaria, may occur from 5 to 10 days after administration of an animal serum to a human being and is apparently due to a violent immune reaction to the foreign protein. The temperature elevation may be considerable—103° to 105° F. Presumably the syndrome is due to the effect of union of large amounts of antigen with its antibody. Fevers characteristically present in many collagen diseases of so-called autoimmunity (lupus erythematosus, polyarteritis, etc.) are perhaps caused by a similar mechanism.

It has been suggested that allergy may cause certain obscure fevers, but there is not a great deal of evidence to support the idea. Rowe, however, has reported a case in which the evidence was strong that a prolonged obscure fever was due to food allergy.[94]

PAROXYSMAL TACHYCARDIA

Patients occasionally have fever during paroxysms of tachycardia, in the absence of any other disease.[95] This may be due to the combined effect of impaired circulation and extra heat production resulting from the muscular activity of the heart.

ANESTHESIA

Because it is usually thought that the body temperature falls during anesthesia, the temperature of operating rooms is usually kept rather warm, and patients are often wrapped in blankets during the immediate postoperative hours. In many cases this practice is illogical. Burford followed the temperature of 50 patients during operations and found that instead of a fall there was a moderate elevation in 33 of them.[96] Dangerous hyperthermia is an occasional complication of anesthesia. This is a special hazard in the case of young children, and the danger is increased in operations about the face, e.g., for cleft palate.[97,98] Burford believes that the production of hyperthermia is as follows: on a warm day the environmental temperature is so high that heat loss can be accomplished only by vaporization; high humidity decreases the efficiency of this mechanism which is further impaired by the patient's mask and drapes. The anesthetic depresses the function of the temperature-regulating centers in the brain. With this combination of circumstances, heat loss cannot keep pace with heat production, and the temperature rises. This aggravates matters, since heat production is increased with a rise in temperature, according to van't Hoff's law. The temperature continues to rise following the operation and within a few hours there is high fever and collapse. This syndrome closely resembles neurogenic hyperthermia, including the absence of sweating and the coldness of the skin of the extremities. Death may ensue. Mangiardi reported on 3 such cases in adults, and advocated therapy with oxygen inhalation, alcohol sponging and continuous intravenous administration of 50 per cent dextrose solution.[99]

DRUG FEVERS

A number of drugs may cause fever after prolonged administration. Some of the important ones are sulfonamides, penicillin, iodides, bromides, barbiturates, atropine, streptomycin, butazolidin, p-aminosalicylic acid (PAS), dilantin and related compounds, and morphine. Drug fevers caused by antibacterial agents may be difficult to identify because they occur in persons who already have fever due to something else. In many cases, drug fevers are associated with the development of skin eruptions, and the simultaneous appearance of rash and fever may make the diagnosis easy.

Temperature elevations of as much as 2° F. may occur when morphine is withheld from an addict.[100]

A syndrome known as ninth-day fever, or ninth-day erythema, sometimes occurs from 7 to 20 days after the first injection of an arsenical drug such as Mapharsen or neoarsphenamine. The syndrome is characterized by fever, erythema, headache, malaise and lymph-node enlargement. It is apparently a manifestation of sensitivity to the arsenical, since it may occur in non-syphilitic individuals, and since further toxic effects are likely to occur if the treatment is continued. Penicillin sensitivity may produce a similar clinical picture.

Another type of febrile reaction that occurs in the therapy of syphilis is known as the Jarisch-Herxheimer reaction. It may result from treatment either with an arsenical or with penicillin and is undoubtedly related to the effect on the syphilitic infection. Within a few hours after the first injection the patient develops fever and malaise; these may be associated with an intensification of a skin eruption or severe pain in a syphilitic lesion of bone. The symptoms seldom last more that 24 to 48 hours.

Other drugs which may induce fever under certain conditions are epinephrine, dinitrophenol (DNP) and lysergic acid diethylamide (LSD), an inhibitor of serotonin.[52,101] Both serotonin and reserpine, though normally nonpyrogenic, cause fevers in animals given monoamine oxidase inhibitors. Presumably the fever is an effect of the high levels of free serotonin in the brain on centers controlling sympathetic nervous activity.[102] Patients with pheochromocytoma characteristically have a moderate elevation in temperature during an attack. Little is known about the mechanism by which these agents produce fever and it seems probable that some are direct stimulants to the central nervous system whereas others, such as DNP and epinephrine, act peripherally rather than on the thermoregulatory center itself. The relationship between central and peripheral roles of endogenous sympathetic amines in modifying body temperature deserves further investigation as does the possibility that these substances contribute (through alterations in their concentration in the brain) to fevers produced by other pyrogenic agents.

Fever Due to Heavy Sedation

It is not unusual for fever to occur in persons who have received heavy sedation (amytal narcosis for psychiatric therapy, barbiturate intoxication in suicide attempt, patients being treated for delirium tremens or tetanus). This temperature elevation suggests the possibility of a pulmonary complication, such as atelectasis or pneumonia, which of course, may be present.[103] Clinical experience shows that the sedation alone may cause fever, since there is frequently no sign of any other complication.

Pyrogens

Chill and high fever occasionally follow the intravenous administration of saline solutions, serums and other biologic preparations, because of the presence of bacterial pyrogens (discussed above), which gained access through contamination of the material at some stage of preparation. Special precautions must be taken to avoid pyrogen contamination of any material that is to be given intravenously. Pyrogens are exceedingly difficult to remove from biologic preparations, because they can pass through bacterial filters and can withstand autoclaving.[50]

Cotton-Dust Fever

Persons who handle raw cotton, in mills or in making mattresses, are subject to a febrile disorder. Toward the end of the day there is malaise, chilliness and fever of 100° to 102° F. The symptoms subside during the night, and the person usually feels well enough to return to work the next day. A tolerance develops within a few days, so that there are no symptoms as long as employment is continued. However, tolerance is lost when the worker takes a short vacation. Studies have indicated that the febrile reaction is related to the presence of a species of *Aerobacter cloacae* in the cotton fibers. This organism has been shown to be a potent pyrogen producer, and the presumption is that the symptoms are caused by absorption of the pyrogen from the respiratory mucosa.[104]

Metal-Fume Fever

Workers in certain metal industries are subject to illness of the type just described for cotton workers, including the development of tolerance. The workers particularly susceptible are those exposed to fumes containing zinc oxide.[105] It has been impossible to produce fever in animals exposed to the same fumes. The suggestion has been offered that in man the metal fumes cause increased absorption of bacterial products from the respiratory mucosa. However, the fever (which also occurs after inhalation of certain polymer fumes)[105a] may be due to an immunologic response[105b] or to absorption of finely divided particles per se, as in some experimental fevers.[56b]

"Catheter Fever"

Occasionally the passage of a catheter or other instrument through an infected urethral tract is followed in an hour or two by the development of fever, sometimes with a chill. It has been shown that this fever is caused by a bacteremia, which is usually transient. A similar fever may follow digital dilatation of a rectal stricture.

Teething

Lay people regard teething as a frequent cause of fever in children, whereas physicians are somewhat reluctant to take this view. However, most pediatricians believe that now and then, especially when there is swelling and inflammation of the gum over the erupting tooth, teething may cause a rise in temperature.

"MILK FEVER"

In the last century, when puerperal infection was more frequent than it is today, physicians were so accustomed to the appearance of fever about the third day after delivery that they came to regard engorgement of the mother's breasts as a process that could cause fever. However, modern obstetricians believe that fever which occurs coincidentally with the onset of lactation is probably due to some undetected infection.

NEUROCIRCULATORY ASTHENIA

Friedman studied a group of soldiers with the syndrome of neurocirculatory asthenia and found that 11 of 30 of these individuals were subject to occasional temperature elevations. The average maximal temperature in the 11 men was 99.8° F., whereas it was 98.6° F. in 11 normal control subjects during the same period of time.[106]

HABITUAL HYPERTHERMIA

Reimann has been interested in the problem of persons whose temperatures are set at a level slightly above the average normal (habitual hyperthermia) and has reported on a group of 16 such cases.[107] Each one was subjected to careful, thorough examination and was observed over a period of years, without the finding of any evidence of organic disease. Reimann believes that persons of this type are not rare and that they are often improperly managed because of the assumption that even a slight fever means disease. He thinks that in certain persons, particularly the neurotic type, the average temperature level may always be slightly above normal, and that long-continued low-grade fever in them should not be interpreted as an indication of infection or other febrile disease. All physicians are familiar with this clinical problem,[108] and, although every precaution must be taken not to overlook the presence of organic disease, it seems advisable to make a positive diagnosis of habitual hyperthermia at times, in order to spare these patients endless examination, treatment and expense.

PSYCHOGENIC FEVER

Most physicians are convinced that under certain conditions an emotional stimulus may induce an elevation of temperature. Dunbar has reviewed the evidence on the subject.[109] The slight rise so often observed at the time of admission to a hospital appears to be an example of psychogenic fever. We have all noticed that occasionally a patient who has no apparent cause for fever will show a slight elevation on the day of admission, but a normal temperature thereafter. Similarly, in pediatric wards it is not unusual to find a number of slight elevations immediately after visiting hours.

Wynn took the temperatures of 40 nurses immediately before and immediately after the writing of a state board examination and found that the average was 98.9° F. before, and 98.3° after the examination. Similarly, he found that among 324 draftees who were awaiting physical examination for the Army, the average temperature was 99.3° F., indeed 17 per cent of the men had temperatures above 100.0° F. He attributed these elevations to anxiety and excitement.[110]

The case described by Falcon-Lesses and Proger[111] is an interesting example of psychogenic fever. These authors kept records on the temperature of a young woman for more than a year. At home her temperature remained normal, except after occasional family quarrels; yet every time she visited the hospital out-patient clinic she developed a low fever. When an operation was suggested, and also when a vaginal examination was performed, her temperature rose approximately 1.0°F. within ten minutes.

Wolf and Wolff[112] reported another interesting example of psychogenic fever; their patient, a man, had had periodic bouts of fever for 13 years. He had suffered from migraine previously, and with the appearance of the fever his migraine ceased. All studies for infectious, neoplastic or metabolic causes of fever were negative. Therapy directed toward certain personality disorders seemed to relieve him of both the fever and the headaches.

Friedman has studied the low-grade fever common in patients with functional cardiovascular disease, and reports its presence in 30 per cent of such individuals.[113] He points out that the fever can be evoked by a variety of stressful situations and that it invariably disappears during sleep.

FEVER OF UNKNOWN ORIGIN

One of the most intriguing and difficult problems of diagnosis in medicine is the fever of unknown origin (F.U.O.). The causes of most of those of short duration are probably infectious diseases, especially viral. Other pyrexic states, which follow a more prolonged course (2 or 3 weeks or longer), are due to a variety of causes, as is evident by the number of diseases which may present at some time or other with fever. A point stressed in a recent series is that most patients with F.U.O. are not suffering from rare diseases but have unusual manifestations of common illnesses.[114] In over one third of the patients in this series the fevers were found after careful study to be of infectious origin and nearly two thirds of these patients recovered or benefited from specific treatment. Although the cause may be obscure one must make every effort to arrive at a correct diagnosis before blindly subjecting such patients to various therapeutical trials.

There appears to be little difference in the relative contribution of various disease categories (infectious, neoplastic and collagen) in the several series of F.U.O. reported over the past 25 years. However, within the fevers of obscure origin due to infectious diseases there has been a diminution of those caused by Gram-positive cocci and a corresponding increase in Gram-negative enteric infections. Tuberculosis continues to be found as the cause of many a chronic obscure fever. Discussions of the problems of diagnosis and treatment of patients with F.U.O. are presented in a number of recent reviews of this subject.[114-118] It seems likely that with our many new diagnostic technics we are today able to remove a higher percentage of cases from the unknown category.

SUMMARY

Maintenance of a relatively constant body temperature is effected largely through central nervous system control by centers located in the hypothalamus. Body heat is derived principally from combustion of food in the liver and voluntary muscles. Heat is lost by radiation, convection and vaporization. Normally the nervous system is able to control body temperature by activating or depressing a number of mechanisms which establish the balance between heat production and heat loss.

There is no set "normal" body temperature. The temperature varies considerably in different parts of the body; furthermore, there are small differences among healthy individuals. In all persons there is a diurnal variation, amounting to as much as 3° F., the peak usually being attained in the evening, the low point during sleep in the early morning hours.

Certain physiologic conditions influence the body temperature; among these are exercise, digestion of food, menstruation and pregnancy. Knowledge of the possible effect of exercise may be of particular importance to clinicians in evaluating "fever" in children.

Elevation of body temperature may be produced in different ways: by increased heat production, impairment of heat elimination, or by an effect on the hypothalamic temperature-regulating centers. In infections, neoplastic diseases and other conditions causing cell injury, it seems probable that some substance which is liberated from the injured tissue affects the hypothalamic centers. A fever-producing substance has been isolated from polymorphonuclear leucocytes and a circulating pyrogen with the same properties (endogenous pyrogen) has been detected in the sera of animals during a variety of experimentally induced fevers.

Many different types of disease cause fever. Among the most important are infections, diseases of the central nervous system, neoplasms and vascular accidents. An understanding of the characteristics and mechanisms of fever is of great value in the study of disease.

REFERENCES

1. Bazett, H. C.: The regulation of body temperatures, *in* L. H. Newburgh, Physiology of Heat Regulation and the Science of

Clothing, pp. 109-192, Philadelphia, Saunders, 1949.

2. Burton, A. C., and Bronk, D.: The motor mechanism of shivering and of thermal muscular tone, Am. J. Physiol. (Proc.) 118: 284, 1937.

3. Burton, A. C.: Range and variability of blood flow in human fingers and vasomotor regulation of body temperature, Am. J. Physiol. 127:437, 1939.

4. Barbour, H. G.: Die Wirkung unmittelbarer Erwärmung und Abkühlung der Wärmezentra auf die Körpertemperatur, Arch. exp. Path. Pharmakol. 70:1, 1912.

5. Isenschmid, R., and Schnitzler, W.: Beitrag zur Lokalisation des der Wärmeregulation vorstehenden Zentralapparates im Zwischenhirn, Arch. exp. Path. Pharmak. 76: 202, 1914.

6. Ranson, S. W.: *in* Hypothalamus and central levels of autonomic function, Nerv. Ment. Dis. Monog. 20:342, 1940.

7. Keller, A. D.: Separation in the brain stem of the mechanisms of heat loss from those of heat production, J. Neurophysiol. 1:543, 1938.

8. Ström, G.: Central nervous regulation of body temperature, *in* Handbook of Physiology, Section 1, Neurophysiology (J. Field, H. W. Magoun, and V. E. Hall, eds.), vol. 2, p. 1173, Washington, D.C., Am. Physiol. Soc., 1960.

9. Benzinger, T. H., Pratt, A. W., and Kitzinger, C.: The thermostatic control of human metabolic heat production, Proc. Nat. Acad. Sci., 47:730, 1961.

10. Sherrington, C. S.: Notes on temperature after spinal transection, with some observations on shivering, J. Physiol. 58:405, 1924.

11. Pickering, G.: Regulation of body temperature in health and disease, Lancet 1:1, 59, 1958.

12. Hammel, H. T., Hardy, J. D., and Fusco, M. M.: Thermoregulatory responses to hypothalamic cooling in unanesthetized dogs, Am. J. Physiol. 198:481, 1960.

12a. Nakayama, T., Hammel, H. T., Hardy, J. D., and Eisenman, J. S.: Thermal stimulation of electrical activity of single units of preoptic region, Am. J. Physiol. 204: 1122, 1963.

13. Hardy, J. D.: Physiology of temperature regulation, Physiol. Rev. 41:521, 1961.

14. Chambers, W. W., Koenig, H., Koenig, R., and Windle, W. F.: Site of action in the central nervous system of a bacterial pyrogen, Am. J. Physiol. 159:209, 1949.

15. Keeton, R. W.: Vaccine fever in rabbits rendered poikilothermous by cervical cord transection, Am. J. Physiol. 71:120, 1924-25.

16. Egdahl, R. H.: Differential response of the adrenal cortex and medulla to bacterial endotoxin, J. Clin. Invest. 38:1120, 1959.

17. Bard, P., and Woods, J. W.: Central nervous region essential for endotoxin fever, Tr. Am. Neurol. Assn. 87:37, 1962.

17a. Thompson, R. H.: Influence of environmental temperature upon pyrogenic fever. Dissertation. Univ. of Penn., 1959. (Quoted in ref. no. 13)

18. von Liebermeister, C.: Handbuch der Pathologie und Therapie des Fiebers, Leipzig, Vogél, 1875.

19. Macpherson, R. K.: The effect of fever on temperature regulation in man, Clin. Sci. 18:281, 1959.

20. Andersen, H. T., Hammel, H. T., and Hardy, J. D.: Modifications of the febrile response to pyrogen by hypothalamic heating and cooling in the unanesthetized dog, Acta Physiol. Scand. 53:247, 1961.

21. Wells, J. A., and Rall, D. P.: Mechanism of pyrogen induced fever, Proc. Soc. Exper. Biol. & Med. 68:421, 1948.

21a. Grant, R.: Nature of pyrogen fever; effect of environmental temperature on response to typhoid-paratyphoid vaccine, Am. J. Physiol. 159:511, 1949.

22. DuBois, E. F.: Fever and the Regulation of Body Temperature, Springfield, Ill., Thomas, 1948.

23. Horvath, S. M., Menduke, H., and Piersol, G. M.: Oral and rectal temperatures of man, J.A.M.A. 144:1562, 1950.

24. Reimann, H. A.: Habitual hyperthermia; a clinical study of four cases with long continued low grade fever, Arch. Int. Med. 55:792, 1935.

25. Gerbrandy, J., Snell, E. S., and Cranston, W. I.: Oral, rectal, and oesophageal temperatures in relation to central temperature control in man, Clin. Sci. 13:615, 1954.

26. Eichna, L. W., Berger, A. R., Rader, B., and Becker, W. H.: Comparison of intracardiac and intravascular with rectal temperatures in man, J. Clin. Invest. 30:353, 1951.

27. Eichna, L. W.: Thermal gradients in man. Comparison of temperatures in the femoral artery and femoral vein with rectal temperatures, Arch. Phys. Med. 30:584, 1949.

28. Rubin, A., Horvath, S. M., and Mellette, H. C.: Effect of fecal bacterial activity on rectal temperature of man, Proc. Soc. Exper. Biol. & Med. 76:410, 1951.

29. Reader, S. R., and Whyte, H. M.: Tissue temperature gradients, J. Appl. Physiol. 4:396, 1951.

30. Horvath, S. M., and Hollander, J. L.: Intra-articular temperature as a measure of joint reaction, J. Clin. Invest. 28:469, 1949.

31. Petrakis, N. L.: Temperature of human bone marrow, J. Appl. Physiol. 4:549, 1952.

32. Bazett, H. C., Love, L., Newton, M., Eisenberg, L., Day, R., and Forster, R.: Temperature changes in blood flowing in arteries and veins in man, J. Appl. Physiol. 1:3, 1948-1949.

33. Mellette, H. C., Hutt, B. K., Askovitz, S. I., and Horvath, S. M.: Diurnal variations in body temperatures, J. Appl. Physiol. 3:665, 1951.

34. Kleitman, N.: Biological rhythms and cycles, Physiol. Rev. 29:1, 1949.

35. Van der Bogert, F., and Moravec, C. L.: Body temperature variations in apparently healthy children, J. Pediat. 10:466, 1937.

36. Searcy, H. B.: Chewing gum fever, J. M. A. Alabama 13:266, 1944.

37. Benedict, F. G., and Slack, E. P.: A Comparative Study of Temperature Fluctuations in Different Parts of the Human Body, Carnegie Institution of Washington, Publication No. 155, 1911.

38. Lee, F. S., and Edwards, D. J.: The action of certain atmospheric conditions on body temperature and the vascular system, Proc. Soc. Exper. Biol. & Med. 12:72, 1915.

39. Whitelaw, M. J.: Hormonal control of the basal body temperature pattern, Fertil. & Steril. 3:230, 1952.

40. Seward, G. H., and Seward, J. P., Jr.: Changes in systolic blood pressure, heart rate, and temperature before, during, and after pregnancy in healthy woman, Human Biol. 8:232, 1936.

41. Smith, L. W., and Fay, T.: Observations on° human beings with cancer, maintained at reduced temperatures of 75°-90° Fahrenheit, Am. J. Clin. Path. 10:1, 1940.

42. Laufman, H.: Profound accidental hypothermia, J.A.M.A. 147:1201, 1951.

43. Kass, G. H.: Hypothermia following cortisone administration, Am. J. Med. 18:146, 1955.

44. Dripps, R. D. (ed.): The Physiology of induced hypothermia: Proceedings of a Symposium, Wash. D.C.: Nat. Acad. Sci.-Nat. Res. Council 1956 (pub. 451).

45. MacNeal, W. J.: Hyperthermia, genuine and spurious, Arch. Int. Med. 64:800, 1939.

46. MacNeal, W. J., Ritter, H. H., and Rabson, S. M.: Prolonged hyperthermia; report of a case with necropsy, Arch. Int. Med. 64:809, 1939.

47. DuBois, E. F.: Why are fever temperatures over 106° F. rare?, Am. J. M. Sc. 217:361, 1949.

48. Cramer, W.: Fever, infections and the thyroid-adrenal apparatus, Brit. J. Exper. Path. 7:95, 1926.

49. Welch, W. H.: The Cartwright Lectures. On the general pathology of fever, Med. News 52:365, 393, 539, 565, 1888.

50. Bennett, I. L., Jr., and Cluff, L. E.: Bacterial pyrogens, Pharm. Rev. 9:427, 1957.

51. Westphal, O.: Pyrogens, in Springer, G. F., (ed.): Polysaccharides in Biology, p. 115, New York: Macy, 1957.

52. Atkins, E.: Pathogenesis of fever, Physiol. Rev. 40:580, 1960.

53. Bennett, I. L., Jr., and Beeson, P. B.: Studies on the pathogenesis of fever. 1. The effect of injection of extracts and suspensions of uninfected rabbit tissues upon the body temperature of normal rabbits, J. Exp. Med. 98:477, 1953.

53a. Atkins, E., and Snell, E. S.: Pyrogenic properties of various tissue extracts in the rabbit, J. Physiol. In press.

54. Atkins, E., and Wood, W. B., Jr.: Studies on the pathogenesis of fever. II, Identification of an endogenous pyrogen in the blood stream following the injection of typhoid vacccine, J. Exp. Med. 102:499, 1955.

55. Snell, E. S., Goodale, F., Jr., Wendt, F., and Cranston, W. I.: Properties of human endogenous pyrogen, Clin. Sci. 16:615, 1957.

56. Herion, J. C., Walker, R. I., and Palmer, J. G.: Endotoxin fever in granulocytopenic animals, J. Exp. Med. 113:1115, 1961.

56a. Snell, E. S.: Pyrogenic properties of human pathologic fluids, Clin. Sci. 23:141, 1962.

56b. Atkins, E., and Freedman, L. R.: Studies in staphylococcal fever, I-III. Yale J. Biol. Med. 35:451, 472, 489, 1963.

56c. Brittingham, T. E., and Chaplin, H., Jr.: Febrile transfusion reactions caused by sensitivity to donor leukocytes and platelets, J.A.M.A. 165:819, 1957.

56d. Jandl, J. H., and Tomlinson, A. S.: Destruction of red cells by antibodies in man.

II. Pyrogenic, leukocytic and dermal responses to immune hemolysis, J. Clin. Invest. 37:1202, 1958.

57. Bennett, I. L., Jr.: Studies on the pathogenesis of fever. V. The fever accompanying pneumococcal infection in the rabbit, Bull. Johns Hopkins Hosp. 98:216, 1956.

58. King, M. K., and Wood, W. B., Jr.: Studies on the pathogenesis of fever. V. The relation of circulating endogenous pyrogen to the fever of acute bacterial infections, J. Exp. Med. 107:305, 1958.

59. King, M. K., and Wood, W. B., Jr.: Studies on the pathogenesis of fever. IV. The site of action of leucocytic and circulating endogenous pyrogen, J. Exp. Med. 107:291, 1958.

60. Kaiser, H. K., and Wood, W. B., Jr.: Studies on the pathogenesis of fever. X. The effect of certain enzyme inhibitors on the production and activity of leucocytic pyrogen, J. Exp. Med. 115:37, 1962.

60a. Berlin, R. D., and Wood, W. B., Jr.: Molecular mechanisms involved in the release of pyrogen from polymorphonuclear leucocytes, Tr. Ass. Am. Phys. 75:190, 1962.

61. Fessler, J. H., Cooper, K. E., Cranston, W. I., and Vollum, R. L.: Observations on the production of pyrogenic substances by rabbit and human leucocytes, J. Exp. Med. 113:1127, 1961.

62. Warren, S. L., Carpenter, C. N., and Boak, R. A.: Symptomatic herpes; a sequela of artificially induced fever; incidence and clinical aspects; recovery of a virus from herpetic vesicles, and comparison with a known strain of herpes virus, J. Exp. Med. 71:155, 1940.

63. Welty, J. W.: Febrile albuminuria, Am. J. M. Sci. 194:70, 1937.

64. Barr, D. P., and DuBois, E. F.: Clinical calorimetry; the metabolism in malarial fever, Arch. Int. Med. 21:627, 1918.

65. Perera, G. A.: Clinical and physiologic characteristics of chill, Arch. Int. Med. 68:241, 1941.

66. Fremont-Smith, F., Morrison, L. R., and Makepeace, A. W.: Capillary blood flow in man during fever, J. Clin. Invest. 7:489, 1929.

67. Altschule, M. D., and Freedberg, A. S.: Circulation and respiration in fever, Medicine 24:403, 1945.

68. Wegman, M. E.: Factors influencing the relation of convulsions and hyperthermia, J. Pediat. 14:190, 1939.

69. Peterman, M. G.: Febrile convulsions, J. Pediat. 41:536, 1952.

70. Lennox, W. G.: Significance of febrile convulsions, Pediatrics 11:341, 1953.

71. Petersdorf, R. G., and Bennett, I. L., Jr.: Factitious fever, Ann. Int. Med. 46:1039, 1957.

72. Bennett, I. L., Jr., and Nicastri, A.: Fever as a mechanism of resistance, Bact. Rev. 24:16, 1960.

73. Futcher, P. H.: The double quotidian temperature curve of gonococcal endocarditis; a diagnostic aid, Am. J. M. Sc. 199:23, 1940.

74. Erickson, T. C.: Neurogenic hyperthermia (a clinical syndrome and its treatment), Brain 62:172, 1939.

75. McKenna, J. B.: The incidence of fever and leukocytosis in multiple sclerosis, Arch. Neurol. & Psychiat. 24:542, 1930.

76. Holmes, G.: Goulstonian lectures on spinal injuries of warfare; II. The clinical symptoms of gunshot injuries of the spine, Brit. M. J. 2:815, 1915.

77. Harsha, W. N.: Fever in malignant disease, Am. Surgeon 18:229, 1952.

78. Clagett, O. T., McDonald, J. R., and Schmidt, H. W.: Localized fibrous mesothelioma of the pleura, J. Thoracic Surg. 24:213, 1952.

79. Browder, A. A., Huff, J. W., and Petersdorf, R. G.: The significance of fever in neoplastic disease, Ann. Int. Med. 55:932, 1961.

80. Boggs, D. R., and Frei, E., III: Clinical Studies of fever and infections in cancer, Cancer 13:1240, 1960.

80a. Silver, R. T., Utz, J. P., Frei, E., III, and McCullough, N. B.: Fever, infection and host resistance in acute leukemia, Am. J. Med. 24:25, 1958.

81. Ferris, E. B., Jr., Blankenhorn, M. A., Robinson, H. W., and Cullen, G. E.: Heat stroke; clinical and chemical observations on 44 cases, J. Clin. Investigation 17:249, 1938.

82. Himwich, H. E.: The metabolism of fever, with special reference to diabetic hyperpyrexia, Bull. New York Acad. Med. 10:16, 1934.

83. Steele, J. M.: Elevation of rectal temperature following mechanical obstruction to the peripheral circulation, Am. Heart J. 13:542, 1937.

84. Stewart, H. J., Evans, W. F., Brown, H., and Gerjuoy, J. R.: Peripheral blood flow, rectal and skin temperature in congestive heart failure: The effects of rapid digital-

ization in this state, Arch. Int. Med. 77:643, 1946.

85. Kinsey, D., and White, P. D.: Fever in congestive heart failure, Arch. Int. Med. 65:163, 1940.

86. Kappas, A., Glickman, P. B., and Palmer, R. H.: Steroid fever studies: physiological differences between bacterial pyrogens and endogenous steroid pyrogens of man, Tr. Ass. Am. Phys. 73:176, 1960.

87. Bondy, P. K., Cohn, G. L., and Castiglione, C.: Etiocholanolone fever: a clinical entity, Tr. Ass. Am. Phys. 73:186, 1960.

88. McCrae, T., and Caven, W. E.: Tertiary syphilis of the liver, Am. J. M. Sci. 172:781, 1926.

88a. Tisdale, W. A., and Klatskin, G.: The fever of Laennec's cirrhosis, Yale J. Biol. Med. 33:94, 1960.

89. Bang, S.: Fever in gastric and in duodenal ulcer, Arch. Int. Med. 41:808, 1928.

90. Dill, L. V., and Isenhour, C. E.: Observations on the incidence and cause of fever in patients with bleeding peptic ulcers, Am. J. Dig. Dis. 5:779, 1939.

91. Schiff, L., Shapiro, N., and Stevens, R. F.: Observations on the oral administration of citrated blood in man; III. The effect on temperature and the white blood cell count, Am. J. M. Sci. 207:465, 1944.

92. Selesnick, S., and White, B. V.: Body temperature in persons with bleeding peptic ulcer, Gastroenterology 20:282, 1952.

93. Woodyatt, R. T.: Ichthyosis, fever and effort syndrome, Tr. A. Am. Phys. 50:105, 1935.

94. Rowe, A. H.: Fever due to food allergy, Ann. Allergy 6:252, 1948.

95. Lian, C., Facquet, J., and Brawerman: Fièvre et tacycardies paroxystiques, Arch. d. mal. du coeur 32:566, 1939.

96. Burford, G. E.: Hyperthermia following anesthesia; a consideration of control of body temperature during anesthesia, Anesthesiology 1:208, 1940.

97. Bigler, J. A., and McQuiston, W. O.: Body temperatures during anesthesia in infants and children, J.A.M.A. 146:551, 1951.

98. Pickrell, H. P.: Hyperpyrexia pallida and its prevention, Australian & New Zealand J. Surg. 21:261, 1952.

99. Mangiardi, J. L.: Experiences with postoperative temperatures above 108° F, Am. J. Surg. 81:189, 1951.

100. Vogel, V. H., Isbell, H., and Chapman, K. W.: Present status of narcotic addiction; with particular reference to medical indications and comparative addiction liability of the newer and older analgesic drugs, J.A.M.A. 138:1019, 1948.

101. von Euler, C.: Physiology annd pharmacology of temperature regulation, Pharm. Rev. 13:361, 1961.

102. Shore, P. A., Pletscher, A., Tomich, E. G., Carlsson, A., Kuntzman, R., and Brodie, B. B.: Role of brain serotonin in reserpine action, Ann. N.Y. Acad. Sci. 66:609, 1957.

103. Swank, R. L., and Smedal, M. I.: Pulmonary atelectasis in stuporous states; a study of its incidence and mechanism in sodium amytal narcosis, Am. J. Med. 5:210, 1948.

104. Ritter, W. L., and Nussbaum, M. A.: Occupational illnesses in cotton industries; "cotton fever," Miss. Doctor, p. 96, Sept., 1944.

105. Sayers, R. R.: Metal fume fever and its prevention, Pub. Health Rep. 58:1080, 1938.

105a. Harris, D. K.: Polymer-fume fever, Lancet 2:1008, 1951.

105b. McCord, C. P.: Metal fume fever as an immunological disease, Industr. Med. Surg. 29:101, 1960.

106. Friedman, M.: Etiology and pathogenesis of neurocirculatory asthenia. I. Hyperthermia as one of the manifestations of neurocirculatory asthenia, War Med. 6:221, 1945.

107. Reimann, H. A.: The problem of long continued, low-grade fever, J.A.M.A. 107: 1089, 1936.

108. Richardson, J. S.: Pyrexia of uncertain origin and psychogenic fever, Practitioner 170:61, 1953.

109. Dunbar, H. F.: Emotions and Bodily Changes, ed. 2, New York, Columbia, 1938.

110. Wynn, F. B.: The psychic factor as an element in temperature disturbance; shown by some observations in the selective draft, J.A.M.A. 73:31, 1919.

111. Falcon-Lesses, M., and Proger, S. H.: Psychogenic fever, New England J. Med. 203: 1034, 1930.

112. Wolf, S., and Wolff, H. G.: Intermittent fever of unknown origin; recurrent high fever with benign outcome in a patient with migraine and notes on "neurogenic" fever, Arch. Int. Med. 70:293, 1942.

113. Friedman, M.: Hyperthermia as a manifestation of stress, in Life Stress and Bodily Disease, Proc. A. Res. Nerv. & Ment. Dis., vol. 29, Baltimore, Williams & Wilkins, 1950.

114. Petersdorf, R. G., and Beeson, P. B.: Fever of unexplained origin: report on 100 cases, Medicine 40:1, 1961.

115. Oppel, T. W., and Berntsen, C. A., Jr.: The differential diagnosis of fevers: the present status of the problem of fever of unknown origin, Med. Clin. N.A. 38:891, 1954.

116. Reid, J. V. O.: Pyrexia of unknown origin: study of a series of cases, Brit. Med. J. 2:23, 1956.

117. Bennett, I. L., Jr., and Hook, E. W.: Fever of unknown origin, Disease-a-Month, Nov. 1957.

118. Keefer, C. S., and Leard, S. E.: Prolonged and perplexing fevers, Boston, Little, Brown, 1955.

23

Lymphadenopathy and Disorders of the Lymphatic System

OTHMAR CHARLES SOLNITZKY AND HAROLD JEGHERS

INTRODUCTION

The lymphatic system is involved in many diseases, both local and systemic, and there are various types of involvement. In addition, lymph nodes are affected by primary disease of both the lymphatic and the reticuloendothelial systems as well as by cancer. The lymphatic system, particularly the lymph nodes, may become involved in the following ways; (1) carcinomatous invasion, (2) infectious adenopathy, (3) infiltration by foreign substances, (4) disturbances of metabolism, especially of lipids (storage type of adenopathy), and (5) primary hematopoietic disease.

Many of the lymph nodes of the body thus affected are amenable to palpation, biopsy and roentgen ray studies. The character of the lymph node enlargement, the degree and extent of the involvement of the nodes and the character of the histologic changes within them are of great importance, not only in diagnosis, but also in treatment.

Diagnostically, involved lymph nodes can give a clue to the site of origin and, in many cases, to the nature of the causative agent.

Therapeutically, a knowledge of the drainage areas of the various regional lymph nodes of the body is essential in planning adequate treatment whether by radiation or by radical surgical dissection.

RELATION OF LYMPHATIC SYSTEM TO OTHER CIRCULATORY SYSTEMS

There are 3 major circulatory systems: (1) the blood vascular, (2) the cerebrospinal, and (3) the lymphatic (Fig. 153). The *blood vascular system* is a closed vascular ring provided with a pump, the heart. The function of this system is to ensure that blood reaches all parts of the body in order that each cell may receive nourishment in accordance with its functional needs. Blood flows away from the heart in the arteries and arterioles to reach the capillaries, which not only permit the escape into the tissue spaces of nutrient fluid but also reabsorb some of the tissue fluid. From the capillaries the blood is returned back to the heart by the veins. Thus, in the blood vascular system, blood flows in two directions: from and to the heart.

The *cerebrospinal fluid circulatory system* is also a closed system of channels containing the cerebrospinal fluid. It consists of the ventricles and the cerebral aqueduct of the brain, the central canal of the spinal cord and the subarachnoid space. Normally, the cerebrospinal fluid, elaborated chiefly by the choroid plexuses of the brain ventricles, flows in one direction: from the ventricles through the foramina of Luschka and Magendie into the subarachnoid space, from which it is transferred across the arachnoid villi into the dural venous sinuses and finally into the internal jugular vein to be returned to the right side of the heart. Thus, cerebrospinal fluid does not enter the venous system directly, but across the meningeal barrier represented by the arachnoid villi and the dura mater.

The *lymphatic system,*[1] unlike the first two, is not closed, but communicates directly with the venous system at the root of the neck. It consists of a system of blindly beginning capillaries, which pick up tissue fluid not absorbed through the blood capillaries, and of a series of collecting vessels of increasing size which eventually drain the contained fluid, called lymph, into the subclavian veins. In the lymphatic system the flow of lymph is always in one direction only, that is, to the heart. A characteristic of the lymphatic system is the interpolation along its main vessels of filters — the lymph nodes — through which lymph must first pass before being transferred to the vein.

FUNCTIONS OF LYMPHATIC SYSTEM

The lymphatic system performs several important functions:[2]

1. Lymphatic vessels furnish preformed tubes for the passage of lymph. These vessels can also serve for the transport of viruses and bacteria. Microorganisms may be introduced directly into lymphatic capillaries or vessels by puncture or incised wounds or they may enter the lymphatics from a suppurative focus. In either case, there may occur a consequent infection of the lymphatic channels (*tubular lymphangitis*) or of the lymph nodes (*lymphadenitis*). If the lymph nodes break down, the infective organism can then enter the blood stream (*septicemia*). At times, infection may be limited to the superficial reticular lymphatics of the skin (e.g., *erysipelas*).

2. Production of lymphocytes. Lymphocytes are produced in the germinal centers of lymph nodes and leave the nodes through their efferent vessels. The ultimate fate of these lymphocytes is not known.

3. Production of antibodies. Immune substances can be extracted from lymphocytes. Lymphocytes contain at least one globulin which is identical with blood globulin. Immune bodies are linked in the blood with globulins.

4. Phagocytosis. This function is performed by the reticuloendothelial cells lining the lymph sinuses of lymph nodes.

5. Hemopoiesis. Under normal conditions, the lymphatic system is concerned

only with production of lymphocytes, but under pathologic conditions, the reticulo-endothelial component of the lymphatic system has the capacity to revert to the function of blood formation.

6. By a process of absorption, on the part of its capillaries, the lymphatic system returns to the blood stream both fluid and chemical substances which escaped from the blood stream across the walls of the blood capillaries. A considerable amount of protein escapes in this manner into the extravascular tissue spaces from which it is partly absorbed into the lymphatic system and thence returned to the blood stream.

7. Absorption of fats and fat-soluble materials from the intestine. This function can be demonstrated easily by giving the patient, by mouth, olive oil stained with Sudan IV or some other dye. The dye will appear in the thoracic duct lymph approximately 1.5 hours after the ingestion of the dye-labeled olive oil. This procedure is utilized as a clinical diagnostic method to locate tears of the thoracic duct in cases of chylothorax.

THE FORMATION OF LYMPH

Tissue fluid is derived both from blood plasma and tissue cells. It represents a balance between the rate of its filtration at the arterial ends of the blood capillaries and its resorption at the venous ends.[3, 4, 5] Ordinarily, there is little tissue fluid.

Substances in true solution in the blood plasma, such as glucose, inorganic salts, amino acids, etc., exert little or no effective osmotic pressure within the blood capillaries. Their molecules are so small that they pass easily through the blood capillary walls into the tissue spaces. As a result, nutritive material from the blood plasma can easily reach the tissue cells, and waste products also can easily reach the blood for excretion. On the other hand, the blood plasma proteins, due to the larger size of their molecules, cannot readily pass through the blood capillary walls. Of the three plasma proteins (albumin, globulin fraction and fibrinogen), albumin has the smallest molecule and hence passes into the tissue spaces in greater amounts than the globulins and fibrinogen. The formation of tissue fluid is regulated by two pressures: the hydrostatic and the osmotic.

The forces which regulate the exchange between blood capillaries and tissue spaces are the same that regulate the formation of lymph. Any condition which enhances the filtration of fluid from the blood capillaries tends to increase the flow of lymph. The lymphatic capillaries are far more permeable than the blood capillaries and offer little resistance to the passage of proteins or crystalloids. The lymphatic capillaries have the very special function of removing extravascular protein which cannot be absorbed by the blood capillaries and which, in the absence of normally functioning lymphatic capillaries, would accumulate in the tissue spaces and lead to edema. From this point of view, the lymphatic capillaries play a major role in protein metabolism and nutrition. The lymphatic capillaries can also take up from the tissue fluid particulate matter, such as microorganisms.

The formation of lymph depends upon: (1) the amount of free fluid in the tissue spaces and (2) influences which empty draining lymphatics and permit further absorption of raw material by lymphatic capillaries.

The formation and flow of lymph can be increased as follows:[3, 4, 5]

1. Increase in capillary pressure consequent to increased venous pressure from venous obstruction. Where the tissues are firm and resistant, little edema develops. In areas with much loose areolar tissue, a considerable degree of edema will develop early.

2. Increase in permeability of the capillary wall by heat or a rise in temperature, reduced oxygen supply, and certain drugs, such as histamine.

3. Increased metabolic activity resulting from both muscular and glandular activity. Little lymph is formed under conditions of absolute rest or anesthesia. Active muscular contractions also exert a pumping effect upon the lymph, driving it along toward the thoracic duct and the blood stream.

4. Passive movement and massage.[6] The bedridden patient with cardiac edema delivers very little edema fluid to the blood vascular system via the lymphatics. Mas-

sage and passive movement not only augment the blood flow and the capillary pressure, but also aid in propelling the lymph along the lymphatic vessels.

5. Hypertonic solutions. Hypertonic solutions of glucose, sodium chloride, or sodium sulfate introduced intravenously, enhance the volume of lymph in the thoracic duct. Isotonic solutions also increase the formation and flow of lymph, since they bring about a dilution of the blood plasma colloids with the resulting rise in filtration through the capillary walls.

ANATOMY AND CHEMICAL COMPOSITION OF LYMPH

Lymph has certain basic similarities with blood. Like the latter, it consists of a fluid medium and certain corpuscular elements.

The fluid portion of lymph, derived from blood plasma by a process of filtration, carries to the tissue spaces both oxygen as well as various nutritive substances (salt, proteins, hormones, enzymes, etc). The tissue cells, in turn, discharge into the tissue spaces various metabolites. Hence, the chemical composition of lymph will necessarily vary at different times and in different parts of the body. Ordinarily, lymph from the greater part of the body is colorless. After a fatty meal, lymph in the thoracic duct contains a high content of absorbed emulsified fat and hence appears milky. Such milky lymph is called chyle.[7]

The proteins of tissue fluid and lymph are derived chiefly from blood plasma. In addition, the liver constantly forms new plasma protein which eventually reaches the blood stream by way of the lymphatics. The proportion of albumin to globulin is greater in lymph than in blood plasma due to the freer passage of the smaller albumin molecule through the walls of the blood capillaries. The chlorides tend to be higher in lymph, while the calcium concentration is lower. Lymph contains fibrinogen in very low concentrations as well as prothrombin. It clots more slowly than blood plasma due to the lack of blood platelets. Like blood plasma, lymph contains 26 to 28 m.Eq./L. carbon dioxide and follows the reaction of the blood.

Cellular elements. The lymph of the thoracic duct contains mostly lymphocytes. The cell count varies from 2,000 to 20,000 lymphocytes per cu. mm. In the case of lymph nodes, the lymphocytes are more numerous in the *efferent* than in the afferent vessels. The cell count can be increased by massage over the lymph nodes. In general, the lymphocyte count of the lymph is greater in the young than in the old.

It has been estimated that under normal conditions an average of 200,000,000 lymphocytes enter the blood stream from the lymphatic system per hour. Nevertheless, the lymphocyte count of the blood remains constant, with the exception of slight fluctuations. The problem of what happens to this large number of lymphocytes has not been solved. There are two main views as to the nature of the lymphocyte: (1) The lymphocyte is an embryonic cell capable of metaplastic transformation into the cellular elements of the blood, such as granulocytes; and (2) the lymphocyte is a special end product of cellular differentiation with specific functions. Most of the evidence so far favors the second view. *Early dissolution under pituitary-adrenal controls seems to be the most likely fate of the lymphocytes.* Such dissolution contributes to the protein content of the blood.

In addition to lymphocytes, lymph may occasionally contain polymorphonuclear leukocytes and macrophages.

Rarely, lymph may contain a few erythrocytes. This occurs in cases where the lymphatic drainage includes areas of inflammation and congestion. In such cases, there is probably direct leakage from blood capillaries which are in direct contact with lymphatic capillaries.

VOLUME OF LYMPH

It has been estimated that in a resting human patient the average flow of lymph from the thoracic duct amounts to 0.93 ml. per minute or 1.38 ml. per Kg. of body weight per hour. The maximum rate of flow induced by a heavy meal was 3.9 ml. per minute, while the minimum was 0.38 ml. per minute.[7] The rate of flow can be increased by the ingestion of food or water, or by abdominal massage. In a recent report of a thoracic duct fistula in another carefully studied patient, the lymph flow varied from 1.06 to 1.86 ml. per Kg. per hour.[8]

FLOW OF LYMPH

Under normal conditions, the direction of the flow of lymph is toward the heart. It resembles the flow of venous blood in that it depends on the presence of neighboring structures, chiefly contracting muscles, which force the flow of lymph in a direction determined by the valves of the lymphatic capillaries, vessels and collecting ducts.[9] The propulsive action of the heart does not directly affect the flow of lymph.

Factors Affecting Movement of Lymph. Specifically, the factors which affect the movement of lymph are the following:[10] (1) The remitting compression of lymph vessels by surrounding structures, especially contracting muscles. (2) Respiratory movements. Through such movements, lymph is propulsed from the cisterna chyli into the thoracic duct. (3) Propulsive action of the smooth muscles contained in the wall of the lymphatic vessels, the lymph nodes and the collecting ducts. (4) Arterial pulsations. Most of the lymphatic vessels course with the regional blood vessels. The deep lymphatic vessels accompany not only the veins but also arteries whose pulsations can be transmitted to the lymph vessels. (5) The negative pressure in the great vessels at the root of the neck determines the flow of lymph from the terminal parts of the jugular, the subclavian, the bronchomediastinal and the thoracic ducts into them. (6) Peristaltic contractions of the intestines. (7) Capillary blood pressure. (8) The force of gravity.

Uncommon Modes of Lymph Flow

Shortcircuiting. While, as a rule, lymph transmitted by the lymphatic vessels must traverse at *least one group of lymph nodes before reaching the thoracic* duct and the blood stream, there are cases where it may by-pass one or more groups of lymph nodes as the result of anastomotic connections between afferent and efferent vessels. Such *anomalous connections* provide the anatomic basis for the tragic cases in which

a small septic scratch results in *rapid septicemia* and death within a short time. This shortcircuiting of lymphatic vessels past lymph nodes also explains the cases of *rapid metastasis* of certain cancers. Thus, while breast cancer usually metastasizes to the axillary nodes, and the enlargement may act as a warning signal to the patient, there are cases in which the lymphatic vessels from the mammary gland by-pass the axillary nodes and drain directly across the costocoracoid membrane to the deeply situated infraclavicular nodes (nodes which are not palpable even when enlarged), hence the cancer emboli can quickly reach the blood stream (see Fig. 166).

Retrograde Lymphatic Spread. The direction of spread of cancer emboli by lymphatics depends on the direction of the lymph flow. When all or a majority of the lymph channels draining a certain area *become blocked,* a *retrograde flow of lymph will take place.*[11,12]

The question of retrograde spread of cancer is an important one since it directly affects the choice of surgical procedures. There is ample evidence to show that radical procedures result in fewer recurrences. The increased incidence of recurrences in less radical operations may be due to a preoperative retrograde spread.

Retrograde spread may not be grossly detectable. In such cases, histologic examination will show distention of intramural lymphatics with cancer cells. Retrograde spread may be indicated grossly by the presence of many hyperplastic nodes, not necessarily invaded by metastases, below the level of the main cancer site or by the presence of actual gross metastases below this level.

Common examples of retrograde spread are the following:

In blockage of the para-aortic abdominal nodes, cancer cell emboli from *ovarian or testicular primary cancer may reach the iliac nodes in a retrograde manner without* involvement of the inguinal nodes, which receive no lymph from the ovary or testis unless cancer in these organs breaks through their capsules.

In case of blockage of the axillary nodes,

cancer cell emboli from mammary cancer may reach the pulmonary lymphatics and thus invade the mediastinal nodes. Conversely, in lung cancer, in the presence of adhesions between the visceral and the parietal pleura, lymph from the lung may pass to the axillary or the para-aortic nodes, with spread of cancer to these locations (see Fig. 164).

In case of cancer of the stomach with blockage of the mediastinal nodes, retrograde flow may lead to annular carcinomatous constriction of segments of the bowel.[11]

Crossed Spread. The spread of cancer cell emboli from one side of the body to the other may occur in one of the following ways.

1. Lymphatic efferents from an organ may terminate in the regional lymph nodes of both sides. This is particularly true of cancer of the tongue and the lip.

2. Communications across the mid-line of cutaneous lymphatics. This is of particular significance in the case of the cutaneous lymphatics of the mammary gland and of the perineum (see Figs. 163, 166).

3. Direct cross anastomoses of the regional lymph nodes of the two sides. Thus, while cancer of the ovary, the testis, the kidney, the bladder and the suprarenal will at first metastasize to the homolateral para-aortic nodes and remain unilateral for a time, eventually it will spread to the other side, since the right and the left para-aortic nodes communicate with each other by cross anastomoses.

4. Anomalous division and termination of the thoracic duct. Thus, the thoracic duct may divide terminally into two or more branches, emptying partly into the left and partly into the right jugulosubclavian junction. Or the thoracic duct may terminally veer to the right and empty wholly into the right jugulosubclavian junction.[13]

LYMPHATICOVENOUS COMMUNICATIONS

For a long time it has been postulated that there are direct communications between the lymphatic system and the venous system other than the termination of the thoracic duct into the internal jugular or the subclavian vein. Recently, Pressman

and Simon[184] demonstrated such communications by the injections of saline into a lymph node, immediately followed by the injection of air at the same site. This method demonstrated direct communications between the lymph node and the immediately adjacent and easily observable veins of the area.

Threefoot, Kent and Hatchett,[185] by means of plastic corrosion models, demonstrated in rats the existence of both lymphaticovenous and lymphaticolymphatic communications.

Under normal conditions, lymphaticovenous communications cannot be demonstrated unequivocally. It is only under conditions of stress, i.e., conditions which impose some obstruction or stress on the lymphatic system, that such connections become evident.

AREAS LACKING LYMPHATIC DRAINAGE

There are large areas of the body which lack lymphatics. The most important of these are:[14]

1. *The central nervous system (brain and spinal cord) and the meninges.* The central nervous system contains a circulatory system peculiar to itself, as described previously.

2. *Nonvascular tissues,* such as the epidermis of the skin, the epithelial lining of mucous membranes, hair, nails and cartilage.

3. *Liver.* While lymphatic vessels accompany the hepatic artery, portal vein and bile ducts, the hepatic lobules are not provided with lymphatic capillaries. The latter are confined to the perilobular connective tissue septa. The hepatic lymphatic capillaries absorb not only material carried by the hepatic artery and portal vein but also protein released directly into the extravascular tissue by the hepatic parenchymal cells.

4. *Spleen.* Lymphatic capillaries and vessels are here confined to the capsule and the larger trabeculae. There is no direct connection between these capsular and trabecular lymphatic channels and the blood sinusoids of the spleen.

5. *Bone marrow.*

6. *Muscles*. Lymphatic vessels here lie only in the intermuscular fascial planes. There is no evidence of their presence within the muscle fiber bundles.

7. *Eyeball*. While there are no true lymphatic vessels in the eyeball, this organ contains in its anterior and posterior chambers a fluid similar to lymph, which is elaborated by the ciliary bodies of the choroid and drained into the canal of Schlemm, which in turn empties its contents into the venous system of the eyeball.

LYMPHATIC CAPILLARIES

In its peripheral portion, the lymphatic system is represented by lymphatic capillaries which begin blindly in the tissue spaces. They have no direct communication with the blood capillaries. They are larger and more variable in caliber than the blood capillaries.

Structurally, lymphatic capillaries consist of endothelial tubes to which are attached externally both reticular and elastic fibers continuous with the surrounding connective tissue. These fibers serve to prevent collapse of the lymphatic capillaries whenever the fluid in the intercellular spaces increases, as in inflammatory states. The pressure of the fluid places tension on the reticular and elastic fibers and thus tends to keep the capillaries open. On the other hand, whenever lymphatic capillaries are damaged, these fibers, by traction, prevent rapid healing, which occurs in the case of tears in blood capillaries. Nevertheless, lymphatic capillaries are highly elastic and can undergo considerable distention without rupture.

Lymphatic capillaries anastomose freely with one another to form lymphatic capillary plexuses. Such plexuses are found in glands and under the body surfaces; the skin, the mucous membranes of the respiratory, the digestive, and the genitourinary tracts, as well as serous membranes (pleura, peritoneum) and synovial membrane (bursae, joints). In the skin and the mucous membranes, these plexuses are usually arranged in a superficial and a deep set.

The lymphatic capillaries of the small intestine particularly are well developed in the villi, where they are called lacteals. These capillaries play an important part in the transportation of fat. Almost two thirds of the fat absorbed from the intestine enters the lacteals and is carried by them as emulsified fat to the lymphatic vessels and eventually to the thoracic duct.

There is no evidence that the caliber of lymphatic capillaries is affected directly by vasoconstrictors such as epinephrine or pituitary hormones.

The lymphatic capillaries are concerned with the primary functional capacity of the tubular portion of the lymphatic system, namely, absorption.

LYMPHATIC VESSELS

Lymphatic vessels are interposed between the lymphatic capillaries and the larger collecting lymphatic ducts. They are characterized also by the interpolation of lymph nodes in their path.

They frequently anastomose and tend to travel in company with veins. Occasionally, veins are surrounded by a web of lymphatic channels. Their walls are made up of collagenous, reticular, and elastic fibers as well as smooth muscle. The proportions and the disposition of these vary considerably depending on the size and location of the vessel. Structurally, they resemble veins, but do not possess clearly defined layers in their walls. They also show less tendency than veins to unite into large vessels. By co-ordinated contraction of circular and longitudinal muscle, effective propulsive movements may result.

A conspicuous feature of lymphatic vessels is the abundance of valves. These are bicuspid, occasionally tricuspid. They project into the lumen in the direction of the flow of lymph. Under physiologic conditions, the intralymphatic pressure is low, so that the valves seem to be the most important factor in controlling direction of lymph flow. They are responsible for the uneven or beaded appearance of lymphatic vessels. The vessel wall is dilated just proximal to the site of the valve. Valves are absent in the superficial capillaries. They usually make their appearance in the deep capillary plexuses. They increase in number in the lymphatic vessels where they are most numerous just before reaching a lymph node.

Usually lymphatic vessels are disposed in

two sets, superficial and deep. This is particularly true of the lymphatic vessels of the extremities. The superficial set lies in the dermis and the superficial fascia. The lymphatic vessels of this set accompany the superficial veins (cephalic and basilic in the upper extremity; lesser and greater saphenous, in the lower). The deep set lies beneath the deep fascia and accompanies the deep arteries and their accompanying veins in the intermuscular planes. Usually there is little communication between the superficial and the deep lymphatic vessels except where the superficial vessels pierce the deep fascia to empty into the deep lymph nodes. Since the lymphatic vessels accompany both the superficial and the deep veins and the deep arteries, the lymphatic and venous drainages coincide closely. This is of practical value from the surgical point of view, since veins and arteries can be seen easily, while lymphatic vessels cannot.

LYMPHANGITIS

Lymph vessels may be affected by acute, subacute or chronic inflammatory processes. Lymphangitis usually arises from superficial wounds, such as punctures, small abrasions, cuts and scratches. Consequently, it affects primarily the superficial lymphatic vessels. Lymphangitis involving the lymphatic capillary plexuses of the skin is called capillary or reticular lymphangitis. Streptococci and pyogenic staphylococci are the most common causative organisms in lymphangitis.

Capillary (reticular) lymphangitis may occur in any part of the body. It is seen most characteristically in erysipelas. Capillary lymphagitis is marked by an intense hyperemia with exudation about the rich cutaneous lymphatic capillary plexuses. The lymphatic capillaries themselves may become plugged by clotting of the lymph within them. There is accompanying intense heat, moderate swelling and redness of the skin. Pain may be present or absent. The face is the area most commonly involved. If the infection occurs in the extremities, the capillary lymphangitis may be the starting point of a tubular lymphangitis. As a rule, the condition is self-limited, ending, after a few days, without suppura-

tion or necrosis. Occasionally it may be very virulent and rapidly fatal.

Tubular lymphangitis occurs almost exclusively in the extremities.[15.16] It is due to infection of lymphatic vessels draining a wounded, infected area. The wound may be very slight and often is not noticed or is forgotten. It is characterized by the appearance, sometime after the infliction of the wound, of subcutaneous red streaks coursing up an extremity, from the area of the wound to the nearest regional lymph nodes. If the involved lymph vessels are large, they may be felt as tender cords on palpation. The lymph nodes into which the inflamed vessels drain also react and become enlarged, tender and painful. Toxemia is often severe in such cases. The lymph node reaction may not occur until the acute tubular lymphangitis has subsided, so errors in diagnosis may arise, particularly if the initial wound has healed.

The involved lymph vessels are surrounded by a zone of hyperemia and exudate. The vessels may become obstructed by an accumulation of desquamated endothelial cells, leucocytes and coagulated lymph. Local abscesses may develop. A diffuse cellulitis may complicate the lymphangitis. Usually, prompt resolution follows the early and adequate treatment of the initial wound. On the other hand, with injudicious treatment or inability of the regional lymph nodes to cope with a particularly virulent organism (usually the streptococcus), the infection may rapidly develop within 48 hours into a serious, often fatal, systemic involvement from the entrance into the blood stream of the infecting organism and its toxins which constitutes the condition known as septicemia.

Chronic tubular lymphangitis may follow acute lymphangitis, but it more often is the result of repeated subacute attacks of infection.

DILATATION OF LYMPHATIC CAPILLARIES AND VESSELS

Dilatation of lymphatic vessels is found as lymphangiectasis, capillary lymphangioma, cavernous lymphangioma and solitary lymph cyst.

Acquired dilatation of lymphatic vessels

is due to obstruction of the main collecting lymphatics.

Lymphangiectasis may involve various parts of the body and lead to enlargement of the affected part. It is most commonly seen in the tongue (macroglossia) [17] and lip (macrocheilia).[18] It may occasionally involve the subcutaneous lymphatics of an extremity (Milroy's disease).[19]

Capillary lymphangioma occurring in the skin is known as lymphatic nevus. This consists of brownish papules covered with small vesicles containing lymph.

Cavernous lymphangioma consists of an aggregation of lymphatic cysts. This condition is found most often in the neck and in the axilla. In the neck it is usually known as cystic hygroma and should be differentiated from lymphadenopathy.[20] Here it appears during early infancy or may be present at birth. Typically, the cystic hygroma occupies the lower part of the neck and may extend upward to the ear or downward behind the clavicle where it comes into relation with the cervical pleura. Cavernous lymphangioma is due to lack of communication, during development, between the primitive lymphatic system and the collecting lymphatic vessels or with the venous system.

OBSTRUCTION OF LYMPHATIC VESSELS

Lymphatic vessels may undergo obstruction from various causes. The end result is lymphatic edema which involves the region drained by the obstructed vessels. Lymphatic edema is characterized by little tendency to pit on pressure (so characteristic of venous obstruction), and by brawny induration of the subcutaneous tissues. Eventually, the skin becomes coarse and rough and the part involved often undergoes tremendous swelling (elephantiasis). Sometimes, lymphatic vesicles develop in the affected area, which may rupture and lead to ulceration and recurrent infection. Leakage of lymph is known as *lymphorrhea*.[21]

Congenital obstruction takes the form of lymphangiectasis, already described. Acquired obstruction[22] may result from:

1. Surgical procedures, such as radical mastectomy, extensive removal of the axillary lymph nodes and the division of lymphatic vessels, may result in massive lymphatic edema of the upper extremity. Similar effects may follow radiation therapy. Factitial proctitis is an example of a localized disorder by which radium therapy of malignancy of the cervix uteri may occasionally, as a complication, destroy the lymphatics of the rectum, producing lymphatic block, lymphedema and an annular type of rectal constriction.[186]

2. Inflammation, followed by fibrosis of the lymphatic vessels. This may occur following an attack of acute lymphangitis, recurring erysipelas, or certain persistent chronic infections, for example, tropical ulcers.

3. Neoplastic invasion of lymphatic vessels. Thus, in the case of breast cancer, obstruction of the subcutaneous lymphatics through their permeation by cancer cells leads to the formation of discrete nodules in the skin (orange peel or *peau d'orange*). Likewise, the brawny arm which develops some months or years after radical mastectomy for cancer may occur from lymphatic permeation by malignant cells. Invasion of the lymphatics of the ligaments of Cooper of the breast eventually results in gross retraction of the skin.

It is well to remember that rarely unilateral lymphedema may be the presenting manifestation of neoplasm, especially in older adults. The most frequent example of this is swelling of one lower extremity as a result of a lymphoma or carcinoma of the prostate.[187]

4. Parasitic infections. The most dramatic form of elephantiasis occurs in connection with infections by *Filaria sanguinis hominis*. The resulting lymphatic edema affects particularly the scrotum or the vulva and the lower extremity and there is enormous thickening of the subcutaneous tissues.

THE MAIN LYMPHATIC DUCTS

ANATOMY

The main lymphatic ducts include the following: (1) the right and the left jugular trunks, (2) the right and the left subclavian trunks, (3) the right and the left bronchomediastinal trunks, (4) the right lymphatic duct, (5) the intestinal trunk, (6) the right and the left lumbar trunks, and (7) the thoracic duct[14,54] (see Figs. 153 and 164).

The jugular trunk is formed on each

side of the *union of the efferents from the inferior deep cervical lymph nodes.* It terminates at the junction of the subclavian and the internal jugular veins. Instead of

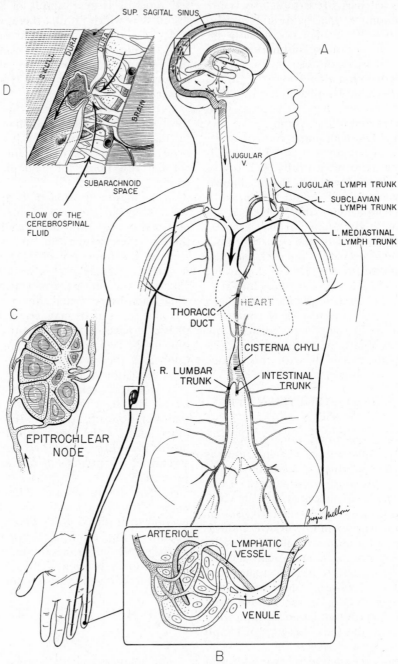

FIG. 153. A. Relation of lymphatic and cerebrospinal fluid systems to venous system. B. Diagram of the magnified view of the peripheral origin of the lymphatic vessels. C. Diagram of enlargement of lymph node intercalated in the lymphatic channels. D. Diagram of magnified view of a subarachnoid villus.

emptying independently into the systemic venous circulation it may join with the subclavian trunk to form the right lymphatic duct; on the left side, it may join the thoracic duct. The jugular trunk receives lymph from the inferior and the superior deep cervical nodes, the axillary nodes, the back of the scalp, the skin of the arm, and the pectoral region. The jugular trunk thus is concerned with the lymphatic drainage of the head, the neck, the arm, and part of the thorax.

The subclavian trunk is formed on each side by the union of the efferents from the apical axillary (infraclavicular) lymph nodes. It terminates, on the right side, in the subclavian vein or joins the right jugular trunk to form the right lymphatic duct; on the left side, it either joins the thoracic duct or empties independently into the left subclavian vein. The subclavian trunk receives lymph by way of the axillary nodes from the upper extremity, the posterior surface of the thorax, the mammary gland, the front of the chest, and the lateral wall of the chest.

The bronchomediastinal trunk is formed on each side by the union of the efferents from the tracheobronchial and the superior mediastinal nodes. While it usually terminates in the subclavian vein, it may join the right lymphatic or the thoracic duct. The bronchomediastinal trunk receives lymph from the lungs, the bronchi, the trachea, the esophagus, and the heart.

The right lymphatic duct is formed on the right side, at the root of the neck, by the junction of the right jugular, the right subclavian and the right bronchomediastinal ducts. It may be absent if one or more of these open independently into the right internal jugular, the right subclavian or the left innominate veins, respectively.

The right lymphatic duct is concerned with the lymphatic drainage of the right half of the head and neck, the right upper extremity and mammary gland and the right half of the thorax. When present, it is about half an inch long. Its tributaries normally communicate with the thoracic duct. Its importance thus lies in the fact that it provides an alternate route for passage of lymph into the systemic venous circulation in cases of obstruction of the thoracic duct.

The intestinal trunk is a single short trunk extending from the celiac preaortic nodes to the cisterna chyli. It may enter the latter independently but often joins the right or the left lumbar trunk. It receives lymph from the preaortic nodes (celiac, superior and inferior mesenteric) and hence is concerned with the lymphatic drainage of the lower part of the esophagus, the stomach, the liver and the gallbladder, the pancreas, the small and the large intestines, exclusive of the anal canal.

The lumbar trunks, right and left, are two short lymphatic vessels extending from the upper para-aortic nodes on each side of the abdominal aorta to the cisterna chyli. The left lumbar trunk passes behind the abdominal aorta. They are concerned with the lymphatic drainage of the lower extremities, the perineum, the pelvis and the pelvic organs, the kidneys, the suprarenals and the deep structures of the abdominal walls.

The thoracic duct is the main collecting duct of the lymphatic system.[2] It transports lymph to the systemic venous system from both lower extremities, the perineum, the pelvic and the abdominal organs, the abdominal walls, and the right half of the body above the xiphisternal junction.

The thoracic duct extends from the cisterna chyli to the root of the neck. The cisterna chyli is a lymph sac about 2 inches long, lying in front of the 1st and the 2nd lumbar vertebrae, beneath the diaphragm. It is formed mainly by the confluence of the intestinal and the two lumbar lymphatic ducts.

The thoracic duct measures 16 to 18 in. (40 to 45 cm.) in length and approximately $\frac{1}{8}$ in. (0.3 cm.) in width. However, its caliber is not uniform.

Structurally, the thoracic duct resembles a vein, differing from the latter by a greater content of smooth muscle and a greater number of bicuspid valves.

In its ascending course from the cisterna chyli, the thoracic duct is in close proximity to large arteries whose pulsations aid considerably in propelling the flow of lymph toward the root of the neck. Thus, the thoracic duct enters the posterior mediastinum by passing through the aortic hiatus of the diaphragm. Here it lies between the azygos vein and the aorta whose right border overlaps it. In the posterior mediastinum, it ascends in or near the midline, lying here on the thoracic vertebrae behind the esophagus and close to the right border of the descending thoracic aorta.

At about the level of the 4th or the 5th thoracic vertebra, it turns to the left and enters the superior mediastinum to ascend along the left border of the esophagus and behind the left subclavian artery. Upon reaching the root of the neck, it curves to the left behind the left common carotid artery, the vagus and the internal jugular vein. After a short downward course, it joins the beginning of the left innominate vein. Near its termination, the thoracic duct is joined by the left bronchomediastinal, the left subclavian and the left jugular lymphatic trunks. The mouth of the thoracic duct is guarded by a sentinel valve which prevents the entrance of blood into it during life. After death this valve no longer functions, so that at autopsy the terminal part of the thoracic duct may contain a variable amount of blood.

The tributaries of the thoracic duct are as follows:

1. In the abdomen it receives the intestinal and the right and the left lumbar trunks, and efferents from the intercostal lymph nodes of the lower six intercostal spaces.

2. In the thorax, it receives: (A) afferents from the right and the left paraortic and the retroperitoneal lymph nodes which enter it after passing through the crura of the diaphragm, (B) efferents from the posterior mediastinal nodes, and (C) efferents from the intercostal lymph nodes of the upper five or six intercostal spaces.

On the other hand, the thoracic duct sends afferents to the superior mediastinal nodes and has communications with the azygos system of veins. Both of these types of anastomoses are found chiefly above the level of the 8th thoracic vertebra. Below this level, the thoracic duct is a single tube. Therefore, traumatic injuries of the thoracic duct below the level of the eighth thoracic vertebra are prognostically far

more serious and may prove fatal unless the torn duct is ligated.

The thoracic duct may show important anomalies.[55] Thus, it may veer to the right and open into the right innominate vein. Or it may bifurcate, one branch opening into the left and the other into the right innominate vein.

Chylous Effusions

Since the thoracic duct drains lymph from the greater part of the body, its severance entails a considerable loss of fluid, fat and protein, and lymphocytes.[56] Hence such injuries are followed by: (1) Dehydration producing excessive thirst, decreasing urinary output and dry skin; (2) loss of weight due to rapid depletion of body fat depots; (3) marked weakness; (4) loss of fat-soluble vitamins A and D absorbed from the gastrointestinal tract; (5) striking drop in number or complete disappearance of lymphocytes in the circulating blood. This marked drop in the lymphocyte count can be of great diagnostic value, especially in accident cases with chest injury but no evidence of injury to the thoracic duct; (6) loss of protein.

To these would be added the effects of compression by the accumulation of the extravasated lymph or chyle.

Extravasated lymph or chyle usually does not clot like blood, hence the wound may not heal. Consequently, life may be endangered unless operative repair or ligation of the duct is carried out. Because of the bacteriostatic action of lymph, severance of the thoracic duct is not accompanied by infection unless this is introduced by the traumatic agent.

Rupture of the thoracic duct may result from trauma, operative procedures, or obstruction. It may occur in the cervical, the thoracic or the abdominal segments of the thoracic duct.

Chylous effusions into the root of the neck may result from trauma and embolism, as well as operations on the neck by the anterior approach. The extravasated lymph or chyle accumulates in the lower part of the neck, and since it does not clot it forms a doughy swelling. Cervical chylous effusions rarely are associated with thrombosis of the neck veins.

Rupture of the duct in its thoracic course may be due to trauma or certain operations such as thoracic sympathectomy, pneumonectomy, rib resection, and thoracolysis. In such cases, the chylous effusion first involves the mediastinum and finally one or both pleural cavities with resulting chylothorax.[56] The chylous effusion usually assumes such proportions that compression of one or both lungs leads to serious embarrassment of respiration. Compression of the thoracic vessels may lead to vascular collapse, resembling shock from hemorrhage. Chyle extravasated into the pleural cavity causes an inflammatory reaction resulting in thickening of the pleura with loss of its elasticity and deposition on its surface of heavy exudate.

In the abdominal cavity, chylous effusions are usually due to obstruction, with consequent increase in the intraductal pressure, dilatation and rupture of the distal afferents of the thoracic duct. The chylous effusion may enter the peritoneal cavity, with resulting chylous ascites (chyloperitoneum), or the urinary passages, with the occurrence of chyluria.[57]

Chylous fluid obtained by aspiration in cases of chylous effusions has the following characteristics; it is a milklike fluid that forms three layers on standing; an upper "cream" layer, a middle "milk" layer and a lower sediment layer, consisting chiefly of cellular elements. On standing for a long time, a small coagulum forms. The specific gravity varies from 1.016 to 1.025. The protein content varies from 3 to 6 Gm. per 100 ml.[56]

STRUCTURE OF LYMPH NODES

A lymph node is made up of (1) a connective tissue framework, (2) lymphoid tissue, (3) reticuloendothelial tissue, and (4) a system of sinuses (see Fig. 154).

The connective tissue framework consists of a capsule, trabeculae and a groundwork of reticular fibers. The capsule forms a dense envelope for the node peripherally. It is particularly well developed at the hilus where it may extend for some distance into

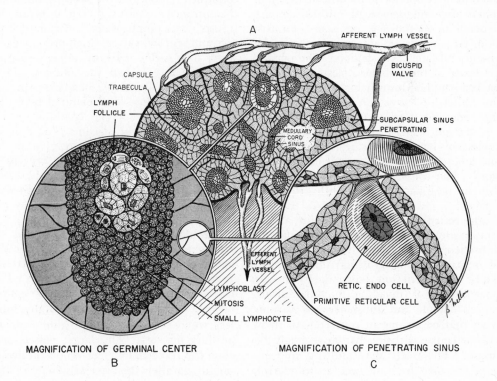

Fig. 154. Diagram of the structure of a lymph node.

the medullary portion of the node. The capsule is made up chiefly of collagenous fibers with some fibroblasts, and a smaller amount of elastic fibers. It also contains smooth muscle, particularly at the sites of entry and exit of the afferent and the efferent vessels. The trabeculae extend into the cortical portion of the node from the deep surface of the capsule. In the medullary portion of the node, the trabeculae anastomose into a meshwork which fuses with the hilar portion of the capsule. The groundwork consists of a fine mesh of reticular fibers which penetrate all parts of the node, forming especially dense networks about the lymph follicles, blood vessels and on the deep surface of the capsule.

The lymphoid tissue of the node is disposed in two forms: the lymph follicles and the medullary cords. The follicles are aggregated under the capsule and constitute the cortex of the node. Each follicle contains a central pale area—the germinal center and a darker peripheral zone. The germinal center contains lymphoblasts, and a few macrophages. It is concerned with the production of lymphocytes by mitotic division. Their size and degree of mitotic activity depends upon the age, the state of nutrition, etc., of the organism. They may be absent and later form de novo. The peripheral part of the follicle consists of densely packed lymphocytes which continually leave the follicle to enter the lymph sinuses of the node and thus leave the node through the efferent vessels. The medullary cords consist of lymphoid tissue. They branch and anastomose to form a wide-meshed network. The cords are continuous with the follicles peripherally; at the hilus they end freely.

The reticuloendothelial cells line all the lymph sinuses of the nodes, covering not only their walls but also the fine trabeculae of reticular fibers crossing their lumen. These cells function particularly in the phagocytosis of invading microorganisms, cancer emboli and substances of various types that may come in contact with them as they course with the lymph through the sinuses. These cells may multiply and enlarge, become free and act as wandering macrophages. Through their phagocytic action they play an important part in the defense of the body against disease.

The lymphatic sinuses of the node consist of (1) subcapsular or marginal sinus, (2) the penetrating or the trabecular sinuses, and (3) the medullary sinuses. All these sinuses communicate with one another. The subcapsular sinus lies just beneath the capsule. It receives lymph from the afferent vessels of the node and transmits it to the penetrating or trabecular sinuses. The latter accompany the trabeculae. The medullary sinuses are particularly wide and surround the medullary cords. From them the lymph passes into the efferent vessels. All the lymph sinuses are traversed by myriads of interconnecting reticular fibers which transform the sinuses into labyrinthine passages in which the flow of lymph is slowed markedly.

Lymph Vessels. Lymph is conducted to the node by afferent and from it by efferent lymph vessels. The afferent vessels, several in number, enter the capsule at various points of its periphery and discharge their contained lymph into the subcapsular sinus, the entrance area for a system of intranodal sinuses. The points of entry are guarded by bicuspid sentinel valves which prevent backward flow. The efferent vessels, one or more, are larger than the afferent. They receive lymph from the medullary sinuses. The speed of flow is accelerated here due to the reduction in the combined cross-sectional area of the stream. The mouths of the efferent vessels also are guarded by bicuspid sentinel valves which prevent a retrograde flow of lymph into the node when the vessels contract by activation of their own musculature or when they are compressed by neighboring muscles.

The blood supply of lymph nodes is derived chiefly from arteries which enter the node through its hilus. Some small arteries enter the node through the capsule. The smaller arteries and the veins course through the medullary cords to the follicles, where they break up into a dense capillary network. The larger vessels pass along the trabeculae. The venous drainage roughly parallels the arterial system.

Nerves to the lymph node are both sensory and motor. Sensory nerves ramify within the capsule; rapid enlargement of a node may produce pain. The motor nerves are postganglionic sympathetic fibers. They enter at the hilus with the blood vessels and follow these throughout. The reader is referred to standard histology texts for more detailed information.

AGE CHANGES IN LYMPHOID TISSUE

The amount of lymphoid tissue and general distribution of lymph nodes bears a definite relation to age.[35] The curve of growth of lymphoid tissue is highest in infancy and continues at a high level throughout childhood. It reaches its peak about puberty and declines thereafter. At 2 years of age the child has 50 per cent of the lymphoid tissue of a 20-year-old person; at 4 years 80 per cent; at 8 years 120 per cent; at 12 years 190 per cent; at 16 years 120 per cent. The maximal development of lymphoid tissue occurs during the time when acute infections of the respiratory and the alimentary tracts are most common and during the period of greatest increase in weight and height. This suggests that it is part of a natural defense mechanism. During infancy and childhood, moreover, lymphoid tissue responds characteristically to infection by prompt and excessive swelling and hyperplasia. With advancing age, such dramatic changes become less frequent.

Lymph nodes are more numerous and larger in children than in adults. There is marked hypertrophy during childhood and involution during adult life. However, there is no real atrophy, as a rule, since at any age local or generalized infections may induce hypertrophy. Involutional changes in the lymph nodes consist of reduction in the size of the nodes and of the germinal centers accompanied by infiltration with fat.

The fact that certain groups of lymph nodes disappear in adult life and that certain areas of lymphoid tissue, while they do not disappear, undergo involution, is of practical significance since it serves to explain the relative incidence of certain pathologic conditions with reference to age.

Perhaps the most significant diseases from this point of view are: adenoiditis, tonsillitis, retropharyngeal abscess, appendicitis and mesenteric adenitis.

Adenoid tissue is present in the nasopharynx at birth. It increases in size and reaches its maximum at 3 to 5 years of age. Hypertrophy during infancy is a normal physiologic process and must not be interpreted as pathologic unless there is evidence of infection (*adenoiditis*). A regressive process eliminates the adenoid tissue of the nasopharynx (pharyngeal tonsil) as a source of obstruction in older children.

The palatine tonsils are present in the newborn. They gradually increase in size during the second and the third years, and become relatively smaller after the age of 5 years. This age corresponds with the marked reduction in the incidence of *tonsillitis* after this age.

Retropharyngeal abscess occurs most commonly in infants up to the age of 2½ or 3 years and more rarely in older children. Such abscesses are due to pyogenic infections of the small retropharyngeal lymph nodes which lie on either side of the midline between the posterior wall of the pharynx and the prevertebral fascia. These nodes undergo involution early in life.

Appendicitis occurs most commonly in childhood, adolescence and early adulthood. In childhood, it is an important pathologic condition, being the most common lesion requiring intra-abdominal surgery. It is rare during infancy but becomes more common after the age of 2 years. This relation between the incidence of appendicitis and age definitely is correlated with the fact that in early life the appendix contains much lymphoid tissue, disposed in the form of a circumferential aggregation of lymph follicles, which is especially prone to infection. The subsequent atrophy of this tissue accounts to a high degree for the markedly reduced frequency of appendicitis in later years.

The mesenteric nodes are more hyperplastic in childhood and adolescence than in adult life. Correspondingly, *mesenteric adenitis,* both acute or chronic, occurs usually between the ages of 3 and 13 years.

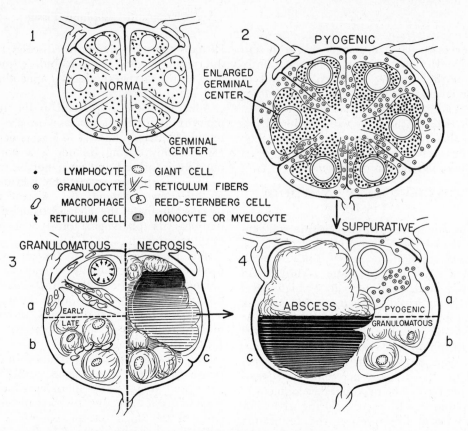

FIG. 155. Diagrammatic schema of lymph node pathology.

1. The normal lymph node shows the subcapsular and the medullary lymphatic spaces that also traverse the cortical zone (in white). The capsule and the fibrous supporting septa are in heavy black. The lymphoid pulp is indicated by dots which represent various stages of lymphocytes from lymphoblasts to small lymphocytes. The germinal centers are shown in the cortex as circles. (See legend for explanation of symbols depicting various types of cells to be referred to later.)

2. Acute pyogenic lymphadenitis. In this diagram the lymphatic sinuses of the node are dilated and engorged with granulocytes (polymorphonuclear leukocytes) represented by small circles with a central dot. The germinal centers are moderately hyperplastic, indicated by double circles. The lymphocytes in the pulp are packed more tightly. The architecture of the lymph node is intact.

3. Granulomatous lymphadenitis. The various stages of development of granulomatous reaction. In segment a, the dilated lymphatics are filled with histiocytes or macrophages. The germinal centers are preserved and enlarged slightly. The pulp contains reticulum cells, the forerunner of the histiocytes, and these also are increased in the germinal centers. Often this is referred to as a reactive lymph node. In segment b, the architecture of the node is replaced entirely by granulomas having a tubercle or tuberclelike structure. These are represented by ball-like masses with a central giant cell (small circles with peripheral dots for nuclei). In segment c, the granulomatous masses are being replaced by caseation necrosis (lighter parallel lines) which, in the upper portion is undergoing liquefaction necrosis (heavier parallel lines).

4. Suppurative lymphadenitis. This usually occurs as an end stage in certain types of acute pyogenic lymphadenitis and perhaps occasionally in granulomatous adenitis as indicated by the arrows. To the left is shown abscess forma-

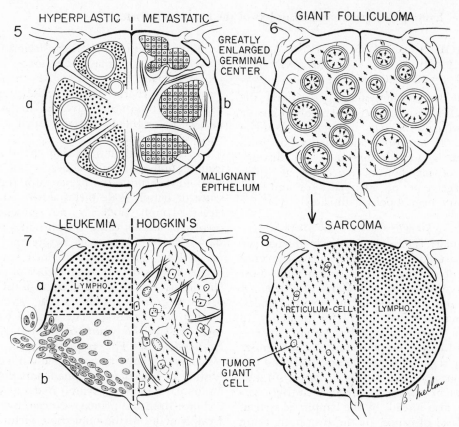

tion. To the right, 4a, is shown the transition of abscess from pyogenic lymphadenitis; below, 4b, from granulomatous lymphadenitis.

5. Chronic hyperplastic lymphadenitis. This represents the hyperplastic response to chronic nonsuppurative infection. The germinal centers are increased in number and enlarged. This is indicated by the double circle. The pulp is increased in amount and crowded with lymphocytes. Polys might occur in the sinuses. b. Metastatic carcinoma. *Above:* An early stage of metastasis is shown with epithelial cells infiltrating the subcapsular lymphatics. *Below:* Islands of malignant epithelial cells are replacing the normal lymphoid architecture and are stimulating fibrosis.

6. Giant folliculoma or Brill-Symmers disease. This is a low-grade malignancy. The germinal centers are increased tremendously in size and number, enlarging the node, at times, to giant size. Reticulum cells are increased in both the germinal centers and the pulp. Ultimately the entire node is replaced by reticulum cells, giving rise to full-blown reticulum-cell sarcoma, as indicated by the arrow. Occasionally the node may assume the character of lymphosarcomatous Hodgkin's disease.

7. This diagram shows leukemic infiltration of the lymph node to the left, and Hodgkin's disease to the right, both of which are malignant. Leukemia. (*Left,* a and b) The entire lymph node is replaced by various types of white cells. These may be myelocytes, lymphocytes, monocytes, or more malignant blast forms, referred to as stem cells. Plasma-cell myeloma or plasma-cell leukemia may also show similar infiltration. The capsule is invaded and the surrounding fat is infiltrated. Hodgkin's Disease. (*Right*) This is the most variable histologic picture seen in the lymph node with destruction of the pre-existing normal architecture. The stromal or ground substance of the lymph node is

(*Continued on p. 486*)

MODES OF INVOLVEMENT OF LYMPHATIC SYSTEM AND PATHOLOGIC CHANGES

The lymphatic system, particularly the lymph nodes, may become involved in the following ways: (1) carcinomatous invasion; (2) infectious adenopathy; (3) infiltration by foreign substance; (4) disturbance of metabolism, especially of lipids (storage type of adenopathy); and (5) primary hematopoietic disease.

CARCINOMATOUS INVASION

Primary carcinoma of the lymphatic system is unknown. Consequently, the presence of carcinoma in a lymph node must be considered as secondary to cancer of some organ drained by the involved nodes. Carcinoma has a special tendency to spread by the lymphatic system, as evidenced by the preponderance of metastases to the regional lymph nodes; therefore meticulous node extirpation is part of surgical treatment. Lymphosarcoma, unlike sarcoma, also spreads by the lymphatic system.

Spread of cancer by the lymphatic route may occur by permeation or cancer cell emboli.[24] In permeation, the cancer cells, after reaching the lymphatic capillaries, invade their lumina and then spread along the lymph streams. Embolic spread is the predominant form of lymphatic spread of cancer. The emboli are filtered from the lymph stream by the lymph nodes. At first, they become arrested in the subcapsular sinus but eventually the metastatic cancer may completely replace the node[25] (Fig. 155). The metastatic cancer has the same morphologic characteristics as the primary cancer. Metastatically involved nodes are subject to secondary changes, such as necrosis and fibrosis.

It must be emphasized that the clinical examination of lymph nodes is not sufficient to determine the presence or the absence of lymph node metastases.[26] An enlarged lymph node is not necessarily involved metastatically; lymph nodes often show reactive hyperplasia before they are invaded by cancer emboli. Such reactive hyperplasia is due to phagocytosis of cellular debris resulting from necrosis of the primary growth. This is the so-called *foreign body reaction.* The affected lymph node presents the picture of *granulomatous lymphadenitis.* The primary cancer may also serve as an entrance site for infection leading to infectious lymphadenopathy. It occurs particularly in lymph nodes at some distance from the primary cancerous focus. Lymph nodes in the immediate vicinity of the cancerous focus may show no reactive hyperplasia and therefore, may not be enlarged and yet contain cancer emboli. Enlarged nodes due to reactive hyperplasia, without cancer emboli, represent a basis for considerable improvement in prognosis.

Atypical lymph nodes may be reached by metastases through lymphatic vessels draining an organ that has become involved

---

FIG. 155. (*Continued*)

increased, as shown by the irregular black bands. Germinal centers and lymphoid pulp are replaced by malignant reticulum cells which differentiate to macrophages or histiocytes, many of them binucleated to form a characteristic tumor giant cell, known as the Reed-Sternberg cell. The latter are indicated in the diagram by double or overlapping cytoplasmic squares with enlarged nuclei. The cytoplasm is often indistinct. The identity of the malignant reticulum cells is disputed, and sometimes they are referred to as retrothelial cells. Typical foreign body giant cells also may be present. An increased number of eosinophils infiltrate the node in a minority of the cases.

8. Reticulum cell sarcoma. The lymph node is replaced completely by a diffuse proliferation of reticulum cells with the occasional formation of tumor giant cells. Lymphosarcoma. The lymph node is replaced entirely by a proliferation of lymphocytes or, at times, lymphoblasts. The identical picture is seen in the lymph nodes in cases of lymphocytic or lymphoblastic leukemia. (Diagrams and legends prepared by Dr. Charles F. Geschickter, Department of Pathology, Georgetown University School of Medicine.)

secondarily by cancer by the hematogenous route.[27]

INFECTIOUS ADENOPATHY

The lymphatic system may be invaded by acute or chronic infectious processes, which may affect both the lymphatic vessels as well as the nodes.

The involvement may be due to the entrance into the lymph stream of viruses, bacteria or parasites or to transportation of toxic substances from foci of infection.

The morphology of the inflammatory reaction depends chiefly on the nature of the infecting organism and the resistance of the patient.

In acute inflammation, the lymph nodes become enlarged, tender, soft and elevated.[28] The overlying skin is reddened and surrounding tissues are edematous and infiltrated. The lymph nodes present the histologic picture of acute pyogenic lymphadenitis (Fig. 155). On section, the nodes are hyperemic and bulge above the cut surfaces. There may be small hemorrhages or areas of necrosis. The lymph sinuses of the involved node contain polymorphonuclear leucocytes from the blood stream and macrophages derived from the reticuloendothelial cells. Both may contain bacteria, dead cells or tissue fragments. If the infection is overcome, regressive changes will take place. On the other hand, the infective process may lead to suppuration and abscess formation.[29] If suppuration occurs, sinuses may open on the surface and the infection may spread to the next group of nodes and eventually reach the systemic venous circulation. Suppurative lymphadenitis may represent the terminal stage of an acute pyogenic lymphadenitis or a granulomatous lymphadenitis (Fig. 155).

In chronic infections, the enlarged lymph nodes are often not accompanied by edema and tenderness. The nodes are more or less firm depending on the degree of fibrosis. The lymph sinuses contain a large number of phagocytes and fewer polymorphonuclears. Among the lymphocytes are found mononuclears and plasma cells. Mitoses are frequent. Reticulum cells also proliferate. There are various degrees of fibrosis. The germinal centers are enlarged.[30]

Granulomatous Lymphadenitis. In various infections caused by bacteria (e.g., tuberculosis, leprosy, typhoid fever), fungi (e.g., histoplasmosis, actinomycosis, blastomycosis, sporotrichosis, cryptococcosis, torulosis and coccidioidomycosis), and viruses (e.g., lymphopathia venereum, ? cat scratch disease), the histologic picture presented by the involved lymph nodes is that of granulomatous lymphadenitis, characterized by the replacement of the architecture of the node by granulomas having a tubercle or tuberclelike structure. The granulomas consist of firm nodules of newly formed connective tissue. Macrophages enlarge to form epithelioid cells, some of which may fuse to form Langhans giant cells. If several granulomas coalesce, the center may undergo necrosis, the surrounding structures being stimulated to form new blood vessels and connective tissue. Eventually, there is scarring.[31]

INFILTRATIVE INVASION

This type of involvement of the lymphatic system occurs prominently in the respiratory system and is associated with the inhaling of dust particles (coal, silica, etc.).[32] Such dust particles are removed from the pulmonary alveoli by macrophages. The dust-laden macrophages then migrate into the interalveolar septa and enter the interlobular and the perivascular lymphatics. In time, the lymphatics of the lung become filled with the dust-laden macrophages with the development of an obstructive lymphangitis. Many of these macrophages eventually migrate to the bronchial lymph nodes. Upon degeneration of the macrophages, the freed dust particles are now taken up by the reticuloendothelial cells of the nodes. Due to reactive changes, a slow proliferation of fibroblasts and formation of a considerable quantity of collagenous fibers follows. Eventually, there is not only more or less extensive replacement of the lung parenchyma, but also obstruction of the pulmonary circulation.

Infiltrative adenopathy is seen particularly in anthracosis, silicosis and chalicosis.

The histologic picture of the affected nodes is that of *granulomatous lymphadenitis* (Fig. 155).

METABOLIC DISTURBANCES

In certain pathologic states associated with disturbances in metabolism of lipids, the reticuloendothelial cells of lymph nodes (and other organs) become engorged with various types of lipids.[33] Such lipoid-storing reticuloendothelial cells are very characteristic. They are large and their cytoplasm is filled with globules of lipid, giving the cell a vacuolated appearance. Hence, these cells are called "foam" cells. The lipids chiefly involved are cerebroside, phosphatide and cholesterol. Since these pathologic states are characterized by hyperplasia of the reticulum cells filled with lipid granules, the condition may be called a lipidosis, lipid histiocytosis or lipid reticulosis. Since the accumulations of lipid-laden macrophages impart to the organs in which they occur a yellow discoloration, the lipidoses also are referred to as xanthomatoses.

The anatomoclinical features of the various types of lipidoses are dominated by the specific lipid involved, by the disturbed fat metabolism and the effects of the xanthomatous accumulations in the tissues of the body. The altered lipid metabolism may be secondary or primary.

In the primary lipidoses the anatomic and functional changes related to the lipoid storage are so constant and specific that they are recognized as disease entities. There are two well-defined primary lipidoses: (1) Gaucher's disease, and (2) Niemann-Pick's disease. Both are congenital and familial and occur almost exclusively in Jewish infants and children. Both pursue a course that is ultimately fatal.

In Gaucher's disease, the essential lipid disturbance affects the metabolism of the galactolipin kerasin.[34] This lipid is a cerebroside and stored in the reticuloendothelial cells of the body. While the accumulation of the foam cells are focal they are generalized in distribution. The foam cells are very large, contain one or more nuclei, and the cytoplasm has a peculiar fibrillary or weblike structure seen in no other lipidosis. Accumulation of foam cells

leads to generalized enlargement of lymph nodes, both superficial and deep. The spleen becomes enlarged enormously. Foam cells fill the lymph sinuses of the nodes. Here they are not distributed diffusely but tend to form nodular accumulations. The germinal centers are hyperplastic. Since the pathologic picture is essentially a storage phenomenon, there are no mitoses visible. The architecture of the nodes is not disturbed. The lipid kerasin cannot be demonstrated histologically by ordinary neutral fat dyes. It also does not rotate the plane of polarized light. Eventually, the foam cells disintegrate, and the liberated kerasin stimulates the proliferation of fibroblasts with consequent development of granulomatous lymphadenitis.

In Niemann-Pick's disease there is a pronounced cholesterolemia (over 500 mg. per 100 ml.). The lipid chiefly and specifically involved in this type of lipidosis is the phosphatide lecithin.[23,33] The foam cells are large and pale yellow. Their cytoplasm is filled with small round drops of lecithin arranged in a typical mulberry-like crustation. The stored lipid stains a dark dirty red with Sudan III and is anisotropic. The foam cells fill the lymph sinuses of lymph nodes.[33] There is no alteration of the architecture of the nodes except that the foam cells are distributed in nodular collections. There is enlargement of the superficial nodes. In addition, the intra-abdominal lymph nodes particularly (especially the hepatic, the pancreatic, the splenic and the mesenteric) are filled with foam cells and hence considerably enlarged. There are no mitoses.

Two other diseases have been classified as lipid storage disease: the Hand-Schüller-Christian and Letterer-Siwe's diseases. In Hand-Schüller-Christian disease the lymph nodes are enlarged moderately, although marked lymphadenopathy may occur.[36] The lesions in the nodes and elsewhere are filled with large mononuclear cells containing much cholesterol and fatty acids. However, there are several factors which indicate that this disease is not a lipid storage disease. Thus, the level of cholesterol in the blood plasma is normal; there is absence of evidence of lipid storage early in the disease; the early lesions are granulomatous in character; and finally the lesions eventually heal by connective tissue replacement. These findings favor the view that Hand-Schüller-Christian disease is an inflammatory granuloma.[37] However, so far no causative organism has been found by bacteriologic and animal inoculation studies.

Letterer-Siwe's disease also is not a true lipid storage disease.[38] While there is generalized lymphadenopathy, the essential pathologic change is a diffuse granulomatous process which is identical in all important respects with the early lesion in Hand-Schüller-Christian disease. Letterer-Siwe's disease is thus apparently a more acute and severe form of Hand-Schüller-Christian disease.

Eosinophilic granuloma[39] is a condition similar in gross pathology and microscopic appearance to Hand-Schüller-Christian disease. The etiology of these three conditions and their relation to each other is not clear.[40]

Secondary lipidosis may occur in connection with diabetes mellitus, jaundice or nephritis. Whenever cholesterolemia occurs in diabetes mellitus, typical foam cells containing cholesterol or cholesterol esters may appear in the lymph nodes and other organs. In obstruction of the biliary passage for a considerable time, as in chronic pancreatitis, the blood cholesterol becomes raised with lipid (cholesterol) storage in the reticuloendothelial cells.

Hypercholesterolemia also can be produced experimentally by the administration of large quantities of cholesterol in the food with the appearance of large depots of cholesterol in the reticuloendothelial cells.

Primary Hematopoietic Disease

Primary disease may involve the lymphatic, the leucocytic or the erythrocytic divisions of the hematopoietic system. Lymph nodes may become involved by primary tumors of lymphoid tissue (primary lymphomas) and by constitutional diseases (leukemias).

Primary tumors of the lymph nodes are all malignant. Such tumors may arise from the lymphoid or the reticuloendothelial elements of the nodes or their derivatives. The tumor may arise from these cells at any stage of their development. Primary tumors derived from the lymphoid elements include lymphosarcoma and Hodgkin's disease. Tumors arising from the reticuloendothelial cells are represented by reticulum cell sarcoma.

Lymphosarcoma is a progressive, eventually fatal neoplasm characterized by invasiveness, destructiveness and the formation of true metastases in various organs.[41,42] It arises not only in lymph nodes but also in the lymphoid tissue (tonsils, lymph follicles of intestines, etc.).[43] Unlike most sarcomas, lymphosarcoma spreads only by the lymphatics. New tumors develop in the direction of lymph flow.

The lymph nodes enlarge and fuse to form a matted chain. Due to invasion of surrounding structures and skin by tumor cells, adherent bulky growths result which may compress neighboring structures and produce embarrassment of respiration, dysphagia, venous obstruction, hydrothorax or intestinal obstruction.

The architecture of the lymph node becomes destroyed (Fig. 155). The germinal centers disappear and the stroma is diminished. The capsule and the trabeculae are infiltrated by neoplastic cells.

The tumor cells are uniform in size. They contain a large round or oval, notched, hyperchromatic, coarsely reticulated nucleus and a small amount of clear cytoplasm. There are numerous mitoses as well as occasional pathologic mitoses.

Giant Follicle Lymphoblastoma (Brill-Symmers Disease).[44,45] In this lymphoma there is a slowly progressive enlargement of a certain regional group of nodes, such as the inguinal or the axillary, or a gradual enlargement of all palpable nodes.

The nodes are characterized by an increase in the absolute number and size of the lymph follicles (Fig. 155). There is a tendency for the germinal centers to coalesce. The germinal centers show a marked proliferation of lymphoblasts and reticuloblasts. The stroma is sparse. The clinical course is often prolonged but is similar to that of malignant lymphoma.

Hodgkin's Disease. In this lymphoma

there is a slow, painless, insidious enlargement of the lymph nodes.[46,47] Most often the first to become involved are the cervical nodes. The next most commonly affected are the axillary, the mediastinal and the mesenteric. The involvement may be unilateral or bilateral. The nodes are at first discrete, movable, smooth, rubbery in consistency and measure 1 to 3 cm. in diameter. Later they become matted together to form large nodular masses. They seldom break down. Local pressure symptoms may arise, especially from enlarged mediastinal nodes (cough, dyspnea, dysphagia, pain, pleural effusions). Herpes may develop along the course of superficial nerves in the area of enlarged nodes.[47] Involvement of the lymphatics of the skin may lead to exfoliative dermatitis and pruritus.

The normal architecture of the nodes is destroyed (Fig. 155). The affected nodes show pleomorphic hyperplasia of lymphocytes and reticuloendothelial elements. The cellular elements include giant cells, eosinophils, polymorphonuclears and plasma cells. The giant cells (Reed-Sternberg cells) are pathognomonic. They are of varying size, with clear cytoplasm and hyperchromatic, irregular or horseshoe-shaped nucleus. They may be mononucleated, binucleated, or multinucleated. There is progressive fibrosis of the nodes due to production of fibroblasts.

When a whole group of nodes becomes involved, the characteristic cellular changes are seen best in a node from the center of the group. A node at the periphery of the group may show only follicular hyperplasia. This is important to remember in connection with biopsy studies.

Reticulum cell sarcoma may occur in diffuse or local form. There is enlargement of the regional and the mediastinal nodes.[48,49] It is often primary in the mediastinum. The architecture of the nodes is destroyed. The malignant cells are proliferating reticulum cells which show cytoplasmic processes forming anastomosing strands. Tumor giant cells may be present. There is an increase in reticular fibers (Fig. 155).

Lymphocytic leukemia is characterized by lymphoid hyperplasia and infiltration. The infiltration involves any part of the body where there is lymphoid tissue. There is also invasion of organs in which lymphoid tissue does not form part of the normal structure.[50] There is generalized lymphadenopathy. The nodes may enlarge singly or in chains. Individual nodes may vary in size from a few millimeters to 3 to 5 cm. Unlike Hodgkin's disease, there is no massive enlargement. The enlarged nodes are firm, rubbery in consistency, movable and not tender, possibly because lymphocytes are softer than red blood cells or fibrous tissue.[51] Since the capsule does not become invaded the nodes remain discrete, do not become matted together nor immobilized. The enlarged nodes may give rise to pressure symptoms from encroachment on neighboring viscera, blood vessels or nerves.

The normal architecture of the nodes is destroyed completely by the uniform dense infiltration with proliferating lymphocytes and lymphoblasts so that the involved nodes assume a homogeneous appearance (Fig. 155).

Monocytic leukemia is a neoplastic disease involving the monocyte. The lymph nodes generally are infiltrated with monoblasts and monocytes.[52] They may or may not be enlarged. However, palpable nodes are found in the majority of cases. The enlargement is not as extensive as in lymphoid leukemia.

Myeloid leukemia is a fatal neoplastic disease of the leukopoietic division of the hematopoietic system and is characterized by enormous proliferation of white blood cells of the myeloid series, originating in the bone marrow. Myeloblasts, premyelocytes and myelocytes dominate the picture at different stages of the disease.[53] There is infiltration not only of lymph nodes but also of almost all other organs and tissues of the body. This infiltration is most likely not mere invasion of the organs of the body by cells originating in the bone marrow and carried by the blood stream, but metaplasia of the reticuloendothelial system, i.e., reversion of this system to its fetal potentialities of producing leukocytes. Infiltration is seen in all lymph nodes, which however do not enlarge until the late stages of the disease. In most cases, the disease runs its entire course without evident enlargement, although infiltration with cells of the myeloid series may be widespread (Fig. 155). Since erythropoietic elements of the bone marrow are crowded out by proliferating myeloid cells, there are bleeding tendencies in the mucous membranes with epistaxis, melena, hematuria, menorrhagia, etc.

DIAGNOSTIC METHODS

LYMPHOGRAPHY

The lymphatic system plays a major role in various diseases, such as infections, metastatic cancer, and lymphomas. Hence, its opacification by radiopaque media and its roentgenographic visualization, known as lymphography, has become an important and useful diagnostic and therapeutic tool.

The term lymphography refers to the visualization of both lymphatic vessels and lymph nodes. Visualization of the lymphatic vessels alone is properly called lymphangiography, while visualization of the lymph nodes is termed lymphadenography. Since the modern method of roentgenographic visualization of the lymphatic system simultaneously demonstrates both lymphatic vessels and nodes, the term lymphography is preferred. This term is less cumbersome than the term lymphangioadenography.

Lymphography, in the past, has been practiced by a direct and an indirect approach. The indirect method consisted of the introduction of vital dyes or radiopaque media into the subcutaneous tissue or peritoneal cavity. While this method was used experimentally, it is of no value in human medical and surgical practice. The direct method has been applied in two forms:

1. The injection of radiopaque material directly into lymph nodes. Although enlarged palpable nodes can be directly injected through the intact skin, such injection into nonpalpable nodes requires surgical exposure, which is often necessarily extensive. Direct intranodal lymphography visualizes only a small portion of the lymphatic vessels and nodes in a particular region studied. There are also accompanying technical hazards associated with the extravasation of radiopaque material due to rupture of the injected node and associated lymphatic trunks, as well as leakage of the medium from the needle.

2. The presently used method of direct lymphography avoids these complications: first a peripheral lymph vessel is made visible by means of a vital dye and then radiopaque material is injected into the lymphatic vessels thus rendered visible. This method was first made practical by Kinmonth, Taylor, and Harper.[188] It has been modified in various ways by Wallace et al.[189] and others.

Technic. Lymphography, as practiced today, consists of the following steps: (1) the intradermal injection of a mixture of a vital dye and a local anesthetic (0.5 ml. of a 1-1 mixture) to make visible the local lymphatic vessels. Various vital dyes have been used, such as, patent blue violet, alphazurine 2G, brilliant blue, etc. The site of injection depends upon the area to be studied. In the lower extremity, the injection is made into the web space between the big and the 2nd toe (this will permit visualization of the lymphatic vessels accompanying the great saphenous vein) or that between the 4th and the 5th toes (for visualization of lymphatics following the lesser saphenous vein), or the injection can be made in each web space on the dorsum of the foot, to demonstrate simultaneously the lymph vessels accompanying the two saphenous veins. Each group of lymphatic vessels drains into its own group of lymph nodes. In the upper extremity, the injection is made in the web space between the thumb and the index finger (to demonstrate lymphatic vessels accompanying the cephalic vein) or that between the 4th and the 5th fingers (to demonstrate lymphatic vessels following the basilic vein). In the head, the injection can be made in two sites: the posterior auricular area for visualization of lymphatic vessels draining into the posterior cervical nodes, and the mental area for visualization of the anterior cervical group of lymph nodes. Since the vital dye is selectively absorbed by the local lymphatic vessels, the latter are thus readily rendered conspicuous. (2) Under aseptic surgical technic, the most

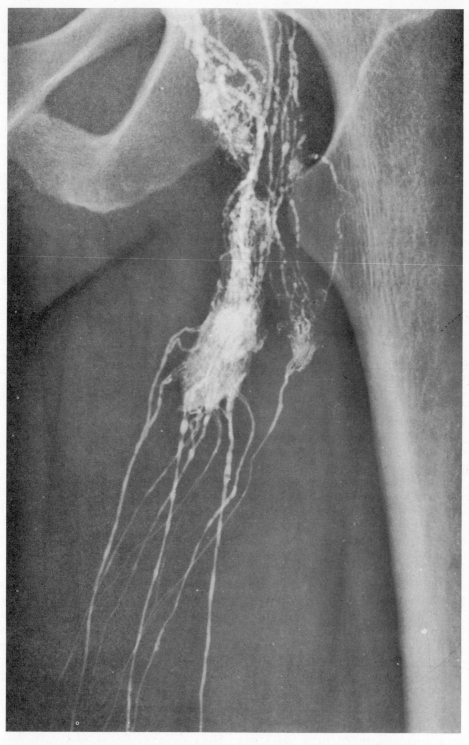

Fig. 156. Magnification radiograph of normal left superficial subinguinal lymph node with afferent and efferent lymphatic channels in a 40-year-old woman. (Isard, H. J., Ostrum, B. J., and Collinan, J. E.: Med. Radiograph Photography 38:92)

conspicuous of the visible lymphatic vessels is exposed by incision and isolated by blunt dissection. (3) The dissected lymphatic vessel is cannulated with a number 25 (or smaller) needle held in place by catgut ligatures. The needle is connected by means of polyethylene tubing to a small syringe, a low-pressure pump or a similar device. (4) Ethiodol (an ethyl ester of fatty acid of poppy seed oil containing 37% iodine) is now introduced into the cannulated lymphatic vessel under slow but continuous pressure. The injection usually takes from 1 to 1½ hours. (5) Following the injection of the Ethiodol, roentgenograms are made. These will show both the regional lymphatic vessels and the lymph nodes into which they drain. Roentgenography is repeated at the end of 24 hours. At this time, the lymphatic vessels are usually empty of the contrast medium, but the lymph nodes are maximally opacified. The contrast medium is retained by normal lymph nodes for 4 to 6 weeks; abnormal lymph nodes retain the contrast medium for a much longer period of time. This feature renders possible repeated roentgenography for a study of the effects of progressive disease or of therapeutic measures. Roentgenograms should be taken both frontally and obliquely. Stereoscopic roentgenograms may be desirable at times.

The normal lymphogram. Normally [190,191] peripheral lymph vessels are fine in caliber (usually less than 1 mm. in diameter), run parallel to the superficial veins (demonstrable by phlebography), and present a characteristic beaded appearance due to the presence of valves (Fig. 156). The lymphatic vessels bifurcate and anastomose with each other. They are of uniform diameter until they reach the pelvis, where they increase slightly in diameter. Ordinarily, when the injection is made unilaterally, lymphatics crossing over to the opposite side are demonstrable in the upper sacral and lumbar regions in the case of the lower extremity. This feature is highly significant in the planning and follow-up of radical surgery and therapy in the retroperitoneal region.

Normal lymph nodes, although usually present singly or in groups at certain locations, do not show a constant pattern. They vary both in number and size from patient to patient. There is also a dissimilarity between the two sides in the same patient. In size, nodes may measure up to 1.5 to 2 cm. in maximum diameter. The peripheral contour is regular and there is usually a slight indentation in the region of the hilus. In shape, normal nodes appear globular or reniform. Usually, 8 to 12 afferent vessels enter the node, the efferent vessels being fewer in number. The opacification of the normal node by the contrast medium is homogeneous, giving the node a fine reticular pattern in the roentgenogram.

Irregularities of nodal architecture, simulating neoplastic disease, may be observed in nodes in the absence of disease. Such irregularities consist primarily of filling defects produced by fatty infiltration or fibrous replacement consequent to previous infections. Such defects are seen most frequently in the femoral and the inguinal lymph nodes, which represent the primary drainage from the lower extremity. However, they may also occur in the iliac and para-aortic nodes. Small defects may be caused by hilar vessels, by superimposition of separate nodes, or by wrapping of the node around a blood vessel. Oblique and stereoscopic roentgenograms can often clarify the situation under such circumstances.

The Abnormal Lymphogram. Abnormalities of the lymphatic channels are observed in primary and secondary lymphedema and in lymphatic obstruction. Kinmonth et al.[197] described four types of lymph vessel abnormality in idiopathic lymphedema; hypoplasia, aplasia, dilatation and varicosity of lymphatic vessels.

Various roentgenographic abnormalities are produced by disease of the lymph nodes. Briefly, these consist of enlargement, filling defects, and irregularities of the marginal outline. These abnormalities are significant not only in the determination of the type of disease, but also of its extent.

Inflammatory Nodes. In nodes involved only by inflammatory processes, the significant roentgenographic findings are: (1) enlargement, the nodes usually measuring 2 to 4 cm. in diameter; (2) regularity of

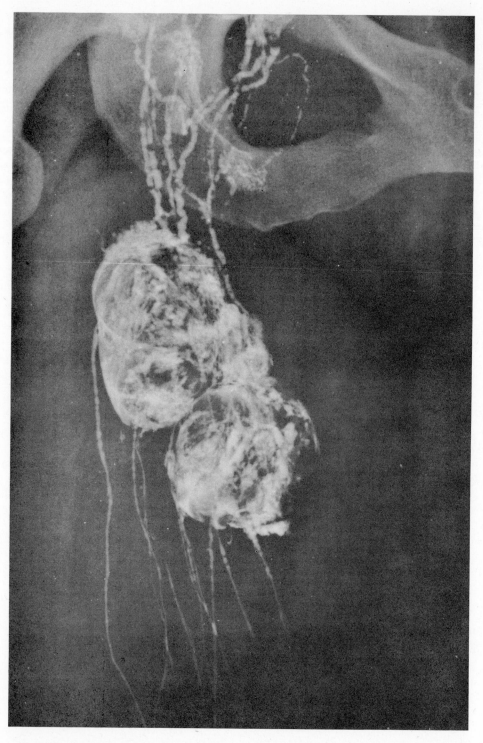

Fig. 157. Magnification radiograph of enlarged right superficial subinguinal lymph node with malignant infiltration secondary to primary melanoma of skin of heel (Same patient as Fig. 156). (Isard, H. J., Ostrum, B. J., and Cullinan, J. E.: Med. Radiography Photography 38:92)

peripheral contours; (3) normality of architecture. While opacification is not homogeneous, as is the case with normal nodes, intrinsically the inflammatory nodes present a finely reticular architecture.

Metastatic Nodes. Early metastatic lesions may not cause any abnormality. As a rule, a metastatic lesion, to be visible on the roentgenogram, must attain a diameter of at least 4 mm. If the node is completely filled with metastases, it is not visualized on the roentgenogram. However, its presence will nevertheless be revealed by deviating afferent vessels. Nodes which are partially occupied by metastases of sufficient size are characterized by: (1) filling defects along the margin of the node, so that the border presents a distinct irregularity in outline; and (2) dilatation of the afferent lymph vessels. Metastatic nodes may be normal in size or only slightly enlarged (Fig. 157). As a rule, not all the nodes of a particular group are visualized. This in itself is indicative of metastatic replacement.

Lymphomatous Nodes. In general lymphomatous nodes are characterized by enlargement and preservation of the normal marginal outlines. Various lymphomas affect the internal architecture differently. Thus, lymphosarcoma is associated with a foamy or lacy pattern, in addition to enlargement and normal peripheral contours. In Hodgkin's disease, enlargement is often great and the internal architecture presents scattered, punched-out areas of replacement within the center of the node. In chronic lymphatic leukemia, the roentgenogram shows areas of increased collection of opaque medium.

Complications.[198,199] As a rule, the use of lymphography is not attended by any significant complications. It has been shown repeatedly that lymphography is not associated with any functional or anatomical changes in the lymphatic vessels and lymph nodes. The minor complications, which may occur occasionally, consist of (1) transient lymphangitis, (2) local wound infection, and (3) fine pulmonary embolization. Perhaps the most serious complication is pulmonary embolization. However, it is rare and can easily be avoided by limiting the quantity of Ethiodol injected.

A possible complication that has been mentioned is the spread of tumor emboli caused by the lymphographic procedure itself. So far no actual case of such a complication has been reported. Its occurrence would be very difficult to substantiate. Iodine sensitivity is another possible complication.

Advantages of Lymphography. Lymphography has these distinct advantages:

1. It makes possible a more exact location of involved lymph nodes and indicates the status of such nodes.

2. It helps to demonstrate involved nodes in case of unsuspected disease.

3. It demonstrates unsuspected extension of malignancy.

4. It determines the feasibility of radical surgery.

5. It helps assess the degree of thoroughness of radical surgery. Here, it may be emphasized that Ethiodol may be combined with chlorophyll if nodal dissection is contemplated. The chlorophyll stains the nodes green. By this distinctive coloration, the dissection can be rendered more thorough than would otherwise be possible.

6. Since opacification of abnormal nodes persists for a long time, lymphography helps to follow the progress of the malignant nodal disease following radiotherapy or chemotherapy.

7. It aids in the detection of metastatic lesions in the absence of palpable nodes.

8. In urologic cases, it demonstrates the cause of displacement of the kidney and the ureters.[200]

9. It aids in the study of abnormalities of the thoracic duct.

10. It aids in differentiating between primary and secondary lymphedema.

SCINTIGRAPHY

Lymph nodes can be studied not only roentgenographically, after the intralymphatic injection of contrast medium, but also by the intralymphatic introduction of various isotopes. The sites of deposition of the isotope, as well as its concentration in the lymph nodes are recorded by means of a moving scintillation counter.[201] The scintigrams (radioisotope patterns of lymph node drainage) thus obtained are useful for the demonstration of anatomic, functional and pathologic pathways of lymphatic drainage. Scintigraphy permits serial or continuous observation of lymph node pickup over a period of at least 7 days. Secondary and variable routes of lymph node drainage can also be demonstrated.

Scintigraphy is of further value in the measurement of lymphatic circulation. This is accomplished by determining the rate of pickup of the isotope by the lymph nodes as well as by the disappearance rate of the isotope from the site of injection.

Compared with lymphography, scintigraphy, according to Lang,[202] is a less reli-

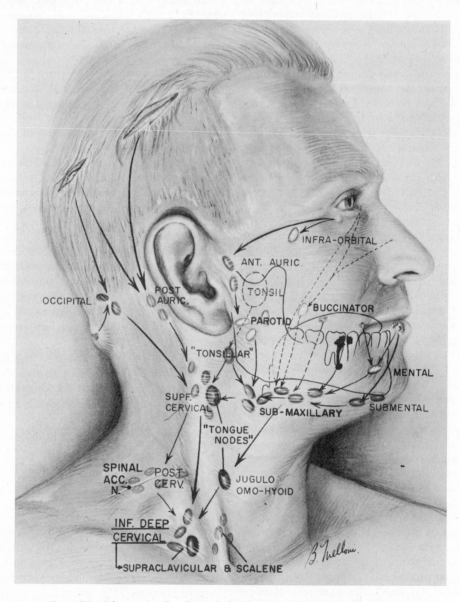

Fig. 158. Diagrammatic view of the lymph nodes of the head and the neck with direction and channels of lymph flow. Nodes indicated in dark color are those generally palpable clinically. Nodes in lighter color (infra-orbital, parotid, buccinator and mental) are either less constant or deeper and generally not detectable clinically.

able tool since lymphography in no instance gave a so-called false-positive result.

RADIOACTIVE LYMPHANGIOGRAPHY

Since it is possible to introduce radiopaque media into the lymphatic system for roentgenographic purposes, attempts have been made to use this method for the introduction into the lymphatic system of radioactive substances with the hope that such a procedure would directly affect local or metastatic malignant lesions. Thus, Fischer,[203] in a preliminary experiment on dogs, introduced radioactive colloid (gold[198] and silver-coated gold[198]) into the lymphatic vessels of the leg. They found that some balance in distribution of radioactive gold among the nodes of a region could be obtained by alternate intralymphatic injection of the colloid and a flushing solution, such as saline.

Seitzman et al.[204] utilized I[131] Ethiodol in cases of testis tumors on the premise that survival rates could be improved by any form of therapy which will increase the adequacy of the lymph node dissection or will destroy tumor cells in the lymphatics prior to their surgical excision. Such therapy would prevent the spillage of viable tumor cells during the dissection and increase the likelihood of death of viable tumor cells contained in lymph nodes left behind during radical surgery. The authors found that lymph nodes exhibited significant histologic effects of radiation. There were no complications. No deleterious effect of such irradiation on the hemopoietic system was observed. All other tissues examined failed to demonstrate significant radioactivity above background. The authors conclude that this technic is applicable in almost all cases of genitourinary tumors, but primarily those of the penis and testis and squamous cell carcinoma of the cervix; also for abdominal lymphomas, or any other malignancy metastasizing to the inguinal or retroperitoneal lymph nodes.

REGIONAL LYMPHADENOPATHY

In the following sections, lymphadenopathy involving various regions will be described, its pathologic physiology analyzed and clinical significance discussed.

LYMPH NODES OF HEAD AND NECK

Group 1—Clinically Important and Readily Palpable

Of the numerous lymph nodes of the head and the neck only the following are easily palpable when enlarged: (1) occipital, (2) posterior auricular, (3) anterior auricular, (4) "tonsillar" and other superior deep cervicals, (5) superficial cervicals, (6) submaxillary, (7) submental, (8) posterior cervical, (9) inferior deep cervicals (including the supraclavicular nodes, jugulo-omo-hyoid (tongue node), etc. The scalene nodes, although not palpable, belong in this group.

Any regional group of nodes may, of course, be involved in a disease producing a generalized lymphadenopathy, which fact will not be mentioned under each region, unless of special importance. Generalized lymphadenopathy will be discussed separately later. The sections under head and neck nodes will stress, instead, the clinical significance of enlargement of nodes in each area or certain combination of areas. Reference to Figure 158 while reading this section will help visualize the anatomic locations of nodes and their drainage areas.

1. The Occipital Nodes. ANATOMY. The occipital nodes, one to three in number, lie midway between the external occipital protuberance and the mastoid process, in close relation to the great occipital nerve, near the occipital insertion of the semispinalis capitis muscle. Enlarged occipital nodes may cause pressure on this nerve and neuralgia in its distribution. These nodes receive afferents from the back of the scalp and the back of the head and drain into the deep cervical nodes.

CLINICAL SIGNIFICANCE. Any infectious lesion in the scalp of this drainage area, whether localized or diffuse, may produce isolated occipital lymphadenopathy which, depending on the nature and the extent of the primary infection, may be unilateral or bilateral. A small primary lesion may be easily overlooked when the hair is heavy. Pediculosis capitis, which may be suspected from the presence of nits in the hair, and ringworm of the scalp are particularly common initiating conditions in children.

Being so readily detectable, occipital lymphadenopathy may be a conspicuous part of a generalized lymphadenopathy and for this reason is often the first node enlargement to be detected. At one time, painless occipital nodes, and also epitrochlear nodes without local reason, were considered suggestive of systemic syphilis. This is now a rare cause. Cancer with primary site in this drainage area is quite rare.

2. The Posterior Auricular Nodes. ANATOMY. The posterior auricular nodes, usually two in number, lie on the mastoid process behind the pinna of the external ear, on the insertion of the sternocleidomastoid muscle. They receive afferents from the external auditory meatus and the skin of the back of the pinna and of the temporal region of the scalp. They drain into the upper part of the superficial cervical nodes.

CLINICAL SIGNIFICANCE. Comments made about the occipital nodes with relation to scalp infections apply also to posterior auricular lymphadenopathy. If the primary scalp lesion of the drainage area is overlooked, pain, fever and local tenderness behind the ear may simulate mastoiditis, especially if the middle ear is injected or chronically infected. The auditory meatus as a site for an infectious process (or rarely, a neoplasm) should not be overlooked. The Ramsay-Hunt syndrome of herpes zoster may involve the auditory meatus with lymphadenopathy.

Enlargement of posterior auricular lymph nodes generally has been considered a characteristic and often diagnostically suggestive finding in rubella, accompanied at times by suboccipital and posterior cervical lymphadenopathy and less commonly by axillary and inguinal adenopathy. This may not always be true, as shown by the study of Kalmansohn[58] who found posterior cervical lymphadenopathy to be more common and often more marked in 100 adults with this disorder. At any rate, the frequent presence of marked posterior auricular lymphadenopathy in rubella (German measles) and the rarity of this sign in regular measles, is a finding of considerable diagnostic value.

3. Anterior Auricular Nodes. ANATOMY. The anterior auricular nodes lie immediately in front of the tragus, superficial to the parotidomasseteric fascia. They receive afferents from the lateral portion of the eyelids and its palpebral conjunctivae, from the skin of the temporal region, the external auditory meatus, and the anterior surface of the pinna of the external ear.

CLINICAL SIGNIFICANCE. The skin drainage area of this node is limited and conspicuously apparent, so that any infectious or neoplastic process is readily detected early. Particularly significant as primary lesions in this area are rodent ulcer, epithelioma, primary syphilitic chancre or any infectious skin disorder of the face. Erysipelas may at times produce significant lymphadenopathy because of its common initiation about the upper cheek and the eyelids.

Herpes zoster ophthalmicus commonly produces unilateral enlargement of the anterior auricular nodes[59] which, in fact, is considered part of the clinical picture. It has been noted at times before the appearance of the skin eruption and results from the primary viral infection, although subject to exacerbation when the skin vesicles become infected secondarily.

Diagnostically peculiar to this area is the association of lesions of eyelids and conjunctivae with anterior auricular lymphadenopathy, a clinical complex known as the *oculoglandular syndrome.*

Kalmansohn[58] noted anterior auricular lymphadenopathy in 52 per cent of adults in a large outbreak of German measles, coupled at times with ocular complaints and palpebral conjunctivitis.

Rice[60] reported a 27 per cent incidence of anterior auricular lymphadenopathy in a large series of 112 cases of trachoma with lid activity.

Oculoglandular Syndrome. It is well known that a wide variety of infecting organisms (especially the gonococcus) may produce acute purulent conjunctivitis endangering sight. The process as a rule is acute and regional lymphadenopathy not prominent. Of particular interest is the ability of the intact conjunctiva to be the site of entrance of a number of infectious agents which may produce a more chronic disorder characterized by involvement of the conjunctiva and significant lymphadenopathy of the anterior auricular nodes. Sometimes these disorders are characterized under the name "oculoglandular syndrome" or "Parinaud's syndrome" (not to be confused with the neurologic syndrome of Parinaud). The early description of a disorder in this group was that of a glandular type of conjunctivitis associated with painful and enlarged anterior auricular nodes with minimal systemic symptoms. A leptothrix organism was demonstrated in some cases by Verhoff[61] in 1913. There may be mild irregular fever, minimal systemic symptoms associated at times with mild blood eosinophilia. Lymphadenopathy commonly is limited to the anterior auricular group, which becomes painfully enlarged and rarely, as is true for all disorders in this group, involves nodes in the neck area, particularly in the submaxillary nodes which drain the inner aspect of the eyelids. Rarely the facial nodes and the infraorbital nodes may become involved also.

The virus of lymphopathia venereum may rarely be a cause of this syndrome.[62] Specific diagnosis by use of the Frei test is possible. Tularemia may occur as a pure oculoglandular syndrome[63] when the *Bacillus tularensis* enters the body through an intact conjunctiva. Nodular conjunctivitis, often ulcerative, followed by marked anterior auricular lymphadenopathy, extending at times to include the cervical nodes, follows. The systemic response and the ocular disability may last for weeks to months. Diagnosis by bacterial culture and agglutination tests usually firmly establishes the etiology. As a rule the systemic response of this form of tularemia is less marked than the usual type, with a consequent lower mortality.

A real advance in explaining obscure instances of the oculoglandular syndrome has been the recent demonstration that *cat-scratch fever*[64,205] may be manifested by conjunctivitis, with granulation, followed by anterior auricular lymphadenopathy and the usual systemic features of this disorder. A history of contact with cats is common. Diagnosis is possible by a specific skin test with antigen prepared from pus. The propensity of this type of lymphadenopathy to suppuration is well known.

Not to be overlooked is the possibility of tuberculosis, syphilis, or sporotrichosis which occasionally produce this syndrome and, more rarely still, other unusual infections such as glanders, chancroid, etc.[65-68] Neoplasm of the eyelid with regional anterior auricular metastasis can closely simulate the oculoglandular syndrome, particularly if the primary lesion on the eyelid is infected.

The viral disorder, *epidemic keratoconjunctivitis*[69] produces an oculoglandular syndrome, commonly unilateral. The more acute form is of about 2 weeks' duration accompanied by conjunctivitis with a watery discharge containing demonstrable lymphocytes. The absence of purulent discharge, in the presence of acute bulbar and palpebral conjunctival inflammation, occasionally with a pseudomembrane, with multiple cases occurring in an epidemic and the absence of a detectable organism in the eye by the usual bacteriologic technics are suggestive diagnostic criteria. A definitive diagnosis depends on special laboratory studies. The edematous erythema of the skin about the eye suggests infection of the reticular lymphatics and resembles erysipelas. In some cases corneal involvement damages sight. Anterior auricular nodes are large and tender in over 90 per cent of cases; such changes are occasionally followed by submaxillary and cervical lymphadenopathy. If present, systemic features are mild but rarely may be marked.[70]

The recently described pharyngoconjunctival fever of adenoidal-pharyngeal-conjunctival (APC) viral etiology is characterized by fever, various systemic complaints, nasopharyngitis and lymphadenopathy of cervical or submaxillary and occasionally anterior auricular groups of nodes.[71] It can be added to the already large group of disorders manifesting the oculoglandular syndrome.

Eyelid edema, occasional enlargement of lacrimal gland, slight conjunctival reaction, anterior auricular and occasionally submaxillary lymphadenopathy, all unilateral, may be an early phase of Chagas' disease of

South America and is known as the oculo-nodal complex (sign of Chagas-Romaña).[72] In this syndrome the eye is apparently the inoculation site for the etiologic agent contained in the excreta of the reduviid bug vector.[73]

In summary, the intact conjunctiva may serve as the portal of entrance for a variety of etiologic infectious agents carried to the area by finger contact, fomites, kissing, spray droplets, contact with cats, etc., producing conjunctivitis and regional anterior auricular lymphadenopathy with spread at times to cervical nodes and with varying systemic features. The submaxillary nodes, draining as they do the inner aspect of the eyelids, often are involved coincidently when the anterior auricular nodes are involved and should be searched for, since they are less conspicuous clinically. The nature of the primary inoculation makes unilateral involvement much more common than bilateral.

4. The Superior Deep Cervical Nodes, Including the "Tonsillar" and the "Tongue" (Jugulodigastric) Nodes. ANATOMY. The tonsillar node, the main node of the tonsil, belongs to the superior deep cervical nodes. This node lies below the angle of the mandible, between the internal jugular and the common facial veins, at the posterior side of the posterior belly of the digastricus.

The jugulodigastric node is an important node in the lymphatic drainage of the tongue, receiving afferents from the greater part of the tongue with the exception of the apex. It lies just below the great cornu of the hyoid bone, close to the bifurcation of the common carotid artery.

CLINICAL SIGNIFICANCE. The tonsillar node undergoes enlargement with infections of the palatine tonsil and, to some degree, of the pharynx. The jugulodigastric node undergoes enlargement due to neoplastic invasion by cancer involving the margins, the central and the posterior portions of the tongue.

5. Superficial Cervical Nodes. ANATOMY. The superficial cervical nodes lie on the external surface of the sternomastoid muscle, in close relationship to the external jugular vein as it emerges from the parotid gland. They receive afferents from the

pinna of the external ear and the parotid region and send efferents around the anterior border of the sternomastoid muscle to the superior deep cervical nodes.

CLINICAL SIGNIFICANCE. The superficial cervical nodes have the same clinical significance as the posterior and the anterior auricular and the parotid nodes.

6. Submaxillary Nodes. ANATOMY. The submaxillary nodes lie within the submaxillary fascial compartment, surrounded by the deep cervical fascia. Some of the nodes are imbedded within and others lie on the submaxillary gland. In cancer, removal of submaxillary nodes necessitates removal of the submaxillary salivary gland. One of the nodes, the node of Stöhr, lying in relation to the external maxillary artery, is concerned particularly in lymphatic drainage of the tongue. These nodes receive efferents from the submental nodes. The submaxillary nodes receive afferents from the sides of the tongue, the gums, the lateral part of the lower lip, the entire upper lip, the angle of the mouth and the cheek, and the medial angle of the eye. Since the submaxillary nodes drain not only cutaneous areas but also parts of the mucous membrane of the lips and the mouth, their efferents drain not only into the superficial but also into the deep cervical lymph nodes.

CLINICAL SIGNIFICANCE. Enlargement follows infection or neoplasm primarily in the drainage area. The initial lesion in the mouth may not always be readily detectable on clinical inspection and may require palpation of the mouth with the gloved hand. Infections of dental origin are very common as a cause of submaxillary lymphadenopathy and may require dental and roentgen examination for evaluation. The lip, the tongue, or the inside of the mouth are common locations for primary syphilitic chancre or for neoplasm. Rarely, the inside of the mouth is the site of primary oral tuberculosis.[206]

Submaxillary lymphadenopathy may be confused readily with mumps of the maxillary salivary glands especially when the parotids are not involved.

One should not overlook that the area of the medial aspects of the conjunctiva and the eyelids drains to the submaxillary lymph nodes which may be enlarged along with the anterior auricular nodes as part of the oculoglandular syndrome.

7. The Submental Nodes. ANATOMY. The submental nodes lie in the submental triangle, bounded by the inferior border of the mandible, the anterior bellies of the two digastric muscles and the hyoid bone. They usually lie near the mid-line. They drain the central part of the lower lip, the floor of the mouth, the tip of the tongue, the skin of the chin, and their efferents pass either to the submaxillary nodes or to the deep cervical nodes.

CLINICAL SIGNIFICANCE. Enlargement follows infection or neoplasm primary in the drainage area. The initial lesion in this area is easily seen or at least detectable by palpation of the mouth with the gloved hand. Infections of dental origin are very common as a cause of submental lymphadenopathy.

Submental lymphadenopathy should not be confused with sublingual mumps. In all instances where the submental and the submaxillary nodes are enlarged the physician should palpate the drainage areas within the mouth with his gloved hand to detect a primary infection or a neoplastic lesion not clinically observable.

8. Posterior Cervicals. ANATOMY. The posterior cervical nodes belong to the deep cervical nodes but often are palpable as a separate group. They are located in the occipital triangle, above the level of the inferior belly of the omohyoid. They are related intimately to the spinal accessory nerve which crosses this triangle.

CLINICAL SIGNIFICANCE. The posterior cervical nodes are commonly involved in scalp infections, pediculosis and tuberculosis. Other infections and neoplasms are more rarely the cause. Due to their close relationship to the spinal accessory nerve, removal of these nodes in the surgical treatment of tuberculous cervical adenitis or biopsy of these nodes in suspected primary or secondary neoplasms often entails damage to this nerve with consequent spinal accessory nerve paralysis.[74]

While generalized lymphadenopathy is common in African trypanosomiasis, bilateral enlargement of the posterior cervical nodes is especially prominent and constitutes a diagnostic feature of this disease, known as Winterbottom's sign.[75]

9. The Inferior Deep Cervicals. ANATOMY. The inferior deep cervical nodes lie in the lower part of the neck, below the level of the inferior belly of the omohyoid muscle. Some of these nodes lie behind the sternomastoid muscle, in the fat covering the anterior scalene muscle; these are known as the scalene nodes. Others lie beyond the posterior border of the sternomastoid muscle in the supraclavicular triangle (the supraclavicular nodes) (Virchow's node).

The inferior deep cervical nodes receive afferents from the back of the scalp and of the neck, from many of the superior deep cervical nodes, from some of the axillary nodes, and even from vessels directly from the skin of the arm and from the pectoral region. Altogether, therefore, the inferior cervical nodes receive a great deal of the lymphatic drainage of the entire head and neck, plus some drainage from the arm and the superficial aspects of the thorax.

CLINICAL SIGNIFICANCE. Because of their wide connections, the inferior deep cervical nodes may be involved in carcinoma originating anywhere in the head or the neck; in addition, the supraclavicular nodes may be involved by carcinoma originating within the abdomen or the thorax. The nodes on the left are involved more frequently, probably because of their relationship to the thoracic duct, while the nodes on the right are usually involved only when there are tumors in the thorax. The supraclavicular and the scalene nodes will be discussed separately.

A number of recent papers present good general information on the problem of cervical lymphadenopathy.[209,210,211,212]

The Jugulo-omohyoid (Tongue Node). The jugulo-omohyoid node belongs to the inferior deep cervical group. It is situated in relation to the internal jugular vein and the common carotid artery, just above the point where these vessels are crossed by the superior belly of the omohyoid muscle. It receives lymph from the apex of the tongue by lymphatics which bypass the submental nodes.

Cancer originating in the apex of the

tongue may spread by lymphatics to the submental nodes, but also by a direct route to the jugolo-omohyoid node (tongue node).[76] This node should not be confused with the large node of the superior deep cervical group, often called the "main tongue node" (jugulodigastric) located at the level of the bifurcation of the common artery, just below the great cornu of the hyoid bone which becomes involved from cancer of the margin and the posterior part of the tongue. (See reference to these two tongue nodes on Fig. 158.)

Supraclavicular Nodes. The supraclavicular nodes on each side are essentially part of the homolateral deep cervical node group and when enlarged are usually palpable behind the clavicular insertion of the sternomastoid muscle. Being intercalated in the drainage system from the head, the arm, the chest wall and the breast, frequently they are involved in infectious and neoplastic processes developing in these drainage areas.

The particular interest of the supraclavicular nodes, especially those on the left, centers in their occasional and peculiar metastatic involvement from neoplasms originating within the abdominal cavity and for that matter, rarely from lesions located anywhere in the drainage area of the thoracic lymphatic duct. Because its lymphatic drainage is from the lungs and the mediastinum, the right supraclavicular node is enlarged primarily from metastases from the lung and the esophagus. It has been reported involved from cancer of the pancreas[77] and rarely from other intraabdominal tumors, probably as a result of lymphatic crossover in the mediastinum.

Excluding a nonvisceral site for a malignancy, metastatic involvement of the supraclavicular nodes has been accepted as diagnostic of distant intrathoracic or intraabdominal neoplasm and is known by various special names such as sentinel node, signal node and the eponyms, Virchow's node and Troisier node.[77] Although this sign was introduced in 1848 by Virchow as associated with cancer of the stomach[78] its present meaning is much broader. In an extensive study of supraclavicular metastases, Viacava and Pack[77] noted them in 28

per cent of 4,365 cases of cancer. The order of the primary site was 13.27 per cent from the lung; 8.1 per cent pancreas; 7.1 per cent esophagus; 6.9 per cent kidney; 6.1 per cent ovary; 4.8 per cent testicle and 2.6 per cent stomach. These figures indicate that this diagnostic sign is not particularly common, and when present is of ominous prognostic interest rather than of helpful early diagnostic value. It is actually infrequent in cancer of the stomach, the neoplasm with which it is usually thought to be commonly associated. McKusick,[78] in an interesting report, stresses that the Virchow-Troisier node may be a noticeable metastatic lesion with cancer of the gallbladder.

In general a *right-sided* or *bilateral* supraclavicular node is suggestive of a *lung* or an *esophageal* lesion while an isolated *left* supraclavicular metastasis suggests a primary site in the *kidney,* the *ovary,* the *testes,* the *gallbladder* or the *stomach.*[77,78]

Controversy has centered in whether tumor spreads to the supraclavicular nodes by lymphatic permeation or by embolization. To support the former view are reports of lymphatic ducts completely filled with tumor cells.[79] Recent interesting experimental studies by Zeidman[80] support the tumor emboli theory and indicate strongly that tumor emboli can reach the supraclavicular node from the thoracic duct through afferent branches and need not be explained by retrograde passage through efferent channels. In one study, there was a positive correlation between supraclavicular metastasis and the presence of neoplastic cells in the thoracic duct lymph.[207]

One should not overlook the fact that any intra-abdominal infection, especially if of chronic nature, such as tuberculous peritonitis, may produce a left supraclavicular infectious lymphadenopathy.[78]

Scalene Nodes and Scalene Node Biopsy. Extensive studies[81-83] have firmly established the value of the scalene node biopsy, a procedure introduced by Daniels[84] in 1949 for the diagnosis of intrathoracic disease. This operation can be performed under local anesthesia and is neither complicated, dangerous nor prolonged. Figure 159 indicates in diagrammatic fashion the anatomic relations of the scalene nodes. This operation permits entrance to a fat-filled space bound medially by the internal jugular vein; laterally by the omohyoid muscle, below by the subclavian vein and overlying the scalenus anticus muscle. The fat pad in this space constantly contains several lymph nodes, even if not enlarged enough to detect on physical examination. The scope of operation can be extended to include exploration of the upper part of the mediastinum.[81]

The report by Harken *et al.*[81] adds much data supporting the diagnostic importance of this procedure and emphasizes especially the value of *exploration of the upper mediastinum* since approximately half of their positive results came from tissue removed from the mediastinum when the scalene node biopsy was negative. The authors reported a positive histologic diagnosis of 45 of 142 cases (31.7%) with the use of this complete technic. Anatomic peculiarities of the lymph drainage of the right and the left lung into the hilar area and to the scalene nodes must be understood to secure the best results (see Fig. 164). Homolateral biopsy can be utilized in all cases with the exception of lesions in the left lower lobe, a point emphasized by Harken *et al.*[81] Figure 164 shows clearly that the left lower lobe has lymphatic drainage via the intertracheal-bronchial nodes to both lateral chains. Bilateral scalene node and upper mediastinal node biopsies are indicated when a primary site is suspected to be in the left lower lobe. Positive results of about 40 per cent in carcinoma of the lung can be expected when these anatomic factors are considered.

Shefts, Terrill and Swindell[82] in a report of 314 biopsies in 293 patients secured a positive histologic diagnosis in 102 patients (35%). Included in their series of cases

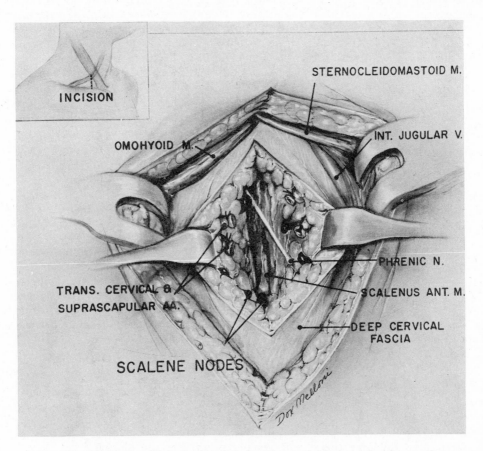

Fig. 159. Diagram to illustrate anatomic location and relations of scalene nodes.

were 60 with Boeck's sarcoid, bronchogenic carcinoma 20, tuberculosis 9, primary lymphoma 7, metastases to lung 4. Cuykendall[83] has reported such biopsies valuable in 41 cases.

Lillington and Jamplis[208] have recently reviewed this subject and the reader is referred to this source for a critical discussion of its present status. Aside from malignancy, the procedure has proved particularly valuable by frequently proving Boeck's sarcoid to be the cause of obscure lung and hilar node pathology. It has also shown that silicosis can involve the scalene node. The curative potential of surgery for lung cancer often can be evaluated more correctly when scalene node biopsy results are available.

Group II—Less Clinically Important and Not Readily Palpable

In the anterior part of the face are several groups of nodes not ordinarily searched for or detectable routinely but which may occasionally become clinically significant and produce signs and/or symptoms. These include the infraorbital, the facial, the parotid and the mental.

Here we shall not discuss other nodes of the head and the neck such as the anterior cervicals, the retropharyngeal, and the many deep neck nodes likely to be encountered only in surgical procedures, especially radical dissections, since such nodes are detectable only indirectly through clinical manifestations or biopsies.

1. Infraorbital Nodes. ANATOMY. The infraorbital nodes lie just below the orbit; they help drain the outer aspect of the eyelids and the conjunctiva. Their efferents join the anterior auricular as well as the submaxillary nodes.

CLINICAL SIGNIFICANCE. This node sometimes becomes enlarged and tender from infections of the conjunctiva and the eyelids and therefore may constitute part of the oculoglandular syndrome.

2. The Facial Lymph Nodes. ANATOMY. The superficial facial lymph nodes (buccinator nodes) lies on the buccinator muscle and are inconstant. They drain the medial aspect of the eyelids, the conjunctiva, the nose and the cheek and send efferents to the submaxillary nodes.

CLINICAL SIGNIFICANCE. These nodes are rarely detectable, since they are inconstant and lie in the deep and not readily palpable areas.[85] If enlarged they may be detected by bimanual palpation of the cheek with one hand gloved for examination within the mouth and are more rarely present as a detectable lump in the cheek which, according to Bailey,[86] must be differentiated from a lipoma of the sucking pad and tumor or cyst of a molar gland.[87] A suppurating gland can leave a scar on the cheek.

3. The Parotid Group. ANATOMY. The parotid group is fairly large, containing usually from ten to sixteen nodes. They lie within the parotid fascial compartment, enclosed by the superficial layer of the deep cervical fascia. Some of the nodes are imbedded within the substance of the parotid, and others are outside of the parotid but within the parotid fascial compartment. The intraparotid nodes receive afferents from the eyelids, the external auditory meatus, the skin of the temporal and the frontal regions, and the tympanic cavity. The deep parotid nodes drain the back of the nose and the nasopharynx, as well as the parotid gland.

CLINICAL SIGNIFICANCE. These nodes are not commonly palpable. Occasionally pain or enlargement in the parotid area may be explained by some infection or tumor in the drainage area, which includes locations not readily accessible to clinical inspection such as the back of the nose and the nasopharynx best studied by endoscopic or mirror examination.

4. Mental Node. ANATOMY. This node lies in relation to the mental foramen of the mandible. It helps to drain the lower lip, the tip of the tongue, and the floor of the mouth. While its efferents drain chiefly into the submaxillary nodes, some of these efferent lymphatic channels enter the mandibular foramen.

CLINICAL SIGNIFICANCE. This node permits cancer emboli to involve the mandible in metastatic cancer from the lip or the tip of the tongue. This is the reason for *combining hemimandibulectomy with radical neck dissection in treatment* of cancer of the lip and the tongue.[88]

Cancerous Metastasis to Head and Neck

Nodes. Any of the head and the neck nodes may be involved with metastatic cancer, the primary site of which lies externally on the scalp or the face, or from the oral, the nasal and the pharyngeal areas. Martin and Morfit[89] have emphasized the importance of always considering this etiology when any of these nodes manifest a chronic enlargement characterized by unilateral location and firmness to touch with absence of pain. Figure 160 from Martin and Morfit[89] shows the more common sites for such metastatic lesions. If an infectious focus can be excluded, the drainage area of the involved node should be searched for a primary site of a neoplasm.

Cancerous lymphadenopathy in the neck may present a difficult diagnostic problem since it must be differentiated from such benign masses as chronic infectious lymphadenopathy, sebaceous cyst, lipoma, thryoglossal cyst, branchiogenic cyst, etc.[90]

THE AXILLARY NODES

Anatomy. The axillary nodes are subdivided into 5 groups: lateral, posterior, central, anterior and apical.

The lateral axillary nodes lie near the junction of the axillary and the brachial veins on the medial aspect of the humerus and constitute the main termination of afferent channels of the superficial and the deep lymphatics of the upper extremity. While their efferents drain mostly into the central and the apical nodes some channels pass directly to the supraclavicular group. *The posterior axillary nodes* lie along the axillary border of the scapula, in relation to the subscapular vein receiving afferent lymph channels from the upper extremity and the posterior thoracic wall and draining efferently into both the lateral and the central axillary nodes. *The central axillary nodes* lie in the deep fat of the axilla or between layers of the axillary fascia at its base, receiving afferents from the lateral, the posterior, and the anterior axillary nodes and terminating their efferents in the apical axillary nodes. *The anterior axillary nodes,* situated along the lower border of

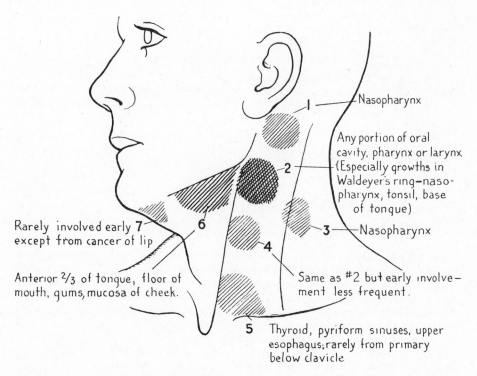

Fig. 160. Various lymph node groups with the most likely sites of the primary lesion which may cause the metastases. (Martin, H. and Morfit, H. M.: Surg. Gyn. & Obst. 78:133-159)

the pectoralis major in relation to the lateral thoracic vein, drain the greater part of the lymph from the mammary gland and also receive efferents from the anterior chest wall. The efferents end in the central and the apical axillary nodes. *The apical axillary or the infraclavicular nodes* lie along the upper part of the axillary vein in the interval between the costocoracoid membrane anteriorly, the axillary vein posteriorly, and the first intercostal space inferiorly. These nodes receive afferents from the other axillary nodes as well as direct afferents from the superior part of the *subclavian trunk* (see Fig. 161, A-A4 lymphatic).

Clinical Significance. Axillary lymphadenopathy is a common clinical problem and suggests mainly an infectious process or neoplasm in the drainage area which includes part of the hand and the arm, chest wall, upper and lateral abdominal wall and part of the breast (Fig. 161). It may follow lesions in the drainage area of the epi-

trochlear nodes if the pathologic condition spreads beyond this lymph node barrier. Evaluation is made more difficult in that nodes may be palpated, at times, in supposedly "normal" persons.[213] There are many reports on the value of careful study of axillary lymphadenopathy.[214,215]

In most instances, infectious lymphadenopathy is responsible for axillary node involvement since the fingers and the arm are subject to so many potentially infected traumatic episodes. Likewise many infectious systemic diseases commence by inoculation in this drainage area, producing axillary lymphadenopathy with one or more satellite nodes prior to systemic invasion. Representative examples include extragenital chancre of syphilis, brucellosis in veterinarians, inoculation tuberculosis, tularemia, cat-scratch disease, sporotrichosis, etc. The axillary nodes are especially likely to be involved in streptococcal infections of the hand with tubular lymphangitis. Axil-

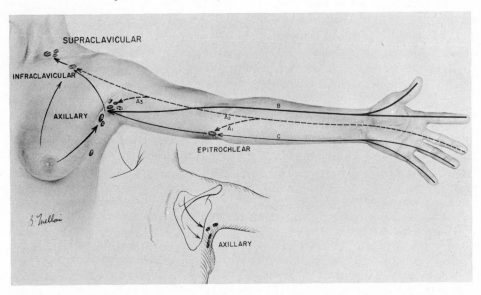

Fig. 161. Lymphatic drainage of the upper extremity. The lymphatic vessels draining the fingers and the hand converge on the dorsum of the hand. From here the lymphatic drainage pursues three courses. The lymph vessels draining the ulnar aspect (little finger and ring finger) accompany (C) the basilic vein and drain into the epitrochlear nodes and thence into the axillary nodes. The lymph vessels draining the thumb and the index fingers (D) bypass the epitrochlear nodes and go directly to the axillary nodes. The lymph vessels (A) draining the middle fingers may drain into the epitrochlear (A_1), the axillary (A_2, A_3) or may bypass both of these groups of nodes to drain directly into the infraclavicular (A–A_4) and thence, into the supraclavicular and finally into the bloodstream. The axillary nodes also receive lymph from the posterior scapular region (insert).

lary nodes commonly suppurate in certain types of infections.

While any skin neoplasm primary in the drainage area, particularly malignant melanoma and epidermoid carcinoma, may metastasize to the axillary nodes, special attention in these nodes centers about the frequency with which they are involved with *carcinoma primary in the female breast.* Presence of axillary nodes gravely influences the prognosis and the type of surgical resection. It is well to note that metastasis to the supraclavicular lymph nodes from carcinoma of the breast is unusual unless the axillary nodes are also invaded.[91] Occasionally, axillary metastasis from breast cancer is striking when the primary lesion is small and readily overlooked.[92,93] Rarely, lymph-node enlargement of infectious nature, if located very anteriorly in the axilla, may simulate a cancer of the breast.

Accessory breast tissue may occur in the axillary area and may be confused readily with axillary lymphadenopathy, especially when such breast tissue is the site of painful enlargement during or after pregnancy.

Prophylactic vaccines, BCG vaccine and serum, are often injected in the shoulder area and may occasionally initiate axillary lymphadenopathy of marked degree on the same side,[94,95] followed rarely by suppuration. BCG vaccine used in infancy may lead to calcification of the axillary nodes, a finding readily detected on the roentgenogram of the chest area.[96]

Also worth noting is the rare presence of Irish nodes;[216] nodes beneath the lateral edge or deeper in the left axilla in the absence of similar nodes on the right side. They have a diagnostic significance for cancer of the stomach similar to the Virchow node.

Rarely an anomalous axillary pectoral muscle (Langer's arch) may present as an axillary mass[217] and cause a diagnostic problem.

Subpectoral Abscess (Suppurative Infraclavicular Lymphadenitis). Acute subpectoral abscess is an unusual and relatively uncommon clinical entity produced by suppuration of the infraclavicular apical axillary nodes on one side of the body, a result usually of infection with a *hemolytic streptococcus.* When infected, these nodes become enlarged and may suppurate to involve the surrounding fat in a suppurative, necrotic process. Because it is enclosed in tight fascia-lined pockets, the infectious process produces a severe disability characterized by high fever, a toxic state, tenderness to palpation over the affected area and much pain in the region of the shoulder, especially on abduction of the arm.[97,98] If not treated, the pus dissects extensively along the fascial planes and may reach the axilla with spontaneous drainage or may cause septicemia.

The infraclavicular nodes are most likely to become involved in those persons with an infection of the middle finger in whom the lymphatic drainage is directly to the infraclavicular nodes without passage through the epitrochlear or axillary nodes (see A-A4 in Fig. 161). It may also follow failure of inadequate defense reaction of the latter nodes in cases where they are intercalated in the lymphatic pathway to the infraclavicular nodes. The initial infection may originate elsewhere on the hands, the arms or the shoulder. There is a close analogy between *acute infraclavicular adenitis* and *deep inguinal adenitis.*

THE EPITROCHLEAR (SUPERFICIAL CUBITAL OR SUPRATROCHLEAR) NODES

Anatomy. The epitrochlear nodes lie on the back of the elbow, in the superficial fascia above the medial epicondyle of the humerus and in relation to the basilic vein. Their afferents drain lymph from the little, the ring and the ulnar half of the middle finger, but not from the thumb and the index fingers, and also from the ulnar part of the palm of the hand and the forearm. Their efferents terminate in the axillary nodes.

Clinical Significance. Acute enlargement of the epitrochlear nodes in one arm as a result of local infection or of neoplasm primary in the drainage area, is common and well understood. More difficulty may be encountered when the drainage area in one arm is the inoculation site for an infectious agent capable of producing a systemic disease, in which the epitrochlear lymph node is only a satellite response in a more complex picture. Representative examples would include lesions such as extragenital chancre of syphilis, tularemia, cat-scratch disease, inoculation tuberculosis, etc.

Being intercalated in the drainage to the axillary nodes, enlargement of the latter nodes may follow epitrochlear adenopathy if the defense mechanism at this level fails.

Of course, epitrochlear nodes may be involved in any disease capable of produc-

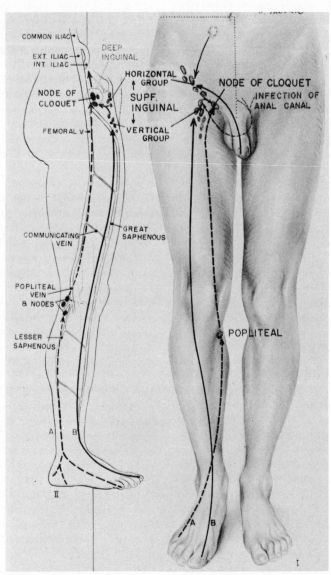

Fig. 162. Lymphatic drainage of lower extremity, genitalia and lower abdomen. I. Lymphatic drainage of medial and middle aspects of foot (B); heel and outer aspect of foot (A), Channel B, superficial drainage of inner and middle aspects of foot, leg, genitalia, perineum and lower abdomen to superficial inguinal nodes.

II. Superficial drainage of small toe and outer aspect of foot, heel and knee to the popliteal nodes with major lymphatic channel deep along femoral vein to deep inguinal nodes.

ing a generalized lymphadenopathy. Being easily palpated, enlargement of these nodes is readily detected clinically. Much interest has centered in the older literature concerning the frequency and the diagnostic significance of bilateral painless epitrochlear lymphadenopathy with regard to the systemic phase of syphilis. [99,100] However, any diagnostic value assigned to this finding must be conditioned by the fact that lymph node enlargement in this region is often a chronic nonspecific lymphadenitis resulting from repeated minor trauma and infections in the drainage area, being more common in men than women and more frequent and striking in those doing manual labor.[100,101] Epitrochlear involvement is said to be minimal or absent with generalized tuberculosis lymphadenopathy,[102] and less frequent in Hodgkin's disease than in lymphosarcoma.[47]

THE INGUINAL LYMPH NODES

Anatomy. The inguinal lymph nodes are arranged in two groups: superficial and deep (Fig. 162). *The superficial inguinal nodes* lie in the superficial fascia and are disposed in an upper horizontal and a lower vertical group. *The horizontal group* lies parallel to the inguinal ligament below the attachment of the fascia of Scarpa to the fascia lata. These nodes drain lymph from the skin of the anterior abdominal wall below the umbilicus, the skin of the penis and the scrotum in the male, the skin of the vulva and the mucosa of the vagina in the female, the skin of the perineum and the gluteal region (Fig. 163), and the lower part of the anal canal. They receive no lymph from the testis or the ovary. *The vertical group* lie on either side of the upper part of the greater saphenous vein. They receive all the superficial lymphatic vessels of the lower extremity which accompany the greater saphenous vein. They do not receive the lymphatic vessels accompanying the shorter saphenous vein; these end in the popliteal nodes. In addition, the vertical group also receives lymph from the penis, the scrotum and the gluteal region. The superficial inguinal nodes drain into the deep inguinal nodes (Figs. 162 and 165).

The deep inguinal nodes, one to three in number, lie beneath the fascia lata, on the medial side of the femoral vein and below the femoral canal. One node (*node of Cloquet*) lies within the fat of the femoral canal. The deep inguinal nodes receive the deep lymphatic vessels accompanying the femoral vein, including those draining the popliteal nodes. They also re-

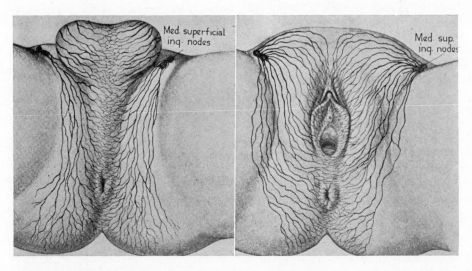

FIG. 163. Diagram of the cutaneous lymphatics of the perineum (*Left*—male, *Right*—female) showing their communication across the mid-line and drainage into the superficial inguinal nodes. (Pack, G. T., and Rekers, P.: Am. J. Surg. 56:545-565)

ceive lymph from the glans penis or the glans clitoris and from the superficial inguinal nodes. They drain into the external iliac nodes by efferents which partly traverse the femoral canal and partly course in front and lateral to the femoral sheath.

Clinical Significance. Persistent enlargement of the superficial inguinal nodes of minimal degree is a common clinical finding, and represents the effect of chronic hyperplasia of these nodes from constant and often unnoticed or forgotten minor infections and irritations in the drainage areas, to which most people are subjected at various times. For this reason, a minimal degree of superficial inguinal lymphadenopathy is difficult to evaluate. Physicians learn to accept a so-called "usual life" baseline degree of groin lymphadenopathy. Diagnostic interest should be aroused when the nodes are (1) increasing in size under observation, (2) larger than expected, (3) painful, or (4) suppurating.

Significant lymphadenopathy of the superficial inguinal nodes is related most commonly to: (1) local infectious process of the drainage area; (2) systemic infection in which the infectious agent enters the body in the drainage region, or (3) primary neoplasm in this area, chiefly a malignant melanoma or an epidermoid carcinoma. The number of disorders possible in the large and anatomically complicated drainage area is infinitely greater than in the axillary node drainage area.

The ease with which a local infection or small primary neoplasm can be overlooked if located on the scrotum, between the buttocks, on the labia, under the prepuce, in the umbilicus, the cutaneous zone of the anus or between the toes is well known, since these areas are not examined as frequently and thoroughly as the upper extremities or head and neck.

Lesions of the penis which are especially important include: syphilitic chancre, gonorrhea, lymphopathia venereum, chancroid and malignancy. Granuloma inguinale is not a lymph node disease but may predispose to secondary infectious lymphadenitis.

Minor but often overlooked causes include pediculosis pubis, tinea crurum of the inguinal area, ringworm between the toes and the irritation incident to wearing a truss to restrain a hernia.

An infectious or neoplastic lesion is not easily overlooked on the legs, the lower abdomen, the buttocks or the lower back but may readily be missed if present on the scrotum, the perineum, the anus, or the labia. Tumors of the testis metastasize directly to the upper para-aortic nodes (Fig. 165) and involve the superficial inguinal nodes only when the tumor breaks through the capsule of the testicle to invade the scrotum (Figs. 162 and 163).

All infections or neoplastic lesions primary in these skin areas do not necessarily involve the superficial inguinal nodes. The skin of the heel and the posterior half of the outer aspects of the foot drain into the popliteal nodes and from these, directly to deep inguinal nodes (see Fig. 162 and discussion in the following section on popliteal nodes). In an occasional anomaly, lymphatics from upper posterior thigh and lower buttocks penetrate the fascia and reach the common iliac nodes along the sciatic nerve sheath,[103] thus permitting lesions in this drainage area to bypass the superficial inguinal nodes. Lesions of the glans penis or the glans clitoris may drain, not only to the superficial inguinals, but also directly into the deep inguinal and the other deep nodes.[103] There is also possibility of drainage of the penis to the prepubic lymph nodes and thence to the external iliac lymph nodes, without passage to the superficial inguinals.[103] Therefore, absence of palpable superficial inguinal nodes does not rule out infections or tumor metastases from these areas. See the excellent paper by Pack and Rekers[103] for a detailed discussion of this subject.

Several infectious systemic diseases, in which the etiologic agent enters the drainage area of the superficial inguinal nodes, may produce a satellite enlargement in these nodes, or if lymphadenopathy is general, exaggeration of the nodes in this location. This is particularly likely to occur with bubonic plague, scrub typhus, rat-bite fever and filariasis. Superficial inguinal adenitis has been noted in swamp fever (due to leptospirae).[104] This suggests the possibility that the infection was acquired through the skin of the leg.

Superficial inguinal adenitis may be noted in infants and small children when the thigh is used as a site for subcutaneous prophylactic inoculation with vaccines against the various diseases of childhood, smallpox vaccination or BCG vaccine.[94,95,105] In infants, suppuration of the superficial inguinal nodes with thigh injections was much more frequent than suppuration of the axillary nodes when comparable injections of BCG vaccine were given in the shoulder area.[105] A possible explanation is that in infants the superficial inguinal nodes are already under continuous phagocytic stress because of constant irritation and soilage from urine and feces in the diaper area and are unable to accept the added phagocytic load resulting from the vaccination.

In contrast with the paucity of subcutaneous masses in the axillary area capable of simulating lymphadenopathy are the variety of conditions present in the groin. Tumefactions in the groin which must be distinguished from lymphadenopathy are: hernia, varix, lipoma, aneurysm, tuberculosis of bursa of short head of rectus femoris muscle, psoas abscess, ectopic testis, ectopic spleen, inguinal endometriosis, etc.[103,106,107,218] For this reason the differential diagnosis of masses in the groin is not always easy and must be considered carefully before a palpable "lump" is called an enlarged node.

In females, a primary lesion of lymphopathia venereum deep in the vagina or the fornix does not produce superficial lymphadenopathy. Instead the lymph drainage is to the lymphatics about the rectum with production of a periproctitis which may eventuate in a rectal stricture.[62]

Acute Iliac Lymphadenitis. Although the nodes are classified as in the retroperitoneal group, suppuration of the external iliacs bears a closer relationship to infections of the extremities and will be better understood if viewed in this light.

Suppuration of the external iliac nodes[108-110] most commonly unilateral, may manifest a striking analogy to subpectoral abscess (suppurative infraclavicular lymphadenitis). These nodes, located retroperitoneally deep in the iliac fossa adjacent to the external and the common iliac vessels and anterior to the psoas muscle, receive drainage from the superficial and the deep inguinals, the penis, the urethra, the prostate, the bladder, the uterus, the deep lymphatics of the abdominal wall and the upper thigh. The nodes enlarge to a clinically significant degree two or three weeks after onset of an infection primary in one of the drainage sites usually due to *hemolytic staphylococcus* or *hemolytic streptococcus*. Such lymphadenitis is most common in children and young adults and may occur without obvious involvement of the superficial inguinal nodes. The clinical picture is one of high fever, leukocytosis, occasionally bacteremia, lower abdominal pain but without sign of peritoneal irritation, psoas muscle spasm limiting extension of the leg on the involved side, abdominal tenderness with rectus muscle spasm. At times the greatly enlarged nodes are detectable as a palpable tender mass just above Poupart's ligament. Often the nodes suppurate to form an extraperitoneal abscess requiring surgical drainage.

THE POPLITEAL NODES

Anatomy. The popliteal nodes, five or six in number, lie under the deep fascia in the fat around the popliteal vessels in the popliteal fossa. They receive lymph vessels from the knee joint and skin of the lateral side of the lower part of the leg, foot and heel. They receive lymph from the deep structures of the leg and foot by lymphatic vessels coursing along the anterior and posterior tibial arteries and veins. Their efferents drain into the deep inguinal nodes by lymphatic vessels which accompany the popliteal and femoral veins. An inconstant anterior tibial node may be intercalated between the heel area and the popliteal node but is only rarely clinically important.

Clinical Significance. Except for the above-described drainage area, infections and neoplasms of the foot and the lower leg spread lymphatically directly to the superficial inguinal lymph nodes without filtering through the popliteal nodes. Infections of the knee joint and lesions on the heel and the outer side of the posterior half of the foot drain into the popliteal nodes (see insert I, Fig. 162). Popliteal nodes are not easy to palpate unless greatly enlarged, because of their subfascial location. It is well to remember that the afferent lymphatic channels from the popliteal nodes course along with the femoral artery to drain directly into the deep femoral and the external iliac nodes, bypassing completely the superficial inguinal nodes.[103] It is a practical clinical point that the absence of enlarged superficial inguinal nodes does not rule out spread beyond the popliteal nodes of a tumor of heel and outer foot. Radical resection of malignant melanoma is influenced by this anatomic fact.

The Mediastinal Lymph Nodes

Anatomy. The mediastinum contains a large number of nodes, the most important of which may be divided into two groups: (1) the superior mediastinal and (2) the tracheobronchial (Fig. 164).

The superior mediastinal nodes lie in front of the aortic arch, in relation to the large arterial trunks arising from the aortic arch and also to the innominate veins. They receive afferents from the thymus, the pericardium, the heart, the esophagus and the trachea as well as from the parasternal nodes. Their efferents join with those from the tracheabronchial, on each side, to form the corresponding bronchomediastinal trunk.

The tracheobronchial nodes include

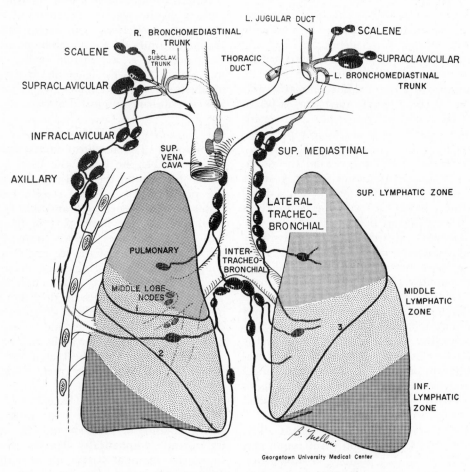

Fig. 164. Lymphatic drainage of lungs and mediastinum.

some of the largest nodes in the body. They may be subdivided into (1) the lateral tracheobronchial, (2) the intertracheobronchial, and (3) the pulmonary.

The lateral tracheobronchial lie in relation to the trachea and lateral to the primary bronchi.

The intertracheobronchial nodes lie at the bifurcation of the trachea, between the primary bronchi.

The pulmonary nodes are both extrapulmonary and intrapulmonary in location. The extrapulmonary nodes lie in the hilum of each lung; these are the so-called *hilar nodes*. The intrapulmonary nodes lie along the secondary branches of the primary bronchi and are related to the lobes of the lungs. Of these, the nodes related to the right middle lobe are of special importance since they drain not only the middle but also the lower lobe of the right lung and almost completely surround the secondary middle lobe bronchus. Consequently, when enlarged these nodes are very likely to compress this bronchus and thus interfere with the drainage of both the middle and the lower lobes.

It is to be noted that the lymphatic drainage of the lung *does not conform* to the anatomic division of the lobes. Hence, in the surgical treatment of cancer of the lung, pneumonectomy and not lobectomy is indicated. The pulmonary nodes drain into the intertracheobronchial and the lateral tracheobronchial nodes, which in turn drain into the superior mediastinal nodes. From the mediastinal nodes of each side, the lymph passes through the corresponding bronchomediastinal trunk into the venous system. Blockage of the mediastinal nodes leads to retrograde flow and in the presence of pleural adhesions, cancer may spread to the axillary nodes. Similarly, with blockage of the axillary nodes, retrograde flow will carry cancer emboli across the chest wall to the mediastinal nodes.

The tracheobronchial nodes drain lymph from lungs, bronchi, thoracic portion of the trachea, heart, esophagus and liver; their efferents join the bronchomediastinal lymphatic trunk.

Clinical Significance—Mediastinal Lymphadenopathy. Only rarely does a clinically significant degree of hilar lymphadenopathy follow ordinary bacterial infections of the lung such as pneumonia or reinfectious type of pulmonary tuberculosis. Diffuse staphylococcal or streptococcal bronchopneumonias or multiple lobe bronchiectasis or abscess formation may rarely produce a bilateral form while unilateral hilar lymphadenopathy may occasionally follow bronchiectasis, lung abscess or viral infection. Tuberculosis, in sharp contrast, whether as a primary complex or hematogenous form, often involves the hilar lymph nodes on one or both sides with persistence for long periods with termination by healing and constriction, calcification or rarely caseation. A lung infection which has cleared may leave a hilar adenitis which persists for a time. Coccidioidomycosis, histoplasmosis and especially sarcoidosis may produce bilateral symmetrical mediastinal lymph-node enlargement, the latter being a particularly common benign type.[111-113]

Silicosis and other pneumoconioses, asbestosis and beryllium intoxication may all manifest by chest roentgenogram evidence of both bilateral lymphadenopathy and pulmonary (lung field) involvement.[112] The pathology of the nodes in these conditions is one of an infiltrative nature.

Bilateral mediastinal lymphadenopathy often without pulmonary involvement, occasionally with arthralgia, commonly is associated with erythema nodosum.[111,114,219] While various etiologies for this syndrome have been proposed, much current attention centers on sarcoidosis as one of the interesting causes.[115,116]

In sarcoidosis the enlarged hilar lymph nodes are bilateral, never calcify, occur early in the course, are harmless as such and generally regress.[220] Rare causes of bilateral mediastinal lymphadenopathy without lung changes are infectious mononucleosis and the collagen diseases.

Metastasis to hilar nodes, irregularly unilateral, especially from the lungs and more rarely from distant organs such as the kidney and the testis, may occur. Lymphatic leukemia and the lymphomata group of disorders are more likely to produce a bilateral but often asymmetrical mediastinal lymphadenopathy.

Mediastinal lymph node hyperplasia may rarely simulate a thymoma.[221,222]

1. ASYMPTOMATIC. The use of routine chest roentgenograms, in miniature or standard size, in mass population surveys for chest disease, pre-employment examination, induction station surveys, on admission to many hospitals, etc., has resulted in detection of many instances of hilar adenopathy which are apparently asymptomatic. Perhaps the majority fall in the asymptomatic group. However, an extensive literature based on the study of certain cases admitted to hospitals indicates that a variety of signs and symptoms may be produced by various forms of hilar lymphadenopathy. A study of these clinical observations is important in understanding the mechanism of their production and often indicates the basic pathology responsible.

2. SYMPTOMATIC. *A. Cough.* Regional nodes about the trachea and the bronchi, when sufficiently enlarged, are said to produce a cough by an irritative process or by pressure; often it is of a type commonly called "brassy." The exact mechanism in any instance is difficult to evaluate since many of these people also have intrinsic lung and bronchial diseases. Pulmonary or bronchial infection, granulation tissue, neoplasm and bronchial lithiasis are other possible mechanisms for the production of the cough.

B. Obstructive phenomena. Early partial bronchial obstruction by lymph nodes may cause obstructive emphysema because the bronchial lumen is greater on inspiration than expiration, and the inspiratory phase is more forceful. Ingress is thus easier than egress. This condition is more common in children because their bronchial structure is compressed more easily and the lymph node enlargement is proportionately greater in that age group. The resulting physical signs are usually lobar in distribution rather than generalized, because of the nature of initiating lymph node enlargement.

Partial obstruction, particularly if persistent for long periods, may lead to bronchiectasis, perhaps by preventing proper ciliary movement of secretions, and thus causing a situation readily predisposing to low-grade persistent infection. Chronicity leads to slow progression of the infectious process, which as in emphysema usually is localized and segmental. More rarely lung abscess may follow partial bronchial obstruction.

Complete bronchial obstruction or partial obstruction with lumen-contained secretions may lead to complete *atelectasis* productive of the usual physical and roentgen findings. At times, atelectasis may result from intraluminal rupture of suppurated mediastinal nodes or extrusion of a broncholith into the lumen. Some feel that atelectasis on this basis may be the explanation for most cases of epituberculosis among infants and children. At this age tuberculosis is especially likely to involve bronchial and hilar nodes primarily, with the lung involvement being atelectatic from mechanical compression of the lumen and not parenchymal.

However, it should be pointed out that edema and inflammation alone of the bronchial wall may lead to bronchial obstruction, and that extrinsic pressure is not necessary.[116]

Although such obstruction from lymph node pressure may occur in any lobe of the lung, the bronchus of the right middle lobe is peculiarly susceptible to compression because it is surrounded by a group of lymph nodes draining both the adjacent lower lobe and the middle lobe, an anatomic situation first stressed by Brock *et al.*[118,119] Therefore, infection in either of these two lobes can predispose to lymph node changes in this particular anatomic group. The small lumen size of the middle lobe bronchus and its almost right angle drainage into intermediate bronchi constitute further peculiar hazards to drainage of this lobe.[117] The clinical features produced by obstruction of the right middle lobe bronchus have become popularly known as the *"middle lobe syndrome"* as the result of the description by Graham, Burford and Mayer.[120] Clinical features are often chronic and most characteristically include obstructive phenomena of the right middle lobe with wheezing, pneumonitis or bronchiectasis, chest pain, periodic hemoptysis and demonstrable roentgen findings.[117,120] This syndrome of extrinsic bronchial obstruction of the right middle lobe should not be confused with obstruction of intraluminal origin such as that produced by a bronchial tumor, granulomatous lesion of the bronchus, etc.

C. *Hemoptysis.* Next to cough, this is probably the most common indirect manifestation of hilar and bronchial lymphadenopathy. Mechanisms include friability of granulation tissue, mechanical erosive process, chronic obstruction with bleeding produced by associated infections (i.e., bronchiectasis, lung abscess, etc.), and the irritating and cutting effects of broncholithiasis with rupture of bronchial pulmonary vessels. Periodic hemoptysis is especially characteristic of the "middle lobe syndrome."[117,120]

D. *Calcification of Lymph Nodes.* A variety of mechanisms may predispose to calcification of intrathoracic lymph nodes. Calcification of lymph nodes is commonly due to tuberculosis or histoplasmosis but may be caused by fungus infection, coccidioidomycosis, etc. Large calcified lymph nodes in the hilar area can produce any of the features discussed in this section. However, there are certain clinical features peculiar to calcified nodes.[121-124] They show a propensity to penetrate the bronchial wall, possibly by erosive action of the calcified node against a bronchial wall in constant motion.[122] Extrusion of the calcified node into the lumen of a bronchus may produce bronchial obstructive symptoms of various types, occasionally an intractable localized wheeze, paroxysms of coughing productive of gritty particles and even of the broncholith itself, hemoptysis and other features. Calcified nodes may compress a bronchus and cause atelectasis, produce a traction diverticulum of the esophagus, cause dysphagia, or even rarely compress the superior vena cava.[223] Bronchoscopic examination and roentgen studies are helpful. Reports of 41 cases by Schmidt, Clagett, and MacDonald[125] indicate that broncholithiasis is by no means rare. Storer and Smith[223]

have recently reviewed this intriguing subject.

Calcification of an entire lymph node should not be confused with peripheral calcification, the so-called "eggshell calcification," considered as diagnostic of silicosis of mediastinal lymph nodes but perhaps very rarely seen in other conditions, such as sarcoidosis.[111]

E. *Caseation* of hilar nodes may lead to traction diverticulum of the esophagus with its attendant disturbance of swallowing and morphology of this organ.[126]

F. *Mediastinitis.* Infectious lymphadenopathy of the hilar area may lead to mediastinitis. However, considering the great frequency of infections of hilar nodes from various pulmonary infections, mediastinitis due to this cause is a rare complication.

G. *Superior Vena Caval Obstruction.* Hilar lymphadenopathy may rarely produce superior vena caval obstruction. This may be a late feature resulting from cicatrization of tissue about the superior vena cava from mediastinal infection of lymph node origin or may result from its compression, particularly from lymph node enlargement as a result of metastasis from a bronchial carcinoma, commonly on the right, because of the peculiar anatomic relationships in that area.

H. *Hoarseness* is an uncommon manifestation. It may occur with lymph node metastasis from cancer, particularly of the breast, compressing the recurrent laryngeal nerve or may possibly result from venous obstruction of the superior vena cava, producing edema of the larynx.

I. *Broncho-esophageal fistula* is an unusual complication which may result from an infectious erosive process originating in tuberculous lymph nodes and resulting in the formation of a fistulous tract between a bronchus and the esophagus. A coughing spell which comes on a short interval after swallowing is diagnostically suggestive. A coughing paroxysm from aspirating food or fluid into the larynx due to an upper esophageal difficulty in swallowing comes on at once without the latent interval necessary for esophageal peristalsis to carry food or fluid to the fistulous opening into the bronchus.

J. Dysphagia is likewise an unusual feature sometimes caused by broncho-esophageal fistula,[127] traction diverticula of the esophagus or enlarged mediastinal nodes.

K. Chest pain has been neither severe nor common with mediastinal lymphadenopathy. It may result from broncholithiasis, traction diverticula of the esophagus or broncho-esophageal fistula.

L. Roentgen studies give much helpful

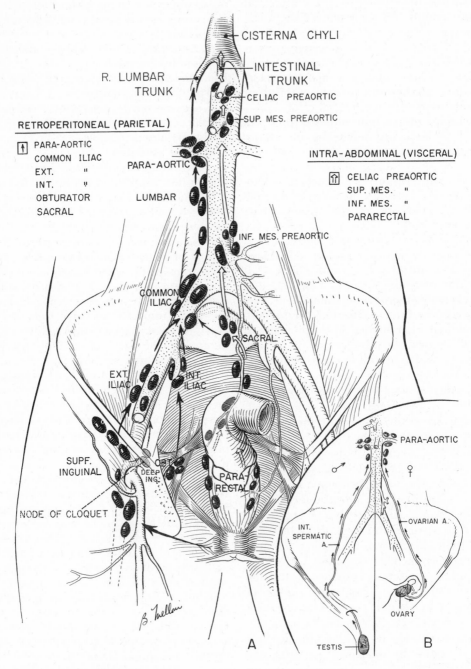

Fig. 165. Lymph nodes of the abdominal cavity. A. Retroperitoneal (parietal) and intra-abdominal (visceral) nodes. B. Lymphatic drainage of ovary or testis directly to upper paraortic nodes without passage through the lower retroperitoneal nodes.

information in evaluating mediastinal lymphadenopathy.[128,129]

M. A palpable swelling of the chest wall in the region of the second and the third intercostal spaces near the sternum may rarely occur when a lymphoma involves the sternal nodes.[47,130]

Occasionally in neoplasm of the breast, and very rarely from primary tumors elsewhere, there may be metastases to the parasternal nodes.[224] It is well to carefully palpate each of the upper five intercostal areas, on both sides, close to the sternum, as part of a search for nodal metastases. This is an area easily overlooked in the physical examination; hence, the reason for the added emphasis.

Abdominal Lymph Nodes

Anatomy. The lymph nodes of the abdominal cavity are divided into two large groups: (1) the intra-abdominal or visceral and (2) the retroperitoneal or parietal.[54] Reference to Figure 165 will be helpful in understanding this section. A more detailed description can be obtained from standard sources.[14]

The intra-abdominal nodes or visceral nodes consist of a large number of nodes which are located in the various peritoneal ligaments (lesser and greater omentum, gastrosplenic ligament, mesentery and mesocolon) and at the root of the large visceral branches of the aorta. The latter are called the preaortic nodes and are subdivided into the celiac, the superior mesenteric and the inferior mesenteric.

The celiac preaortic nodes are disposed about the origin of the celiac artery. They receive lymph from the organs supplied by the branches of the celiac artery, namely, the lower part of the esophagus, the liver, the gallbladder, the stomach, the spleen, the pancreas and the duodenum. Lymph from these organs first passes through nodes which are located close to these organs within the peritoneal ligaments traversed by the nutritive branches of the celiac artery. Such nodes include the gastric nodes (in the lesser and the greater omenta), the hepatic and the cystic nodes (in the lesser omentum), the pancreaticolienal nodes (in the gastrosplenic ligament).

The superior mesenteric preaortic nodes lie about the origin of the superior mesenteric artery. The inferior mesenteric preaortic nodes surround the origin of the inferior mesenteric artery. These two groups of nodes receive lymph from the small and the large intestines, not directly but indirectly after its passage through a series of nodes located within the mesentery and the mesocolon. The latter nodes are collectively known as the mesenteric nodes. They are arranged in two groups: (1) the proximal, lying about the arterial arcades formed by the branches of the superior and the inferior mesenteric arteries, and (2) the distal, located along the wall of the gut along the vasa recta, branches of the arterial arcades.

The efferents of the preaortic nodes unite to form a single trunk, the intestinal trunk, which joins the cisterna chyli.

The retroperitoneal or parietal nodes comprise (1) the sacral, (2) the internal iliac, (3) the external iliac, (4) the common iliac, and (5) the para-aortic.

The sacral nodes lie in the hollow of the sacrum, in relation to the middle and the lateral sacral arteries. They receive lymph from the rectum, the posterior wall of the pelvis, the prostate, and the cervix of the uterus. Their efferents join the internal iliac and the para-aortic nodes.

The internal iliac nodes are disposed about the internal iliac vessels and their branches. A special group is located about the obturator canal and constitutes the obturator nodes. They receive a large part of the lymph from the rectum, the bladder, the urethra, the prostate, the uterus and the buttocks. Their efferents drain into the common iliac nodes.

The external iliac nodes are located about the external iliac vessels, just behind the inguinal ligament, and in relation to the genitofemoral nerve. They receive lymph from superficial and deep inguinal nodes, internal iliac nodes, deep structures of the anterior abdominal wall below the level of the umbilicus, glans penis or glans clitoris, bladder, cervix and body of the uterus, upper part of the vagina, prostate and membranous urethra. Their efferents join the common iliac nodes.

The common iliac nodes are disposed about the common iliac vessels. They receive afferents from the external iliac, the internal iliac and the sacral nodes. In addition they also receive lymph directly from the rectum, the vagina, the uterus and the prostate. Their efferents empty into the right and the left para-aortic nodes.

The para-aortic nodes form an almost continuous chain on each side of the abdominal aorta. They rest on the psoas major muscle. Those on the right side also are related to the inferior vena cava. They receive the efferents of the common iliac nodes (hence the lymph from the lower extremities, the external genitalia and most of the lymph from the pelvis). In addition, they receive lymph from the lateral abdominal wall by lymphatics accompanying the lumbar arteries, the kidneys, the suprarenals, the testes, the ovaries, the fallopian tubes and the body of the uterus. Their efferents unite on each side to form the right and the left lumbar lymphatic trunks which unite to form the cisterna chyli. Some of the efferents join the preaortic nodes as well as some relatively unimportant nodes behind the abdominal aorta (retro-aortic nodes). Still other efferents, instead of joining the lumbar trunks, pass through the crura of the diaphragm to join the thoracic duct directly.

Clinical Significance. The lymph nodes of the abdomen and the pelvis constitute the largest group of nodes of the body. These nodes drain lymph not only from the lower extremities, but also from all the pelvic and the abdominal organs which are frequently subject to infectious and neoplastic processes. Because of their anatomic proximity to blood vessels and nerve plexuses of the abdominal cavity and to the various segments of the gastrointestinal tract, their enlargement, due to neoplastic or infectious involvement, produces a rich symptomatology,[131-134] the analysis of which is of great value in diagnosis.

Clinically, the most important symptoms are: abdominal discomfort, digestive disturbances, abdominal pain, backache and fever. Less frequent in occurrence, but nevertheless significant, are the following: constipation, ascites, edema, chyloperitoneum, urinary disturbances, jaundice and intestinal obstruction. While the clinical picture is characterized by a variety of symptoms, the physical signs of neoplastic involvement of the abdominal nodes are few and consist of demonstration of palpable nodes, localized tenderness and occasionally of abnormal bruits.[131,132]

1. ABDOMINAL DISCOMFORT occurs as soreness, sense of heaviness or fullness in the epigastric region after meals and inability to eat a full meal. It is caused by the crowding of the stomach and the intestine by enlarging para-aortic and intra-abdominal nodes. The stomach and intestines are unable to expand as their contents increase with the ingestion of meals. There is also delay in emptying of the stomach and passage of food down the intestine due to impaired peristaltic activity.[132]

2. DIGESTIVE DISTURBANCES. *Bloating* and *belching* may be the only symptoms and may be misinterpreted as due to cholecystitis, peptic ulcer, neurasthenia, or even malingering. *Nausea* and *vomiting* are less frequent and may occur irregularly or become constant and progressive with rapid loss of weight. Generally, nausea and vomiting appear with other digestive disturbances. *Diarrhea* is not common. When it occurs, it may be irregular or may continue indefinitely. It has a tendency to increase progressively in severity. It is associated with loss of weight and strength in spite of a normal or ravenous appetite. Usual therapeutic measures are unavailing, and whatever improvement may be obtained proves to be only temporary. Diarrhea may be associated with melena. Diarrhea usually sets in when the intramural lymphoid tissue of the bowel (solitary lymph follicles, patches of Peyer and annular follicles of the appendix) become involved by the neoplastic process.[131,132]

3. ABDOMINAL PAIN. The para-aortic and the pelvic retroperitoneal, as well as the preaortic intra-abdominal lymph nodes are associated intimately with the abdominal autonomic nervous system, which contains parasympathetic, sympathetic and pain fibers. The parasympathetic fibers regulate the motility and the secretory activity of the gastrointestinal tract. The sympathetic fibers are concerned especially with regulation of vasomotor tone of the blood vessels of the gut. The pain fibers relay pain im-

pulses from all the abdominal and the pelvic organs. After passing through the abdominal autonomic nervous system, which is intimately related to the whole length of the abdominal aorta and its branches, the pain impulses are finally transmitted to the spinal cord by the lumbar and the thoracic splanchnic nerves.

The intra-abdominal lymph nodes, located within the lesser and the greater omenta, the mesentery and the mesocolon, also are related intimately to the branches of the celiac, the superior and the inferior mesenteric arteries, which are accompanied throughout their course by the peripheral fibers of the parasympathetic and sympathetic nerves and by pain fibers.

Enlarged retroperitoneal, as well as intra-abdominal lymph nodes, may irritate both autonomic and pain fibers and thus lead not only to impairment of the secretory and motor activity of the gastrointestinal tract but also to pain. Pain may be caused also by the effects of direct neoplastic infiltration of the wall of the digestive tube, gaseous distention and excessive motor activity ("spastic" pain).

Pain due to compression by enlarged lymph nodes is at first characteristically dull in character and felt as soreness. Its distribution depends entirely on the nerves involved by the pressure. Thus, enlarged para-aortic or preaortic nodes compressing the pain fibers coursing through the abdominal autonomic nerves related to the aorta may produce pain suggestive of disease of various organs such as the gallbladder, the pancreas or the appendix. If the pain is severe, the clinical picture may suggest an acute abdominal emergency. Surgery in such cases may bring temporary relief. However, the underlying neoplastic process is relentless in its progress so that the pain may recur with even greater intensity. With progressive enlargement of the nodes the pain may be so severe as to simulate the intractable pain of interstitial pancreatitis. The distribution of the pain will become more extensive as more and more of the para-aortic and the preaortic nodes become enlarged.

"Spastic pain" is cramplike or colicky and occurs in waves. Pressure on the ureter may lead to ureteral spastic pain, simulating ureteral stone.[135] In mesenteric adenitis, the spastic pain occasionally may be due to ileocecal intussusception.[134]

4. BACKACHE. This type of pain is especially characteristic of pressure by enlarged para-aortic and mesenteric nodes on branches of the lumbar and the sacral plexuses and may be felt at various levels of the trunk or in the lower extremities. Depending on the particular nerve irritated, it may be localized in the hip, the thigh, the knee, the ankle or the feet. It may first be felt in the hip and then extend to the foot, simulating sciatic neuritis. It may be unilateral or bilateral. At first, the pain is dull in character. Later, when the nerves become infiltrated with cancer metastases or when metastases to the pubic bones or to the bones of the lower extremities have occurred, the pain becomes boring and severe.[132]

5. FEVER. Often enlargement of the para-aortic and intra-abdominal nodes in Hodgkin's disease and lymphosarcoma is characterized by fever, which is conspicuously absent if the lymphadenopathy in these diseases is confined to the cervical nodes. Fever also develops with involvement of mediastinal nodes. Usually the fever is continuous but occasionally may be of the relapsing or intermittent Pel-Ebstein type. Irradiation of the abdomen may cause the fever to diminish or disappear within 1 to 3 weeks. This therapeutic test is helpful in the diagnosis of abdominal lymphadenopathy due to Hodgkin's disease or lymphosarcoma.

6. CONSTIPATION. Enlargement of both para-aortic and intra-abdominal (mesenteric) nodes may lead to mechanical interference with the motor activity of the gut and thus cause constipation which is proportional to other preceding or concomitant symptoms, such as abdominal pain, backache, bloating and belching. It is characteristic of this type of constipation that it often diminishes or disappears with retrogression of the enlarged nodes following irradiation, to reappear when the nodes enlarge again with advance of the neoplastic process.

7. ASCITES. Ascites may be caused by por-

tal vessel compression from lymph nodes or by metastases to peritoneal surfaces, the latter being more common.

8. EDEMA. Enlargement of the iliac and the pelvic retroperitoneal nodes may compress the iliac veins, especially the external iliac, with resulting edema of the lower extremities. However, this is rarely of a degree to involve an entire lower extremity. Usually, the edema first appears in the feet and the ankles. Compression of the common iliac vein by enlarged common iliac nodes results in edema not only of the lower extremity, but also of the scrotum, penis, pubic region and lower abdomen. Deep palpation of the iliac region may reveal a nodular mass of enlarged nodes or a matted mass, tender to pressure.

9. CHYLOPERITONEUM. Marked enlargement of the celiac preaortic or of the para-aortic nodes in the immediate vicinity of the celiac artery may block the cisterna chyli with the production of chyloperitoneum. At the same time, such blockage, due to retrograde flow, may result in cancerous infiltration of the stomach and the duodenum associated with gastro-intestinal bleeding.

10. URINARY DISTURBANCES. Such disturbances, when present, usually take the form of increased frequency of urination and hematuria. Urinary disturbances are not a common complication. They may be due to compression of the ureter by enlarged iliac nodes resulting in hydronephrosis or pyonephrosis. However, urinary disturbances may also result from cancerous infiltration of the ureter by the lymphatic spread from the primary cancer or by direct extension from involved adjacent para-aortic nodes.

11. JAUNDICE. Jaundice occurring with intra-abdominal lymphoid tumors or lymph node metastases usually indicates liver metastases and only rarely results from lymph node obstruction of extrahepatic biliary passages as indicated by paucity of even isolated case reports in the literature.[136,137]

12. INTESTINAL OBSTRUCTION. Such obstruction may involve the duodenum, the cecum or the other parts of the intestine and is due either to compression by enlarged nodes adjacent to these structures or to actual infiltration of the bowel by the neoplastic process affecting the nodes. The intestinal obstruction is accompanied by pain of increasing severity, nausea and vomiting.

13. PHYSICAL SIGNS. The physical signs associated with enlarged retroperitoneal and intra-abdominal nodes are scanty and usually consist of the demonstration of the enlarged nodes by palpation and the elicitation of tenderness on pressure over the nodes. Occasionally, abnormal bruits may be heard.

Physical signs are conspicuously absent in the early stages and may also be absent in cases where the clinical symptoms are marked. Evidence of nodes may be obscured by cancerous involvement of the gastro-intestinal tract, the liver and the spleen as well as by peritoneal carcinomatosis.

As a rule, the physical signs do not become apparent until the involved nodes have reached a certain size. Under such conditions, by careful palpation, through relaxed abdominal walls, over the iliac region or over the course of the abdominal aorta, the enlarged nodes can be felt as nodular masses of irregular size. Should the nodes be matted together, only a deep resistance may be felt on deep palpation. This must not be mistaken for muscular rigidity. The palpable nodes or resistance may be confined to one side. This is particularly true with lymphadenopathy associated with cancer of the testis or the ovary. In such cases the palpable nodes are always confined to one side or the other depending on the site of the primary cancer, since with cancer of these organs, the spread is always to the homolateral nodes at first. The enlarged nodes are situated high in the abdomen at the level of the renal vessels, because the lymphatics from the testis or the ovary follow the internal spermatic or the ovarian vessels, respectively, and drain into the upper para-aortic nodes (see Fig. 165). Later, with retrograde involvement of the iliac para-aortic nodes, the palpable nodular mass extends vertically toward the iliac region.

Palpable, enlarged para-aortic nodes are

fixed characteristically and show practically no mobility, not even with respiration. By contrast, enlarged intra-abdominal nodes, particularly the mesenteric or the mesocolic, display a noticeable degree of mobility and shifting and may give the impression of a pedicled mass. At the same time, the mass gives a sensation of solidity and lack of resilience. If these physical aspects of enlarged para-aortic and intra-abdominal nodes are kept in mind, their confusion with enlarged liver, spleen or kidney can be avoided. The liver and the spleen may be displaced forward and downward by greatly enlarged para-aortic nodes.

The palpable enlarged nodes may vary in size at intervals. This is particularly true in cases of abdominal lymphadenopathy due to Hodgkin's disease or lymphosarcoma. In these diseases there is an abnormal predisposition to respiratory infections. With each infection there occurs a rapid enlargement of the nodes. With subsidence of the infection, the nodes may regress in size, but the enlargement seldom disappears. Eventually, there is progressive enlargement, although there are cases in which the nodes remain small throughout the disease.

In lymphoblastoma, there may be enlargement of all retroperitoneal and intra-abdominal nodes, but also all aggregations of lymphoid tissue of small and large bowel may become infiltrated with neoplastic cells. Also there is a marked tendency for retroperitoneal nodes of the two sides to become matted together along the whole length of the abdominal aorta. In the majority of cases of lymphoblastoma, however, definite masses cannot be felt.

Enlarged nodes may be demonstrated not only by abdominal palpation, but also by rectal or vaginal examination. In women, enlarged pelvic nodes must be differentiated from uterine fibroids, ovarian cysts or pyosalpinx. At the same time, it must be remembered that these conditions may be coincidental.

In palpating for enlarged retroperitoneal and intra-abdominal nodes, careful attention must be paid to certain procedural details. The patient must be placed in the recumbent position; the head should be flexed on the chest; and the arms should be relaxed and placed by the side of the body. In order to relax the anterior wall as completely as possible, the patient should be encouraged to breathe through the mouth. Further relaxation may be achieved by placing a pillow under the small of the back.

The second significant physical sign of enlarged nodes is tenderness elicited by pressure. Such tenderness is usually slight or moderate.

Abnormal Bruits. Enlarged para-aortic nodes may interfere with normal expansion of the aorta and thus produce abnormal bruits. Constriction of the abdominal aorta may also result from either bilateral or unilateral enlargement of the para-aortic nodes.

Clinical Syndromes of the Intra-abdominal Nodes. 1. THE SPRUE SYNDROME. Lymphomatous involvement of the lymphatic system of the abdomen may lead to the syndrome of secondary sprue in several ways.[138,139]

Infiltration of the wall of the gastrointestinal tract may block the intestinal lacteals and result in malabsorption with the development of a nutritional deficiency state.

Enlarged lymphomatous nodes, through pressure on the gut or the pain fibers, may produce pain related to meals. Under such circumstances, often the patient will resort to a simple monotonous diet, usually low in proteins, and again suffer from nutritional deficiency.

The lymphomatous process may interfere with the motor functions of the gut and lead to diarrhea. If this is marked, there will be loss of fluid, electrolytes and nutritive elements.

2. SYNDROME OF CALCIFIED INTRA-ABDOMINAL LYMPH NODES. Calcified intra-abdominal nodes may produce no symptoms and be discovered on routine x-ray examination or as an incidental finding in x-ray studies of the urinary or the genital tracts. Such asymptomatic calcified nodes may cause confusion in the presence of renal, ureteral and vesical calculi.

However, calcified intra-abdominal nodes in the mesentery may cause symptoms which suggest the advisability of x-ray studies of the gastrointestinal tract.

Such nodes are particularly the mesenteric nodes near the ileocecal junction. Almost invariably such symptomatic calcified nodes are due to tuberculosis. In addition to the calcified nodes, the patient may show evidences of a tuberculous process involving the wall of the gut itself. The calcified nodes are tender on pressure, usually slightly movable. Since they are associated intimately with blood vessels and nerves coursing through the mesentery, there is usually distortion of the affected segments of the blood vessels. The mesentery itself often shows scarring and puckering, interfering with normal motor function of the intestine.[140]

Clinically, the syndrome of calcified mesenteric nodes is characterized by repeated attacks of abdominal pain in the right lower quadrant, accompanied by nausea, vomiting and weakness. There is no elevation of temperature and no leukocytosis during the attack. There is usually a history of underweight and lack of endurance in spite of a good appetite, of repeated visits to a physician and of slow convalescence following various attacks of infections.

Roentgenographic studies show not only the calcified nodes, but barium studies demonstrate spasm of the loop of the intestine at the site of the calcified nodes, delay in emptying of the ileum, and reversed peristalsis.[141]

3. SYNDROME OF TUBERCULOSIS MESENTERIC LYMPHADENITIS. This condition is usually secondary to tuberculosis elsewhere. The process begins in the patches of Peyer and the solitary lymph follicles of the ileum. These lymphoid structures enlarge, fuse, caseate and ulcerate. The ulcers enlarge laterally since the tuberculous process follows the intestinal lymphatics which course at right angles to the longitudinal axis of the bowel. Accompanying this process there is massive involvement of the mesenteric lymph nodes.[142,143] As a rule, tuberculous mesenteric lymphadenitis is confined to the ileum. However, in some cases, it may also involve the jejunum and the duodenum as well as the cecum and the colon. The nodes may remain discrete or become matted together to form large masses. Eventually, gradual calcification of the involved nodes takes place.

Some cases are asymptomatic. Calcified nodes may be seen on routine roentgenograms of the gastrointestinal or urinary tracts. When the infection is active there is fever, malaise, loss of weight and abdominal pain. Since the mesenteric nodes near the ileocecal junction are involved most often, the pain and associated tenderness in the right iliac fossa may simulate that of appendicitis. The nodes are usually not palpable unless they are enlarged considerably.

The tuberculous nodes may break down and discharge their contents into the peritoneal cavity, with resulting localized (cold abscess) or generalized tuberculous peritonitis. Fistulas may develop between different segments of the small intestine. The enlarged, fused nodes may also produce multiple obstructions of the bowel.[144,145]

4. SYNDROME OF ACUTE NONSPECIFIC MESENTERIC LYMPHADENITIS. This syndrome is characterized by recurring abdominal pain and tenderness in the right iliac fossa, associated with enlarged mesenteric (intra-abdominal) nodes.[146,147] It is seen most commonly in children and subsides by the time of puberty. Since it simulates acute appendicitis, diagnosis is usually made at laparotomy.

In the early stages there is discrete enlargement only of the nodes within the mesentery. It is characteristic of this condition that the mesenteric nodes near the ileocecal junction are involved constantly. This is not true of acute appendicitis. The nodes are red and swollen. On culture, they prove to be sterile.[147] Histologically, the nodes show a nonspecific inflammatory reaction and cellular hyperplasia. While many cases of nonspecific mesenteric adenitis are associated with upper respiratory tract infection, the reactive lymphadenopathy probably is due to absorption of toxins from the intestinal tract. Gambill[225] has recently discussed its status as a clinical entity. Suppuration of the affected nodes occurs rarely.

There is generalized abdominal pain, intermittent and colicky in nature and centered about the umbilical region. Usually, it is more severe than the initial pain in acute appendicitis. There is tenderness in the right iliac fossa. The point of tenderness shifts to the left when the patient is turned on the left side (Brennan's sign). This shift in tenderness does not occur in acute appendicitis and is due to the positional shift of the mesentery and its contained enlarged nodes. There is also moderate elevation of temperature and occasionally nausea, vomiting and anorexia. There is an initial polymorph leukocytosis which, however, subsides rapidly in 2 to 3 days.

5. SYNDROME OF PERITONITIS FROM LYMPH NODE SUPPURATION. Very rarely, peritonitis may follow suppuration of an intra-abdominal lymph node.[148]

LYMPH NODE SYNDROMES

A considerable literature attests to the wide interest in lymph node disease. In the section to follow a number of characteristic lymph node syndromes are briefly described. The reader is also referred elsewhere for representative papers which discuss various classifications and clinical features of and give fuller details about various types of lymphadenopathy.[149-156]

In addition to the regional types of lymphadenopathy, related mostly to local area disease as already described, are other clinical states not so easily classified. The following groupings of syndromes has been found by us to be a helpful method of presenting certain of the lymphadenopathies.

SYNDROME OF PRIMARY SORE OR
ENTRANCE LESION ON AN EXTREMITY,
REGIONAL LYMPHADENOPATHY,
FEVER AND SYSTEMIC SYMPTOMS

A number of diseases, mostly infections, fit into a clinical pattern or syndrome characterized by a primary sore or entrance lesion on an extremity, regional (satellite) lymphadenopathy, fever and systemic symptoms with or without a rash. The initial inoculation of the infectious agent, although much more common on the more exposed limb, may occur occasionally on the chest or the abdomen with axillary or superficial inguinal lymphadenopathy, respectively, with a similar clinical picture.

The best-known syndrome consists of a wound or abrasion at site of entry, tubular lymphangitis and septicemia, due to *Streptococcus hemolyticus*[157] referred to in the past by the old-fashioned term "blood poisoning." It is now rare since the advent of sulfa and antibiotic therapy. The unusual occurrence of a primary syphilitic chancre and regional lymphadenopathy, not yet subsided, simultaneously with the presence of the systemic features of the secondary stage of syphilis fits into this category. The nonvenereal site of extragenital chancre (e.g., the finger of a dentist or a physician) often makes the diagnosis confusing.[158] Rarely, primary inoculation of tuberculosis in the skin of an extremity, in a person tuberculin-negative, may produce an indolent ulcer at the inoculation site, lymphangitis and satellite lymphadenopathy, with usually only minimal systemic reaction and fever but causing transition of the tuberculin test to positive as healing occurs.[159,160] In a sense this constitutes, by analogy with the primary lung infection, a dermatologic, Ghon tubercle with a primary skin complex.[160]

Sporotrichosis of the lymphangitic type may commence as indolent ulcers at the inoculation site, with chronic nodular and often painless lymph channel involvement but without marked regional lymphadenopathy or systemic symptoms.[161]

Anthrax usually commences as a firm red papule, progressing through vesicular formation to a painless ulcer surrounded by a zone of erythema and edema followed by tender regional lymphadenopathy with severe systemic symptoms, often with bacteremia.[162,163]

Inoculation of the skin by the *Erysipelothrix rhusiopathia,* commonly from handling fish or dead animal matter, may produce a local lesion, lymphangitis and regional adenitis with variable systemic symptoms and constitute the clinical picture of the occupational disease known as *erysipeloid* of Rosenbach.[164]

A sensitive ulcer on a finger, regional lymphadenopathy, fever, systemic symptoms, with or without a rash, often with bacteremia in a person who has handled rabbits, constitutes a picture classic for the ulceroglandular type of *tularemia.*[165,166]

Bubonic plague is another classic example of this syndrome. A vesicle forms at the site of bite of an infected flea, followed by very large painful regional adenitis, often suppurative or hemorrhagic, with severe systemic symptoms.[167]

Several rickettsial diseases fit into this pattern. Best known, as a result of World War II experiences, is *scrub typhus* due to *R. orientalis*.[168] A black eschar forms at the site of a mite bite, followed by regional adenopathy (usually without lymphangitis), systemic spread, fever and rash. At times lymphadenopathy becomes generalized. *Boutonneuse fever* (due to *R. conorii*) carried by a dog tick, *South African tick bite fever* and possibly *Kenya typhus* have an initial sore, lymph node enlargement and a systemic picture similar to scrub typhus.

Rickettsialpox (due to *R. akari*), a relatively new American rickettsial disease, is somewhat similar, manifesting an initial painless lesion at the site of the infecting mite bite, painful regional adenitis, systemic spread, fever and a characteristic rash.[169]

Filariasis does not entirely fit this syndrome. Usually the legs are involved but fail to show a primary entrance lesion. However, lymphangitis, regional lymphadenopathy and various systemic symptoms may occur.

Rat-bite fever is characterized by a late local lesion at the rat-bite site followed by lymphangitis, regional lymphadenopathy, systemic symptoms, rash and fever, all of which may show remissions and relapses.[170,171] The *Spirillum minus* organism does this more strikingly than the *Streptobacillus moniliformis*.

Cat-scratch disease (nonbacterial regional lymphadenitis) is now known to be a frequent cause of this syndrome. Commonly, but not always, a cat scratch causes a local inoculation lesion (? due to virus), regional lymphadenitis (often large and suppurating), and systemic symptoms with occasional transitory rash.[172] Absence of bacteria in the pus and a positive skin test with "cat-scratch antigen" help establish the diagnosis.

While all these syndromes are infectious, one never should overlook the fact that a *primary neoplasm* may occur on an extremity, cause regional metastasis and manifest systemic symptoms and fever as a result of visceral metastases.

Syndrome of Diseases Originating in the Oropharynx with Cervical Satellite Lymphadenopathy, Fever and Systemic Symptoms

In a sense, the usual bacterial infections of the throat (especially of the tonsils) such as streptococcal sore throat, scarlet fever, diphtheria, etc., belong to this category. Lymphadenopathy in throat infections of viral etiology is usually less striking than for bacterial infections. Most characteristic of diseases illustrating this syndrome is infectious mononucleosis when associated with a severe sore throat. Weil's disease occasionally produces cervical adenopathy as part of the total clinical picture.

Cat-scratch disease[172] occasionally may have an oropharyngeal site of origin with striking lymph node enlargement of the neck, progressing at times to suppuration. An oral cavity syphilitic chancre with regional neck lymphadenopathy followed by the secondary systemic phase is especially classic of this syndrome. Likewise is cervical node tuberculosis, which may rarely manifest a systemic spread.

Syndrome of a Genital Lesion, Groin Lymphadenopathy, Fever and Systemic Symptoms

Of course, many of the diseases described under the first section for an extremity site of origin could occur if the inoculation site of the infectious agent is on the genitalia instead of an extremity. In general, however, infectious disorders with a primary genital site are of venereal origin and include primarily syphilis, gonorrhea, chancroid and lymphopathia venereum. Rarely, a tuberculous infection may be responsible. Cancer of the penis with regional groin metastases and systemic metastatic spread fits into this pattern quite readily.

Generalized Lymphadenopathy

Generalized lymph node enlargement obviously can occur as a result of various diffuse skin disorders which permit infectious and toxic multiple regional lymph node involvement of a chronic reactive type. A specific syndrome (lipomelanotic reticular hyperplasia of lymph nodes) usually related to erythematous and exfoliative types of pruritic dermatosis, in which the lymphadenopathy is characterized by lipid and melanin infiltration and reticulum cell reaction (at times suggesting a lymphoma),[173,174] can be identified specifically in this general category.

Superficial lymphadenopathy is one of the features of the Sézary syndrome, a rare disorder, presenting with an exfoliative erythroderma in association with some striking systemic clinical manifestations as well as a characteristic cell in the peripheral blood.[226]

By common understanding, the term "generalized lymphadenopathy" has come to mean involvement of 2 and preferably 3 regionally separated lymph node groups in which enlargement results from a systemic disorder acting on lymphoid tissue generally by one of the mechanisms described previously under modes of involvement. Although the basic stress is generalized, enlargement of nodes often occurs in irregular fashion and need not appear simultaneously and to an equal degree in all body areas.

Generalized lymphadenopathy of infectious origin may occur in addition to a more prominent regional adenopathy in the drainage area of the inoculation site in a number of the disorders described in the preceding sections 1, 2 and 3, such as cat-scratch disease,[172] infectious mononucleosis, tularemia,[166] plague,[167] secondary syphilis, etc. Children often manifest a greater degree of generalized lymph node response to a particular infection than adults for reasons commented upon previously (e.g., in measles, rubella, rheumatic fever, scarlet fever, etc.). While some of the infectious diseases which produce a generalized type of lymphadenopathy are well known, others are less understood: for example, brucellosis,[175,176] generalized peripheral lymphadenopathy of tuberculous origin,[177] and certain tropical diseases.[178]

Generalized lymph node enlargement may be primary in lymphoid or reticular endothelial tissue of lymph nodes, as in Hodgkin's disease, lymphosarcoma and lymphatic leukemia; or secondary to primary involvement of the hemopoietic system as in myelogenous or monocytic leukemia, sickle cell and hemolytic anemia. General lymph node enlargement may be of metabolic origin, as in Niemann-Pick's disease, Gaucher's disease, etc. These are all well known and adequately described in many excellent articles and standard texts.

Less well understood is the generalized lymphadenopathy so common in sarcoidosis,[179] serum sickness[180] and status lymphaticus. Generalized lymphadenopathy may occur in some of the disorders of the collagen tissues. Particularly well-documented are rheumatoid arthritis,[181] Still's disease,[181] dermatomyositis and disseminated lupus erythematosus.[182,183]

Particular attention should be paid to patients with suspected systemic disease if the original biopsy diagnosis of a superficial lymph node is reported as hyperplasia. One should carefully follow the clinical course of this type of patient, whether the nodes are regional or generalized, for possible development of a recognizable serious illness, particularly a disease of collagen tissue or malignancy.[227] This sequence appears to be rather common when looked for.

Generalized lymphadenopathy may occur occasionally in the adult acquired form of toxoplasmosis and the entire syndrome may resemble, to a remarkable degree, acute infectious mononucleosis. One should suspect toxoplasmosis especially if this picture occurs in a person exposed to certain birds and mammals, including the domestic dog. The diagnosis can be confirmed by the toxoplasma dye test and toxoplasma complement fixation test.[228] At times, the lymphadenitis may be relapsing.[229] Rarely, leishmaniasis may be localized to lymph nodes and cause enlargement at multiple sites.[239] Generalized adenopathy occurs in "Ardmore disease,"[231] characterized also by upper respiratory infection, enlarged and painful liver, splenomegaly and a prolonged course of several months. Posterior cervical nodes were reported as enlarged in 95 per cent of cases with this disease.

Rarely, some of the hydantoin type of anticonvulsant drugs may cause lymphadenopathy, mimicking a lymphoma clinic-

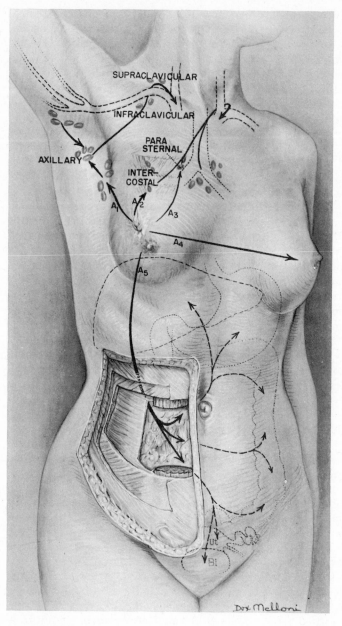

Fig. 166. Lymphatic drainage of the mammary gland. Metastases from cancer of the mammary gland may follow several lymphatic pathways: A_1. Upper outer quadrant to axillary, infravicular, supraclavicular nodes, etc. A_2. Upper inner quadrant to intercostal and parasternal nodes. A_3. Upper inner quadrant directly to parasternal nodes. A_4. Directly across mid-line to opposite breast. A_5. Lower quadrants, particularly inner aspect, through pectoralis major, external oblique and linea alba to subperitoneal lymphatic plexus, followed by abdominal and pelvic spread.

ally and even pathologically, but reversible upon cessation of their use.[232,233] Histiocytic medullary reticulosis, a rapidly fatal reticuloendothelial proliferative disorder, should be included among the unusual causes of generalized lymphadenopathy. A characteristic clinical picture, coupled with bone marrow findings, may serve to establish antemortem diagnosis.[234,235] "Rademacher's disease," as recently described, is

another rare condition capable of causing generalized lymphadenopathy.[236]

SYNDROMES OF LYMPHATIC METASTASES FROM CANCER OF BREAST

Cancer of the mammary gland may metastasize by several lymphatic pathways (see Fig. 166). Cancer arising in the upper outer quadrant of the gland metastasizes to the axillary nodes (A_1), the infraclavicular and the supraclavicular nodes. From here, cancer emboli can reach the venous system via the jugular trunk. Cancer, metastasizing in this manner has the most favorable prognosis.

In the upper inner quadrant it may metastasize first to the intercostal, then to the parasternal nodes (A_2) or may reach the parasternal nodes directly (A_3). The parasternal nodes drain into the mediastinal nodes from which cancer emboli can reach the venous system by way of the bronchomediastinal trunk. Due to the involvement of the mediastinal nodes, cancer spreading by this route has a dangerous prognosis. Parasternal nodes (A_3) should

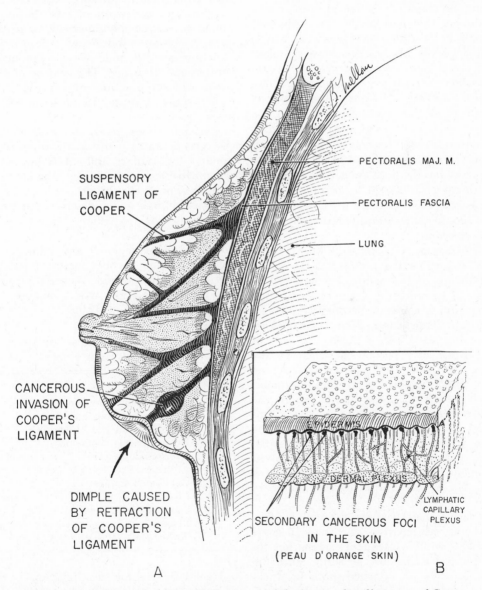

SUSPENSORY
LIGAMENT OF
COOPER

PECTORALIS MAJ. M.

PECTORALIS FASCIA

LUNG

CANCEROUS
INVASION OF
COOPER'S
LIGAMENT

DIMPLE CAUSED
BY RETRACTION
OF COOPER'S
LIGAMENT

EPIDERMIS

DERMAL PLEXUS

LYMPHATIC
CAPILLARY
PLEXUS

SECONDARY CANCEROUS FOCI
IN THE SKIN
(PEAU D'ORANGE SKIN)

A

B

Fig. 167. A. Retraction of the skin in cancer of the breast when ligaments of Cooper contract following cancer invasion. B. Secondary cancerous foci in skin producing *peau d'orange* skin.

be searched for by careful palpation in the upper 5 intercostal spaces, on both sides, close to the sternum.[224]

The lymphatics of the skin of one mammary gland communicate directly across the mid-line (A_4). with those of the opposite side. Hence, unilateral cancer may become bilateral by this lymphatic route.

Cancer developing in the lower quadrants, particularly the lower inner, may spread by lymphatics which traverse the pectoralis major, the external oblique and the upper thin part of the linea alba and communicate with the subperitoneal lymphatic plexus (A_5). Thus cancer emboli may reach the peritoneal cavity and set up secondary foci on any of the abdominal organs. Cancer cells may also drop by gravity from the peritoneal cavity into the pelvic cavity and thus give rise to secondary pelvic metastases. Due to the possibility of invasion of the peritoneal cavity, this type of spread has the most dangerous prognosis. Furthermore, due to this possible mode of metastasis, every patient with breast nodules should have careful rectal and vaginal examination.

The mammary gland and its overlying skin is anchored to pectoral fascia, covering the pectoralis major, by bands of fibrous tissue called the ligaments of Cooper. When these ligaments become invaded by cancer emboli, contraction occurs along these ligaments. As a result, the skin of the breast may become attached to the subjacent neoplastic growth so that the skin cannot be pinched up from the tumor. With further extension of the cancer, the entire breast may be bound to the pectoral fascia so that it can no longer move in the long axis of the pectoralis major. Finally, with continued contraction of the involved ligaments of Cooper, there is dimpling of the skin or the nipple of the mammary gland (Fig. 167A).

The lymphatic vessels draining the skin over the mammary gland may become blocked with consequent stagnation of lymph and edema of the skin. Since the hair follicles are attached more firmly to the underlying superficial fascia, the edematous skin projects in between the hair follicles. This skin thus presents pitting. This condition is called *peau d'orange* (Fig. 167B). *Peau d'orange* may occur in other parts of the body where blockage of the skin lymphatics occurs, e.g., ischiorectal abscess.

SUPPURATION OF LYMPH NODES

A distinctive phenomenon which occasionally follows infectious lymphadenopathy occurs when the infecting organism overwhelms the local defensive mechanism within the node to produce excess cellular reaction and collection of pus. Suppuration may subside spontaneously, or it may require incision and drainage or lead to destruction of the node with spontaneous rupture and drainage. This may occur in a single node or lead to coalescence of multiple nodes with suppuration, at times from several sites.

The nodes most likely to suppurate are the cervical and superficial inguinal, occasionally the axillary and much less often the epitrochlear or popliteal. The rarity of suppuration of the intrathoracic and the intra-abdominal nodes deserves comment, considering the frequency of involvement of these nodes.

Of the many regional and systemic infections leading to adenopathy, relatively few produce lymph node suppuration with any regularity. Those most commonly responsible are listed in Table 22.

TABLE 22. IMPORTANT CAUSES OF SUPPURATION OF LYMPH NODES

Streptococcal pharyngitis
Streptococcal wound infection
Tuberculous lymphadenitis
Staphylococcal lymphadenitis
Lymphopathia venereum
Coccidioidomycosis
Anthrax
Cat-scratch disease
Chancroid
Sporotrichosis
Plague
Tularemia

Hemolytic streptococcus infections of the pharynx and tonsils producing cervical and more rarely retropharyngeal suppuration (most commonly in children under age 5) were the most common forms prior to the sulfonamide era. There is some question whether the occasional peritonsillar abscess or cellulitis of the neck complicating tonsillitis is due to another superimposed bacterial infection. Streptococcus infections in extremity wounds often produce tubular lymphangitis (characterized by painful red streaks) and suppurative regional lymphadenotis, the pus often being thin, possibly because of the presence of the enzymes, streptokinase and streptodornase. Staphylococcus infection is manifested by a thick yellow-white type of pus. Lymphopathia venereum (of viral origin), especially in the male, and chancroid (due to *Bacillus ducrei*) are common genital infections predisposing to suppurative superficial inguinal adenitis. Cervical tuberculous lymphadenitis with suppurative scrofula, now rare in Europe and America, was in past years a classic and common form of cervical node suppuration with localization at a lower level in the neck than streptococcus adenitis. Pediculosis of the scalp, probably by permitting secondary infection, occasionally may produce suppuration of occipital and posterior neck nodes.

Anthrax and plague represent serious systemic disorders with regional nodes draining the entrance area manifesting marked suppuration, which occasionally may be hemorrhagic or manifest necrotic liquefaction. Fungus infections, especially sporotrichosis (usually on an extremity) and coccidioidomycosis (cervical area), occasionally may produce suppuration. In recent years, cat-scratch disease (nonbacterial regional lymphadenitis) of probable virus etiology, has been found to be a common cause of lymph node suppuration, most common in the groin or the axilla, occasionally epitrochlear and rarely cervical.[172] Early, the enlarged nodes may simulate a lymphoma. Following suppuration they simulate tularemia. Bacteriologically negative pus, history of contact with cats and use of the cat-scratch antigen skin test assist in diagnosis.

An unusual cause is the recently described disorder of serious prognosis which occurs in infants and young children, with a possible genetic predilection for males.

It is characterized by chronic suppurative lymphadenitis (cervical in location), along with pulmonary infiltrations, hepatosplenomegaly, and a characteristically distributed eczematoid dermatitis. Pathologically, there is a generalized granulomatous process and hypergammaglobulinemia.[237]

BCG vaccination in infants may lead to suppuration of the axillary nodes when the shoulder is the site of injection, and suppuration of the superficial inguinal nodes when the thigh is the injection site. Suppuration may not take place until months following the injection and appears related to the dosage. Groin suppuration is much more common than axillary suppuration for reasons explained in the section on inguinal adenitis.

REFERENCES

1. Drinker, C. K., and Yoffey, J. M.: Lymphatics, Lymph and Lymphoid Tissue: Their Physiological and Clinical Significance, Cambridge, Mass., Harvard, 1941.
2. Drinker, C. K.: The functional significance of the lymphatic system, Bull. New York Acad. Med. 14:231-251, 1938.
3. Landis, E. M., Jonas, L., Angevine, M., and Erb, W.: The passage of fluid and protein through the human capillary wall during venous congestion, J. Clin. Invest. 11:717-734, 1932.
4. Markowitz, C., and Mann, F. C.: The role of the liver in the formation of lymph, Am. J. Physiol. 96:709-712, 1931.
5. McMaster, P. D.: Condition in skin influencing interstitial fluid movement, lymph formation and lymph flow, Ann. New York Acad. Sc. 46:743-787, 1946.
6. Ladd, M. P., Kottke, F. J., and Blanchard, R. S.: Studies of effect of massage on flow of lymph from foreleg of dog, Arch. Phys. Med. 33:604-612, 1952.
7. Bierman, H. R.: Characteristics of the thoracic duct lymph in man, J. Clin. Invest. 32:632-649, 1953.
8. Crandall, L. A., Jr., Barker, S. B., and Graham, D. G.: A study of the lymph flow from a patient with thoracic duct fistula, Gastroenterology 1:1040-1048, 1943.
9. Henry, C. S.: Studies on the lymphatic vessels and on the movement of lymph in the ear of the rabbit, Anat. Rec. 57:263-278, 1933.
10. Smith, R. O.: Lymphatic contractility; possible intrinsic mechanism of lymphatic

vessels for transport of lymph, J. Exp. Med. 90:497-509, 1949.

11. Heller, E. L.: Carcinoma of the stomach with multiple annular metastatic intestinal infiltrations, Arch. Path. 40:392-394, 1945.

12. Glover, R. P., and Waugh, J. M.: The retrograde lymphatic spread of carcinoma of the "rectosigmoid region"; its influence in surgical procedures, Surg. Gynec. & Obst. 82:434-448, 1946.

13. Pernis, van, P. A.: Variations of the thoracic duct, Surgery 26:806-809, 1949.

14. Rouvière, H.: Anatomy of the Lymphatic System (Transl. by M. J. Tobias), Ann Arbor, Mich., Edwards Brothers, Inc., 1938.

15. Weeks, A., and Delprat, G. D.: Superficial abrasion with secondary infection and lymphangitis, Surg. Clin. North America 14:1537-1545, 1934.

16. Steel, W. A.: Acute lymphangitis, Am. J. Surg. 36:37-43, 1937.

17. Hendrick, J. W.: Macroglossia or giant tongue, Surgery 39:674-677, 1956.

18. Archer, W. H.: Lymphangioma of lips; report of 2 cases, Oral Surg. 5:170-171, 1952.

19. Allen, E. V.: Lymphedema of the extremities: classification, etiology and differential diagnosis: a study of three hundred cases, Arch. Int. Med. 54:606-624, 1934.

20. Gross, R. E., and Goeringer, C. F.: Cystic hygroma of the neck, Surg. Gynec & Obst. 69:48-60, 1939.

21. Fishback, F. C.: Lymph leakage (lymphorrhea) : a complication of saphenous vein ligation, with suggestions for treatment, Surgery 22:834-836, 1947.

22. Martorell, F.: Chronic edema of the lower limbs, Angiology 2:434-460, 1951.

23. Menten, M. L., and Welton, J. P.: Lipid analysis in a case of Niemann-Pick disease, Am. J. Dis. Child. 72:720-727, 1946.

24. Gilchrist, R. K., and David, V. C.: Lymphatic spread of carcinoma of the rectum, Ann. Surg. 108:621-642, 1938.

25. Black, M. M., Kerpe, S., and Speer, F. D.: Lymph node structure in patients with cancer of the breast, Am. J. Path. 29:505-521, 1953.

26. Lachman, E.: Common and uncommon pathways in the spread of tumors and infections, Surg. Gynec. & Obst. 85:767-775, 1947.

27. Batson, O. V.: Function of the vertebral veins and their role in the spread of metastases, Ann. Surg. 112:138-149, 1940.

28. Edwards, H. C., Acute lymphangitis and acute lymphadenitis, Practitioner 136:281-288, 1936.

29. Price, L. W.: The pathology of lymph node enlargement, Post. Grad. M. J. 23:401-425, 1947.

30. Hadfield, G.: General pathology of lymphadenopathies, Ann. Roy. Coll. Surgeons England 5:89-105, 1949.

31. Quinland, W. S.: Some types of lymphadenopathy with emphasis on lymphosarcoma, J. Nat. M. A. 43:113-121, 1951.

32. Lanza, A. J.: Silicosis and Asbestosis, New York, Oxford, 1938.

33. Thannhauser, J.: Lipidosis; Disease of the Cellular Lipid Metabolism, ed. 2, New York, Oxford, 1950.

34. Medoff, A. S., and Bayrd, E. D.: Gaucher's disease in 29 cases: Hematologic complication and effect of splenectomy, Ann. Int. Med. 40:481-492, 1954.

35. Scammon, R. E.: A summary of the anatomy of the infant and child, in Abt, I. A. (ed.) : Pediatrics, vol. I, Ch. 3, pp. 277-278, Philadelphia, Saunders, 1923.

36. Freund, M., and Ripps, M. L.: Hand-Schüller-Christian disease: a case in which lymphadenopathy was a predominant feature, Am. J. Dis. Child. 61:759-769, 1941.

37. Hansen, P. B.: Relationship of Hand-Schüller-Christian syndrome, Letterer-Siwe's disease and eosinophilic granuloma of bone with report of five cases, Acta radiol. 32:89-112, 1949.

38. Abt, A. F., and Denenholz, E. J.: Letterer-Siwe's disease. Splenohepatomegaly associated with widespread hyperplasia of non-lipoid-storing macrophages; discussion of so-called reticulo-endothelium, Am. J. Dis. Child. 51:499-522, 1936.

39. Jaffe, H. L., and Lichtenstein, L.: Eosinophilic granuloma of bone, Arch, Path. 37:99-118, 1944.

40. Lichtenstein, L.: Histiocytosis: X. Integration of eosinophilic granuloma of bone, "Letterer-Siwe disease," and "Schüller-Christian disease" as related to manifestations of a single nosologic entity, Arch. Path. 56:84-102, 1953.

41. Pund, E. R., and Stelling, F. H.: Lymphosarcoma, Am. J. Surg. 52:50-54, 1941.

42. Sugarbaker, E. D., and Craver, L. F.: Lymphosarcoma: a study of 196 cases with biopsy, J.A.M.A. 115:17-23, 112-117, 1940.

43. Clarke, R. G., and Simonds, J. P.: Primary lymphosarcoma of the appendix, Cancer 4: 994-998, 1951.

44. Currie, D. J., and Luke, J. C.: Giant follicular hyperplasia of the rectum showing malignant degeneration, Can. M. A. J. 63: 150-152, 1950.

45. Baehr, G., and Klemperer, P.: Giant follicle lymphoblastoma; benign variety of lymphosarcoma, N. Y. State J. Med. 40:7-11, 1940.

46. Jackson, H., Jr., and Parker, F., Jr.: Hodgkin's disease: clinical diagnosis, New England J. Med. 234:103-110, 1946.

47. Goldman, L. B.: Hodgkin's disease: An analysis of 212 cases, J.A.M.A. 114:1611-1616, 1940.

48. Warren, S., and Picena, J. P.: Reticulum-cell sarcoma of lymph nodes, Am. J. Path. 17:385-394, 1941.

49. Wilkie, D.: Reticulum-cell sarcoma of small intestine with perforation, Brit. J. Surg. 41:50-53, 1953.

50. Wintrobe, M. M.: Clinical Hematology, ed. 5, Philadelphia, Lea & Febiger, 1961.

51. Isaacs, R.: Correlation of clinical and laboratory data in diseases of lymph nodes, J. Michigan M. Soc. 37:1072-1073, 1938.

52. Herbert, P. A., and Miller, F. R.: Histopathology of monocytic leukemia, Am. J. Path. 23:93-123, 1947.

53. Whitby, L. E. H., and Britton, C. J. C.: Disorders of the Blood, ed. 9, London, Churchill, 1963.

54. Solnitzky, O.: Anatomical factors influencing the spread of cancer, Bull. Georgetown Univ. M. Center 3:176-193, 1950.

55. Davis, H. K.: A statistical study of the thoracic duct in man, Am. J. Anat. 17:211-244, 1915.

56. Hoffman, E., Ivins, J. L., and Kern, H. M.: Traumatic chylothorax, A.M.A. Arch. Surg. 64:253-268, 1952.

57. Little, J. M., Harrison, C., and Blalock, A.: Chylothorax and chyloperitoneum, Surgery 11:392-401, 1942.

58. Kalmansohn, R. B.: Rubella (German measles); observations on an epidemic, with particular reference to lymphadenopathy, New England J. Med. 247:428-429, 1952.

59. Edgerton, A. E.: Herpes zoster ophthalmicus: report of cases and review of literature, Arch. Ophth. 34:45-64, 114-153, 1945.

60. Rice, C. E.: A note on the frequency of involvement of the anterior auricular lymph nodes in trachoma, Am. J. Ophth. 18:651, 1935.

61. Verhoeff, F. H., and King, M. J.: Leptothricosis conjunctivae (Parinaud's conjunctivitis), Arch. Ophth. 9:701-714, 1933.

62. Koteen, H.: Lymphogranuloma venereum, Medicine 24:1-69, 1945.

63. Francis, E.: Oculoglandular tularemia, Arch. Ophth. 28:711-741, 1942.

64. Cassady, J. V., and Culbertson, C. S.: Cat scratch disease and Parinaud's oculoglandular syndrome, A.M.A. Arch. Ophth. 50:68-74, 1953.

65. Tassman, I. S.: The Eye Manifestations of Internal Diseases (Medical Ophthalmology), St. Louis, Mosby, 1951.

66. Sorsby, A.: Systemic Ophthalmology, St. Louis, Mosby, 1951.

67. Allen, J. H.: Lids, lacrimal apparatus and conjunctiva: review of recent literature, A.M.A. Arch. Ophth. 45:100-119, 1951.

68. Hartmann, K.: Ectogenous conjunctival tuberculosis due to bovine tubercle bacilli; treatment by electrocoagulation; contribution to Parinaud's symptom complex, Klin. Monatsbl. Augenh. 113:20-28, 1948.

69. Sanders, M., Gulliver, F. D., Forcheimer, L. I., and Alexander, R. C.: Epidemic keratoconjunctivitis; clinical and experimental study of an outbreak in New York City; further observations on the specific relationship between a virus and the disease, J.A.M.A. 121:250-255, 1943.

70. Curry, J. J., and Lowell, F. C.: Epidemic keratoconjunctivitis: report of a case with marked systemic manifestations, New England J. Med. 231:11-13, 1944.

71. Ryan, R., O'Rourke, J. F., and Iser, G.: Conjunctivitis in adenoidal-pharyngeal-conjunctival virus infection, A.M.A. Arch. Ophth. 54:211-216, 1955.

72. Weinman, D.: Chagas' disease, Oxford Syst. Med. 5:860 (55) -860 (107), 1950.

73. Moseley, V., and Miller, H.: South American trypanosomiasis (Chagas' disease), Arch. Int. Med. 76:219-229, 1945.

74. Munslow, R. A., and Capps, J. M.: Droop shoulder following cervical node biopsy, Texas J. Med. 48:706-707, 1952.

75. Strong, R. P.: Stitt's Diagnosis, Prevention and Treatment of Tropical Diseases, p. 187, Philadelphia, Blakiston, 1942.

76. Looney, W. W.: Lymphatic drainage of the head and neck—emphasizing special structures, Ann. Otol. Rhinol. & Laryng. 44:33-41, 1935.

77. Viacava, E. P., and Pack, G. T.: Significance of supraclavicular signal node in patients with abdominal and thoracic cancer: a study of one hundred and twenty-two cases, Arch. Surg. 48:109-119, 1944.

78. McKusick, V. A.: Virchow-Troisier node: an occasional conspicuous manifestation of gallbladder cancer, South. M. J. 46:965-967, 1953.

79. Willis, R. A.: The spread of tumours in the human body, p. 32, London, Butterworth, and St. Louis, Mosby, 1952.

80. Zeidman, I.: Experimental studies on the spread of cancer in the lymphatic system. III. Tumor emboli in thoracic duct, the pathogenesis of Virchow's node, Cancer Res. 15:719-721, 1955.

81. Harken, D. E., Black, H., Clauss, R., and Farrand, R. E.: A simple cervicomediastinal exploration for tissue diagnosis of intrathoracic disease with comments on the recognition of inoperable carcinoma of the lung, New England J. Med. 251:1041-1044, 1954.

82. Shefts, L. M., Terrill, A. A., and Swindell, H.: Scalene node biopsy, Am. Rev. Tuber. 68:505-522, 1953.

83. Cuykendall, J. H.: Use of prescalene lymph node biopsy in absence of palpable supraclavicular nodes: report of forty-one cases, J.A.M.A. 155:741-742, 1954.

84. Daniels, A. C.: A method of biopsy useful in diagnosing certain intrathoracic diseases, Dis. Chest. 16:360-366, 1949.

85. Bailey, H.: Demonstrations of Physical Signs in Clinical Surgery, ed. 12, p. 88, Baltimore, Williams & Wilkins, 1954.

86. Bailey, H.: Adenitis of facial lymph gland, Practitioner 125:618-620, 1930.

87. Fifield, L. R.: Mixed tumours of the molar glands, Lancet 2:652, 1927.

88. Polya, A. E., and Navrath, D. V.: Untersuchungen über die Lymphbahnen der Wangenschleimhaut, Deutsche Ztschr. Chir. 66:122-175, 1902.

89. Martin, H., and Morfit, H. M.: Cervical lymph node metastasis as the first symptom of cancer, Surg. Gynec. & Obst. 78:133-159, 1944.

90. Martin, H., and Romieu, C.: The diagnostic significance of a lump in the neck, Postgrad. Med. 11:491-500, 1942.

91. Carey, J. M., and Kirklin, J. W.: Extended radical mastectomy: a review of its concepts, Proc. Staff Meet. Mayo Clin. 27:436-440, 1952.

92. Weinberger, H. A., and Stetten, D. W.: Extensive secondary axillary lymph node carcinoma without clinical evidence of primary breast lesions, Surgery 29:217-222, 1951.

93. Cogswell, H. D.: Hidden carcinoma of the breast, Arch. Surg. 58:780-789, 1949.

94. Lapin, J. H., and Tuason, J.: Immunization adenitis, J.A.M.A. 158:472-474, 1955.

95. Guld, J., Magnus, K., Tolderlund, K., Biering-Sørensen, K., and Edwards, P. O.: Suppurative lymphadenitis following intradermal B.C.G. vaccination of the newborn: a preliminary report, Brit. M. J. 2:1048-1054, 1955.

96. Stein, S. C., and Sokoloff, M. J.: Calcification of regional lymph nodes following B.C.G. vaccination, Am. Rev. Tuber. & Pul. Dis. 73:239-245, 1956.

97. Lawrence, K. R., and Anglem, T. J.: Acute subpectoral abscess: A surgical emergency, New England J. Med. 237:390-395, 1947.

98. Straus, D. C.: Subpectoral abscess (suppurative infraclavicular lymphadenitis, with report of 3 cases), Internat. Surg. Digest 20:259-273, 1935.

99. Evans, G.: Palpable epitrochlear glands: their value as a physical sign, Lancet 2:256-257, 1937.

100. Beeson, P. B.: Epitrochlear adenopathy in secondary syphilis, Arch. Dermat. & Syph. 32:746-749, 1935.

101. Martin, L.: Palpable epitrochlear gland: incidence and relation to syphilis, Lancet 1:363-364, 1947.

102. Chanarin, I.: Epitrochlear adenopathy in the Bantu, South African M. J. 23:960-962, 1949.

103. Pack, G. T., and Rekers, P.: The management of malignant tumors in the groin: a report of 122 groin dissections, Am. J. Surg. 56:545-565, 1942.

104. Spain, R. S., and Howard, G. T.: Leptospirosis due to leptospira grippotyphosa, J.A.M.A. 150:1010-1012, 1952.

105. Gaisford, W., and Griffiths, M.: B.C.G. Vaccination in the newborn, preliminary report, Brit. M. J. 2:702-705, 1951.

106. Cole, P. P.: Inguinal swellings, M. Press 207:91-96, 1942.

107. Cohn, I.: Masses in groin, Internat. Clin. 2:229-256, 1935.

108. Carson, M. J., and Hartman, A. F.: Diagnosis and management of severe infections in infants and children: A review of experiences since the introduction of sulfonamide therapy; VI. Acute iliac lymphadenitis, J. Ped. 29:183-188, 1946.

109. Irwin, F. G.: Acute iliac adenitis, Arch. Surg. 36:561-570, 1938.

110. Hyman, A.: Suppurative retroperitoneal pelvic lymphadenitis, Ann. Surg. 91:718-723, 1930.

111. Hodgson, C. H., Olsen, A. M., and Good, C. A.: Bilateral hilar adenopathy: Its significance and management, Ann. Int. Med. 43:83-99, 1955.

112. Dawber, T. R., and Hawer, L. E.: Diseases of the Chest, pp. 123-145, 363-375, Baltimore, Williams & Wilkins, 1952.

113. Katz, S.: The etiology of mediastinal lymphadenopathy, GP 8:64-65, 1953.

114. Favour, C. B., and Sosman, M. C.: Erythema nodosum, Arch. Int. Med. 80:435-453, 1947.

115. Wynn-Williams, N., and Edward, G. F.: Bilateral hilar lymphadenopathy; its association with erythema nodosum, Lancet 1: 278-280, 1954.

116. Löfgron, S., and Lundback, H.: The bilateral hilar lymphoma syndrome: a study of the relation of tuberculosis and sarcoidosis of 212 cases, Acta med. scandinav. 142:265-273, 1952.

117. Lindskog, G. E., and Spear, H. C.: Middle-lobe syndrome, New England J. Med. 253: 489-495, 1955.

118. Brock, R. C., Cann, R. J., and Dickinson, J. R.: Tuberculous mediastinal lymphadenitis in childhood. Secondary effects on lungs, Guy's Hosp. Rep. 87:295-317, 1937.

119. Brock, R. C.: The Anatomy of the Bronchial Tree with Special Reference to the Surgery of Lung Abscess, New York & London, Oxford, 1946.

120. Graham, E. A., Burford, T. H., and Mayer, J. A.: Middle lobe syndrome, Postgrad. Med. 4:29-34, 1948.

121. Ziskind, M. M.: Effects of calcified lymph nodes perforating the bronchial tree, New Orleans M. & S. J. 104:640-644, 1952.

122. Halle, S., and Blitz, O.: Eroding calcified mediastinal lymph nodes, Am. Rev. Tuberc. 62:213-218, 1950.

123. Maurer, E. R.: The surgical significance of calcified parabronchial and paratracheal lymph glands, J. Thoracic Surg. 23:97-110, 1952.

124. Head, J. R., and Moen, C. W.: Late non-tuberculous complications of calcified hilus lymph nodes, Am. Rev. Tuberc. 60:1-14, 1949.

125. Schmidt, H. W., Clagett, O. T., and McDonald, J. R.: Broncholithiasis, J. Thoracic Surg. 19:226-245, 1950.

126. Katz, H. L.: Traction diverticula of the esophagus in middle lobe syndrome, Am. Rev. Tuberc. 65:455-464, 1952.

127. Coleman, F. P., and Bunch, G. H., Jr.: Acquired non-malignant esophagotracheobronchial fistula, J. Thoracic Surg. 19:542-558, 1950.

128. McCort, J. J.: Radiographic identification of lymph node metastases from carcinoma of the esophagus, Radiology 59:694-711, 1952.

129. McCort, J. J., and Robbins, L. L.: Roentgen diagnosis of intrathoracic lymph node metastases in carcinoma of lung, Radiology 57:338-359, 1951.

130. Sicher, K.: Sternal swelling as presenting sign of Hodgkin's disease, Brit. M. J. 2:824, 1948.

131. Wilensky, A. O.: General abdominal lymphadenopathy; with special reference to non-specific mesenteric adenitis, Arch. Surg. 42:71-125, 1941.

132. Desjardins, A. U.: Retroperitoneal lymph nodes; their importance in cases of malignant tumors, Arch. Surg. 38:714-754, 1939.

133. Webster, D. R., and Madore, P.: Mesenteric lymphadenitis; a clinical and experimental study, Gastroenterology 15:160-165, 1949.

134. Ferguson, G.: Acute non-specific mesenteric lymphadenitis: possible mechanism pain illustrated by 2 cases, A.M.A. Arch. Surg. 65:906-911, 1952.

135. Marshall, V. F., and Schnittman, M.: Iliac lymphadenopathy as a cause of ureteral obstruction, Surgery 23:542-549, 1948.

136. Bower, J. S., and Coca-Mir, R.: Jaundice in acute subleukemic-lymphatic leukemia due to obstruction of the common duct by portal nodes, J.A.M.A. 146:987-988, 1951.

137. Berkowitz, D., Gambescia, J. M., and Thompson, C. M.: Jaundice with signs of extra-hepatic obstruction as presenting symptom of bronchogenic carcinoma, Gastroenterology 20:653-657, 1952.

138. Sleisinger, M. H., Almy, T. P., and Barr, D. P.: Sprue secondary to lymphoma of the small bowel, Am. J. Med. 15:666-674, 1953.

139. Adlersberg, D., and Schein, J.: Clinical and pathological studies in sprue, J.A.M.A. 134: 1459-1467, 1947.

140. Auchincloss, H.: Clinical study of calcified nodes in mesentery, Ann. Surg. 91:401-415, 1930.

141. Golden, R.: Observations on small intestinal physiology in the presence of calcified mesenteric lymph nodes, Am. J. Roentg. 35:316-323, 1936.

142. Blacklock, J. W. S.: Tuberculosis in infancy and childhood, Brit. Med. J. 2:324-328, 1936.

143. ————: Surgical tuberculosis of bovine origin, Ann. Roy. Coll. Surg. 2:93-103, 1948.

144. Marshak, R. H., and Dierling, D.: Duodenal obstruction due to tuberculous lymphadenitis, Radiology 44:495-497, 1945.

145. Culligan, J. M.: Intestinal obstruction due to calcified mesenteric glands, Minnesota Med. 21:482-483, 1938.

146. Klein, W.: Nonspecific mesenteric adenitis, Arch. Surg. 36:571-585, 1938.

147. Postlethwait, R. W., and Campbell, F. H.: Acute mesenteric lymphadenitis, Arch. Surg. 59:92-100, 1949.

148. Studley, H. O.: Intra-abdominal rupture of retroperitoneal tuberculous lymph node, Ann. Surg. 115:477-480, 1942.

149. Held, I. W., and Goldbloom, A. A.: Lym-

phadenopathy, a clinical interpretation, M. Clin. North America 18:633-702, 1934.

150. McGuinness, A. E.: The significance of lymphadenopathy, Med. J. Australia 1:285-288, 1953.

151. McGovern, V. J.: The significance of generalized lymph node enlargement. M. J. Australia 1:288-330, 1953.

152. Poncher, H. G., and Pierce, M.: Chapter 57, pp. 583-596 in Grulee, G. G., and Eley, R. C., eds.: Child in Health and Disease, Baltimore, Williams & Wilkins, 1952.

153. Craver, L. F.: The significance of enlarged lymph nodes, Am. J. Digest Dis. 11:65-70, 1944.

154. Wiseman, B. K.: The lymphadenopathy question, Publ. No. 13, pp. 20-26, Washington, D. C., Am. Assoc. Advancement Science, 1940.

155. Murray, N. A., and Broders, A. C.: Pathology of lymph nodes: diagnosis and prognosis, Am. J. Clin. Path. 13:450-463, 1943.

156. Kastlin, G. J.: A clinical résumé of cervical lymph gland disease, Pennsylvania M. J. 43:801-808, 1940.

157. Ghormley, R. K., and Hoffmann, H. O.: Lymphangitis and lymphadenitis, Am. J. Surg. 50:728-731, 1940.

158. Tobias, N.: Extragenital chancres: A clinical study, Am. J. Syph. & Neur. 20:266-274, 1936.

159. Carter, B. N., and Smith, J.: Tuberculous lymphadenitis secondary to inconspicuous healed traumatic cutaneous tuberculous lesions, J.A.M.A. 105:1839-1842, 1935.

160. O'Leary, P. A., and Harrison, M. W.: Inoculation tuberculosis (Review), Arch. Dermat. & Syph. 44:371-390, 1941.

161. Gastinean, F. M., Spolzar, L. W., and Haynes, E.: Sporotrichosis: Report of six cases among florists, J.A.M.A. 117:1074-1077, 1941.

162. Gold, H.: Studies of anthrax (Clinical report of ten human cases), J. Lab. & Clin. Med. 21:134-152, 1935-36.

163. Lebowich, R. J., McKillip, B. G., and Conboy, J. R.: Cutaneous anthrax; pathologic study with clinical correlation, Am. J. Clin. Path. 13:505-515, 1943.

164. Klauder, J. V.: Erysipeloid as an occupational disease, J.A.M.A. 111:1345-1348, 1938.

165. Pullen, R. L., and Stuart, B. M.: Tularemia, analysis of 225 cases, J.A.M.A. 129:495-500, 1945.

166. Kavenaugh, C. N.: Tularemia (123 cases), Arch. Int. Med. 55:61-85, 1935.

167. Meyer, K. F.: Plague, M. Clin. North America 27:745-765, 1943.

168. Sayan, J. J., Pond, H. S., Forrester, J. S., and Wood, F. S.: Scrub typhus in Assam and Burma, 616 cases, Medicine 24:155-214, 1946.

169. Greenberg, M., Pellisseri, O., Kleim, J. F., Huebner, R. J.: Rickettsialpox (clinical description), J.A.M.A. 133:901-906, 1947.

170. Brown, T. M., and Nunemaker, J. C.: Ratbite fever; review of American cases with reevaluation of etiology; report of cases, Bull. Johns Hopkins Hosp. 70:201-327, 1942.

171. Watkins, C. G.: Ratbite fever, J. Pediat. 28:429-448, 1946.

172. Daniels, W. B., and MacMurray, F. G.: Catscratch disease, J.A.M.A. 154:1247-1251, 1954.

173. Laippy, T. C., and White, C. J.: Dermatitis with lipomelanotic reticular hyperplasia of lymph nodes, A.M.A. Arch. Dermat. & Syph. 63:611-618, 1951.

174. Nairn, R. C., and Anderson, T. E.: Erythrodermia with lipomelanic reticulum-cell hyperplasia of lymph nodes (dermatopathic lymphadenitis), Brit. M. J. 1:820-824, 1955.

175. Spink, W. W., and Anderson, D.: Studies relating to the differential diagnosis of brucellosis and infectious mononucleosis; clinical, hematologic, and serologic observations, Tr. A. Am. Physicians 64:428-434, 1951.

176. Bloomfield, A. L.: Enlargement of the superficial lymph nodes in brucella infection, Am. Rev. Tuberc. 45:741-750, 1942.

177. Rosencrantz, E.: Generalized tuberculous lymphadenitis, Am. Rev. Tuberc. 41:806-808, 1940.

178. Ash, J. E.: The lymph node in tropical diseases, Am. J. Trop. Med. 27:483-491, 1947.

179. Longcope, W. T., and Freiman, D. G.: A study of sarcoidosis (based on a combined investigation of 160 cases including 30 autopsies from the Johns Hopkins Hospital and Massachusetts General Hospital), Medicine 31:1-132, 1952.

180. Kojis, F. G.: Serum sickness and anaphylaxis, Am. J. Dis. Child. 64:93-143, 313-350, 1942.

181. Motulsky, A. G., Weinberg, S., Saphir, O., and Rosenberg, E.: Lymph nodes in rheumatoid arthritis, A.M.A. Arch. Int. Med. 90:660-676, 1952.

182. Fox, R. A., and Rosahn, P. P.: The lymph nodes in disseminated lupus erythematosus, Am. J. Path. 19:73-99, 1943.

183. Harvey, A. M., Shulman, L. E., Tumulty, P. A., Conley, C. C., and Schoenrick, E. H.: Systemic lupus erythematosus; review of

the literature and clinical analysis of 138 cases, Medicine 33:291, 1954.

184. Pressman, J. J., and Simon, M. B.: Experimental evidence of direct communications between lymph nodes and veins, Surg. Gynec. & Obst. 113:537-541, 1961.

185. Threefoot, S. A., Kent, W. T., and Hatchett,, B. F.: Lymphaticovenous and lymphaticolymphatic communications demonstrated by plastic corrosion models of rats and by post-mortem lymphangiography in man, J. Lab. Clin. Med. 61:9-22, 1963.

186. Wenzel, J. F.: Factitial proctitis: the role of lymphatic destruction, Am. J. Surgery 92: 678-682, 1956.

187. Spittell, J. A., Jr., Smith, R. D., Harrison, E. G., Jr., and Schirger, A.: Unilateral secondary lymphedema. A clue to malignant disease, Proc. Staff Meetings Mayo Clinic 38:139-144, 1963.

188. Kinmonth, J. B., Taylor, G. W., and Harper, K.: Lymphangiography; technique for its use in lower limbs, Brit. Med. J. 1:940-942, 1955.

189. Wallace, S., Jackson, L., Schaffer, B., Gould, J., Greening, R. R., Weiss, A., and Kramer, S.: Lymphangiograms: their diagnostic and therapeutic potential, Radiology 76:179-199, 1961.

190. Fischer, H. W., Lawrence, M. S., and Thornbury, J. R.: Lymphography of the normal adult male. Observations and their relation to the diagnosis of metastatic neoplasm, Radiology 78:399-406, 1962.

191. Ditchek, T., Blahut, R. J., and Kittleson, A. C.: Lymphadenography in normal subjects, Radiology 80:175-181, 1963.

192. Malamos, B., Moulopoulos, S. A., and Sarkas, A.: Lymphadenography: its uses in haematology, Brit, Med. J. 2:1360-1361, 1959.

193. Wallace, S., Jackson, L., and Greening, R. R.: Clinical applications of lymphangiography, Am. J. Roentg. 88:97-109, 1962.

194. Viamonte, M., Jr., Altman, D., Parks, R., Blum, E., Bevilacqua, M., and Recher, L.: Radiographic-pathologic correlation in the interpretation of lymphangioadenograms, Radiology 80:903-916, 1963.

195. Pomerantz, M., and Ketcham, A. S.: Lymphangiography and its surgical applications, Surgery 53:589-597, 1963.

196. Greening, R. R., and Wallace, S.: Further observations in lymphangiography, Radiol. Clin. N. Amer. 1:157-173, 1963.

197. Kinmonth, J. B., Taylor, G. W., Tracy, G. D., and Marsh, J. D.: Primary lymphoedema: clinical and lymphangiographic studies of a series of 107 patients in which the lower limbs were affected, Brit. J. Surg. 45:1-9, 1957.

198. Fuchs, W. A.: Complications in lymphography with oily contrast media, Acta Radiol. 57:427-432, 1962.

199. Bron, K. M., Baum, S., and Abrams, H. L.: Oil embolism in lymphangiography. Incidence, manifestations, and mechanism, Radiology 80:194-202, 1963.

200. Schaffer, B., Gould, R. J., Wallace, S., Jackson, L., Iuker, M., Leberman, P. R., and Fetter, T. R.: The urologic applications of lymphangiography, J. Urol. 87:91-96, 1962.

201. Sage, H. H., Kizilay, D., Miyazaki, M., Shapiro, G., and Sinha, B.: Lymph node scintigrams, Am. J. Roentg. 84:666-672, 1960.

202. Lang, E. K.: Demonstration of blockage and involvement of the pelvic lymphatic system by tumor with lymphangiography and scintiscanograms, Radiology 74:71-73, 1960.

203. Fischer, H. W.: Intralymphatic introduction of radioactive colloids into the lymph nodes; Preliminary study, Radiology 79: 297-301, 1962.

204. Seitzman, D. M., Wright, R., Halaby, F. A., and Freeman, J. H.: Radioactive lymphangiography as a therapeutic adjunct, Am. J. Roentg. 89:140-149, 1963.

205. Margileth, L. M.: Cat scratch disease as a cause of oculoglandular syndrome of Parinaud, Pediatrics 20:1000-1005, 1957.

206. Editorial: Primary tuberculosis of the mouth, Brit. M. J. 2:147, 1956.

207. Watne, A. L., Hatiboglu, I., and Moore, G. E.: A clinical and autopsy study of tumor cells in the thoracic duct lymph. Surg., Gynec. & Obst. 110:339-345, 1960.

208. Lillington, G. A., and Jamplis, R. W.: Review: Scalene node biopsy, Ann. Int. Med. 59:101-110, 1963.

209. Sage, H. H.: Palpable cervical lymph nodes, J.A.M.A. 168:496-498, 1958.

210. Snapper, I.: The bedside diagnosis of cervical lymphadenopathies. Med. Clin. N. Am. 46:627-639, 1962.

211. Brandow, E. C., Jr., Volk, B. M., and Olson, K. B.: The significance of a lump in the neck, Postgrad. Med. 2:401-410, 1957.

212. Jones, P. G.: Swellings in the neck in childhood, Med. J. Austral. 1:212-214, 1963.

213. McNair, T. J., and Dudley, H. A. F.: Axillary lymph nodes in patients without breast carcinoma, Lancet 1:713-715, 1960.

214. Pierce, E. H., Gray, H. K., and Dockerty, M. B.: Surgical significance of isolated axillary adenopathy, Ann. Surg. 145:104-107, 1957.

215. Atkins, H., and Wolff, B.: The malignant

gland in the axilla, Guy's Hospital Reports 109:1-6, 1960.

216. Aaron, A. H., in the discussion of Bacon, H. E.: Extra-rectal metastatic growths from upper abdominal and mammary cancer: report of seventeen cases, J.A.M.A. 112: 808-814, 1939.

217. Saitta, G. F., and Baum, V.: Langer's axillary arch: an unusual cause of axillary mass, J.A.M.A. 180:690, 1962.

218. Dormandy, T. L.: Inguinal endometriosis, Lancet 1:832-834, 1956.

219. Winn-Williams, N.: On erythema nodosum, bilateral hilar lymphadenopathy and sarciodosis, Tubercle 42:57-63, 1961.

220. Smellie, H., and Hoyle, C.: The hilar lymph-nodes in sarcoidosis: with special reference to prognosis, Lancet 2:66-70, 1957.

221. Castleman, B.: Localized mediastinal lymph node hyperplasia resembling thymoma, Cancer 9:822, 1956.

222. Inada, K., and Hamajaki, M.: Localized mediastinal lymph-node hyperplasia resembling thymoma: a case report, Ann. Surg. 147:409-413, 1958.

223. Storer, J., and Smith, R. C.: The calcified hilar node: its significance and management, Am. Rev. Resp. Dis. 81:853-867, 1960.

224. Smithies, D. W., and Rigby-Jones, P.: Clinical evidence of parasternal lymph node involvement in neoplastic disease, Acta Radiol. Suppl. 188:235-247, 1959.

225. Gambill, E. E.: So-called mesenteric adenitis—a clinical entity or wastebasket diagnosis? Minn. Medicine 43:614-616, 1960.

226. Taswell, H. F., and Winkelmann, R. K.: Sézary syndrome—a malignant reticulemic erythroderma, J.A.M.A. 177:465-472, 1961.

227. Moore, R. D., Weisberger, A. S., and Bowerfind, E. S., Jr.: An evaluation of lymphadenopathy in systemic disease, Arch. Int. Med. 99:751-759, 1957.

228. McCreanor, J. D.: Lymphadenopathy in toxoplasmosis, New Zealand Med. 61:18-20, 1962.

229. Harrison, R. J., Broomfield, B. E., and Kippax, P. W.: Toxoplasmosis with relapsing lymphadenitis, Lancet 1:247-248, 1963.

230. Bell, D. W., Carmichael, J. A. G., Williams, R. S., Holman, R. L., and Stewart, P. D.: Localized leishmaniasis of lymph nodes: report of four cases, Brit. M. J. 1:740-744, 1958.

231. Wilson, W. L., Williams, C. D., Sanders, S. L., and Warner, R. P.: Ardmore disease, Arch. Int. Med. 100:943-950, 1957.

232. Saltzstein, S. L., and Ackerman, L. V.: Lymphadenopathy induced by anticonvulsant drugs and mimicking clinically and pathologically malignant lymphomas, Cancer 12:164-182, 1959.

233. Bajoghli, M.: Generalized lymphadenopathy and hepatosplenomegaly induced by diphenylhydantoin, Pediat. 28:943-945, 1961.

234. Greenberg, E., Cohen, D. M., Pease, G. L., and Kyle, R. A.: Histiocytic medullary reticulosis, Proc. Staff Meetings Mayo Clinic 37:271-283, 1962.

235. Zak, F. G., and Rubin, E.: Histiocytic medullary reticulosis, Am. J. Med. 31:813-819, 1961.

236. Clinicopathologic Conference: Recant, L., and Hartroft, W. S. eds.: Rademacher's disease: diminished immunity of an unusual form complicated by lymphadenopathy, Am. J. Med. 32:80-95, 1962.

237. Bridges, R. A., Berendes, H., and Good, R. A.: A fatal granulomatous disease of childhood: the clinical, pathological and laboratory features of a new syndrome, Dis. Child. 97:387-408, 1959.

24

Pathologic Bleeding

ROBERT GOLDSTEIN

Definition. For the purpose of this chapter pathologic bleeding is defined as hemorrhage resulting from impaired hemostatic mechanisms with consequent loss of the normal ability to terminate blood loss.

Obviously, the mechanisms of hemostasis may be normal but yet inadequate to meet the demands imposed by trauma or disease. Examples of such situations are: bleeding peptic ulcer, ruptured aneurysm, laceration of major vessels, erosions of vessels by ma-

lignant tumor or other pathological processes. Although in most such instances, the causes of bleeding are usually evident, the physician is not infrequently called upon to distinguish such conditions from those in which the hemostatic mechanisms are primarily at fault or to determine whether or not any derangement of the hemostatic mechanisms is contributing to the hemorrhages. Hemostasis is a complex phenomenon, and although our understanding of the mechanisms involved is far from complete and concepts are still the subject of considerable controversy, notable advances in our knowledge have been made so that the patient with disordered hemostasis can benefit enormously by a rational approach to his disease.

NORMAL HEMOSTASIS

The various mechanisms concerned in hemostasis may be considered as involving extravascular, vascular, and intravascular factors all of which are interrelated. For more detailed and extensive reviews of hemostasis and hemorrhagic diseases the reader is referred to recent monographs and reviews.[1-10]

Extravascular and Anatomic Factors. The extent of hemorrhage which follows a vascular injury is dependent not only upon the severity of the injury and the size of the vessel involved, but also upon the blood pressure within the vessel (Fig. 168) and the counter-pressure which is built up in the adjacent extra-vascular tissue by the accumulation of extravasated blood (Fig. 169). Bleeding into firm tissue or a "solid" organ rapidly results in progressively increasing extravascular pressure, which in turn decreases the flow of blood from the injured vessel, enabling other mechanisms of hemostasis to function more effectively. The degree of tamponade developed depends upon the distensibility, denseness and elasticity of the surrounding tissues. Thus, in bone, hemorrhage into the matrix is practically impossible, whereas injury to a vessel of similar size in muscular tissue would result in more hemorrhage but still considerably less than that which would occur in regions where structures are loose, as in the subcutaneous tissues of the infraorbital regions, of the neck or the axillae. An injury to a vessel of comparable size in the mucous membrane of hollow organs, such as the gastrointestinal, the respiratory, or the genitourinary tracts, might be life-endangering, since there is so little supporting tissue that blood can escape freely. Conditions affecting supporting tissue, such as debility, advanced age, Ehlers-Donlos syndrome, or prolonged corticosteroid therapy will also increase blood loss.

Most, if not all, tissues contain clot-promoting substances called tissue thromboplastin. It is probable that injury to the vessel wall and extravasation of blood into surrounding tissues results in the release of this thromboplastic substance which may play a role in hemostasis by accelerating platelet massing at the site of injury (described below) and coagulation of the extravasated blood, both of which aid in sealing the injured vessel. Since there is wide variation in thromboplastic activity among tissues, the relative amounts of thromboplastin released may account in part for the differences noted in bleeding tendency in different areas of the body.

Vascular Factors. The importance of vascular factors in hemostasis deserves special emphasis, since all too often blood coagulation has been considered synonymous with the hemostatic mechanism. Actually, the majority of patients with pathologic bleeding show no abnormality in clotting and it should be pointed out that subjects with profound coagulation disturbances such as hemophilia, Christmas disease, or afibrinogenemia, usually have a normal bleeding time and may experience long intervals of freedom from spontaneous hemorrhage, indicating that hemostasis is satisfactory in the absence of obvious trauma. Furthermore, Factor XII (Hageman) deficiency, which causes a profound defect in coagulation, is not characterized by abnormal bleeding, either spontaneous or posttraumatic.

The vascular factors which are concerned in hemostasis are vessel size, elasticity, strength, tone and contractility. By virtue of their thick walls containing muscular and elastic tissue, arteries can withstand more stress and trauma than arterioles, capillaries, venules or veins. Once perforated or ruptured, however, the egress of blood is great, due to the high intravascular pressure in relation to the low extravascular tissue tension. Under such circumstances, hemostatic mechanisms must act rapidly to prevent catastrophe. The vessel retracts longitudinally and circularly, undergoes segmental spasm, which decreases blood flow, and the aperture is decreased by puckering of the intima. In addition, drop in blood pressure and vascular collapse may supervene. Though temporary, these reactions may retard blood flow sufficiently to permit initiation and completion of coagulation which will plug the hole. It is thus evident that, at this level of the circulation, losses in elasticity of the artery from any cause—arteriosclerosis, aneurysms, etc.—may seriously jeopardize hemostasis. Also, it is clear that hypertension may impose an additional increment of strain on the hemostatic mechanism when arterial bleeding occurs.

The situation regarding veins is quite different. They, too, react to trauma with spasm and retraction. But since venous pressure is low, tamponade from extravascular tissue pressure is more effective in stemming the flow of blood, provided sufficient tissue surrounds the open vessel. However, under some pathologic conditions, such as portal obstruction, congestive heart failure, phlebarteriectasia or varicose veins, venous pressure may be abnormally high, which may lead to excessive hemorrhage. Also, veins are more easily traumatized than arteries because of the relative thinness of the venous wall.

At the microscopic level of the vascular tree there is proportionally much less muscle and elastic tissue in the vessel walls than in the large vessels, and it decreases progressively from arterioles, to venules, to capillaries. Therefore, in these smaller vessels and particularly in the capillaries, vascular strength is dependent in large part upon the endothelial structure and basement membrane plus support from surrounding tissue. It is these vessels whose strength is so impaired by vitamin C deficiency, allergic, immunologic, inflammatory and drug reactions, infectious diseases, and thrombocytopenia. The role of platelets in the maintenance of the strength of the capillary wall remains unknown, and equally unexplained is the mechanism by which corticosteroids can decrease the capillary fragility seen in thrombocytopenia without increasing the platelet level. Clinically, capillary fragility is determined by subjecting the capillaries to increased physical stress either by means of a tourniquet (thus increasing intracapillary pressure to a predetermined level for a measured period of time) and noting the number of petechiae, or by application of negative pressure for a one minute period and determining the relative pressure which first produces petechiae.[13]

Extravascular tissue pressure is most effective in controlling bleeding from these small vessels because of the relatively low intravascular pressures. (Figs. 168 and 169). At the arteriocapillary junction pressure is approximately 30 mm. of mercury and at the capillary venule junction about 10 mm. It should be pointed out that in the instances of an arteriole supplying a plexus of capillaries, obstruction of the flow in one or several of the capillaries by the increase in tissue pressure will result in back-pres-

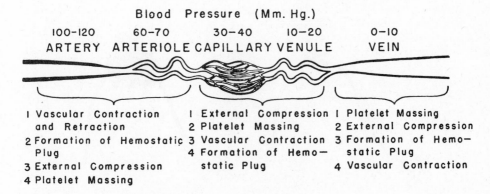

Blood   Pressure   (Mm. Hg.)

| 100-120 | 60-70 | 30-40 | 10-20 | 0-10 |
| ARTERY | ARTERIOLE | CAPILLARY | VENULE | VEIN |

1 Vascular Contraction and Retraction	1 External Compression	1 Platelet Massing
2 Formation of Hemostatic Plug	2 Platelet Massing	2 External Compression
3 External Compression	3 Vascular Contraction	3 Formation of Hemostatic Plug
4 Platelet Massing	4 Formation of Hemostatic Plug	4 Vascular Contraction

Fig. 168. Probable order of importance of the components of hemostasis in different vessels. (Tocantins: Ann. Surg. 125:292)

sure equal only to that of the arteriole—approximately 30 mm. of mercury. However, if all the capillaries from arterioles are obstructed, the pressure within the capillaries rises until it either overcomes the obstruction or becomes equal to that of the arterial supply. Thus, capillary bleeding may become very extensive despite high tissue pressures unless the break in the vessel is repaired.

The response of arterioles, venules and capillaries to trauma is very important in the mechanism of hemostasis, since by far the greatest number of traumatic incidents —cuts, bruises, abrasions, puncture wounds, etc.—involve this region of the vascular tree. It has been emphasized by Macfarlane,[12] Tocantins[11] and others that under normal conditions puncture of a capillary is followed by prompt disappearance of the vessel (Fig. 170) and cessation of bleeding. Since this occurs even in the presence of increased intracapillary pressure, it is unlikely that it is due to passive collapse of the punctured vessel. It is felt by some observers[12] that disappearance of the capillaries represents an active constriction of the capillaries in response to the stimulus mediated through the Rouget cells in the capillary wall. However, microscopic evaluation would indicate that true capillaries are simple endothelial tubes with no contractile ability, which branch from the meta-arterioles and have a sphincter at their origin. Trauma could cause constriction of the meta-arterioles or of the "precapillary sphincter" which would reduce the flow of blood into the capillaries and cause "plasma skimming" in which fluid without red cells traverses the capillary, with the result that the vessel becomes invisible. Whether or not there is true constriction of the capillaries, or only constriction of the meta-arterioles and venules in reponse to injury,

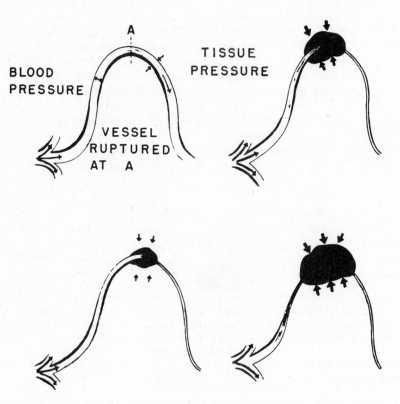

Fig. 169. Diagram showing hydrostatic dynamics of hemorrhage from small blood vessels. (Tocantins: Ann. Surg. 125:292)

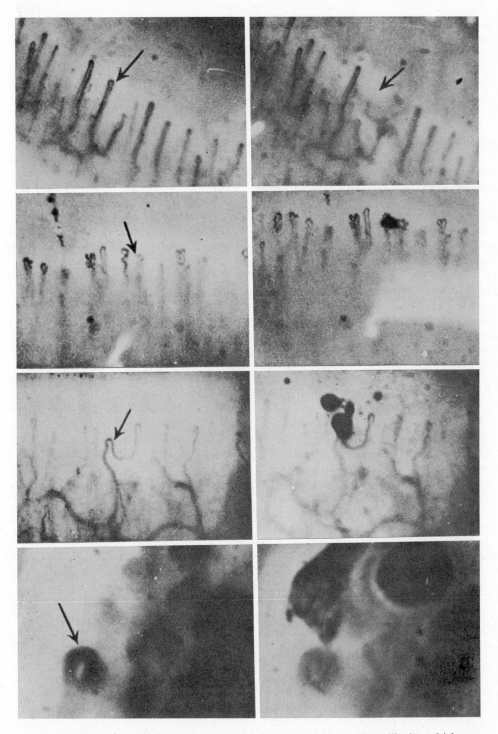

Fig. 170. Response of capillaries to trauma. (*Top row*) Normal capillaries, which constrict and disappear promptly after needle puncture. (*Second row*) Distorted bizarre-shaped capillaries in idiopathic thrombocytopenic purpura, which fail to constrict. (*Third row*) Similar defect in a patient with thrombasthenia. (*Bottom row*) Dilated vessels in a telangiectasis of a patient with multiple telangiectasia; bleeding had to be stopped by pressure. (Macfarlane: Quart. J. Med. 34:1)

certain findings are difficult to explain. Disappearance of capillary loops following trauma fails to occur in the absence of platelets (thrombocytopenia). The role platelets play in vasoconstriction remains obscure, for although they do contain serotonin, a vasoconstrictor, which is released when they are damaged or take part in coagulation, and which may be released when platelets adhere to the vessel wall at the point of injury, it has been reported that both the bleeding time and capillary fragility remained normal despite prolonged depletion of platelet serotonin induced by reserpine.[14] Recently it has also been reported that a plasma protein which has no coagulation activity also plays some role in the vascular response to injury. The prolonged bleeding time found in patients with von Willebrand's disease has been thought to be due to a primary vascular defect characterized by capillaries which may appear distorted and which fail to disappear in response to trauma. Nilsson et al.[15] have reported that the bleeding time can be reduced to normal by injection of fraction I-O from both normal and hemophilic plasma but not with a similar fraction obtained from the plasma from a patient with von Willebrand's disease. The mode of action of this fraction is not known. The active material is distinct from fibrinogen and AHF (factor VIII) and has no corrective effect upon the prolonged bleeding time of thrombocytopenia.

It has been generally accepted that the bleeding time, whether done by the Duke[16] or Ivy[17] method, reflects the hemostatic response of the capillaries to trauma. However, it is more than likely that arterioles and venules are also involved and that the bleeding time primarily reflects their hemostatic response to trauma.

Intravascular Factors—Platelets and Coagulation. That coagulation is important in the hemostatic mechanism is amply demonstrated by the hemorrhagic manifestations encountered in patients with disturbances of their coagulation. However, its exact role and relative importance is still controversial. Although it can be readily demonstrated, as described above, that platelets have a profound effect upon capillary fragility and the bleeding time, it is still not clear what role, if any, coagulation plays in these functions of the platelets. Indeed patients with profound deficiencies of one or more of the plasma coagulation factors, as noted above, usually exhibit no increase in capillary fragility, have normal bleeding times, and may experience long intervals of freedom from "spontaneous" hemorrhage. In addition to their vascular action, platelets also have a number of coagulation activities and whether or not these are related to their action on blood vessels is not known.

Platelets. The importance of platelets in hemostasis and coagulation has been recognized for many years, but only recently has the complexity of these small cellular structures been appreciated. It is apparent now that they are viable, active, metabolic units as complex as any other cell. The activities of platelets which appear to be concerned with hemostasis and blood coagulation are listed in Table 23. Some of these are intrinsic constituents of the platelet (these are platelet factors 2, 3, 4 and the clot-retracting factor), others are taken up by an active transport mechanism (for example, serotonin, adrenalin and histamine), and still others are probably simply ab-

TABLE 23. PLATELET FACTORS OR ACTIVITIES WHICH MAY PLAY A ROLE IN HEMOSTASIS

1. Platelet factor 1: Plasma factor V-like activity
2. Platelet factor 2: Accelerator of the conversion of fibrinogen to fibrin by thrombin-fibrinoplastic activity
3. Platelet factor 3: Platelet thromboplastin activity
4. Platelet factor 4: Anti-heparin activity
5. Platelet factor 5: Clottable factor, fibrinogen or fibrinogen-like protein clotted by thrombin
6. Platelet factor 6: Anti-fibrinolytic activity
7. Platelet factor 7: ? factor VII-like activity
8. Clot retraction activity—probably due to a contractile protein in platelets similar to actomyosin of muscle, contracts in the presence of Ca++ or Mg++ and ATP
9. Vascular factor—action on capillary fragility and vasoconstriction
10. Serotonin

sorbed onto the surface of the platelet or diffuse into it from the plasma (these are factor 1, fibrinogen, and antifibrinolysin). Other plasma coagulation factors, which are claimed by some investigators and denied by others, to be in or on platelets, are plasma coagulation factors II, VII, VIII, IX and X (see Table 24). Whether or not these clotting factors are found in platelets probably depends on how thoroughly the platelets are washed before testing, for platelets do adsorb proteins to their surface probably, in part, due to the negative charge on their surface. What role these various platelet activities play in hemostasis is not clear.

Platelets are produced in the bone marrow by the megakaryocytes and normally are maintained at a level of 150,000 to 350,000 per mm.³ in the peripheral blood. Relatively little is known about the regulation of platelet production. Recently, evidence[19,20] has been obtained to indicate that a factor or factors present in plasma accelerate the maturation rate of megakaryocytes and increase the production and liberation of platelets. Under normal conditions platelet life span, as determined by a variety of radioisotope tagging technics, is from 9 to 11 days.[20-25] There is disagreement amongst investigators as to whether the platelet survival experiments indicate a linear or an exponential loss of platelets from the peripheral circulation. If there is a linear loss, this would be consistent with the concept of a finite platelet life span and removal of senescent platelets similar to what happens with red cells. On the other hand, if there is an exponential survival curve, this would be indicative of random platelet loss, and would be supportive evidence for the concept that normally platelets are constantly being utilized within the body for repair of injured vessels and by slow continuous intravascular clotting.

How the platelets affect the strength of the capillary wall and reduce capillary fragility is not known, nor is it understood how corticosteroids decrease capillary fragility in the absence of platelets. However, there is considerable experimental data on the role of platelets in the formation of the hemostatic plug in vascular injury.[26-28]

When a small vessel such as an arteriole or venule is severed or lacerated, constriction occurs within a few seconds, but this is not sufficient to stop the flow of blood, and in the absence of platelets the vasoconstriction does not persist. Almost immediately platelets begin to adhere to the injured vascular wall and to each other. Thus, a loose platelet aggregate is formed both inside and outside the vessel wall, the so-called white thrombus. Such an aggregate of platelets may suffice to stop bleeding from a smaller vessel with low intravascular pressure. However, on the arterial side of the circulation parts of the platelet plug may be carried away by the blood stream but these are rapidly replaced. In these vessels blood continues to ooze through the loose platelet plug until it is made more solid by changes which take place within it (viscous metamorphosis of the platelets, the laying down of fibrin by the process of coagulation, and clot retraction). What causes the platelets to adhere to the damaged vessel and then to each other is not known. It has been postulated that: (1) injury to the vascular wall causes a change in its physicochemical properties which attracts the platelets[34] (if a positive charge occurred, this would attract the negatively charged platelets), (2) an unidentified substance is released by the vascular endothelium which causes an alteration in the platelets and makes them sticky,* and (3) a small amount of tissue thromboplastin, liberated by the injury, converts a small amount of prothrombin to thrombin, which causes the platelets to adhere and to clump, and also initiates platelet viscous metamorphosis.[27-29] Whatever the mechanism, once the platelet aggregates form, a series of events takes place that stops the bleeding and firmly seals the injured vessel. Some of the platelets swell and rupture and liberate materials which cause acceleration of coagulation, continued vascular constriction and clot retraction. Platelet factor 3 (platelet thromboplastic activity), is a lipoprotein, the active lipid portion of which is phosphatidylserine and phosphatidylethanola-

---

* Recently it has been shown that ADP causes platelets to adhere to each other. Whether or not this substance plays a role in vivo is not known.

mine.[31,32] When liberated it accelerates blood coagulation (see below) thus increasing the production of thrombin which in turn converts fibrinogen to fibrin within and around the platelet plug and strengthens it. Thrombin also causes further clumping and lysis of platelets resulting in the release of more platelet factor 3 and further acceleration of clot formation. Other factors in or on the surface of the platelets favor fibrin formation within the platelet aggregates. Platelet factor 2 accelerates the conversion of fibrinogen to fibrin by thrombin. The clottable protein in the platelets, which by immunologic tests closely resembles fibrinogen[33] and the fibrinogen on their surface ensures the presence of fibrinogen for conversion to fibrin within the hemostatic plug. The presence of plasma coagulation factors in or on the surface of the platelets (platelet factor 1, and Factors II, VII, VIII, IX and X) whether they are intrinsic constituents of the platelets or not ("plasmatic atmosphere of platelets") favors

TABLE 24. PLASMA COAGULATION FACTORS

PRO-COAGULANTS

INTERNATIONAL NOMENCLATURE	TERMINOLOGY FREQUENTLY USED IN LITERATURE
Factor I	Fibrinogen
Factor II	Prothrombin
Factor III	Thromboplastin, Thrombokinase, Prothrombinase
Factor IV	Calcium
Factor V	Labile Factor, Proaccelerin, Plasma Accelerator Globulin (AC-G), Plasma Prothrombin Conversion Accelerator, Plasmatic Co-factor of Thromboplastin
Factor VI	not used
Factor VII	Serum Prothrombin Conversion Accelerator (SPCA), Proconvertin, Stable Factor, Cothromboplastin, Autoprothrombin I
Factor VIII	Antihemophilic Factor (AHF) Antihemophilic Factor A (AHFA) Antihemophilic Globulin (AHG) Platelet Co-factor I, Thromboplastinogen
Factor IX	Plasma Thromboplastin Component (PTC), Christmas Factor, Antihemophilic Factor B (AHFB), Platelet Co-factor II, Autoprothrombin II
Factor X	Stuart Factor*, Prower Factor*
Factor XI	Plasma Thromboplastin Antecedent (PTA), Antihemophilic Factor C (AHFC)
Factor XII	Hageman Factor, Antihemophilic Factor D (AHFD), Glass Factor, Contact Factor

INHIBITORS

Anti-thromboplastin, Antithrombin, ? Heparin, Heparin Co-factor

---

* Factors VII and X were first clearly differentiated in 1957. Prior to that time the terms listed for Factor VII actually could refer to either Factor VII or X or both.

coagulation by supplying the necessary factors for both intrinsic and extrinsic coagulation (see below). The clot-retracting factor which is probably the actomyosinlike protein in platelets that contracts in the presence of divalent cations (Ca^{++}, Mg^{++}) and adenosine triphosphate,[35] causes retraction of the fibrin clot when released by the platelets, thus strengthening the hemostatic plug. The antiheparin activity neutralizes any heparinlike substances which may be released from the injured vessel wall (thus favoring coagulation) and the antifibrinolytic activity of the platelets may well prevent premature dissolution of the hemostatic plug by the normal mechanism of clot lysis. The vasoconstriction caused by vascular injury is of short duration, but with the aggregation of platelets there is reinforcement and prolongation of the vasoconstriction.

Whether this is due to the release of serotonin or some other factor from the platelets or to the formation of some vasoconstrictor during coagulation is not known.

Blood Coagulation. Although the bleeding time may be normal and minor injuries (such as that inflicted for the determination of the bleeding time) may not cause immediate excessive loss of blood in patients with severe coagulation defects other than thrombocytopenia, delayed or secondary bleeding often occurs, indicating a defect in the hemostatic plug which is probably due to faulty fibrin formation. When somewhat larger vessels are injured in which platelet aggregates (white thrombi) alone are ineffective, bleeding may continue indefinitely or until the coagulation defect is corrected. Identification of such defects is, therefore, important both in the diagnosis and the

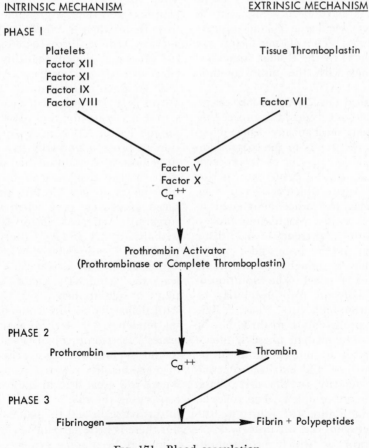

FIG. 171. Blood coagulation.

treatment of pathologic bleeding. For a rational approach to diagnosis and treatment, an understanding of present concepts of the coagulation mechanism is fundamental.

The coagulation of blood is a complex phenomenon, and although many aspects of it are poorly understood, recent advances have brought about considerable agreement in and clarification of our concepts. At the present time 9 plasma factors, which are believed by most investigators to be distinct and separate plasma proteins, have been identified as procoagulants that interact with each other, and with calcium and platelets in the process of coagulation. Considerable confusion has arisen in the past from the multiplicity of terms used to identify these factors. Recently an International Committee on Nomenclature has attempted to bring some order to this chaos and has suggested the use of Roman numerals to identify the plasma clotting factors (some platelet factors have been designated by Arabic numbers, see Table 23, and this may cause confusion). The plasma factors are listed in Table 24 by the Roman numerical system together with the most common synonyms.

For a practical clinical approach, coagulation can best be considered as proceeding by two different mechanisms. One, designated as *intrinsic,* refers to the coagulation of whole blood or plasma as it proceeds without the addition of tissue extracts (tissue thromboplastin) which accelerate coagulation whereas the other designated as *extrinsic* refers to the coagulation process as it proceeds in the presence of such tissue extracts. Both the intrinsic and extrinsic mechanisms may be thought of as occurring in three phases. Phase 1: The evolution of prothrombin activator (prothrombinase or "complete" thromboplastin). Phase 2: The conversion of prothrombin to thrombin by the activator developed in phase 1. Phase 3: Conversion of fibrinogen to fibrin by thrombin. Intrinsic and extrinsic coagulation differ primarily in the first phase, which is the most complex. The coagulation scheme in Figure 171 illustrates the differences between the intrinsic and extrinsic pathways by which prothrombin activator (prothrombinase) is formed.

Intrinsic Mechanism. In spontaneous coagulation (intrinsic) as studied in vitro, plasma Factors XII, XI, X, IX, VIII and V interact with each other and platelets, in the presence of ionized calcium, to produce the activator of prothrombin. A deficiency of any one of these factors will cause either a delay in the formation of activator or a decrease in the amount of activator formed, or both, and will result in a delay and a decrease in the conversion of prothrombin to thrombin, and thus a delay in the conversion of fibrinogen to fibrin and in clot formation. The exact role of each of the coagulation factors in the complex reaction is not known, but considerable information has accumulated from studies on blood and plasma from patients with congenital deficiencies of a single coagulation factor and from partially purified preparations of coagulation factors derived from serum and plasma. For many years it has been recognized that blood or plasma exposed to foreign surfaces, such as glass, clots more rapidly than when exposed to nonwettable surfaces such as silicon-coated glass or plastics. It is now evident that this acceleration effect of surface is mediated entirely, or at least in great part, through activation of Factor XII, the Hageman factor. Calcium is not necessary for this reaction.[36-41] (Although Factor XII is necessary for coagulation to proceed normally in vitro, its role in hemostasis is questionable, since patients with marked deficiency of this factor, exhibiting prolonged clotting times, do not bleed excessively even when subjected to surgery.) Activated Factor XII interacts with Factor XI (PTA) to form activation product[36-41] (also referred to as contact activation product or activated PTA). In contrast to Factor XII, Factor XI obviously plays a role in hemostasis since subjects with deficiency of this factor have a bleeding tendency.[42,43] Activation product accelerates a reaction involving Factors VIII, IX, X and calcium which gives rise to an intermediary activity referred to as Product I. There is a great deal in the literature[3,44-48] concerning the role of each of these factors in this reaction and the sequence of events, but there is little agreement. More recently there has been some evidence to indicate that Product I may be activated Factor X.

The available evidence indicates that Product I reacts rapidly with platelet factor 3 and Factor V in the presence of calcium to form a potent activator or prothrombin (prothrombinase). It is still not clear whether or not Factor V is also involved in Product I formation and whether it reacts with Product I before or after the latter reacts with platelet factor 3. These reactions are summarized in Figure 172, but it should be pointed out that the last two reactions could be in reverse order.

In vitro the most time-consuming phase of coagulation is the formation of activation product. The rate of formation of Product I appears to vary directly with the level of activation product,[38-41] and the reaction of Product I with platelet factor 3 and Factor V is a very rapid one.[49] During coagulation of normal human blood certain changes take place in the activity of the various plasma coagulation factors so that there are considerable differences between the coagulation activities of plasma and serum. Most of the prothrombin disappears either by conversion to thrombin or to some inactive form. Fibrinogen is converted to fibrin. Factors V and VIII are activated early in coagulation but then these activi-

ties rapidly diminish so that little or none remains in serum. Factors VII and IX are also thought to be activated early in coagulation but this activation persists in serum. Factors X, XI, and XII may go through changes during coagulation but their activity in plasma and serum are about the same.[48,51,55,57]

When blood clots in vitro there is a latent period during which the blood remains fluid and there is no conversion of prothrombin to thrombin. Once a small amount of prothrombin activator is formed, thrombin begins to appear at a slow rate and visible clotting begins. If the conversion of prothrombin to thrombin is followed, it is found to proceed very slowly at first and then to accelerate until conversion proceeds at a very rapid rate. This has been referred to as the autocatalytic nature of thrombin formation. Since the hemostatic effectiveness of coagulation depends more upon the velocity of thrombin evolution than its final yield, considerable attention has been focused on the autocatalytic reaction and various mechanisms have been postulated to explain this phenomenon. As outlined in Figure 172 the formation of prothrombin activator is a time-consuming

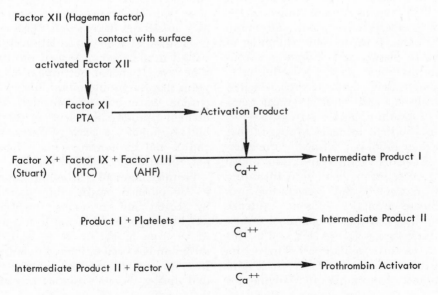

FIG. 172. First phase of coagulation: intrinsic mechanism.

process. At first only small amounts of prothrombinase are formed, which will slowly convert prothrombin to thrombin, but as the reaction proceeds, more and more of this prothrombin activator is formed. The accumulation of activator obviously will increase the velocity of thrombin formation from prothrombin. The development of prothrombinase activity also does not proceed at a steady rate, but it first develops slowly and then there is a period of a rapid acceleration of its formation, which also might be referred to as autocatalytic. Since the development of prothrombinase activity is dependent upon a chain of reactions, one catalyzing another, the velocity of each reaction would increase as the product of the preceding reaction increased. This would lead, of course, to an increasing velocity of prothrombinase production. In addition, there is also evidence that end products of certain reactions in coagulation can accelerate preceding reactions. Thus, there is evidence that minute amounts of thrombin activate Factor V (increase activity 3 to 5 fold) and that an increase in Factor V activity occurs early in the clotting of whole blood, before there is any evidence of fibrin formation or decrease in prothrombin content as determined by the available procedures.[50,51] Activation of Factor V by thrombin or other intermediary products accelerates production of prothrombinase, and in turn, of thrombin. This activated Factor V in humans is more labile and the activity disappears fairly rapidly. Thrombin also has been shown to cause clumping of platelets in plasma and to induce viscous metamorphosis and platelet lysis, thus making available more platelet factor 3, which in turn results in a more rapid and greater evolution of prothrombinase activity.[29,52,53,54] There is also some evidence to suggest that intermediate product I, formed by the interaction of Factors VIII, IX, and X, may have a lysing effect on platelets, thus liberating platelet factor 3[44] and accelerating prothrombinase formation. Recent evidence also indicates that trace amounts of thrombin activate Factor VIII (AHF), and by this means accelerate coagulation.[55] This occurs only at the stage of coagulation where minute amounts of thrombin are available, for higher activities of thrombin destroy Factor VIII. Factor VII activity is also increased in the early phase of coagulation before conversion of prothrombin to thrombin. How this is brought about is not known, since it is now generally agreed that Factor VII does not play a role in the intrinsic pathway of coagulation, but that it is essential for rapid coagulation of blood by tissue thromboplastin. An increase in Factor VII activity will accelerate coagulation induced by tissue thromboplastin, and this may be of importance in hemostasis.[56,57]

Extrinsic Mechanism. As illustrated in Figure 171 certain of the plasma coagulation factors (XII, XI, IX and VIII) essential in the intrinsic mechanism of prothrombinase formation, are not necessary in the extrinsic pathway in which tissue thromboplastin is present in excess or optimal concentration. Factors V and X are necessary in both pathways for rapid prothrombinase formation and Factor VII plays a role only in the extrinsic pathway.[3,56-58] Tissue thromboplastin, Factors V, VII and X interact in the presence of ionized calcium to form a potent prothrombin activator. The sequence of events is not known, but the most recent evidence suggests that an early reaction involving tissue thromboplastin and Factors VII, X, and calcium leads to the formation of an intermediate product which then reacts with Factor V.[59] An increase in Factor VII and Factor V activity occurs during the process and probably accelerates the reaction. This extrinsic mechanism of blood coagulation is that involved in the commonly used prothrombin time test. It should be emphasized at this point that the prothrombin time, as the discussion above shows, is dependent not only upon the prothrombin level of the plasma but also upon the levels of Factors V, VII and X and fibrinogen. This is frequently not appreciated by the physician.

Prothrombin and Thrombin. From studies on purified prothrombin preparations by Seegers and coworkers, the molecular weight of prothrombin has been estimated to be from 62,000 to 69,000 and that of thrombin has been estimated to be 31,000.[60] It is also maintained by the Seegers group that during the activation of prothrombin to thrombin other coagulation activities also are formed from prothrombin and accelerate the formation of thrombin.[61] These have been designated as autoprothrombin I, similar to or identical with Factor VII activity, and autoprothrombin II, similar to or identical with Factor IX activity. Whether or not Factors VII and IX exist as separate entities in plasma or are formed from prothrombin during the process of prothrombin activation awaits clarification.

Thrombin is a proteolytic enzyme which acts upon fibrinogen by splitting off two small polypeptides probably by disruption of arginyl-glycine bonds in the fibrinogen molecule.[62,63] The large fibrin monomers formed then polymerize, apparently taking up end to end alignment to form fibrils. Later these fibrils become arranged side to side to form the coarser strands of fibrin which form the clot. The polymerization depends on conditions such as pH and ionic strength but not on the presence of thrombin. Calcium is not essential for the action of thrombin on fibrinogen or for polymerization but it does affect the rate of these reactions.

Clot Retraction. It is now quite generally agreed that a minimal system for clot retraction must contain fibrinogen, intact platelets, calcium or magnesium, and thrombin, all reacting in a solution of appropriate pH and ionic strength. Glucose will enhance the retraction but is not essential with fresh normal platelets. When platelets are stored in vitro, their clot-retracting activity decreases and this loss of activity more or less parallels the loss of platelet ATP. Platelets that have been disrupted or have been repeatedly washed also lose their clot-retracting activity. Removal of calcium and magnesium completely inhibits retraction; inhibition thus caused can be reversed by the addition of either or both of these cations. With the isolation of a contractile protein from platelets,[35] similar to actomyosin, which contracts in the presence of divalent cations (Ca^{++}, Mg^{++}) and adenosine triphosphate, much of the mystery of clot retraction has been clarified. When this protein contracts, ATP decreases. Platelets have a high content of ATP and during the early phase of retraction when glucose is present there is a rapid accumulation of lactic acid, and ATP first increases, then as clot retraction proceeds, ATP decreases. When the glycolytic system is impaired by storage or an enzymatic defect which interferes with ATP synthesis, clot-retraction activity of the platelets is reduced. Platelets have a very active metabolism and contain the enzymes essential for anerobic glycolysis, the tricarboxylic acid cycle and the hexosemonophosphate shunt. Gross and his colleagues[64] have found that in congenital thrombasthenia with disturbed clot retraction, the platelets had considerable decrease of ATP and a marked decrease in glyceraldehyde phosphate dehydrogenase and pyruvate kinase activity, enzymes which are essential for normal ATP production.

Fibrin-stabilizing Factor. Clots derived by clotting purified fibrinogen with thrombin with or without the presence of calcium are readily soluble in 5M urea or 1 per cent monochloracetic acid. When plasma is clotted by thrombin in the presence of calcium, the fibrin clot is not soluble. The increased "strength" of the clot is apparently due to a plasma protein (globulin) which has the action of producing a more strongly cross-linked fibrin clot.[65] The role this factor plays in hemostasis is not known, but it has been reported that a deficiency of this factor has been found in a patient with a delayed bleeding tendency after injury and poor wound healing.[66]

Inhibitors of Coagulation. One of the most provocative and as yet unsolved questions concerning coagulation is how the fluidity of the blood is maintained in vivo. No matter how carefully blood is withdrawn and handled, and no matter in what type of container it is stored, if maintained at 37°C it will clot within minutes to several hours. Blood within a carefully isolated vascular segment will show small fibrin clots within 20 to 30 minutes although complete clotting out of the fibrin may take longer than 8 hours.[67] These findings plus the short in vivo half life of many of the coagulation factors (Factor VIII 6 to 12 hours, Factor VII less than 12 hours, Factor IX 20 to 24 hours, fibrinogen 4 to 5 days, platelets 3 to 4 days) have suggested to many investigators that coagulation is going on continually in vivo, but that it progresses very slowly and that there are mechanisms which prevent massive deposition of fibrinogen. The mechanisms involved may be considered under vascular, plasmatic, and clearing of intermediate products from the blood stream.

VASCULAR. It has been postulated that the vascular endothelium may inhibit clotting either by the nature of the surface (negative charge) or by production of some as yet unidentified anticoagulant. That such a mechanism could not suffice by itself is evident by the fact that stasis of blood within vessels due to partial obstruction frequently results in intravascular clot formation.

PLASMATIC. There are specific inhibitors of coagulation in normal blood which are directed primarily against intermediary products or activation products of coagulation. 1. *Antithromboplastin,* prothrombin activator or the prothrombinase developed during coagulation is slowly neutralized by plasma. In vitro this inhibitor does not prevent clotting, but potent prothrombinase activity which develops during clotting is not found in serum, nor does complete conversion of prothrombin to thrombin occur even during in vitro clotting. In vivo, where the production of prothrombin activator would be very slow, the small amounts formed could be neutralized before being able to convert much if any prothrombin to thrombin. 2. *Antithrombin.* There is a protein in plasma which neutralizes the clotting activity of thrombin. This has been referred to as *antithrombin III.*[68] When large amounts of thrombin are added to plasma the thrombin-fibrinogen reaction occurs more rapidly than the thrombin-antithrombin reaction, and fibrin forms. However, trace amounts of thrombin may be neutralized before the thrombin reacts with large amounts of fibrinogen, so that, in vivo, if very slow thrombin evolution occurs, fibrin formation could be limited by this mechanism, and massive fibrin accumulation prevented. Thrombin has also been found to be adsorbed on to fibrin and under these circumstances is not readily available to react with fibrinogen. This has been

referred to as *antithrombin I.* It is possible that the adsorption of thrombin onto fibrin is another mechanism whereby massive fibrin formation is prevented in vivo. *Antithrombin II* refers to the plasma cofactor of heparin, which acts with heparin to interfere in the action of thrombin on fibrinogen. It is still not clear whether or not the heparin cofactor and antithrombin III are identical. *Heparin* itself is a very potent inhibitor of coagulation, for it interferes in all three phases of coagulation. It inhibits the formation of prothrombin activator, it inhibits the action of prothrombin activator in the conversion of prothrombin to thrombin, and it also interferes with the action of thrombin on fibrinogen. Whether or not heparin enters into the blood stream in man and plays a role in the prevention of intravascular coagulation is still controversial. *Antithrombin IV,* as described by Seegers and coworkers,[68] is an activity which arises in plasma during the conversion of prothrombin to thrombin and inactivates thrombin as it is being formed.

CLEARING MECHANISM. The inhibitors described above, although they may limit coagulation, could hardly be expected to maintain the fluidity of the blood in vivo. That there must be some mechanism by which accelerators or intermediate activators of coagulation are cleared from the blood stream is suggested by the findings that serum and certain intermediary products of clotting, when administered intravenously, will cause intravascular thrombi in vessels in which stasis is produced by complete or partial obstruction within a few minutes of their administration. However, such thrombi are not formed if stasis is produced five to ten minutes later. These findings indicate that the clot-producing activity has been lost from the blood stream. Furthermore, there is little evidence of intravascular coagulation when thromboplastic materials are slowly administered intravenously,[67,69,70] although rapid administration of such potent materials can cause generalized fibrin deposition. Spaet *et al.* have reported evidence to indicate that clearance of such material may be a function of the reticuloendothelial system particularly in the liver.[70]

Fibrinolysis. There exists in plasma a mechanism by which fibrin can be lysed.[71] The body therefore, has a means for disposing of fibrin or fibrin clots within the vascular tree. Undoubtedly this mechanism plays a role in dissolving intravascular thrombi and in recanalization of vessels, and it may be important in disposing of small amounts of fibrin formed during continuous intravascular coagulation, if this indeed does occur.

Plasminogen (profibrinolysin), the inactive precursor of a potent proteolytic enzyme plasmin (fibrinolysin), is present in plasma in sufficient concentration so that when fully activated it is capable of digesting the total fibrinogen in the body in a few minutes. Normally there is little or no fibrinolytic activity in blood, but under certain circumstances it can be activated. The fibrinolytic mechanism is a compli-

cated one, and as yet not fully understood. There are both activators and inhibitors of this system as indicated diagrammatically in Figure 173. Under certain conditions plasminogen is activated and this may occur by two mechanisms. Substances (lysokinases) may be released into the blood stream from tissues which convert an inactive material (proactivator), a normal protein constituent of plasma, to its active form, referred to as activator. This in turn converts plasminogen to plasmin. Direct activators of plasminogen may also be liberated into the blood stream from tissues or secretions (fibrinokinases). Once activated, plasmin, a proteolytic enzyme, can digest both fibrin and fibrinogen, the latter at a slower rate. It also can digest other proteins such as casein and gelatin, and it is known to inactivate at least two coagulation factors, Factor V and Factor VIII. Certain end

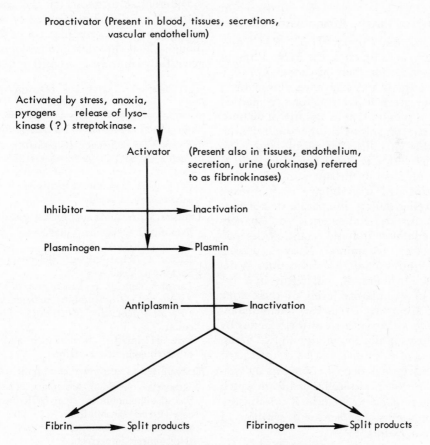

Fig. 173. Diagrammatic scheme of fibrinolysis.

products of the lysis of fibrinogen and fibrin interfere with the thrombin-fibrinogen reaction (this has been referred to as antithrombin VI) apparently by interfering with polymerization of fibrin monomers. Not only does the clot form more slowly but under these conditions it is more spongy and fragile than a normal clot. Other products of fibrinolysis act as inhibitors of thromboplastin generation.[72,73]

Streptokinase, a bacterial product, activates the human fibrinolytic system and for this reason has been used therapeutically, as a thrombolytic agent. Exactly how streptokinase activates plasminogen is controversial. Some investigators feel that it accomplishes this by activating the normal plasma proactivator to activator, which in turn activates plasminogen, whereas others believe that streptokinase reacts with plasminogen to form a complex which then activates plasminogen.

SYNTHESIS OF PLASMA COAGULATION FACTORS

Prothrombin, Factors VII, IX (PTC), and X (Stuart) are formed in the liver. Vitamin K is essential for their synthesis. Approximately 1 mg. of this substance, abundant in eggs and green leafy vegetables, is needed daily. Also important as a source of vitamin K are the organisms in the small bowel. Since this vitamin is fat-soluble and is assimilated with fats, deficiency of vitamin K may result from disturbances in fat absorption associated with biliary tract disease, sprue, celiac disease, idiopathic steatorrhea, pancreatitis, regional enteritis, etc. Changes in bacterial flora induced by antibiotics may also produce avitaminosis K by decreasing the amount available for absorption. A deficiency of vitamin K will result in a decrease in the plasma levels of these four factors. Coumarin drugs and phenylindandione block the synthesis of these factors by competitive inhibition of vitamin K. Thus, the effect of vitamin K can be counteracted by coumarin and that of coumarin by vitamin K. Severe hepatocellular disease which will not respond to vitamin K administration also results in a decrease in synthesis of these four factors.[74]

Factor V and fibrinogen are probably also synthesized in the liver, but vitamin K is not involved. Plasma Factor V activity, which is depressed in severe hepatocellular disease, is not depressed in biliary tract obstruction,[74] vitamin K deficiency or Dicumarol intoxication. Fibrinogen levels may be moderately depressed in severe liver disease, but the evidence for fibrinogen formation in the liver rests upon the findings of the fall in fibrinogen following hepatectomy in animals.[75]

Although there are reports of some diminution of Factors XII[2] and XI[76] in severe liver disease, there is no other evidence that the liver is involved in the synthesis of these factors or that vitamin K plays a role in their synthesis. There is no information in regard to the sites of synthesis of the other plasma coagulation factors.

INHERITED HEMORRHAGIC DISEASES: GENETIC FACTORS

Differential diagnosis of the congenital hemorrhagic disorders is aided by a knowledge of the usual genetic patterns seen. Although these disorders are assumed to be genetically controlled, a positive family his-

TABLE 25. INHERITED HEMORRHAGIC DISEASES

Transmitted as sex-linked recessive traits
  Factor VIII deficiency (Classical hemophilia)
  Factor IX (PTC) deficiency (Christmas disease)
  Congenital thrombocytopenia with repeated infections and eczema

Transmitted as autosomal recessive traits
  Factor XII (Hageman) deficiency
  Factor XI (PTA) deficiency
  Factor X (Stuart-Prower) deficiency
  Factor VII deficiency
  Factor V deficiency (Parahemophilia)
  ? Factor II (Prothrombin) deficiency
  ? Factor I deficiency (Congenital afibrinogenemia)
  Familial aplastic anemia with and without other congenital anomalies

Transmitted as autosomal dominant traits
  Hereditary hemorrhagic telangiectasia
  Vascular hemophilia (von Willebrand's Disease—Pseudohemophilia)
  Ehlers-Danlos syndrome
  Osteogenesis imperfecta

tory can be obtained in only about 60 to 70 per cent of the cases. This may be due either to inadequacy of the history or to mutation. Three types of genetic transmission are seen (1) the sex-linked recessive, (2) the autosomal recessive, and (3) the autosomal dominant. Table 25 classifies the hemorrhagic disorders according to the type of genetic transmission and Figure 174 illustrates the different patterns of inheritance.

In the conditions transmitted through a recessive sex-linked gene abnormality, as for example classical hemophilia and Factor IX deficiency, the disease is seen almost exclusively in males, and the female carriers are usually not symptomatic. The synthesis of Factors VIII and IX depend upon the presence of a gene located in the X chromosome which has no counterpart in the Y chromosome. A hemophilic male inherits an X chromosome from his carrier mother

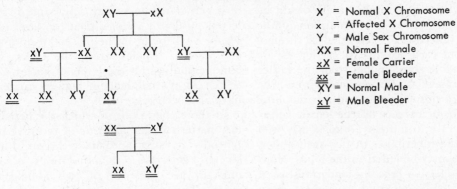

SEX-LINKED RECESSIVE PATTERN

X = Normal X Chromosome
x = Affected X Chromosome
Y = Male Sex Chromosome
XX = Normal Female
xX = Female Carrier
xx = Female Bleeder
XY = Normal Male
xY = Male Bleeder

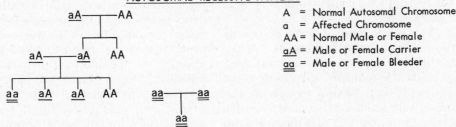

AUTOSOMAL RECESSIVE PATTERN

A = Normal Autosomal Chromosome
a = Affected Chromosome
AA = Normal Male or Female
aA = Male or Female Carrier
aa = Male or Female Bleeder

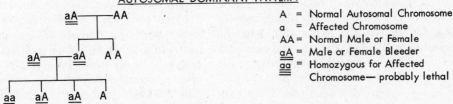

AUTOSOMAL DOMINANT PATTERN

A = Normal Autosomal Chromosome
a = Affected Chromosome
AA = Normal Male or Female
aA = Male or Female Bleeder
aa = Homozygous for Affected
     Chromosome— probably lethal

FIG. 174. Inheritance in hemorrhage diseases.

which has the abnormal allele, and from his normal father a normal Y chromosome. Half the male offspring of a union between a normal male and carrier female will inherit the normal X chromosome from the carrier mother and will be normal, and half will inherit the abnormal X chromosome and be hemophiliacs. Half the daughters will be carriers and half will be normal. A hemophilic male married to a normal female will have all normal sons, since they inherit their X chromosome from their mother, but all his daughters will be carriers, since they must inherit his abnormal X chromosome. The union of a female carrier with a hemophiliac male would be expected to produce a true hemophilic female (inherting an abnormal X chromosome from each parent), a carrier female (abnormal X chromosome from the father and normal X chromosome from the mother), a normal male, and a hemophilic male. The occurrence of true female hemophilia is rare in humans[77] and it may well be that the inheritance of two such abnormal genes may be lethal to the fetus. However, by selective breeding and transfusion therapy Brinkhous and coworkers have been able to produce female hemophiliac dogs by mating carrier females with hemophilic males. The bleeding manifestations in the females were similar to those seen in the males.[78]

If the average normal level of plasma antihemophilic factor is taken as 100 per cent, the levels among the normal male population are found to vary from about 70 to 150 per cent. Normal females are also found to have levels ranging from 70 to 150 per cent despite the fact that they have two normal X chromosomes and the male only one X chromosome. Recent studies report that the antihemophilic factor level in female carriers tends to run lower than that of the normal female or male, varying from 20 to 130 per cent[79,80] with an average of about 60 per cent. It is not clear why the normal female with two X chromosomes and therefore two genes for antihemophilic factor has the same plasma level of this factor as males who have only one X chromosome and therefore only one such gene, whereas the female carrier of hemophilia

with one normal gene and one abnormal allele tends to have a lower level than the male. The low level in the female carrier may be due to some modifying genes or it may be due to the production of an inhibitor controlled by the abnormal gene. The Factor VIII levels in both the normal and carrier female in relation to what is present in the normal male could also be explained if only one X chromosome is functional in the female and the other, forming the chromatin body seen on microscopy, is inactive; or the part of the chromosome containing the hemophilic or Factor VIII gene is inactive. Assuming that the X chromosome of a cell slated to be the active one is selected purely by chance, then the levels of Factor VIII found in the plasma of normal and carrier females would be expected. Similar findings for the levels of Factor IX (PTC) in normal females and in carriers have also been reported.[81,82]

In those conditions in which the hereditary pattern is characteristic of recessive or partially recessive autosomal transmission, severe hemorrhagic manifestations occur only in the presence of two abnormal genes. The carrier can be either male or female and may have a slight to moderate depression of the level of the coagulation factor in question which may or may not be associated with a mild bleeding tendency. Variation in the carrier state may be due to the variability of the recessiveness or penetrance of the abnormal gene. In these disorders the appearance of the homozygous individual, which would necessarily mean inheriting one abnormal gene from each parent, is frequently associated with consanguinity in the preceding generation. A carrier male or female married to a normal individual can transmit the carrier state to one half of the progeny, whether male or female. All the children of a male or female homozygous for the abnormal gene married to normal individual will be carriers. Both the parents of a homozygous individual must either be carriers (heterozygous) or one must be a carrier and the other homozygous for the abnormality. There is fairly good evidence that the hereditary deficiencies of Factors XII,[83] XI,[84] X,[85] VII,[86] and V[87] fall into this group. The evidence for hereditary deficiency of prothrombin and fibrinogen belonging to this group is not as good.

In the pattern of dominant inheritance, only one abnormal autosomal gene occurring in either sex is necessary for the abnormality to manifest itself. In all probability the homozygous state for the abnormal dominant gene is not compatible with survival of the fetus. The abnormality is transmitted to half the male and female children by the single parent who is heterozygous for the abnormal gene. None of the single congenital coagulation deficiencies are inherited by this mode of transmission. In von Willebrand's disease, in which there is a mild Factor VIII deficiency and some vascular abnormality, inheritance appears to be of this type. Since in this syndrome the transmission is not sex linked, it is evident that Factor VIII (antihemophilic factor) synthesis is affected by more than the one gene on the X chromosome. Synthesis must also be affected by a gene on an autosomal chromosome. It would also appear that in this condition one is dealing with a double heterozygosity for a dominant autosomal gene, one affecting Factor VIII synthesis and another affecting the vasculature.[88] Also typical of this type of dominant inheritance is hereditary hemorrhagic telangiectasia. It is evident from clinical observations in this condition that there is considerable variation in the severity of the syndrome and the distribution of lesions from patient to patient,[71] indicating the variable penetrance of the dominant gene or a number of alleles.

HEMORRHAGIC DISEASES

The clinical and laboratory manifestations of pathologic bleeding depend largely upon which component or components of the hemostatic mechanisms are deranged. The classification of hemorrhagic diseases that follows (Table 26) is intended solely as a guide and is based upon present knowledge of the defects underlying the various disorders. An attempt has been made to classify according to whether the disturbance is of the coagulation mechanism, the vasculature, the supporting tissue, or any combination of these, and as far as possible

upon the pathogenesis of these disturbances. While considerable progress has been made in elucidating the pathogenesis of many hemorrhagic states, there are still areas of ignorance and controversy, consequently, certain categories in the classification may be questioned. However, any such classification should be considered flexible and should be altered as new information becomes available so that it remains a useful guide to the differential diagnosis of pathologic bleeding.

CONGENITAL HEREDITARY PLASMA COAGULATION DEFECTS

HEMOPHILIA

Hemophilia was first recognized as a distinct clinical entity in 1803 by Otto,[89] who delineated the conditions governing its transmission. It is now well established, as described above, that hemophilia is transmitted as a sex-linked recessive characteristic, although approximately one third of the cases fail to give a positive family history. It is thought that sporadic cases do arise as a result of mutation of the controlling gene on the X chromosome. It is undoubtedly the occurrence of mutations that maintains the incidence of hemophilia, otherwise one would have anticipated that the incidence would have steadily declined to the point of disappearance of the disease, since relatively few of the males with hemophilia have children. It is of interest that the clinical severity of the disease and of the coagulation defect is approximately the same for all the members of a given family or pedigree. Severe, moderate, and mild cases (see below) do occur, and it has been suggested that such variation may be due to the fact that there are several alleles of the hemophilia gene[90] which result in different degrees of deficiency of the antihemophilic factor. It is also evident from the studies on patients with a vascular defect and varying degrees of antihemophilic factor deficiency that at least one gene on an autosomal chromosome has an effect upon the production of this factor. The true incidence of hemophilia is not known and in the countries where it has been most extensively studied (United States,

TABLE 26. CLASSIFICATION OF HEMORRHAGIC DISEASES

I. DEFECTIVE COAGULATION–DERANGEMENT
IN PLASMA CONSTITUENTS

FIRST PHASE DEFECTS: DEFECTIVE THROMBOPLASTIN FORMATION

Deficiencies of plasma factors involved in intrinsic thromboplastin formation only:

Factor VIII deficiency
1. Congenital-hereditary (Classical hemophilia)
2. Acquired: intravascular coagulation

Factor IX deficiency
1. Congenital-hereditary (Christmas disease)
2. Acquired: vitamin K deficiency, drugs of coumarin and phenylindanedione types, hepatocellular disease, obstructive jaundice, neonatal

Factor XI (PTA) deficiency
1. Congenital-hereditary
2. Acquired: hepatocellular disease, neonatal

Deficiencies of plasma factors involved in both intrinsic and extrinsic thromboplastin formation:

Factor V deficiency (pseudohypoprothrombinemia)
1. Congenital-hereditary (parahemophilia)
2. Acquired: severe hepatocellular disease, severe sepsis, intravascular fibrinolysis or coagulation

Factor X deficiency (pseudohypoprothrombinemia)
1. Congenital-hereditary
2. Acquired: vitamin K deficiency, drugs of coumarin and phenylindanedione type, hepatocellular disease and obstructive jaundice, neonatal

Deficiencies of plasma factors involved in extrinsic thromboplastin formation only:

Factor VII deficiency (pseudohypoprothrombinemia)
1. Congenital-hereditary
2. Acquired: vitamin K deficiency, drugs of coumarin and phenylindanedione type, hepatocellular disease and obstructive jaundice, neonatal

Circulating anticoagulants inhibiting thromboplastin formation:

Inhibitors of specific coagulation factors
1. antifactor VIII
2. antifactor IX
3. antifactor V
4. others

Nonspecific inhibitors
1. acquired: dysproteinemias (hyperglobulinemia, macroglobulinemia, cryoglobulinemia, multiple myeloma, lupus erythematosus)
2. drugs (heparin, protamine, polybrene)

SECOND PHASE DEFECTS: DEFECTIVE THROMBIN FORMATION

Factor II (Prothrombin) deficiency
1. Congenital (hypoprothrombinemia)
2. Acquired: vitamin K deficiency, drugs of coumarin and phenylindanedione type, hepatocellular disease, and obstructive jaundice, neonatal

Thromboplastin inhibitors
1. Acquired: dysproteinemias (hyperglobulinemia, macroglobulinemia, cryoglobulinemia, multiple myeloma, lupus erythematosus)
2. Drugs: heparin and protamine

THIRD PHASE DEFECTS: DEFECTIVE FIBRIN FORMATION

Hypofibrinogenemia (Factor I deficiency)

Congenital-hereditary

Acquired
1. decreased production: liver disease, polycythemia vera
2. increased utilization: intravascular coagulation with defibrination (complication of pregnancy: premature separation of the placenta, intrauterine retention of a dead fetus, amniotic fluid embolism, septic abortion; carcinoma of prostate and stomach; pulmonary and cardiac surgery).

TABLE 26. CLASSIFICATION OF HEMORRHAGIC DISEASES (*Continued*)

3. Increased destruction: increased fibrinolytic activity (complications of pregnancy as mentioned above: carcinoma of prostate, liver disease, polycythemia vera, leukemia, shock, anoxia, severe exertion, pulmonary and cardiac surgery, secondary to fibrinolytic therapy—streptokinase, plasmin).

Inhibition of thrombin-fibrinogen interaction:

1. Increased antithrombin activity: dysproteinemias, liver disease, products of fibrinogenolysis and fibrinolysis.
2. Drugs: heparin

Circulating anticoagulants directed against fibrinogen

II. DEFECTIVE COAGULATION PLUS VASCULAR ABNORMALITIES

THROMBOCYTOPENIC PURPURA

Megakaryocytic thrombocytopenia:

Conditions in which the life-span of platelets is predominantly reduced

Conditions in which an immune mechanism probably plays a role

1. Idiopathic thrombocytopenia (Werlhof's disease), acute and chronic primary thrombocytopenia
2. Sensitivity to drugs (Sedormid, Phenobarbital, Quinine, Quinidine, Sulfonamides, Penicillin, Chlortrimeton, Benadryl, Antazoline, Thiouracil, Propylthiouracil, organic arsenical compounds, Amidopyrine, Salicylates, Chlorothiazide compounds, Digitoxin, Chlorpropamide, DDT)
3. Infections, (Viral or probably viral: measles, rubella, chicken pox, mumps, cytomegalic inclusion disease, infectious hepatitis, infectious mononucleosis, upper respiratory tract viral infections; bacterial: particularly streptococcal infection but can occur in any bacterial infection; rickettsial: typhus)
4. Thrombotic thrombocytopenic purpura
5. Systemic lupus erythematosus
6. In association with auto-immune hemolytic anemia (Evans syndrome)
7. In lymphoproliferative diseases (chronic lymphatic leukemia, lymphosarcoma)
8. Neonatal thrombocytopenia (In babies born of mothers with idiopathic thrombocytopenia; in erythroblastosis, secondary to isoantibodies formed in the mother to the infant's platelets)

Conditions in which the platelets are sequestered, destroyed or utilized excessively

1. Splenomegaly with hypersplenism (Gaucher's disease, sarcoidosis, tuberculosis, congestive splenomegaly, myeloid metaplasia, lymphosarcoma, amyloidosis)
2. Congenital hemangiomatosis
3. Massive hemorrhage with replacement of blood loss by transfusion of platelet-poor blood
4. Intravascular coagulation

Conditions in which production of platelets is predominantly reduced (megakaryocytes present)

1. Nutritional deficiencies (vitamin B_{12}, folic acid, ? vitamin C, Kwashiorkor)
2. Infiltration of marrow with abnormal cells (leukemia, metastatic carcinoma, multiple myeloma)
3. Splenomegaly of any cause, particularly congestive splenomegaly
4. Renal failure with severe azotemia
5. Lack of thrombopoetin

Pathogenesis of thrombocytopenia unknown

1. Congenital thrombocytopenia with eczema
2. Onyalai
3. Paroxysmal nocturnal hemoglobinuria

Amegakaryocytic thrombocytopenia:

1. Congenital-hereditary conditions (congenital hypoplastic anemia, Fanconi's anemia, congenital thrombocytopenia with other congenital abnormalities)
2. Aplastic anemia with thymoma
3. Idiopathic aplastic anemia

TABLE 26. CLASSIFICATION OF HEMORRHAGIC DISEASES (*Continued*)

4. Secondary to drugs, chemicals, or ionizing radiation (nitrogen mustard and related components; antimetabolites such as folic acid antagonists, 6 mercapto-purine; organic solvents such as benzene; arsenicals; gold; mercury; antithyroid drugs such as thiouracil; anti-convulsants such as Mesantoin and Tridione; insecticides such as DDT and chlordane; antibiotics such as chloramphenicol and less commonly the tetracyclines; carbutamide; barbiturates; promazines; meproba-mate; Pyribenzamine; hair dyes; x-radiation, P^{32}, etc.)
5. Displacement by other cells as in acute leukemia, chronic leukemia, multiple myeloma, myelofibrosis with and without myeloid metaplasia.

QUALITATIVE PLATELET ABNORMALITY PLUS (?) VASCULAR ABNORMALITY:
1. Hereditary hemorrhagic thrombasthenia (Glanzman's disease, thrombocytopathic purpura with impaired clot retraction)
2. Familial thrombocytopathic purpura due to deficiency in platelet factor 3
3. Acquired platelet factor 3 defect or other abnormality of platelets:
   Uremia
   Polycythemia vera
   Myeloid metaplasia
   Primary hemorrhagic thrombocytosis

VASCULAR ABNORMALITY (? DEFICIENCY OF A PLASMA FACTOR) PLUS A PLASMA COAGULATION DEFECT:
1. Vascular hemophilia, von Willebrand's disease, pseudohemophilia: vascular abnor-mality plus Factor VIII deficiency.
2. Vascular abnormality plus plasma deficiency of coagulation Factors other than VIII (IX, XI, etc.).

III. VASCULAR ABNORMALITIES

Hereditary
  Hereditary hemorrhagic telangectasia (Rendu-Weber-Osler disease)
Acquired
  Vitamin C deficiency—scurvy
  Anaphylactoid purpura
  1. Idiopathic (Henoch-Schönlein purpura)
  2. Secondary to drugs, chemicals and infections (purpura fulminans, Shwartzman reaction)
  Probable vascular abnormality: Shamberg's disease, Majocchi's disease.
  Purpura associated with hypertension, atherosclerosis, diabetes mellitus, and infec-tions.

IV. CONNECTIVE TISSUE ABNORMALITIES
(VASCULAR AND EXTRAVASCULAR ABNORMALITIES)

Hereditary
  Ehlers-Danlos syndrome
  Osteogenesis imperfecta
  Pseudoxanthoma elasticum

Acquired
  Pulmonary hemosiderosis

V. PATHOGENESIS UNCERTAIN

Purpura senilis, purpura in Cushing's disease and with corticosteroid therapy, auto-erythrocyte sensitization, auto-DNA sensitization, and other as yet unsolved hemor-rhagic disorders which cannot at present be categorized.

England, Sweden, France, Switzerland, etc.) the estimated incidence varies from 1 in 10,000 to 20,000 to 1 in 100,000. Hemo-philia has been reported in the negroid and mongoloid as well as in the caucasian races.

Most observers believe that hemophilia is due to a deficiency of a single plasma pro-tein factor, the antihemophilic factor or Factor VIII, which is an essential component of the coagulation mechanism. This pro-tein has been partially purified by a variety of technics from normal human and animal plasma and has been found to effectively correct the coagulation defect of hemophilia in vitro and in vivo.[91-93] Factor VIII has many chemical characteristics similar to fibrinogen, so that it is concentrated in fraction I of the Cohn fractionation procedures and is difficult to separate from fibrinogen. However, it is not identical to fibrinogen as is indicated by the normal levels of Factor VIII in the blood of patients with congenital afibrinogenemia,[53] and recent methods have been found to at least partially separate Factor VIII from fibrinogen. Purification has not progressed to the point at which the protein can be accurately characterized. It has not been possible to isolate a protein from hemophilic plasma which has factor VIII activity, whether this is due to failure of the hemophilic to produce this protein or to the production of an abnormal protein with no Factor VIII activity has not been determined. It is also not clear whether a deficiency of Factor VIII is the sole etiologic factor in the pathogenesis of hemophilic bleeding. Tocantins[94] and others believe that hemophilic blood contains all the procoagulant factors present in normal blood in normal amounts and that the coagulation defect is due to the presence of an excess of a lipid inhibitor, frequently referred to as *antithromboplastin*. Most other investigators believe that such an inhibitor is present only in those hemophilics who have developed a resistance to the corrective effects of normal plasma and Factor VIII concentrates. That a vascular factor may also play a role in bleeding is suggested by the findings that although the Factor VIII plasma level in a given hemophilic shows no significant variations, the ease with which hemorrhage develops varies considerably, from periods of complete freedom even with appreciable trauma, to periods in which only mild trauma will elicit major hemorrhage, or bleeding appears to start spontaneously, frequently at multiple sites. It has also been noted that capillary fragility may be increased at such times. Nevertheless, hemorrhage can be controlled even at such periods, if the circulating Factor VIII level is raised to 30 per cent of normal or above by the administration of plasma or of Factor VIII concentrates. Usually the severity of the clinical manifestations parallels the degree of Factor VIII deficiency. In severe hemophilia, hemorrhagic manifestations are frequent, occuring with minor trauma or spontaneously, the clotting time is markedly prolonged, usually greater than 45 minutes, prothrombin consumption is poor, and the Factor VIII level is less than 1 per cent. In those classified as moderate, the hemorrhagic manifestations are usually less extensive, rarely appear to be spontaneous but occur after mild to moderate trauma, the clotting times vary from normal to prolonged, the prothrombin consumption is almost always impaired, and the Factor VIII level ranges from 1 to 5 per cent of normal. In mild hemophilia, hemorrhage does not occur spontaneously, the abnormal hemostasis usually manifests itself as excessive bleeding only after moderate to severe trauma, the clotting times are almost always in the normal ranges, prothrombin consumption is usually normal, and the Factor VIII level ranges from 5 to 25 per cent of normal.

Clinical Manifestations. Episodic and persistent bleeding from or into various parts of the body constitutes the outstanding clinical feature of hemophilia. Certain areas of the body are particularly susceptible, notably the joints, the subcutaneous tissues, the muscles, and the mucous membranes of the mouth, the nose and the genitourinary tract. Curiously, intracranial bleeding is not as frequent as one might anticipate, probably because the brain is well protected against trauma. Petechiae are not characteristic, but may appear at times at the height of or preceding a bleeding episode. Usually the bleeding follows injury, which frequently is trivial. Sometimes it appears spontaneously, but there is always the possibility that the precipitating trauma may have passed unnoticed. Usually the bleeding is of the persistent oozing type, lasting for days or weeks, although it occasionally may be massive and accompanied by shock.

Hemophilia may be manifest at birth, for the defect is demonstrable in cord blood and occasionally the infant bleeds from injuries sustained at childbirth. Bleeding from the umbilical stump is unusual. The disease may first become evident because of severe bleeding at the time of circumcision although surprisingly some undergo this procedure without difficulty. Hemorrhagic episodes are uncommon during infancy, probably because the infant is not so liable to trauma. However, once the child begins moving around, and particularly when he begins to creep and try to walk, thus subjecting himself to trauma, "unexplained" hematomas may appear and may reach large proportions. Hemorrhagic manifestations are usually most severe during childhood and adolescence when it is difficult to restrict the affected child's activities, since he cannot readily appreciate or accept his abnormalities. If the hemophilic, as he matures, can learn to accept his limitations and if he can adjust his activities accordingly, hemorrhagic episodes are usually less frequent and less severe.

Hemarthrosis generally involves the knees, the elbows, the ankles, the hips and the shoulders, joints which are most subject to trauma. At first, the joint is stiff and painful, but as bleeding continues, it becomes swollen, warm to the touch, and when the capsule is distended, exquisitely tender. There is usually no discoloration around the joint except when subcutaneous ecchymosis is present due to the original trauma. The muscles crossing the joint may be in protective spasm. Bleeding is usually self-limited, arrest of the hemorrhage resulting largely from tamponade. When bleeding stops, the blood within the joint is gradually absorbed and mobility is slowly regained. However, damage to the joint occurs as a result of atrophic changes induced by high intra-articular pressure from the tamponaded blood and by disturbance in blood supply to the joint structure. Once a joint has been the site of hemarthrosis it is more likely to bleed again and with repeated hemorrhage permanent joint deformities occur. Vascular hyperplasia of the synovia and thickening of capsular and pericapsular tissue may develop, resulting eventually in scarring and contracture. The synovial tissues become impregnated with iron and thickened, the cartilages become thin and are invaded by hyperplastic synovial and subsynovial tissues. Cysts form in the subchondral bone due to the destruction of bone by vascular connective tissue. Bony proliferation, lipping, contractures and eventually ankylosis may occur. In children the epiphysial areas may become involved leading to premature closure of the epiphysis and eventual shortening of the bone. Each episode of hemarthrosis imposes an additional burden on both involved and uninvolved parts of the skeletal system. Locomotion becomes difficult, balance is impaired, other joints are subjected to unusual strain, and the likelihood of a new "spontaneous" or traumatic incident is enhanced. The clinical, pathologic and roentgenographic features of hemophilic arthropathy have been extensively reviewed.[95-97]

Intramuscular bleeding may also appear to occur spontaneously or following minor trauma particularly that which causes sudden tension or twisting of a muscle. Crippling often results from destruction of muscle, replacement by fibrous tissue, and subsequent contracture. Bleeding frequently continues until it is stopped by the effect of tamponade and this may result in embarrassment of blood supply to an extremity with subsequent contractures (Volkman's contracture) or gangrene. Paralysis may be produced by pressure on nerve trunks, such as the branches of the femoral plexus. Bleeding retroperitoneally into the psoas muscles may produce symptoms simulating acute appendicitis. Hemorrhage into muscular areas such as the chest wall, the buttock, the neck or the thigh may dissect widely as may retroperitoneal bleeding, resulting in a marked fall in circulating blood volume and shock, or encroachment on such structures as airways, esophagus, and ureters. With the accumulation of blood in muscular areas or in joints, the problem frequently arises whether one should relieve tension by aspiration. This poses a difficult problem to resolve because of the important role tamponade plays in the hemostatic mechanism, especially when clotting is deranged. Each case must be considered individually, but usually aspiration should not be attempted unless a sufficient quantity of plasma or of a potent Factor VIII preparation is available for adequate therapy (i.e. to maintain a Factor VIII level between 20 and 30 per cent of normal) for a period of several days to a week, depending upon the lesion. Hemorrhage into muscle may also result in the formation of cysts which can grow to such size that they become incapacitating.

Bleeding from the mucous membranes is one of the most common and serious hemorrhagic manifestations of hemophilia. The most trivial trauma (e.g. a cut tongue, loss or extraction of deciduous teeth, or trauma from ingestion of a relatively sharp object) can induce persistent oozing which may prove fatal despite all therapeutic measures when the bleeding point is not readily accessible, since the effect of tamponade is not operative in such bleeding. Epistaxis is very common in children. Melena, hematemesis and hematuria occur in about 30 per cent of the cases, are apt to recur and may last from days to weeks. There may be associated local manifestations such as distention, abdominal pain and increased peristalsis, or in case of genitourinary hemorrhage, symptoms of renal colic.

Bleeding into the nervous system probably occurs more frequently than is generally described. Besides hematomas in soft tissues that may compress or damage peripheral nerves, epidural, subdural, subarachnoid hemorrhage or focal bleeding into the central nervous system may occur. Signs and symptoms will depend upon the location and extent of such hemorrhage, and permanent damage of the central nervous system may occur.

LABORATORY. The laboratory abnormalities are confined to alterations of the clotting mechanism of the blood except that bleeding may cause melena, hematuria, anemia, etc. As indicated above, the capillary fragility (tourniquet test) and bleeding times are usually normal. All test procedures which measure the formation of plasma thromboplastin or prothrombinase by the intrinsic mechanism or the overall coagulation via the intrinsic mechanism will be abnormal if the deficiency of Factor VIII is great enough. The tests commonly employed which will reveal this first phase defect are the clotting time, recalcification time, partial thromboplastin time, prothrombin consumption and thromboplastin generation. Each of these tests has a different sensitivity to deficiency of Factor VIII. Thus, although a *prolonged clotting time* is generally considered one of the classical findings in hemophillia, it is a rather insensitive test for Factor VIII deficiency, for it is significantly prolonged only when the Factor VIII level is less than 1 to 2 per cent of normal. It is therefore not surprising that severe hemorrhagic manifestations may occur in a hemophilic with a normal clotting time. The *plasma recalcification time* is somewhat more sensitive but is even more prone to variation due to nonspecific factors than the whole-blood clotting time. The manner of collection of blood, the centrifugal force used to prepare the plasma, the amount of exposure to glass surface, all have an effect on the recalcification time which makes determination of the normal range difficult, and the test less reliable. The determination of residual prothrombin in the serum after 1 hour of clotting or the *prothrombin consumption test* is somewhat more sensitive than the whole blood clotting time, and will be abnormal (poor prothrombin consumption or increased residual serum prothrombin) when the Factor VIII level is below 5 to 10%. It is evident that the mild to moderately severe form of hemophilia may be missed with these procedures. Both the *partial thromboplastin time*[98] (with or without the addition of surface activating agents such as kaolin or celite) and the *thromboplastin generation tests*[3] are much more sensitive to Factor VIII deficiency and are almost always abnormal when Factor VIII is reduced to levels (30% or lower) which interfere with normal hemostasis.

Other coagulation tests such as the prothrombin time, stypven (Russel Viper Venom) time, thrombin time and clot retraction are usually normal. However, the presence of hemophilia does not preclude the coexistence of other hemostatic defects. Scurvy and vitamin K deficiency may result from malnutrition. Decreased levels of Factors II (prothrombin), V, VII, IX and X may be present because of liver disease,

TABLE 27. CHARACTERISTIC LABORATORY FINDINGS IN HEMORRHAGIC DISORDERS

DISORDER	CAPILLARY FRAGILITY	BLEEDING TIME	CLOTTING TIME	PROTH.* TIME	PTT†	PROTH. CONSUMP.	TGT‡	STYPVEN TIME	THROMBIN TIME	COAGULATION CORRECTED BY NORMAL			
										PLASMA	ADSORBED PLASMA	SERUM	ADSORBED SERUM
XII Deficiency	Normal	Normal	Long	Normal	Long	Decreased	Abnormal	Normal	Normal	Yes	Yes	Yes	Yes
XI (PTA) Deficiency	Normal	Normal	Long	Normal	Long	Decreased	Abnormal	Normal	Normal	Yes	Yes	Yes	Yes
X (Stuart) Deficiency	Normal	Normal	Long	Long	Long	Decreased	Abnormal	Long	Normal	Yes	No	Yes	No
IX (PTC) Deficiency	Normal	Normal	Long	Normal	Long	Decreased	Abnormal	Normal	Normal	Yes	No	Yes	No
VIII Deficiency Classical Hemophilia	Normal	Normal	Long	Normal	Long	Decreased	Abnormal	Normal	Normal	Yes	Yes	No	No
VII Deficiency	Normal	Normal	Normal	Long	Normal	Normal	Normal	Normal	Normal	Yes	No	Yes	No
V Deficiency	Normal	Variable	Normal–Long	Long	Long	Decreased	Abnormal	Long	Normal	Yes	Yes	No	No
II (Proth.) Deficiency	Normal	Normal	?	Long	?	—	? Abnormal	Long	Normal	Yes	No	No	No
I Deficiency (Afibrinogenemia)	Normal	Normal– ?Prolong.	Long– Infinite	Long– Infinite	Long– Infinite	Normal	Normal	Long– Infinite	Long– Infinite	Yes	Yes	No	No
Thrombocytopenia	Increased	Prolonged	Normal–Long	Normal	Normal	Decreased	Normal	Normal	Normal	No	No	No	No
Von Willebrand Syndrome	Increased– Normal	Prolonged	Normal– Long	Normal	Long	Normal– Decreased	Abnormal– Normal	Normal	Normal	Yes	Yes	No	No
Anaphylactoid Purpura	Normal; Occ. Increased	Normal	Normal	Normal	Normal	Normal	Normal	Normal	Normal	—	—	—	—
Fibrinolysis	Normal– Increased	Normal– Prolonged	Normal– Long	Long	Long	Decreased	Abnormal	Normal– Long	Long	Variable			

* Proth. = Prothrombin
† PTT = Partial Prothrombin Time
‡ TGT = Thromboplastin Generation Test

since serum hepatitis is a common complication among patients receiving multiple transfusions. Also, hypoprothrombinemia may arise as a consequence of prolonged severe bleeding, prothrombin regeneration failing to keep pace with the losses incurred. The platelets are rarely if ever reduced. More often they are increased, especially following active bleeding.

DIFFERENTIAL DIAGNOSIS. In general it is not difficult to differentiate hemophilia from most other disturbances of the hemostatic mechanism by: (1) the type of hemorrhagic manifestations, (2) the absences of vascular abnormalities (prolonged bleeding times, increased capillary fragility, and petechiae), (3) the normal platelet levels and the normal prothrombin and thrombin times, and (4) prolonged clotting times (poor prothrombin consumption), increased partial thromboplastin times, or abnormal thromboplastin generation with the use of normal platelets or a platelet substitute. Such findings are characteristic of deficiencies of Factors XII, XI, IX and VIII. Deficiencies of Factors V, VII, X, prothrombin and fibrinogen are eliminated by the normal prothrombin time. Since Factor XII (Hageman) deficiency is not associated with a hemorrhagic diathesis, a deficiency of this factor can be eliminated from consideration of the cause of hemorrhage. Deficiencies of Factors VIII, IX and XI can be differentiated from each other by determining the corrective effect of normal plasma, serum, adsorbed plasma and adsorbed serum on the prolonged clotting time, poor prothrombin consumption, prolonged partial thromboplastin time, or the abnormal thromboplastin generation (Table 27). The coagulation defect in classical hemophilia (VIII deficiency) is corrected by normal plasma and adsorbed normal plasma but not by normal serum or adsorbed serum, whereas that of Factor IX deficiency is corrected by normal plasma and serum but not by adsorbed plasma or adsorbed serum and that of Factor XI deficiency is corrected by all four. It should be noted that because of nonspecific activators present in serum the clotting time and partial thromboplastin time of hemophilic blood may be shortened by serum despite the lack of Factor VIII in serum, but there is little corrective effect upon prothrombin consumption or thromboplastin generation. For final identification of a Factor VIII defect, the corrective effect of the patient's blood or plasma upon the coagulation defect of the blood or plasma from a subject with known classical hemophilia should be determined. In true hemophilia the corrective effect is always markedly decreased as compared to normal.

FACTOR IX OR PLASMA THROMBOPLASTIN COMPONENT DEFICIENCY

(CHRISTMAS DISEASE)

It is now clear that about 10 to 20 per cent of the cases which would have been classified as hemophilia prior to 1952 are not due to Factor VIII deficiency but rather to a deficiency of another coagulation factor, Factor IX. The hemorrhagic manifestation and complications, and the hereditary pattern (sex-linked recessive) in congenital Factor IX deficiency or Christmas disease are identical to those of classical hemophilia.[99-101] As in classical hemophilia the severity of the hemorrhagic manifestations varies from patient to patient and roughly correlates with the degree of the deficiency of the clotting factor.

All the affected members of a family have approximately the same degree of deficiency of Factor IX. The diagnosis of Factor IX deficiency is made by the laboratory findings. The platelet count, the bleeding time, the capillary fragility, the prothrombin time, and the thrombin time are normal. The clotting time, recalcification time and prothrombin consumption are abnormal if the deficiency is great enough (plasma IX levels less than 5%), but the partial thromboplastin time and thromboplastin generation tests are much more sensitive and become abnormal when the Factor IX level falls below about 30 per cent of normal, a level at which hemorrhage may occur with trauma. The coagulation defect is corrected by plasma or serum but not by adsorbed plasma or adsorbed serum since the adsorbing agents such as barium sulfate and aluminum hydroxide remove Factor IX. Whereas Factor VIII appears to be consumed or inactivated during coagulation so that it is not present in serum, Factor IX is not and indeed it is felt by many investigators that Factor IX is activated during the clotting process, since normal serum has considerably greater corrective activity than plasma. Whether this is actually due to the activation of Factor IX or some intermediary product or nonspecific accelerator present in serum has not been adequately ascertained. The diagnosis ultimately depends upon demonstrating that the coagulation defect of the plasma from a patient with known Christmas disease is not corrected by the plasma of the patient. The impression that Christmas disease is not as severe a hemorrhagic disease as, and has better prognosis than classical hemophilia is probably due to the fact that the percentage of milder cases is higher than in classical hemophilia. It has been the author's experience that in cases of profound deficiency of Factor IX (clotting times greater than 1 hour) the hemorrhagic manifestations are as severe as those seen in hemophilias with comparable clotting times. However, it should be pointed out that in both deficiency states, the severity of hemorrhagic manifestations vary considerably in patients who appear to have the same degree of deficiency.

Factor XI (Plasma Thromboplastin Antecedent) Deficiency

In 1958 Rosenthal and coworkers[42] described a new hemorrhagic syndrome which they postulated was due to a deficiency of a previously unrecognized clotting factor designated first as plasma thromboplastin antecedent (PTA) and more recently as Factor XI. Patients with Factor XI deficiency have a relatively mild hemorrhagic diathesis even when the deficiency is severe enough to prolong the clotting time to 30 or 40 minutes. Epistaxis is relatively common but other types of spontaneous hemorrhage are uncommon. Easy bruising is occasionally seen, but hematomas and hemarthrosis are rare. Menorrhagia is uncommon but may occur. The most frequent hemorrhagic manifestation is bleeding after surgery, dental extractions, or injuries. Rarely does death occur from hemorrhage.

Although cases have been seen by many investigators, there is a great variation in the reported frequency. Rosenthal has observed as many cases of this deficiency as of classical hemophilia but most others have found it to be much less common. In my own experience it is about one tenth as frequent as hemophilia.

The diagnosis is made by the laboratory findings. Bleeding time, capillary fragility, platelet count, prothrombin time, stypven time, and thrombin time are normal. In severe cases the clotting time in glass is prolonged, as is the recalcification time. The most frequently observed abnormality has been an *impaired prothrombin consumption*. This has been the only abnormality noted in some cases labeled as PTA deficiency, even when such tests as the thromboplastin generation test and partial thromboplastin time, which are much more sensitive in most other coagulation defects, are normal. It is still questionable under such circumstance whether or not a true deficiency exists. In unquestionable cases the *partial thromboplastin time* is prolonged and the *thromboplastin generation test* is abnormal. These abnormalities are corrected by normal plasma, adsorbed plasma, normal serum or adsorbed serum. The adsorbing agents remove some of the Factor XI activity but not sufficient to impair the corrective effects. This pattern of correction by both unadsorbed and adsorbed plasma and serum differentiates Factor XI deficiency from all other deficiency states except Factor XII (Hageman) deficiency. Final identification rests upon demonstrating that the defect in the blood of the patient is not corrected by the blood or plasma from a subject with known Factor XI deficiency, and that it is corrected by blood or plasma from a subject with known Factor XII deficiency. One of the difficulties encountered in studying the clotting defect has been the lability of the defect in plasma on storage either at 4°C. or in the frozen state. The deficient plasma behaves like normal plasma after storage under such conditions, unless the blood is collected and the plasma is prepared platelet-poor and is frozen using nonwettable surfaces throughout.[102]

The clinical course is usually mild, with excessive bleeding occurring only after severe trauma and surgery. Transfusion therapy has always been effective in my experience, correcting the coagulation defect and the hemostasis. Rosenthal has reported the effectiveness of plasma transfusions on hemostasis, but frequently found little or no correction of the abnormal prothrombin consumption.[103]

Factor XII Deficiency (Hageman Trait)

Despite the fact that this factor is essential for normal in vitro blood clotting, patients lacking Factor XII have few if any hemorrhagic manifestaitons, and can even undergo surgery without excessive bleeding.[3,36,37] This phenomenon emphasizes the inadequacies of our present concepts of hemostasis. The characteristic abnormal laboratory findings are similar to those found in Factor XI deficiency; prolonged clotting, recalcification and partial thromboplastin times, decreased prothrombin consumption, and abnormal thromboplastin generation. These abnormalities can be corrected by normal plasma and serum and adsorbed normal serum and plasma. Since the blood and plasma in severe Factor XII deficiency is not activated by glass surfaces, the clotting time and recalcification time in glass and silicon-coated glass (nonwettable) are much less different than in other coagulation defects or normal blood. Since the hemorrhagic tendency in Factor XII deficiency is for all practical purposes nonexistent, it is important to differentiate this defect from Factor XI deficiency, and this can best be done by determining the corrective effect upon the abnormal coagulation of the patient's blood by the addition of plasma from subjects with known Factor XII or Factor XI deficiency.

Factor X (Stuart) Deficiency and Factor VII Deficiency

From 1951, when Factor VII deficiency was first reported,[104] until 1957 when Factor X was first distinguished from Factor VII,[58] all cases of Factor X deficiency were considered to be deficiencies of Factor VII. The hemorrhagic manifestations of both these deficiency states are quite similar

and tend to be rather mild when compared to hemophilia. Easy bruising, epistaxis, occasional gastrointestinal bleeding and menorrhagia occur, but other forms of spontaneous bleeding are unusual. Hemarthrosis following trauma may occur and excessive bleeding after surgery or trauma is common. Since both Factors X and VII are essential for the formation of prothrombinase from tissue thromboplastin (i.e. for the conversion of prothrombin by tissue thromboplastin) both deficiency states are characterized by *prolonged prothrombin times.* Since Factor VII is not involved in the formation of prothrombinase in the intrinsic mechanism of blood clotting,[56] the clotting time, prothrombin consumption, recalcification time, partial thromboplastin time, and thromboplastin generation are *normal* in a Factor VII deficiency. However, since Factor X is essential for prothrombinase formation via the intrinsic mechanism, all these tests are *abnormal* in Factor X deficiency. In addition Factor X, but not Factor VII, is essential for the rapid conversion of prothrombin to thrombin by Russel viper venom (Stypven), so that the Stypven time is prolonged only with X deficiency. By these characteristics, it is possible to distinguish Factor X deficiency from Factor VII deficiency. Although Factor V also affects the intrinsic clotting mechanism, and is essential for the conversion of prothrombin to thrombin by both tissue thromboplastin and Stypven, thus resembling Factor X, it is not adsorbed from plasma by barium sulfate or aluminum hydroxide as are Factors X and VII, also it is consumed during the clotting process in human blood and therefore is not present in human serum as are Factors VII and X. Thus, by determining the corrective effect of adsorbed plasma and serum on the prothrombin time and the Stypven time, it is possible to differentiate Factor V deficiency from that of Factor VII or X. The prolonged prothrombin and Stypven times of Factor X deficiency differentiate it from deficiencies of Factors XII, XI, IX and VIII. As in all coagulation deficiency states, conclusive identification of the deficient factor rests on demonstrating that the blood or plasma from the patient does not correct the coagulation defect on the blood from a subject with a known deficiency of Factor VII or X (Table 27).

FACTOR V DEFICIENCY (PARAHEMOPHILIA)

Since Owren first described this hereditary hemorrhagic disease[105] in 1947, about 30 families have been reported. The hemorrhagic manifestations vary from case to case, but in general the greater the deficiency state the more severe the bleeding tendency, although there are remarkable exceptions just as in the other deficiency states. Bleeding usually does not occur unless the Factor V level is below 20 per cent. The common manifestations are epistaxis, easy bruising, hematomas, menorrhagia, and excessive bleeding after surgical procedures or injury.[87,106,107] In some cases prolonged bleeding time has been reported whereas in others it is normal. Whether or not prolonged bleeding time in some cases is due to the Factor V deficiency or to an associated "vascular abnormality" similar to that seen in von Willebrand's syndrome is not clear. Shortening of the bleeding time has been reported with partial correction of the Factor V deficiency after transfusion of fresh plasma.[106] Capillary fragility is normal. The most characteristic laboratory finding is a prolonged prothrombin time which is corrected by adsorbed plasma, but not significantly by aged plasma or serum. If the deficiency is severe enough, the clotting time is prolonged, the prothrombin consumption is impaired and the partial thromboplastin time, the thromboplastin generation and the Stypven time are also abnormal. Probably the most sensitive screening test is the prothrombin time. Factor V deficiency can be differentiated from other deficiencies, as indicated in the preceding section. In addition, the prolonged prothrombin time of aged normal plasma, which is due to Factor V deficiency, is not corrected by plasma from a patient with this deficiency. Although in some cases the hereditary pattern appears to be that of the autosomal recessive type, since both parents show a partial deficiency,[87] in others no abnormality can be found in the parents.[106] It has been postulated that a deficiency of Factor V may be caused by each of several genes. Cases have been described in association with congenital cardiovascular disease, syndactylism, epidermolysis bullosa congenitalis[2,106] and Factor VIII deficiency.

FACTOR II (PROTHROMBIN) DEFICIENCY

Congenital deficiency of prothrombin is rare. Of 6 or 7 cases so far reported, only in the two most recently reported have deficiencies of all the other known coagulation factors been eliminated.[108,109] Hemorrhagic manifestations reported are mild to moderate and consist of epistaxis, easy bruising, menorrhagia, bleeding after surgery or trauma and hemarthrosis. Laboratory tests have varied considerably. Of interest is the finding that the prothrombin time is only slightly to moderately prolonged (1 to 10 seconds longer than control time), apparently being less abnormal than that encountered in severe Factor VII, V or X deficiency. The clotting time may be normal or prolonged, and the partial thromboplastin time and thromboplastin generation tests have been reported to be normal in some cases and abnormal in others. These variations do not seem to be related to the prothrombin level, and it is still questionable whether these cases actually represent only prothrombin deficiency. The diagnosis is made by specific measurement of the prothrombin, or by the finding that the prolonged prothrombin time is not corrected by adsorbed plasma or aged serum.

FACTOR I (FIBRINOGEN) DEFICIENCY

Congenital afibrinogenemia is an inherited disease of both sexes which is probably transmitted as a recessive trait on an autosomal chromosome. In the homozygous state only traces of fibrinogen (1 to 5 mg.%) are found in the plasma and studies indicate that this deficiency is not due to destruction or rapid turnover but rather to a failure of production of fibrinogen.[110] In the heterozygous state (parents of individuals with the severe deficiencies) the fibrinogen levels are usually normal although in some instances lower than normal levels have been reported.[111]

Although the blood of the affected individuals appears to be completely incoagulable, the hemorrhagic manifestations are much milder than those of severe hemophilia or Christmas disease. "Spontaneous" ecchymosis, epistaxis, hematemesis, hemoptysis, bleeding into the gastrointestinal tract or central nervous system have all been reported, but most common is excessive bleeding after trauma or surgery. Bleeding from the umbilical cord shortly after birth is quite frequent. Hemarthrosis is *not* characteristic. Normal menses have been reported in one patient.[112] The characteristic laboratory findings are infinite prolongation of the clotting time, prothrombin time, partial thromboplastin time, and thrombin time in the absence of any evidence of fibrinolysis. These abnormal tests are all corrected by the addition of fibrinogen or adsorbed plasma but not by serum. Heating the plasma to 53° to 56° C. does not cause any flocculation and the sedimentation rate is always very low. Platelet counts and plasma levels of all the other known coagulation factors are normal. The clotting mechanism, except for the final phase of the conversion of fibrinogen to fibrin, is normal, and if anything, the conversion of prothrombin to thrombin takes place at a more rapid rate than normal.[53] Capillary fragility and bleeding times are characteristically normal although a few cases have been reported to have had prolonged bleeding times.

ACQUIRED PLASMA COAGULATION DEFECTS

Acquired Hypofibrinogenemia or Afibrinogenemia. Acquired states of fibrin deficiency may result from (1) poor production of fibrinogen, (2) excessive consumption of fibrinogen by intravascular clotting, or (3) excessive destruction of fibrinogen by fibrinogenolysin or other proteolytic enzymes circulating in the blood system.

REDUCED PRODUCTION of fibrinogen occurs in severe parenchymatous liver disease (cirrhosis, acute yellow atrophy), in advanced metastatic involvement of the liver, in some cases of polycythemia vera or of secondary polycythemia, and in advanced tuberculosis of the lung.[4] The fibrinogenopenia which

occurs in these conditions is usually not severe enough (not down to plasma fibrinogen levels below 75 mg.%), to cause a break in the hemostatic mechanism. However, not infrequently it is associated with other coagulation deficiencies and the combined defects may result in a hemorrhagic diathesis. Thus in parenchymatous liver disease there may be significant reduction in the plasma levels of Factors II, V, VII, IX, X and XI and platelets, as well as an increase in fibrinolytic activity.[74] In polycythemia vera there may be similar but usually milder plasma coagulation defects, increased fibrinolytic activity, a qualitative platelet abnormality and perhaps some vascular abnormality.

INCREASED UTILIZATION of fibrinogen by intravascular coagulation or destruction of fibrinogen by activation of the *fibrinolytic mechanism* are far more frequent causes of marked hypofibrinogenemia and severe bleeding than failure of production of fibrinogen. Both intravascular coagulation and fibrinolysis produce other coagulation defects. During coagulation of blood, as pointed out above, Factor VIII and V activity as well as prothrombin decreases and platelets clump, lyse and are enmeshed in the fibrin clot. Thus intravascular clotting can produce marked depression of Factors VIII, V, prothrombin and platelets as well as of fibrinogen. The proteolytic enzyme plasmin (fibrinolysin), which hydrolyzes fibrinogen, also acts upon Factors VIII and V, destroying their coagulation activity. Thus, intravascular activation of the fibrinolytic mechanism may also produce a decrease in Factor VIII and V activity as well as fibrinogenopenia. In addition certain products of fibrinogenolysis or fibrinolysis interfere with the polymerization of fibrin monomers formed by the action of thrombin on fibrinogen and delay clot formation. Other products inhibit thromboplastin (prothrombinase) formation by the intrinsic pathway, thereby also delaying coagulation.[72,73] Even in the presence of adequate fibrinogen levels, these inhibitors can produce a coagulation defect resulting in prolonged prothrombin times, thrombin times and delayed thromboplastin generation.

It would appear that it should be relatively simple to differentiate fibrinogeno-penia caused by intravascular coagulation from that produced by fibrinolysis. However, in practice this is often not easy. In many patients both processes may be going on concurrently, either because they are both initiated by the underlying condition, or because, as some investigators believe, intravascular coagulation activates the fibrinolytic mechanism and intravascular fibrinolysis is always accompanied by some degree of intravascular coagulation. Since intravascular coagulation may cause shock, anoxia, or stress reaction, all of which are states known to activate the fibrinolytic system, it may be this mechanism which is responsible for the appearance of fibrinolysis in some patients with extensive intravascular coagulation.[113,114] Since there is a difference in therapy depending upon whether coagulation or fibrinolysis is playing the dominant role, every effort should be made to determine this point, particularly since therapy with antifibrinolytic agents such as epsilon aminocaproic acid may be harmful in the presence of intravascular coagulation.

There are no specific coagulation tests which can identify intravascular coagulation as the sole cause of rapidly acquired hypofibrinogenemia. Such a conclusion can only be reached by elimination of other causes, particularly fibrinolysis. If fibrinogen is still present in the blood, fibrinolysis is readily recognized by the complete dissolution of the whole blood clot which is formed in vitro either by spontaneous coagulation or after the addition of thrombin. Normally such a clot persists for at least 24 hours when incubated at 37° C. Lysis in less than 24 hours indicates the presence of excess fibrinolytic activity, and the shorter the lysis time the greater the fibrinolytic activity. Experience indicates that severe and spontaneous hemorrhage due to fibrinolysis occurs only when clot lysis occurs in less than an hour, and that when lysis times are longer than this, bleeding is moderate if present at all. Severe bleeding when lysis times range from 2 to 24 hours indicates that in all probability some other abnormality of the hemostatic mechanism is also present. In observing clots for lysis it must be borne in mind that the clots formed in the presence of fibrinogenopenia are inadequate, for as the clot retracts the red cells are extruded and the clot shrinks to a small nub which may fall to the bottom of the tube and be covered by the extruded red cells. This type of imperfect clotting may be erroneously taken for clot dissolution unless care is taken to examine the contents of the tube carefully. In polycythemia vera there may also be a marked degree of red cell "fall out" from the clot even when the plasma fibrinogen level is normal and there is no increased fibrinolytic activity. The very small clot which remains may be missed. *Only complete lysis of the whole blood clot incubated at 37° C can be interpreted with certainty as indicating increased fibrinolytic activity.* Visually, it is not possible to differentiate clot retraction from partial clot lysis. Other more complex technics are available to measure fibrinolytic activity, and they are particularly useful in identifying situations in which there is slight to moderate increase of fibrinolytic activity.[71,113,115] When fibrinogen has been completely destroyed by a severe fibrinolytic episode, clot lysis of the patient's blood cannot, of course, be used to determine the presence of fibrinolytic activity. Other technics must be used. The simplest and most rapid maneuver consists in mixing normal blood with freshly drawn patient's blood, clotting the mixture with thrombin and observing for clot lysis. Afibrinogenemia or hypofibrinogenemia caused by a fibrinolytic episode may still be present when the blood shows no evidence of fibrinolytic activity, because the plasmin (fibrinolysin) has been inactivated by the antiplasmin (antifibrinolysin) of the blood. Under these circumstances determination of the plasma plasminogen (profibrinolysin) and antiplasmin levels may be helpful since reduction of either or both would be indicative of a preceding fibrinolytic episode.

COMPLICATIONS OF PREGNANCY. There are a number of conditions in which acquired hypofibrinogenemia and hemorrhage due to intravascular coagulation or fibrinolysis or both may be encountered. Such states occur most frequently and dramatically in certain complications of pregnancy. *Premature separation of the placenta* occurs in about 0.5 to 1.0 per cent of pregnancies and in a few it is accompanied by serious and even fatal bleeding. In these cases the vaginal bleeding is associated with a generalized hemorrhagic tendency. The most characteristic finding is hypofibrinogenemia or afibrinogenemia but other coagulation factors are usually reduced also. These include prothrombin, Factor V, Factor VIII and platelets.[116] In the majority of cases reported no increased fibrinolytic activity has been found, but in many instances complete studies were not done. In some cases definite increased fibrinolytic activity has been demonstrated.[117] It is generally believed that the primary process is defibrination by coagulation. Some investigators hold that the fibrinogen is utilized by formation of clots at the placental site[118] whereas others believe that fibrinogen is consumed by coagulation within the mother's blood vessels produced by the introduction of thromboplastic materials from the placenta into the mother's circulation.[117,119,120] It is probable that fibrinolysis plays a secondary role in most cases and that activation of this mechanism results either from shock and anoxia induced by hemorrhage or intravascular coagulation. On the other hand, it is also conceivable that fibrinolysis may be the primary mechanism in some cases caused by introduction of activators of the fibrinolytic enzymes from the placenta. *Amniotic fluid and meconium embolism* may produce a severe hemorrhagic diathesis which is principally due to defibrination.[121] Other defects of blood clotting are usually demonstrable and include thrombocytopenia, decreased levels of plasma prothrombin, Factor V and Factor VIII. In addition, increased fibrinolytic activity and a heparinlike inhibitor (probably a product of fibrinolysis) have been described.[122] Amniotic fluid has been shown to have a thromboplastinlike activity and can cause defibrination in animals. In this syndrome the primary event probably is intravascular coagulation induced by introduction of amniotic fluid into the maternal circulation. This hypothesis is substantiated by the finding of multiple pulmonary thrombi along with constituents of amniotic fluid in fatal cases. Fibrinolysis seems to play a secondary role in the pathogenesis of the bleeding phenomena and may represent activation of the mechanism by shock and anoxia although activation by kinases of amniotic origin could also play a role. *Intrauterine fetal death* may also produce a hemorrhagic tendency characterized by ecchymosis, mucosal bleeding and bloody uterine discharge. The most consistent and characteristic change in the coagulation mechanism is fibrinogenopenia, but in addition thrombocytopenia, decreases in prothrombin and Factor V, increased fibrinolytic activity and circulating inhibitor activity have been reported.[122-124] The cause of the fibrinogenopenia is not known. In many cases of fetal death there is a slow gradual drop in fibrinogen without other coagulation changes, and the fall in fibrinogen does not proceed to levels which cause hemorrhage. In others there may be a sudden decrease in fibrinogen and hemorrhage ensues. It is usually in these cases that the other coagulation defects are noted. Whether or not the sudden fall in fibrinogen is caused by intravascular coagulation or fibrinolysis secondary to the introduction of fetal or placental materials into the maternal circulation is not known.

Self-induced abortion may be complicated by a generalized hemorrhagic diathesis. This complication usually occurs when caustic chemicals have been introduced into the uterus or sepsis occurs. Hypofibrinogen or afibrinogenemia is the most consistent defect noted, but thrombocytopenia, deficiencies of prothrombin, Factor V, and Factor VIII, and increased fibrinolytic activity have also been reported.[120,124] In some cases the primary mechanism appears to be an activation of the fibrinolytic system[120] whereas in others coagulation induced by entrance of fetal or placental materials into the maternal circulation appears to be the primary event. In the presence of infection the underlying mechanism may be similar to a generalized Shwartzman reaction.

TRANSFUSION REACTIONS, BURNS, SURGERY. Generalized hemorrhagic manifestations with hypofibrinogenemia and the other coagulation defects (decrease in prothrombin and in Factors V and VIII, thrombocytopenia, and increase in circulating anticoagulants) associated with intravascular coagulation or fibrinolysis may occur in hemolytic transfusion reactions,[4] with severe burns,[4] during thoracic surgery[125] in which there is manipulation of the lung, in pancreatic and prostatic surgery, and after open-heart surgery with use of a pump oxygenator bypass.[126] In these acute syndromes the fibrinolytic factor usually predominates but it is difficult to assess to what extent intravascular coagulation may play a role.

CHRONIC FIBRINOLYTIC STATES. Fibrinolysis of a chronic nature associated with mild to severe hemorrhagic manifestations may be seen in a variety of conditions. It is occasionally encountered in acute leukemia,[127] polycythemia vera, multiple myeloma,[128] sarcoidosis,[129] cirrhosis of the liver[2] and disseminated carcinoma, particularly of the prostate.[130] In these chronic states bleeding into the skin, hematuria, and melena are the common manifestations. Even minor surgical procedures may precipitate severe hemorrhage. Fibrinogen, plasminogen, and antiplasmin levels may be reduced, the degree of deficit depending upon the severity of the fibrinolytic process. In the more severe cases Factors V and VIII may be reduced and inhibitors of coagulation may be present. The occurrence of hemorrhagic manifestations in the absence of significant changes in coagulation tests or platelet levels should suggest the possibility of a fibrinolytic mechanism.

Acquired Deficiencies of Vitamin K–Dependent Coagulation Factors. Prothrombin, Factor VII, Factor IX, and Factor X all require vitamin K for their synthesis, so that a lack of this vitamin or interference with its action in the synthesis will result in a decrease of these factors in blood. The character and severity of the hemorrhagic manifestations and the alterations of coagulation tests which may occur depend upon the extent to which each of these factors is decreased. Dietary deficiency of vitamin K is unusual in the adult, since the daily requirement of the vitamin is only 1 milligram per day and it is abundant in many foods (green leafy vegetables, butter, cow's milk), and synthesis of vitamin K by the normal bacterial flora of the gastrointestinal tract is also an important source of the vitamin. Accordingly, deficiency results more frequently from pathologic conditions which interfere with absorption rather than from dietary insufficiency. Vitamin K in its naturally-occurring form is fat-soluble and its absorption is impaired in those conditions in which *fat absorption is decreased.* Thus, any pathologic process which curtails the flow of bile into the small bowel, such as common duct obstruction, biliary fistulae, cholangitis, or biliary atresia, may induce deficiency of vitamin K as well as of other fat-soluble vitamins. Other causes of impaired fat absorption will do the same, e.g. sprue, celiac disease, pancreatic fibrosis, gastrocolic fistulae and extensive resection of the small bowel. Diseases associated with *increased intestinal motility* may also result in reduced absorption of vitamin K, (ulcerative colitis, regional enteritis and polyposis of the bowel). *Antibiotics,* whether administered orally or parenterally, may decrease the available vitamin K for absorption by altering the bacterial flora of the intestinal tract and thus inducing vitamin K deficiency. This is most apt to occur with the use of broad-spectrum antibiotics, especially in infants and children.

Another cause for deficiency of the vitamin K-dependent clotting factors is *deficient utilization* of the vitamin. This occurs in severe parenchymatous liver disease and with the administration of coumarin drugs, phenylindandione, and salicylates. It is assumed that the effect of coumarin therapy upon the plasma levels of the affected coagulation factors is similar to that of vitamin K-deficiency. Factor VII appears to be the most sensitive and its plasma level falls after coumarin administration before there are significant changes in the levels of the other factors. However, there have been conflicting reports concerning the rate at which the concentration of each of these factors decreases and the extent to which each decreases with the same drug and with different coumarin drugs.[4,131,132] The discrepancies in these reports reflect both the individual variability of the subjects studied and differences in technics used to determine plasma levels of these factors. It is generally agreed that Factor VII falls more rapidly than any of the other factors and that prothrombin itself falls more slowly than the other factors and usually does not decrease to the same extent as Factors VII and X. There is considerable difference of opinion as to how rapidly, and to what extent Factors IX and X fall. In my own experience with the usual therapeutic doses of Dicumarol and Warfarin, Factor IX falls to levels of 20 to 40 per cent within 48 to 72 hours and usually remains at this level with continued therapy. Factor X falls at about the same time and usually reaches levels of 10 to 20 per cent. Factor VII reaches levels of 10 to 20 per cent in 24 to 48 hours, whereas prothrombin usually does not fall below levels of 30 per cent, which is reached on the fourth to fifth day. With prolonged coumarin therapy, although the prothrombin time may not change significantly, the levels of the different coagulation factors may vary considerably and this may account for unexpected bleeding. With excessive doses of anticoagulant and in severe vitamin K-deficiencies all factors may fall to very low levels (0 to 10%).

Hematuria, melena, epistaxis, and easy bruising are the early hemorrhagic manifestations of the hemostatic defect caused by vitamin K-deficiency or coumarin administration. These manifestations may occur when the prothrombin time is 2 to 3 times as long as normal, a prolongation which is considered to be in the therapeutic range for anticoagulant therapy. With more profound alteration in coagulation there may be spontaneous ecchymosis, hematomas, severe gastrointestinal bleeding, bleeding into the central nervous system, hemarthrosis, prolonged bleeding after trauma or menorrhagia. The most characteristic laboratory finding is *prolongation of the prothrombin time*. Since Factor VII is the first coagulation factor to fall, the prothrombin time is prolonged before alteration of any tests which depend upon the intrinsic clotting mechanism. With depression of prothrombin, Factors IX and X, the partial thromboplastin time and thromboplastin generation test become ab-

normal. Whole blood clotting times and recalcification times also become prolonged when these deficiencies are great enough, but these tests are less sensitive than the partial thromboplastin time and thromboplastin generation. The bleeding time is usually normal. However, when there is marked depression of the clotting factors, it becomes prolonged. Whether the prolonged bleeding time is due to the coagulation defect or to an effect upon the vasculature or platelets is not known. Recently it has been demonstrated that platelet adhesiveness is decreased in Dicumarol therapy,[133] and loss of adhesiveness may delay the formation of the platelet plug.

Hemorrhagic disease of the newborn also represents a deficiency of the vitamin K-dependent coagulation factors. The normal newborn infant, although exhibiting no hemorrhagic diathesis, does have coagulation deficiencies when compared to the adult. At birth prothrombin and Factors VII, IX and X are found to be about 30 to 60 per cent of the normal adult levels.[4,134] Factors XI[135] and XII[2] have also been reported to be reduced, whereas Factor V[136] is elevated. During the first two to three days of life there is normally a further fall in prothrombin and in Factors VII, IX and X and the plasma levels may fall to 10 to 20 per cent of normal. The levels then rise to their original values in about one week, and without supplementary vitamin K it may take 6 to 10 weeks before they reach normal adult levels. There is still some question whether or not vitamin K can accelerate this secondary rise, although there is evidence that the administration of the vitamin will accelerate the recovery from the low values reached on the second or third day. In premature infants even lower plasma levels of these factors are encountered, and vitamin K administration does not accelerate their rise towards normal. The failure of the premature infant to respond to vitamin K and the initial drop in coagulation factors in both the premature and the full term infant are probably due to incomplete development of the enzyme systems necessary for the synthesis of these proteins as well as due to low vitamin K levels in the liver. The higher plasma levels initially seen probably represent passage of these factors from the mother's plasma through the placenta to the infant's circulation. Hemorrhagic disease of the newborn represents an exaggeration of these abnormalities of the clotting mechanism ordinarily found in the newborn. Why these severe defects occur in some newborns is not clear. Certainly they occur when the mother is normal and it is still not certain that administration of vitamin K to the mother prior to delivery will prevent their occurrence.

Symptoms usually appear suddenly upon the second or third day after delivery, at the time when the newborn usually exhibits the greatest alteration in coagulation. However, they may occur at the time of birth. Bleeding is usually not massive but is characterized by persistent oozing from the stump of the umbilical cord, and from mucosal surfaces. Hemoptysis, hematemesis, melena, hematuria, vaginal bleeding and ecchymosis are common. Fatal hemorrhage into the central nervous system, the adrenals, the kidneys, and the liver may occur. The coagulation findings are those described in vitamin K-deficiency or coumarin administration. Unless associated with severe liver disease, the hemorrhagic manifestations and the coagulation defects respond within a matter of hours to vitamin K.

It should be pointed out that administration of *water-soluble vitamin K analogues* (menadione bisulfate, Synkayvite, Hykinone) may cause a *hemolytic anemia* in the infant with resulting kernicterus when given either to the mother shortly before delivery or to the infant. They should therefore be avoided in treating infants. The sensitivity of the infant's red cells to these drugs is due to the low content of glucose-6-phosphate dehydrogenase of these cells. The naturally occurring fat-soluble vitamin K_1 or K_1 oxide does not seem to have this hemolytic effect and probably the newer aqueous colloidal solutions of K_1 (Aqua Mephyton) do not. Therefore, these are the drugs of choice in infants, but overdosage should be avoided. In vitamin K-deficiency in the adult, whether due to malabsorption or dietary

deficiency, the water-soluble vitamin K preparations are effective, but they appear to have little or no effect in counteracting the action of Dicumarol and related drugs. Vitamin K_1 and vitamin K_1 oxide intravenously or orally and Aqua Mephyton intravenously or intramuscularly will have a corrective effect within 2 to 3 hours and usually will raise the vitamin K-dependent clotting factors to safe levels within 4 to 12 hours. When very large doses of these preparations are used the patient may become resistant for a considerable period to the action of the coumarinlike drugs.

Deficiencies Associated With Liver Disease. Obstruction of the common duct, or cholangitis which is not associated with extensive parenchymatous liver disease but causes biliary stasis, results in poor absorption of vitamin K and of deficiency of the vitamin K-dependent clotting factors only. Such deficiencies respond to vitamin K administration. Extensive hepatocellular disease may also result in a marked deficiency of these clotting factors because there is inability to utilize vitamin K. However, other clotting factors may also be depressed, depending upon the severity of liver impairment. Factor V[74] and Factor XI[76] are frequently decreased and less frequently fibrinogen may be decreased. A progressive fall in Factor V is an ominous prognostic sign and a rise in Factor V frequently heralds the recovery phase of severe hepatitis. Occasionally, increased fibrinolytic activity is evident, but this usually is rather mild and not persistent. Not infrequently in viral hepatitis and more frequently in cirrhosis of the liver there may be an associated thrombocytopenia. Although the cause of this thrombocytopenia is not known, it apparently is not due directly to any alteration of liver function, but is related in cirrhosis to the associated congestive splenomegaly and in viral hepatitis to some extrahepatic effect of or reaction to the virus. A qualitative change in the platelets (a decrease in platelet factor 3 activity) has been reported in cirrhosis but this has not been confirmed. In addition to the depression of coagulation factors, a circulating anticoagulant or inhibitor may be present which interferes with the thrombin-fibrinogen reaction and may also interfere with thromboplastin generation.[137] In parenchymal liver disease, in contrast to biliary obstruction, there is little or no improvement of the coagulation defects after the administration of vitamin K.

Circulating Anticoagulants. Circulating anticoagulants may be defined as "abnormal endogenous components of blood which inhibit the coagulation of normal blood."[138] In general they may be divided into two groups, one group in which the inhibitor is directed against a specific coagulation factor and appears to destroy the activity of this factor; and a second group in which the inhibitor blocks or interferes with one of the reactions of coagulation but is not directed against a specific coagulation factor. Anticoagulants have been described against every clotting factor and against several of the recognized intermediary steps of coagulation. In addition, there are numerous case reports in which a circulating anticoagulant has been demonstrated, but its mode of action not identified. The reader is referred to an extensive and excellent review of the whole subject for more detailed information.[138] The hemorrhagic manifestations which are seen depend upon the level of the circulating anticoagulant and to some extent the nature of the anticoagulant. Inhibitors which are directed against a single specific clotting factor produce the type of bleeding seen in hereditary deficiencies of these factors.

ANTICOAGULANTS DIRECTED AGAINST A SPECIFIC CLOTTING FACTOR. Perhaps the most frequently encountered acquired anticoagulant is that directed against the antihemophilic factor. This type has been observed in four groups of patients: (1) patients with classical hemophilia; (2) women who develop a bleeding disorder resembling hemophilia within a year postpartum; (3) middle aged or elderly men and women with no history of hemophilia or any other hemorrhagic diathesis and in whom no other disease process can be found; and (4) middle aged or elderly men and women with no previous history of a hemorrhagic tendency but who have some other pathologic process. In this last group the anti-

coagulant has appeared after penicillin reactions, in the course of lupus erythematosus, rheumatoid arthritis, tuberculous adenopathy, and various dysproteinemias. The anticoagulants in these various groups of patients cannot be distinguished by their action or physiochemical characteristics.

The incidence of circulating anticoagulant in classical hemophilia has varied widely in various reports, ranging from 0 to 21 per cent. Of 84 cases of hemophilia reported from Johns Hopkins 18 (21%) were found to have an anticoagulant on one or more occasions,[138] and Lewis and her associates reported an incidence of 5 cases out of a total of 52.[139] In my own series of 35 cases, 5 developed or had an anticoagulant during observation. Although the occurrence of this type of anticoagulant is almost entirely in the severe hemophilic, it has been reported in mild hemophilics also. The mechanism of development of an anticoagulant is not known, but since it is seen almost always in patients who have had repeated transfusions, it is considered by many to be a result of such therapy. In favor of this concept is the observation that in a number of cases the titer of anticoagulant activity rises after transfusion and gradually decreases when transfusions are withheld. These findings have suggested that the anticoagulant actually is an antibody against the antihemophilic factor, which could be considered a foreign protein to the hemophilic. This concept is also supported by reports of positive ring precipitin reactions between the patient's plasma or serum and normal plasma. However, more recent studies do not support this concept. The kinetics of the anticoagulant-antihemophilic reactions have been found not to be characteristic of an antibody-antigen reaction but are more characteristic of an enzyme reaction.[140,141] In most cases precipitin reactions are not present. The anticoagulant has been reported in at least one hemophilic who did not receive transfusions,[142] and the anticoagulant which appears in non-hemophilics has the same physiochemical and kinetic characteristics as that of hemophilics.[140,141]

The severity of the hemorrhagic manifestations usually does not increase or change in character with development of an inhibitor in the hemophilic. However, transfusion becomes ineffective, since it no longer corrects the clotting defect. In vitro it can also be demonstrated that the amounts of normal plasma which are usually sufficient to correct the clotting defect in classical hemophilia have little or no corrective effect upon clotting and recalcification times, prothrombin consumption, partial thromboplastin times and thromboplastin generation tests. When the inhibitor activity is sufficiently high, the patient's blood will inhibit the clotting of normal blood. Incubation of the patient's plasma with normal plasma destroys the Factor VIII activity of the latter. All coagulation factors other than Factor VIII are present in the patient's plasma at normal levels. Prothrombin times and thrombin times remain normal. If the anticoagulant is present in high titer when severe hemorrhage occurs, the usual transfusion therapy is ineffective and in order to get even transient restoration of hemostasis it may be necessary to use exchange transfusions or very large amounts of Factor VIII-rich plasma fractions. Corticosteroids and ACTH are of questionable value even in large doses. The titer of inhibitor may gradually drop over the course of months or years and the patient again becomes responsive to transfusion therapy but in many instances the titer rises following such therapy.

Although the Factor VIII inhibitor which appears in nonhemophilics has the same physiochemical characteristics there is considerable variation in the clinical course. If women who develop such an inhibitor following pregnancy survive the initial hemorrhagic episode, the inhibitor gradually disappears. It does not seem to be increased by transfusion therapy and in at least one instance it did not recur following a subsequent pregnancy.[138] The anticoagulant which makes its appearance following a penicillin reaction also may not be increased in titer by transfusion therapy and usually disappears within the relatively short time of three to six months. In some

previously normal individuals and in patients with a chronic disease process, the level of the inhibitor may remain elevated with little variation for months and years, whereas in other persons there may be significant improvement, with disappearance of the inhibitor.

The incidence of the development of an inhibitor in patients with Factor IX deficiency is probably about the same as that in classical hemophilia, however in these individuals the anticoagulant is directed against Factor IX. All the other coagulation factors are normal. The inhibitor again appears to be related to transfusion therapy since the titer rises after transfusion and gradually decreases when transfusions are withheld.[138,143] It is of interest that it is rare to find this type of inhibitor appearing in patients without pre-existing Factor IX deficiency, which is in contrast to the inhibitor of Factor VIII.

Anticoagulants directed against Factors V, VII, XI and fibrinogen have been reported but these are extremely rare and in most instances have occurred in patients with a pre-existing deficiency of the factor against which the anticoagulant is directed. The hemorrhagic manifestations are those seen in the corresponding deficiency state.

ANTICOAGULANTS DIRECTED AGAINST A REACTION IN COAGULATION. Of the inhibitors which appear to be directed at a reaction in coagulation rather than against a specific factor, an *inhibitor of thromboplastin or prothrombinase* is the most common. This occurs most frequently in disseminated lupus erythematosus but is also seen in other collagen diseases and occasionally in patients with abnormal plasma proteins (macroglobulin, cryoglobulin, and hypergammaglobulinemia). The hemorrhagic manifestations are usually mild, but ecchymosis, hematuria, bleeding from mucous membranes and menorrhagia have been reported. The most characteristic laboratory finding is a prolonged prothrombin time, particularly with diluted thromboplastin, in the presence of normal levels of all known clotting factors. In most cases the clotting time is only slightly to moderately prolonged, but the recalcification time of platelet-poor plasma is markedly prolonged.[138,144,145] The exact nature or mechanism of action of this type of anticoagulant is not known. It should also be added that some patients with systemic lupus have in addition a significant decrease of prothrombin without other evidence of liver disease.

An anticoagulant which *inhibits the action of thrombin on fibrinogen* has been reported in liver disease and in patients with either hypergammaglobulinemia or abnormal plasma proteins as seen in multiple myeloma. The characteristic finding is a prolonged thrombin time which can be shortened by the addition of calcium or protamine in concentration greater than that needed to neutralize heparin.[138,146,147] This inhibitory activity has been referred to as antithrombin V. The mechanism of action is not known. As discussed above the products of fibrinolysis also produce prolonged thrombin times and although this is frequently referred to as an antithrombin VI, the inhibition is against the polymerization of fibrin rather than the action of thrombin.

Although a number of reports have appeared describing *heparinlike* anticoagulants, it is doubtful that any of these cases, with the exception of one, represent true hyperheparinemia.[138,148] Since heparin is known to interfere with all three phases of coagulation, the characteristic findings should include prolonged clotting times, prothrombin times, and thrombin times. The clotting abnormality should be corrected both in vivo and in vitro by protamine, toluidine blue, or polybrene. However, in interpreting the results, it must be borne in mind that protamine in concentrations higher than that necessary to neutralize heparin will shorten the thrombin time of normal blood or of blood with nonheparin inhibitors of the thrombin-fibrinogen reaction as well as that of heparinized blood.

THROMBOCYTOPENIA

Thrombocytopenia is probably the most common cause of pathologic bleeding encountered by the physician. The characteristic hemorrhagic manifestations are a reflection of the unique role of platelets in hemostasis, particularly in relation to the small blood vessels. The platelets, by a mechanism that is not understood, contribute to the maintenance of the integrity and strength of these vessels. Platelets are also involved in the first response to injury of a vessel, that is platelet massing at the site of injury followed by formation of the platelet plug, which by itself is sufficient to control bleeding from small arterioles and capillaries. It is therefore not surprising that the most characteristic hemorrhagic lesions in thrombocytopenia are the petechiae, which are due to rupture of or bleeding from the smallest arterioles or the arterial end of the capillary loop. Although the platelets also play a very important role in coagulation, large ecchymoses, hematomas and hemarthroses, so common in coagulation deficiencies, are usually not present except in the most severe cases. Two classical findings in thrombocytopenia, increased capillary fragility and prolonged bleeding time, are manifestations of the loss of platelet function in small blood vessels, and are usually not present in coagulation deficiency states.

In general, no matter what the etiology of the thrombocytopenia, the hemorrhagic manifestations are the same. Petechiae may be widely distributed but are most apt to occur in dependent areas, in areas overlying bony structures and in the mucous membranes of the mouth. These lesions are usually not palpable nor do they have an associated erythema as is noted in anaphylactoid purpura. Bleeding from mucous membranes is very frequent (epistaxis, gingival bleeding, bleeding into the gastrointestinal tract, and hematuria), although massive hemorrhage rarely occurs. In women there is usually a history of prolonged and profuse menses. Ecchymoses may occur without obvious trauma and prolonged and excessive bleeding from abrasions or minor lacerations is generally noted. In the severe cases hemorrhagic blisters frequently appear on the mucous membranes of the lips, the mouth, the tongue, the nose and the pharynx. Intracranial bleeding is not common (particularly in children) and is most apt to occur in patients with associated aplastic anemia and acute leukemia. The typical laboratory findings are a prolonged bleeding time, increased capillary fragility, normal clotting time, poor prothrombin consumption and poor clot retraction. However, since all the plasma clotting factors are usually normal, there is normal partial thromboplastin time, prothrombin time and thrombin time. The diagnosis of thrombocytopenic purpura rests upon demonstrating a decreased number of platelets in the peripheral blood. Bleeding and derangement in coagulation rarely occurs until the platelets fall below 75,000 per cubic mm. Below this level there is no strict correlation between the severity of the clinical picture and the platelet level, although in general the lower the platelet count, the more severe the bleeding tendency. This suggests that other factors beside the number of platelets must play a role in the pathogenesis of purpuric bleeding. In some types of thrombocytopenia there may well be vascular damage due to antibody-antigen reaction or by abnormal proteins. There is also evidence that there may be qualitative differences in platelets in thrombocytopenia which could account, at least in part, for the clinical variability.[149]

Thrombocytopenia can occur in a large variety of conditions, many of which appear to have little in common except a decrease in the number of circulating platelets. Since the prognosis and therapy are often dependent upon the pathogenesis of the thrombocytopenia or at least upon the associated pathologic process, it is of importance for the physician to investigate the pathogenesis thoroughly. Any meaningful classification of the conditions which may be associated with or produce thrombocytopenia is limited by our inadequate knowledge of the mechanisms involved. However, a logical approach can be made by starting with the simple concept that the numerical level of circulating platelets will depend upon the rate of production of platelets versus the rate of destruction of platelets. Since the megakaryocytes of the bone marrow are the primary site for the production of circulating platelets, the initial consideration is the status of the megakaryocytes in the bone marrow. This can be determined from bone marrow aspiration or biopsy. Thrombocytopenic states can thus be classified into two major groups: (1) amegakaryocytic, and (2) megakaryocytic. In addition, the marrow may show abnormalities which point to a definitive diagnosis which may or may not have been suspected, such as leukemia, metastatic carcinoma, myeloma, Gaucher's disease, folic acid or vitamin B_{12} deficiency, etc.

Amegakaryocytic Thrombocytopenia. In amegakaryocytic thrombocytopenia decreased production of platelets is the obvious cause of the thrombocytopenia, although increased destruction of platelets may play a minor role. The hypoplasia of the megakaryocytes may be congenital or acquired, the latter being much more frequent.

The *congenital variety* may show a marked reduction of megakaryocytes without disturbance of other bone marrow elements. This type is sometimes associated with absence of the radii.[150] More frequently there is also hypoplasia of the myeloid and erythroid elements and sometimes this type is also associated with other congenital abnormalities (Fanconi Syndrome).[151] It is of particular importance to differentiate the amegakaryocytic from the megakarocytic type in infants since the prognosis and treatment are significantly different.

The *acquired form* is most frequently due to replacement of the marrow tissue with abnormal cells (leukemia, myeloma, etc.) with crowding out of the normal elements or to a generalized hypoplasia of the bone marrow secondary to chemicals, medications, or irradiation. The agents which have been reported to induce such changes are listed in Table 26. The sensitivity of individuals to these agents varies considerably. In some persons the same chemicals and drugs may produce thrombocytopenia by a different mechanism, that is, by peripheral destruction of the platelets, without hypoplasia. This will be discussed later. Idiopathic aplastic anemia with hypoplasia of the marrow is almost always associated with thrombocytopenia. Not infrequently in aplastic anemia it is the hemorrhagic complications which cause death.

Megakaryocytic Thrombocytopenia. The megakaryocytic type of thrombocytopenia may result from a variety of pathogenic mechanisms but they all cause the thrombocytopenia either by decreasing production of platelets or by increasing their peripheral destruction or both. A classification of megakaryocytic thrombocytopenia on this basis certainly has more logic and is more useful than the older classification of idiopathic and secondary or symptomatic thrombocytopenia. Recently Cohen et al.[23] have proposed such a classification based on the life span of platelets determined by the Cr^{51} labeling technique. From their studies they divided cases of thrombocytopenia into three broad groups: (1) those that had a normal platelet survival and reduced production; (2) those with predominantly decreased production but with some decrease in life span; and (3) those in which shortened survival predominated but decreased production might be present. Since the division between the first and second groups and the second and third groups may be somewhat arbitrary, it is perhaps more useful clinically to divide the thrombocytopenias into two groups depending on whether the major factor is shortened survival or decreased production.

FACTORS REGULATING NUMBER OF CIRCULATING PLATELETS

Little is actually known concerning the normal regulatory mechanism of the level of circulating platelets. However, evidence has accumulated in the past decade to indicate that a number of factors are involved.

Plasma Factor. Shulman et al.[19] have recently described a plasma factor which promotes megakaryocytic maturation and platelet production in an orderly and sequential manner. Lack of this factor can be responsible for thrombocytopenia in the presence of megakaryocytes in the bone marrow. This factor is apparently distinct from erythropoietin and has been referred to as thrombopoietin. A lack of this factor has so far been described in only one case and studies indicate that it is present in

normal or excessive levels in the plasma of patients with so-called idiopathic thrombocytopenia and in patients with thrombocytosis.

Folic acid deficiency and vitamin B_{12} deficiencies are frequently associated with thrombocytopenia. Megakaryocytes are either somewhat decreased or normal in number in the marrow. Cohen and Gardner[23] have found normal survival of platelets in such patients, indicating that folic acid and B_{12} are essential for normal production. Treatment with folic acid or B_{12} will result in restoration of platelet levels to normal. Vitamin C has also been implicated in platelet production, particularly in relation to folic acid metabolism.[152]

Hormones seem to have an effect upon platelet levels which is probably related to platelet production rather than destruction. In normal women there is usually a slight to moderate fall in circulating platelets during the last two weeks of the menstrual cycle and a rapid return to normal after the onset of menses.[153] Whether or not this is related to changes in the levels of estrogens, progesterone or FSH is not known. A few cases of cyclic thrombocytopenia occurring in women at the time of the menses have been reported.[154,155] Corticosteroids and ACTH may also produce an increase in platelets when administered to patients without thrombocytopenia. What role they play in the normal regulatory mechanism is not known.

The role of the spleen still remains an enigma. An old observation that has been confirmed countless times is that following splenectomy for reasons other than thrombocytopenia, the platelet count rises above normal levels and remains elevated for weeks to months or even for years. This may also occur after splenectomy for "idiopathic" thrombocytopenia, and it is not unusual to find the platelets rising to levels three to five times normal within a week to ten days after splenectomy, and the patient, who but a few days before was having serious hemorrhagic manifestations, now suffers from thromboembolic phenomena. Although any surgical procedure may be followed by a moderate increase in circulating platelets, persistence of thrombocytosis for more than a few days occurs only after splenectomy. The effect of splenectomy can be interpreted as evidence either that the spleen has an inhibitory effect upon platelet production or that the spleen removes platelets from the peripheral blood by a process similar to its action in regard to red cells. Thrombocytopenia might therefore result from an increase in splenic activity regardless of which of these interpretations is correct. Recent studies have indicated that under certain circumstances the spleen at least when enlarged does have an inhibitory effect upon platelet production. In rats fed methyl cellulose splenomegaly is induced and thrombocytopenia occurs. It has been shown that under these circumstances there is no change in the life span of the platelets, indicating a reduced production as the cause of the thrombocytopenia. In such animals, splenectomy results in a thrombocytosis even greater than that seen in splenectomized normal animals.[156] Cohen and Gardner[23] have found that in thrombocytopenia associated with congestive splenomegaly caused by portal hypertension the platelet survival time is only slightly reduced, whereas production is significantly reduced. Thus the thrombocytopenia would appear to be due in large part to a decrease in platelet production, possibly caused by a humoral factor produced in the chronically congested spleen. Relief of portal hypertension by portacaval shunt without splenectomy is almost always followed by a rise in the platelet count.[157] The role of the spleen in platelet survival in normal persons is far from clear. Controversy still exists as to whether most platelets are removed from the blood stream by the spleen as they become senescent, as suggested by some platelet survival data,[20,22,25] or are utilized in a random manner in hemostasis as is suggested by the curvilinear survival curves reported by others.[21,23,24] That thrombocytopenia may result from increased utilization of platelets in intravascular coagulation has been demonstrated in animals and also is evident in certain clinical syndromes. It has also been shown that excessive platelet loss, as produced by plateletphoresis in animals[158] or by severe hemorrhage in man treated with a large volume of bank blood containing nonviable platelets,[159] will result in thrombocytopenia when the capacity of the bone marrow to produce platelets is exceeded, and that such thrombocytopenia may persist for three to four days after platelet loss stops and then the platelet count begins to rise. It is therefore evident that continued sequestration or destruction of platelets, by whatever means, can induce a severe thrombocytopenia and can also result in secondary decrease in platelet production due to bone marrow exhaustion. The thrombocytopenia which occurs in patients with giant hemangiomas is thought to be due to sequestration and destruction of the platelets within the abnormal vessels. In such cases splenectomy, corticosteroids and ACTH are ineffective and only a decrease in size of the hemangioma by surgery, radiation or spontaneous regression results in a rise in the number of circulating platelets.[160] In many seemingly unrelated thrombocytopenias it has been suggested that increased sequestration or destruction of platelets occurs in the spleen[161] with splenomegaly such as is seen in Gaucher's disease, sarcoid, lymphoproliferative syndromes, tuberculosis, etc. It has been postulated that hyperplasia or abnormality of the reticuloendothelial system causes an increase in this activity of the spleen, and that in "idiopathic" thrombocytopenia it occurs for some unknown reason. More recent developments would indicate that when increased destruction of platelets takes place in any of these conditions there may be more than one mechanism, and that a similar mechanism may be operative in different pathologic processes. In the past few years evidence has accumulated to indicate that thrombocytopenia may be of immunological origin in many of these cases and that the spleen may play a role both in production of platelet antibodies and in clearing the blood of platelets which have been coated with an antibody.

Immunologic origin of thrombocytopenia has been definitely proved in certain types of thrombocytopenia and there is suggestive and controversial evidence in others. In drug-induced megakaryocytic thrombocytopenia (Sedormid, quinine, quinidine, etc.) it has been demonstrated that an antibody exists in the plasma which in the presence of the offending drug and platelets will fix complement and lyse platelets, and when complement is not present will agglutinate platelets in vitro. It is thought that the drug acts as a hapten and enters into a chemical union with some portion of the platelet to form an antigen to which the body reacts with the formation of an antibody. The antibody will react only against platelets when the specific drug is present although the platelets may be from normal individuals or from the patient. When the offending drug is given to a sensitized person with circulating antibody there is a marked fall in circulating platelets within an hour, indicating a peripheral destruction of platelets.[162,163] Recovery usually follows in these cases within one week following removal of the responsible agent.

It has long been known that blood platelets are isoantigenic. Serum antibodies which react with platelets have been demonstrated in patients who have received mutiple blood transfusions and in multiparous women.[164,165,167] Plasma or blood from these individuals can produce acute thrombocytopenia in appropriate recipients. The demonstration of isoantibodies by the usual immunologic technics (agglutination, antihuman globulin consumption, indirect Coombs, and complement fixation) in patients receiving multiple transfusions is rather low (3% to 14%), probably because these technics are relatively insensitive. Recent studies on platelet survival by the Cr[51] labeling technic after repeated transfusions of platelets into normal recipients indicate a much higher incidence of platelet antibody formation, as demonstrated by decreased survival times.[167,23] Such shortened survival times are found in the absence of positive results with the usual immunologic tests. How many platelet groups actually exist still remains controversial. At least two major antigen systems have been identified and probably more exist.[168] It has been definitely established that neonatal thrombocytopenic purpura, which occurs in otherwise normal children of healthy mothers, can be caused by maternal antibodies formed against fetal platelets.

Shulman[166] et al. have also presented evidence that an isoantibody provoked by mismatched platelet transfusion may destroy platelets in the sensitized individual. The mechanism suggested is that foreign platelet antigen survives in vivo longer than the period of antibody induction and that antibody, complexed with foreign antigen, is adsorbed by autologous platelets making them more susceptible to processes of in vivo sequestration. It is also possible than antigen-antibody complexes in which the antigen is not related to platelets may induce thrombocytopenia since it has been demonstrated that adsorption of such complexes by platelets is a common immunologic phenomenon.[169] At present there is no definite evidence to indicate that this mechanism is involved in thrombocytopenic purpura.

In many thrombocytopenic states an immunologic process is suspected as the underlying mechanism. Supportive evidence for such a mechanism in "idiopathic" thrombocytopenia has been the demonstration that plasma from a fairly high percentage of such cases (40% to 70%) when transfused into a normal individual will induce thrombocytopenia in the recipient within the course of an hour or two.[164] Such reactions may also occur from plasma of patients with thrombocytopenia in the course of systemic lupus erythematosus and lymphatic leukemia. The spleen is not essential for the production of thrombocytopenia under these circumstances, but the evidence indicates that it is one of the areas of sequestration and destruction of the platelets in the recipient. The data that have been reported on the presence of platelet antibodies in the serum or plasma of patients with thrombocytopenia other than that due to drug sensitivity or in patients who have had multiple transfusions have been confusing and contradictory. Harrington[170] and Tullis[171] using different technics have reported positive tests for circulating antiplatelet antibodies in 50 to 60 per cent of patients with idiopathic thrombocytopenic purpura (ITP). However, as pointed out by Cohen et al.,[23] these two technics frequently give conflicting results in a given patient and are often negative in cases of idiopathic thrombocytopenia in which platelet life span is markedly reduced. Others[172] have not been able to demonstrate platelet antibodies in ITP by immunologic technics. Data have also been reported which indicate that platelet agglutination tests may give false positive results because of the presence of nonspecific abnormal proteins[170] or because of the coagulation factors remaining in a serum which can lead to the formation of thrombin, a very potent agglutinator of platelets.[173] Despite these rather disappointing results of immunologic technics to demonstrate conclusively platelet antibodies, the concept of an immunologic mechanism as the cause of thrombocytopenia in megakaryocytic thrombocytopenia with increased platelet destruction has continued to gain popularity.

IDIOPATHIC THROMBOCYTOPENIA

At the present time this term refers to a thrombocytopenia which cannot be attributed to or associated with some other disease process. Characteristically, the marrow contains adequate or increased numbers of megakaryocytes, the spleen is not palpable, and the patient's symptoms are limited to manifestations of the bleeding tendency. Idiopathic thrombocytopenic purpura as defined above undoubtedly encompasses more than one disease entity or etiology. Although the platelet survival time is very short in most such cases, some cases have been shown to have normal platelet survival time,[23,164] indicating different mechanisms (decreased production) for the thrombocytopenia in patients who appear similar clinically. The thrombocytopenia-producing agent is not present in the plasma of all cases. Thrombocytopenia indistinguishable clinically from the idiopathic type may be the first manifestation of systemic lupus erythematosus.[174] The thrombocytopenia which occurs following measles, rubella, mumps, chickenpox, or infectious mononucleosis is very similar to the so-called acute form of idiopathic thrombocytopenia in the abruptness of onset, sex distribution, and the limited duration of a few weeks or months. Since many cases of "acute idiopathic" thrombocytopenia do occur after upper respiratory infections, particularly in children, it is questionable whether or not there is any significant difference between such cases and those that occur after known viral infections. In all those instances the thrombocytopenia may be secondary to sensitization of the platelets to sequestration by the absorption of antigen-antibody complexes to the platelet surface.

Clinically two types of idiopathic thrombocytopenic purpura are recognized, the acute and chronic forms. The *acute* form is characterized by an abrupt onset without previous history of a bleeding tendency, equal sex distribution, greater frequency in children and young adults, spontaneous recovery in a few weeks to six months. When thrombocytopenia persists for longer than six months, the case is usually classified as chronic. However, the usual *chronic* type is characterized by a more gradual onset of hemorrhagic manifestations so that the patient may have a history of easy bruising, excessive bleeding after dental extraction, or menorrhagia dating back for several months or years before the appearance of purpura. This form is characterized by remission and exacerbation. The remissions are rarely complete, the platelet counts returning to 50 to 60 per cent of normal, which is usually sufficient to correct the hemostatic defect, and the relapses vary in severity. In contrast to the acute form, the chronic form occurs more commonly in females (3:2 to 3:1) and in adults. The distinction between acute and chronic is not always evident at the time a patient is first seen, since a chronic case may start out acutely and a relapse in a chronic case may give as severe hemorrhagic manifestations as those seen in the acute form. The response of both the acute and the chronic forms to various types of therapy is not predictable from the clinical course. Although the acute form usually goes into complete remission spontaneously, a remission may be induced much sooner with corticosteroids or splenectomy. However, both of these forms of therapy may fail. In the chronic form response to corticosteroid therapy and splenectomy is also variable, and in a certain percentage of cases (this varies in the different series reported from 10 to 30%), relapse occurs after an initial response to splenectomy or corticosteroids. Patients who fail to respond to steroids may respond to splenectomy and the reverse may also occur. The variability of the clinical course, and the varied response to therapy in ITP are further indications that this is not a single disease entity, and that there is more than one pathogenic mechanism. Although ITP is frequently referred to as auto-immuned thrombocytopenia, it should be pointed out that at the present time there is no substantiating evidence for this concept, since the evidence for platelet antibodies in any of these cases, as discussed above, is still controversial. The occurrence of thrombocytopenia in other diseases considered as autoimmuned, such as systemic lupus erythematosus and auto-immuned hemolytic anemia, does lend weight to this concept as one cause of ITP.

It should be pointed out that neonatal thrombocytopenia occurs in about half the newborn infants of mothers who have idiopathic thrombocytopenic purpura or who have had a remission subsequent to splenectomy; whereas it does not occur if the mother has had a spontaneous remission.[164,175] Hemorrhagic phenomena are most pronounced in the first few days of life and then decrease as the platelet count usually starts rising, however it may not reach normal levels for two to three months.

Thrombotic Thrombocytopenic Purpura

This syndrome, first described by Moschcowitz,[176] is characterized by the triad of thrombocytopenia, hemolytic anemia, and transient bizarre neurologic signs and symptoms. The majority of cases have an abrupt onset and a rapid downhill course, death occurring within one to six weeks. Only recently have a few chronic cases been reported. The purpuric manifestations are the same as those of any severe thrombocytopenia. The bone marrow has many megakaryocytes, and platelet survival is probably very short. The cause of the short platelet life span is obscure. It is probably not due to the utilization of the platelets in the multiple small vessel thrombi seen in this disease, as was originally postulated. These thrombi appear to be composed primarily of fibrin with little platelet material as determined by immunofluorescent technic.[177] The initial lesion is in all probability a vascular one involving the small arterioles and is characterized by a proliferation of the vascular endothelium and an infiltration of the vascular wall with a homogeneous acidophilic fibrinoid material, with little or no inflammatory reaction. The thrombi are thought to occur secondary to the vascular lesion, since they are found in relation to changes in the vessel, whereas vascular lesions can be seen in the absence of thrombosis.[178] The purpuric manifestations are due to the thrombocytopenia. However, the neurologic abnormalities are usually due to the occlusive vascular lesions in the brain rather than to hemorrhage into the brain. So far no platelet antibodies have been identified, nor has a thrombocytopenia-producing factor been identified in the plasma of such patients.

The anemia seen in this disease is moderate to severe and is characterized by normochromic normocytic red cells, increase in reticulocytes, increase in serum bilirubin, shortened life span of the red cells, and in most cases a negative Coombs test. The bone marrow in addition to having numerous megakaryocytes, shows erythroid hyperplasia. The cause of the hemolysis is not known.

The etiology of the complex syndrome remains unknown. It has been suggested that thrombotic thrombocytopenia may represent (1) an autoimmuned process involving platelets, red cells and vascular endothelium; (2) a Shwartzman-like phenomenon in the human; (3) a hypersensitivity reaction to an infectious agent or drug; (4) a variation of systemic lupus erythematosus.

Qualitative Platelet Abnormalities

Qualitative abnormalities of platelets occur both on a congenital and an acquired basis and may be associated with hemorrhagic manifestations. Considerable confusion has arisen, particularly concerning the congenital variety, because of the indiscriminate nomenclature used in the literature. Rather than use complex terms with no specific meaning such as thrombocytasthenia and thrombocytopathia, to classify these platelet abnormalities, it is more reasonable to classify them according to the platelet factor which is affected. At the present time two types have been definitely distinguished, one in which the *clot-retracting activity* of the platelets is decreased and the other in which the *thromboplastic activity* or platelet factor 3 is abnormal.

Defect in clot-retracting activity of the platelets in patients with a bleeding tendency was first described by Glanzmann,[179,180] and he called this syndrome hereditary hemorrhagic thrombasthenia. The hemorrhagic manifestations are easy bruising, excessive bleeding after surgical procedures, epistaxes, menorrhagia, and bleeding from the gums. Blood clotting other than impaired clot retraction is normal. The platelets may show morphologic abnormalities but for the most part appear normal by light microscopy. The bleeding time is usually prolonged and capillary fragility may be increased. Recently Gross[64] has reported an enzymatic defect in the platelets of such patients. Two key enzymes of glycolysis were found diminished, glyceraldehyde phosphate dehydrogenase and pyruvate kinase. These enzymes are necessary for the maintenance of ATP, and, as might be expected, it was found that this important energy source necessary for clot retraction was low in these platelets.

The symptomatology in the second type of qualitative platelet abnormality is the same. The bleeding time is prolonged and capillary fragility is increased. However, in contrast to the type described previously, clot retraction is normal but prothrombin consumption is abnormal. This is not due to a deficiency or abnormality of any of the plasma coagulation factors but to a defect in the platelet factor 3 or thromboplastic activity. The abnormality apparently is not a decrease in this platelet factor but a *failure to release it* during the clotting process, since freezing and thawing of such platelets or lysing in distilled water

restores their factor 3 activity to normal.[181] This type of qualitative abnormality has been referred to as *thrombocytopathia* in the literature.

Cases have been reported in which both the clot-retracting activity and the factor 3 activity of the platelets have been affected. Others have been reported in which neither of these platelet factors is affected, but a hemorrhagic diathesis has been present which was thought to be due to some type of platelet abnormality.

Qualitative abnormalities of platelets have been reported in many diseases and it is questionable as to whether or not they contribute to any hemorrhagic diathesis which may be present, since such changes are also found when there is no bleeding tendency. This type of acquired platelet change involves a decrease in platelet factor 3 activity and has been reported in uremia, liver disease, leukemia, myeloid metaplasia, polycythemia vera, and macroglobulinemia.

Vascular Abnormality Plus a Plasma Coagulation Defect

In 1926 von Willebrand described a hereditary bleeding disorder prevalent among both the male and female inhabitants of the Äland Island.[182] The characteristic finding was a prolonged bleeding time and a normal clotting time. The symptoms varied considerably from case to case and were similar to, but milder than, those of classical hemophilia. Hemarthrosis was much less common and joint deformities did not occur. Severe bleeding after operative procedures, menorrhagia, and bleeding at parturition were prominent features. In this first description of the syndrome it was referred to as pseudohemophilia, but later it was referred to in the literature as von Willebrand's disease. Considerable confusion has arisen concerning this syndrome because of continuing changes in the concept of the defect in hemostasis. Many conflicting reports are found in the literature, but with improvement in methodology and advancement of our knowledge of hemostasis, the hemostatic defect in this syndrome has been considerably clarified although not completely worked out. After the initial report Jurgen and von Willebrand[183] concluded from further studies that the bleeding tendency was due to a qualitative defect of the platelets. Macfarlane[12] and others, however, believed that the bleeding tendency was due to a vascular abnormality in which the capillaries reacted abnormally to injury. Bizarre and tortuous capillary loops were also described.

In 1953 Alexander and Goldstein[184] reported the reduction in antihemophilic factor in two patients with prolonged bleeding times, normal platelets and irregular and distorted nail bed capillaries. This reduction in Factor VIII was soon reported in many other patients considered to fall into this syndrome, and finally re-examination of the Äland Island patients revealed that they also had a deficiency of Factor VIII.[185] The Swedish group in addition reported that there was a factor in plasma which could correct the prolonged bleeding time. Fractionation of normal plasma revealed that this factor was not Factor VIII or fibrinogen although it was concentrated in Fraction I. Further studies revealed that this factor was present in at least normal levels in the plasma of patients with clasical hemophilia. (To date it has not been possible to purify this factor to the extent that its physicochemical characteristics can be determined. It is, however, believed to be a protein.) Nilsson et al.[185] were able to correct the prolonged bleeding time without significantly increasing the Factor VIII level of the patient's blood by use of hemophilic plasma, or they could correct the Factor VIII level to normal without correcting the bleeding time by the use of certain purified Factor VIII fractions from normal blood. Cornu et al.[186] have recently confirmed these findings. From such data and studies on platelet adhesiveness it has been postulated that this plasma protein may play a role in platelet adhesion or massing at the site of vascular injury. Biggs,[187] on the other hand, found in the four patients she studied that the bleeding time was never reduced to normal with the materials she used (fresh frozen plasma, several Factor VIII-rich plasma fractions, serum, and fibrinogen fractions). Although

reduction in bleeding did occur in some instances it was of brief duration and the control of traumatic bleeding appeared to be correlated with the increase in Factor VIII levels rather than with the correction of the bleeding time.

Of interest in this syndrome is the finding that Factor VIII levels not only vary greatly from patient to patient but may vary significantly from one time to another in a given individual, which is distinctly different from what is found in classical hemophilia. In addition, exercise and the administration of adrenalin produce a much greater rise in the plasma Factor VIII activity than in the hemophilic. The effect of transfusion therapy upon the plasma Factor VIII levels is also significantly different in these two groups. In classical hemophilia the rise in plasma Factor VIII activity in response to transfusion reaches its peak immediately after completion of transfusion, the increase in activity is directly related to the total Factor VIII in the transfused material, and fall-off of activity begins immediately with a half-life variously estimated as 10 to 20 hours. In contrast in the von Willebrand group the peak of Factor VIII activity occurs from several to 24 hours after completion of transfusion. The rise in activity is greater than that expected from the total amount of Factor VIII administered. It has also been found that serum devoid of Factor VIII activity[187] and hemophilic plasma[186] will induce a delayed rise in Factor VIII which is equivalent to that produced by normal plasma. The fall-off rate is slower than that seen in hemophilia. From these findings, it appears that the Factor VIII deficiency in von Willebrand's syndrome is not due to an inability to produce Factor VIII but rather to the absence or deficiency of a stimulating factor for Factor VIII production. The concept is compatible with the difference in the inheritance pattern between hemophilia and von Willebrand's disease, the former exhibiting a sex-linked recessive pattern and the latter an autosomal dominant pattern.

At the present time most investigators define von Willebrand's disease as a hemorrhagic disease characterized by a prolonged bleeding time, reduced Factor VIII plasma levels, and normal platelets both in quality and quantity (although qualitative abnormality of platelets have been reported in some patients, most investigators have found the platelets to be normal). Bizarre and tortuous capillary loops may or may not be present. The bleeding time may vary from slightly above normal to markedly prolonged, and Factor VIII levels may vary from low normal to one to two per cent of normal. In general, the Factor VIII levels are not as low as those found in the moderate to severe classical hemophilics. In the untreated patient there is no correlation between the decrease in Factor VIII and the prolongation of the bleeding time, and some cases which undoubtedly belong to this syndrome have been reported in whom the bleeding time was prolonged but the Factor VIII level was within the normal range. In all probability the reverse findings may also occur. Whether or not there is a decrease in a plasma protein which has no function in coagulation but which plays some role in vascular integrity or platelet function remains to be clarified.

The variability of the clinical findings and symptoms and the conflicting reports in the literature concerning the nature of the hemostatic defect have led to the use of a number of terms in the literature, in addition to von Willebrand's disease, to refer to this syndrome: pseudohemophilia, pseudohemophilia B, angiohemophilia, and vascular hemophilia. It is still not clear what the relationship is between von Willebrand's disease as defined above and certain cases described in the literature. Cases have been reported in which abnormal platelet morphology or a decrease in platelet factor 3 was found in addition to prolongation of the bleeding time with or without reduction of Factor VIII or increased capillary fragility.[188] Cases have also been reported in which the prolonged bleeding time was associated with a decrease in Factor IX or XI rather than VIII.

HEREDITARY VASCULAR ABNORMALITIES

Hereditary hemorrhagic telangiectasia (Rendu-Osler-Weber disease) is a vascular disorder in which sporadic pathologic bleeding arises from localized, discrete vascular lesions which are usually widely distributed. This clinical entity, first recognized by Rendu in 1896,[189] was more clearly delineated by Osler in 1901[190] and somewhat later by Weber.[191]

This vascular abnormality is transmitted as an autosomal dominant trait so that either parent if affected may transmit it to half the progeny both male and female. It is probable that the homozygous form of hereditary hemorrhagic telangiectasia is lethal. The vascular lesions, which may occur in any organ or tissue of the body, tend to be particularly prominent in the skin and mucous membranes. They are rarely evident in infancy or early childhood but usually tend to appear during the 2nd to 5th decade. In most affected individuals new lesions continue to appear throughout their life time, but lesions may also disappear over a period of months to years leaving no visible vascular abnormality.[7] The lesions seen in the skin and mucous membranes are of three types: macules, spiders, and nodules. The macule is the most common and earliest type and usually is a pinpoint, red to purple spot which is not elevated and may even be depressed. The spider superficially resembles the vascular spider of cirrhosis but in contrast to the latter it usually does not blanch completely with pressure. This type of lesion does not make its appearance before the more characteristic macules. The nodules are red, or violaceous to purple lesions which may reach 5 to 8 mm. in diameter and are elevated above the surrounding skin. These too are usually a late manifestation. The vascular lesions may be distributed over the entire skin but are notable for their frequency on the palmar surface of the fingers and the hands, the fingernails, the lips, the ears, the face, the lower portion of the arms and the toes. The trunk and the abdomen are less often affected. From the point of view of pathologic bleeding, the more serious lesions are those in the mucous membranes of the nose, the tongue, the pharynx, the larynx, the trachea and the bronchi, gastrointestinal tract, and the genitourinary tract. The basic histologic defect in the vascular lesions is the failure of muscle and connective tissue to develop properly in the wall of the vessel. The lesions consist of dilated small vessels (arterioles, capillaries, and venules) whose walls may be nothing more than a layer of endothelial cells with little or no muscular or elastic elements. Atrophy of the skin or mucous membranes overlying these lesions occurs, thus reducing the mechanical protection ordinarily afforded. The involved vessels fail to contract normally when traumatized.[12] The frequent hemorrhages result only from the vascular lesions, the hemostatic mechanism in unaffected vessels is normal and there is no coagulation or platelet abnormality. Accordingly, the clotting time, platelet count, bleeding time, tourniquet test, etc. are all normal.

Hemorrhage often begins spontaneously. Epistaxis is most common, frequently precipitated by sneezing or blowing the nose. Gastrointestinal hemorrhage is fairly frequent and is probably the most serious, since it is not possible to apply local measures to stop the bleeding. Hemoptysis is not unusual and may be fatal. It arises from the vascular lesions of the bronchi rather than from the arteriovenous fistulae. In the classical case, the triad of a familial background, episodic bleeding, and obvious multiple telangiectasia make diagnosis relatively simple. However, in some instances diagnosis may be difficult, particularly when lesions are not apparent and no family history of bleeding is elicited. Hemorrhage may be frequent and severe, often originating repeatedly in the same location, and may induce profound anemia. Since more and more lesions appear with advancing years, the frequency of hemorrhagic episodes usually increases with age. Lesions occurring in certain organs may complicate the picture. Pulmonary arteriovenous fistulae may occur. Such lesions are usually found only in adults and when they occur are very frequently multiple.[7] They may, of course, result in cyanosis, polycythemia, clubbing of the fingers, and heart failure. Vascular lesions may occur in all organs including the brain, the spleen, and the liver. In the liver and spleen these lesions may expand into cavernous hemangiomas.[192] Aneurysms of systemic arteries, such as the

splenic and mesenteric arteries, have been reported.[7] It has also been reported that a specific form of cirrhosis of the liver may be associated with this disease.[7] As would be expected from consideration of the underlying pathology, effective therapy consists in local application of pressure when the angioma is accessible, followed by its extirpation surgically or by electrocautery. Systemic therapy has little to offer other than treatment of iron deficiency anemia when it is present. Estrogens[193] which have been reported as helpful are in general of little use.

Angiokeratoma Corporis Diffusum (Fabrey's Syndrome). Although this syndrome is not associated with pathologic bleeding, it is mentioned here because the vascular lesions which occur may be mistaken for petechiae or the lesions of hereditary hemorrhagic telangiectasia. However, careful examination of the lesions and their distribution usually is sufficient to distinguish them. In Fabrey's syndrome the lesions vary in size from barely visible to 2 to 4 mm. in diameter. The small ones are flat and the larger ones are elevated slightly above the surface of the skin. They range in color from deep red to black. The smaller ones are usually the lightest in color and can be partially blanched by pressure. Since thrombosis may occur in a given lesion, it may closely resemble a petechial lesion, however, there are always lesions present which will blanch and which do not disappear in a few days as petechiae do. The lesions usually appear in clusters, and in contrast to hereditary telangiectasia, the most prominent clusters are between the level of the umbilicus and the knees, and in particular over the hips, the iliac crests, the genitalia, the lumbosacral area, the buttocks, and around the umbilicus. The palms and soles are rarely involved and lesions on the face, the scalp and the ears have not been reported. The lesions may appear on the mucous membranes of the mouth and the pharynx, but rarely if ever on the dorsum of the tongue. This is a diffuse disease process which involves many organs. The renal lesion is probably the most serious one and uremia usually supervenes by the 4th or 5th decade. Premature cerebral vascular and coronary artery disease resulting in strokes and myocardial infarctions are prominent manifestations. Superficial corneal opacities are common as well as varicosities of the retinal veins. From histopathologic studies, it would appear that this disease process may be one of the "lipid storage" disorders but its exact nature remains to be determined. The condition is hereditary and appears to be transmitted as a sex-linked recessive trait. However, it has been reported in females, but this is thought to represent a function of penetrance of the gene. There is no abnormality in hemostasis or coagulation. An excellent review on the subject by Wise *et al.* has recently been published.[194]

ACQUIRED VASCULAR ABNORMALITIES

Vitamin C Deficiency (Scurvy). Ascorbic acid deficiency causes a defect in intercellular collagenous cement substance which in turn results in increased permeability and fragility of the small blood vessels (arterioles, capillaries, and venules). Although this effect upon the vasculature is undoubtedly the principal cause of the hemorrhagic tendency of scurvy, it may not be the only factor. In some cases thrombocytopenia may also occur and may contribute to the hemorrhagic diathesis.[4,152] It is thought that the thrombocytopenia is due to decreased production of platelets. Qualitative platelet changes of questionable significance have also been described in patients with scurvy[195] and recently findings in scorbutic guinea pigs indicate that a coagulation defect (decreased Factors XI and XII) might play a role in bleeding. The coagulation defects have not as yet been demonstrated in humans.

Hemorrhagic manifestations consist of follicular and perifollicular purpura, ecchymoses, large subcutaneous extravasations of blood, and oozing from the gums. The gum bleeding is frequently associated with peridontal sepsis, loosening of the teeth, and gum retraction. In infants subperiosteal bleeding and petechiae are outstanding features. The subperiosteal bleeding causes severe pain made worse by movement. Since the hemorrhages occur most frequently at the lower end of the femur

and the upper end of the humerus, the child refuses to move his limbs and tends to lie absolutely still with his legs flexed and widely abducted.

Usually the only test of hemostasis which is abnormal is the tourniquet test, which is often strikingly positive. The bleeding time and all coagulation tests are most often normal. If thrombocytopenia is present, a prolonged bleeding time, poor prothrombin consumption and poor clot retraction may occur. However, it is rare that the thrombocytopenia is of a severe enough degree to produce such changes. Both the increased vascular fragility and the thrombocytopenia are corrected within a few days by the administration of ascorbic acid (200 to 300 mg. daily).

Anaphylactoid Purpura. Anaphylactoid, allergic or Henoch-Schönlein purpura is a generalized disturbance of the small blood vessels in which purpura is but one of a wide variety of manifestations. Because of the widespread involvement of the small vessels, signs and symptoms referable to many organs (skin, mucous membranes, joints, gastrointestinal tract, urinary tract, central nervous system and heart) may be present. The characteristic vascular lesion is an angiitis of the arterioles and capillaries in which there is perivascular cuffing with varying numbers of polymorphonuclear, lymphocytic, histiocytic and eosinophilic cells. There may be swelling and proliferation of the endothelial cells which at times may be so marked as to occlude the vessel. The vascular wall may be necrotic and collagen fibers in the areas of intensive cellular reaction may be distorted and stain abnormally. In the areas of purpura extravasated erythrocytes are seen about the affected vessels. In the dermis and the mucous membranes there may be evidence of edema. The early renal lesions have many similarities to those of disseminated lupus erythematosus[197] whereas the older lesions are difficult to differentiate from subacute or chronic glomerulonephritis.[198]

The etiology of the syndrome is unknown. Osler was probably the first to attribute its pathogenesis to an anaphylactic or allergic mechanism because of its similarity to serum sickness. Although the concept has fallen out of favor from time to time, recent advances made in the study of the relation of the immune mechanism to disease states suggest that this syndrome is a result of an immune reaction involving blood vessels. Certain clinical and pathologic aspects of Henoch-Schönlein purpura give support to this theory. The joint manifestations and some of the skin lesions (urticaria, edema, erythema) are similar to those seen in serum sickness and known allergic reactions. Some cases with classical clinical and pathologic findings have been shown to be due to reactions to specific foods and drugs. In such cases recovery occurs when the offending agent is withdrawn and reappears when it is again given to the patient. Among the offending agents reported are milk, chocolate, wheat, beans, penicillin, barbiturates, quinine, chlorothiazide, salicylates, and influenza vaccine.[8,198,199] About 70 to 90 per cent of cases follow an upper respiratory infection occurring one to three weeks before onset of purpura.[198,200] In only about 25 to 30 per cent is the preceding infection due to beta hemolytic streptococci as determined by culture or antistreptolysin titers, in contrast to the infections more regularly preceding rheumatic fever and glomerulonephritis. None the less, the high incidence of recent upper respiratory infections is impressive. It is of course possible that antibodies formed in response to an infection might cross-react with vascular tissue, thus producing a generalized vascular lesion, but a more likely explanation in view of recent experimental findings in animals, is that soluble antigen-antibody complexes of various types produce the injury to blood vessels. Dixon *et al.*[201] were able to produce vascular lesions in the kidney of rabbits by repeated injection of antigen (foreign protein), and the critical factor determining whether or not an animal would develop renal disease was the amount of antibody the animal formed. Vascular lesions have also been produced in animals by intravenous administration of a number of antigen-antibody complexes made soluble by the presence of excess antigen.[202] It is possible therefore that the lesions in this disease process are caused by

"immunologic pathogens" which are without immunologic specificity for vascular tissue. Although Henoch-Schönlein purpura has been referred to as an "autoimmuned" disease, and lesions have been produced in animals which are similar to those seen in the human by the administration of heterologous antivascular serum, there has been no convincing demonstration of circulating antibodies in the serum of patients against any antigen in blood vessels or of tissue localizing antibody in the vessels of patients as determined by fluorescent technics.[203]

The onset and course of the disease is quite variable. It may begin with fever, headache and anorexia, or purpura, arthralgia, abdominal pain or hematuria may be the first manifestation. Although it occurs commonly in children under the age of eight, it may occur at any age. The sexes are probably affected equally since in some series males were found to predominate, whereas in others it occurred more frequently in females.[198] Each episode usually lasts no more than a few weeks, but recurrent attacks occur in about 50 per cent of the cases.

Skin involvement has been reported in almost all cases, probably because without it the diagnosis is rarely if ever made. A wide variety of lesions occur which may or may not be hemorrhagic. The rash is often urticarial at first and is then replaced by a red macular or maculopapular lesion. These lesions, which can occur without the preceding urticaria, may remain small and discrete but usually they enlarge and often become confluent. Hemorrhages occurring in these lesions give the characteristic purpura of the disease. Frequently, hemorrhage occurs early in the formation of the lesion so that the underlying erythema is not apparent. In such instances the purpura may be confused with that of thrombocytopenia, although certain characteristics help differentiate it. The purpuric lesions are usually larger and more confluent than those seen in thrombocytopenia and small round petechiae are uncommon. The distribution is also different, since in allergic purpura the purpura is most prominent over the lower extremities and buttocks and may be limited to these areas; however, the arms, face and rarely the lower trunk may become involved. The lesions are more prominent on the extensor surfaces of the extremities and in the joint areas. Other skin lesions such as blebs, bullae, and erythema nodosa may appear. Localized areas of edema, particularly on the hands, the feet, and around the face, the eyes, the neck, the lips and the penis are often present.

Joint symptoms are a very common manifestation. The joints most frequently affected are the ankles and the knees. Joint pains often seem excessively severe, out of proportion to the objective evidence. The involved joint is usually slightly to moderately swollen and tender, but rarely red or warm. Roentgenographic examination reveals periarticular soft tissue swelling without any change in the joint space. Joint involvement is usually transient and not migratory, but may recur during the course of the illness and does not respond well to salicylates.

Gastrointestinal symptoms consist of colicky abdominal pain, vomiting, melena and hematemesis. The abdominal pain is the most common symptom and is thought to be due to edema and/or bleeding into the intestinal wall. Intussusception is the most serious gastrointestinal complication and occurs most often in children under the age of eight.

In about 40 to 60 per cent of the cases there is evidence of renal involvement as indicated by hematuria, proteinuria, or elevation of blood urea. In most cases there is complete recovery, but in about 20 to 25 per cent of cases some abnormality of renal function persists for years, and in a small percentage it progresses to renal failure and death.[198]

Involvement of the central nervous system may result in transient attacks of paresis, epileptiform convulsions, chorea, and subarachnoid bleeding.

Hemorrhage in Henoch-Schönlein purpura is rarely severe enough to endanger life. There is no generalized breakdown of the hemostatic mechanism, and bleeding occurs only at the site of vascular damage. There is no alteration in the coagulation mechanism and platelets are usually qualitatively and quantitatively normal. Occasional cases with an associated thrombocytopenia have been described. The tourniquet test is usually negative and the bleeding time normal.

PURPURA PROBABLY DUE TO AN ACQUIRED VASCULAR DISORDER

This group is composed of syndromes characterized by mild hemorrhagic skin lesions associated with other vascular abnormalities and pigmentary disorders.

Shamberg's Disease (progressive pigmentary dermatitis) is characterized by appearance of reddish pin-head-sized lesions on the lower extremities. These coalesce to form larger irregular-shaped lesions which gradually fade and become brown to yellow in color. Histologically there is a proliferation of capillaries and of endothelial cells and some vessels become dilated, allowing diapedesis of red cells. The brownish color which develops is in part due to accumulation of hemosiderin in phagocytes in the skin. *Majocchi's disease (purpura annularis telangiectodes)* is characterized by purpuric and pigmented macules and rings which do not fade on pressure and which usually begin in the lower extremities but subsequently involve the arms and trunk. Telangiectasia may occur. Histologically the lesions reveal atrophy of the epidermis, perivascular inflammatory reaction of small vessels with polymorphonuclear and lymphocytic cells, thickening of the vascular wall with occlusion occurring in some vessels. The etiology of these two conditions is not known nor is their relationship to each other or to syndromes such as Henoch-Schönlein purpura clear. There are several other similar conditions described in the dermatologic literature. However, all of these are rare, and none are associated with any severe bleeding or a generalized disturbance of the hemostatic mechanism.

DISEASES OF CONNECTIVE TISSUE WITH HEMORRHAGE PROBABLY DUE TO VASCULAR DEFECTS AND ABNORMALITY OF SUPPORTING TISSUE

There are a number of syndromes which appear to be hereditary disorders of connective tissue or collagen in which hemorrhagic manifestations are common.[204] In these cases the abnormal bleeding tendency is thought to be due to a vascular defect which may be enhanced by a defect of the supporting tissue.

Ehlers-Danlos syndrome is a hereditary disorder of both sexes which is inherited as a simple dominant trait. It is characterized by hyperelasticity of the skin, hyperextensibility of the joints, increased fragility of the skin and blood vessels, dislocation of the lens and increased incidence of dissecting aneurysm of the aorta. Hemorrhagic manifestations are easy bruising, petechiae, epistaxis, bleeding from the gums, hematuria, melena, menorrhagia and excessive bleeding after surgical procedures. In most cases the only test of the hemostatic mechanism which is abnormal is the tourniquet test. Occasionally the bleeding time is slightly prolonged and in scattered cases mild thrombocytopenia, qualitative defect of platelets, or low Factor IX has been reported. These defects have usually been rather mild and ordinarily would not be expected to cause any serious defect in hemostasis. In all probability the bleeding tendency is due to the abnormal formation of elastic tissue in the blood vessels and surrounding tissue.

Osteogenesis imperfecta is thought to be an hereditary disorder of collagen formation and may be associated with hemorrhagic manifestations such as ecchymosis, hematoma, melena, subconjunctival hemorrhages, etc. The bleeding tendency is assumed to be due to a vascular defect caused by abnormal collagen formation. However, qualitative abnormalities of platelets (decreased platelet factor 3 activity) has recently been reported in this syndrome. Whether or not this platelet defect is always present and is responsible for the hemorrhagic diathesis has not been determined.

Pseudoxanthoma elasticum may be associated with bleeding from virtually any organ. The cause remains obscure. As yet, no abnormality in coagulation has been reported. The pathologic abnormality (which is a hereditary one, although its hereditary pattern is as yet not certain) appears to be a defect of either the elastic

tissue or collagen. The small and medium-sized arteries may show degenerative changes in the elastic membrane, and capillaries and small veins may be widely dilated. These vascular changes may well be responsible for the bleeding tendency.

Pulmonary hemosiderosis[205] is characterized by recurrent, subacute episodes of pulmonary hemorrhage and progressive pulmonary insufficiency. About 80 per cent of the cases occur in children and the remainder in young adults. The onset is often insidious. The pulmonary bleeding may be mild, giving rise only to blood-tinged sputum. However, at some time during the course of the disease frank hemoptysis usually occurs. Dyspnea and cough are almost always present and become much more pronounced during episodes of bleeding, at which time cyanosis also becomes prominent. With recurrent pulmonary hemorrhages, pulmonary symptoms increase and become more persistent. Pulmonary fibrosis progresses and cor pulmonale may occur eventually, giving rise to signs of right-sided heart failure. Frequently a moderate to severe anemia develops due to iron deficiency, for although there is a great deal of iron in the pulmonary tissue, it is not available for hemoglobin synthesis. The accumulation of iron in the lung results in the appearance of hemosiderin-laden histiocytes in the sputum, an important diagnostic finding. The hemorrhagic tendency is confined to the lungs. All coagulation studies are normal, and there is no evidence of any platelet or generalized vascular disorder.

The etiology of this syndrome is obscure. There is no evidence of an increased familial incidence. It is classified here in the group of connective tissue disorders because the characteristic pathologic findings have been considered to be a degeneration of the alveolar, interstitial and vascular elastic fibers. However, these changes are now thought to be secondary to the hemosiderin deposited in the lung from repeated bleeding. Three postulations have been advanced: (1) A defective vasomotor control of the pulmonary vessels gives rise to pulmonary hypertension with subsequent diapedesis of red cells. (2) An autoimmuned process or some immunologic reaction affects the pulmonary vessels leading to hemorrhage. (3) This disease represents primarily an abnormality of alveolar epithelial growth and function which critically affects the mechanical stability of the alveolar capillaries. As yet none of these theories have been substantiated. What the relation is between this syndrome and *Goodpasture's syndrome* (pulmonary hemorrhage and extensive glomerular disease) also is obscure.

PURPURA AND BLEEDING OF OBSCURE ETIOLOGY

Autoerythrocyte Sensitization. In 1955 Gardner and Diamond first described a peculiar chronic recurrent purpura which occurred in women.[206] It usually first makes its appearance shortly after an injury or surgical procedure. The lesions arise spontaneously or following minor trauma and are most frequently limited to the extremities. Characteristically, the patient first notes a tingling or painful sensation and within a few minutes an urticarial or erythematous skin lesion appears in the area. Within minutes or hours the area becomes ecchymotic and painful. The ecchymotic area may be ringed by an area of erythema. After a week or two the ecchymosis disappears. At irregular intervals new lesions appear. Associated with such episodes left upper quadrant pain similar to that of a splenic infarct, or melena, hematuria, hemiparesis or hemiplegia may occur. Gardner and Diamond demonstrated that these lesions could be induced by intradermal administration of the patient's own red cell stroma, but not by plasma, white cells or hemoglobin, and postulated autoerythrocyte sensitization as the mechanism producing the purpura. Histamine has also been shown to produce the lesions in such patients. Most of the affected persons have rather severe emotional disturbances. Agle and Ratnoff[207] have emphasized this and have reviewed the relationship of emotional disturbance and hemorrhagic phenomena. Although no definite conclusion can be drawn, the author suggests a trial of psychiatric therapy for treatment of patients with this type of purpura.

A somewhat similar condition has recently been reported in which the purpuric lesions appear to be due to *autosensitization to desoxyribonucleic acid*.[208,209] The lesions begin as erythematous swelling which increases in size over a period of a few hours, after which ecchymosis replaces the erythema. Chloroquin is effective in treatment.

Polycythemia Vera. That thromboembolic phenomena occur in polycythemia vera is not surprising in view of the increased viscosity of the blood, the resulting decrease in velocity of blood flow, and the thrombocytosis which is frequently present. However, the cause of the hemorrhagic diathesis, which is often present even when there is evidence of intravascular coagulation, is for the most part obscure. Increased fibrinolytic activity, marked hypofibrinogenemia, or severe liver damage with resulting decrease in coagulation factors produced in the liver can account for bleeding in an occasional case. In the remainder a variety of mechanisms have been suggested. Because of the increased red cell mass and high hematocrit, the level of plasma coagulation factors per volume of whole blood is reduced even though the plasma levels may be normal. However, studies do not indicate that such reduction is usually sufficient to account for hemorrhage, and in addition the hemorrhagic tendency remains even after reduction of red cell mass and hematocrit to normal levels by venesection. It is possible that the clot formed is inadequate because of the increased number of red cells or because of some qualitative abnormality in the fibrin clot which is suggested by the abnormally high red cell fallout observed in vitro. The increased fallout may occur even when the hematocrit and platelet levels have been reduced to normal by therapy. Decreased platelet 3 activity has been reported but is rarely if ever of sufficient degree to account for bleeding. It has also been postulated that there is a vascular defect perhaps caused by prolonged over-distention of the vascular tree by the increased blood volume, which results in the loss of vascular response to injury.

Hemorrhagic Thrombocythemia. As

might be anticipated, intravascular thrombosis is one of the complications of thrombocytosis. However, a hemorrhagic diathesis, which is characterized by easy bruising and excessive bleeding following trauma or surgery, also occurs.[210] The mechanism by which thrombocythemia leads to bleeding has been the subject of much speculation, but there is little to support any of the suggested theories. The underlying cause of the thrombocytosis, (whether polycythemia vera, myeloid metaplasia, chronic granulocytic leukemia, or idiopathic) does not seem to be a determining factor in whether or not a bleeding tendency is present. Although in patients with bleeding there seems to be a relationship between the level of the platelet count and the tendency to bleed, other patients with equally high counts have no bleeding tendency. It has been suggested that the bleeding is due to: (1) a defect in platelet factor 3, which has been demonstrated in some patients (This defect, however, is not always present nor does it ever seem severe enough to be the cause of bleeding) (2) a vascular defect which may or may not be related to the thrombocythemia (There usually is no evidence by the tests available of a defect in vascular integrity.) (3) A defect in plasma coagulation factors. (Such a defect may be present because there frequently is involvement of the liver by the underlying disease process; however, it rarely is severe enough to account for the bleeding.) (4) The anticoagulant effect of excessive platelets, a phenomenon which can be demonstrated in vitro. (In the majority of cases the platelet elevation does not appear to be of sufficient magnitude to cause this coagulation defect.)

Hemorrhagic Manifestation in Association With Plasma Protein Abnormalities

Hyperglobulinemic purpura is a clinical entity first reported by Waldenström in 1943. It is characterized by episodic purpura and an increase in serum gamma globulin.[211, 212] The increased gamma globulin is of the 7S type and, unlike myeloma globulin, migrates as a broad band on paper electrophoresis. This syndrome has been observed most frequently in middle-aged women but has been reported in males. The condition usually begins insidiously with occasional attacks of purpura over the distal lower extremities but over the course of years the attacks become more frequent and more extensive, involving the entire lower extremity and occasionally the trunk. The purpura usually occurs after prolonged standing or exercise and may be heralded by burning or stinging and may be preceded or accompanied by edema of the legs, pain in the knees or ankles, and low grade fever. Most often no underlying disease can be found, but it has been described in patients with sarcoid, lupus erythematosus, Sjögren's syndrome and Mikulicz's disease. The bleeding tendency is limited to the skin. The purpuric lesions consist of small petechiae or ecchymoses ranging from a few mm. to 2 cm. in diameter. The rash gradually fades over a week or two and at first disappears without a trace, but after repeated bouts, persistent pigmentation develops. The purpura is not associated with any significant disturbance of blood coagulation. All the usual coagulation tests are normal and although in some cases a mild thrombocytopenia or a moderate decrease in platelet factor 3 activity has been reported it is unlikely that such changes play any role in the purpura. The bleeding time is normal and the tourniquet test is normal in most cases. Pathologic examination reveals a vasculitis which is limited to the areas of the purpuric lesion. Vessels in normal-appearing skin either from the lower extremities or elsewhere seem histologically normal. The early pathologic changes are found in the capillaries and small arterioles and consist of perivascular edema, and infiltration with leukocytes, plasma cells and histiocytes. Proliferation of the endothelial cells also occurs and may completely occlude the vessel. Later changes consist of fibrinoid degeneration of the collagen fibers and loss of elastic fibers. The purpura obviously is secondary to the vascular lesion. However, the etiology of these lesions and role of the hypergammaglobulinemia remains obscure. There is no good evidence to implicate antibodies against the vascular wall or sensitization to altered gamma globulin. However, immunologic mechanisms cannot be ruled out, for as discussed in the previous section on Henoch-Schönlein purpura recent studies have demonstrated the vascular toxicity of soluble antigen-antibody complexes; such a mechanism has not been ruled out in this condition. It is of interest that it was recently reported that thioguanine therapy resulted in marked improvement in two patients with hyperglobulinemic purpura without significantly altering the plasma proteins by the parameters used.[213]

Hyperglobulinemia Associated With Multiple Myeloma. In multiple myeloma a bleeding tendency characterized by ecchymoses, petechiae, epistaxis, gingival bleeding, hematemesis, and excessive bleeding at surgery is commonly encountered. The pathogenesis of the hemorrhagic diathesis varies from patient to patient. In some it is due to thrombocytopenia, and in a rare case increased fibrinolysis is the cause. However, in most cases the pathogenesis is not so clear cut. In some instances the abnormal protein may delay clotting by acting as an inhibitor of the action of thrombin or fibrinogen or of the polymerization of fibrin monomers. Whether or not this activity of the protein is ever responsible for bleeding is not clear. In other cases no explanation for bleeding has been found.

Cryoglobulinemia. Cryoglobulins are proteins which precipitate or gel when whole blood or plasma is cooled, and at body temperature increase the viscosity of the blood if present in high enough concentrations. They may have the molecular weight of normal gamma globulin, or may be macroglobulins. In most cases there is an underlying disease process such as multiple myeloma, lymphoproliferative disease, Hodgkin's disease or lupus erythematosus, but an essential or idiopathic variety has also been reported. There is considerable variation not only in the level of these proteins from one case to another but also in their physical properties. In some cases lowering the temperature of the blood just a few degrees below body temperature results in gel formation or precipitation whereas in others this does not take place unless the temperature is dropped considerably below room temperature. Symptoms vary depending upon the concentration and physical properties of the protein. Slowing of the circulation is caused by the increased viscosity of the blood and as the temperature drops, there may be complete cessation of the flow of blood in the small vessels. The circulatory alterations result in cyanosis, particularly of the exposed portions of the body and may cause Raynaud's phenomenon. Complete obstruction of vessels may lead to injury of the vessel with thrombosis and/or hemorrhage. Ecchymosis, epistaxis, melena, retinal hemorrhage and excessive bleeding after trauma or surgery have been reported. The mechanism of the bleeding is not clear. However, several abnormalities in coagulation have been noted: prolonged prothrombin times, decreased prothrombin and Factor VII and V levels, increased clotting and partial thromboplastin times may occur. Many of these findings are felt to be due to the interference of the abnormal protein in the clotting process. It has also been postulated that these proteins may form complexes with certain of the coagulation factors and thus make them unavailable. They also may interfere with the thrombin-fibrinogen reaction and clot retraction. The clots that are formed are friable, and this may contribute to the defect in hemostasis. Coating of the platelets with these proteins, particularly when they are macroglobulins, may interfere with platelet function and in particular with release of platelet factor 3.

Macroglobulinemia. Normally about 2 to 5 per cent of the plasma proteins have a molecular weight of 1,000,000 or more. Occasionally the concentration of these macroglobulins is high. Such an increase may be associated with some underlying disease process such as cirrhosis, lymphoproliferative diseases, myeloma or lupus, but in other instances it appears to be part of a distinct syndrome referred to as Waldenström's macroglobulinemia.[214,215] In this syndrome there are many peculiar cells in the bone marrow, and at times in the spleen and lymph nodes which have features of both lymphocytes and plasma cells and may represent some transition form between the lymphocyte and plasma cell.

It is believed that these cells produce the macroglobulin. Subjects with high levels of macroglobulin may have a severe hemorrhagic diathesis characterized by bleeding from mucous membranes, particularly of the gums and nose. These mucosal surfaces frequently show persistent oozing which is difficult to control. Minor surgery may be complicated by severe and persistent hemorrhage. Bleeding into the skin and subcutaneous tissues (petechiae and ecchymoses) occur much less commonly as does bleeding into the eye, the central nervous system and the gastrointestinal tract. Typically the bleeding time is prolonged and the tourniquet test it normal. Coagulation studies have produced a remarkable variety of findings. The clotting time of whole blood may be prolonged, particularly if carried out in siliconized tubes. Decreased prothrombin, Factor V and VII levels have been reported as well as inhibitors directed against thromboplastin formation, the action of thrombin on fibrinogen, or the polymerization of fibrin. Prothrombin consumption may be markedly decreased during coagulation. In some patients thrombocytopenia does occur but it is usually not of a severe enough degree to produce prolonged bleeding times or poor prothrombin consumption. It has been reported that at least in some patients poor prothrombin consumption can be due to a lack of release of platelet factor 3. Although the platelets of the patients reported contained normal amounts of this factor, it appeared that macroglobulin on the surface of the platelets seemed to inhibit the release of factor 3. The macroglobulin in these patients was also shown to coat red cells and white cells.[216] Despite all these reports there are cases in which none of these abnormalities appear to adequately explain the bleeding tendency. It has been postulated that the macroglobulins in some way impair the function of the small vessels. That the macroglobulins are in some way directly responsible for the hemorrhagic diathesis would appear to be substantiated by the decrease in the bleeding tendency following reduction of the level of macroglobulin by plasmapheresis.[217]

SUMMARY

Pathologic bleeding occurs when there is impairment of the hemostatic mechanism, in which extravascular, vascular, and intravascular factors all play a role. Study of the various components involved has helped to clarify the pathogenesis and explain the clinical manifestations of many hemorrhagic disorders. In this chapter an attempt has been made to summarize our present knowledge of the hemostatic mechanism and to indicate how it is altered in various hemorrhagic states. Although our present knowledge is far from complete, it does permit a rational approach to the study, diagnosis, and treatment of pathologic bleeding.

REFERENCES

1. Quick, A. J.: Hemorrhagic Diseases, Philadelphia, Lea & Febiger, 1957.
2. Ratnoff, O. D.: Bleeding Syndromes, A Clinical Manual, Springfield, Ill., Thomas, 1960.
3. Biggs, R., and Macfarlane, R. G.: Human Blood Coagulation and Its Disorders, ed. 3, Oxford, Blackwell Scientific Publ., 1962.
4. Stefanini, M., and Dameshek, W.: The Hemorrhagic Disorders. A Clinical and Therapeutic Approach, ed. 2, New York, Grune & Stratton, 1962.
5. Macfarlane, R. G.: The Reactions of the Blood to Injury: Blood Coagulation and Hemostasis; Changes in the Blood Cells and the Activation of Fibrinolysis, in General Pathology, Florey, H., ed., Philadelphia, Saunders, 1958.
6. Alexander, B.: Coagulation, hemorrhage and thrombosis, New England J. Med. 252:432, 1955.
7. Bean, W. B.: Vascular Spiders, and Related Lesions of Skin, Springfield, Ill., Thomas, 1958.
8. Harrington, W. J.: The Purpuras, Disease-a-Month, Chicago, Year Book Pub., 1957.
9. Budtz-Olsen, O. E.: Clot Retraction, Oxford, Blackwell Scientific Pub., 1951.
10. Brinkhous, K. M., ed.: Hemophilia and Other Hemorrhagic States. Chapel Hill, N. C., U. North Carolina Press, 1959.
11. Tocantins, L. M.: The mechanisms of hemostasis, Ann. Surg. 125:292, 1947.
12. Macfarlane, R. G.: Critical review: the mechanisms of hemostasis, Quart. J. Med. 34:1, 1941.

13. Kramár, J.: The determination and evaluation of capillary resistance—a review of methodology, Blood 20:83, 1962.

14. Chambers, R., and Zweifack, B. W.: Vasomotion in the hemodynamics of the blood capillary circulation, Ann. N. Y. Acad. Sci. 49:549, 1948.

15. Weiner, M., and Udenfriend, S.: Relationship of platelet serotonin to disturbances of clotting and hemostasis, Circulation 15:353, 1957.

16. Nilsson, I. M., Blömback, M., and Blömback, B.: Von Willebrand's disease in Sweden: its pathogenesis and treatment, Acta med. scandinav. 164:263, 1959.

17. Duke, W. W.: The relation of blood platelets to hemorrhagic disease, J.A.M.A. 55: 1185, 1910.

18. Ivy, A. C., Shapiro, B. F., and Melnick, P.: The bleeding tendency in jaundice, Surg. Gyn. & Obst. 60:781, 1935.

19. Shulman, I., Pierce, M., Lukens, A., and Currimbhog, Z.: Studies on thrombopoiesis. I. A factor in normal human plasma required for platelet production; chronic thrombocytopenia due to its deficiency, Blood 16:943, 1960.

20. Odell, T. T., and Kniseley, R. M.: The Origin, Life Span, Regulation and Fate of Blood Platelets. Progress in Hematology, vol. 3, p. 203, Tocantins, L. M., Ed. New York, Grune & Stratton, 1962.

21. Adelson, E., Rheingold, J. J., and Crosby, W. H.: Studies of platelet survival by in vivo tagging with P[32], J. Lab. & Clin. Med. 50:570, 1957.

22. Leeksma, C. H. W., and Cohen, J. A.: Demonstration of the life span of human blood platelets using labeled diisopropylfluorophosphate, J. Clin. Invest. 35:964, 1956.

23. Cohen, P., and Gardner, F. H.: Reclassification of thrombocytopenias by Cr[51] labeling method for measuring platelet life span, New England J. Med. 234:1294, 1350, 1961.

24. Adelson, E., Rheingold, J. J., and Lear, A. A.: Continuous in vivo coagulation, the determinant of platelet survival, Blood 18:796, 1961.

25. Baldini, M., Costea, N., and Dameshek, W.: The viability of stored human platelets, Blood 16:1669, 1961.

26. Roskam, J., Hughes, J., Bounameaux, Y., and Salmon, J.: The part played by platelets in the formation of an efficient hemostatic plug, Throm. et Diath. Hem. 3:510, 1959.

27. Lüscher, E. F.: Blood platelets—their relationship to the blood clotting system and to hemostasis, Vox. Sang. 5:259, 1960.

28. Berman, J. B., and Fulton, G. P.: Platelets in the Peripheral Circulation, in Blood Platelets, International Symposium, Johnson, S. A., Monto, R. W., Rebuck, J. W., and Horn, R. C. eds. Boston, Little Brown, 1961.

29. Zucker, M. B., and Borrelli, J.: Viscous metamorphysis, clot retraction and other morphologic alterations of blood platelets, J. Appl. Physiol. 14:575, 1959.

30. Mason, R. G., Hocutt, E. J., Wagner, R. H., and Brinkhous, K. M.: Evolution and decay of platelet-agglutinating activity in normal and pathological human plasma, J. Lab. & Clin. Med. 59:645, 1962.

31. Marcus, A. J., and Spaet, T. H.: Platelet phosphatides: their separation, identification and clotting activity, J. Clin. Invest. 37:1836, 1958.

32. Troop, S. B., Reed, C. F., Marinetti, G. V., and Swisher, S. N.: Thromboplastic factors in platelets and red blood cells: observations on their chemical nature and function in in vitro coagulation, J. Clin. Invest. 39:342, 1960.

33. Salmon, J., and Bounameaux, Y.: Etude des Antigens Plaquettes et en particulier du Fibrinogène, Thromb. Diath. Hem. 2:93, 1958.

34. Bounameaux, Y.: L'Accolement des Plaquettes aux Fibres Sous-endothéliales, Compt. Rend. Soc. Biol. 153:865, 1959.

35. Bettex-Galland, M., and Lüscher, E. F.: Extraction of an actomyosin-like protein from human platelets, Nature 184:276, 1959.

36. Ratnoff, O. D., and Colopy, J. E.: A familial hemorrhagic trait associated with a deficiency of a clot promoting fraction of plasma, J. Clin. Invest. 34:602, 1955.

37. Ratnoff, O. D., and Rosenblum, J. M.: Role of Hageman factor in the initiation of clotting by glass, Am. J. Med. 25:160, 1958.

38. Ratnoff, O. D., Davie, E. W., and Mallett, D. L.: Studies on the action of Hageman factor: evidence that activated Hageman factor in turn activates plasma thromboplastin antecedent, J. Clin. Invest. 40:803, 1961.

39. Margolis, J.: Initiation of blood coagulation by glass and related surfaces, J. Physiol. 137:95, 1957.

40. Soulier, J. P., Prou-Wartelle, O., and Ménaché, D.: Hageman trait and PTA de-

ficiency. The role of contact of blood with glass, Brit. J. Hemat. 5:121, 1959.

41. Soulier, J. P., and Prou-Wartelle, O.: New data on Hageman factor and plasma thromboplastin antecedent. The role of contact in the initial phase of blood coagulation, Brit. J. Hemat. 6:88, 1960.

42. Rosenthal, R. L., Dreskin, O. H., and Rosenthal, N.: New hemophilia-like disease caused by deficiency of a third thromboplastin factor, Proc. Soc. Exp. Biol. & Med. 82:171, 1953.

43. Rosenthal, R. L.: Plasma thromboplastin antecedent (P.T.A.) deficiency in man; clinical, coagulation, hereditary, and therapeutic aspects, J. Clin. Invest. 33:961, 1954.

44. Bergsagel, D. E., and Hougie, C.: Intermediate stages of the formation of blood thromboplastin, Brit. J. Hemat. 2:113, 1956.

45. Hougie, C.: The role of Factor V in the formation of blood thromboplastin, J. Lab. & Clin. Med. 50:61, 1957.

46. Biggs, R., and Bidwell, E.: Kinetics of Blood Thromboplastin Formation, Proc. 4th International Congress of Biochemistry, Vienna, p. 172, 1959.

47. Fisch, U., and Duckert, F.: Some aspects of kinetics of the first stages of blood thromboplastin formation, Throm. Diath. Haem. 3:98, 1959.

48. Yin, E. T., and Duckert, F.: The formation of intermediate product I in a purified system. The role of Factor IX or of its precursor and of a Hageman-PTA fraction, Thromb. Diath. Haem. 6:224, 1961.

49. Horowitz, H. I., and Spaet, T. H.: Generation of coagulation product I and its interaction with platelets and phospholipids, J. Appl. Physiol. 16:112, 1961.

50. Ware, A. G., Murphy, M. C., and Seegers, W. H.: The Function of AC-globulin in blood clotting, Science 106:617, 1947.

51. Lewis, J. H., Didisheim, P., Ferguson, J. H., and Hattori, K.: Changes occurring during coagulation in glass. 1. Normal human blood, Thromb. Diath. Haem. 4:1, 1959.

52. Quick, A. J., Shanberge, J. N., and Stefanini, M.: The role of platelets in the coagulation of blood, Am. J. Med. Sci. 217:198, 1949.

53. Alexander, B., Goldstein, R., Rich, L., LeBolloc'h, A. G., Diamond, L. K., and Borges, W.: Congenital afibrinogenemia: a study of some basic aspects of coagulation, Blood 9:843, 1954.

54. Mason, R. G., Hocutt, E. J., Wagner, R. H., and Brinkhous, K. M.: Evolution and decay of platelet-agglutinating activity in normal and pathologic human plasmas, J. Lab. & Clin. Med. 59:645, 1962.

55. Rapaport, S. I., Schiffman, S., Patch, M. J., and Ames, S. B.: Rapid clotting in the presence of activation product plus traces of thrombin, Proc. IX Congress Int. Society of Hemat. 1962.

56. Goldstein, R., and Alexander, B.: Coagulation factors concerned with thromboplastin generation, Fed. Proc. 14:219, 1955.

57. ———: Further studies on proconvertin deficiency and the role of proconvertin, in Hemophilia and Hemophilioid Diseases, p. 93, Brinkhous, K. M., ed. Chapel Hill, U. North Carolina Press, 1957.

58. Hougie, C., Barrow, E. M., and Graham, J. B.: Stuart clotting defect. Segregation of hereditary hemorrhagic state from heterogeneous groups heretofore called "stable factor" (SPCA, proconvertin, Factor VII) deficiency, J. Clin. Invest. 36:485, 1957.

59. Straub, W., and Duckert, F.: The formation of extrinsic prothrombin activator, Thromb. Diath. Haem. 5:402, 1961.

60. Seegers, W. H., Levine, W. G., and Shepard, R. S.: Further studies on the purification of thrombin, Can. J. Biochem. Physiol. 36:603, 1958.

61. Mammen, E. F., Thomas, W. R., and Seegers, W. H.: Activation of purified prothrombin to autoprothrombin I or autoprothrombin II (platelet co-factor II) or autoprothrombin II-A, Thromb. Diath. Haem. 5:218, 1960.

62. Gladner, J. A., Folk, J. E., Laki, K., and Carroll, W.: Thrombin-induced formation of cofibrin I. Isolation, purification and characterization of co-fibrin, J. Biol. Chem. 234:62, 1959.

63. Scheraga, H. A.: Thrombin and its interaction with fibrinogen, Ann. N.Y. Acad. Sci. 75:189, 1958.

64. Gross, R.: Metabolic Aspects of Normal and Pathological Platelets, p. 407, in Blood Platelets, Boston, Little, Brown, 1961.

65. Lorand, L., and Jacobsen, A.: Studies on the polymerization of fibrin, The role of the globulin: fibrin-stabilizing factor, J. Biol. Chem. 230:421, 1958.

66. Duckert, F., Jung, E., and Shmerling, D. H.: A hitherto undescribed congenital hemorrhagic diathesis probably due to fibrin stabilizing factor deficiency, Thromb. Diath. Haem. 5:179, 1960.

67. Wessler, S.: Studies in intravascular coagulation. I. Coagulation changes in isolated venous segments, J. Clin. Invest. 31:1011, 1952.

68. Fell, C., Ivanovic, N., Johnson, S. A., and Seegers, W. H.: Differentiation of plasma antithrombin activities, Proc. Soc. Exp. Biol. & Med. 85:199, 1954.

69. Wessler, S., Ward, K., and Ho, C.: Studies in intravascular coagulation. III. The pathogensis of serum-induced venous thrombosis, J. Clin. Invest. 34:647, 1955.

70. Spaet, T. H., Horowitz, H. I., Zucker-Franklin, D., Cintron, J., and Biezenski, J. J.: Reticuloendothelial clearance of blood thromboplastin by rats, Blood 17: 196, 1961.

71. Sherry, S., Fletcher, A. P., and Alkjaersig, N.: Fibrinolysis and fibrinolytic activity in man, Physiol. Rev. 39:343, 1959.

72. Niewiarowski, S., Kowalski, E., and Stachurska, J.: Influence of fibrinogen derived antithrombin (antithrombin VI) on the blood coagulation, Acta. Biochem. 6:45, 1959.

73. Fletcher, A. P., Alkjaersig, N., and Sherry, S.: Pathogenesis of the coagulation defect developing during pathological plasma proteolytic (fibrinolytic) states. I. The significance of fibrinogen proteolysis and circulating breakdown products, J. Clin. Invest. 41:896, 1962.

74. Finkbiner, R. B., McGovern, J. J., Goldstein, R., and Bunker, J. P.: Coagulation defects in liver disease and response to transfusion during surgery, Am. J. Med. 26:199, 1959.

75. Jones, T. B., and Smith, H. P.: The blood fibrinogen level in hepatectomized dogs and an outline of a method for the quantitative determination of fibrinogen, Am. J. Physiol. 94:144, 1930.

76. Rapaport, S. I.: Plasma thromboplastin antecedent levels in patients receiving coumarin anticoagulants and in patients with Laennec's cirrhosis, Proc. Soc. Exp. Biol. & Med. 108:115, 1961.

77. Merskey, C.: Hemophilia occurring in the human female, Proc. Int. Soc. Hemat. p. 441, 1950.

78. Brinkhous, K. M., and Graham, J.: Hemophilia in the female dog, Science 111:723, 1950.

79. Nilsson, I. M., Blömback, M., Thelin, A., and Von Francken, I.: Carriers of hemophilia A: a laboratory study, Acta Med. scand. 165:357, 1959.

80. Rapaport, S. I., Patch, J. M., and Moore, F. J.: Anti-hemophilic globulin levels in carriers of hemophilia A, J. Clin. Invest. 39:1619, 1960.

81. Barrow, E. M., Bulloch, W. R., and Graham, J. B.: A study of the carrier state for PTC deficiency utilizing a new assay procedure, J. Lab. & Clin. Med. 55:936, 1960.

82. Didisheim, P., and Vandervoort, L. E.: Detection of carriers for Factor IX (PTC) deficiency, Blood. 20:150, 1962.

83. McCain, K. F., Chernoff, A. I., Graham, J. B.: Establishment of the inheritance of Hageman defect as an autosomal recessive trait. Hemophilia and other hemorrhagic states, p. 179, Chapel Hill, U. North Carolina Press. 1959.

84. Rapaport, S. I., Proctor, R. R., Patch, M. J., and Yettra, M.: The mode of inheritance of PTA deficiency: evidence for the existence of major PTA deficiency and minor PTA deficiency, Blood. 18:149, 1961.

85. Graham, J. B., Barrow, E. M., and Hougie, C.: Stuart clotting defect: genetic aspects of a "new" hemorrhagic state, J. Clin. Invest. 36:497, 1957.

86. Kupfer, H. G., Hona, L. B., and Kennie, D. R.: Congenital Factor VII deficiency with normal Stuart activity: clinical, genetic and experimental observations, Blood. 15, 146, 1960.

87. Friedman, I. A., Quick, A. J., Higgens, F., Hussey, C. V., and Hickey, M. E.: Hereditary labile factor (Factor V) deficiency, J.A.M.A. 175:116, 1961.

88. Graham, J. B.: The inheritance of "vascular hemophilia" a new and interesting problem in human genetics, J. Med. Ed. 34:385, 1959.

89. Otto, J. C.: An account of hemorrhagic disposition existing in certain families, Med. Reposit. 61:1803.

90. Graham, J. B., McLendon, W. W., and Brinkhous, K. M.: Mild hemophilia, an allelic form of the disease, Am. J. Med. Sci. 225:46, 1953.

91. Wagner, R. H., Richardson, B. A., and Brinkhous, K. M.: A study of the separation of fibrinogen and antihemophilic factor in canine, porcine and human plasmas, Thromb. Diath. Haem. 1:1, 1957.

92. Blömback, M.: Purification of antihemophilic globulin. I. Some studies on the stability of the antihemophilic globulin activity in fractions I-0, and a method for its partial separation from fibrinogen, Arkiv. F. Kemi. 12:387, 1958.

93. Bidwell, E.: The purification of antihemophilic globulin from animal plasma, Brit. J. Haemat. 1:386, 1955.

94. Tocantins, L. M.: Hemophilic syndromes and hemophilia, Blood. 9:281, 1954.

95. DePalma, A. F., and Colter, J.: Hemophilic arthropathy, Clin. Arthop. 8:163, 1956.

96. Ivins, J. C.: Bone and Joint Complications of Hemophilia, p. 225, *in* Hemophilia and Hemophilioid Diseases. Chapel Hill, U. North Carolina Press, 1959.

97. Jordan, H. H.: Hemophilic Arthropathies, Springfield, Ill., Thomas, 1958.

98. Nye, S. W., Graham, J. B., and Brinkhous, K. M.: The partial thromboplastin time as a screening test for the detection of latent bleeders, Am. J. Med. Sci. 243:279, 1962.

99. Aggeler, P. M., White, S. G., Glendenning, M. B., Page, E. W., Leake, T. B., and Bates, G.: Plasma thromboplastin component (PTC) deficiency, a new disease resembling hemophilia, Proc. Soc. Exper. Biol. & Med. 79:692, 1952.

100. Biggs, R., Douglas, A. S., Macfarlane, R. G., Dacie, J. V., Pitney, W. R., Merskey, C., and O'Brien, J. R.: Christmas disease, a condition previously mistaken for hemophilia, Brit. M.J. 2:1378, 1952.

101. Aggeler, P. M., White, S. G., and Spaet, T. H.: Deuterohemophilia. Plasma thromboplastin component (PTC) deficiency, Christmas disease, hemophilia B, Blood 9:246, 1954.

102. Rapaport, S. I., Shiffman, S., Patch, M. J., and Ware, A. G.: A simple specific one-stage assay for plasma thromboplastin antecedent activity, J. Lab. & Clin. Med. 57:771, 1961.

103. Rosenthal, R. L.: The Present States of Plasma Thromboplastin Antecedent Deficiency, p. 116, *in* Hemophilia and Hemophilioid Diseases. Brinkhous, K., *ed.* Chapel Hill, U. of North Carolina Press, 1957.

104. Alexander, B., Goldstein, R., Landwehr, G., and Cook, C. D.: Congenital SPCA deficiency: a hitherto unrecognized coagulation defect with hemorrhage rectified by serum and serum fractions, J. Clin. Invest. 30:596, 1951.

105. Owren, P. A.: Parahemophilia: hemorrhagic diathesis due to absence of a previously unknown clotting factor, Lancet 1:446, 1947.

106. Alexander, B., and Goldstein, R.: Parahemophilia in three siblings (Owren's disease), Am. J. Med. 13:255, 1952.

107. Fantl, P.: Parahemophilia (Proaccelerin Deficiency) Occurrence and Biochemistry, p. 79, *in* Hemophilia and Hemophilioid Diseases. Brinkhous, K., ed., Chapel Hill, U. North Carolina Press, 1957.

108. Borchgrevink, C. F., Egeberg, O., Pool, J. G., Skulason, T., Stormorken, H., and Waller, B.: A study of a case of congenital hypoprothrombinemia, Brit. J. Hemat. 5:294, 1959.

109. Pool, J. G., Desai, R., and Kropatkin, M.: Severe congenital hypoprothrombinemia in a Negro boy, Thromb. Diath. Haem. 7:235, 1962.

110. Gitlin, D., and Borges, W. H.: Studies on the metabolism of fibrinogen in 2 patients with congenital afibrinogenemia, Blood 8:679, 1953.

111. Frick, P. G., and McQuarrie, I.: Congenital afibrinogenemia, Pediat. 13:44, 1954.

112. Lawson, H. A.: Congenital afibrinogenemia, report of a case, New England J. Med. 298:552, 1953.

113. Sherry, S., Lindmeyer, R. I., Fletcher, A. P., and Alkjaersig, N.: Studies on enhanced fibrinolytic activity in man, J. Clin. Invest. 38:810, 1959.

114. Tagnon, H. J., Levenson, S. M., Davidson, C. S., and Taylor, F. H. L.: The occurrence of fibrinolysis in shock, with observation on the prothrombin time and the plasma fibrinogen during hemorrhagic shock, Am. J. Med. Sci. 211:88, 1946.

115. Sawyer, W. A., Fletcher, A. P., Alkjaersig, N., and Sherry, S.: Studies on the thrombolytic activity of human plasma, J. Clin. Invest. 39:426, 1960.

116. Ratnoff, O. D., Pritchard, J. A., and Copley, J. E.: Hemorrhagic states during pregnancy, New England J. Med. 254:63, 1955.

117. Weiner, A. E., Reid, D. E., and Roby, C. C.: Incoagulable blood in severe premature separation of the placenta. A method of management, Am. J. Obst. & Gynec. 66:475, 1953.

118. Pritchard, J. A., and Wright, M. R.: Pathogenesis of hypofibrinogenemia in placental abruption, New England J. Med. 261:218, 1959.

119. Schneider, C. L.: Fibrin embolism (disseminated intravascular coagulation) with defibrination as one of the end results during placenta abruptio, Surg., Gynec. & Obst. 92:27, 1951.

120. Gollub, S., Ulin, A., Paxson, N. F., Winchell, H. S., O'Riordan, J., Black, M., and Ambrus, J. L.: Obstetrical hemorrhage in criminal abortion and abruptia placentae, J. Lab. & Clin. Med. 53:765, 1959.

121. Reid, D. E., Weiner, A. E., and Roby, C. C.: Intravascular clotting and afibrinogenemia: the presumptive lethal factors in the syndrome of amniotic fluid embolism, Am. J. Obst. & Gynec. 66:465, 1953.

122. Albrechtsen, O., Storm, O., and Troll, D.: Fibrinolytic activity in circulating blood following amniotic fluid infusion, Acta Hemat. 14:309, 1955.

123. Pritchard, J. A., and Ratnoff, O. D.: Studies of fibrinogen and other hemostatic factors in women with intrauterine death and delayed delivery, Surg., Gynec. & Obst. 101: 467, 1955.

124. Jackson, D. P., Hartman, R. C., and Busby, T.: Fibrinogenopenia complicating pregnancy: clinical and laboratory studies, Obst. & Gynec. 5:223, 1955.

125. Chalnot, P., Michon, P., and Lochard, M.: Afibrinémie Mortelle à L'occasion d'une Intervention Endothoracique, Rev. Hemt. 7:27, 1952.

126. von Kaulla, K. N., and Swan, H.: Clotting deviations in man during cardiac by-pass: fibrinolysis and circulating anticoagulant, J. Thoracic Surg. 30:519, 1958.

127. Pisciotta, A. V., and Schulz, E. J.: Fibrinolytic purpura in acute leukemia, Am. J. Med. 19:824, 1955.

128. Sirridge, M. S., Bowman, K. S., and Garber, P. E.: Fibrinolysis and changes in fibrinogen in multiple myeloma, Arch. Int. Med. 101:630, 1958.

129. Nilsson, I. M., Skanse, B., and Gydell, K.: Fibrinolysis in Boeck's sarcoid. Acta Med. scand. 159:463, 1957.

130. Tagnon, H. J., Schulman, P., Whitmore, W. F., and Levine, L. A.: Prostatic fibrinolysis: study of a case illustrating role in hemorrhagic diathesis of cancer of the prostate, Am. J. Med. 15:875, 1953.

131. Bachmann, F., Duckert, F., and Koller, F.: The Stuart-Prower factor assay and its clinical significance, Thromb. Diath. Haem. 2:24, 1958.

132. Owren, P. A.: Control of anticoagulant therapy, Arch. Int. Med. 111:249, 1963.

133. Murphy, E. A., and Mustard, J. F.: Dicumarol therapy and platelet turnover, Circulation Research 9:402, 1962.

134. Aballe, A. J., Banus, V. L., de Lamerens, S., and Rosengvaig, S.: Coagulation studies in the newborn period. Alterations of thromboplastin generation and effects of vitamin K in full-term and premature infants, Am. J. Dis. Child. 94:589, 1957; III. Hemorrhagic disease of the newborn, Am. J. Child 97:524, 1959; IV. Deficiency of Stuart-Prower factor as a part of the clotting defect of the newborn, Am. J. Dis. Child. 97:549, 1959.

135. Hilgartner, M. W.: Personal communication.

136. Fresh, J. W., Ferguson, J. H., Stamey, C., Morgan, F. M., and Lewis, J. H.: Blood prothrombin, proconvertin, and proacceleran in normal infancy. Questionable relationship to vitamin K, Pediatrics 19: 241, 1957.

137. Shanberge, J. N., and Regan, E. E.: The thromboplastin generation heparin tolerance test (TGHTT) in hypocoagulable states, Fed. Proceed. 19:3, 1960.

138. Margolius, A., Jr., Jackson, D. P., and Ratnoff, O. D.: Circulating anticoagulants: a study of 40 cases and a review of the literature, Medicine 40:145, 1961.

139. Lewis, J. H., Ferguson, J. H., Fresh, J. W., and Zucker, M. B.: Primary hemorrhagic diseases, J. Lab. & Clin. Med. 49:211, 1957.

140. Biggs, R., and Bidwell, E.: A method for the study of antihemophilic globulin inhibition with reference to six cases, Brit. J. Hemat. 5:379, 1959.

141. Breckenridge, R. T., and Ratnoff, O. D.: Studies of the nature of the circulating anticoagulant directed against antihemophilic factor: with notes on an assay for antihemophilic factor, Blood 20:137, 1963.

142. Masure, R.: Les Inhibiteurs Normaux et Pathologiques de la Coagulation Sanguine, Brussels, Arscia S.A. 1960.

143. Goldstein, R., Gelfand, M., Sanders, M., and Rosen, R.: Anticoagulant appearing in plasma thromboplastin component (PTC) deficiency, J. Clin. Invest. 35:707, 1956.

144. Conley, C. L., and Hartman, R. C.: A hemorrhagic disorder caused by circulating anticoagulant in patients with disseminated lupus erythematosus, J. Clin. Invest. 31:621, 1952.

145. Lee, S. L., and Sanders, M.: A disorder of blood coagulation in systemic lupus erythematosus, J. Clin. Invest. 34:1814, 1955.

146. Frick, P. G.: Inhibition of the conversion of fibrinogen to fibrin by abnormal proteins in multiple myeloma, Am. J. Clin. Path. 25:1263, 1955.

147. Wayne, L., Goldsmith, R. E., Glueck, H. I., and Berry, H. K.: Abnormal calcium binding associated with hyperglobulinemia, clotting defects, and osteoporosis: a study of this relationship, J. Lab. Clin. Med. 54:958, 1959.

148. Heni, F., and Krauss, I.: Angeborene Familiare Gerinnungsstorung durch Heparintige Hemmkorper, Klin. Wschr. 34:-747, 1956.

149. Czernobilsky, H., and Alexander, B.: Some Qualitative Aspects of Platelet Function in

Normal, Thrombocytopenic and Thrombocytopathic States, p. 565, *in* Blood Platelets, Henry Ford Hospital International Symposium, Boston, Little, Brown, 1961.

150. Emery, J. L., Gordon, R. R., Rendle-Short, J., Varadi, S., and Warrack, A. J. N.: Congenital amegakaryocytic thrombocytopenia with congenital deformities and leukemoid blood picture in newborn, Blood 12:567, 1957.

151. Reinhold, J. D. L., Neumark, H., Lightwood, R., and Carter, C. O.: Familial hypoplastic anemia with congenital abnormalities (Fanconi's syndrome), Blood 7:915, 1952.

152. Cox, E. V., Meynell, M. J., Cooke, W. T., and Gaddie, R.: Scurvy and anemia, Am. J. Med. 32:240, 1962.

153. Pohle, F. J.: Blood platelet counts in relation to menstrual cycle in normal women, Am. J. Med. Sci. 197:40, 1939.

154. Pepper, H., Liebowitz, D., and Linsay, S.: Cyclical thrombocytopenic purpura related to the menstrual cycle, Arch. Path. 61:1, 1956.

155. Minot, G. R.: Purpura hemorrhagica with lymphocytosis. An acute type and an intermittent type, Am. J. Med. Sci. 192:445, 1936.

156. Hjort, P., and Paputchis, H.: Platelet life span in normal, splenectomized and hypersplenic rats, Blood 15:45, 1960.

157. Ekman, C.: Portal hypertension, diagnosis and surgical treatment, Acta Chir. scandinav. Supp. 222:1, 1957.

158. Craddock, C. G., Jr., Adams, W. S., Perry, S., and Lawrence, J. S.: Dynamics of platelet production as studied by depletion techniques in normal and irradiated dogs, J. Lab. & Clin. Med. 45:906, 1955.

159. Jackson, D. P., Krevans, J. R., and Conley, C. L.: Mechanism of the thrombocytopenia that follows multiple whole blood transfusions, Trans. Ass. Am. Physicians 69:155, 1956.

160. Sutherland, D. A., and Clark, H.: Hemangioma associated with thrombocytopenia. Report of a case and review of the literature, Am. J. Med. 33:150, 1962.

161. Wright, C. S., Doan, C. A., Bouroncle, B. A., and Zollinger, R. M.: Direct splenic arterial and venous blood studies in hypersplenic syndromes before and after epinephrine, Blood 6:195, 1951.

162. Ackroyd, J. B.: Pathogenesis of thrombocytopenic purpura due to hypersensitivity to Sedormid, Clin. Sci. 7:249, 1949.

163. Shulman, R. R.: Immunoreactions involving platelets. I. A steric and kinetic model for formation of a complex from a human antibody, quinidine as a haptene, and platelets: and for fixation of complement by the complex, J. Exp. Med. 107:665, 1958.

164. Harrington, W. J., Sprague, C. C., Minnick, V., Moore, C. V., Aulvin, R. C., and Dubach, R.: Immunologic mechanisms in idiopathic and neonatal thrombocytopenic purpura, Ann. Int. Med. 38:433, 1953.

165. Dausset, J., Colin, M., and Colombani, J.: Immune platelet iso-antibodies. Vox. Sang. 5:4, 1960.

166. Shulman, R., Aster, R. H., Leitner, A., and Hiller, M. C.: Immunoreactions involving platelets. V. Post-transfusion purpura due to a complement-fixing antibody against a genetically controlled platelet antigen. A proposed mechanism for thrombocytopenia and its relevance in "autoimmunity", J. Clin. Invest. 40:1597, 1961.

167. Baldini, M., Costea, N., and Ebbe, S.: Studies in the Antigenic Structure of Blood Platelets, p. 378, Proc. VIII Cong. Europ. Soc. Hemat. 1961. Basel and New York, S. Karger, 1962.

168. Shulman, R., Aster, R. H., Pearson, H. A., and Hiller, M. C.: Immunoreactions involving platelets. VI. Reactions of maternal isoantibodies responsible for neonatal purpura. Differentiation of a second platelet antigen system, J. Clin. Invest. 41:1059, 1962.

169. Miescher, P., and Cooper, N.: The fixation of soluble antigen-antibody-complexes upon thrombocytes, Vox. Sang. 5:138, 1960.

170. Harrington, W. J., and Arimura, G.: Immune Reactions of Platelets, p. 659, *in* Blood Platelets, Henry Ford Hospital International Symposium, Boston, Little, Brown, 1961.

171. Tullis, J. L.: Identification and significance of platelet antibodies. New England J. Med. 255:541, 1956.

172. Corn, M., and Upshaw, J. D., Jr.: Evaluation of platelet antibodies in idiopathic thrombocytopenic purpura, Arch. Int. Med. 109:117, 1962.

173. Jackson, D. P., Schmid, H. J., Zieve, P. D., Levin, J., and Conley, C. L.: Nature of a platelet-agglutinating factor in serum of patients with idiopathic thrombocytopenic purpura, J. Clin. Invest. 42:383, 1963.

174. Rabinowitz, Y., and Dameshek, W.: Systemic lupus erythematosus after "idio-

pathic" thrombocytopenic purpura: a review, Ann. Int. Med. 52:1, 1960.

175. Epstein, R. D., Lozner, E. L., Coffey, T. S., and Davidson, C. S.: Congenital thrombocytopenic purpura. Purpura hemorrhagica in pregnancy and in the newborn, Am. J. Med. 9:44, 1950.

176. Moschcowitz, E.: An acute pleiochromic anemia with hyaline thrombosis of the terminal arterioles and capillaries, Arch. Int. Med. 36:89, 1925.

177. Craig, J. M., and Gitlin, D.: The nature of the hyaline thrombi in thrombotic thrombocytopenic purpura, Am. J. Path. 33:251, 1957.

178. Orbsin, J. L.: Morphology of thrombotic thrombocytopenic purpura with demonstration of aneurysms, Am. J. Path. 28:129, 1952.

179. Glanzmann, E.: Hereditare Hammorrhagische thrombasthenie. Ein Beitrag zur Pathologia der blutplattchen, J. Kinderheills 88:113, 1918.

180. Braunsteiner, H., and Pakesch, F.: Thrombocytasthenia and thrombocytopathia—old names and new diseases, Blood 11:965, 1956.

181. Ulutin, O. N.: The Qualitative Platelet Diseases, p. 553, in Blood Platelets, Henry Ford Hospital International Symposium, Boston, Little, Brown, 1961.

182. von Willebrand, E. A.: Hereditare Pseudohemofili, Finska Lab.-sallsk. hande. 68:87, 1926.

183. von Willebrand, E. A., and Jurgens, R. I.: Ueber eine neue Bluterkrankheit, die konstitutionelle Thrombopathie, Klin. Wschr. 12:414, 1933.

184. Alexander, B., and Goldstein, R.: Dual hemostatic defect in pseudohemophilia, J. Clin. Invest. 32:551, 1953.

185. Nilsson, I. M., Blömback, M., Jorpes, E., Blömback, B., and Johansson, S. A.: von Willebrand's disease and its correction with human plasma fraction I-O, Acta Med. scand. 159:179, 1957.

186. Cornu, P., Larrieu, M. J., Caen, J., and Bernard, J.: Transfusion studies in von Willebrand's disease: effect on bleeding time and Factor VIII, Brit. J. Hemat. 9:189, 1963.

187. Biggs, R., and Matthews, J. M.: The treatment of hemorrhage in von Willebrand's disease and the blood level of Factor VIII (AHG), Brit. J. Hemat. 9:203, 1963.

188. Baccuglia, G., and Neel, J. V.: Congenital vascular defect associated with platelet abnormality and antihemophilic factor activity, Blood, 15:807, 1960.

189. Rendu, M.: Epistaxis répétees chez un Sujet Sufferant Pour Angiomes Cutanés et Muquex, Bull. Mem. Soc. Med. Hosp. Paris 13:731, 1896.

190. Osler, W.: On a familial form of recurring epistaxis associated with multiple telangiectases of the skin and mucous membrane, Bull. Johns Hopkins Hosp. 12:333, 1901.

191. Weber, F. P.: A case of multiple hereditary developmental angiomata (telangiectasis) of the skin and mucous membrane associated with recurring hemorrhages, Lancet 2:160, 1907.

192. Bird, R. M., and Jaques, W. E.: Vascular lesion of hereditary hemorrhagic telangiectasia, New England J. Med. 260:597, 1960.

193. Koch, H. J., Jr., Escher, G. C., and Lewis, J. S.: Hormonal management of hereditary hemorrhagic telangiectasia, J.A.M.A. 149:1376, 1952.

194. Wise, D., Wallace, H. J., and Jellinek, E. H.: Angiokeratoma corporis diffusum, a clinical study of eight affected cases, Quart. J. Med. 31:177, 1962.

195. Cetingil, A. I., Ulutin, O. N., and Karaca, M.: A platelet defect in a case of scurvy, Brit. J. Hemat. 4:350, 1958.

196. Flute, P. T., and Howard, A. M.: Blood coagulation in scorbutic pigs: a defect in acceleration by glass contact, Brit. J. Hemat. 5:421, 1959.

197. Vernier, R. L., Farquhar, M. G., Brunson, J. G., and Good, R. A.: Chronic renal disease in children, J. Dis. Child. 96:306, 1958.

198. Allen, D. M., Diamond, L. K., and Howell, D. A.: Anaphylactoid purpura in children (Schönlein-Henoch syndrome) review and a follow-up of the renal complications, J. Dis. Child. 99:833, 1960.

199. Ackroyd, J. F.: Allergic purpura including purpura due to foods, drugs and infections, Am. J. Med. 14:605, 1953.

200. Bywaters, E. G. L., Isdole, I., and Kempton, J. J.: Schönlein-Henoch purpura, Quart. J. Med. 26:161, 1957.

201. Dixon, F. J., Feldman, J. D., and Vasquez, J. J.: Experimental glomerulonephritis. The pathogenesis of a laboratory model resembling the spectrum of human glomerulonephritis, J. Exp. Med. 113:899, 1961.

202. Benacerrai, B., Patter, J. L., McCluskey, R. T., and Miller, F.: The pathologic effects of intravenously administered soluble antigen-antibody complexes. II. Acute glomerulonephritis in rats, J. Exp. Med. 111:195, 1960.

203. Cruichshank, B.: The role of auto-anti-
bodies in anaphylacoid purpura, Immunol.
2:123, 1959.
204. McKusick, V.: Heritable Disorders of Connective Tissue, St. Louis, Mosby, 1960.
205. Soergel, K. H., and Sommers, S. C.: Idiopathic pulmonary hemosiderosis and related syndromes, Am. J. Med. 32:499, 1962.
206. Gardner, F. H., and Diamond, L. K.: Auto-
erythrocyte sensitization: a form of purpura producing painful bruising following
autosensitization to red cells in certain
women, Blood, 10:675, 1955.
207. Agle, D. P., and Ratnoff, O. D.: Purpura
as a psychosomatic entity, Arch. Int. Med.
109:89, 1962.
208. Levin, M. B., and Pinkus, H.: Autosensi-
tivity to desoxyribonucleic acid (DNA)
report of a case with inflammatory skin
lesions controlled by chloroquin. New
England J. Med. 264:533, 1961.
209. Schwartz, R. S., Lewis, B., and Dameshek,
W.: Hemorrhagic cutaneous anaphylaxis
due to autosensitization to deoxyribonucleic acid, N. England J. Med. 267:1105,
1962.
210. Gunz, F. W.: Hemorrhagic thrombocythemia. A critical review, Blood 15:706,
1960.

211. Strauss, W. G.: Purpura hyperglobulinemia of Waldenström: report of a case and
review of literature, New England J. Med.
260:857, 1959.
212. Goetz, R. W., and Good R. A.: Benign
hyperglobulinemic purpura. Relation to
Mikulicz's disease, Sicca syndrome and
epidermolysis bullosa dystrophica, Arch.
Dermat. 83, 26, 1961.
213. Weiss, H. J., Demis, D. J., Elgart, M. L.,
Crawford, S. B., and Crosby, W. H.: Treatment of two cases of hyperglobulinemic
purpura with thioguanine, New England
J. Med. 268:753, 1963.
214. Rosen, F. S.: The macroglobulins, New
England J. Med. 267:491, 1962.
215. Ritzman, S. E., Thurm, R. H., Truaz, W.
E., and Levin, W. C.: The syndrome of
macroglublinemia. Review of the literature and a report of two cases of macroglobulinemia, Arch. Int. Med. 105:939,
1960.
216. Pachter, M. R., Johnson, S. A., Neblett,
T. R., and Truant, J. P.: Bleeding, Platelets, and macroglobulins, Am. J. Clin. Path.
31:467, 1959.
217. Schwab, P. J., and Fahey, J. L.: Treatment
of Waldenström's macroglobulinemia by
plasmapheresis, New England J. Med.
263:574, 1960.

25

Nervousness and Fatigue

EDWIN F. GILDEA

INTRODUCTION

Nervousness and fatigue have so many literary and popular meanings that it is important to define them from the medical point of view.

Nervousness. This word implies a state of either mental or bodily restlessness in which capacities for purposeful activity have become impaired. The subjective components are important. The patient feels uneasy and frequently uncertain as to his abilities, does not know which way to turn and is usually apprehensive.

Fatigue. The term fatigue includes a wide variety of conditions which involve a decrement in potential or actual capacity of a person for work. The patient usually reports a loss of interest and ambition, a disinclination as well as an inability to work or even to play.

Nervousness and fatigue are among the commonest complaints that patients make to their physicians. It is remarkable that textbooks in medicine usually omit any serious discussion of these symptoms. The Cecil-Loeb *Textbook of Medicine*[1] does not list the word fatigue or any discussions under this heading in the index. In Harrison's *Principles of Internal Medicine* there is a good discussion of the subject under a special section and the index refers to fatigue in association with a number of other conditions. Fulton avoids a discussion of fatigue in its broader aspects in his otherwise remarkably thorough *Physiology of the Nervous System*. The people who have encouraged the serious investigation of fatigue have been those concerned with industrial workers, athletes and soldiers. The military problems of World War I gave considerable impetus to the study of fatigue. This special interest lasted for a few years and died away. More recent wars have again thrust the problems of fatigue on the medical profession and on psychologists. Wide variation in the ability of military recruits to withstand the stress of special army tasks has led to a frantic effort to improve the methods of selecting men.[2] The common use of the expressions "combat fatigue," "pilot fatigue," etc., indicate the pressing reality of this complex condition.[3] Bartley's *Fatigue and Impairment in Man,*[3] is a cautious and critical review of the literature and of his own work. It has an excellent bibliography.

In the past the biochemical and biologic investigations of fatigue have been limited by the rigidity of classical biology and biochemistry. With the development of the concepts of biologic relativity one achieves a new view of living organisms. Martin[4] and others have pointed out that there are no sharp boundaries between phenomena. Even the ancient and classical example of life and death has given way to a study of degrees of being alive which correlates with the same relativity for death. There is a general plan or pattern and a hierarchy of complexity in biologic systems extending from the proton to total organisms, from ion to intelligence. There can be no alteration in totality which does not in some measure modify the components thereof.

When the phenomena of fatigue are considered from this relativistic point of view, fatigue becomes *degrees of fatigue* which will correlate with *degrees of capacity* to perform special functions. In the case of the laborer or athlete it is the amount of weight lifted or of distance run in a given time.

The psychological facets of fatigue will be presented as a part of this biologic continuum. We are encouraged to do this by Bartley[5] who, after years of study in this field, has recently recognized the limitations of severely compartmentalized psychology and has suggested that recent discoveries of the remarkable biochemical changes that occur in animals in response to stress should be included in attempts to comprehend the phenomena of fatigue in man.

While we plan to focus our attention on the whole organism and to evaluate what methods are available for measuring degrees of fatigue and capacities of performance we recognize in advance that the problem is infinitely complex and that we will achieve only partial answers at best. In fact the neurophysiologists have found the problem of fatigue in experiments on comparatively simple and isolated units of the nervous system so baffling that many investigators have abandoned the term entirely. The monumental three-volume *Handbook of Neurophysiology*[6] published in 1960 omits fatigue from an otherwise comprehensive index.

In spite of this scientific rejection, fatigue is a phenomenon that controls daily living and is of the utmost importance to employers and workers in industry, to athletics and finally to the military services.

The capacity to experience and to adapt to fatigue is as essential to the growth and development of animals as is the capacity to experience thirst, hunger for food or air, or to experience and adapt to changes in temperature. It is remarkable to find that many of the leading texts in physiology and medicine ignore the phenomena of fatigue while they devote sections to thirst, appetite, hunger, etc. Yet even the most superficial study of the development of young animals, and particularly children, will reveal that the capacity to recognize and adapt to the experience of fatigue is as important as adapting to the experience of appetite, hunger and thirst, heat or cold.

Elsewhere in this book are presented discussions which link various centers in the hypothalamus to temperature regulation, to thirst, appetite, state of consciousness, etc. It seems likely that hypothalamic centers are also concerned in energy regulation and in the sensations of nervousness and fatigue. Apparently these centers receive impulses from higher levels (cerebral) and also from lower levels (somatic and visceral).

The Diencephalon. In recent years, Hess[40] has advanced a plan of functional organization of the diencephalon on the basis of extensive experimental studies, largely in the cat. Although admittedly these concepts have not gained universal acceptance, nonetheless they are of sufficient theoretical interest to be reviewed briefly at this point. Hess subdivides the diencephalon into two fundamentally distinct zones: (1) the *ergotrophic,* or *dynamogenic* zone, extending from the anterior midbrain into the posterior hypothalamus, and (2) the *endophylactic-trophotrophic* zone, encompassing the anterior and lateral hypothalamus, septum, supraoptic and preoptic areas and the ventral nuclei. Stimulation in the *ergotrophic* field produces pupillary dilatation, rise in the blood pressure, tachycardia, and an increased respiratory rate and depth, along with a state of heightened motor excitability. In the trophotrophic field, the opposite effects are observed—pupillary constriction, hypotension, diminished respiratory activity and a state of relative adynamia and lethargy, as well as a variety of other phenomena including salivation, retching, vomiting, urination and defecation. The activity of the ergotrophic field is considered to be sympathetic in nature, that of the trophotrophic field parasympathetic. Exteroceptive mechanisms (visual, auditory or painful stimuli) are considered to play a significant role in the activation of the ergotrophic system; enteroceptive stimuli from a variety of viscera activating the trophotrophic system. Thus, Hess postulates two mutually antagonistic systems, one oriented toward *catabolic* events and energy utilization, the ergotrophic, the other toward *anabolic* mechanisms and the preservation of energy, the trophotrophic.

Neurohumoral Transmission, Tranquilizers, Psychic Energizers. Brodie[41] and Baker[42] have advanced this scheme still further by relating the action of various psychotherapeutic agents to neurohumoral transmission within these two systems. The neurohumoral transmitting agent within the ergotrophic system is considered to be *norepinephrine*: in the trophotrophic system, *serotonin*. The tranquilizing and parasympathetic, or cholinergic, effects of the Rauwolfia alkaloids are thought to be due to a direct stimulation of the trophotrophic system by releasing the stored mediator substance serotonin, whereas the similar clinical effects of the phenothiazine derivatives are due to a direct blockage of the norepinephrine-ergotrophic system (a so-called adrenergic blockade). Stimulants such as amphetamine and mescaline are adrenergic agents and activate the ergotrophic system, probably by virtue of the phenylethylamine grouping common to these drugs as well as to norepinephrine itself. LSD-25 also activates the ergotrophic system, presumably because it too contains a phenylethylamine grouping. Since an indole group is also part of its chemical structure, LSD-25 may in addition compete with the indole-containing serotonin for reactor sites. The monoamine-oxidase inhibitors, the "psychic energizers," similarly have an adrenergic, ergotrophic action, but the mechanism here is still different in that these compounds appear to act by interfering with the destruction of norepinephrine by enzymatic activity.[43]

Nutrition. In addition to the concepts of homeostasis the recognition that animals, including man, are essentially energy-capturing devices[7] will aid in our study of fatigue. To live, the organism must continually drain energy from its environment. Living organisms take up energy of higher potential and give it off at a lower potential. Fundamentally the amount of energy that the human organism is capable of producing depends largely on food-energy intake.

The discoveries of the modern science of nutrition have become so generally accepted that often it is forgotten that the amount and the chemical composition of the diet determine a man's capacity to perform work. Deficits of calories are quickly manifested by a decrease in work capacity, i.e., fatigue. More subtly and after lapse of time deficits of protein, vitamins and minerals result in increasing fatigability.

The science of nutrition has reached a point where a balanced diet can be prescribed that makes it possible for man and animals to achieve a predictable optimum work output. Furthermore, such diets can be provided in most civilized countries and consequently food deficiencies are rarely a factor in producing fatigue in this country. The effects of the balance or lack of balance in various dietary components appear also to be important in developing maximum capacity for work, but the data on this subject are controversial.[8]

PATHOLOGIC PHYSIOLOGY OF NERVOUSNESS

Nervousness arises as the result of almost any break in the complex integrations that are necessary for maintaining normal human behavior. These symptoms appear particularly when the source of the disturbance of integration is not obvious to the patient. For example, in the prodromal period of a chronic disease, such as tuberculosis or cancer, the patient notes that he is not able to work the way he used to, that he is "lazy." This disturbs his confidence in his ability. He becomes uncertain as to whether he should give in to the laziness or drive himself to work, and in this conflict he loses confidence, his former ambitions seem unattainable—in short, he summarizes this trouble as nervousness. Some order can be brought out of this generalization with regard to the various origins of nervousness by outlining the various levels of personality organization that may be impaired.

The psychological level is the one in which disturbances of integration most frequently produce the symptoms of nervousness. Frustrations in attaining the common goals of life are the most frequent origin of nervousness. The prodromal symptoms of the major psychoses, particularly in manic-depressives and schizophrenics, may appear as mere nervousness.

At the **neurologic level** various injuries to the brain such as encephalitis and sequelae of head trauma result in nervousness.

Diseases of endocrines probably would be the next most common occasion for nervousness.

Nutritional deficiencies may produce these symptoms.

Finally, a **miscellaneous group** of diseases including infections, toxic conditions, drugs and poisons must be considered. Alcoholism is the commonest cause of drug-induced fatigue. A wide variety of drugs may produce easy fatigability. For example, barbiturates, bromides, morphine or arsenic taken over a long period may produce chronic fatigue.

Psychopathology of Nervousness. Only a brief outline of the psychodynamics of nervousness can be included in this chapter. Certain general rules of examination, if followed, will reveal the fact that mental and emotional difficulties are probably at the root of the symptoms of nervousness in the majority of patients.[9] If it is found that the patient has failed or is failing to achieve the status in the community that is in keeping with his age, family and cultural background and his ambitions, psychologic conflicts are probably the leading factors in the nervousness. Each component of the patient's development as a person should be investigated. Of particular importance is the level of development of the patient's psychosexual life. If he is an adult, he should have achieved independence of his family, both psychologically and economically. If the person has not married and established congenial relations with his wife leading to children, such a person will nearly always be a frustrated individual, and these frustrations usually produce symptoms of nervousness. If an adult does not have a job that he respects, with an economic return approximating his needs and ambitions, these frustrations may be the source of his nervousness.

In general, the lack of specific goals, plans for the future and the absence of a feeling of belonging to a social group in a community and to a family are basic sources of nervousness that should be looked for. It should also be remembered that the symptoms of nervousness may arise only in specific situations. For example, some people will be free of nervous symptoms when they are on vacation; others may have the symptoms only when they are at home or, more specifically, for example, when a mother- or a father-in-law is in the home. On the other hand, the personality disorganization may reach the point where there are practically no life situations in which the patient is not nervous.

Although it may be difficult to differentiate nervousness due to psychologic disorders from that due to other factors, the problem is usually a simple one if a careful history is obtained with attention to precise chronology. The exact time of the onset of the nervousness should be determined. In the case of the patient who has been reasonably competent in life it will be found that the nervousness has begun comparatively recently, and it will be possible to demonstrate that specific symptoms of disease have begun to appear not long after the onset of the nervousness. For example, in patients who report seasonal attacks of nervousness, it can be shown that there was a definite change in dietary habits with season, and further investigation establishes that in these periods food intake was deficient in one or more essential elements. On examination of the patient specific evidence of dietary deficiency may be demonstrated. The administration of the deficient elements will then produce a fairly prompt and striking relief of symptoms.[10]

PATHOLOGIC PHYSIOLOGY OF FATIGUE

Like nervousness, susceptibility to fatigue depends on the degree of stability and integration of the whole person. Fatigue may occur as a result of exhaustion of metabolic reserves.[8,11,12] It may also arise as a symptom of physiologic disorganization. Cannon's conception of homeostasis is useful in understanding the problem of susceptibility to fatigue. It can also be extended to the psychological sphere. It is noteworthy that fatigability as seen in patients arises uncommonly from exhaustion of metabolic reserves[12,14] A study by Allan[13] of 300 consecutive cases admitted to the Lahey Clinic with the chief complaint of weakness and fatigue discovered physical disorders as etiologic factors in only 20 per cent of the patients. The great majority, 80 per cent, proved to be suffering from nervous disorders of various kinds. The physical disorders responsible for fatigue were: chronic infections, 4.3 per cent; metabolic disorders, 4.0 per cent; neurologic, 5.5 per cent; heart disease, 2.7 per cent; anemia from five causes, 1.7 per cent; and nephritis, 1.0 per cent. Miscellaneous (1.3 per cent) included lung tumor, one case each of vitamin deficiency, Hodgkin's disease and unclassified fever. Pathologic fatigue should be distinguished from "normal fatigue." Normal fatigue appears only after strenuous work, and a rest period rapidly restores the patient's feeling of well-being as well as his capacity for work.

In the case of pathologic fatigue the patient frequently arises from a long rest period feeling more fatigued than ever. The psychopathology and the psychodynamics of pathologic fatigue are similar to those of nervousness. Again, the diseases that produce symptoms of fatigue are similar to those for nervousness. Injuries to the brain or the nervous system may result in easy fatigability. In the sequelae of head injuries easy fatigability may be the leading symptom. In the case of endocrine disorders, Addison's disease constitutes one of the dramatic examples. The prodromal symptoms of diabetes mellitus and thyroid disease may well be those of easy fatigability. This is true also of nutritional disorders, chronic and infectious diseases, toxic states and poisons. The results of the search for a specific fatigue toxin have been negative. At the present time it is thought that the normal human being possesses a comfortable margin of metabolic reserve and develops symptoms of fatigue only when activity is prolonged well beyond the usual civilian level.

The studies of metabolic function in industrial workers[8,14,15,16] and in athletes have served to establish this principle. Through the findings of these investigators, which actually depend on our knowledge of biochemistry and metabolism, some of the disorders that produce pathologic fatigue are known. It has been established that the amounts of the constituents in the blood are maintained continually within a relatively narrow range. Variation in these constituents above or below these narrow limits frequently results in the patient's experiencing a sense of fatigue as well as an actual decrement in capacity to perform work. The brain is particularly dependent on a continual and stable supply of *oxygen* and *glucose*. Consequently, conditions that impair this supply most frequently produce easy fatigability. Congenital defects of the heart that may impair circulation can be responsible for chronic easy fatigability in spite of the fact that other evidences of circulatory failure are absent. Various kinds of anemia decrease the oxygen supply of the brain and are common conditions encountered by the clinician. The disturbances in carbohydrate metabolism that are most commonly encountered are the hypoglycemia due to hyperinsulinism and the hyperglycemia associated with diabetes mellitus. Disturbances in the regulation of the hydrogen ion concentration and the amount and the nature of serum calcium, sodium and potassium probably come next in importance. Deficiencies of the blood proteins are not infrequently found in a variety of conditions. The accumulation of metabolic waste products in the blood, such as ketone bodies in diabetes mellitus and the protein residues that accumulate in kidney disorders, are important in causing states of chronic fatigability. The frequent ingestion of many drugs and of alcohol produces chronic fatigability and nervousness. Any imbalance in the complex integration of the endocrines may produce pathologic fatigue. Disorders of the thyroid, the ovaries, the pancreas and the adrenals are the best known. The pituitary is probably extremely important in this connection. For example, large doses of adrenocorticotropic hormone, when injected intramuscularly, produce a marked feeling of well-being in most patients and occasional states of elation and excitement. Much remains to be learned about the mechanism of its action.

Most people experience fatigue as the result of mental and emotional conflicts, and particularly as a result of frustration in the pursuit of one or more of their fundamental interests. While these statements hold true in the statistical sense, there are such marked individual differences that caution has to be employed in applying them to individual patients. For example, there are apparently healthy people who actually develop symptoms of fatigue and nervousness if they postpone a meal for even as much as an hour; they also develop these symptoms whenever they go beyond their usual amount of physical activity. They can be relieved of these symptoms by the ingestion of small amounts of carbohydrate-containing food. Such patients may or may not always have remarkably low blood sugar at the time their symptoms are severe. The same problems are encountered in evaluating the significance of a moderate degree of anemia in producing symptoms of fatigue. Individual differences in the effects of alcohol, hypnotics and other drugs and poisons are not uncommon.[17]

The recent advances in the knowledge of the chemistry of muscles and nerves have given us insight into many of the steps in metabolism that are essential to normal nerve and muscle function. The importance of high energy bonds of phosphorus have been particularly stressed as essential sources of energy. For this reason, adenosine triphosphate[44] has been tried in the treatment of patients suffering from acute and chronic fatigue. Albeaux-Fernet and associates treated a series of 45 patients with intramuscular injections of ATP and reported a significant relief in symptoms.

Laborit[45] and his associates made an extensive exploratory study of many of the chemical components of the Krebs cycle. They used rats exposed to forced swimming as a standard test. A number of chemical substances were found that improved the rats' capacity to survive the test. Potassium and magnesium aspartates were found to be particularly effective. Comparison with controls were strikingly significant. They went on to try aspartates on soldiers and reported both prevention and relief of fatigue after strenuous exercise in a significantly large series or men. Shaw et al.[46] repeated this work on a wide variety of patients suffering from pathologic fatigue and reported favorable effects. Out of this work a standard preparation of potassium and sodium salts of aspartates was developed and named Spartase. Lasagna et al.[47] set up a carefully designed and controlled experiment to evaluate the effects of Spartase. They used athletes who were also prisoners and who were highly motivated to participate in specific standardized strenuous athletic activities. No differences were found between placebos and Spartase. There have been many other clinical trials with Spartase that confirm its efficacy. Unfortunately, a recent review of this subject by the Council on Drugs of the American Medical Association[48] concluded that the efficacy of Spartase had not been convincingly established.

Finally, there are people[18] who manifest marked susceptibility to fatigue early in childhood. Exercise, minor frustrations and excitement produce nervousness, palpitation, fatigue, sweating, breathlessness, muscle tremor and weakness. Some of these people seem to have been defective from birth, others developed the condition after severe head trauma or after encephalitis.

DIFFERENTIAL DIAGNOSIS

The first problem of diagnosis[19] in cases with nervousness and fatigue lies in determining which symptoms came first.

Nervousness can be an important factor in producing fatigue. On the other hand, a person who is chronically fatigued frequently becomes nervous because of his inadequacy and his apprehension over the future. The fatigue occurring in organic disease often results in fears and frustrations expressed as nervousness. A detailed and discriminating history is essential in solving this problem. If the nervousness clearly appeared before symptoms of fatigue occurred, the probabilities are that the source of the difficulty will prove to be psychological. On the other hand, if easy fatigability appeared some time before the nervousness some disease like tuberculosis, Addison's disease, diabetes, or dietary deficiency should be looked for.

Another useful generalization is that if nervousness and fatigue have lasted for a year or two it is improbable that any known physical disorders in prodromal stage will prove to be responsible for the symptoms. Denker[20] found in a study of a large series of insurance disability claims for psychoneuroses that by the end of a year physical factors missed when the first diagnosis was made had developed to a point where they were readily observed and diagnosis corrected. He also noted that 73 per cent of the psychoneurotic patients had recovered from their psychoneuroses sufficiently to terminate disability claims within two years of onset. Therefore, when nervousness and fatigue have persisted for more than two years chronic psychoneuroses, or less frequently other mental disorders, such as depression or schizophrenia are usually responsible for these symptoms.

MENTAL DISORDERS

As all major mental disorders may begin with symptoms of nervousness or in their abortive form may reveal only nonspecific symptoms of nervousness, the possibility of these conditions should be considered.

It is a remarkable fact that in spite of much work on the part of biochemists and psychiatrists no consistent biochemical or physiologic abnormality has been found in patients with the common mental disorders. This statement is made in spite of the fact that many investigators have claimed and are claiming to have found abnormal metabolites or errors in metabolism in the blood and the urine of schizophrenic,[21,22] depressive,[23] or neurotic patients. However, these claims have not as yet been corroborated by other competent investigators. Therefore, we still have to depend on the history and the symptoms for diagnosis and indications for treatment.

This is the place to point out that the world-wide enthusiasm for the new "tranquilizers and energizers" has produced a new group of patients with drug-induced consequences ranging from fatigue and nervousness, and parkinsonism, to stupor and sometimes death.[24]

When properly used, however, the new drugs such as chlorpromazine, meprobamate and many others have proved effective in ameliorating the symptoms of severely psychotic patients.[22] They also have promise as tools in investigation but at present our knowledge of them is entirely empirical. The most effective drugs are those that control nervousness, agitation and overactivity.[24] The most commonly used are the phenothiazines. The drugs for reducing depression and relieving fatigue are not nearly so effective. In fact, in double-blind studies they appear to be little if any more effective than the placebos.[25-29]

The possible relationships of tranquilizing or of energizing drug actions to "ergotrophic" and "trophotrophic" centers in the hypothalamus has been discussed in the Introduction to this chapter, with comment upon evidence that drugs, like certain metabolites, nutrients, toxins, etc., may influence the neurohumoral transmitting agents norepinephrine and serotonin.

PSYCHOSES

Manic-depressive psychosis, depressed phase, is the mental disorder most frequently overlooked as the cause of nervousness and fatigue. For practical purposes, the terms *melancholia* and *mental depression* are synonymous. The psychoneuroses are much more common and they are generally recognized as an etiologic factor in symptoms of fatigue and nervousness. Manic-depressive tendencies may be discovered by investigating the stability of the patient's mood and his work record. If it is found that the patient has been subject to occasional periods of "blue spells" that broke into his otherwise cheerful outlook on life, the possibility of manic-depressive psychosis should be considered. Again, if there are unexplained periods when the patient did little or no work for two or three months or more, in contrast with his usual high work accomplishment, this fact is evidence in favor of such a disorder. Many patients are unaware of these swings of activity and whenever they experience the inability to work they seek for some respectable reason for their incapacity. They often merely state that they are nervous because their eyes are bothering them. In spite of the fact that they have consulted many of the leading ophthalmologists and have been repeatedly reassured about their eyes, they persist in this complaint. Any other part of the body may be fixed on in this way. The symptoms reported by the patient may be surprisingly specific for a particular disorder and lead to extensive medical investigations and even to surgery. It is important to recognize these manic-depressive disorders because they tend to be self-limited, and the patient will recover if he is not mistreated due to the failure of the physician to recognize the source of his disorder.

Stone and Burris[30] have reported on 50 cases of mental depression or melancholia that were misdiagnosed and mistreated for from three months to three years before their correct condition was recognized. The incorrect diagnoses were diabetes mellitus, hypertension, arteriosclerosis, thyroid disease, menopause, peptic ulcer, gallbladder disease, brucellosis, hysteria and senility. It is noteworthy that 95 per cent of these cases recovered on treatment with electroshock. The following case history illustrates this commonly neglected disease:

Case 1. A male, aged 52, was referred to the psychiatric clinic complaining of several frontal headaches, nervousness, easy fatigability, right-sided pain which extended into the urethra, frequent and painful micturition. If questioned further, he complained of symptoms referable to almost every system in the body.

PRESENT ILLNESS. Onset of symptoms occurred 8 months previously, with nervousness shortly followed by easy fatigability. He noticed that he could not read for more than a few minutes without feeling tired and having the letters blur. He then noted the frontal headaches. He had numerous changes of his glasses, although the ophthalmologist told him that his only difficulty lay in a moderate degree of farsightedness, which was adequately corrected with reading glasses. He was then treated for chronic sinusitis. Fatigability increased and he gave up working. He was more tired in the morning than he was when he went to bed in the evening. He had his tonsils removed, but fatigability and nervousness became more marked. He then was referred to a genitourinary specialist because by this time he was complaining of frequency. Pyelograms and repeated urine examinations were made. Frequency and difficulty of micturition became more marked. A circumcision was performed in the hope that it would improve his condition. Finally the patient began to think that he was making his wife ill, that there was no use in his living any longer, and he found it practically impossible to get out of bed before noon. He lost weight rapidly and at the time of admission this loss amounted to 30 pounds. His weight when well was 170 pounds.

PHYSICAL EXAMINATION. On admission, physical examination revealed a well-developed man, who showed evidence of recent weight loss and malnutrition. He looked discouraged, was slow in his movements and answered questions slowly in monosyllables. The other positive findings were slight tremor of outstretched hands, ill-defined abdominal tenderness on palpation, and flat feet.

MENTAL EXAMINATION. The patient looked as though he felt extremely sad, was slow in his movements and in his speech. He stated that he was sure he had some hopeless disease, that he probably had given it to his wife, that there was no use in his living any longer. Except for slowness in response, his intellectual functions were not impaired. He was well oriented in all spheres.

PAST HISTORY. The patient had been a healthy young man, who graduated from high school and had been a successful athlete. He played semiprofessional baseball. In high school he had partly worked his way. On leaving school he entered a small machine shop and worked up to the position of foreman in a large plant. Just after he had received his first promotion at the age of 21, he suffered from sleeplessness and insomnia and easy fatigability. He went to a number of physicians who stated that they were unable to find anything wrong with him. Finally one man pointed out to him that he had been working overtime for many years in addition to playing semiprofessional baseball and that he rarely allowed himself more than six hours sleep at night. This physician stated that he had nervous exhaustion and all he needed was a long rest. He gave up his job and went to Florida where he spent the winter with some relatives. The patient volunteered that he had the same kind of nervousness at that time as with his present illness except that it was not so bad. By spring he felt as well as ever, returned to the old job and also became an officer in a union and joined a number of clubs.

When he was 31, his mother died. He was terribly upset, his nervousness returned and he was unable to work. It required a year for him to recover from this tragedy. Subsequently the patient resumed his high level of work and social activity and was in excellent health until the present illness.

SUBSEQUENT COURSE. It was easy to persuade the patient that his present illness was similar to his previous illnesses, that although it was a little more severe he could be as sure of recovery this time as formerly. This reassurance helped the patient considerably. He responded well to hydrotherapy, his nervousness subsided and he gradually became able to do a little work in occupational therapy. In 6 weeks he recovered sufficiently to be discharged. Two weeks after discharge he returned for a checkup, at which time he was practically recovered. He was working again and had begun to take up his activities as a union officer. He stated that he could not understand what had made him feel so bad.

This type of history is not uncommon. Almost any variation of such an illness can occur. Many patients who are thought to have brucellosis or malaria or chronic appendicitis belong to this manic-depressive group. The diagnosis is often suggested by the evidence of previous similar attacks of loss of ability to work and depression in mood that have been followed by complete recovery. Most of these patients are able and vigorous people in between their attacks.

Symptoms of nervousness and multiple physical complaints may be used by some patients to cover up their disturbed mental content.

Some schizophrenics may actually have many delusions or hallucinations that are making them very uncomfortable. They try to attribute them to their physical disabilities. One striking example of this sort of condition is given:

Case 2. A young woman 28 years of age with a complaint of nervousness went to the State Capitol to inquire where she could go for an honest appraisal of her health. She was referred to the psychopathic hospital. During the first two interviews in the outpatient clinic she gave a long history that included difficulty in swallowing, attacks of palpitation, diarrhea, weight loss and intolerance to heat. She had consulted many of the leading medical centers on the Atlantic seaboard. At one place she was advised to have her thyroid removed, but she eloped from the hospital before the operation. The early impression from the first three interviews was that the patient had sufficient symptoms to warrant the tentative diagnosis of hyperthyroidism. A basal metabolic rate determination was attempted, but the patient was convinced that the apparatus would choke her to death, and a satisfactory test was not obtained. On the fourth interview she was even more nervous than before. An effort was made to discover what was troubling her. It was only at the end of the hour when she was about to leave that she suddenly turned and said, "Oh, those people—they are trying to strangle me." She was persuaded to sit down again and with a little urging poured out the complex story of the way her stepmother had hired people to persecute her. The choking feelings came when she felt that these people came up behind her and were strangling her. She thought her thyroid was diseased and was the cause of her troubles. She stated, however, that many times when she was under observation in various hospitals she had been on the point of telling the doctor about the persecutions when the doctor would terminate the interview. The ultimate diagnosis proved to be schizophrenia.

Cases like this are more commonly overlooked for years than is generally realized. Some investigation of the patient's content of thought would prevent these mistakes.

PSYCHONEUROSES

The commonest instances of nervousness and fatigue, however, arise not from major mental illnesses such as psychoses but from acute or chronic psychologic and emotional maladjustments. These conditions are usually grouped under the term psychoneurosis. A brief personal history usually will make the diagnosis evident.

Neurocirculatory Asthenia. This group of psychoneurotic patients[18] appears to have been extremely susceptible to fatigue from childhood. They are thought to have a fundamental defect in their vasomotor regulatory mechanisms. Moderate exercise brings on symptoms of fatigue, sweating, breathlessness, palpitation and nervousness. During exercise the blood lactic acid rises much more rapidly than in normal controls. Unlike patients with other forms of neuroses who were healthy and vigorous children and whose symptoms appeared only after severe emotional conflicts or life crises, the patients with neurocirculatory asthenia have usually developed symptoms under moderate stress or no stress at all.

Anxiety States, Hysteria, Obsessive-Compulsive States, Hypochondriasis. These terms include diagnoses made in the great majority of psychoneurotic patients. In most patients these symptoms have begun in adolescence and the afflicted person has never been completely free from them. In other cases the symptoms date from the beginning of marriage or from the delivery of the first baby. Situations under which human beings may become frustrated and maladjusted are too numerous to enumerate here. It should be sufficient to emphasize that enough personal history should be taken on each patient to provide information as to whether or not there were frustrations or disappointments or changes in the patient's life at the time of the onset of the illness. When such a connection can be demonstrated it is almost certain that the nervousness and fatigability are due to this situation. Obtaining evidence of this type is something of an art. The patient who has been hurt by failures or unresolved conflicts frequently "forgets" that the events transpired. Such experiences gather emotional energy about them and become like a deep-seated abscess that builds up pressure, discharges toxic elements into the blood stream and makes the whole person ill. These repressed distressing experiences tend to build

up emotional or nervous tension that finds psychopathologic expression by making the patient feel vaguely uneasy, anxious, tense, guilty, and leading him to compensatory forms of ineffective behavior. He knows there is something wrong. He thinks "Perhaps I have a focus of infection." The job for the physician is to discover whether the focus is psychologic or pyogenic. Adequate drainage in either case will bring about a remarkable improvement in the symptoms of fatigue and nervousness. This does not mean that people with psychoneurotic illnesses cannot also develop tuberculosis, brucellosis or other diseases. The fact that a patient is a psychoneurotic should not prevent the physician from making a thorough medical examination.

In Allan's study of the Lahey Clinic patients whose chief complaint was fatigue, the 80 per cent group of nervous disorders included 15 per cent with psychoneuroses and 63 per cent with "benign nervous states." This latter group by definition belongs with the psychoneuroses. The fact that a neurotic reaction is mild does not mean that the patient is not psychoneurotic. Many apparently benign neuroses turn out to be severe when neglected. It is noteworthy that only 2 per cent in this series were considered depressions, i.e., manic-depressive depressed. From the experience of psychiatrists there should also have been one or two schizophrenic patients in a series as large as 300. The figures thus revised indicate that 78 per cent of nervous disorders producing fatigue as first complaint were psychoneuroses, while 2 per cent were psychoses. This figure approximates estimates of the comparative frequency of neuroses in the psychiatric literature.

After one has established the diagnosis of psychoneurosis, an attempt should be made to evaluate the severity and type of neurosis. If the symptoms began in childhood or adolescence and there have been only partial remissions and many kinds of situations produce exacerbations, the prognosis is poor.

Anorexia Nervosa. These cases are so dramatic (see Fig. 200) due to the extremeness of malnutrition that they are officially classified independently of the psychoneuroses. This is in spite of the fact that the cases almost uniformly have been shown to be caused by a rejection of food because of emotional conflicts. Adjustment to or relief of these conflicts has repeatedly resulted in recovery. Recurrence of symptoms may come with reactivation of the conflict, thereby confirming the importance of the psychological components back of the psychoneurosis. These patients are usually young women who are sensitive, immature and dependent. The symptoms have arisen because of fancied or real deprivation of love or because food has come to represent something disgusting.

The following examples may be cited:

Case 3. A 16-year-old girl had grown up with an only brother. The parents both worked and paid little attention to the extreme dependence this girl had on her brother. His going away to college precipitated the illness. The patient weighed only 60 pounds on admission to the hospital. Intravenous and tube feedings kept the patient alive but her brother had to return home before her appetite returned.

Case 4. A girl of 14 suffered a moderate degree of anorexia after father's death. She recovered in two months. At 16 she returned to the hospital in a severely emaciated condition. She was a very shy, sensitive girl who had always kept her thoughts to herself. The mother was a talkative, busy woman who never understood the child. "She is like her father's sisters." The patient was slow in recovering. The psychologic factors were difficult to get from the patient. Ultimately after two months it was revealed that a maternal uncle lived with the family. He was a big, gross creature and an enormous and messy eater. The patient would lose her appetite watching him eat. She usually would try to finish eating before he sat down at the table. The crisis came when the patient surprised this uncle having sexual intercourse with her favorite older sister. Her sister, although embarrassed, laughed and said that they would "teach her how" some day. This patient not only lost her ideal of a sister whom she formerly thought to be perfect but also had associated any thought of food with the uncle and gross sex behavior.

Anorexia nervosa should be differentiated from Simmonds' disease (pituitary cachexia). This is usually not difficult because Simmonds' disease usually occurs in older people, sometimes after pregnancy, or after tumor, trauma or vascular lesions with acute injury of the pituitary. (Chap. 33.)

NEUROLOGIC CONDITIONS

The neurologic conditions that must be considered are cerebral vascular disorders, the sequelae to head injuries, postencephalitic disorders, cerebral syphilis, multiple sclerosis, subacute combined system disease and tumors of the brain. These cases are often not recognized because a neurologic examination has not been done and no one has thought of them as a possibility where nervousness and fatigue are leading features.

ENDOCRINE DISORDERS

Many patients with endocrine disorders complain of fatigue and nervousness, sometimes to an incapacitating degree. Differential diagnosis as to the relative importance of the endocrine dyscrasia versus psychologic conflicts can be made only with the aid of a careful personal history in addition to physical and special metabolic examinations. It should be stated that, even with all the information available and the most careful psychiatric investigation, many of these patients remain unsolved problems.

Thyroid Disorders

Hyperthyroidism of various degrees is not uncommon. Easy excitability, apprehensiveness and every type of "nervousness" are characteristic of hyperthyroidism. Fatigue is a prominent symptom. Whenever palpitation, tremor, eye signs, perspiration, heat intolerance, etc., are seen with or without thyroid enlargement, hyperthyroidism must be considered.

One often sees persons with many of the symptoms commonly attributed to hyperthyroidism who do not have overactive thyroids. However, the recognition of the importance of thyroid disorders in producing symptoms of nervousness and easy fatigability is one of the brilliant contributions of medicine. Patients with rapidly developing states of hyperthyroidism usually do not present a problem in diagnosis and treatment, but there is a considerable group of patients whose symptoms began insidiously and apparently were precipitated and aggravated by emotional difficulties. These patients are nervous, complain of easy fatigability and may or may not have tremor, tachycardia, sweating and diarrhea. They are so tense and restless that it is difficult to interpret the results of basal metabolic tests. The administration of iodides usually results in uncertain degrees of improvement. Until quite recently, thyroidectomy remained the only certain method of differential diagnosis. A number of patients were not improved by thyroidectomy; in fact, although their basal metabolic rates fell to and below normal limits, they remained nervous and easily fatigued. Recently methods for determining serum iodide have been improved to a point where they can be used in differential diagnosis. Man, Riggs and associates[31] have devised a practical method for determining protein-bound iodine in serum and have shown that this fraction can be employed as a measure of active thyroid hormone. This method has proved effective in differential diagnosis. High protein-bound serum iodine indicates overactivity of the thyroid.

The development of the radioactive iodine uptake methods have greatly refined the means of evaluation of thyroid activity.[32] The discovery of active fractions of thyroid hormone has suggested a solution to atypical low metabolism patients who did not respond to thyroxin. For example, much has been claimed for triiodothyronine in treatment of borderline cases of thyroid deficiency. Early promising results suggesting superiority to thyroxin have not been confirmed.

Hypothyroidism, when it develops insidiously, may produce marked increase in fatigability in the absence of signs of myxedema. Moderate bradycardia, dry skin and sensitivity to cold may be present. The patient reacts to this decreased capacity for work by becoming irritable and apprehensive about the future and often says that he is nervous. Occasionally, such a patient may be so nervous that the test of the basal metabolic rate may not be reliable. Measurement of the serum cholesterol is helpful in this problem. A high cholesterol will almost invariably be found if the patient has thyroid deficiency. Protein-bound serum iodine determination is also of value, a low value indicating hypothyroidism. Normal serum protein-bound iodine levels range from 4 to 8 μg. per 100 ml. of serum. Values of 4 or below suggest deficient thyroid hormone secretion.

PITUITARY DISORDERS

Pituitary disease is a rare but striking cause of fatigue. Hypopituitarism of pituitary cachexia type (Simmonds' disease) produces extreme debility. Late stages of acromegaly often are characterized by easy exhaustion which belies the falsely robust appearance. Low thyroid function, adrenal cortical deficiency and gonadal failure contribute to the muscle atrophy, weakness and fatigue of pituitary deficiency.

OVARIAN DYSFUNCTION

This subject constitutes a difficult and controversial field. Loss of both ovaries by a woman before the normal age for the menopause practically always produces nervousness and easy fatigability in addition to other symptoms. Few women who have been castrated prematurely ever recover their former stability or capacity for work. The effects of partial ovarian dysfunction are extremely variable. Most of the symptoms attributed to hypofunction of the ovary are similar to those complained of by psychoneurotics. Suggestion, reassurance and special attention from the physician can do much to alleviate these symptoms. The actual effect of replacement therapy under these circumstances has proved extremely difficult to evaluate. One has only to look back in the older literature to be aware of these difficulties. At that time what are now known to be inactive ovarian preparations were reported as being therapeutically effective. Today physicians realize that one must establish the presence of the characteristic hot flashes and other more definite symptoms, usually including amenorrhea, before one accepts the diagnosis of ovarian deficiency. When these symptoms are not present, the nervousness may well be due to other conditions.[30]

Now that potent oral estrogens are available, the psychotherapeutic effects of injections and of trips to the doctor's office can be eliminated. It is possible to establish the diagnosis of estrogen deficiency by vaginal smears and hormone assays. Estrogen therapy may be of great value in relieving nervous tension, irritability and fatigue when a true estrogen deficiency is present.

TESTICULAR DEFICIENCY

Prepubertal males who are castrated or who have deficient testicular development suffer from nervousness, have poor muscular development and fatigue easily. The "male climacteric" is less well-defined, much less frequent, usually less severe, and comes on some 10 to 15 years later than the menopausal syndrome in women. Nervous symptoms and fatigue occurring in men 50 to 60 years old may be due to declining androgen secretion. Irritability, depression, loss of memory, hot flashes and sweating are suggestive manifestations.

Diagnosis may be confirmed by (1) high urinary gonadotropin assay or (2) definitive relief from androgen therapy.

PANCREATIC DISORDERS

Hypoglycemia from a functional disorder or an adenoma of the islands of Langerhans of the pancreas should be considered as a possibility in all patients with easy fatigability and nervousness, particularly when the symptoms come on before breakfast or 2 or 3 hours after meals.[33] The fasting blood sugar may be abnormally low. Diagnosis can usually be established by following the blood sugar after the administration of a measured amount of glucose. In patients suffering from functional hypoglycemia, the blood sugar will usually fall far below normal within 2 to 4 hours. It is well to follow the blood sugar for 6 hours after glucose administration because there are rare patients in whom the hypoglycemia does not appear until late.

Hypoglycemia provoked by fasting is more characteristic of insulinoma, sugar tolerance tests in this condition being notoriously variable. A steady fall, or sometimes a precipitous decline in blood glucose levels after a fast of 12 to 36 hours is highly suggestive of islet-cell insulin-producing tumor.

Diabetes mellitus causes fatigue as characteristically as it causes polyuria. Typical early symptoms may be nervousness and easy fatigability. In some patients there may be a story of a number of years of these symptoms before some physician actually takes the trouble to make a urine examination and find glycosuria.

Carcinoma. The earliest symptom of disease (particularly carcinoma) of the parenchyma of the pancreas[34] may be easy fatigability. Dull pain deep in the midabdomen and depression in mood usually appear next. The objective evidences of pancreatic disorder may not appear for months. For example, in one case, a man of 56 with symptoms of depression had surgical exploration because of severity of abdominal pain, but nothing was found. A few months later metastases in the neck appeared. The patient finally died of carcinoma of the pancreas. This syndrome is fortunately rare, and physical findings and laboratory evidence of pancreatic disease usually appear shortly after onset of fatigability and deep abdominal pain.

ADRENAL CORTEX DEFICIENCY

This disorder produces striking increases in fatigability. The recent interest in Addison's disease has made these symptoms common knowledge. In this chapter it is important only to point out that Addison's disease, adrenal tumors and partial deficiency of adrenocortical hormones are relatively rare conditions. The efforts to establish minor disorders of adrenal cortical functions as etiologic factors in common conditions of easy fatigability have not been convincing. The estimation of the value of adrenal steroids in the treatment of these unclassified conditions of easy fatigability and nervousness is still in the experimental stage. One can be certain of adrenal cortical deficiency only when symptoms of Addison's disease can be demonstrated, or when one finds extremely low blood pressure with decreased sodium and increased potassium in the blood, when 17-OH steroid levels in blood or urine are below normal, or when response to diagnostic tests is specific.[35]

Neurasthenia and the asthenia of adrenocortical deficiency may be difficult to distinguish at times. Not all patients with Addison's disease are typically pigmented. Weakness and easy fatigability with or without adrenocortical deficiency may be associated with hypoglycemia or gastrointestinal symptoms, or dizziness and syncopal attacks, or nervousness and mental symptoms.

Many fatigue states are associated with low blood pressure levels. Whenever such a combination is seen, and the patient is questionably pigmented or has other signs or symptoms suggestive of possible adrenocortical deficiency, determination of urinary steroids should be done. The 24-hour 17-ketosteroid level will be below the normal of 15 ± 5 mg. for males and 10 ± 5 mg. for females, if adrenocortical deficiency is present. However, various other disorders associated with inanition and debility also give low levels. More specific is a low output of 17-hydroxy-corticosteroid (below the normal of 9 ± 3 mg. for males and 7 ± 4 mg. for females). A value below 3 mg. suggests adrenal insufficiency. This is confirmed if ACTH given intravenously or intramuscularly fails to provoke a rise in 17-hydroxy-corticosteroid secretion and excretion.[36] Methods to measure blood plasma levels of 17-hydroxy-corticosteroid have been developed.

OTHER ORGANIC DISEASES

As shown above in the section headed Pathologic Physiology of Fatigue, about 80 per cent of cases of fatigue are due to mental disorders, only about 20 per cent to physical disorders. We have discussed the neurologic conditions accounting for about 5 per cent, and the metabolic and endocrine disorders accounting for another 5 per cent. About half of the remaining 10 per cent are due to chronic infections, of which tuberculosis and brucellosis are probably the most common in this country; other frequent causes are malaria, amebiasis, urinary-tract infections and the rheumatic group of diseases.

Over half of the remaining 5 per cent of cases of fatigue are due to circulatory disease, particularly heart disease. The various types of anemia account for 1 or 2 per cent, nephritis for perhaps 1 per cent. The last fraction of 1 per cent is due to malignant disease and nutritional disorders. The above figures are based on the study by Allan.[13] It must be realized that other series of patients would give different figures, depending upon the locality and the type of institution. The figures for malignant disease and for nutritional disease would probably be considerably higher as causes of fatigue in the general population.

Pain, from whatever cause, is a potent producer of fatigue and of nervousness. Probably the commonest conditions causing chronic pain are rheumatoid arthritis and osteoarthritis. Other frequent causes of chronic discomfort, and thus of fatigue (and often of nervousness), are gastrointestinal diseases, such as cholecystitis and cholelithiasis, peptic ulcer and affections of the colon.

The mechanisms by which the various types of organic disease produce fatigue and nervousness are analyzed in the sections on pathologic physiology at the beginning of this chapter.

NUTRITIONAL DISORDERS

It should be emphasized that minor degrees of malnutrition and dietary deficiency can produce fatigability and nervousness. This happens particularly in deficiencies of the vitamins A, D, the B complex and C. Easy fatigability and nervousness may also be symptoms of deficiencies in protein, iron or calcium intake. Deficiencies in the unsaturated fatty acids also probably produce easy fatigability, but this subject has not been studied in the case of human beings.

It is obvious that fatigue especially (but also nervousness) can result from the simple failure to take in sufficient calories. Mild degrees of starvation may produce these symptoms, or just missing a meal or two may cause symptoms. Occasionally, it can be demonstrated that hypoglycemia is an important factor when caloric intake is inadequate. In other instances, the weakness and inability to carry on mental and physical activities can be explained by nervous reactions to the failure of supply of "quick energy" which seems to come after the intake of food. Even when hypoglycemia cannot be demonstrated, it seems likely that during fasting not only glucose but other nutritive elements may be supplied to the tissues at a slower than normal rate.

DRUG ADDICTION AND POISONS

Although it is well known that chronic alcoholism, addiction to morphine, cocaine, bromides and barbiturates can produce easy fatigability and nervousness, this possibility is often overlooked in making a diagnosis. An accurate history that will usually reveal the diagnosis is frequently unobtainable in these cases. While the symptoms of some degree of mental confusion, disorientation and loss of memory, if present, should suggest this diagnosis, they are not specific enough to be conclusive. When drug addiction is suspected it would be helpful if it were possible to determine the amount of the drug in the blood. The only practical clinical test for poisonous drugs that has been developed to date is that for blood bromides.[17] This test is simple and should be carried out in all patients suffering from unexplained easy fatigability and nervousness who have been taking many kinds of medicine. Tests for the other drugs have not reached the point where they are practical for clinical purposes.

AGING

Aging is the commonest and the inevitable cause of increasing fatigability. This process is frequently but not inevitably accompanied by increased nervousness.

The aging process begins in some organs of the body even before growth stops in the rest of the body—the thymus for example.

In most persons diminished capacity in performance begins early in certain sense organs. Night vision begins to decline in some people at age 30. Eye accommodation for distance begins to fail at 40 years. Astrand[37] in a good review, documents the many physiologic functions that begin to decline after 30. It is a rare athlete that does not note the beginning stages of loss of youthful vigor after 30, the decline often being chiefly in the legs. Some persons retain powers and functions for decades beyond the usual age of decline but these people are exceptional.

Although much work has been done on the physiology and chemistry of aging, the process is not well understood. The organ systems of various persons age at different rates and begin aging at different times. Most body constituents decline at varying rates after age 40. There is loss of muscle mass and with it strength, agility, etc. In some people and some families the central nervous system begins to deteriorate at an early age. The numerous studies that have been done on aging are well summarized in the *Psychopathology of Aging*.[38]

Delay of aging processes is now thought to be possible through regular "moderate" exercise and a well-balanced diet sufficiently low in calories to prevent obesity. There is some evidence that predominance of unsaturated fats over saturated in the diet may prevent atherosclerosis. This controversy is still unsettled.

DIET AND EXERCISE IN THE PREVENTION OF DISEASE AND IN RELIEF OF FATIGUE

The nutritionists claim that the increased size of American young people, and the ability of the people from Western Europe, United States and Australia to continue to break athletic records are primarily due to improved nutrition. On the other hand, overindulgence in eating produces obesity and easy fatigability and probably predisposes to atherosclerosis and other ills. In the past decade the medical profession has joined the nutritionists in advocating carefully balanced diets sufficiently low in calories to prevent even moderate overweight. Dieting has undoubtedly become a fad.

The physical education experts are also having their day. They seem to claim that regular exercise is good for everything, including prevention of easy fatigability, obesity, atherosclerosis, etc. Did not regular golf prevent a recurrence of President Eisenhower's heart disease?

The data and the lack of data in support of the importance of diet and exercise are well summarized in Science and Medicine of Exercise and Sports, 1960.[8]

CONCLUSION

Symptoms of fatigue and nervousness are among the most common complaints. They are not of value in diagnosis unless the specific circumstances under which they arose are determined. The establishment of the circumstances under which fatigability and nervousness first appeared and the exact chronology of subsequent disabilities may give the leading clue to the correct diagnosis. Only when physical signs and laboratory findings indicate clearly a specific causative process can one estimate the significance of nervousness and fatigue without a detailed personal history. In addition, the patient's prevailing mood and the content of his thoughts should be investigated. Much loss of time and mistreatment of patients can be avoided if the careful personal history is obtained in the beginning of the first physician's initial contact with these patients.

It should also be noted that although important advances have been made in the biochemistry of intermediary metabolism and the chemistry of muscle and nerve, these findings are still a long way from aiding the clinician in evaluating the fatigued or nervous patient. The energy-rich phosphorus and ribose nucleic acid bonds have been studied in isolated enzyme mixtures. What these basic discoveries mean for patients has not yet been disclosed.[39]

REFERENCES

Bibliographies on various aspects of Nervousness and Fatigue may be found in the books and papers of Mayer-Gross, Johnson, Dill, Mayo, Whitehead and Karpovitch.

1. Cecil-Loeb: Textbook of Medicine, Beeson, P. B. and McDermott, W. (eds.), Ed. 11 Philadelphia, Saunders, 1963.
2. Sayers, R. R.: Findings from Major Studies of Fatigue, Bureau of Mines Information Circular 7209, U. S. Dept. Interior, Washington, D. C., 1942.
3. Bartley, S. H., and Chute, E.: Fatigue and Impairment in Man, New York, McGraw-Hill, 1949.
4. Martin, G. J.: Clinical Enzymology, Boston, Little Brown, 1958.
5. Bartley, S. H.: Fatigue and inadequacy, Physiol. Rev. 37:301-324, 1957.
6. Field, J., Magoun, H. W. and Hall, V. E.: Handbook of Neurophysiology, Amer. Physiol. Soc. Vols. 1, 2, 3: Washington, D. C., 1960.
7. White, Leslie A.: The Evolution of Culture, p. 40, New York, McGraw-Hill, 1959.
8. Johnson, W. (ed.): Science and Medicine of Exercise and Sports, New York, Harper, 1960.
9. Mayer-Gross, V., Slater, E., and Roth, M.: Clinical Psychiatry, Ch. 2, Baltimore, Williams & Wilkins, 1960.
10. Frostig, J. P., and Spies, T. D.: Initial nervous syndrome of pellagra and associated deficiency diseases, Am. J. Med. Sci. 199:268-274, 1940.
11. Dill, D. B.: Fatigue, Indust. Med. 8:315-318, 1939.
12. ———: Applied Physiology, Ann. Rev. Physiol. 1:551-576, 1939.
13. Allan, F. N.: Differential diagnosis of weakness and fatigue, New England J. Med. 231:414-418, 1944.
14. Karpovitch, P. V.: Physiology of Muscular Activity, Ch. 15, Philadelphia, Saunders, 1959.
15. Mayo, E.: The Human Problems of Industrial Civilization, New York, Macmillan, 1933.
16. Whitehead, T. N.: The Industrial Worker, Cambridge, Harvard Univ. Press, 1938.
17. Preu, P. W., Romano, J., and Brown, W. T.: Symptomatic psychoses with bromide intoxication; their occurrence in southern New England, New England J. Med., 214:56-62, 1936.
18. Cohen, M. E., White, P. D., and Johnson, R. E.: Neurocirculatory asthenia, anxiety neurosis or the effort syndrome, Arch. Int. Med. 81:260-281, 1948.
19. Ulett, G. A., and Goodrich, D. W. (eds.): A Synopsis of Contemporary Psychiatry, St. Louis, Mosby, 1960.

20. Denker, P. G.: Prognosis and life expectancy in psychoneuroses; study of 1,000 disability insurance claims, Proc. A. Life Insur. M. Dir. America (1937), 24:179-211, 1938.

21. Robins, E., Smith, K., and Lowe, I. P.: Attempts to Confirm the Presence of "taraxein" in the Blood of Schizophrenic Patients. Neuropharmacology, H. A. Abramson, ed. Trans. 4th Conf., pp. 123-135, New York, Josiah Macy, Jr. Foundation, 1959.

22. Gildea, E. F.: Present status of the schizophrenia problem, Amer. J. Med., 25:942-949, 1958.

23. Gildea, E. F., Ronzoni, E., and Trufant, S. A.: Results from the use of ACTH and cortisone in psychoses, in Biology of Mental Health and Disease, p. 600-613, New York, Hoeber, 1952.

24. Spiegel, E. (ed.): Progress in Neurology and Psychiatry, Ch. 33, New York, Grune & Stratton, 1960.

25. Beecher, H. K.: The powerful placebo, J.A.M.A.. 159:1602-1606, 1955.

26. Frank, J. D., Gliedman, L. H., Imber, S. D., Stone, A. R., and Nash, E. H.: Patients' expectancies and relearning as factors determining improvement in psychotherapy, Am. J. Psychiat. 115:961-968, 1959.

27. Gliedman, L. H., Nash, E. H., Imber, S. D., Stone, A. R., and Frank, J. D.: Reduction of symptoms by pharmacologically inert substances and by short-term psychotherapy, Arch. Neurol. & Psychiat. 79:345-351, 1958.

28. Hampson, J. L., Rosenthal, D., and Frank, J. D.: A comparative study of the effects of mephenesin and placebo of the symptomatology of a mixed group of psychiatric outpatients, Bull. Johns Hopkins Hosp. 95:170-177, 1954.

29. Lasagna, L., Mosteller, F., von Felsinger, J. M., and Beecher, H. K.: A study of the placebo response, Am. J. Med., 16:770-779, 1954.

30. Stone, T. T., and Burris, B. C.: Melancholia, J.A.M.A. 142:165-168, 1950.

31. Man, E. B., Smirnow, A. E., Gildea, E. F., and Peters, J. P.: Serum iodine fractions in hyperthyroidism, J. Clin. Invest. 21:773-780, 1942.

32. Berson, S. A.: Symposium on Thyroid disease, Am. J. Med., 20:651, 1956.

33. Howland, G., Campbell, W. R., Maltby, E. J., and Robinson, W. L.: Dysinsulinism; convulsions and coma due to islet cell tumor of pancreas, with operation and cure, J.A.M.A. 93:674-679, 1929.

34. Ulett, G. A., and Parsons, E. H.: Psychiatric aspects of carcinoma of the pancreas, J. Missouri State M. A. 45:490-493, 1948.

35. Williams, R.: Textbook of Endocrinology, Philadelphia, Saunders, Ed. 3, pp. 319-333, 1962.

36. Perkoff, G. T., et al.: Clinical usefulness of determination of 17-hydroxycorticosteroid levels, Arch. Int. Med., 93:1-8, 1954.

37. Astrand, P. O.: Human physical fitness with special reference to sex and age, Physiol. Rev. 36:307-333, 1956.

38. Hoch, P. H., and Zubin, J. (eds.): Psychopathology of Aging, New York, Grune & Stratton, 1961.

39. Gaebler, O. H. (ed.) : Enzymes; Units of Biological Structure and Function, pp. 573-583, New York, Acad. Press, Inc., 1956.

40. Hess, W. R.: The diencephalic sleep centre, in Delafresnaye, J. F. (ed.); Brain Mechanisms and Consciousness, Oxford, Blackwell Scientific Pub., 1954;
——: The Functional Organization of the Diencephalon, New York, Grune & Stratton, 1957.

41. Brodie, B. B., Prockop, D. J., and Shore, P. A.: An interpretation of the action of psychotropic drugs, Postgrad. Med. 24:305, 1958.

42. Baker, W. W.: Pharmacology of the central nervous system, Prog. Neurol. & Psychiat. 14:103, 1959.

43. Alpers, B., and Mancall, E.: The Nervous System, in Sodeman, W., ed.: Pathologic Physiology, ed. 3, p. 1105, Philadelphia, Saunders, 1961.

44. Albeaux-Fernet, M., Bugard, P. et Romani, J. D.: Traitement de la fatigue chronique par l'acide adenosine triphosphorique, La Presse Medicale 66:1265-1268, 1958.

45. Laborit, H.: Stress and Cellular Function, p. 76, Philadelphia, Lippincott, 1959.

46. Shaw, D. L., Chesney, M. A., Tullis, I. F., and Agersborg, H. P.: Management of fatigue: a physiological approach, Am. J. Med. Sci. 243:758-769, 1962.

47. Fallis, N., Wilson, W. R., Tetreault, L. L., and Lasagna, L.: Effect of potassium and magnesium aspartates on athletic performance, J.A.M.A. 185:129, 1963.

48. New Drugs and Developments in Therapeutics. Council on Drugs: Potassium and Magnesium Aspartates (Spartase), J.A.M.A. 183:362, 1963.

26

Coma and Convulsion

JAMES L. O'LEARY AND WILLIAM M. LANDAU

INTRODUCTION

Coma and convulsion, outstanding symptoms of cerebral disorder, occupy the extremes of an excitability gradient which extends from a zone of hypoexcitability at one end of the normal range to one of hyperexcitability at the other. Coma develops as the state of neural excitability enters either of these end-zones. Thus, suspension of consciousness can occur either during a generalized epileptic attack (hyperexcitability) or when trauma, anoxia, infection, systemic metabolic disturbance, toxin, poison, or drug markedly depresses neural functioning (hypoexcitability).

We digress to discuss certain rudiments of neurophysiology. The human brain contains some ten billion nerve cells arranged in an intricate communication net roughly analogous to a telephone system or a computer but infinitely more intricate than either. Each single cell component functions both as a receiver-transmitter (cell body and dendrites) and as a conductor (axon). The axon terminals of one nerve cell are applied to the cell body or dendrites of others to produce circuits of vary-

ing complexity. Information is propagated along axons as variations in the spacing between a quick succession of *all-or-none* impulses. At the synapses the digital all-or-none information carried by axons is transformed into an analogical *graded* process. Two basic kinds of information are thus transmitted—excitatory and inhibitory. Naturally, it is the excitatory processes upon which the nervous system depends chiefly for its operations, the inhibitory either preventing over-action or slowing or stopping action in progress. The richness of the interconnections between neurons makes for ready distribution of coded information through the neural net. However, inhibitory controls restrict normal activity to purposive channels. Under conditions of *exalted excitability* (i.e., epileptic states) distribution of information is far too permissive, particularly when inhibitory brakes are also ineffective. In such circumstances a few neurons discharging at frequencies up to 100 per second (a speed not uncommon at the site of epileptogenic lesions) may transmit impulses which rapidly infiltrate neighboring neurons poised on the thresh-

619

old of discharge, drawing them into the orbit of excessive firing from a small start. Thus a convulsion may avalanche across wide areas of the cerebral gray matter.

The depressed functioning of the *hypo-excitable state* is occasioned by elevation of the synaptic threshold and subnormal responsiveness of the membrane which invests the nerve cell, the former being one specific expression of the properties of the latter. Upon the relative reactivity of the membrane depend the important functions of synaptic transfer and impulse propagation: impaired excitability of the membrane greatly slows the operations of the system as a whole. Such slowing may cause abnormal scarcity of circulating impulses within the neural net and abolition of all but the most vital activities. Thus unconsciousness results. The state of hyperexcitability, a prelude to convulsion, is manifested by low resistance at the synaptic bridges and a high tide of irritability. The latter leads to the discharge of spurts of impulses of excessive length and astonishingly high frequency. This has the effect of overloading the system with a jam of circulating signals, and, through resultant overaction, suspending the logistics of normal functioning. Besides interrupting consciousness, the impulses discharge outward through avenues of diminished synaptic resistance, massively invading the nerve routes leading to skeletal muscle and producing the overt signs of convulsion. Since the nervous system depends largely upon energy sources transported via the blood supply, the time is relatively brief during which the chaotic over-action of convulsion can be maintained. As a result, more likely than not, a convulsion will terminate with the brain in a depressed state. Thus, during and after a generalized seizure the accompanying unconsciousness can occur for two reasons which appear in succession, the first that of overactivity associated with the convulsion proper, and the second (postictal parasomnia) with terminal underactivity.

By unconsciousness we mean a void of consciousness. The range of consciousness extends from the alert wakefulness (vigilance) of the expectant mind through clouding (obtundity) and stupor to precoma and coma. Any loss implies the prior existence of a state of *normal consciousness,* the introspective yardstick the experienced observer uses to estimate the severity of the loss. It is the definition of normal consciousness that is most difficult. Its meanings are obscured in a haze of metaphysics, and Brain[1] has pointed out that to different savants it can mean six things: forms of behavior by which we distinguish the unconscious from the conscious individual; psychological terms used to describe conscious states such as sensory and perceptual experiences; consciousness as related to the activity of the nervous system; role of consciousness in the biological functions of the living organism; the logical terms which can be applied to conscious experience; and the metaphysical status of consciousness. The notion of distinguishing between *content of consciousness* and the *state of awareness* in which it exists is also prevalent, the phrase *spontaneity of consciousness* being used for the latter. Sartre,[2] for example, alludes to consciousness as a pure spontaneity, "confronting the world of things which is sheer inertness." James[3] challenged its very foundations in an essay, "Does Consciousness Exist?"

HISTORICAL RÉSUMÉ

Efforts to comprehend how brain and mental states conjoin go back some 2,400 years. Viewed in retrospect they signify man's most prolonged struggle to comprehend his own nature. One lesson taught is that speculations based upon erroneous structural and physiologic information can long persist as a habit of thinking even though challenged occasionally during the passage of centuries. The ancients certainly knew something of the brain, recognizing at the least that the ventricles contained fluid, for in several instances hydraulic terms were applied to brain parts which adjoined ventricular channels, such as pons, aqueduct and valve. Thus the erroneous view that the ventricles contain a "pneuma" (air, gas or vapor) arose as speculation after a fair start had already been made in the right direction. The error resulted from sheer laziness to observe, reliance being placed instead upon the transmission of book knowledge. Such speculation continued to be accepted as fact until near our own time when Magendie (1825) proved the fluid content of the brain ventricles in freshly dead bodies.

Aristotle viewed the seat of animal spirits as existing in the heart. However, Hippocrates formed a more correct opinion of the importance of the brain to mental states. Erasistratus, a student of Aristotle, taught also that animal spirits derive from the head. Plato recognized three mental faculties of which the rational was related to the brain. Most of the ancients, including Galen, believed that the ventricles received a pneuma through nose and sphenoid bone and that this mixed in the ventricles with vital spirits brought upwards from the heart by the arteries. The animal spirits there produced were supposed to be transmitted downward through the ventricles to be distributed over the nerves. Galen also conceived of the brain as having movements of diastole and systole. In the former he supposed that it receives air and vital spirits into the ventricles, and in the latter distributes animal spirits via the nerves. Later, it was denied that animal spirits were formed in the ventricles, and taught instead that they were generated in the substance of the brain, since dissections showed that nothing macroscopic could pass inward through channels in sphenoid and ethmoid bones. Nevertheless, the view long persisted that the ventricles had an excretory function, dispelling to the outside effete material that arises as a waste product during nutrition of the brain.

The modern era began with the phrenologists who, in addition to fathering an outlandish theory of brain localization related to cranial protuberances were masters of brain dissection. Their rivals of the more orthodox school were forced to seek corresponding proficiency as dissectors, and thus emphasis turned inevitably to reestablishing the science of observation. Prochaska,[4] for example, supported the view (based in dissection) that the nerves of sensation and of motion met and communicated in the medulla oblongata, giving rise there to a "seat of the sensorial consciousness." Later (about 1850) that seat was moved forward to the thalamus where we leave it to take up work of our own time which also appears to support a thalamic center for consciousness.

Theoretical considerations arising out of the modern studies dominate today's thinking upon the subject, and are in opposition to the view that the whole brain acting together performs the function of consciousness. This dichotomy of thinking was recognized long before the present epoch, and is stated clearly in the following quotation from Richerland.[5]

The existence of a centre, to which all the sensations are carried, and from which all motions spring, is necessary to the unity of a thinking being, and to the harmony of the intellectual functions. But is this seat of the principle of motion and of sensation circumscribed within the narrow limits of a mathematical point? or rather should it not be considered as diffused over the whole brain?

THE NEURAL BASIS OF CONSCIOUSNESS

CONTRIBUTION OF STUDIES UPON SLEEP

The vagueness of our concept of consciousness was alluded to above, as was the behavioral significance of *awareness* or *vigilance* as expressions of the state, if not the content, of mind. Any stimulus which usurps the attention of animal or man simultaneously produces vigilance and "activates" the scalp- (or brain-) recorded electroencephalogram (EEG); that is, it converts the usual spontaneous rhythm of the waking brain into an irregular tracing of low voltage in which no remainder of usual activity is evident. From that change we deduce the importance of the sensory paths to the cortex in the maintenance of awareness. Sensory monotony, or deprivation, has the opposite effect, lending itself to sleep.

In animals a brainstem severance at the mesodiencephalic junction, which permanently deprives the cerebral cortex of a sensory inflow, leads to perpetual slumber along with the ocular and EEG manifestations of sleep.[6] Analysis of the phenomena of normal sleep in animals and man has aided importantly in the neurologic appraisal of consciousness and unconsciousness, recognizing, of course, that in sleep the mental operations of animal and man most closely approach equivalence. Hereafter we examine sleep as a prelude to matters which concern the pathological suspension of consciousness.

The notion of a sleep center did not originate with von Economo[7] the German neurologist who is credited with describing the form of encephalitis called sleeping sickness, but he gave it a strong impetus by concluding that a *wakefulness center* exists in the hypothalamic wall of the third ventricle because the destructive lesions of encephalitis center there. He also described a *sleep center* situated just ahead of that area, verging upon the preoptic region. Lesions at the latter site were characterized by wakefulness (asomnia) and von Economo theorized that it produced sleep by inhibition of the remainder of the brain. Between them, these half-centers were presumed to establish the diurnal sleeping-waking cycle. Later, W. R. Hess,[8] stimulating a corresponding region of the ventralmost thalamus with slowly repetitive electrical pulses of long duration, also produced sleep. He, too, proposed a more posteromedially situated wakefulness center.

Bremer[6] is credited with replacing this older static view of a sleep center with the more dynamic one that sleep is due to an interruption of a continuous stream of afferent impulses which flows past the mesodiencephalic junction upwards and outwards to cerebral cortex. He believed the lemnisci to be the channels of flow, whereas later workers describe instead a collateral path (derived from the lemnisci) which filters more gradually through the in-lying brainstem tegmentum to connect at the level of the centre median thalamic nucleus with a diffuse thalamocortical system to be described next.

Bremer showed that severance of the brainstem at the mesodiencephalic junction produced a state closely akin to sleep, and replaced usual waking frequencies of the EEG with diffusely slow (delta) activity interrupted by spindles closely similar to those recorded in human EEG sleep tracings. Dempsey and Morison[9] proved the origin in the midline thalamus of a fiber system which distributes diffusely to the cortex. Through repetitive electrical stimulation at the thalamic source they produced generalized wave sequences (recruiting response) in the cortex, which closely resemble the spontaneously repetitive spindles of light sleep. Later, Moruzzi and Magoun[10] showed that rapidly repetitive stimulation in the brainstem tegmentum can convert the sleep type EEG with spindles (such as is produced during barbiturate anesthesia) to the low voltage desynchronized tracing characteristic of a just awakened alert animal. Tonic drive feeding into the diffuse thalamocortical system of Dempsey and Morison[9] is presumed responsible for maintenance of the waking state. When the tonic drive is interrupted sleep intervenes. Thus the origin of the term *reticular activating system* used by the followers of Moruzzi and Magoun.

For a long time deepest sleep was associated with very slow delta EEG activity and spindles as observed by Bremer in his animals with brainstem transection. It came as a surprise, therefore, when a still deeper stage of sleep was recognized in the cat (Dement,[11] Jouvet[12]). It was dubbed *paradoxical sleep* because the EEG closely resembles that of the awake, alert animal. Nevertheless, if the cat is stimulated during paradoxical sleep it only reverts to the stage of sleep with slow waves and spindles, not to full awakening. It is known that the nervous system is peculiarly sensitive to auditory arousal. Thus it is not surprising that responses of single tegmental neurones to auditory clicks are reduced during usual deep sleep and are practically absent during paradoxical sleep. However, in curious contrast is the fact that the spontaneous activity of the same neurone is greatest during paradoxical sleep.[13] It has recently been shown that usual sleep with slow waves and spindles depends upon the integrity of cerebral mechanisms, whereas paradoxical sleep requires the operation of rhombencephalic mechanisms. The latter has also been called archisleep suggesting more archaic origin than has telecephalic sleep.

Out of modern studies upon sleep and activation has come a renewed interest in a mesodiencephalic center of consciousness. Penfield[14] theorizes that the highest level of integration in the brain of man, "to which all the sensations are carried and from which all motions spring," is situated in the mesodiencephalic region.[5] Penfield incorporates into his hypothesis much of the evidence just presented and other data based upon evaluation of the unconscious state associated with brain lesions in man. Walshe[15] has reviewed the Penfield evidence critically and with enviable lucidity. His easily accessible account should be read by everyone interested in the problems of mind and brain.

UNCONSCIOUSNESS IN BRAINSTEM LESIONS IN MAN

Much has been learned of the site of origin of comatose states from study of patients with lesions of the brainstem or the superstructure. One important source has been observations upon anencephalic and hydrocephalic monsters.[16,17]

It appears that such mesodiencephalic subjects sleep and wake, react to hunger, loud sounds and crude visual stimuli by movement of eyes, eyelids and facial muscles. Such an infant may see and hear, taste and smell, reject the unpalatable and accept such food as it likes, utter sounds, show displeasure when hungry and pleasure when sung to. They may also perform crude limb movements spontaneously. All this can perhaps be described collectively as rudimentary awareness, or indeed as crude consciousness, if we could somehow make ourselves aware of its content.

Cairns[18] analyzed the effect upon consciousness of lesions at lower and upper brainstem levels, the latter, of course, including involvement of thalamic centers. He found that a disturbance of the medulla or the pons can produce sudden loss of consciousness, ordinarily with associated disturbance of breathing and circulation. The question arises as to whether anoxia resulting from the cardiorespiratory deficit might not be the cause of coma in lower brainstem lesions. However, in some instances loss of consciousness has been shown to precede the drop in blood pressure and respiratory change. Howell[19] analyzed the case histories of 6 patients who showed foraminal impaction of the brainstem at postmortem. He found the most common feature of this syndrome to be the hydrocephalic attack, consisting in its mildest form of a brief *agonizing headache* (often lasting only a minute or two) with or without transitory confusion, deafness or amaurosis. Inconstant features were bilateral cranial nerve palsies (involving nerves 7 to 10 inclusive), neck rigidity and sustained hydrocephalus developing insidiously. Between attacks patients were found to be alert, in contrast to the global impairment of consciousness seen with upper brainstem compressions. In fact, Howell says, global impairment is no part of this syndrome, and that with medullary compression a patient alert one moment may be dead the next. When coma occurred it lasted a minute in one case, several hours in three others with possible upper brainstem compression as well.

Two main varieties of loss of consciousness occur in upper brainstem and thalamic lesions, one intermittent and the other continuous.[18] The former is exemplified by petit mal epilepsy, the latter by coma with decerebrate rigidity, coma with hyperthermia, hypersomnia and akinetic mutism. In hypersomnia persistent unconsciousness may resemble sleep with quiet breathing, muscular relaxation, and loss of the expression which characterizes the waking state. The patient can be aroused temporarily, and the EEG is of the sleep type with diffuse delta activity, as is also true with other kinds of unconsciousness. In akinetic mutism the eyes may follow the observer about but the patient is otherwise unresponsive.

Because of their acute development the signs of coma associated with downward pressure from supratentorial mass lesions may be significantly more dramatic. Two possible sequences of brainstem dysfunction may accompany such conditions.[20] In one, the signs of uncal herniation occur, including 3rd nerve involvement and lateral midbrain compression. The other reflects bilateral diencephalic impairment,

Cheyne-Stokes respiration, "doll's head" eye movements and bilateral motor involvement. Howell,[19] whose study upon brainstem and foraminal impaction has already been mentioned, examined some 150 cases of upper brainstem compression. He reports that the main features of the syndrome are sufficiently constant for it to be distinguished from other conditions causing coma. Increased headache, vomiting, and stiffness of neck develop at the onset. The most constant feature is a global impairment of all mental functions progressing, rapidly or slowly, from lethargy to a semicomatose state. Patients in his series might die before they became fully comatose, and thus death could only be attributed to coma when severe aspiration or hypostatic pneumonia developed. Bradycardia occurred less frequently than tachycardia. Hyperpyrexia was common. In rapidly developing compression sudden respiratory arrest might be seen, and this could follow a phase of slow, shallow, grunting respiration. Loss of pupillary light reflex was very constant, although it might not be observed until compression is far advanced. Dilatation of the pupil is usual but the pupils may remain small or even contracted. Decerebrate rigidity is common and it is exceptional not to detect extensor spasm of the limbs in response to painful stimulation at some stage of the illness.

Ingvar and Lundberg[21] recorded EEG and ventricular fluid pressure (VFP) simultaneously in patients showing increased intracranial pressure associated with brain tumor. Paroxysmal variations in the VFP were observed in the form of large, suddenly appearing plateau waves with peaks of 100 mm. Hg. and rhythmically recurring VFP variations showing a frequency of 1 to 2 per minute. It is important to note that high plateau waves can be accompanied by loss of consciousness and tonic-clonic movements. Only subtle EEG changes are found to accompany plateau waves. The onset of such a wave can be accompanied by the arousal type of EEG change; its termination with hyperventilation shows an increase in slow activity. However, despite the loss of consciousness and obvious tonic-clonic movements, no convulsive activity appears in the electroencephalogram. They conclude that the convulsive phenomena observed resulted from brainstem seizures.

The evidence from organic lesions of brainstem and thalamus points to the consciousness inherent in this region as being essentially a *crude consciousness*. This leaves the cerebral cortex essential for the manifestation of higher levels of consciousness, even though a healthy cerebral cortex cannot of itself maintain the conscious state. Massive bifrontal lesions in man, for example, have been shown not to disturb crude consciousness but instead to impair will, initiative, foresight and judgment.[18]

ABNORMAL STATES OF CONSCIOUSNESS AND THEIR ETIOLOGIES

Figure 175 presents a scheme of the relationships of the waking state to normal sleep and to coma of a variety of etiologies as taken up in the ensuing account.

In a 1933 survey of patients who entered Boston City Hospital in coma, alcohol was held responsible for 50 per cent, trauma for 13 per cent, and cerebrovascular disorder for 10 per cent.[22-24] Other causes, each accounting for 3 per cent or fewer patients, were poisoning, epilepsy, diabetes, meningitis, pneumonia, cardiac decompensation, exsanguination, CNS syphilis, uremia and eclampsia. Those causes in which prompt diagnosis and emergency treatment are imperative were diabetes, hyperinsulinism, poisoning, traumatic shock, exsanguination, subdural hematoma, brain tumor, abscess, meningitis, and eclampsia. History was of immediate importance in 60 per cent of cases, and ambulance drivers were instructed to bring in a relative, or other witness whenever possible to facilitate obtaining a history. Depth of coma, state of reflexes and pupils were not found to be of great diagnostic importance although of course neurological signs ordinarily depended upon the depth of the coma. Table 28 A & B, from Solomon and Aring,[22] provide excellent summaries of physical and laboratory observations helpful in the differential diagnosis of coma and of the conditions in which it occurs (pages 626 and 627).

Hereafter we outline the salient features of a variety of conditions which cause coma. The discussion is necessarily far from complete.

HEAD TRAUMA

The best possible history and neurologic appraisal are always obtained. For future reference Symonds[25] advises us to distinguish between patients who are never unconscious, those unconscious but a few

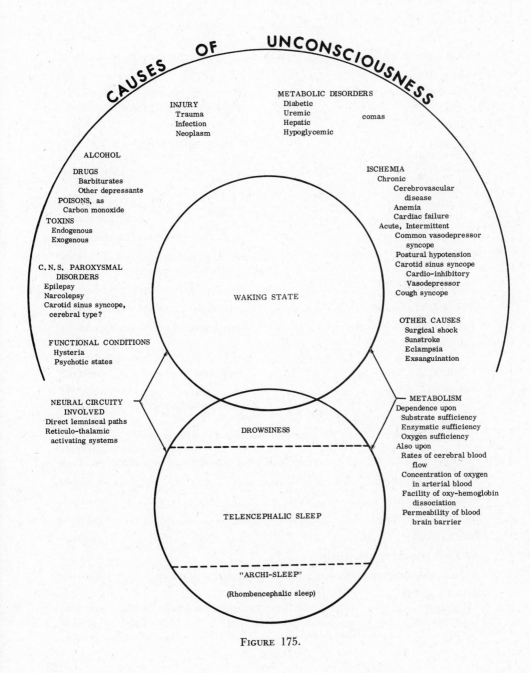

FIGURE 175.

PHYSICAL CHANGES HELPFUL IN THE DIAGNOSIS OF COMA AND THE CONDITIONS IN WHICH THEY OCCUR*

Odor of breath
  Alcohol ....alcoholism
  Acetone ....diabetes, uremia
  Illuminating gas ....carbon monoxide poisoning

Color of skin and mucous membranes

  Hyperemic ....alcoholism
  Cherry red ....carbon monoxide poisoning
  Cyanosis ....cardiac decompensation, pneumonia
  Pallor ....hemorrhage, pernicious anemia
  Jaundice ....cholemia

Local signs of injury ....trauma, burns, hemorrhage, epilepsy, erysipelas

Temperature
  Increased ....pneumonia, meningitis, encephalitis
  Decreased ....carbon monoxide poisoning, diabetes

Pulse
  Rapid ....diabetes, pneumonia, meningitis, eclampsia
  Irregular ....cardiac decompensation
  Slow ....Stokes-Adams disease

Respiration
  Kussmaul ....diabetes
  Increased ....pneumonia

Hemiplegia ....cerebral vascular lesions

Observation of convulsions ....epilepsy, cerebral vascular lesions, central
                                   nervous system syphilis, alcoholism

Vomiting ....cerebral hemorrhage, poisoning

Stiffness of the neck ....meningitis, cerebral vascular lesions

Kernig's leg sign positive ....meningitis, cerebral vascular lesions

Chest signs
  Consolidation ....pneumonia
  Fluid ....empyema, ruptured aortic aneurysm

Pulmonary congestion ....ascites, enlarged liver, distended
                                      neck veins, cardiac decompensation

Distention and spasticity of
    the abdomen ....ruptured esophageal varix, carcinomatous erosion
                                         of the gastrointestinal tract,
                          ruptured ectopic pregnancy, miliary tuberculosis

Muscular twitchings ....uremia

Abdominal tumor ....eclampsia

Bulging fontanels ....meningitis

Soft eyeballs ....diabetes

Wounds or scars on the tongue ....epilepsy

Vaginal examination abnormal ..pelvic malignancy, ruptured ectopic pregnancy

Blood pressure
  Increased ....cerebral vascular lesions, uremia, eclampsia
  Decreased ....trauma

LABORATORY OBSERVATIONS HELPFUL IN THE DIAGNOSIS OF COMA
AND THE CONDITIONS IN WHICH THEY OCCUR*

Lumbar puncture: spinal fluid

Pressure

Increased ....cerebral vascular lesions,
meningitis, trauma,
central nervous system syphilis

Decreased ....diabetes
Bloody fluid ....cerebral vascular lesions, trauma
Purulent fluid ....meningitis
Organisms by smear and culture ....meningitis

Sugar

Low ....meningitis
High ....diabetes
Protein high ....meningitis; central nervous
system syphilis
Spinal fluid Wasserman positive ....central nervous system syphilis

Blood examination

Sugar

High ....diabetes
Low ....insulin shock

Nonprotein nitrogen high ....uremia
Wassermann test positive ....central nervous system syphilis
Low red blood count,
abnormal smear ....pernicious anemia, leukemia
Culture positive ....pneumonia, meningitis, septicemia
Spectroscopy ....carbon monoxide poisoning,
methemoglobinemia

Urine examination

Sugar ....diabetes
Gross albuminuria ....eclampsia, uremia, cardiac
decompensation

Gastric lavage
examination of gastric contents ....poisoning

Roentgenogram
Skull ....fracture across middle meningeal
artery in extradural hemorrhage
Lungs ....pneumonia, empyema, miliary
tuberculosis
Heart ....cardiac decompensation

Electrocardiogram ....heart block, cardiac decompensation

Courtesy of Solomon and Aring: J.A.M.A., 105:7.

moments, and those who exhibit prolonged periods of unconsciousness. Patients with cerebral contusion may show focal neurologic signs. Those with severe head injury (as in automobile accidents), who come to postmortem often show severe laceration of the orbital surfaces of the frontal lobes and the tips of the temporal lobes.[26] In middle meningeal hemorrhage (epidural hematoma) a brief interval of unconsciousness following the accident may be succeeded by lucidity and several hours later a rapidly deepening coma may develop. Subdural hematoma may be acute or chronic. In the latter instance gradually increasing coma and progressive paralysis may develop even when there is no history of an accident. In all cases of head injury, proved or suspected, a careful watch should be made for signs of increased intracranial pressure (as estimated from repeated recordings of blood pressure), respiration and pulse. Roentgenograms are important as early as the condition of the patient will permit. An excellent brief survey of post-traumatic epilepsy is available.[27]

In prolonged unconsciousness due to head injury with brainstem impairment it is important not to discuss prognosis in the presence of the patient, for such cases may recover and remember what went on about them.

NEOPLASM AND BRAIN ABSCESS

Either neoplasm or abscess may cause coma with or without paralysis. The history is that of progressive neurologic deficit of variable duration. Important historical data concern headache, vomiting, convulsion, paralysis or incoordination with failing vision or personality change in the background. Papilledema is an important sign. In possible abscess inquiry should be made about past lung, ear or sinus disease with or without operative intervention. A history of skull fracture may also be important. In tumor suddenly developing coma may result either from secondary hemorrhage or tentorial or foramen magnum herniation due to increased pressure.

MENINGITIS AND ENCEPHALITIS

In meningitis severe headache may develop acutely followed by loss of consciousness. The important diagnostic signs are nuchal rigidity, Kernig and Brudzinski signs. Dissociation in ocular movements, pupillary abnormalities, convulsion, and focal neurologic signs may be seen. Tuberculous meningitis is gradual in onset and isolated cranial nerves may be affected.

There are several types of encephalitis, any of which may show hypersomnia as an acute symptom. However, lethargic encephalitis is outstanding for producing hypersomnia. Demyelinating encephalitides are associated with vaccinia, smallpox, measles and antirabies treatment. Dissociated eye movements may feature viral encephalitis. Diagnosis of specific viral etiology may be sought through neutralization and complement-fixation tests. These may be done on successive serum samples obtained during the course of the illness, seeking a rise in titer.[28] Hemagglutination of cells is used in the case of arthropod viruses. It may be possible to isolate virus from the spinal fluid.

CEREBROVASCULAR DISEASE

Coma may occur at the onset of cerebral hemorrhage, but often it develops gradually. It is uncommon with cerebral thrombosis. Associated hemiplegia is frequent. Sudden loss of consciousness in cerebral hemorrhage is due to massive explosive injury to the cerebrum and to accompanying neural shock. Cerebral embolism shows a sudden onset, but loss of consciousness is far less likely than with cerebral hemorrhage. Subarachnoid hemorrhage is distinguished by sudden onset of intense headache, often following exertion. Coma may come on more gradually. The pulse may be slowed, and meningeal signs are observed. Coma may also develop in hypertensive encephalopathy, either with or without convulsions; there is usually a history of severe hypertension.

When vascular lesions involve the lesser brainstem vessels, as the branches of the vertebrobasilar system, localizing signs and symptoms commonly occur without loss of consciousness unless the lesion is hemorrhagic. However, symptoms of attacks of vertebrobasilar and carotid insufficiency may appear as the prodrome of a massive cerebral thrombosis with unconsciousness. For that reason we list below principal symptoms of the two main types of insufficiency drawn from a USPHS cerebrovascular survey report.[29]

Vertebrobasilar Insufficiency
   Dizziness
   Diplopia
   Blurred vision
   Blindness
   Pupillary change
   Memory lapses
   Confused behavior
   Unilateral or bilateral numbness
   Unilateral or bilateral weakness
   Dysarthria
   Dysphagia
   Impaired hearing
   Numbness of face
   Staggering gait
   Hiccuping

Carotid System Insufficiency
   Unilateral weakness or numbness
   Dysphasia
   Confusion
   Ipsilateral monocular blindness
   Homonymous field defects
   Headache
   Possibly focal epileptic seizures

BRAIN METABOLISM AND METABOLIC COMA

The brain derives most of its energy from the oxidation of glucose, although it can also oxidize certain amino and fatty acids which are synthesized within its cells. However, the total energy which comes from this restricted source would not last for an appreciable time, and thus the brain is almost entirely dependent upon the glucose delivered to it across the blood-brain barrier. Hence the adult brain (which comprises only 2 per cent of total body mass) utilizes 20 per cent of the total oxygen and 65 per cent of the total glucose consumed by the body, and requires 15 to 20 per cent of the total blood circulation per minute to deliver the high requirements for oxygen and glucose. Thus when supplies of

one or both are cut off, neural function fails with disastrous rapidity.[30] It has been estimated that the cerebral blood flow of a recumbent normal man is 750 ml. per minute. At any moment the blood circulating through the brain contains 7 ml. oxygen, an amount sufficient to supply its needs for less than 10 seconds. However, under conditions of reduced systemic blood pressure, as little as 32 ml. of blood per minute per 100 Gm. of brain can maintain consciousness—a little over half the usual supply. In experiments of Rossen, Kabat and Anderson,[31] in which the human brain was deprived of oxygen by sudden and complete arrest of cerebral circulation, consciousness was lost in 6 seconds. Restoration within 100 seconds was followed by rapid return of consciousness and without objective evidence of brain injury.

Diabetic Coma is usually attributed to the gradual accumulation of aceto-acetic and beta-hydroxybutyric acids in the blood. However, Fazekas and Bessman[32] note that in diabetic coma cerebral oxygen consumption is greatly depressed, although cerebral blood flow, vascular resistance and oxygen delivery may be normal and glucose supply far greater than normal. They attribute the condition to inhibition of cerebral enzymatic activity, adding that they find no support for the contention that diabetic coma is due to the accumulation of ketone bodies, or to changes in water or electrolyte metabolism.

Hypoglycemic Coma. Arteriovenous oxygen differences in the brain are closely related to the blood sugar level, and intense hypoglycemia causes severe impairment in oxygen uptake by the brain. The almost sole dependence of the brain upon the constant delivery of glucose makes it particularly vulnerable to hypoglycemic states.

Uremic Coma is due to the accumulation of noxious substances as a result of impaired excretory and detoxifying mechanisms as well as to disturbances in water and electrolyte metabolism.[32] The coma is believed due to impairment of cerebral enzymatic activity.

Hepatic Coma. Depth of hepatic coma appears to be related to blood ammonia level. Ammonia is produced in the intestine by bacterial action and conveyed to the liver by the portal vein. In the presence of either liver failure or extensive collateral circulation such as develops in hepatic cirrhosis, ammonia accumulates in the blood in increasing amounts.[33] The slowing of the EEG correlates well with the extent of neurologic and mental disturbance. Reduction of dietary protein and administration of neomycin for gut sterilization may improve the character of the EEG. Increasing protein intake or administering methionine or ammonium chloride cause the EEG to deteriorate.[34]

Electrolyte Disturbances. Variation in either the potassium or the sodium level of plasma is said not to affect the brain wave tracing.[35] However, in hypokalemia with familial periodic paralysis the EEG has been reported normal in some instances and disordered in others. Severe sodium depletion has also been said to slow the EEG and produce sleepiness leading into coma.[36] Calcium deficit leads to convulsions and also produces EEG slowing. Excessive hydration in combination with sodium depletion can lead to convulsions and also slows the EEG or transforms it into a convulsive pattern. Impaired consciousness can also result. Uncomplicated acidosis does not produce an unusual EEG effect, although that occasioned by inhalation of CO_2 brings about some increase in background fast activity and lowers the voltage of the EEG. Temporary alkalosis, as produced by hyperventilation, slows the EEG trace and produces amplitude build-up, especially in the frontal leads. More prolonged alkalosis (from vomiting, for example) occasions clouding of consciousness and produces runs of high voltage rhythmic slow activity.[35]

SYNCOPAL ATTACKS

Pathophysiologic factors in the various kinds of faints have been systematized by Engel[37] who classifies them under broad categories of peripheral circulatory inadequacy, cardiac arrhythmias, and respiratory or pulmonary disorders. Such brief periods of unconsciousness can be brought about in one of three ways: by cerebral ischemia, localized or generalized; by change in composition of the blood; by reflex cerebral dysfunction.[38]

Ischemia is the most important of these, and the site most vulnerable is believed to be the upper brainstem, a locus already discussed with respect to brain lesions which are prone to cause suddenly developing unconsciousness in the experimental animal or man. With prompt restoration of blood supply such lost consciousness is readily reversible. The EEG is a very sensitive indicator of anoxia, and the rapidity with which a slow delta pattern replaces usual background activity during an attack is intimately related to the abruptness of onset of unconsciousness. If ventricular stand-still occurs (as may happen in Adams-Stokes attacks), brain wave slowing can be closely related to alterations in pulse and blood pressure. Under these circumstances the pulseless period which precedes the onset of unconsciousness may be variable, extending from a few to 10 or more seconds.

Vasodepressor syncope[37] is the commonest form of fainting, and can be precipitated by fear, anxiety, pain or injury. It practically never occurs except in the erect posture, and symptoms are usually relieved by lying down. At the onset of an attack pulse and blood pressure may be somewhat elevated, blood pressure falling thereafter, systolic more rapidly than diastolic. Ordinarily recovery is rapid. Slowing of the EEG has been observed as consciousness is lost. An important factor is said to be the shunting of blood from brain to muscle by vasodilation mediated through the cholinergic vasodilator system.

Postural hypotension can develop in several ways, the common denominator being the repeated occurrence of fainting upon a rise from bed. Limited capacity for postural adjustment is important, and micturition or post-micturition syncope occurring in the middle-aged man who arises from a deep sleep to hurry to the bathroom may have this precipitating base. In chronic orthostatic hypotension, the classical form of postural hypotension, blood pressure falls rapidly upon assumption of the erect posture. Both systolic and diastolic pressures fall but there is little or no pulse alteration.[37] Consciousness is also lost rapidly, and restored rapidly upon correction of the precipitating postural change. Diffuse disease of the autonomic nervous system is often held responsible.

Adams-Stokes syndrome is the most widely known of the episodic syncopal attacks which occur in cardiac conditions. Such instances are divisible into two categories, one associated with permanent complete heart block and slow pulse (Adams-Stokes syndrome) and the other rising from reflex and/or metabolic factors with or without structural changes.[37] In Adams-Stokes syndrome the attacks of syncope are believed to be due to decrease in cerebral blood flow resulting from ventricular standstill, tachycardia, or fibrillation. The duration of asystole may be long, and convulsion caused by cerebral hypoxia may occur. High voltage slow EEG activity occurs during asystole, and if the standstill persists the tracing may flatten out. Among the instances which arise in individuals with reflex and/or metabolic factors are those with transient and paroxysmal heart block. Afferents of vagal reflexes arising from the upper gastroenteric tract, respiratory tract, mediastinum and external auditory canal may contribute to causation, as may afferent paths arising in eye or nasopharynx and carried in trigeminal and glossopharyngeal nerves.[37] Increased activity of the vagus nerves resulting from such heightened afferent impulses may cause sinoatrial standstill or atrioventricular block. This is true especially if associated with metabolic or organic changes affecting the mechanisms controlling origin and conduction of the stimulus to the heart beat. Reflex cardiac standstill and syncope can result in patients with intense paroxysmal pain in the glossopharyngeal distribution (glossopharyngeal neuralgia).

Carotid Sinus Hypersensitivity. Syncope associated with hypersensitivity of the carotid sinus also utilizes an afferent arm which passes over a branch of the glossopharyngeal nerve. In this disorder the specific nerve endings in the carotid sinus may be the major source of activation but summate with overly-sensitive afferents from other sources which augment vagal outflow. Significantly more persons show carotid sinus hypersensitivity to massage than ever show spontaneous fainting of this origin. Engel[37] advocates demonstration of identity between induced (by massage) and spontaneous faints, differentiation between massage of the sinus and of the carotid below it, and abolition of the hypersensitivity by atropine as criteria for establishing the carotid sinus as the source of troubles. He points out that the sinus region in such cases is usually exquisitely sensitive to stimulation. Besides prolonged asystole, there is a vasodepressor type of response in which fall of blood pressure is independent of change in heart rate. According to Wayne[38] this is abolished by epinephrine administration only.

A cerebral type of carotid sinus syncope is also described in which fainting is not related to change in blood pressure or pulse and is uninfluenced by either atropine or ephedrine.[39] Gurdjian et al.[40] believe this form to be misinterpreted and to result instead from partial or complete occlusion involving components of the contralateral arterial supply. They believe, of course, that a carotid sinus inhibitory reflex may be associated with the ischemic response. Engel has contraverted this evidence using the criteria set forth above. He found that the cerebral type of carotid sinus reflex may be elicited by very gentle and brief non-occlusive stimulation of the sinus. Recently Reese, Green and Eliott[41] have reported a case in which the features of the cerebral type of hypersensitivity were observed and yet panarteriography failed to show significant disease of the cervical arteries.

RESPIRATORY AND PULMONARY

Among forms of syncope associated with respiratory and pulmonary disorders, two are selected for brief mention, cough syncope and Pickwickian syndrome.

Cough syncope is prone to occur in robust middle-aged men, the stimuli which promote coughing leading to attacks resulting from rapidly repeated inspiration, incomplete expiration, and rapidly repeated very forceful expiratory effort against a closed glottis. Increased intrathoracic pressure in turn obstructs the return of blood from the cranium.

In Pickwickian syndrome the association of obesity with hypersomnolence, hypoventilation and polycythemia occurs, and in this instance attention is directed to somnolence instead of to syncope. Drachman and Gumnit[42] showed by intensive investigation of a single case that oxygen lack was the predominant factor in driving the subject's respiration and in awakening her from the somnolent state she might fall into.

ALCOHOL, DRUGS AND POISONS

Alcohol is by far the most frequent cause of hospital admissions for coma. The signs and symptoms of *acute alcoholism* are too well known to need emphasis here. For medicolegal purposes the concentrations of alcohol in blood, urine, saliva or exhaled air can be determined. As in other kinds of unconsciousness brain rhythms are slowed by alcohol, the degree of slowing being roughly related to the severity of intoxication.

About 20 per cent of hospital admissions for acute drug intoxication are for *barbiturate* poisoning. When the subject is discovered in acute poisoning deep sleep or coma is characteristic. Cyanosis may be prominent and Cheyne-Stokes respiration evident. The involvement of superficial and deep reflexes relates to the degree of central depression, and toe signs may be obtained. Pupils tend to be somewhat constricted, although they may dilate late in the course of the poisoning. The EEG shows the high-voltage slow delta activity which is a general characteristic of brain activity in comatose patients. Identification can be made of barbiturates in the stomach contents, blood and urine. For treatment Plum and Swanson[43] believe there is no substitute for the direct physiological treatment of depressed respiration or circulation; the use of analeptic drugs in their hands provided little additional help. The immediate dangers to the patient admitted in a comatose state are generally respiratory. The airway must be cleared scrupulously and one must ensure adequate intake of oxygen. Circulatory treatment should include starting venoclysis at the time of admission to provide an immediate route if plasma expanders or vasopressor drugs become necessary.

Opium, morphine and other opium derivatives should also be remembered as possible causes of coma. Diacetylmorphine (heroin) is 5 times as potent as morphine and is especially apt to cause addiction. It is not an official drug in the United States and its importation into or manufacture in this country is prohibited by law. Not uncommonly *salicylate* poisoning may occur (especially in children) and need consideration in differential diagnosis.

Among the poisonous gases causing coma *carbon monoxide* is important,[44] most often from automobile exhaust or from gases used in the home or produced in industry. Skin, lips and nail beds may be a cherry-red color, pupils dilated, temperature subnormal, and respirations irregular, rapid or shallow. Blood chemistry studies for carbon monoxide and for methemoglobin may be diagnostic.

Dinitro-ortho-cresol, a weed killer, should be considered where poisoning is suspected, as should pesticides which are DFP congeners. The latter inactivate cholinesterases.

HYSTERIA

Considered as a cause of unconsciousness, hysteria usually occurs in females with chronic multiple system complaints often starting at adolescence. By age 30 such women frequently have had several surgical operations. When periods of unconsciousness are of brief duration they may have been preceded by difficulty in breathing at a time of emotional stress with subsequent hyperventilation, and respiratory alkalosis (with numbness, muscle cramps, etc.).

CONVULSIVE DISORDERS

ANALYTIC VALUE OF BRAIN WAVES AND CLASSIFICATION

The electroencephalogram is the most important adjunct we have to the clinical appraisal of convulsive states. In general, we believe that refractoriness to anticonvulsant drugs correlates positively with excessive, persistent disorder of brain rhythm.

Certain types of seizures known to respond effectively to one medication but not to another can often be identified from unique characteristics of a disordered EEG, when other bases of clinical appraisal leave the issue in doubt. Examples are the 3 per second generalized spike-wave EEG of petit mal epilepsy and the asynchronous spikes which arise from a background of suppression (called hypsarhythmia). In the latter

EEG CLASSIFICATIONS

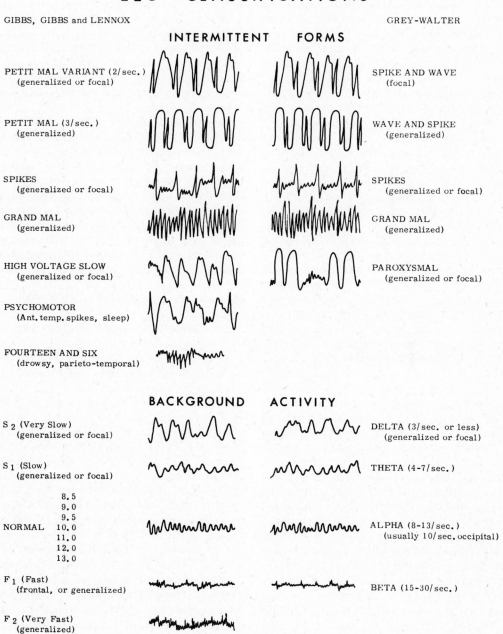

GIBBS, GIBBS and LENNOX   GREY-WALTER

INTERMITTENT   FORMS

PETIT MAL VARIANT (2/sec.)
(generalized or focal)

SPIKE AND WAVE
(focal)

PETIT MAL (3/sec.)
(generalized)

WAVE AND SPIKE
(generalized)

SPIKES
(generalized or focal)

SPIKES
(generalized or focal)

GRAND MAL
(generalized)

GRAND MAL
(generalized)

HIGH VOLTAGE SLOW
(generalized or focal)

PAROXYSMAL
(generalized or focal)

PSYCHOMOTOR
(Ant. temp. spikes, sleep)

FOURTEEN AND SIX
(drowsy, parieto-temporal)

BACKGROUND   ACTIVITY

S 2 (Very Slow)
(generalized or focal)

DELTA (3/sec. or less)
(generalized or focal)

S 1 (Slow)
(generalized or focal)

THETA (4-7/sec.)

NORMAL

8.5
9.0
9.5
10.0
11.0
12.0
13.0

ALPHA (8-13/sec.)
(usually 10/sec. occipital)

F 1 (Fast)
(frontal, or generalized)

BETA (15-30/sec.)

F 2 (Very Fast)
(generalized)

FIGURE 176.

condition steroids may provide the base for successful treatment of a severely incapacitated infant. In adults, when an aura or signal symptom (Fig. 176) points to a focal seizure originating at a particular site upon one side of the brain, the electroencephalogram may confirm the supposition in an interseizure interval by producing evidence of an associated spike or slow wave focus. Finally, if a generalized seizure first occurs in middle adult life, the EEG may yield the first evidence localizing a brain tumor. For these reasons it is profitable to consider EEG rhythms and their classification as a prelude to discussion of the pathophysiology of seizure.

Background Activity. The first recordings of spontaneous brain rhythms in animals were obtained long before the electronic era produced a technology capable of coping with the clinical aspects of electrical recording. Berger is credited with the first indubitable records of brain activity in man. His clinical success activated a universal interest in brain recording. At the start, Adrian and Buytendijk[45] were able to show that the isolated brainstem of the goldfish gives forth a rhythm which has the same frequency as the movement of the gills in the intact fish. Ever since, spontaneous rhythms have been accepted as another manifestation of the essential rhythmicity which sustains many of life's processes. Adrian also confirmed Berger's interpretation of the 10 per second adult alpha rhythm which is recorded from the parieto-occipital scalp area in the relaxed subject who has his eyes closed. A variety of other electrical manifestations of the activity of the human brain can also be recorded through scalp electrodes, differences appearing in individuals awake and asleep and at different stages of life from infancy to old age. At birth the electroencephalogram shows only low, slow waves of 4 per second or lower frequency. For the first year of life these slow patterns increase in amplitude and are then replaced by intermediate slow frequencies at 4 to 7 per second. Finally (in a small percentage of infants beginning as early as the 10th month) the precursor of the adult alpha

rhythm in turn replaces the intermediate frequencies as the principal background pattern of the human electroencephalogram. In old age metabolic letdown again introduces slow activity into the normal tracing, and the ravages of cerebrovascular disease can markedly hasten this process. As with animals, rhythm at 1 per second characterizes the human brain asleep, and it is also the principal pattern associated with pathologic loss of consciousness for whatever reason. This rhythm (called delta and assigned limits of 1 to 4 per second) also appears focally as a pathological process over sites of cerebral infarct, contusion, abscess or tumor.

Intermittent Forms Characteristic of Convulsive States. Beside the spontaneous background activity described above intermittent wave patterns also occur. Often these show a voltage 4 to 20 times greater than that of the background activity. They signify abnormally synchronized electrical disturbance of unique wave form which has a very high correlation with seizure state, and can be recorded in interseizure traces. Such intermittent forms can occur as single wave complexes, or repeat the identical wave shape continuously over intervals extending from seconds to minutes. When diffusely recorded from scalp (that is, showing no localization) they are presumed to signify a generalized cortical disturbance projected from a limited central source situated at the mesodiencephalic origin of the diffuse thalamic projection system. Grand and petit mal seizure discharges of the usual idiopathic variety belong in this category, and Penfield and Jasper[46] would list them as *centrencephalic seizures*. In the case of repetitive spike-wave disturbance it is important that brief runs lasting 4 to 6 seconds can occur without either a petit mal seizure or lapse of consciousness intervening. Such are called *subclinical* or *electrical* seizures. When closely repetitive large spikes occur at 12 to 24 per second they correlate with grand mal seizures and complete loss of consciousness. Such are difficult to record during an attack because electrodes are easily torn off. However, very adequate records have been obtained recently using immobilizing drugs. There are also other unique intermittent wave forms such as single spikes or spike waves which appear focally over an underlying epileptogenic focus of the brain. Such indicators of the site of a focal seizure may often be recorded in the interseizure period. Thus they are a valuable asset to the electroencephalographer because he does not have to depend upon recording a seizure. Presumably when a seizure spreads widely from such a focus these spikes become a confluent series which spread as an avalanche to the remotest areas of the brain, producing generalized seizure manifestations.

It is important to understand that EEG classifications developed simultaneously in several different parts of the world. Those of Gibbs, Gibbs and Lennox[47] and Grey-Walter[48] are in commonest use (Fig. 176). They agree in general principles but differ in detail of subclassification of both background and intermittent forms. In interpretation one must understand that even in the absence of the intermittent types of activity which have a high correlation with convulsive state, the degree of departure of background activity from the expected normal for age also has use in establishing an unknown electroencephalogram as obtained from a subject with a convulsive disorder. Thus the S-2 (very slow) pattern of the adult electroencephalogram[47] occurs 20 times as frequently in epileptics as compared with normal controls. By contrast, a mildly slow tracing occurs only twice as often.

During sleep several unique intermittent (convulsive) features can appear which are not evident in the waking state. Outstanding among these are the anterior temporal spikes which derive from the tips of the temporal lobes in psychomotor epilepsy. Another such pattern is the "14 and 6" pattern of the drowsy state. This is most easily recorded from the temporo-parietal areas in monopolar records, and is believed by some authorities to correlate highly with behavior disorder, abdominal epilepsy, etc. However, these relations have not been firmly established.

THE BROAD SPECTRUM OF CONVULSIVE DISORDER

Convulsions are of common occurrence, appearing, for example, in one of two hundred draftees and in a significantly higher incidence of still younger individuals. Attacks are far more diversified than can be encompassed under the combined symptoms of loss of consciousness and massive generalized spasm. The term *epilepsy* also includes a variety of focal seizure patterns in which consciousness is either not lost at all or (at most) is altered, and those others which show fleeting but complete interruption of consciousness attended by a minimum of rhythmic movement. Features common to all attacks are episodic occurrence, brief duration, and coincidence in the EEG of the unique wave forms mentioned in the last section. Such are the inseparable accompaniments of the epileptic attack, and their occurrence as brief interludes of the interseizure EEG trace caused Gibbs, Gibbs and Lennox[47] to refer to epilepsy as a *paroxysmal cerebral dysrhythmia*. There may be instances in which seizure develops without concomitant scalp-recorded EEG change. However, if it does, its site of origin is either at a considerable distance from the scalp leads through which it might be recorded or else it is so exquisitely small as not to spread to even a nearby electrode. Undoubtedly both circumstances arise rarely.

The causes of epileptic attacks are multiple and can be systematized in a number of ways. One classification sets generalized against focal attacks. The origin of the latter are ascribed to one discrete area of the brain, and the sequence of development of the seizure somehow exemplifies the function attributed to parts through which it spreads. Focal seizures are usually symptomatic of an organic brain lesion and fall into the group called *symptomatic epilepsy*. Thus only secondarily do they signify a pathophysiologic process. By contrast, generalized seizures of the kind referred to as *idiopathic* (or by Penfield as centrencephalic) represents a primary pathophysiologic process arising through some predisposition, genetically determined or otherwise.

It is important to remember that instances of symptomatic epilepsy are not infrequent among generalized seizures. The perinatal period particularly abounds in contributory causes. Among them are changes in the uterine environment such as predispose to congenital malformations (as viral or bacterial infections of the mother), kernicterus, anoxia and mechanical birth trauma. Encephalitis and meningitis occurring in the postnatal period also take a significant toll, and postnatal trauma is the precipitating cause in some instances. In later life, the residuals of CNS infectious processes, cerebrovascular disease and neoplasm precipitate the condition. Thus the relative proportion of the remainder of generalized seizures attributable to *genetic predisposition* remains moot. Lennox[49] estimated that in a group of 2,000 epileptics a family history was obtained in about 20 per cent. However, the same writer has pointed out the similarity in detail of spike and wave discharges as they occur in uniovular twins. As in other disorders of paroxysmal recurrence, heredity and environment are not mutually exclusive determinants but interact considerably.

Generalized Seizures

We restrict the term generalized to seizures in which there is an interruption of consciousness, however fleeting, and in which the EEG discharge appears simultaneously or successively from leads over the two hemispheres.

Grand Mal. Onset is usually sudden and may be ushered in by an expulsion of air through a partially closed glottis giving rise to an epileptic cry. Ordinarily the convulsion is of the tonic-clonic type. Loss of control of bladder or bowels and biting of the tongue are common. During and immediately following a seizure the pupils may be fixed and positive toe signs may be found. Postictal drowsiness or automatism can occur and last for several hours. While repetitive spike activity of the type called grand mal is the commonest seizure finding, tracings from young children may show a high amplitude synchronized slow pattern instead.

Petit Mal. A momentary stare or blank look, (indicative of a suspension of consciousness) is the minimal finding, and not unusually such lapses occur for some time before being discovered by teacher or parent. The episodes may be called spells, blackouts, trances, day-dreaming, even thinking, by distracted parents. They are of abrupt onset and ending, often occur very frequently, and are of brief duration. However, *petit mal status* may occur. Status attacks consist of longer lapses from consciousness, sometimes lasting for many seconds or even several minutes, without a fall or convulsion. Gibbs and Gibbs[50] detected a history of status in approximately one quarter of their petit mal cases. The diagnosis can be established by detection of the classical 3 per second spike and wave pattern in the electroencephalogram. When such sequences are more than a few seconds long they are invariably accompanied by a typical lapse. Hyperventilation producing alkalosis, ingestion of large amount of alkali, hydration, anoxia, hypoglycemia, or emotional disturbance may precipitate attacks. Facial twitches and jerks of the limbs may accompany a lapse, individual twitches correlating in time with the spikes of the spike-wave pattern. Sometimes there are also minor automatisms such as licking the lips or shuffling the feet. The subject remains erect if standing.

Other seizure types related to petit mal by the similar occurrence of generalized spike and wave activity are myoclonic attacks, ranging from small jerks to mass spasms, and falling spells sometimes called *akinetic epilepsy*.

Psychomotor Seizures. There is confusion between authorities as to the exact limits of psychomotor seizure phenomena, and terminology for and site of origin of the seizures. Attacks with which they may be confused are automatisms of frontal or temporal origin,[45] uncinate attacks, and psychic equivalents of temporal lobe origin (as *déjà vu* and *déjà pensée*). It would appear that a nuclear pattern of automatism can attach to a variety of reported psychic experiences, including those of fear, rage and the dream state. We are concerned, however, with the pattern of attack associated with anterior temporal spikes in the sleep electroencephalogram. That is best described by Gibbs and Gibbs.[50] For hours or days before a seizure the patient may be irritable. A seizure commences with a wild look, an inappropriate phrase, or a peculiar gesture. The movements during an attack may appear purposeful but are poorly co-ordinated. To a degree they are automatic and repetitive. They may consist of simple

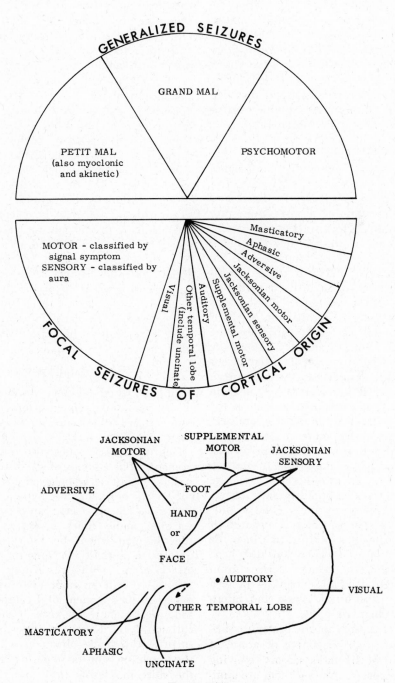

FIGURE 177.

acts like lip smacking, hand wringing or clutching or plucking at objects. In some cases they consist in more elaborate posturing or movements which have the appearance of being purposive, such as undressing or sweeping with a broom. Content of speech is commonly affected, and may be rambling or tangential. Inability to recollect events points toward a sufficient suspension or diversion of the stream of consciousness to mark the seizures as generalized. EEG traces which we have recorded during such seizures also show bilateral disorder, even though interseizure spiking during sleep may be principally unilateral.

FOCAL SEIZURES

It is the sensory aura or the motor signal symptom (Fig. 176) which lends distinctive character to a focal seizure. In the case of the *jacksonian motor seizures* there are three predominant foci in the motor cortex: for movements of thumb and the index finger, the angle of the mouth and the hallux (great toe). All such attacks spread from these parts in an ordered march of convulsion which as a rule corresponds fairly closely with the localization of motor control in the cortex.[50] However, the march need not invariably follow the points indicated upon the familiar charts of cerebral localization. A jacksonian motor seizure, of course, may spread from an exquisitely localized source such as the thumb or hallux to become generalized. Other seizures with more massive signal symptoms derive from other areas of the frontal lobe. For example the *frontal adversive seizure,* combining head and eye turning toward the opposite side derives from the premotor territory. The *supplemental motor seizure,* which is initiated by the assumption of a posture in which the contralateral arm is raised and the head turned toward the arm,[51] derives from frontal marginal cortex extending posteriorly to the paracentral lobule and inferiorly to the cingulate gyrus.

Seizures of *sensory* origin present a variety of auras, each suggestive of a site of origin in one of the major sensory receiving areas of the cortex. Among them are auditory, visual, olfactory (uncinate), and sensory jacksonian types (Fig. 177). The last is the sensory replica of the motor jacksonian seizure with march, arising instead in the general sensory cortex just behind the major central sulcus which divides the frontal from the parietal lobes. Spread of the disturbance from any one of these may eventuate in a generalized motor seizure. Other focal seizure types are the masticatory and the aphasic (of which speech arrest is one kind), arising respectively from temporal and frontal regions of the brain. Evaluation of the epileptic significance of episodic psychic aberrations rests upon uncertain ground unless indisputable neurologic concomitants occur. Such seizures pass through an intervening shadowland into mental experiences which would only engage the attention of a psychiatrist.

On occasion sensory stimuli are known to precipitate seizures, instances of such activation by touch, pain, smell, noise and music having been recorded. *Reading epilepsy* is a special variety of the latter,[52] about 20 cases having been reported to date. Seizures occur during reading precipitated by intermittent brief involuntary movements of the jaw. Several types of EEG abnormalities have been observed in such cases.

NARCOLEPSY

In cases where narcolepsy occurs with all of its commonly related symptoms, recurrent attacks of sleepiness are associated with cataplexy (attacks of tonelessness), "sleep paralysis," and hallucinatory phenomena. The etiology of the disturbance is unknown but it is believed to center in the sleep areas of the hypothalamus, if such exist. Sleep attacks can occur without warning many times a day. Ordinarily they happen when the subject is sitting quietly in a chair or lying in bed. The attack occurs without warning and may last up to half an hour. Normal persons experience a fragment of a cataplectic episode every time their "knees become weak" through fear. Laughter, anger, fright, or surprise can bring on an attack. Besides the tonelessness of the somatic musculature, the voice may grow weak and the eyelids droop. After about a minute recovery occurs. "Sleep paralysis" is a corresponding state of tonelessness which occurs when the subject is falling asleep or awakening. Frightening hallucinations also occur in some narcoleptics.

SUMMARY

The chapter commences with a review of the pathophysiology of coma and convulsion. Sleep is used to illustrate a normal, reversible kind of unconsciousness which has its pathologic counterpart in lesions that destroy the rostral brainstem tegmentum. Coma can also result from a sufficient general depression of brain metabolism. The brain is almost entirely dependent for its energy upon the delivery of oxygen and glucose across the blood-brain barrier. For example, at any moment the blood circulating through the brain carries only enough oxygen to sustain functioning for a matter of 10 seconds. Even a brief failure of delivery of these important energy sources through ischemia (for example in common vasodepressor syncope or in an Adams-Stokes attack) can produce a corresponding suspension of consciousness. It is estimated that a complete arrest of cerebral circulation for 100 seconds can still be followed by rapid return of consciousness without objective sequelae of brain injury. Disordered systemic metabolism may produce a more prolonged, although a less drastic effect upon the brain than arrest of circulation does. Uremia, diabetes, hypoglycemia and liver disease can produce coma through interference with the delivery of glucose or by suppression by toxins of the cerebral enzymatic activity necessary to convert glucose and oxygen to energy.

Coma also accompanies generalized seizures. In fact a brief suspension of consciousness is the outstanding symptom in one type of generalized seizure called petit mal. In another type (grand mal) loss of consciousness is of longer duration and accompanied by massive tonic-clonic spasm of the somatic musculature. In a third type a diversion of the stream of consciousness occurs coupled with an episode of automatism (psychomotor). Electroencephalograms of these three principal types have dis-tinguishing characteristics which are very useful diagnostically.

A variety of focal seizures also occur. These arise at a spot of cortical damage which results from invasion by neoplasm, anoxia, or scarring due to injury. The seizure process is the same as in the generalized seizure and the focal attack may spread to produce one. It is the sensory aura or the motor signal symptom which lends a distinctive character to a focal seizure, pointing to the site of origin in the plan of cerebral localization. Seizures of sensory origin present a variety of auras, each suggestive of a site of origin in one of the major sensory receiving areas of the cortex. Among these seizures are auditory, visual, olfactory, and sensory jacksonian types. Focal motor seizures commence in the motor cortex ahead of the central sulcus as jacksonian motor seizures with signal symptoms in thumb and index, hallux or side of mouth. Other types of focal motor seizure are "adversive" and "supplemental motor" which arise from other areas of the frontal lobe. In all instances it is important to discover the etiology of a focal seizure, for it may be caused by a surgically remediable condition.

REFERENCES

1. Brain, R.: The physiological basis of consciousness, Brain 81:426, 1958.
2. Sartre, J. P.: Imagination. A psychological critique, *translated by* F. Williams. Ann Arbor, U. of Mich. Press, 1962.
3. James, W.: A Pluralistic Universe, New York, Longmans, Green & Co., 1932.
4. Prochaska, G.: Dissertation on the Functions of the Nervous System, *translated and edited by* Thomas Laycock, London, Sydenham Society, 1851.
5. Richerland, A.: Elements of Physiology, *translated by* G. J. M. de Lys, Phila., Dobson & Son, 1813.
6. Bremer, F.: Cerveau isolé et physiologie du sommeil. Compte Rendus Biol., Paris, 118:1235, 1935.
7. von Economo, C. J.: Sleep as a problem of localization, J. Nerv. & Ment. Dis. 71:249, 1930.
8. Hess, W. R.: The Functional Organization of the Diencephalon, New York, Grune & Stratton, 1957.

9. Dempsey, E. W., and Morison, R. S.: The production of rhythmically recurrent cortical potentials after localized thalamic stimulation, Am. J. Physiol. 135:293, 1942.

10. Moruzzi, G., and Magoun, H. W.: Brain stem reticular formation and activation of EEG, EEG Clin. Neurophysiol. 1:455, 1949.

11. Dement, W.: The occurrence of low voltage, fast, electroencephalogram patterns during behaviorial sleep in the cat, EEG Clin. Neurophysiol. 10:291, 1958.

12. Jouvet, M.: Telencephalic and rhombencephalic sleep in the cat, in The Nature of Sleep, a Ciba Symposium ed. by G. E. W. Wolstenholme and M. O'Connor, Boston, Little, Brown, 1960.

13. Huttenlocher, P. H.: Evoked and spontaneous activity in single units of medial brainstem during natural sleep and waking, J. Neurophysiol. 24:451, 1961.

14. Penfield, W.: Centrencephalic integrating system, Brain 81:231, 1958.

15. Walshe, F. M. R.: The brain-stem conceived as the "highest level" of function in the nervous system; with particular reference to the automatic apparatus of Carpenter (1850) and to the "centrencephalic integrating system" of Penfield, Brain 80:510, 1957.

16. Puetsch, P., Guilly, P., Fischgold, H., and Bounes, G.: Un cas d'anencephalie hydrocephalique, Revue Neurol. 79:117, 1947.

17. Nielsen, J. M., and Sedgwick, R. P.: Instincts and emotions in an anencephalic monster, J. Nerv. & Ment. Dis. 110:387, 1949.

18. Cairns, H.: Disturbances of consciousness with lesions of the brain stem and diencephalon, Brain 74:109, 1952.

19. Howell, D. C.: Upper brain-stem compression and foraminal impaction with intracranial space-occupying lesions and brain swelling, Brain 82:525, 1959.

20. McNealy, D. E., and Plum, F.: Brain-stem dysfunction with supratentorial mass lesions, Arch. Neurol. 7:10, 1962.

21. Ingvar, D. H., and Lundberg, N.: Paroxysmal symptoms in intracranial hypertension, studied with ventricular fluid pressure recording and electroencephalography, Brain 84:446, 1961.

22. Solomon, P., and Aring, C.D.: The causes of coma in patients entering a general hospital, Am. J. Med. Sci. 188:805, 1934.

23. ———: The differential diagnosis in patients entering the hospital in coma, J.A.M.A. 105:7, 1935.

24. ———: A routine diagnostic procedure for the patient who enters the hospital in coma, Am. J. Med. Sci. 191:357, 1936.

25. Symonds, C. P.: Concussion and contusion of the brain and their sequelae, in S. Brock, ed., Injuries of the Skull, Brain and Spinal Cord, ed. 4, Baltimore, Williams & Wilkins, 1960.

26. Courville, C. B.: Pathology of the Central Nervous System, Mountain View, Calif., Pacific Press Pub. Ass., 1937.

27. Walker, A. E.: Posttraumatic Epilepsy, Springfield, Ill., Thomas, 1949.

28. Robbins, F. C.: The clinical and laboratory diagnosis of viral infections of the central nervous system, in W. S. Fields and R. J. Blattner, eds.: Viral Encephalitis, Springfield, Ill., Thomas, 1958.

29. Survey Report: Cerebrovascular Study Group, Institute of Neurological Diseases and Blindness, National Institutes of Health, Bethesda, Md. and St. Louis, Mo., Bardgett Printing & Publishing Co., 1961.

30. Tower, D. B.: Neurochemistry, Report of an Extramural Survey and Program Committee, Neurological & Allied Sciences, U.S. Public Health Service, Bethesda, Md. and St. Louis, Mo., Bardgett Printing & Publishing Co., 1960.

31. Rossen, R., Kabat, H., and Anderson, J. P.: Acute arrest of cerebral circulation in man, Arch. Neurol. & Psychiat. 50:510, 1943.

32. Fazekas, J. F., and Bessman, A. M.: Coma mechanisms, Am. J. Med. 15:804, 1953.

33. McLagen, N. F.: The biochemistry of coma, in Biochemical Aspects of Neurological Disorders, Oxford, Blackwell Scientific Pub., 1959.

34. Parsons-Smith, B. G., Summerskill, W. H. J., Dawson, A. M., and Sherlock, S.: The electroencephalogram in liver disease, Lancet 2:867, 1957.

35. Kiloh, L. G., and Osselton, J. W.: Clinical Electroencephalography, London, Butterworths, 1961.

36. Moyer, C. A.: Fluid Balance, Chicago, Ill., Year Book, 1953; Personal communication.

37. Engel, G. L.: Fainting, Springfield, Ill., Thomas, 1962.

38. Wayne, H. H.: Syncope, Am. J. Med. 30:418, 1961.

39. Weiss, S., and Baker, J. P.: The carotid sinus reflex in health and disease. Its role in the causation of fainting and convulsions, Medicine 12:297, 1933.

40. Gurdjian, E. S., Webster, J. E., Hardy, W. G., and Lindner, D. W.: Nonexistence of the

so-called cerebral form of carotid sinus syncope, Neurology 8:818, 1958.

41. Reese, C. L., Green, J. B., and Elliott, F. A.: The cerebral form of carotid sinus hypersensitivity, Neurology 12:492, 1962.

42. Drachman, D. B., and Gumnit, R. J.: Periodic alteration of consciousness in the "Pickwickian" syndrome, Arch. Neurol. 6:471, 1962.

43. Plum, F., and Swanson, A. G.: Barbiturate poisoning treated by physiological methods with observations on effects of betamethylglutarimide and electrical stimulation, J.A.M.A. 163:827, 1957.

44. Polson, C. J. and Tattersall, R. N.: Advances in clinical toxicology, Practitioner 187:549, 1961.

45. Adrian, E. D., and Buytendijk, F. J.: Potential changes in the isolated brain stem of the goldfish, J. Physiol. 71:121, 1931.

46. Penfield, W., and Jasper, H.: Epilepsy and Functional Anatomy of the Brain, Boston, Little, Brown, 1954.

47. Gibbs, F. A., Gibbs, E. L., and Lennox, W. G.: Electroencephalographic classification of epileptic patients and control subjects, Arch. Neurol. & Psychiat. 50:111, 1943.

48. Grey-Walter, W.: Normal rhythms—their development, distribution and significance, in Electroencephalography, a Symposium on its Various Aspects, London, MacDonald, 1950.

49. Lennox, W. G.: Epilepsy and Related Disorders, vol. 1, Boston, Little, Brown, 1960.

50. Gibbs, F. A., and Gibbs, E. L.: Atlas of Electroencephalography, vol. 2, Cambridge, Mass., Addison-Wesley, 1952.

51. Walshe, F. M. R.: On the mode of representation of movements in the motor cortex with special reference to "convulsions beginning unilaterally," Brain 66:104, 1943.

52. Ajmone Marsan, C. and Ralston, B. R.: The Epileptic Seizure: its functional morphology and diagnostic significance. Springfield, Ill., C. C. Thomas, 1957.

53. Bickford, R. G., Whelan, J. L., Klass, D. W., and Corbin, K. B.: Reading epilepsy: clinical and electroencephalographic studies on a new syndrome, Trans. Amer. Neurol. Ass., pp. 100-102, 1956.

27

Disturbances of Movement

WILLIAM M. LANDAU AND JAMES L. O.'LEARY

Because the distribution of activity in the neuromuscular system is readily appraised by visual inspection, manipulation and palpation, both in spontaneous behavior and reflex activation, clinical observation alone has proved to be a remarkably successful analytic method. By 1900 most of the major disorders mentioned in this chapter were well described, and in many cases correlated with neuropathologic findings. Most of the groundwork had been laid during the time that Cajal and Sherrington were developing our modern concepts of the neuron doctrine, the synapse, the reflex, and the final common path. In fact, many of the important early studies in neuroanatomy were derived from clinical material. In physiology, as Walshe has pointed out, the experiments demonstrating the electrical excitability of the motor cortex in animals were based upon the clinical observations and inferences of Hughlings Jackson.

The fact that Jackson's early studies upon the natural experiments of disease proved accurate and valid warrants more than an historical footnote because the integrative theory of nervous functioning which he developed remains important. These ideas are the philosophical premises of most modern thinking and investigation in neurology (not of the motor system alone) and, though not often admitted, of experimental neurophysiology and psychology as well.

Here, as a framework for discussion of the pathophysiology of movement, we only have space to assert principles. For a better understanding of their derivation, the interested reader is referred to Walshe's review,[1] and thence to some of the classical studies upon the subject.

Symptoms may be due simply to the absence of function following a destructive lesion, as when, for example, a muscle is completely paralyzed by transection of its motor nerve. In contrast, a discharging lesion is one in which diseased elements are abnormally active, as when the anterior horn cells fire spontaneously in fasciculation, or the motor cortex, in convulsion.

There are both negative and positive results of central nervous system lesions. The negative aspect of a lesion in the motor cortex may be the loss of skilled movement, while a positive aspect would be the organization of remaining neural tissue into activity patterns which produce simpler, less variably adaptive movements and hyperactive reflexes. This is also called release of function. It is inferred that neural connections which become hyperactive are normally controlled and regulated by the regions damaged. Whether or not this regulation includes direct inhibition is seldom clear.

Jackson emphasizes the view that both normal and injured nervous systems perform adaptive functions as an integrated whole. This does not mean that functional analysis is impossible, or that all regions are equipotential. It means rather that behavioral function can be best analyzed in terms of levels of complexity. The nervous system clearly is not like a system of electrical relays, the higher triggering the lower. Rather it is the ultimate organ of adaptation: its flexibility and variability of response are a function of the available multiplicity of connections. Jackson put it most simply "the more gray matter, the more movements."

This leads to his concept of levels of neural integration. The lowest level of representation of movement in Jackson's language is the anterior horn cell and the local segmental reflex connections. This stump of the nervous system is capable of mediating stereotyped protective and ambulatory movements. A higher level of adaptive response in organized behavior is possible when the organism has available brainstem and motor cortical connections. The highest level of behavior is available with the complete nervous system.

A specific example of the levels of CNS dysfunction may be presented for the tongue. If the motor nerve is damaged, there is complete paralysis. If the pyramidal tract and brainstem connections are damaged, the motoneuron and the muscle remain intact, and can be activated in some reflexes, but most complex organized movement is not possible. If the motor cortex is relatively spared, the tongue may move quite well in complex movements of swallowing and purposeful movements of the tongue on command. But if the region around the left Sylvian fissure is damaged, the patient will be aphasic and still unable to use the tongue in the most complex movements of speech.

Many movement disorders have several aspects of malfunction. Thus their arbitrary assignment in the classification that follows is only for convenience of presentation.

IMPAIRED MOVEMENT
MUSCULAR DYSTROPHY

The primary symptom of muscle disease is the weakness in the movements of affected muscles. Clinical definition depends upon the distribution and the course of impairment. Distortions of movement may result from compensatory efforts to overcome weakness.

There are several varieties of progressive muscular dystrophy.[2,3] The majority have their onset early in life, with progression slowly over a period of years, and with impairment of the proximal musculature early and most severely. The most common type is inherited as a sex-linked recessive. It probably occurs only in boys, begins during the first few years of life, and leads to severe disability before maturity. The early symptoms are difficulty in climbing stairs and in arising from the recumbent position. Observation of this performance shows that the patient uses his hands to climb up the furniture or his own extremities in order to overcome the weakness of his trunk and pelvic girdle muscles. There is usually a swayback posture. The gait is waddling because of gluteal weakness. Stretch reflexes and response to direct muscle percussion are decreased. The calf muscles are prominently spared early in the course of the disease, and may be enlarged by increased size of muscle fibers. However, true "pseudohypertrophy" due to fatty infiltration, with or without weakness, is rare.

Other varieties may affect either sex, may be inherited as dominant or recessive characters, usually start in the later first to third decades, progress less rapidly, and may primarily affect the face and shoulder girdles or both limb girdles. There are rare families afflicted with dystrophy of distal limb muscles. Hereditary extraocular muscle dystrophy presents symptoms in adult life.

The most common cause of distal myopathy in early adult life is myotonic dystrophy. In addition to slowly progressive involvement of the forearms and legs, along with the diagnostic myotonic phenomenon (see below), there are prominent atrophy of the sternomastoid and facial muscles, baldness, early lenticular cataracts, gonadal atrophy, and other endocrine hypofunction.

The hypotonic, floppy infant is a complex diagnostic problem.[3,4] Many such patients suffer from diffuse brain damage, either congenital or progressive, and are generally severely retarded. When such processes are excluded, the most common disease of floppy babies is infantile motoneuron disease (Werdnig-Hoffman). Also progressive is an infantile variety of progressive muscular dystrophy. A nonprogressive hereditary myopathy, central core disease, is characterized by a unique central histologic abnormality of the muscle fibers. A benign congenital myopathy is characterized by retarded improvement in muscle strength, some preservation of stretch reflexes, and histologically by uniformly small or normal fibers. Infantile varieties of polyneuritis, polymyositis, and myasthenia gravis may also occur.

POLYMYOSITIS

This is one of the collagen diseases. When there is associated skin or gastrointestinal involvement, it is called dermatomyositis. The disease may develop at any age but appears most commonly in adult life and then is often associated with a malignant neoplasm. Symmetrical muscle wasting and weakness, usually in a proximal distribution, develop over periods of weeks to years. Muscle tenderness and pain may occur but are relatively uncommon. The clinical and even the biopsy findings may be quite similar to those of hereditary dystrophy, and only the age of onset, the clinical course, and the absence of family history may be distinctive.[5] Since many cases respond well to steroid therapy, clinical distinction is of practical importance. The EMG often shows fibrillation potentials and small motor units. Several serum enzymes may also be increased. Rare causes of localized or diffuse myositis are sarcoidosis and trichinosis.

METABOLIC MYOPATHIES

Rarely myopathy is related to endocrine malfunction. Weakness is usually diffuse, but sometimes more prominent proximally or distally.

Hyperthyroid myopathy may be proximal or general. Fasciculation, bulbar weakness, and eye muscle involvement may occur along with wasting. Thus there may be confusion with motoneuron disease or with myasthenia gravis. Indeed, the latter may also be present. Hypothyroidism is characterized by weakness, sometimes muscle enlargement, and a unique slowed relaxation due to abnormality of the contractile mechanism. This may be clinically evident in the tendon jerks. A proximal or diffuse weakness and wasting has been reported with hyperparathyroidism.

A proximal or generalized myopathy may occur in Cushing's syndrome, spontaneous or induced. A myopathy in Addison's disease is associated with joint contractures that are thought to relate to primary affection of fascial tissue.

Hyperinsulinism may produce a distal, or less often proximal muscle impairment. Evidence for both primary myopathy and neuropathy has been recorded. There is controversy concerning the occurrence of a primary myopathy in diabetes mellitus.

Congenital deficiency of muscle phosphorylase (McArdle) results in inability to metabolize muscle glycogen. The patient suffers painful muscle cramping leading to muscle contracture and weakness when he attempts to exercise beyond a minimum rate. These patients may also have myoglobinuria following excessive exercise. Muscle wasting is not conspicuous.

PERIODIC PARALYSIS

This is a recurrent acute familial syndrome of severe weakness leading to paralysis which comes on over a period of minutes to hours. Each episode lasts a few hours to a day or more. The originally described periodic paralysis is usually associated with hypokalemia during attacks which may be reversed by potassium therapy. The paralysis is characteristically ascending and tends to spare the respiratory muscles. A unique feature of the disease is the electrical inexcitability of both motor nerves and muscles during an attack. Muscle membrane potentials have been shown to be normal during an attack.

Gamstorp has described a familial periodic paralysis associated with hyperkalemia or normokalemia. Paramytonia congenita is a hereditary disease related to myotonia in which symptoms of stiffness and paralysis are provoked by exposure to cold or occur spontaneously. Several authors think this is essentially the same as Gamstorp's disease. A periodic paralysis syndrome is often one of the symptoms of hyperaldosteronism, with depletion of body potassium, and paradoxically also may occur with potassium intoxication.

A subacute syndrome of generalized weakness may be due to poisoning of the neural portion of the muscle endplate by botulinus toxin. The toxin secreted by some species of ticks produces progressive paralysis by poisoning of the motor neuron fiber. Simply by removing the tick the paralysis is reversed.

MYASTHENIA

Myasthenia gravis is the archetype of disease at the muscle endplate. Classically this has been considered to be a disorder of neuromyal transmission, analogous to poisoning by competitive acetylcholine blocking agents like curare. Because individual muscles vary in their degree of clinical and pharmacologic impairment, it has been postulated that there is a localized defect in acetylcholine metabolism or the endplate membrane with curarelike poisoning by a metabolic product like choline.[6,7] Recent evidence has distinctly implicated a presynaptic hypofunction as well.[8] Other studies have implicated an autoallergic mechanism involving the entire muscle structure.[9]

The hallmark of the clinical picture is fatiguability, particularly affecting the extraocular and bulbar muscles, limb muscles being involved in the more severe generalized cases. Symptoms of diplopia or dysarthria are typically worse later in the day and are diagnostically relieved by injection of Tensilon or Prostigmin. Stretch reflexes are intact though sometimes fatiguable, and muscle wasting occurs only rarely in severely affected muscles. Characteristically there are spontaneous exacerbations and remissions. Severe generalized weakness with respiratory paralysis is called myasthenic crisis. Myastheniclike symptoms with some response to Prostigmin have been described in association with carcinoma of the lung and with motoneuron disease.[10]

PERIPHERAL NEUROPATHY

The basic motor symptom of peripheral nerve disease is weakness. Following section of nerve the motor axons become electrically inexcitable in a few days and undergo Wallerian degeneration. The muscle fibers supplied by the nerve atrophy, and gross muscle atrophy may be apparent in two to three weeks. Affected muscles are flaccid, and although stretch reflexes are absent, myotatic response to direct muscle percussion may be increased. Sensory impairment and distortion of sensation are appropriate to the superficial distribution of mixed motor and sensory nerves.

If the gross nerve structure remains intact, or after surgical anastomosis when the nerve is severed, the central motor axons grow out toward the denervated muscles at a rate of 1 to 3 millimeters a day. If reinnervation occurs, the muscle mass may be restored to a varying degree. Functional recovery may be diminished if some nerve axons grow back into muscles other than those originally supplied.

Acute contusion of a nerve may produce a physiologic block for a period of days to weeks without degeneration of the distal axons. The distal axons remain electrically excitable, there is no significant muscle wasting, and recovery is usually excellent. Even when a lesion in continuity is severe enough to produce degeneration of the distal axons, the recovery is usually better than that following surgical anastomosis because the nerve sheath relationships which guide axon growth are better preserved.

Chronic trauma may be produced by compression in several entrapment syndromes, the most common of which is carpal tunnel compression of the median nerve. In addition to symptoms of pain and sensory loss or distortion, there may be weakness and wasting in the muscles of the thenar eminence. In many cases there is a significant delay of conduction of nerve impulses under the compressed region when the motor nerve is stimulated electrically.[11] This test is of diagnostic value; the physiologic explanation of delay is uncertain, but it is probably due to inactivation of one or more nodes of Ranvier.

Other commonly vulnerable loci are the peroneal nerve at the fibula (as affected in habitual leg crossing), the ulnar nerve at the elbow, and the brachial plexus at the first rib. Spinal roots are commonly compressed by herniated intervertebral disks near the intervertebral foramina. The anatomic distribution of muscle involvement defines the level at which a population of motoneurons is affected. Mononeuropathies are particularly prone to occur with trivial mechanical insult when there is systemic disturbance, as alcoholism, malnutrition or diabetes.

Multiple mononeuritis may occur in diabetes, polyarteritis nodosa and other conditions. The more common polyneuritis is a syndrome of diffuse involvement of those motor and sensory axons which extend farthest from their cell bodies. Thus weakness, wasting, loss of stretch reflexes and proprioception are usually most marked in a diffuse distal pattern particularly in the legs and the feet. The time course of neuropathies may vary from months and weeks in metabolic disturbances to an acute or subacute picture in toxic, porphyric, or postinfectious polyneuritis, lupus erythematosus, etc.

Anterior Horn Cell Disease

Amyotrophic lateral sclerosis is a disease of adults in which there is a progressive degeneration of anterior horn cells in the spinal cord along with the homologous cranial motor neurons, excepting those to the extraocular muscles. In addition there is an ascending degeneration of pyramidal tract fibers, the symptoms of which overlap those of the lower motor neuron process. Thus instead of the decreased stretch reflexes that might be expected with the muscle wasting and weakness of motoneuron damage, there are paradoxically increased stretch reflexes (as long as some motoneurons survive) and often extensor plantar responses (see below). Hyperirritable surviving motoneurons fire spontaneously, resulting in muscle fasciculation. The clinical picture is defined by the diffuse craniospinal involvement. An infantile variety of anterior horn cell disease (Werdnig-Hoffman) is not associated with corticospinal tract involvement.

Upper Motor Neuron Syndrome

This expression is generally used in reference to the corticospinal tract, for this is the largest single efferent internuncial pathway. There is considerable controversy about which effects of upper motor neuron lesions are pyramidal, and which, if any, are extrapyramidal. The distinction is probably less important than the polemics about the matter would indicate.

Spinal shock is a condition of severe reflex depression in the distal spinal cord following acute transection. This lasts for several weeks in man, with gradual recovery of both nociceptive and stretch reflexes. The former, although they are polysynaptic, recover first, and may be present in depressed form immediately after the lesion is made. At this time the two neuron stretch reflex is severely depressed. Yet the same motoneurons *can* be excited by electrical stimulation of stretch receptor nerve fibers (H reflex). This suggests that depression occurs at the stretch receptor end organs, which are less sensitive because of temporarily decreased activity in the fusimotor (gamma efferent) system.[12]

The shock phenomenon seems to be reasonably explicable on the basis of the sudden diminution of synaptic barrage at both interneuron and motoneuron synapses. The recovery of reflexes not only to the normal level, but to the hyperactive state has not been satisfactorily explained.

It has been suggested that postsynaptic membranes, thus partially denervated, become hyperexcitable to the transmitter substance from surviving presynaptic terminals.[13] Another explanation for the development of increased reflexes over a long period of time is that dorsal root neurons develop additional collateral branches which increase the number of synaptic connections in the reflex pathway.[14] The suggestion that hyperreflexia is due to increased fusimotor tone has not been confirmed.[15]

A transient period of hyporeflexia with flaccid paralysis also occurs with massive lesions of the upper motor neuron in a cerebral hemisphere. This is thought to be homologous to spinal shock, but less severe and prolonged because of the larger proportion of surviving efferent connections.

The classical model of chronic upper neuron lesion is the condition evolving from a lesion of the internal capsule. If the lesion develops slowly, the hyperreflexic state evolves continuously without the initial depressed phase of acute lesions. The paralysis is characterized by being most severe in the fine dexterous movements of the extremities. Thus finger movement is more impaired than forearm, and forearm more than shoulder. Muscle strength is usually reduced, but severe disability may be present even with good strength of individual muscles because the repertoire of performance is greatly limited. Thus the hemiplegic patient may be limited to a movement including flexion of the fingers, the wrist and the elbow and protraction and elevation of the arm regardless of which movement of the fingers he is attempting to perform.

Long ago Beevor[16] showed that trunk muscles may be functionally weak for postural maintenance in one position in space and quite strong in another. Thus with a right hemispheral lesion the sitting patient

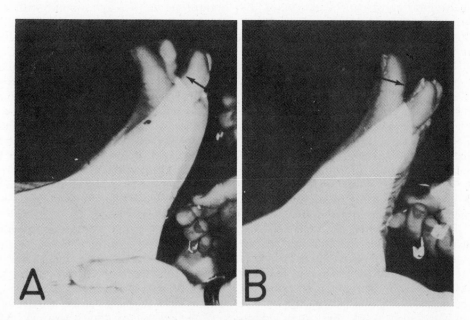

Fig. 178. Extensor plantar reflex (Babinski sign). (A) Superposed motion picture frames showing dorsiflexion of the hallux along with dorsiflexion of the foot. (B) Same subject after block of the peroneal nerve which paralyzes foot and toe dorsiflexors. The prime movement of hallux plantar flexion is apparent. In *A* this movement is overcome by the stronger contraction of extensor hallucis longus.

falls to the left and the *right* paraspinal muscles are weak in the effort to sit up straight. The same muscles are quite strong in abducting from the upright position toward the right. Conversely, the *left* trunk muscles are strong in adduction from right to midline and weak in continuation of the movement to abduction from midline toward the left. Beevor concluded that motor cortex is concerned primarily in contralateral *movements,* not simply related to contralateral muscles in the fashion of marionette strings.

After an acute capsular lesion, the phasic stretch reflexes (tendon jerks) on the affected side are slightly decreased or normally active for several days. They then become more and more hyperactive. When the hyperactivity becomes extreme, a steady stretch stimulus applied to the muscle will result in 4 to 7 rhythmic contractions per second, each followed by a silent period, and the renewed stretch response. This is clonus. Increased resistance to passive limb movement manifests spasticity (see below).

Associated with the development of hyperactive reflexes is a functional recovery of behavioral movement conditioned by proprioceptive stimuli. If movement evolves toward complete recovery, there is also return of the stretch reflexes toward the normal level and, according to Twitchell,[17] the grasp reflex may appear transiently as evidence of the facilitatory influence of contactual stimuli.

The plantar reflex elicited by nociceptive stimulation of the lateral planta normally produces a reflex withdrawal of the foot from the stimulus. The prime movement is plantar flexion of the hallux, along with dorsiflexion of the ankle and irregular flexion at the hip and the knee. When the upper motoneuron is damaged, this reflex becomes hyperactive in a very special way: the extensor hallucis longus, which is silent in the normal plantar reflex, becomes by reflex irradiation a synergic cocontractor of the neighboring ankle dorsiflexors, tibialis anticus and extensor digitorum longus. As a result, the hallux *dorsiflexes* even though there is active contraction of the hallux flexors. This is the *extensor toe sign of Babinski* (Fig. 178).[18]

The pathologic reflex usually has a lower threshold for response than the normal; increased excitability is also indicated by the spatial irradiation of the afferent arc so that stimuli applied elsewhere on the extremity than the lateral planta may be effective. On the efferent side, the extensor reflex tends to recruit a more vigorous generalized limb muscle synergy than does the normal flexor pattern.

The plantar reflex has great clinical value because it often becomes abnormal early in the course of disease before other signs or symptoms of pyramidal tract damage are apparent. Extensor toe signs may occur in transient conditions of cortical depression and coma.

In progressive paraparesis due to spinal cord disease hyper-reflexia in the extensor muscles is more prominent; the resting posture is one of extension. With progression this commonly evolves into paraplegia in flexion where the lower extremities tend to remain flexed at the hip, the knee and the ankle. This is also the end stage of the phasic hyperactive flexion reflex or flexor spasm, an exaggerated plantar reflex. The paraplegic limb may respond with vigorous transient flexion to a slight movement of the bed sheets, to the stimulation of trophic skin lesions, or (apparently) spontaneously. Since, it has been possible to maintain patients with complete cord transection for an indefinite period of time, it has been found that some remain in extension most of the time, and some in flexion, without significant relationship to the level of the cord lesion. Flexor spasms may occur in either circumstance. There is no clear understanding why some patients with complete section assume one posture and others another.

A transient upper motor neuron paralysis (Todd) may be associated with the period immediately following a focal convulsive seizure. Although it has usually been assumed that this represents postconvulsive fatigue and decreased tonic activity in the appropriate motor cortex, critical analysis indicates that there may also be an element of active inhibition.[19]

Highest level paralysis occurs with cortical lesions in the motor region and is

Table 29. Conditions Causing Muscular Weakness

Disease	Distribution	Atrophy	Fasciculation	Tendon Jerks	Tone	Direct Myotatic Response	Plantar Reflex	Associated Sensory Loss
Myopathy	Usually proximal	Usual except hypertrophic calves	None	Decreased	Decreased	Decreased	Normal	None
Myasthenia gravis	Eye and throat, variable in limbs	Rare	None	Normal or fatiguable	Normal	Normal	Normal	None
Periodic paralysis	Ascending	None	None	Absent	None	None	None	None
Root or Nerve disease	In root or nerve innervation	Present	Rarely evident	Decreased	Decreased	Increased or normal	Normal or depressed	Often in nerve or root distribution
Lower motor neuron syndrome	Usually distal; can be generalized	Prominent	Present	Decreased	Normal or decreased	Increased or normal	Normal or depressed	None
Upper motor neuron syndrome (chronic)	Movements of distal parts more affected	Minimal, if any	None	Increased	Spasticity	Normal	Extensor	Sometimes as a result of other cerebral damage
Parkinsonism	Generalized hypokinesia	None	None	Normal	Rigidity; often cog-wheeling	Normal	Normal	None
Cerebellar disease	Ataxia, most prominent in limbs. Weakness is mild	None	None	Normal (pendular)	Hypotonic	Normal	Normal	None

called apraxia. Here the patient may have preserved the capacity to use muscles in complex coordination for automatic or associated movements, and yet be unable to perform a skilled act purposefully, as using a key, a fountain pen or a comb. The grasp reflex and instinctive grasp reactions are generally correlated with frontal or diffuse cortical lesions.

DISTORTIONS OF MOVEMENT AND POSTURE

SPASTICITY*

The tendon jerk is the most sensitive measure of stretch reflex excitability because the synchronous activation of muscle spindle stretch receptors results in temporal summation at the spinal cord. Spasticity is evident when the reflex synapses are so sensitive that even asynchronous afferent impulses, ineffective in a normal subject, result in muscle contraction. Thus when excitability is high, even slow passive extension of a muscle will result in reflex contraction which increases in intensity as the stretch increases and then suddenly gives way (lengthening reaction). This whole reaction is the *claspknife phenomenon which, by definition, is clinical spasticity.* The release of the claspknife tension is attributed to the autoinhibitory action of high tension on the muscle tendon (Golgi) stretch receptors.

Between a stage of increased tendon jerks and that of fully developed spasticity, varying degrees of incremental-decremental plastic resistance to passive movement may be observed. In human subjects these tend to be variable and are often difficult to dis-

---

*The terms flaccid and spastic are confusing because they denote different methods of observation. *Muscle tone is determined by evaluating the resistance to passive stretch.* In normal relaxed subjects this resistance is slight but significant as compared with the hypotonia of severe neuropathy, myopathy, or cerebellar disease. Hypertonia in spasticity, as well as in some other conditions, is due to muscle contraction *induced* by the act of passive muscle lengthening. *Flaccidity is an observation of visual inspection and palpation of the muscle at rest;* this term properly contrasts with contraction. Thus a muscle affected by tetanus toxin or parkinsonism will show activity at rest by inspection and palpation which can also be shown by passive joint movement.

tinguish from poor cooperation. True spasticity *never* occurs except in association with hyperactive phasic stretch reflexes. In spite of the reflex hyperexcitability, spastic muscles are flaccid and electrically silent when the limb is positioned so that there is no passive muscle stretch.

Although such terms as spastic hemiparesis are in common usage, the disturbance of movement is more the result of loss of control (negative effect) that it is a manifestation of increased stretch reflexes (positive release effect). To be sure, in hemiparesis the flexed posture of the upper extremity and the extended posture of the lower one reflect the effect of stretch reflexes. But the shoulder-arm synergy of the upper extremity and the coarse circumducting movement of the lower extremity in walking, accomplished largely with the proximal musculature, are essentially the same regardless of the degree of hyperreflexia. The tendency of the extremities to cross in the gait of upper neuron paraparesis does indicate a disability due to exaggeration of the stretch reflex in the thigh adductors.

Decerebrate rigidity in animals was originally defined by Sherrington as a state of hyperactivity of antigravity (extensor) stretch reflexes in all limbs resulting from midbrain transection. The homologous condition occurs with similar lesions in man and the reflex behavior is that of spasticity. Thus spasticity and decerebrate rigidity are physiologically synonymous. However, there is a significant difference, in that decerebrate rigidity occurs immediately after brainstem transection without the transient period of reflex depression seen with lesions either rostral or caudal to this level. It seems probable therefore that the midbrain lesion somehow releases in the brainstem an excessive downstream discharge to the motoneurons even though the pyramidal tract section might be expected to produce a shocklike state.

Some confusion exists about the position of the upper extremity. This has been attributed to the fact that it is the upper extremity flexors that are stretched by gravity in the biped. Moreover, the flexors are mechanically stronger. It has also been observed that the hemiplegic flexed forelimb may extend in the quadrupedal position. When the flexed forelimb posture develops acutely with deep cerebral lesion, the condition may be called decorticate or high decerebrate rigidity. With more noxious or more caudal midbrain lesions, the forelimbs pronate and extend as in the animal; the lower extremities are more rigid in extension. This is called decerebrate or low decerebrate rigidity. The relationship between these postures has not been adequately explained; brainstem vestibular and tonic neck reflex pathways may be involved.

Parkinsonian Rigidity

The pathologic basis of this syndrome is still controversial, although many authors believe that lesions in the substantia nigra are the most significant ones. There are also lesions of the basal ganglia, particularly the pallidum, and Denny-Brown emphasizes the damage to corticopallidal and striopallidal fibers.[20] There are two major aspects to the clinical syndrome: (1) constant innervated contraction of most of the musculature at rest, and (2) generalized weakness and difficulty in starting movements (hypokinesia). The abnormal resting tone may sometimes be relaxed by careful positioning of limbs, but it is practically always present in the waking state and is much exaggerated by emotional stress or attention. Although the generalized rigidity seriously interferes with motor activity, fine movements of the fingers may be relatively well preserved compared with the syndrome of the upper motoneuron. Afflicted patients move slowly with stooped posture, short steps, and lack of associated movements in the upper extremities.

Passive movement at affected joints reveals a continuous resistance throughout the excursion tested. Most often this rigidity has a rhythmic phasic quality (*cogwheeling*) which is clearly related to the tremor (*paralysis agitans*) that many patients have. Rigidity is partially sustained by proprioceptive reflex drive since desensitization of muscle stretch receptors by anesthetic block of fusimotor fibers can abolish the hypertonicity.[21] An abnormality of fusimotor tone is unlikely. Although there is controversy about the relationship between rigidity and tremor we think it most probable that tremor represents a reciprocal organization at the spinal level of the increased tonic neural drive from above, somehow released by the primary lesions (cf. tremor).

It has not been possible to produce a convincing parkinson-like picture in experimental animals, but previously unaffected human subjects may develop the syndrome (or less often a choreic picture) reversibly (rarely permanently) on large doses of reserpine or phenothiazine drugs. The mechanism of this phenomenon is not understood, but localized differences in neural transmission mechanism and drug reactivity in various forebrain structures are suspected. Neither is it known how the drugs that improve the pathologic syndrome accomplish the result. Most useful drugs are related either to antihistamines (Benadryl) or to the belladonna alkaloids.

Myotonia

This is a hereditary disturbance of muscle excitability and structure in which individual fibers are hyperirritable and may fire repetitively and produce prolonged contraction in response to physiologic activation by motoneurons, or mechanical stimulation by percussion.[22] In addition, myotonic muscle continues to contract throughout the flow of threshold stimulation by direct electrical current instead of firing only when the cathodal current is turned on, as in normal muscle. Electromyographic (EMG) recording indicates that individual muscle fibers may even go into high frequency activity without any apparent triggering stimulus. Intracellular recording has shown spontaneous oscillations of membrane potential similar to those seen in experimentally hypersensitive membranes like that of hypocalcemic nerve.[23] Involuntary muscle contraction after a handgrasp or percussion may last 10 to 30 seconds. Associated with this hindrance to normal movement there may be innervated contraction of both the primarily affected and associated muscles (afterspasm).

In myotonia congenita the stiffness of the proximal muscles of the lower extremities results in an unusual stiff gait resembling that associated with hip joint disease. The myotonic phenomenon usually improves with exercise (warming up) and may be helped to some degree by quinine or procaine amide therapy. Most adult patients with this condition are unaware of the muscle stiffness and come to medical attention because of the distal muscle wasting and weakness (see Myotonia Dystrophica above).

ATAXIA

Irregular failure of coordination in purposeful movement is generally attributed to disease of the cerebellum or its tracts. Limbs affected by cerebellar lesions have some degree of hypotonia and weakness, and difficulty in maintaining a stable position against gravity. When the hand is directed toward a target, the movement tends to be decomposed into oscillations toward either side of the target with a crescendo increase of amplitude, finally arrested to greater or less degree when the target is reached. This is called intention tremor. Similar dysfunction in respiratory and bulbar musculature produces explosive, scanning, dysarthric speech.

Stretch reflexes are normal in amplitude but the hypotonic state may be seen in pendulous oscillations following the initial contraction. This is particularly evident for the knee jerk.

Although Sherrington defined the cerebellum as the head ganglion of the proprioceptive system, more recent studies have shown that afferent pathways from skin, ear and eye also project to the cerebellum. Patients with cerebellar lesions have no sensory loss and the function of these projections is unknown.

Walshe[24] has emphasized that cerebellar symptoms are not present when there is superposed affliction of the cerebrospinal pathways, and this has also been shown when a pyramidal tract lesion is superposed on a cerebellar lesion in monkeys.[25] In the monkey improvement is reported following lesions of the pallidum, and in man following contralateral thalamic lesions.[26] Thus the cerebellum is implicated in motor behavior in relation to forebrain

projection rather than directly in organization at the spinal level. The theory that cerebellar symptoms are due to fusimotor hypotonia has not been confirmed.[21] Some current theories of the mechanism of cerebellar symptoms reduce to the absurd position that the function of the normal cerebellum is to prevent cerebellar ataxia. No more satisfactory explanation has been brought forward.

There is some degree of somatotopic localization of the cerebellum, in that midline lesions of the vermis tend to be related to instability and ataxia of the trunk, while lesions of the medial anterior lobe produce predominance of lower extremity symptoms and the upper extremities may be involved by more lateral posterior lesions. If the dentate nucleus is spared, large ablations of neocerebellum may produce very little disability. Because the major cerebellar afferent paths and its efferent tract in the superior peduncle as far as the midbrain are uncrossed, unilateral cerebellar lesions produce ipsilateral ataxia.

Behavior resembling cerebellar symptomatology may also occur in other conditions. The fact that frontal lobe tumors may simulate contralateral cerebellar lesions has not been satisfactorily explained. The fact that ablation of the frontal lobe does not produce such symptoms has led to the argument that the phenomenon is due to distortion of brainstem structures by the mass of the tumor. Occasionally a cerebral lesion which affects both precentral and parietal regions, associated with loss of position and localization sense, may also result in ataxia, whether the eyes are open or not. Proprioceptive loss due to lesions of peripheral nerves or spinal dorsal columns produces ataxia which is much worse when visuomotor control is subtracted by closing the eyes. Occasionally too, the weakness associated with neuropathy affecting the motor nerves, or even with debilitating systemic disease, may simulate true ataxia.

DYSTONIA

This term, indicating disordered muscle tone, is usually used more specifically to define conditions like *dystonia musculorum deformans* where there are severe tonic distortions of posture and movement most conspicuously affecting truncal, neck, and proximal limb musculature. Jung and Hassler[27] have called the dystonic syndrome proximal athetosis. Denny-Brown[20] uses the term in a more literal and general sense as a relatively fixed attitude, emphasizing early distortions of limb movement as the disease develops. Degenerative lesions seem to be primarily but not exclusively in the putamen along with thalamic and cortical involvement. Dystonic rigidity may be the major finding in some patients with Huntington's chorea, where the most impressive degeneration is in the caudate nucleus. The pathophysiology of dystonia is poorly defined. Denny-Brown believes that this released activity is a common feature of the advanced stages of the other basal ganglia conditions, and that it represents released contactual reflexes.

ATHETOSIS

Denny-Brown has defined this term in relation to its literal meaning of lack of fixation or stability of position, but it is generally used to define a condition with bizarre, wormlike distortions of movement, particularly affecting the hands, distal limb segments, and face. When quiet, there is no resistance to passive movement in affected extremities. The abnormal movements are usually irregular and tend to be stereotyped, e.g. hyperextension of the fingers with hyperflexion at the wrists. Lesions affect the putamen predominantly. Denny-Brown believes that the instability represents the competition for expression of an approach reaction to cutaneous stimulation released by lesions of the precentral cerebral system, with avoidance reaction released by lesions of the parietal lobe system. Usually the symptoms are present from birth, although rarely the condition develops progressively. Athetosis is often associated with the spontaneous movements of chorea.

Tabetic athetosis is associated with severe loss of proprioceptive sense due to dorsal root and dorsal column disease. Irregular small movements of the distal extremities, particularly the fingers, are observed during posture maintenance, and sometimes at rest. It has been suggested that the phenomenon represents denervation sensitization of motoneurons.[28]

SPONTANEOUS MOVEMENT

FIBRILLATION

Spontaneous, often rhythmic, contractions of individual muscle fibers constitute fibrillation.[29,30] Since normal muscle fibers are less than one tenth of a millimeter in diameter, and atrophied fibers even smaller, it is obvious that these contractions are not usually visible. Occasionally fine vermicular movements can be seen when the affected muscle is in the tongue or underlies thin skin over portions of the hand. Elsewhere they are detected by EMG as brief (1 msec.), low voltage potentials uninfluenced by voluntary effort.

The most common cause of fibrillation is separation of muscle fibers from their motoneuron, whether the lesion occurs at cord, root or peripheral nerve. The orphaned muscle fibers undergo progressive atrophy for a month or more during which there are also progressive physiologic changes. Instead of the normal localized sensitivity to acetylcholine at the endplate the fiber becomes equally sensitive over its entire surface.[31] There are also changes in the electrical characteristics of the membrane so that adaptation to a continuous stimulating electric current does not occur. Whereas normal muscle fibers will contract only at the make of a continuous threshold current, denervated fibers will fire repetitively throughout the flow of current and at lower threshold. There is also an increase in mechanical excitability; fibrillations are readily stirred up by movement of an EMG recording needle electrode. They are diminished by cooling. Although they may persist for many years after nerve section, they may not be present if there is excessive fibrosis. When motor axons grow back into a denervated muscle and begin to form effective contact, threshold for electrical stimulation rises and fibrillation disappears before spontaneous innervated movement occurs.

Increased muscle fiber irritability and frank persistent fibrillation are seen sometimes in primary myopathies, particularly those that develop very rapidly like polymyositis.[32] The diffuse inflammatory reaction may produce direct changes in muscle membrane irritability and may also effectively produce denervation by the destruction of muscle fiber segments between motor endplates and surviving segments. Fibrillations are observed quite rarely in muscular dystrophy. Disappearance of previously observed fibrillations in polymyositis may serve as a measure of therapeutic clinical improvement.

FASCICULATION

Fasciculation is defined as the spontaneous isolated contraction of individual motor units. The muscle fibers supplied by a single motoneuron produce a brief twitch of a muscle fascicle, the size being larger in large muscles. Normal motor units in limb muscles may include many hundreds of muscle fibers, while those of the extraocular muscles contain only a few. Fasciculations usually occur irregularly at slow frequencies ranging from once every several seconds to two or three a second.

Fasciculations are most notorious as a sign of diffuse motoneuron disease in amyotrophic lateral sclerosis. Curiously, these patients practically never complain of fasciculation and come to medical attention because of muscle weakness. By EMG the fasciculation units in this disease are often several-fold larger and more polyphasic than normal.[33] This seems to be due to the fact that surviving motoneurons put out collateral axon branches to reinnervate orphaned muscle fibers. The hyperexcitability of the motoneuron in this condition extends beyond the cell body, for fasciculations have been observed to persist when the motor nerve is blocked or even severed. This hyperirritability, plus that related to newly growing axonal sprouts, may explain why muscle percussion is a useful technic for bringing out latent fasciculation.

Fasciculations also occur with other varieties of spinal cord disease. They may be seen associated with the early inflammatory reaction of poliomyelitis, or chronically, when the cord is damaged by neoplasm, compression or scar.

Benign fasciculation is commonly seen in normal subjects, often when they are tense and anxious or overfatigued. Neurologists in a medical school are accustomed to visits from medical students who become concerned about themselves after hearing a lecture about amyotrophic lateral sclerosis. In middle age and beyond, benign fasciculations of the calf muscles are common. Benign twitches are not intrinsically different from those seen with motoneuron disease, except that the giant, more irregularly shaped fasciculation potentials are not seen in the EMG. Nor are there muscle fibrillations, atrophy or weakness.

Nerve root compression may give rise to localized fasciculation more often, it seems, than does peripheral nerve compression. These fasciculations may be single, or they may be brief tetani of two to several action potentials at a rate of 60 to 100 per second. These fasciculations may appear more prolonged to visual inspection than do the usual single twitches.

Myokymia is a benign condition of unknown mechanism in which the patient may complain of spontaneous muscle twitching which characteristically occurs in the multiple high frequency pattern.[34] This symptom is usually present in the calf muscles, but it may be generalized.

The involuntary muscle contraction of shivering looks like, and is by definition, fasciculation, although the discharge rate is faster. Thus it is important that the patient be examined for pathologic fasciculation in a warm environment. Fasciculations are often seen with electrolyte disturbance in toxic states like uremia. Contraction fasciculation is purposeful movement in muscles reduced to a very few motor units by the decimation of disease.

SPASM

This is a marked, if not violent, contraction of a muscle or group of muscles which is often but not always painful. The most common variety is common muscle cramp. It may occur in normal subjects when a muscle is contracted maximally, especially if it is in the shortened position, as when the triceps surae is strongly contracted with the foot plantar-flexed. Once the cramp is set up, it cannot be stopped by relaxation but may be resolved by massage and passive extension. The EMG during cramp shows high frequencies of unit discharge, several times the 20 to 30 per second seen in normal movement.[35] Cramp may occur more readily after excessive exercise, and in patients with peripheral vascular disease and those with motoneuron disease. Its mechanism is not known.

The spasm of tetany occurs predominantly in the distal extremities (carpopedal spasm) with the characteristic flexion of fingers and hands and flexion of toes with inversion of feet. It is due to low concentration of ionized calcium. Spontaneous overventilation may produce such spasm in otherwise normal subjects. That the hyperirritability of hypocalcemia resides in the nerve axon is shown by the provocation of tetany by ischemia (Trousseau's sign).

Tetanus toxin may provoke localized sustained muscle contraction, in the beginning only as a prolongation of normal movement, later as sustained contraction. Such a condition may last for many days. Systemic spread of the toxin will early affect the muscles of mastication and produce trismus.

Postdenervation muscle spasm most commonly affects the facial musculature after nerve regeneration from Bell's palsy. Here there may be background activity of single motor units in the multiple fasciculation pattern of myokymia along with intermittent high frequency bursts of one or more units associated with the clinical spasm. Here, as in nerve root compression, one suspects a primary hyperirritable state in the proximal portion of the motor axon.

Generalized recurrent muscle spasm may be seen with many varieties of diffuse neuronal irritation such as virus infection (rabies), strychnine poisoning and various subacute degenerative neuronal diseases.

TREMOR

This term implies a relatively continuous state during which individual muscle contraction varies in a rhythmic pattern. Parkinsonian tremor (paralysis agitans) is characteristically a tremor of rest. There is a regular contraction at 4 to 7 per second which is most prominent in the upper extremities, producing the characteristic pill-rolling movement in the hand with spread to involve proximal muscles. Less often tremor may involve the lower extremities and the facial muscles. During active movement the silent periods between motor unit bursts may be filled in by contraction of the same and other motor units as the tremor becomes less evident or disappears, only to reappear as the limb comes to a new resting position.[36] However, sometimes this filling-in does not occur, and movement may be produced by increased amplitude of tremor bursts. In most cases there is reciprocal relaxation of antagonistic muscles, but there may be "overflow" contraction in the antagonists which is obviously a handicap to movement. Thus muscle contraction may occur in agonists and antagonists without gross movement. Cogwheel rigidity observed with passive movement in parkinsonian patients reflects a basic tremor, whether or not visually apparent. Tremor frequency may increase during active movement, and may vary spontaneously, or even independently in antagonistic muscles.

As noted above, we believe that resting tremor is essentially a segmental phenomenon of reciprocal reaction to a tonic efferent discharge released by forebrain lesions. The rhythm and reciprocal relationships are like those of clonus released by corticospinal tract damage. Unlike clonus, the stretch reflexes are not increased, but stretch receptor function is essential for the maintenance of both conditions, for both are stopped by local anesthetic block of fusimotor fibers and consequent desensitization of muscle spindles, or by dorsal root section.[21] Shivering provides a useful physiologic model, for the involuntary hypothalamic discharge produced by cooling leads first to diffuse muscle contraction and thence to alternating reciprocal clonus.[37] Liberson[38] has shown that when the median nerve is stimulated electrically in a patient with parkinsonian tremor, the tremor rhythm in that hand is reset so that the next burst after the shock comes at the same interval as that between preceding and succeeding spontaneous bursts. This resetting could hardly occur if the tremor pattern were established elsewhere than in the segmental level concerned. Moreover, although tremor may be affected by stimulation of various deep brain structures, the tremor rhythm has been recorded from none.

Denny-Brown[20] has observed in some patients with hepatolenticular disease the evolution of less regular athetosis into regular tremor. He believes that tremor, like athetosis, represents antagonistic movement patterns released by deranged forebrain mechanisms. He also believes that tremor primarily relates to lesions of the inner globus pallidus. However, concerning neuropathologic findings in parkinsonism it is fair to say that there is no widely accepted correlation of symptoms with specific lesions. It is certain that parkinsonian symptoms may be associated with various degrees and distributions of pathologic findings among several basal forebrain structures.

Parkinson himself observed that resting tremor disappears in the limbs affected by hemiplegia, only to return if there is sufficient recovery of voluntary movement. Thus, it may be presumed that some pyramidal tract tonic activity is necessary for the maintenance of the abnormal movement. Indeed, Bucy[39] suggests that therapeutic lesions aimed at the globus pallidus or thalamus to relieve tremor do so by inadvertent damage to the internal capsule. Lesions in the thalamus seem more likely to produce good results. Whatever the mechanism, it is not specific to resting tremor, for symptoms of dystonia, chorea, essential tremor, and ataxic intention tremor are also said to be improved by the same lesion.[40-43] When the underlying disease process is progressive, relief of symptoms by brain lesions is usually transient.

Purdon-Martin[26,44] believes that the pallidum is released to excessive activity by lesions of the substantia nigra, that the pallidum is the major efferent path of the basal forebrain neuronal complex, and that this explains why lesions of the pallidum may be helpful.

Senile tremor may be related to the parkinsonian variety. Head tremor is conspicuous and the hand tremor may be exaggerated by movement. It is seldom disabling and rigidity is not significant. Essential or heredofamilial tremor usually becomes evident in adolescence. There is a regular alternating tremor of the outstretched hands, usually somewhat faster than that of parkinsonism, and not present at rest. The tremor may be exaggerated during movement, diminishing at termination. Patients afflicted with this condition can often do remarkably fine work in spite of the tremor during limb transit. The condition is usually not progressive and there is no rigidity. Pathologic and physiologic bases are unknown.

Flapping or wing-beating tremor of the outstretched hands in hepatolenticular degeneration (Wilson's disease) is slower than parkinsonian tremor, is less prominent or absent at rest but has both clinical and pathologic features related to parkinsonism and athetosis. The lesions are most prominent in the putamen. A similar type of "liver flap" has been described in patients suffering from other varieties of hepatic disease.

Tremor attributed to midbrain lesions has features related to both the parkinsonian and cerebellar syndromes.[20] The resting tremor tends to be variable and includes pronation and supination of the forearm and protraction of the shoulder. With movement the tremor may resemble the intention pattern of cerebellar disease.

The tremor of hyperthyroidism is irregular, rapid and fine; it is maintained by tonic contraction of active muscles. It is not easily confused with those due to neurologic lesions. The tremor of anxiety states may be similar or more coarse, but it is faster than parkinsonian tremor, and usually does not show the parkinsonian alternation in antagonists. The tremulousness seen in various chronic alcoholic conditions is manifest during movement, is irregular, unsteady and slow, but not ataxic in the usual sense.

Chorea

The name of this symptom is derived from the Greek word for dance. Involuntary movements at rest are irregular, jerky and highly varied; a finger or hand may twitch or flick in any direction. Often minor movements are covered up by the patient's concealing them beneath some quasipurposeful movement like scratching.

Irregular twitching movements of the tongue, the face, and the lower extremities are usual. In advanced cases the movements involve whole extremities and the patient may be bedridden.

Symptomatic relief may be obtained from reserpine and phenothiazine derivatives, which can produce the parkinsonian syndrome. Other sedatives may also be helpful.

In hereditary chorea (Huntington) there is progressive degeneration of the striatum, particularly the caudate nucleus, but degeneration is also more widespread. Muscle tone and the ability to move purposefully between abnormal movements are normal, as are the reflexes. Denny-Brown emphasizes a continual flow of motion in chorea, but this is not present in early cases. He proposes that choreic movement, like athetosis, is a manifestation of conflicting movement biases triggered by sensory input, and released by the striatal lesions. Others propose damage to an inhibitory system with consequent release of abnormal function. The possibility of a discharging lesion is not excluded.

In rheumatic chorea (Sydenham) the pathologic findings that have been described are quite diffuse and nonspecific. Possibly the choreic symptoms are due to anoxia related to rheumatic arteritis. Chorea or parkinsonism may result from carbon monoxide poisoning. Some authors believe that the movements of this disease can be distinguished from Huntington's chorea.

Chorea sometimes develops in the older age group without a family history. The lesions are thought to be similar to those of the hereditary variety. Hemichorea may occur following a vascular lesion in the internal capsule region. As the patient recovers from hemiparesis, the permanent lesion of the striatum manifests itself in the abnormal movements.

BALLISM

This symptom is usually present unilaterally following a contralateral lesion in or near the subthalamic nucleus of Luys.[26,44] Affected extremities undergo extreme flinging movements with such vigorous involvement of proximal muscles that the patient may injure other portions of his body or head. There may be slight weakness. Purposeful movement can be carried out between the abnormal ones. Whether these movements differ from those of Huntington's chorea more than in degree has been debated. Denny-Brown emphasizes the rotatory movements in ballism together with internal rotation at elbow and wrist.[20] This syndrome can be reproduced by experimental lesions in the monkey, and as in man, it can be relieved by secondary lesions in the pallidum or thalamus. Such movements are also diminished by motor cortex or pyramidal tract lesions.[25] Again the symptoms are explained as a manifestation of released inhibitory control.

OCULOGYRIC CRISES

These are involuntary tonic upward movements of the eye which may last minutes to hours. The patient may be able to look downward briefly but the abnormal movement soon overcomes his effort. The condition is seen in post-encephalitic parkinsonism and also in the parkinsonian syndrome due to phenothiazine drugs. It is presumably due to a disorder of upper brainstem function. Some varieties of torticollis and tic may also relate to undefined brainstem and basal ganglia lesions. The majority of these disorders are believed to be psychogenic but they are notoriously resistant to psychiatric treatment.

PALATAL MYOCLONUS

This is a regular rhythmic elevation of the palate at a frequency of 1 to 2 per second, persisting even during sleep in many cases. Concomitant synchronous or asynchronous movements may occur in facial, extraocular and respiratory muscles. Lesions of various etiologies have been associated, but always in the brainstem region bounded by the inferior olivary nucleus, dentate nucleus, and red nucleus. The mechanism is unknown.

CLONIC CONVULSIVE MOVEMENTS

Focal motor seizures most often affect the thumb and fingers, the great toe, or the perioral region. The strong muscle contractions are brief tetani, rhythmic or irregular and impossible to control by effort. The movements are produced by sudden bursts of high frequency discharge into the pyramidal tract. In general such seizures connote abnormal discharge in motor cortex rather than in subcortical regions. Clonic jerks may sometimes build up into tonic prolonged contractions, usually with spread to other areas (jacksonian seizure).

Short rhythmic bursts of muscle jerks (myoclonus) at the brain wave rhythm of 2 to 3 per second may involve whole limbs or parts of limbs in children with convulsive disorder. Such myoclonic seizures occur with diffuse neuronal disease at any age.

SUMMARY

Disturbances of function of striated muscle are related to disease of muscle, the motoneurons, the spinal cord, or the brain. Varieties of dysfunction include weakness, distortions of posture, movement and co-ordination, abnormal reflexes, distortions of muscle tone, and spontaneous movements which occur in various relationships to normal posture and spontaneous movement. Pathophysiologic analysis must include consideration of the function of uninjured tissue when normal structures are destroyed or become pathologically overactive. In many areas pathophysiologic understanding lags far behind clinicopathologic correlation.

REFERENCES

1. Walshe, F. M. R.: Contributions of John Hughlings Jackson to Neurology. A brief introduction to his teachings, Arch. Neurol. 5:119, 1961.
2. Walton, J. N. and Nattrass, F. J.: On the classification, natural history and treatment of the myopathies, Brain 77:169, 1954.
3. Adams, R. D., Denny-Brown, D. E., and Pearson, C. M.: Diseases of Muscle. A study in Pathology, ed. 2, New York, Hoeber-Harper, 1962.
4. Greenfield, J. G., Cornman, T., and Shy, G. M.: The prognostic value of the muscle biopsy in the "floppy infant," Brain, 81:461, 1958.
5. Greenfield, J. G., Shy, G. M., Alvord, E. C., and Berg, L.: An Atlas of Muscle Pathology in Neuromuscular Diseases, London, Livingstone, 1957.
6. Grob, D., Johns, R. J., and Harvey, A. M.: Studies in neuromuscular function. IV. Stimulating and depressant effects of acetylcholine and choline in patients with myasthenia gravis and their relationship to the defect in neuromuscular transmission, Bull. Johns Hopkins Hosp., 99:153, 1956.
7. Churchill-Davidson, H. C., and Richardson, A. T.: Neuromuscular transmission in myasthenia gravis, J. Physiol. 122:252, 1953.
8. Dahlback, O., Elmqvist, D., Johns, T. R., Radner, S., and Thesleff, S.: An electrophysiologic study of the neuromuscular junction in myasthenia gravis, J. Physiol. 156:336, 1961.
9. Strauss, A. J. L., Seegal, B. C., Hsu, K. C., Burkholder, P. M., Nastuk, W. L., and Osserman, K. E.: Immunofluorescence demonstration of muscle binding complement-fixing globulin fraction in myasthenia gravis, Proc. Soc. Exper. Biol. Med. 105:184, 1960.
10. Eaton, L. M., and Lambert, E. H.: Electromyography and electric stimulation of nerves in diseases of motor unit. Observations on myasthenic syndrome associated with malignant tumors, J.A.M.A. 163:1117, 1957.
11. Lambert, E. H.: Clinical Examinations in Neurology, Chap. 15, Philadelphia, Saunders, 1957.
12. Weaver, R. A., Landau, W. M., and Higgins, J.: Fusimotor function: II. Evidence of fusimotor depression in human spinal shock, Arch. Neurol. 9:127, 1963.
13. Teasdall, R. D., and Stavraky, G. W.: Responses of deafferented spinal neurons to cortico-spinal impulses, J. Neurophysiol. 16:367, 1953.
14. McCouch, G. P., Austin, G. M., Liu, C. M., and Liu, C. Y.: Sprouting as a cause of spasticity, J. Neurophysiol. 21:205, 1958.
15. Meltzer, G. E., Hunt, R. S., and Landau, W. M.: Fusimotor function: III. The spastic monkey, Arch. Neurol. 9:133, 1963.
16. Beevor, C.: Remarks on paralysis of the movements of the trunk in hemiplegia, and and the muscles which are affected. Brit. Med. J. 1:881, 1909.
17. Twitchell, T. E.: The restoration of motor function following hemiplegia in man, Brain 74:443, 1951.
18. Landau, W. M., and Clare, M. H.: The plantar reflex in man, with special reference to some conditions where the extensor response is unexpectedly absent, Brain 82:321, 1959.

19. Efron, R.: Post-epileptic paralysis: Theoretical critique and report of a case, Brain 84:381, 1961.

20. Denny-Brown, D. E.: The Basal Ganglia and their Relation to Disorders of Movement, London, Oxford, 1962.

21. Landau, W. M., Weaver, R. A., and Hornbein, T. F.: Fusimotor nerve function in man: differential nerve block studies in normal subjects and in spasticity and rigidity, Arch. Neurol. 3:10, 1960.

22. Landau, W. M.: The essential mechanism in myotonia. An electromyographic study, Neurology 2:369, 1952.

23. Norris, F. H., Jr.: Unstable membrane potential in human myotonic muscle, EEG Clin. Neurophysiol. 14:197, 1962.

24. Walshe, F. M. R.: The significance of the voluntary element in the genesis of cerebellar ataxy, Brain 50:377, 1927.

25. Carpenter, M. B.: Brainstem and infratentorial neuraxis in experimental dyskinesia, Arch. Neurol. 5:504, 1961.

26. Martin, J. P.: Further remarks on the functions of the basal ganglia, Lancet 1:1362, 1960.

27. Jung, R., and Hassler, R.: The Extrapyramidal Motor System, in Handbook of Physiology, vol. 2, sec. 1, Ch. 35, p. 863, Washington, American Physiological Society, 1960.

28. Moldaver, J.: Contribution a l'étude de la regulation réflexe des movements, Arch. Int. Med. Exper. 11:405, 1936.

29. Denny-Brown, D., and Pennybacker, J.: Fibrillation and fasciculation in voluntary muscle, Brain 61:311, 1938.

30. Landau, W. M.: Synchronization of potentials and response to direct current stimulation in denervated mammalian muscle, EEG Clin. Neurophysiol. 3:169, 1951.

31. Thesleff, S.: Effects of motor innervation on the chemical sensitivity of skeletal muscle, Physiol. Rev. 40:734, 1960.

32. Lambert, E. H., Sayre, G. P., and Eaton, L. M.: Electrical activity of muscle in polymyositis, Tr. Am. Neurol. Ass. 79:64, 1954.

33. Erminio, F., Buchthal, F., and Rosenfalck, P.: Motor unit territory and muscle fibre concentration in paresis due to peripheral nerve injury and anterior horn cell involvement, Neurology 9:657, 1957.

34. Denny-Brown, D., and Foley, J. M.: Myokymia and the benign fasciculation of muscular cramps, Trans. Ass. Am. Physicians 61:88, 1948.

35. Norris, F. H., Jr., Gasteiger, E. L., and Chatfield, P. O.: An electromyographic study of induced and spontaneous muscle cramps, EEG Clin. Neurophysiol. 9:139, 1957.

36. Bishop, G. H., Clare, M. H., and Price, J., Patterns of tremor in normal and pathological conditions, J. Appl. Physiol., 1:123, 1948.

37. Denny-Brown, D., Gaylor, J. B., and Uprus, V.: Note on the nature of the motor discharge in shivering, Brain 58:233, 1935.

38. Liberson, W. T.: In press.

39. Bucy, P. C.: The Cortico-spinal Tract and Tremor, in Pathogenesis and Treatment of Parkinsonism, p. 271, Springfield, Ill., Thomas, 1958.

40. Cooper, I. S.: Neurosurgical Alleviation of Parkinsonism, Springfield, Ill., Thomas, 1956.

41. ———: Neurosurgical alleviation of intention tremor of multiple sclerosis and cerebellar disease, New England J. Med. 263:441, 1960.

42. ———: Heredofamiliar tremor abolition by chemothalamectomy, Arch. Neurol. 7:129, 1962.

43. ———: Dystonia reversal by operation on basal ganglia, Arch. Neurol. 7:132, 1962.

44. Martin, J. P.: Remarks on the functions of the basal ganglia, Lancet 1:999, 1959.

28

Fainting (Syncope)

EUGENE A. STEAD, JR.

DEFINITION

Fainting and syncope are terms commonly used interchangeably to describe a transient loss of consciousness caused by reversible disturbances in cerebral function from (1) transient ischemia, (2) change in composition of blood perfusing the brain, and (3) changes in the pattern of central nervous system activity by stimuli entering the central nervous system.[1] Loss of consciousness accompanied by the clinical or electroencephalographic features of epilepsy is excluded.

PATHOGENESIS

The words *fainting* and *syncope* imply brief loss of consciousness and suggest that the fundamental disturbance must be quickly reversible. Fainting must be dis-

tinguished from more prolonged, less quickly reversible losses of consciousness which are discussed in Chapter 26. The most common cause of syncope is a sudden decrease in the blood supply to the higher nerve centers, the centers of *consciousness*. For a discussion of these centers, see Chapter 26.

Among the physiologic disturbances which may cause a decrease in the blood supply to the brain are (1) peripheral arteriolar vasodilatation, (2) failure of normal peripheral vasoconstrictor activity, (3) sharp fall in cardiac output from heart disease or from a decrease in blood volume, (4) occlusion or narrowing of internal carotid or other arteries to the brain, and (5) ventricular asystole.

Less frequent in the pathogenesis of

true syncope are reflex effects upon the cerebral centers of consciousness. Whether these act directly on the nervous system or indirectly, by local changes in blood supply, remains to be determined.

Also less frequent in syncope (more common in other unconscious states), but predisposing and associated factors, are: changes in the constituents of the blood (chemical and metabolic causes, such as hypocapnia, hypoxia, alkalosis, acidosis, hypoglycemia, etc.).

FAINTING FROM ARTERIOLAR DILATATION
THE COMMON FAINT
(Vasodepressor Syncope)

The benign faint, produced by such stimuli as bad news, the sight of blood, hypodermic injection or venipuncture, commonly occurs while the subject is standing or sitting. The signs and the symptoms of the faint result from reflex activity from a variety of sensory stimuli. The afferent impulses producing the faint may arise from the emotional content of thought or from any sensory nerve endings. Whether or not a subject faints from a given stimulus depends to a great degree upon the amount of anxiety mobilized in him by the stimulus. The intensity of the stimulus and the organ stimulated are less important.

In a few subjects a given stimulus will cause fainting no matter how often it is repeated. More commonly, the same stimulus causes less and less reaction each time. Many persons faint at the time of their first venipuncture, but never have any reaction to subsequent ones.

Clinical Picture. The clinical picture of the common faint is well known. The patient complains of a feeling of warmth in his neck and face; he becomes deathly pale and beads of sweat appear on his forehead. Yawning, belching, nausea, increased peristalsis of the gut, dilatation of the pupils, coldness of the hands and the feet and profound weakness are noted. The heart rate is usually increased. Then the arterial pressure falls rapidly. The radial pulse becomes weak and may be imperceptible, though the femoral and the carotid

pulses remain full. The heart rate frequently slows dramatically. If the subject is standing he usually becomes unconscious. When the head is lowered, consciousness returns quickly. Occasionally there may be a short period of disorientation. The arterial pressure usually rises immediately when the patient is placed in the recumbent position, but at times it remains depressed for minutes or hours. Pallor, nausea, weakness and sweating frequently persist for from 30 minutes to 2 hours; occasionally they persist for 24 hours. If the patient stands up before recovery is complete, a precipitous fall in arterial pressure with syncope may again occur. If the subject remains upright after the loss of consciousness, clonic movements of the hands and the legs are not infrequent.

In many instances all of the phenomena usually preceding and following the loss of consciousness occur, although the patient remains conscious. To these signs and symptoms, which frequently but not necessarily terminate in syncope, the term *fainting reaction* has been applied.[2]

The fainting reaction without loss of consciousness is frequently seen in patients who are in the horizontal position when an appropriate stimulus occurs. In the blood-donor centers an occasional person loses consciousness in the recumbent position. In some of these instances convulsions with tonic and clonic phases and urinary incontinence occur in persons who never have had seizures before.

The circulatory dynamics during the fainting reaction induced in blood donors by venesection have been studied intensively during the last few years.[3,4] The reaction is reflex in nature and may occur before anything is done to the donor. It may occur before the needle is inserted; after the venipuncture, but before any blood is drawn; or it may occur during or shortly after the venesection. The sharp fall in arterial pressure, the feeble radial pulse and the intense pallor suggest a sudden marked fall in cardiac output. Studies of the cardiac output indicated that the cardiac output did not fall as the fainting reaction occurred. The sudden fall in arterial pressure without a corresponding fall in cardiac output indicated a great decrease in peripheral resistance, as would be expected to occur with widespread arteriolar dilatation. Studies of the blood flow in the forearm demonstrated *an increase in blood flow to the muscles* in spite of the low arterial pressure and the decrease in blood flow in the skin.[4] Vasoconstriction in the skin with vasodilatation in the muscles is not an unusual response. Epinephrine reduces the blood flow to the skin and increases it in the muscles.

The mechanism of the loss of consciousness in patients in the upright position during a precipitous fall in arterial pressure is easily understood. The arterial pressure reaches such a low level that it is insufficient to maintain the blood flow to the head against the force of gravity. Complete unconsciousness is always accompanied by high voltage, slow waves in the electroencephalogram. When the patient is placed in the recumbent position, the arterial pressure is sufficient to restore the cerebral circulation and consciousness returns.

Detailed observations have not been made on persons who have lost consciousness while in the recumbent position. It is not known whether the entire reaction represents a more profound degree of arteriolar dilatation, with a drop in arterial pressure to such a low level that the circulation cannot be maintained even with the head level with the heart, or whether some other factor such as reflex ventricular asystole occurs in these severe reactions.

The demonstration that the *cardiac output is well maintained in the fainting reaction* accounts for the fact that the fall in arterial pressure in this condition does not usually lead to serious complications. In spite of the appearance of the patient and the low arterial pressure, the overall blood flow to the tissues remains relatively normal.

This reaction of generalized activity of the autonomic nervous system with a precipitous fall in blood pressure has been called *primary shock* or *acute circulatory collapse* when it has occurred in injured persons. It may occur with any type of injury. At times it complicates the circulatory failure produced by a small blood volume. In patients with broken bones or severe injuries manipulation of the parts or movement of the patient may be followed by circulatory failure.

It is of interest to note that signs of stimulation of both the sympathetic and the parasympathetic systems are present in the person with the fainting reaction. From a theoretical point of view the activity of the autonomic nervous system might result from the fall in arterial pressure, or the fall in arterial pressure might be one of the manifestations of an over-stimulated nervous system. In the first instance, the signs and the symptoms of the fainting reaction would result from the fall in arterial pressure; in the second, they would be part of the response to the afferent stimulus producing the fall in arterial pressure, but not caused by the fall in pressure itself. The signs and the symptoms of the fainting reaction frequently occur without the fall in arterial pressure and may persist long after the pressure has returned to normal. They may not occur when the blood pressure falls profoundly in patients with postural hypotension. These observations suggest that they are not caused by the fall in arterial pressure, but are responses to the same stimulus as that producing the fall in arterial pressure.

The relationship between the intensification of the fainting reaction and the upright position of the subject is of interest. After a patient has apparently recovered in the recumbent position, assumption of the upright position often causes a recurrence of the entire reaction. After venesection blood donors frequently have no symptoms until they stand. Acute infections, chronic illnesses, acute or chronic blood loss, fever, high external temperature, dehydration, and ingestion of nitrites are frequently associated with fainting when the patient assumes the upright position. The upright position causes pooling of blood by gravity in the portions of the body below the heart, with a reduction of cardiac output because of a decrease in venous return to the heart and a progressive fall in arterial pressure. The upright position is a strong stimulus to increased activity of the autonomic nervous system and greatly increases the number of visceral afferent stimuli entering the nervous system. This combination of a decreased pressure head and increased nervous system activity results in a precipitous fall in arterial pressure, the final sharp break in pressure being caused by reflex arteriolar dilatation.

In at least one situation, fainting may be precipitated by lying down and relieved by standing. The writer has made observations on two pregnant women near term who fainted if they were placed on their backs in the recumbent position. The clinical picture was that of reflex vasodepressor syncope. They were able to lie on their sides without difficulty.

CAROTID SINUS DEPRESSOR REFLEX

Pressure on the carotid sinus may rarely cause a striking fall in arterial pressure, with or without the other signs and symptoms of the fainting reaction, which cannot be accounted for by slowing of the heart rate.[5] Pressure on the carotid sinus may cause a precipitous fall in arterial pressure after cardiac slowing has been eliminated by atropinization. If the subject is upright, unconsciousness may occur. Epinephrine prevents the fall in arterial pressure when the carotid sinus is stimulated and syncope does not occur (Fig. 179).

DISEASE OF THE SYMPATHETIC NERVOUS SYSTEM (POSTURAL HYPOTENSION)

Syncope, occurring only when the patient is in the upright position, and without any

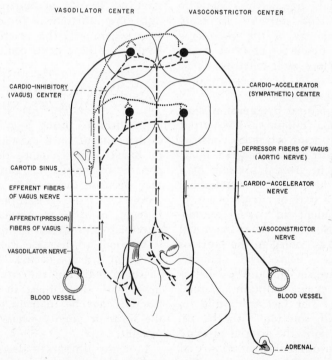

FIG. 179. Diagrammatic representation of the cardiovascular reflex mechanisms. Afferent vagal fibers are shown by broken lines; sinus nerve fibers, by a dotted line; efferent fibers to the heart and to the blood vessels, by a continuous line. The afferent fibers are represented as causing reciprocal effects upon the medullary centers. (Best, C. H., and Taylor, N. B.: The Physiological Basis of Medical Practice, ed. 7, Baltimore, Williams & Wilkins)

of the unpleasant symptoms that are characteristic of the common faint, may be caused by postural hypotension.[6] In this condition the arterial pressure is normal or elevated when the patient is horizontal, but falls precipitously on standing. It is usually seen in middle-aged or elderly people, but may occur much earlier. Syncope is more likely to occur in the morning and often follows exercise. There are frequently signs and symptoms of disturbance in the central or peripheral nervous systems. Pupillary abnormalities, fixed heart rate, bladder disturbances, diarrhea, impotence, loss of sweating over a part of the body, loss of vasoconstriction and vasodilatation in the extremities when the body is cooled or heated are frequently seen singularly or in any combination.

Postural hypotension is usually the result of a disease of the autonomic nervous system. It is seen most frequently in *diabetic neuropathy* and *tabes dorsalis*. In many instances, the etiology of the neurologic disease remains obscure. Postural hypotension also develops after extensive *bilateral sympathectomy* has been performed to relieve hypertension.

Persons with postural hypotension show either an abnormal fall in cardiac output on standing with good arteriolar constriction or an inability to vasoconstrict in response to a fall in arterial pressure or a combination of the two. These abnormal responses reflect a state of circulatory incoordination dependent on partial autonomic paralysis. No more than the usual amount of blood is pooled in the portions of the body below heart level. The response to the average amount pooled is abnormal and does not maintain a normal arterial pressure. The fact that rapid infusion of albumin solution with the patient standing restores the arterial pressure to normal demonstrates the importance of the postural shift in blood volume. The ability of the heart to respond normally to a fall in arterial pressure, the ability of the veins to constrict in response to usual stimuli, and the ability of the arterioles to constrict when the cardiac output falls may all be impaired in varying degrees. The lack of coordination in the circulation is caused by loss of function of the autonomic nervous system. This may be peripheral, as in the postural hypotension caused by sympathectomy; it may be in the spinal cord, as in patients with transverse myelitis, or it may be in the medulla or the hypothalamus.[7]

Postural hypotension resulting from disease of the sympathetic nervous system must be differentiated from the vasodepressor syncope precipitated by standing which is common in persons with Addison's disease, with febrile illnesses, with blood loss and with chronic wasting diseases. In these patients the vasodepressor reaction with the accompanying signs and symptoms of the fainting reaction improve as the general condition of the patient improves. In the patient with postural hypotension from disease of the autonomic nervous system, the fall in arterial pressure on standing is not accompanied by other signs of stimulation of the autonomic nervous system and the reaction persists regardless of the general condition.

FAINTING FROM A SHARP FALL IN CARDIAC OUTPUT WITHOUT CARDIAC STANDSTILL

Conditions causing a great decrease in cardiac output, such as a marked decrease in blood volume, acute pericardial tamponade, or massive myocardial infarction, may decrease the cardiac output to such a degree that the arterial pressure is greatly lowered, in spite of normal or increased arteriolar tone. When the drop in pressure is sufficient to decrease the circulation to the brain, syncope occurs. A pressure adequate to maintain the circulation to the brain with the subject in the horizontal position may be inadequate to overcome the force of gravity when the subject is upright.

In many illnesses a decrease in venous tone leads to excessive venous pooling in the erect position. When inadequate filling of the heart is present, syncope follows.

In certain patients with diabetic neuropathy, a marked fall in arterial pressure occurs in spite of normal or excessive arteriolar constriction. The cardiac output is strikingly reduced and returns to normal when the blood volume is increased. Whether this represents a loss of venous tone common to many illnesses or whether it represents disease of the autonomic nerves supplying the veins remains to be determined.

Fainting at times occurs at the onset of an attack of paroxysmal tachycardia. The tachycardia may cause a sufficient fall in cardiac output to cause fainting on the basis of cerebral ischemia. Other mechanisms may be operative, however. Awareness of a disturbance in cardiac function may cause sufficient anxiety to precipitate an attack of vasodepressor syncope in an anxious subject. Comeau[8] described a patient with paroxysmal atrial fibrillation in whom attacks of syncope were caused by complete cardiac arrest between the cessation of normal rhythm and the establishment of atrial fibrillation. Carefully taken histories reveal that this is a common sequence of events in fainting associated with atrial tachycardia.

FAINTING FROM VENTRICULAR STANDSTILL (ADAMS-STOKES ATTACKS)

When the ventricles stop pumping blood for a few seconds, consciousness is lost. The effects of brief periods of acute arrest of the cerebral circulation in normal subjects have been reported by Rossen and his collaborators.[9] Arrest of the cerebral circulation was accomplished by means of a cervical pressure cuff (a constricting band about the subject's neck). These patients showed fixation of the eyes, tingling, constriction of the visual fields, loss of consciousness and, immediately after the restoration of blood flow, a brief, mild tonic and clonic seizure. The average time from arrest of the cerebral circulation to loss of consciousness was 7 seconds. The corneal reflex may disappear in less than 10 seconds. They found that arrest of the circulation for 100 seconds may be followed by rapid recovery of consciousness and no objective evidence of injury.

Weiss and Baker[5] observed that, after complete arrest of the heart, syncope usually occurred in 8 seconds and regularly within 12 seconds. Rossen *et al.*[9] point out that the somewhat longer maintenance of consciousness following cardiac asystole than with the cervical cuff may be explained on the basis that arrest of the heart fails to arrest cerebral circulation as rapidly as does occlusion of the arteries supplying blood to the brain.

The ventricle may cease pumping blood as the result of (1) sinus standstill or heart block and (2) ventricular fibrillation. Heart block may be caused either by abnormal reflex activity or by organic disease in the conduction system of the heart.

Stimulation of the efferent endings of the vagus causes ventricular asystole either by sinus standstill or auriculoventricular block. Pressure on the carotid sinus is frequently an effective afferent stimulus. Less frequently, pressure on the eyeball causes cardiac standstill. Stimulation on the pharynx, the esophagus, the duodenum and the bronchi may produce the same effect. Less often afferent stimuli from other areas may cause sinus standstill or atrioventricular block.

Patients with organic heart disease frequently have periods of ventricular asystole sufficient to produce syncope. These periods of cardiac standstill characteristically occur when the rhythm of the heart shifts from normal sinus rhythm or partial heart block to complete heart block. When the impulses from the atria are completely blocked several seconds may elapse before a site of impulse formation becomes active in the ventricles. In some patients, however, with constant complete atrioventricular block, syncope will occur because of periods during which the idioventricular rhythm fails. The diagnosis of syncope due to heart block is easy if the patient has some evidence of block at the time that he is seen. In certain patients normal sinus rhythm will be present the majority of the time and repeated observations must be made before characteristic abnormalities are detected and the diagnosis of heart block can be definitely established.

The symptoms caused by ventricular standstill are the same regardless of the cause of the standstill. The patient has none of the unpleasant symptoms of overactivity of the autonomic nervous system so characteristic of the common faint. He notices only blurring of vision and loss of consciousness. On inspection slight pallor may be noted, followed by a flush as the ventricles begin to pump blood. Apnea is common. If the period of asystole is prolonged, hyperventilation and convulsive movements follow. Recovery is usually prompt when the ventricles begin to contract.

In the writer's experience, patients with ventricular standstill from heart block because of disease of the conduction system often have attacks in their sleep, while patients with ventricular standstill from reflex activity do not. The intravenous injection of atropine will restore normal sinus rhythm if the block is caused by reflex activity.

Patients with serious heart disease may rarely have attacks of asystole caused by short periods of ventricular fibrillation.[10] On physical examination no evidence of ventricular activity can be detected. The electrocardiogram shows the characteristic bizarre pattern of ventricular fibrillation. At times in patients with complete heart block the syncope is caused by ventricular fibrillation rather than ventricular standstill.

REFLEX FAINTING OF CEREBRAL TYPE

Pressure on the carotid sinus may cause syncope by inducing ventricular standstill or by causing a precipitous fall in arterial pressure. In certain persons syncope is produced by pressure on the carotid sinus without a change in pulse rate or arterial pressure.[11] Focal neurologic signs and symptoms with or without syncope may occur on the opposite side of the body from the carotid sinus that was stimulated. Ten patients with this cerebral type of carotid sinus syncope have been studied by Engel and Romano[12] and they find that slow electroencephalographic waves always accompany unconsciousness of more than one or two seconds. These authors point out that hysterical syncope may easily be confused with the cerebral type of carotid sinus syncope, if the specificity of the carotid sinus as the sensitive zone is not controlled.

The mechanism of the production of unconsciousness in these patients with the cerebral type of carotid sinus syncope has not been definitely determined. Engel, Romano and McLin[13] found that when focal neurologic signs and symptoms occur without loss of consciousness they are associated with slow waves which arise from the corresponding hemisphere. When unconsciousness occurs the slow waves arise diffusely and subsequently focal manifestations do not lead to any further change. Abnormally slow waves arising from one cortex might result either from a local reflex vasoconstriction or from a direct cortical reflex mediated through the midbrain.

TUSSIVE FAINTING WITH OBSTRUCTIVE EMPHYSEMA, TRACHEAL OR LARYNGEAL OBSTRUCTION

Patients who have uncontrolled violent attacks of coughing may lose consciousness if they are unable to collapse their lungs in a normal manner.[14] Hysterical closure of the glottis, obstructive emphysema or tracheal obstruction most commonly from aneurysm may prevent normal collapse of the lungs. When strong pressure is exerted by the chest wall and diaphragms on noncollapsible lungs, a very high intrathoracic pressure results. This pressure is transmitted to the systemic arteries. The rise in pressure is buffered by the elastic qualities of the systemic arteries outside the thorax and the abdomen, and the increase in arterial pressure is less than the increase in intrathoracic and intra-abdominal pressures. The aorta and the large vessels within the thorax and the abdomen are collapsed. The cerebrospinal pressure rises as blood is forced into the extradural venous plexus, and soft tissues are displaced inward through the vertebral foramina. This rise in cerebrospinal pressure is not buffered as is the arterial pressure, and the cerebrospinal pressure becomes equal to the intrathoracic pressure and greater than the arterial pressure, thus forcing blood from the cranium. In cough syncope, the circulation is interfered with at two levels: (1) at the capillary level in the brain, and (2) at the lung and heart level by direct compression.[15] Subjects who stretch vigorously with the glottis closed may occasionally faint.

FAINTING FROM EXTERNAL COMPRESSION OF THE THORAX WITH GLOTTIS CLOSED

Fainting may occur during external compression of the thorax, or on release of the compression.[16] It is assumed that the thoracic compression interferes with the flow of blood through the lungs, causing a fall in cerebral blood flow and loss of consciousness. If syncope does not occur during the compression it may occur when it is released. On removing the compression, the blood from the right heart fills the empty lungs. This may cause a temporary fall in the rate of filling of the left heart and result in a sharp fall in cardiac output. The importance of reflex changes as accessory or primary factors in this type of fainting has not been determined.

FAINTING FROM CEREBRAL ANOXEMIA IN TETRALOGY OF FALLOT

Patients with tetralogy of Fallot may become unconscious on exertion. It has been shown that during exercise the oxygen content of the arterial blood becomes much lower than it is at rest.[17] The exercising muscles extract nearly all of the oxygen from the blood passing through them. This dark, unoxygenated blood enters the systemic arteries through the interventricular septal defect without passing through the lungs. The oxygen content of the arterial blood falls sharply, and the patient becomes unconscious because of cerebral anoxemia.

FAINTING FROM EXTRACRANIAL OBSTRUCTION OF THE CEREBRAL VESSELS

Atherosclerosis may cause various degrees of obstruction of all the major vessels to the head and upper extremities as they leave the aorta.[18] The carotid and brachial pulses may be absent. If one vessel is partially open, a systolic and diastolic murmur will be present. A diastolic murmur over a partially occluded artery occurs only when the collateral circulation is greatly reduced. On standing, the patient may lose consciousness, not because the arterial pressure in the aorta falls but because in the presence of occlusive disease the normal aortic pressure cannot perfuse the head against the increased force of gravity produced by the upright position.

In extracranial disease of the internal carotid arteries, syncope, intermittent paralysis and transient blindness may occur. A systolic stenotic murmur can frequently be heard over the area of the carotid bifurcation, over the mastoid process, or over the eyeball. When one internal carotid is completely occluded, the murmur will be heard over the open vessel. No murmur on one side and a systolic and diastolic murmur over the opposite side is an ominous sign. It means that the collateral circulation from the carotid and vertebral arteries is severely impaired and that there is a large pressure gradient during systole and diastole. A loud systolic murmur at the bifurcation of the common carotid may indicate localized narrowing of the external rather than internal carotid artery.

When the subclavian vessel is occluded just proximal to the vertebral vessel, an interesting syndrome may develop. Vigorous exercise of the arm on the occluded side may cause weakness in the opposite side of the body. The sharp fall in peripheral resistance caused by the exercise of the arm reverses the direction of blood flow in the vertebral artery and blood is channeled from the circle of Willis into the exercising arm. This syndrome has been called the "vertebral steal."

FAINTING FROM OBSTRUCTION OF MITRAL VALVE THROMBUS OR TUMOR

Intermittent obstruction of mitral valve by myxoma or ball thrombus in the left atrium causes sudden loss of consciousness. Peripheral embolization is common in both conditions.

FAINTING FROM EMBOLUS LODGING IN A CEREBRAL ARTERY

Transient periods of unconsciousness without focal neurologic signs are occasionally seen in patients in whom small vessels of the brain are being occluded by emboli. In one patient with subacute bacterial endocarditis these episodes recurred frequently over several days. Usually emboli produce focal neurologic signs rather than syncopal attacks.

FAINTING FROM HYPERVENTILATION

An increase in ventilation above that required by metabolic needs of the body results in alkalosis because of the loss of CO_2 from the body. Numbness and tingling of the mouth, the face and the extremities, coldness of the extremities, feeling of lightheadedness and confusion and, at times, tetany are characteristic symptoms. The overventilation may be voluntary or reflex in origin. Anxiety is the most common cause of involuntary hyperventilation, but stimuli from any sensory organ or nerve may be the cause.

The disturbance in the level of awareness results from changes in cerebral metabolism produced by alkalosis. The electroencephalogram shows slow large waves. Consciousness is usually not lost when the subject remains in the recumbent position, but when he is upright typical vasodepressor reaction may develop with a sudden fall in arterial pressure and loss of consciousness.

FAINTING FROM ANOXEMIA

Loss of consciousness may result from an inadequate supply of oxygen to the brain when the blood supply is adequate but the blood transport of oxygen is deficient. This may occur in anemia; thus persons with severe anemia are especially apt to faint whenever any of the other possible causes are added to this predisposing cause. Carbon-monoxide poisoning may lower the ability of the red cells to carry oxygen.

Inadequate oxygen concentration in the inspired air or interference with access of oxygen through the lungs to the blood may result in oxygen want in the tissues. Since the cerebral centers are particularly sensitive to lack of oxygen, a tendency to syncope may be an early evidence of such a condition.

FAINTING FROM HYPOGLYCEMIA

The symptoms produced by a decrease in blood sugar are strikingly similar to those produced by anoxia. In both instances cerebral metabolism is interfered with: in one case by oxygen lack, in the other by the lack of fuel to utilize the oxygen.

Hypoglycemia affects the function of both the autonomic and the central nervous systems. Weakness, sweating, flushing, pallor and trembling are evidence of disturbance in the autonomic nervous system. Anxiety, difficulty in concentrating, lightheadedness, disorientation, amnesia, unconsciousness and convulsions result from disturbance in cerebral metabolism. Administration of glucose by vein results in prompt recovery.

The signs and the symptoms of hypoglycemia are most frequently seen in patients with diabetes who have received an overdose of insulin. Hypoglycemia occurs spontaneously in patients with insulin-secreting adenomas of the isles of Langerhans or with functional hyperactivity and hyperplasia of the islets. It is seen also in patients with adrenal cortical insufficiency, hypophyseal deficiency and liver disease. Evidences of hypoglycemia may appear in some otherwise normal subjects a few hours after the ingestion of a large carbohydrate meal. Profound heart failure is occasionally associated with severe hypoglycemia. In most instances this occurs in irreversible situations, but we have seen one patient with pericardial tamponade from purulent pericarditis in whom the recognition of the hypoglycemia was lifesaving.

Sudden transient loss of consciousness without any other symptom has not in my experience been caused by hypoglycemia. Mental confusion, with abnormal behavior, occurring when no food has been ingested for several hours, with or without loss of consciousness, suggests hypoglycemia. Many apparently normal persons complain of weakness, tremor and lightheadedness when the interval between meals is prolonged. Although in such instances the clinical symptoms suggest hypoglycemia, the blood sugar level is usually normal.

HYSTERICAL FAINTING

Certain patients seem to lose consciousness without any changes in the circulation or respiration. The differentiation between hysterical fainting and syncope associated with altered cerebral metabolism has been discussed by Romano and Engel.[12] Hysterical fainting tends to occur more often in women. Other hysterical manifestations are frequently present and the patient may manifest little concern about the repeated faints. The loss of consciousness, which usually occurs in the presence of other people, is abrupt and not preceded by premonitory symptoms of nausea, sweating and pallor. There are no changes in the heart rate, the respiration, the arterial pressure or the electroencephalogram. All types of syncope except hysterical syncope are accompanied by alteration in cerebral metabolism which can be demonstrated by changes in the electroencephalogram.

LESS WELL UNDERSTOOD CAUSES OF FAINTING

NONCYANOTIC HEART DISEASE

Persons with heart disease and left ventricular failure are prone to syncope. The combination of angina pectoris, dyspnea and syncope is not uncommon. Syncope occurs with unusual frequency in three obstructive lesions of the heart and the pulmonary circulation—aortic stenosis, isolated pulmonic stenosis and primary pulmonary hypertension. The mechanism of the syncope has not been determined. While one or more of the causes of syncope discussed previously may be operative, when the patient is examined after recovery the responses to motionless standing, carotid sinus pressure and hyperventilation are normal.

PLEURAL SHOCK

Syncopal attacks have occurred on introduction of a needle into the pleural space. In rare instances such syncope has proved fatal. In many instances the faint has occurred while air was being introduced to produce a pneumothorax, but in some the reaction has occurred before the introduction of air. The reactions appear to be of two types: (1) vasodepressor syncope from stimulation of the pleura; and (2) air embolus from introducing air into the pulmonary veins. Air normally in the lungs may enter the pulmonary veins through a tear in the lung, or it may be injected directly into the pulmonary veins.

FAINTING FROM REMOVING FLUID FROM BLADDER OR BODY CAVITIES

Transient loss of consciousness, and, rarely, even death have occurred after draining a distended bladder or after removing fluid from the pleural or the peritoneal cavities. When this has occurred with drainage of a distended bladder or after the removal of a large quantity of ascitic fluid, the syncope has been attributed to the pooling of blood in the venous system as the result of the decrease in the pressure of the urine or fluid. This hypothesis has never been tested experimentally. The role of reflex responses in this type of reaction has not been investigated.

MICTURITION SYNCOPE

During or immediately after micturition, syncope may occur. It usually happens in the night and is more common in males. The loss of consciousness is brief, and there is no postsyncopal confusion or weakness.

DIAGNOSTIC APPROACH IN REFERENCE TO CHIEF COMPLAINT OF FAINTING

HISTORY

Diseases that Predispose to Vasodepressor Syncope. Hemorrhage, dehydration, or any condition that lowers the blood volume, febrile illnesses, chronic wasting diseases and trauma are important. Pregnancy and high external temperatures must be considered. Determine the relation of the attacks to minor respiratory illnesses and fatigue, as these predispose to vasodepressor syncope.

Circumstances Attending the Fainting Attacks. Vasodepressor syncope is very common in situations that cause anxiety. Vasodepressor syncope, with its characteristic changes in brain metabolism demonstrated by altered electroencephalographic activity, must be differentiated from hysteria in which the metabolism of the brain is unaltered and the electroencephalogram unchanged.[19]

Relation to Posture. Syncope produced by vasodepressor reaction, by cardiac standstill from reflex causes and by fall in arterial pressure from stimulation of the carotid sinus occurs only rarely when the patient is recumbent. Mental confusion from hyperventilation in the recumbent position is common, but loss of consciousness rarely occurs except when the patient sits or stands. The patient with postural hypotension never has any syncopal symptoms when recumbent. A person with sensitive carotid sinus reflex may have attacks varying from a feeling of lightheadedness to loss of consciousness on turning the head sharply, particularly if he wears a tight collar.

Heart Rate and Nature of Pulse During Attack. A very slow heart rate with a strong radial pulse suggests heart block. A slow rate with a very weak radial pulse suggests vasodepressor syncope.

Relation of Loss of Consciousness to Exercise. Syncope in patients with postural hypotension and aortic stenosis frequently occurs during exercise.

Presence of Other Symptoms Typical of the Fainting Reaction. These are absent in patients with ventricular standstill and postural hypotension. They do not occur with hyperventilation unless this reaction is accompanied by vasodepressor syncope. They are present in vasodepressor syncope and hypoglycemia.

Duration of the Unconsciousness. Unconsciousness from syncope usually lasts only a few seconds, *except in patients with aortic stenosis, left ventricular failure, hypoglycemia, and hysteria.* Patients with vasodepressor syncope characteristically have persistence of weakness, sweating, pallor and nausea after recovering consciousness; those with ventricular asystole or postural hypotension have no residual symptoms. The somnolence and headache which are so frequently seen after an epileptic seizure are not often present after fainting.

Symptoms of Heart Disease. Syncope may accompany attacks of angina pectoris; syncope may occur with left ventricular failure.

Relation to Sleep. Ventricular standstill from disease of the conduction system may cause syncopal attacks during sleep. Seizures during sleep are common in patients with epilepsy.

Presence of Incontinence and Tonic and Clonic Movements. Rhythmic jerking movements of the upper and lower extremities commonly occur in persons who faint and do not fall to the floor. A tonic and clonic convulsion with incontinence is rare in vasodepressor syncope, but does occur. Convulsive seizures with incontinence and biting of the tongue strongly suggest the diagnosis of epilepsy.

Symptoms Produced by Hyperventilation. Was the attack accompanied by numbness, tingling and coldness of the extremities? Did tetany develop? These are the characteristic symptoms of hyperventilation.

Relation to Meals. Patients with hypoglycemia may be found unconscious after sleeping through the night (prolonged fasting). After fasting they may develop abnormalities of behavior and amnesia which are promptly relieved by food.

Occurrence of Abnormal Behavior and Amnesia. Transient loss of consciousness may be preceded or followed by peculiar behavior or amnesia not only in hypoglycemia but also in patients with "epileptic equivalents."

PHYSICAL EXAMINATION AND SPECIAL TESTS

1. Look for evidence of diseases considered at the beginning of History.

2. Listen for systolic murmurs of localized arterial stenosis over common carotids, at the carotid bifurcation, over the mastoid processes and over the eyeballs. Stenotic murmurs over the aorta, renal vessels, iliac and femoral vessels are frequently present in patients with extracranial vascular occlusion.

3. Have the subject sit in chair; massage first the right and then the left carotid bulb. Note any change in color, heart rate, arterial pressure, level of awareness, or focal neurologic signs.

4. While the patient remains sitting have him hyperventilate maximally for 2

minutes. Question him as to any similarity between his spontaneous attacks and the symptoms produced by hyperventilation.

5. Determine the arterial pressure and the pulse rate with the patient recumbent and after he has stood leaning against the wall for one minute.

6. Examine heart for evidence of block, both by auscultation and by the electrocardiograph. Look for the physical signs of aortic stenosis and insufficiency.

7. Look for evidence of diffuse neurologic damage. Postural hypotension may accompany tabes dorsalis, combined system disease, or diabetic peripheral neuritis.

8. Feel radial pulse and take arterial pressure while the patient coughs. Repeat during forced expiration against closed glottis.

9. Determine the blood sugar concentration in the fasting state.

SUMMARY

Fainting (syncope) implies a brief, quickly reversible loss of consciousness. It is usually caused by diminution suddenly occurring in the blood supply to the centers of consciousness in the brain. It may be of no clinical importance, or it may be the first symptom of occlusion of the extracranial circulation. Less frequently syncope may result from changes in the constituents of the blood. Other causes include primary neurophysiologic disorders.

Fainting with unconsciousness lasting only a few seconds may occur in aortic stenosis or left ventricular failure. These two conditions and others such as hypoglycemia and hysteria, however, are apt to produce longer lapses. Such longer periods of unconsciousness, with the pathogenic mechanisms involved, are discussed in Chapter 26.

It is important to recognize syncope and to find its cause; also to be able to distinguish it from other unconscious states, since upon such differential diagnosis the choice of therapy depends, and proper therapy may prevent permanent impairment or death.

REFERENCES

1. Wayne, H. H.: Syncope. Physiological consideration and an analysis of the clinical characteristics in 510 patients, Am. J. Med. 30:418, 1961.
2. Engel, G. L.: Mechanisms of fainting, J. Mt. Sinai Hosp. 12:170-190, 1945.
3. Warren, J. V., Brannon, E. A., Stead, E. A., Jr., and Merrill, A. J.: Effect of venesection and pooling of blood in extremities on atrial pressure and cardiac output in normal subjects with observations on acute circulatory collapse in 3 instances, J. Clin. Invest. 24:337-344, 1945.
4. Barcroft, H., Edholm, O. G., McMichael, J., and Sharpey-Schafer, E. P.: Posthemorrhagic fainting; study by cardiac output and forearm flow, Lancet 1:489-490, 1944.
5. Weiss, S., and Baker, J. P.: Carotid sinus reflex in health and disease; its role in causation of fainting and convulsions, Medicine 12:297, 1933.
6. Bradbury, S., and Eggleston, C.: Postural hypotension, Am. Heart J. 1:73-86, 1933.
7. Stead, E. A., Jr., and Ebert, R. V.: Postural hypotension; disease of sympathetic nervous system, Arch. Intern. Med. 67:546-562, 1941.
8. Comeau, W. J.: Mechanism for syncopal attacks associated with paroxysmal auricular fibrillation, New Eng. J. Med. 227:134-136, 1942.
9. Rossen, R., Kabat, H., and Anderson, J. P.: Acute arrest of cerebral circulation in man, Arch. Neurol. Psychiat. 50:510-528, 1943.
10. Levine, S. A.: Clinical Heart Disease, ed. 5, Philadelphia, Saunders, 1958.
11. Ferris, E. B., Jr., Capps, R. B., and Weiss, S.: Carotid sinus syncope and its bearing on mechanism of unconscious state and convulsions; study of 32 additional cases, Medicine 14:377, 456, 1935.
12. Romano, J., and Engel, G. L.: Studies of syncope; differentiation between vasodepressor and hysterical fainting, Psychosom. Med. 7:3-15, 1945.
13. Engel, G. L., Romano, J. and McLin, T. R.: Vasodepressor and carotid sinus syncope; clinical, electro-encephalographic and electrocardiographic observations, Arch. Intern. Med. 74:100-119, 1944.
14. McCann, W. S., Bruce, R. A., Lovejoy, F. W., Jr., Yu, P. N. G., Pearson, R., Engel, G., and Kelly, J.: Trans. Ass. Amer. Physicians 62:116, 1949.

15. McIntosh, H. D., Estes, E. H., and Warren, J. V.: Circulatory effects of cough; the mechanism of cough syncope, Clin. Res. Proc. 3:82, 1955.

16. Weiss, S.: The Oxford Medicine, vol. 2, Chicago, Oxford, 1943.

17. Blalock, A., and Taussig, H.: J.A.M.A. 128:189, 1945.

18. Conference on Vascular Disease of the Brain, Neurology 11: No. 4, Part 2, pp. 1-176, 1961.

19. Karp, H. R., Weissler, A. M., Heyman, A.: Vasodepressor syncope: electroencephalogram and circulatory changes, Arch. Neurol. 5:94, 1961.

29

Vertigo and Dizziness

H. H. Hyland

DEFINITIONS

The word *vertigo* is used in medical practice to imply a symptom which has certain specific characteristics. However, this word is rarely used by patients; the layman refers to it as "dizziness" or "giddiness," two terms that are commonly used to describe a wide variety of sensations as well as vertigo.

Dictionaries include among the synonyms of *dizziness* "foolish" or "stupid" and of *giddiness* "insane" or "possessed by a god," showing that originally these words implied a mental as well as a physical disturbance of equilibrium. To some extent this conception still exists, and the words are used interchangeably by patients to describe many symptoms, such as feelings of mental confusion, a general sense of insecurity, swimming or spinning sensations within the head, lightheadedness with or without brief visual impairment, a feeling of unsteadiness on the feet, a subjective sensation of movement of the individual or of his surroundings, etc.

Analysis of these abnormal sensations makes it evident that they vary in their pathogenesis, since they include symptoms accompanying psychogenic disorders and syncope as well as disturbed vestibular function. Because vertigo comes within the meaning of dizziness and giddiness, it would avoid much confusion if physicians would confine their use of these words to the symptom of vertigo and to those sensations which while not truly vertigo are related to it.

The physician should always obtain a detailed description of the actual sensations that have been experienced by the patient in order to be sure whether or not vertigo exists. This may take time and patience because many people find difficulty in describing accurately abnormal sensations of this nature. Those symptoms which are clearly not vertigo or related to it must be evaluated in the light of the history and findings on examination. The necessity of careful inquiry from the patient was stressed by Hughlings Jackson[1] years ago: "The term vertigo is often used somewhat loosely. I do not take the explanation giddiness from the patient's mouth always to mean true giddiness. We have to put down not his name for, but the description he gives of the sensation he calls giddiness."

Vertigo is derived from the Latin verb *vertere* meaning "to turn," so that by its derivation it implies a sensation of turning either of the body or its surroundings.

However, it is generally agreed that the word should not be restricted to the sensation of rotation but should be used to describe a hallucination of movement in any plane. The observations of McNally and Stuart[2] give justification for not interpreting vertigo too narrowly, since they found that the descriptions given by patients following vertigo induced by caloric tests indicate a variety of other sensations as well as that of turning.

Vertigo has been defined concisely by Russell Brain[3] as "the consciousness of disordered orientation of the body in space." The essential symptoms are a *hallucination of movement either of the surroundings or of the person himself.* In the former objects may seem to move in a rotary, horizontal, vertical or oblique fashion. In the latter the false feeling of movement may consist of sensations of the body spinning, falling or being pushed in various directions. Sometimes the sensation is confined to the head which is felt to be revolving, swaying or rocking. Observation of the patient during an attack of vertigo may reveal no objective movement of his body, but if the vertigo is at all severe he will stagger and may even fall to the ground.

Symonds[4] has emphasized that following all attacks of true vertigo there is a sensation of unsteadiness of the legs, usually lasting some hours. Another sensation which may occur as a common accompaniment or independently is a general sense of uncertainty in equilibrium on walking with sometimes a vague sense of movement of the surroundings. The patient often relates it to movement, particularly of the head. Although not necessarily implying a hallucination of movement, these two symptoms are closely akin to vertigo since they are common and sometimes persistent complaints from patients with vestibular disorders. Their regular occurrence as the aftermath of an acute attack of vertigo is helpful in identifying atypical attacks in which the patient may fall with little or no awareness of preceding vertigo.

It is not clear what determines whether the false sense of movement in vertigo will be related to the surroundings or to the patient himself. The former occurs more commonly than the latter. Brain[3] considers that for consciousness the orientation of the body in space is normally an orderly dynamic relation between the bodily schema and the schema of the external world. Vertigo is the state of consciousness which arises when this relation becomes disordered. He points out that electrical stimulation at the cortical level has shown that a hallucination of rotation either of the body in one direction or the environment in the other direction may be evoked from the same region.[5] This suggests to him that what is evoked primarily is the functional relation between the body schema and the schema of the external world, thus indicating relative movement between them. Which is felt to be moving and which is felt to be stationary probably depends upon the pre-existing background provided by the proprioceptors of the body. This could be determined by their past conditioning relative to movement.

ANATOMIC AND PHYSIOLOGIC CONSIDERATIONS

The maintenance of equilibrium depends on the integration by the brain of various afferent stimuli from the periphery that operate (for the most part) without entering consciousness. These include afferent impulses from the retinae, the skin and the labyrinths, together with proprioceptive impulses from the ocular muscles, the neck, the trunk and the lower limbs. Vertigo is the false sense perception which develops in consciousness when a disturbance or imbalance occurs in these peripheral mechanisms or their central connections. The most important of the peripheral mechanisms in maintaining orientation in space are the labyrinths; the most severe and clearly defined vertigo occurs if their function is disturbed.

The membranous labyrinth, filled with a fluid known as *endolymph,* lies inside the bony labyrinth, surrounded by perilymph, and consists of three semicircular canals known as the anterior and posterior (vertical) and the lateral (horizontal). These canals lie in planes approximately at right angles to one another. The cavities of the three canals open by both extremities into the wall of a small saclike structure known as the utricle which in turn connects with a similar structure called the saccule, by way of the ductus endolymphaticus. The utricle and the saccule are situated in the ovoid bony chamber known as the vestibule. The saccule communicates with the cochlea through the cochlear duct. Part of the epithelium forming the walls of the utricle and saccule is specialized for sensory reception. These structures, called the *macula utriculi* and the *macula sacculi,* each consist of a plaque of sensitive hair cells covered by a layer of gelatinous material upon which is situated a mass of tiny crystals of calcium carbonate. The maculae, which lie in different planes in relations to each other, are known as the otolith organs, and impulses from them are transmitted by branches of the vestibular nerve (Fig. 180). The function of the saccule is not completely understood, but it is thought to be mainly involved in cochlear function and to have relatively little to do with the maintenance of posture. This neural mechanism may serve to record bony vibrations as distinct from vibration through air. The appreciation of

the sound of one's own voice therefore may depend upon saccular as well as upon cochlear function. The utricle appears, from experimental study, to be an organ of static sense influencing muscle tone and serving to maintain posture. It registers the position of the head in space and governs the statotonic reflexes, the righting reflexes and the compensatory positions of the eyes. An additional function suggested for the otolith structures is that they are the receptor organs concerned with linear acceleration.[6]

A branch of the vestibular nerve passes to the ampulla of each semicircular canal where it terminates in a receptor organ called the *crista.* This also consists of specialized epithelium (hair cells) imbedded in a gelatinous fluid material. The crista has to do with kinetic sense, in contrast to the utricle, and is responsible for the statokinetic reflexes which are the compensatory movements of eyes and limbs brought about by movements of the head. The crista responds to changes in the velocity and in the direction of movement. The response is accomplished through the effect which movements of the head exert upon the endolymph in the particular

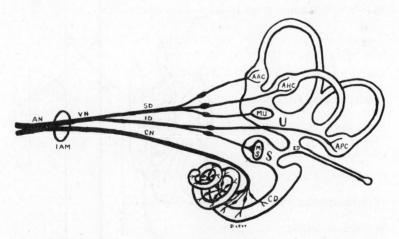

Fig. 180. Diagram of membranous labyrinth showing nerve distribution. AN, acoustic nerve; IAM, internal auditory meatus; VN, vestibular nerve; SD, superior division of vestibular nerve; ID, inferior division of vestibular nerve; CN, cochlear nerve; AAC, ampulla of anterior semicircular canal; AHC, ampulla of horizontal semicircular canal; APC, ampulla of posterior semicircular canal; U, utricle; MU, macula utriculi; S, saccule; MS, macula sacculi; CD, cochlear duct; ED, endolymphatic duct.

canal whose plane is involved in the movement.

The sensory impulses from the cristae of the semicircular canals, along with those from the maculae of the utricle and the saccule, proceed by way of the vestibular nerve, which originates from the bipolar cells of the vestibular ganglion. It passes through the internal auditory meatus, as the median part of the eighth nerve, to the cerebellopontine angle, then separates from the cochlear division on entering the brain stem. Apart from some fibers passing directly to the cerebellum, the nerve terminates in four cellular masses constituting the vestibular nuclei, which extend from the pons to the upper part of the medulla, located in the floor and the lateral wall of the fourth ventricle.

From the vestibular nuclei secondary tracts are given off to the cerebellum, the oculomotor nuclei, the spinal cord and the cortex (Fig. 181). The fibers to the cerebellum, including those coming directly from the vestibular nerve and the secondary fibers from the vestibular nuclei, pass primarily into the flocculonodular lobe, according to Larsell and Dow.[7] This structure, consisting of the nodulus in the mid-line and paired lateral parts known as the flocculi, is situated in the postero-inferior part of the posterior lobe of the cerebellum. Secondarily, fibers pass to adjacent parts which include the uvula, the lingula and the fastigial or roof nuclei. It is possible that secondary vestibular fibers also reach other parts of the cerebellar cortex.[8] In addition to receiving only vestibular fibers, the flocculonodular lobe sends efferent fibers only to the vestibular nuclei.[7] Therefore, the *flocculonodular mechanism* is entirely vestibular in function and is concerned with the maintenance of equilibrium. The uvula, lingula and fastigial nuclei also send fibers to the vestibular nuclei.

Axons from the medial, spinal and superior vestibular nuclei go to form a large

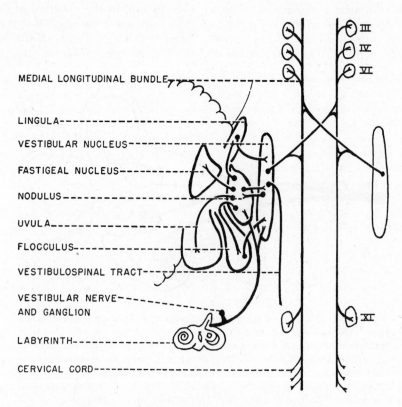

Fig. 181. Diagram of the vestibular pathways.

portion of the median longitudinal bundle of the same and opposite sides. This tract passes up the brain stem to the nuclei of the oculomotor, trochlear and abducens nerves. Thus, each vestibular nucleus is able to influence ocular movement of both eyes. The tract passes downward to the nuclei of the spinal accessory nerve and to the anterior horn cells of the cervical portion of the spinal cord. Therefore, the median longitudinal bundle constitutes a pathway for the reflex control of movement of the head, the neck and the eyes in response to vestibular stimulation. From the lateral vestibular nucleus (Deiters' nucleus) arises the vestibulospinal tract which descends to the motor neurons of the spinal cord conveying impulses concerned with the maintenance of tone and equilibrium.

The course of the connections between the vestibular nuclei and the cortex is not definitely established as yet, but it is believed that the thalamus lies on the route.[9] Clinical and experimental evidence shows that certain parts of the cortex are capable of initiating vertigo and respond by increased activity to the stimulation of the labyrinth. As a result of observations on epileptics, including stimulation experiments on the exposed cortex, Penfield[10] considers that area 22 in the first temporal convolution is the end station of the vestibular tract, the auditory and the vestibular representations lying close together. With stimulation of this region, he found that the sensation of vertigo may occur as an aura of an induced seizure; or it may occur alone; or it may be associated with a humming sound (auditory vertiginous seizure). Penfield[11] has concluded from his studies that the pathway of vestibular sensory information makes a detour from the thalamus out to the cortex, where the vestibular area is next to the auditory area in the superior temporal convolution on both sides. From there, the pathway probably returns to the higher brain stem where it enters the centrencephalic integrating system. He has found that removal of the superior temporal convolution on either side is not followed by any defect of vestibular function or auditory acuity.

Spiegel[12] showed experimentally that, following application of strychnine to the posterosuperior parts of the temporal lobe, labyrinth stimulation may result in convulsions. Using electrocortigrams, Spiegel found that abnormal stimulation of the labyrinth produces an increase in cortical potentials from the posterosuperior part of the temporal lobe. On the other hand, Foerster[5] induced severe vertigo by stimulation of the superior lip of the interparietal sulcus. His description of the result indicates that true vertigo with either a subjective or objective sensation of movement may occur. "The patient sees the objects before him moving towards the side of stimulation, or he has the sensation of turning towards the contralateral side," although objectively no movement of the head or trunk is observed. Foerster refers also to cases of epilepsy, where the lesions proved to be in the above situation (area 5), which showed an aura of sudden vertigo. These various observations suggest that there are areas of cortex in the temporal and parietal regions which are concerned with the reception of vestibular impulses. These impulses provide conscious information about the position and movements of the head and interference with them is likely to cause vertigo.

Vertigo that occurs with lesions involving the labyrinth may be accompanied by incoordination of movement and nystagmus as well as by certain visceral symptoms, including pallor, sweating, nausea and vomiting, and occasionally diarrhea. These visceral symptoms point to a spread of abnormal impulses from the vestibular nuclei to other centers, including the vagus nuclei. It has been suggested that there are connections direct or indirect between the vestibular nuclei and the vagus nuclei.[13] Incoordination of movement, including falling and past pointing, is the result of abnormal motor impulses transmitted to the skeletal muscles from the vestibular nuclei by way of the vestibulospinal tracts. The nystagmus that accompanies vertigo is caused by abnormal impulses transmitted from the vestibular nuclei to the oculomotor nuclei by way of the median longitudinal bundle.

It has two components, a quick and a slow. The latter is the more important, being of vestibular origin, and is a reflex response resulting from abnormal stimulation of the semicircular canals. The direction of the slow component of the nystagmus, together with the falling and the past pointing, during an attack of labyrinthine vertigo, are all to the side of the more active labyrinth, while the quick component is directed toward the opposite side. Vertigo, together with the other signs of labyrinthine imbalance, can be produced physiologically by means of the caloric and the rotation tests as well as by disease. When the caloric test is carried out with cold water on a normal subject the labyrinth on the tested side becomes the more active one. The direction of the vertigo is toward the opposite side but the objective signs, such as falling, past pointing, and the slow (vestibular) component of the nystagmus are to the side stimulated. When a subject is rotated with the head erect, the vertigo induced will be in the horizontal plane, that is in the plane of the horizontal canals, its direction being opposite to his previous rotation and therefore opposite to the direction of the endolymph movement. The falling, past pointing, and the slow component of the nystagmus will be to the side corresponding to the direction in which he was rotated.

CLINICAL SIGNIFICANCE OF VERTIGO AND DIZZINESS

There will follow a consideration of various pathologic conditions in which vertigo and dizziness occur. The mechanism of production of these symptoms, their character with lesions in different anatomic sites and the diagnostic features concerned will be discussed.

AURAL VERTIGO

Inflammatory. A common form of vertigo is that which usually is referred to as "acute labyrinthitis." It is acute in onset, benign in course, and occasionally occurs in small epidemics in a community.[14,15] The vertigo usually is induced or aggravated by movements of the head or change in posture. There is no deafness and rarely any tinnitus although occasionally a transitory tinnitus has been noted. Vague sensations of fullness may be referred to an ear, and mild reduction in responses to caloric testing is occasionally found. Nausea, vomiting and nystagmus may be present during acute episodes of vertigo. Recovery is usually gradual over a period of a few days or weeks and, although sometimes relapses occur, it is always ultimately complete. Diplopia with actual ocular muscle paresis has been found in some of the epidemic cases and this has led to the assumption that these patients may be suffering from a form of encephalitis, although the cerebrospinal fluid has usually been found normal. In some instances, where an increase in cells has been recorded, it is slight.[17] Sometimes the onset of the vertigo is preceded by a respiratory or other systemic infection and hence it has been assumed to be due to an infectious agent, probably a virus. However, in many cases there is no evident infection and no premonitory malaise.

Dix and Hallpike[16] studied 100 cases similar to the above except in regard to duration of the symptoms. They state that in their patients recovery generally took place in the course of a few years. The patients presented with vertigo, usually, but not always, paroxysmal, and were entirely free of cochlear signs or symptoms. Investigations showed that acute or quiescent focal infection, in the nose and throat particularly, was commonly present and such infection is believed by the authors to play an important part in the pathogenesis. The caloric responses consistently were reduced. This was unilateral in 53 per cent and bilateral in 47 per cent. Since there was no evidence of involvement of the cochlear apparatus, the authors believe that the lesion is central to the labyrinth involving the vestibular nervous pathways up to and including the vestibular nuclei in the brain stem. They have called the condition "vestibular neuronitis." They consider it to be essentially benign and state that it responds well to treatment of focal infection when this is present. In a few cases they have observed the re-establishment of caloric responses with recovery from symptoms.

Cawthorne[17] regards the condition of vestibular neuronitis as due to sudden failure of one vestibular end organ. He points out that the onset is sudden and severe and that the vertigo and nystagmus, which are intense at the onset, gradually diminish so that after three weeks the nystagmus has disappeared and vertigo is only likely to occur on sudden movements of the head. This recovery is due to compensation within the central nervous system for the loss of one set of end organs. In his experience, the only physical sign is the absence or reduction of the normal response to caloric stimulation on one side. While the lesion can be anywhere in the vestibular nerve from the end organ to the vestibular nuclei in the brain stem, he thinks it is quite possible that Scarpa's ganglion is the site.

Vertigo may develop in the presence of middle ear suppuration, indicating labyrinthine involvement. Another cause for the onset of attacks of vertigo in patients with longstanding middle-ear disease is the development of a cholesteatoma extending to involve the inner ear. Vertigo may appear also during certain specific febrile illnesses, notably mumps, indicating the complication of a neurolabyrinthitis. In the above disorders the vertigo is due to the resulting imbalance between the two labyrinths.

Noninflammatory. The condition of spontaneous aural vertigo was first recognized as being of labyrinthine origin by Ménière in 1861. Since that time it has been called Ménière's syndrome or Ménière's disease, the former term having been preferred because the etiology was unknown, and cases were considered due to a variety of causes. Numerous conditions have been suggested as playing a part in the etiology. These include abnormalities of fluid metabolism,[18] sodium retention in the body,[19] local alterations in capillary permeability resulting in local edema,[20] vasomotor disturbance in the inner ear,[21] angioneurotic crisis,[22] allergic responses of the inner ear,[23,25] stenosis of the eustachian tube,[26] hypothyroidism,[26-28]

focal sepsis,[3,29] psychogenic disturbances,[30] etc. Autopsy studies had been lacking until some light was shed on the problem through the demonstration of a pathologic condition common to a number of cases with Ménière's syndrome. In 1938, Hallpike and Cairns[31] found in two cases a marked dilatation of the endolymphatic system of the inner ear, suggesting the existence of increased endolymphatic pressure. Since that time other cases have been described, although the scarcity of pathologic material in this disease makes the number small. In 1945, Altman[32] collected 14 cases from the literature, in 9 of which the involvement was unilateral. The cochlear duct was dilated in all, the saccule in most, the utricle in many, but the semicircular canals were dilated in none. No inflammatory changes were demonstrated, and it is assumed that the disorder is due to an overproduction or a diminished resorption of the endolymph, or to a combination of both. The cause of this condition of an obstructive distention of the endolymph system is unknown. It has been called *idiopathic hydrops of the labyrinth* to distinguish it from the hydrops associated with serous labyrinthitis which shows more widespread degenerative change.

These pathologic observations have provided some basis for understanding the syndrome but it is disturbing that the main changes are in the cochlear apparatus and no pathologic lesions in the semicircular canals have been recorded. Thus, the fundamental etiology is still obscure, and the explanation of the signs and symptoms remains controversial. Hallpike and Cairns[31] believe that the attacks of vertigo are due to a sudden rise of the endolymphatic pressure with "rapidly initiated bouts of asphyxia" of the vestibular end organs. Lindsay[33] explains the attacks as due to herniation of the utricle or saccule into the semicircular canals, with subsequent distortion of the walls of the ampullae. The distortion would interfere with the normal function of the crista which could explain both the attacks of vertigo and the depression of caloric excitability in the late stages.

The syndrome consists of attacks of vertigo in an otherwise healthy adult, accompanied by deafness and tinnitus. The attacks occur spontaneously (bearing no relation to activity) at intervals which may vary from a few hours to several years. In most instances there is no warning before an attack, but sometimes there may be an increase in the intensity of the tinnitus and perhaps also of the deafness preceding the onset. In some cases cephalic sensations occur before an attack, such as sensations of fullness, pressure or stiffness in the back of the head, or in the region of the ear, which may last throughout the attack and persist for some time afterward. The attacks of vertigo characteristically come on abruptly, last usually a matter of minutes (rarely for an hour or more) and terminate abruptly. During the attack the patient is prostrated, desiring to remain motionless, with pallor, sweating and spontaneous nystagmus, either horizontal or rotatory. He is liable to be nauseated throughout, and commonly vomits repeatedly in the later stages of the attack. Recovery is usually rapid, although the patient is likely to have a sensation of unsteadiness on standing lasting up to several hours, and abrupt movements of the head may result in brief vertiginous sensations. The nystagmus subsides with the cessation of vertigo or shortly afterward. Occasionally transitory loss of vision without unconsciousness may occur in an attack. Diplopia has also been described and attributed to skew deviation, a disorder of ocular posture emanating from the labyrinth.[3]

Loss of consciousness has occasionally been observed in severe attacks but it is not common. In such cases epilepsy always has to be excluded although the loss of consciousness may be due to vasovagal syncope resulting from the vasomotor disturbance which accompanies severe vertigo. Rarely patients with long-standing Ménière's disease may develop epileptic attacks that seem to be a product of the labyrinthine disorder. The writer has had such a case under observation. This middle-aged man developed convulsive seizures 8 years after the onset of perceptive deafness, tinnitus and attacks of vertigo. The seizures were infrequent and took place without warning but on recovery of consciousness he experienced vertigo lasting 10 to 15 minutes. The interictal electroencephalogram was normal. The convulsive attacks ceased after a period of 5 years coinciding with a spontaneous remission of the attacks of vertigo. The remission lasted for the next 3 years that he was under observation. During this time, he had no attacks of any kind. This case conforms with what has been called "vestibular epilepsy," i.e., a form of epilepsy in which seizures are provoked by excessive spontaneously arising discharge from the vestibular apparatus. Occasionally patients with Ménière's disease are subject to sudden brief attacks, without loss of consciousness in which the limbs go limp and they fall. These attacks may occur with no accompanying vertigo and they have been attributed to a disorder of the otolith organs ("the otolithic catastrophe" of Tumarkin).[34]

Subjective deafness, with or without tinnitus, commonly precedes the onset of attacks of vertigo, sometimes by many years. This is not surprising since the observed pathologic change appears to have its initial expression in the cochlear structures. It has been suggested that Ménière's disease may have loss of hearing as its only clinical symptom[35] but probably, if the patients survive long enough, attacks of vertigo will occur in the great majority. In a smaller number of patients the deafness and tinnitus appear at approximately the time of onset of the first attack of vertigo and in occasional instances they are not manifest for a considerable time after the attacks commence. The patient usually notices the deafness and tinnitus only in one ear at the start and often for a long time afterward. If these symptoms become bilateral they tend to preponderate on one side, being often relatively slight in the other ear. Cawthorne, Fitzgerald and Hallpike[36] studied 50 cases of Ménière's disease finding objective impairment of cochlear function in all. They were able to show that this was bilateral in 86 per cent of the cases.

A characteristic feature of the deafness in this disease is its variability, particularly in the early stages when sudden changes are common. It is likely to be more marked at a time when attacks of vertigo are occurring, and it may lessen materially between attacks, suggesting that—in the early stages at least—a reversible factor must be present in its causation. It is a perceptive deafness showing either a uniform loss of hearing throughout the entire scale in the affected ear, or a predominant loss for low tones. Distortion of sounds (diplacusis) and hypersensitivity to loud sounds (subjective recruitment) occur, as well as the hearing loss, and may be very distressing to the patient. Lindsay[33] considers the auditory disturbances to be caused by the distortion of the saccule and the membrane of Reissner, associated with the hydrops, thus interfering with the sound transmission in the column of fluid in the cochlea.

The tinnitus likewise is usually more marked at the time when attacks of vertigo occur. It commonly consists of a high-pitched ringing or hissing sound with a low-pitched roaring or pounding which is continuous even in the quiescent periods between attacks.[37] The tinnitus has been explained on the basis of irritation of the nerve endings by increased endolymph pressure, but the fact that section of the eight nerve does not usually abolish the tinnitus makes it necessary to postulate a central factor in its causation, in some cases at least.

Tests for vestibular function in Ménière's disease reveal abnormal reactions in a large proportion of the cases if the tests are properly carried out. According to Altman,[32] there are abnormal caloric reactions in 90 per cent of the cases, with the majority showing a decrease in vestibular irritability on the affected side. Cawthorne,[38] who studied 400 cases, states that the method of caloric testing used rarely failed to reveal a lack of balance between the two labyrinths, the commonest finding being a depression of function on the side of the deafness. He points out that it affords almost the only and the most consistent physical sign of a vestibular disorder, and as each labyrinth is tested separately, it gives valuable information as to whether or not the disorder is limited to one labyrinth, a point of great importance if operative treatment is being considered. In contrast to what was found in testing cochlear functions, definite bilateral vestibular involvement was revealed in less than 5 per cent of these cases. Usually, but not always, the more affected labyrinth is on the side with the greater hearing loss. As in the case of the deafness, there may be considerable variation in the amount of labyrinthine response where tests are carried out at intervals and the latter usually parallels the deafness in degree.[37]

Between attacks the patient is characteristically well and free of symptoms, except deafness and tinnitus which gradually become less variable and more severe over the years. In some cases the fear of attacks may lead to an anxiety state with resulting tension symptoms which add materially to the disability. In Ménière's disease, as in other paroxysmal disorders, emotional maladjustments with morbid anxiety may aggravate and precipitate attacks of vertigo.

A feature of Ménière's disease which has not received the attention it merits is the frequent tendency to spontaneous remissions of the vertigo. Patients who have had many attacks of vertigo for months or years may experience periods of lessened frequency, whether they are receiving treatment or not. In about 50 per cent of long-standing cases a history can be obtained of attacks having stopped spontaneously for months or years, although they tend to recur eventually.[39] It is important to consider this characteristic of the disease in evaluating any method of therapy. The removal of an abscessed tooth, eliminating a food from the diet, administering thyroid extract, inflating an eustachian tube, removing a plug of wax from the ear, etc., if carried out at the time a spontaneous remission is due to occur, may be considered of therapeutic value, and lead to false conceptions about causal relationship. The auditory symptoms are likely to continue and may progress during these periods of remission of the vertigo, indicating that although a temporary balance may have developed in labyrinthine function, the underlying disorder is not quiescent.

Aural vertigo occasionally results from a vascular accident such as hemorrhage within the otic labyrinth or perhaps more commonly thrombosis or embolism of the internal auditory artery. Such lesions cause explosive attacks of vertigo, usually accompanied by a high degree of permanent deafness.[40] It has been anatomically established that the internal auditory artery separates into branches which supply the cochlea and the labyrinth respectively, the branch to the labyrinth being commonly an end artery. Milliken et al.[41] have suggested that certain patients who have an instantaneous onset of severe vertigo associated with nausea and vomiting but no pain, tenderness, or hearing loss, nor any symptoms or signs or neurological dysfunction, have suffered an occlusion of the labyrinthine division of the internal auditory artery. Caloric studies in such patients reveal a dead labyrinth which appears to be permanent. Vertigo and nystagmus are severe for weeks with ultimate gradual recovery.

Acute unilateral obstruction of the eustachian tubes often is stated to be a cause of vertigo as well as conductive deafness but the mechanism of the production of vertigo is not entirely clear. Usually it is attributed to an alteration of the pressure relationship that exists in the middle ears since normally this is kept equal to the outside atmosphere by the passage of air through the eustachian tubes. Tubal catarrh may occur as a result of infection or in the presence of adenoids.

In aviation medicine the term "baratrauma" has come into frequent use. It implies the middle ear damage that can result from violent and tremendous pressure changes caused by climbing and power diving. Deafness and tinnitus are the most common symptoms, but vertigo may be an occasional accompaniment.

VERTIGO AND DIZZINESS WITH LESIONS OF THE EIGHTH NERVE

Vertigo occurring in attacks and comparable in severity to that of Ménière's disease is uncommon with lesions which are confined to the eighth nerve. The usual site of involvement of this nerve is in the cerebellopontine angle. Tumors, particularly acoustic neuroma, are the commonest lesions, but vascular anomalies, including aneurysms and abnormally distributed arteries undergoing arteriosclerotic change, may occasionally affect the eight nerve directly. Chronic syphilitic pachymeningitis, arachnoiditis and platybasia are uncommon causes. Vertigo, deafness and tinnitus occasionally accompany the herpes oticus, facial palsy and pain of the Ramsay Hunt syndrome. They are considered to be due to an associated neuritis of the eighth nerve.

Several statistical studies have been made on cases with verified lesions (mainly tumors of the eighth nerve) to estimate the frequency of vertigo.[4,39,42,43,44] Combined figures from the various sources show that vertigo occurred in about 22 per cent of 293 verified cases. Thus it is not common and, when present, it is usually a late manifestation accompanied by other neurologic signs and symptoms which help to distinguish it from labyrinthine disease. Very rarely vertigo occurring in attacks may be the first or an early symptom in acoustic neuroma.[4,42,45] The inconstancy of true vertigo in lesions affecting the eighth nerve and its tendency to appear as a late symptom if at all, suggest that when it occurs in cerebellopontine angle tumors it may be the result of involvement of the vestibular nuclei in the adjacent brain stem either by the lesion directly or through changes resulting from internal hydrocephalus.

The rather surprising finding that lesions of the vestibular nerve itself rarely produce vertigo, in any way comparable to what occurs with lesions of the end organ, receives support from the observations of Dandy.[46] He sectioned the eighth nerve for labyrinthine vertigo in three cases under local anesthetic. In two there were no sensations when the nerve was being liberated or divided. The third patient experienced transient vertigo when the nerve was being manipulated, but this stopped when it was divided. These observations provide a great contrast to the results from stimulation or sudden destruction of the labyrinth itself.

In the rare instances in which vertigo is an early symptom with tumors in the cerebellopontine angle, there may be difficulty in differentiation from Ménière's disease, since unilateral perceptive deafness and tinnitus are likely to be present in both conditions. However, with a few exceptions, a careful neurologic examination is likely to show evidence of involvement of the fifth and possibly the seventh cranial nerve, persistent nystagmus and signs of cerebellar dysfunction when tumor is the cause. A fluctuating tendency in the deafness and tinnitus, together with the presence of loudness recruitment and diplacusis, which are attributed to disease of Corti's organ, favors Ménière's disease. The degree of impairment of vestibular function by caloric test is likely to be much greater with acoustic neuroma than is usually found in Ménière's disease. While verified cases of acoustic neuroma have been recorded which are said to have shown good vestibular reactions on the affected side prior to operation, Dix and Hallpike[45] found abnormal caloric responses in 100 per cent of their large series using the particular method of testing they employ.

Brief dizziness, consisting of sensations of unsteadiness in walking and uncertainty of equilibrium occurring on change of posture, is much more common than true vertigo with tumors involving the eighth nerve. These symptoms are most prone to occur when signs of increased intracranial pressure are present and it is possible that they are caused by edema and altered vascularity in the central vestibular pathways resulting from distention of the fourth ventricle associated with hydrocephalus.

VERTIGO AND DIZZINESS WITH LESIONS IN THE BRAIN STEM

Lesions which involve the vestibular nuclei in the brain stem are likely to cause very severe vertigo comparable to that seen in labyrinthine disease. Atkinson[21] considers that only lesions in this situation will produce true objective vertigo other than those in the labyrinth itself. Lesions of the brain stem most prone to

cause vertigo are those that occur acutely, such as vascular accidents.

Important vestibular pathways, including the large part of the vestibular nuclei situated in the pons, receive blood supply from the anterior inferior cerebellar arteries and a thrombosis of one of these vessels or a hemorrhage arising from a pontine branch, would be expected to cause vertigo. Much more commonly occlusion of a posterior inferior cerebellar artery occurs, giving rise to severe vertigo at the onset together with the other characteristic findings due to involvement of certain structures in the dorsolateral portion of the medulla. Both the posterior inferior cerebellar and the anterior inferior cerebellar arteries show considerable variation in their relative sizes and distributions, but ordinarily the major part of the descending vestibular nucleus is included in the distribution of the posterior inferior cerebellar artery.[47] The severity and duration of the vertigo with thrombosis or embolism affecting this vessel doubtless depend on the degree and extent of the occlusion and the corresponding amount of damage to the vestibular structures in the upper medulla.

Vertigo may occur with acute exacerbations of multiple sclerosis, since plaques are not uncommonly situated in the brain stem—particularly in the pontine reticular substance. The vertigo in multiple sclerosis is often transitory, but sometimes it is very severe and protracted, accompanied by vomiting and lasting for days. Alpers[48] analyzed 156 cases, finding vertigo the first, or early, symptom in 26 and a late symptom in 11. He points out that when it occurs as an early symptom, other findings characteristic of multiple sclerosis may be absent, rendering diagnosis difficult. However, careful inquiry in such cases will often reveal mild subjective symptoms accompanying the vertigo, like numbness on one side of the face or brief diplopia, which aid in their recognition.

Gradually developing lesions, such as *tumors,* situated in the brain stem occasionally give rise to vertigo, as a prominent and early symptom. Fifty-seven verified cases of tumor involving the brain stem were analyzed at the Toronto General Hospital.[49] Vertigo occurring in spontaneous attacks or on change of posture was an initial or very early symptom in 8 patients. Two other patients had less specific dizziness as a presenting symptom. In 8 of these cases the tumors arose primarily in the brain stem; the other 2 arose in the fourth ventricle. In Cairns' series of 9 verified cases of brain-stem tumor vertigo was present in 2.[50] The reason vertigo does not occur more often with tumors in this situation is probably because slowly developing lesions enable adjustments to take place. Symonds[4] suggests that when vertigo is a symptom of a brain-stem tumor, it is probably due to a phase of congestion or edema of rapid development. Episodes of vertigo accompanied by headache and visual disturbance on movements of the head occasionally occur with tumors and cysts situated in the fourth ventricle (Brun's syndrome). Syringobulbia may very rarely cause severe and prolonged vertigo.

Symptoms of dysequilibrium on change of posture, similar to those described with tumors of the eighth nerve, occur commonly with tumors in this region, particularly those arising in the fourth ventricle. They are probably due to changes in the vestibular connections in the brain stem caused by the tumor directly or as a result of the associated hydrocephalus.

The differentiation between vertigo originating in the brain stem and that of labyrinthine origin is occasionally difficult. If headaches and vomiting precede the onset of vertigo a central cause must be suspected. The vertigo with brain-stem lesions has the same quality as labyrinthine vertigo but it is very sensitive to movements of the head which may precipitate or aggravate it. Both peripheral and central vertigo may be influenced by change in posture but, according to Denny-Brown,[51] this is more common with central lesions. In contrast to labyrinthine lesions, central causes may give rise to vertigo which is nonepisodic and persistent. With lesions in the brain stem, deafness and tinnitus characteristically associated with vertigo of labyrinthine origin are lacking. Although the absence

of associated findings (such as evidence of involvement of other cranial nerves, the long tracts and cerebellar connections) does not exclude a brain-stem lesion, they are commonly present and enable correct localization to be made.

Spontaneous nystagmus does not as consistently accompany vertigo due to brain-stem lesions as it does labyrinthine lesions. When present in the former, it is likely to persist after the vertigo has ceased, which is not the case with labyrinthine nystagmus. The nystagmus encountered may be horizontal, rotatory or vertical in direction. Horizontal and rotary nystagmus may be present with lesions in either situation, but if spontaneous vertical nystagmus is found it points to a lesion in the brain stem near the vestibular nuclei[48] and it is not seen in lesions confined to the labyrinth. In contrast with spontaneous nystagmus, which remains unchanged with changes in the position of the head, there is another variety of nystagmus known as positional nystagmus. The latter is elicited only in certain positions of the head or else it is influenced greatly by the position of the head and it commonly accompanies postural vertigo. When present it suggests a central lesion, particularly if it is irregular in direction or changes direction with alteration in position.[52] In this connection Dix and Hallpike[16] recently have produced clinical and pathologic evidence to show that in certain patients suffering from a benign disorder characterized by transient vertigo with paroxysmal positional nystagmus, the site of the lesion is in the otolith organs. In such cases it is not head movement per se but some critical position of the head in space which precipitates the vertigo and the nystagmus. The positional nystagmus in these patients does not change direction with changes in the position of the head.

Vestibular tests are sometimes of value in distinguishing a central from a peripheral cause of vertigo. Phillips[53] points out that the caloric tests may be relied upon as regards nystagmus, past pointing, falling, and induced vertigo when only the labyrinth is in question. When disease affects the central nervous system, the manifestations with caloric tests may be dissociated according to the tracts involved. A dissociation of responses may be helpful as indicative of a central rather than a peripheral lesion, but it is often impossible to be more specific. With a lesion in the brain stem involving the vestibular structures and the cerebellar connections there may be an absence of induced past pointing and vertigo on caloric test, with the nystagmus persisting. On the other hand, nystagmus is likely to be absent, with vertigo and past pointing persisting, if the lesion is confined to the median longitudinal bundle in the brain stem.

VERTIGO AND DIZZINESS WITH LESIONS OF THE CEREBELLUM

Although vertigo may be present in many conditions where the cerebellum is affected, there is considerable doubt as to whether a lesion entirely confined to the cerebellum will cause the subjective sensation of vertigo in addition to the characteristic objective disturbance of equilibrium that occurs. A clinical decision on this question is difficult because the majority of the pathologic conditions that affect the cerebellum also involve other structures, particularly the brain stem. This applies to vascular lesions such as thrombosis of the posterior inferior cerebellar artery and to many inflammatory and degenerative lesions. In tumors and abscesses the problem is even more complicated. In Cairns[50] series of 38 verified cases of cerebellar tumor, there were 17 patients who complained of vertigo, the majority having tumors mainly confined to the middle lobe. However, with subtentorial expanding lesions, increased intracranial pressure is an early manifestation and, in addition to the local pressure effects of the tumor on the brain stem, there is likely to be considerable physiologic disturbance in the region of the fourth ventricle as a result of the associated hydrocephalus. Thus, the vertigo can be explained by pressure alterations causing the rapid development of congestion and edema in the region of the vestibular nuclei. Dizziness of a less specific nature and related to change of posture, which is common with tumors in this situation is more likely due to involvement of the vestibular connections in the cerebellum.

If indeed true vertigo does occur from lesions confined to the cerebellum it would be assumed that the flocculonodular mechanism in the region of the posterior vermis, which is connected so intimately with the vestibular apparatus, should be involved. Discrete lesions in this part of the cerebellum are not common, but what evidence is available suggests that gross impairment of equilibrium is the principal manifestation without the subjective accompaniment of vertigo. Fulton[54] points out that in midline medulloblastomas, which are common tumors in children, the cells have been shown to develop from primitive embryologic cells arising in the nodulus of the cerebellum. The patients show disturbance of equilibrium and gait early, and these symptoms are often the first signs of the presence of the tumor. Experimental work on this region gives confirmation that the main vestibular connections in the cerebellum are concerned in the maintenance of bodily equilibrium. Dow[55] removed the nodulus from various animals, including chimpanzees. He found a striking syndrome of disturbed equilibrium unassociated with any other symptom. The animals walked on a broad base and required support from two sides to stand but appeared undisturbed when seated.

Thus, there is no substantial evidence that cerebellar lesions per se give rise to true vertigo, although they may be accompanied by a disturbance of bodily equilibrium, which is apt to be very severe, when the vestibular connections in the posterior vermis, particularly the nodulus, are involved. Vertigo is a frequent symptom when the cerebellum is affected by vascular, inflammatory or neoplastic lesions, but this is most probably due to the effect of the lesions, either by direct involvement or indirectly as a result of hydrocephalus, on the vestibular structures in the brain stem.

VERTIGO AND DIZZINESS WITH DISORDERS OF THE FOREBRAIN INCLUDING EPILEPSY AND MIGRAINE

True vertigo is uncommon with supratentorial lesions. When it occurs it lacks many of the features seen when the peripheral part of the mechanism is involved. The attacks are not of the clear-cut prostrating type, there is no nystagmus, no deafness or tinnitus, and the characteristic aftermath sensations of disturbed equilibrium do not occur. At the onset of supratentorial vascular accidents where consciousness is retained, dizziness is an occasional complaint. This is often a poorly described light-headed or unsteady sensation rather than true vertigo.

Vertigo is rarely a prominent symptom in patients with supratentorial tumors. Cairns[50] analyzed 242 cases, finding vertigo in only 13. In 5 of these the tumor was situated in the frontal region and vertigo was the first symptom in one patient, who proved to have a left frontal meningioma. There is fairly general agreement that vertigo has no localizing value when it occurs with supratentorial tumors, although Spiegel and Alexander[56] found the incidence increased with tumors close to the sylvian fissure. In subdural hematoma vertigo may occur occasionally but it is rarely an outstanding complaint. Abbott and Kaump,[57] reviewing 51 cases, found it to be a subjective symptom in 20 per cent. Personal experience indicates a much lower frequency than this.

Dizziness, similar to that described with subtentorial tumors, consisting of transitory vertiginous sensations and sensations of unsteadiness related to change of posture, may be a symptom with supratentorial expanding lesions when the intracranial pressure is high. These symptoms are probably not the direct result of destructive changes in the pathways between the brain stem and the cortex but are more likely due to remote changes, associated with increased intracranial pressure, including edema and altered vascularity, affecting the vestibular structures in the brain stem. The uncommon instances where true vertigo is a prominent symptom might be similarly explained. Cloake[58] has pointed out that lesions involving the hypothetical pathways between the vestibular nuclei and the cortex would be expected to produce depression of function making it more difficult to become vertiginous. This view is supported by the fact that vertigo is not a recognized symptom of purely destructive lesions of the temporal and the parietal lobes.

Occasionally in both *epilepsy* and *migraine* the attacks may be accompanied by vertigo. In epilepsy a vertiginous aura is not infrequent,[59] and the observations of Penfield[10] and Foerster,[5] previously referred to, indicate that this type of aura may occur with epileptic seizures originating in the temporal and parietal lobes. In this event the aura of vertigo may be the forerunner of a convulsion or on occasions it may occur alone, as is commonly the case with all types of aura in epilepsy. When this aura takes place and is not followed by a convulsion, it must be distinguished from vertigo due to other causes, since it implies the existence of an organic cerebral lesion and represents one type of "temporal lobe epilepsy." If a history is obtained that interference with consciousness has occurred on previous occasions preceded by the brief aura of vertigo, the source of the presenting attack of vertigo can be identified. There may also be the accompaniment of dreamy states, automatisms, or some other types of hallucinatory experience which aid in the diagnosis. In addition to electroencephalogram and other diagnostic measures, lesions of the temporal lobe may sometimes be recognized by an induced nystagmus on caloric testing in which the response is of longer duration towards the side of the lesion, so-called directional preponderance.

Rarely, in epilepsy the patient experiences vertigo on regaining consciousness after the seizures. Behrman[60] has reported a number of cases of epilepsy showing a recurrent transient postictal vertiginous state. Some but not all of these patients had in addition clinical evidence of functional labyrinthine disorder. Postictal vertigo did not occur in patients he surveyed who had cerebral lesions giving rise to epileptic seizures with a vertiginous aura. He suggests therefore that postictal vertigo is not an integral part of the epileptic phenomenon but is rather of vestibular origin and that this syndrome of seizures with postictal vertigo is a variant of vestibular epilepsy. Reference has been made to vestibular epilepsy when discussing Meniere's disease. It is one type of sensorily precipitated epilepsy, i.e., epilepsy provoked under certain circumstances in constitutionally predisposed individuals by the stimulation of various types of receptors. Vasovagal syncope occurring in the course of an attack of vertigo may sometimes be difficult to distinguish from epilepsy if judgment has to be based on history alone. Syncope is only likely to occur in severe attacks and then some considerable time after the onset. The loss of consciousness tends to be gradual, in contrast to epilepsy, and vertigo may still exist when consciousness returns.

Vertigo is an occasional accompaniment of migraine. In some patients it occurs regularly as the aura of each attack while in others it may replace the headache in certain of their attacks. Occasionally it is present throughout each migraine attack but is only made manifest by change of posture. The abrupt alterations in the caliber of the cerebral and the meningeal arteries which are presumed to give rise to the manifestations of migraine can explain the association of vertigo with the attacks. The patients in whom it occurs probably have arteries involved in the process which contribute to the supply of the vestibular mechanism either peripherally in the labyrinth or centrally in the brain stem.

Post-Traumatic Vertigo and Dizziness

Next to headache, dizziness is the most common complaint following head injury. Statements by various authors show a frequency ranging from 90 per cent[61] to 10 per cent.[62] This wide variation is probably due to the differences in material and in the interpretation of the symptoms. Most investigators find the frequency to fall within a range from 30 per cent to 60 per cent.[63-67]

Analysis of the complaint reveals that true vertigo is not common. Studies on large series of cases after head injury have shown it to be present in less than 10 per cent.[64,68] Much more commonly the symptom consists of less specific sensations which patients may have difficulty in describing but which often indicate a subjective disturbance of equilibrium without hallucination of movement of self or surroundings. These include feelings of unsteadiness and movement within the head, sometimes accompanied by the necessity of seeking support, and "blackouts" consisting of visual impairment with a feeling of confusion or even clouding of consciousness. Symonds[68] believes that in some cases there is a transition between this latter symptom and epilepsy. However, in most instances in which momentary loss of consciousness occurs on change of posture, the premonitory symptoms, including light-headedness, sweating and impaired vision suggest that it is syncopal and vasovagal in origin.

Dizziness and vertigo after head injury often occur in attacks not accompanied by nausea or vomiting which tend to last from one to ten minutes. These are likely to be precipitated by a change of posture such as arising from reclining, stooping and straining and not by movements of the head alone. Much less commonly emotional stress may be the precipitating factor. Relief is sought from the attacks by lying or sitting down. Headaches, emotional lability and difficulty in mental concentration are other features of the post-traumatic syndrome which may be associated with the attacks of dizziness, but the latter may occur alone.[64]

There has been much controversy about the nature of the underlying mechanism responsible for post-traumatic vertigo and dizziness. Attacks of true vertigo after head injury point definitely to organic damage and their occurrence and persistence bear a relationship to the severity of the injury. There has been speculation as to whether they are the result of injury to the labyrinth either directly through cranial fracture, or through concussion, or whether they are a product of traumatic lesions in the brain stem affecting the vestibular connections.

Although a disorder of vestibular function shown by caloric tests has been found in a large number of cases[65] and a proportion of cases show bleeding from the ears, deafness and tinnitus after the injury,[64,68] yet the correlation between this suggestive evidence of labyrinthine damage and the occurrence of post-traumatic vertigo or dizziness is not absolute. In such cases lesions of the labyrinth and of the vestibular pathways in the brain may be indistinguishable if one uses times of nystagmus response to caloric stimulation as the sole criterion.[65]

Friedman et al.[64] found that in cases with bleeding from the ears and deafness, the latter symptoms usually cleared rapidly and they question that the common traumatic hemorrhage from the meatus implies equivalent damage to the labyrinth. Even where there was clear evidence of direct damage to the bony labyrinth by cranial fracture these observers did not find the frequency of dizziness and vertigo to be increased after head injury. Contrary to the usual opinion, their findings do not indicate that the occurrence of post-traumatic vertigo and dizziness bears a direct relation to damage to the vestibular end organ. Their observations suggest that in most instances true vertigo following head injury is caused by traumatic lesions affecting the vestibular structures in the brain stem. Harrison,[69] on the other hand, concludes from his studies that "serious, persistent dizziness following head injuries, not necessarily associated with skull fracture, is very frequently, particularly if it is of a rotational character, due to traumatic lesions of the otolithic apparatus." Caloric tests, using the technic described by Fitzgerald and Hallpike, showed abnormalities in most but not all of his cases. The diagnosis depends upon the demonstration of paroxysmal vertigo and nystagmus when the head is placed in certain critical positions. The nystagmus, accompanied by vertigo, lasts less than a minute and dies away. Even if the position is resumed, it does not reappear for several minutes.

The mechanism of production of the less specific type of dizziness that follows cerebral trauma is not clearly understood, although its occurrence on change of posture, like true vertigo after head injury, suggests a causal relationship. Most observers are agreed that two elements are involved in causation of the dizziness: these are the *physical effect* of the injury on the structures inside the skull and the *psychogenic factors* arising out of the circumstances associated with the head injury. It is very difficult and, in many instances, impossible to be sure of the relative parts these play in a given case. However, the finding of positional nystagmus in a patient complaining of post-traumatic postural dizziness is positive evidence of organic disorder. This observation may be of great value in assessing cases involving litigation where all other tests are negative.

The degree and persistence of this type of dizziness do not bear so clear a relationship to the severity of the head injury as does true vertigo. Its nature and close association with change of posture has given rise to speculation as to whether it could be due to a defect in vasomotor adjustment,[65,68,70] perhaps resulting from medullary concussion.[62,71] It seems possible that this may be an important factor in causing the dizziness as well as the headache in the first few months after head injury, but the evidence available is not conclusive.

When dizziness persists for many months or years after head injury it is usually accompanied by headaches and evidence of an anxiety state. Such patients often show no signs of structural damage from the trauma on neurologic investigation. Inquiry frequently reveals evidence of nervous instability in the past history of the patient, with varying degrees of maladjustment, resentment arising out of the circumstances of the injury or the compensation received, pending litigation, anxiety regarding future employment, etc. Although the foregoing factors are important in many cases with prolonged post-traumatic dizziness, there is not always a consistent relationship between the occurrence of the symptoms and the emotional disturbances. In addition, the incidence of prolonged dizziness is decidedly higher in patients with more severe head injuries.[64] Therefore, there is reason to believe that impairment of function resulting from primary injury to some part of the vestibular mechanism from the peripheral end organ to the cortex, or secondary to post-traumatic vasomotor disturbance, is a fundamental basis of all post-traumatic dizziness, but it seems probable that emotional factors when present may aggravate and prolong the symptoms.

Vertigo and Dizziness in Cardio-Vascular and Cerebrovascular Disease

In cardiovascular and blood diseases true vertigo is a rare complaint but sensations described as dizziness related to change of posture or to sudden exertion occur more frequently. The sensations include unsteadiness, a swimming feeling, visual blurring and light-headedness, which are usually transitory and often immediately relieved by lying down. Among the conditions in which this type of dizziness may be a complaint are postural hypotension, severe anemia, aortic valvular disease (particularly aortic stenosis), Stokes-Adams syndrome, the carotid sinus syndrome, severe cardiac dysrhythmias and, rarely, coronary thrombosis. In these disorders it is likely that cerebral *anoxia* due to transitory ischemia is the usual cause of the symptoms since they are more often allied to syncope than to vertigo. As a rule such patients experience no hallucination of movement of themselves or of objects, and nystagmus does not accompany the postural dizziness. In certain cases, however, there is degenerative disease of the cerebral arteries present as well. In this event the location of the latter may determine that the maximum anoxia resulting from the circulatory disorder is somewhere in the vestibular pathways, thus causing more specific vertiginous sensations.

Brief dizzy sensations, often of a vertiginous type, are a common complaint of the elderly and usually prove to be a manifestation of cerebrovascular disease. They are induced or aggravated by change of posture and less commonly by exertion, suggesting that they are due to imperfect vasomotor adjustment as a result of diseased blood vessels. It is movement and not position alone that is the provoking factor, so the symptoms can often be lessened by changing posture slowly and also avoiding excessive physical activity, which these patients soon learn to do.

Patients with hypertension sometimes complain of dizziness or vertigo but it is difficult to see how hypertension per se could cause these symptoms, unless possibly through sudden marked fluctuations occurring in the blood pressure. It is more probable that the symptoms are due to the underlying state of the blood vessels causing recurrent local circulatory insufficiency in some part of the vestibular system, perhaps the result of vasospasm associated with hypertensive vascular disease.

In cases where deafness is associated with the attacks of vertigo in hypertensive vascular disease it can be inferred that the internal auditory artery is one of the vessels at fault.

Stenosis of the vertebral and basilar arteries may lead to intermittent vascular insufficiency with relative ischemia of the brain stem, causing periodic vertigo which is often accompanied by other manifestations indicating interference with the basilar circulation. These include blurred vision, frank diplopia, obscuration of vision, tingling in the face, ataxia, weakness of the legs, and even loss of consciousness. The diagnosis is based on the periodic return of symptoms after intervals of time. A transient diminution of blood flow causing symptoms, of which vertigo is the most constant, may be brought about by such factors as fluctuations in blood pressure or recent dehydration associated with diarrhea. The vestibular nuclei far out in the pons are especially vulnerable under these circumstances because they are supplied by tenuous, long branches of the vertebral and basilar arteries. The parent vessels of the basilar, the vertebral arteries, are also long, ascending through the foramina in the transverse processes of the upper six cervical vertebrae. They are extremely subject to congenital anomaly as well as to pressure from osteophyte formation and they are particularly liable to atherosclerosis.[72] Apart from involvement of the vestibular nuclei in the brain stem in cases of stenosis of the vertebral-basilar system, there may be intermittent vascular insufficiency, affecting the labyrinth directly, resulting from impaired blood flow through the internal auditory branches of the basilar. Attacks of vertigo due to this cause will not be accompanied by signs of brain stem involvement.

In addition to intermittent, spontaneous vertigo resulting from insufficiency of the vertebral-basilar arterial system as described

above, atherosclerotic individuals may suffer vertigo produced mainly by neck-turning
in a right or left backward direction. Radiologic studies after injections of opaque substances into the vertebral arteries of cadav-
ers, have demonstrated narrowing of the
lumen of the contralateral vertebral artery,
at the level of the joint between the atlas
and the axis, on rotation movements of the
neck.[73] In normal individuals symptoms
do not occur because there is adequate circulation from the opposite side. However
when the blood flow is impaired through
atherosclerosis, perhaps accompanied by
obstruction from without due to cervical
spondylosis and/or by a vascular anomaly
with one vertebral artery being extremely
small, then symptoms and signs are liable
to occur with neck turning. Evidence that
symptoms produced in this way are more
common than is generally believed is obtained from the observations of Biemond[74]
who investigated a series of patients over
60 years of age with signs of arteriosclerosis.
Twisting the neck in a right or left lateral
direction resulted in the repeated appearance of a horizontal-rotatory type of nystagmus as well as the frequent occurrence
of pathologic plantar responses and a slight
dysarthria.

Other conditions that will cause vertigo
and nystagmus with turning movements
or retraction of the head have to be differentiated from vertebral artery insufficiency but this is usually not difficult. The
syndrome may occur in primary labyrinthine disease but the lack of a history of
previous *spontaneous* attacks of vertigo and
the absence of cochlear symptoms, together
with normal caloric responses, usually enables this to be excluded. More difficulty
may be experienced with what is known as
positional nystagmus of the benign paroxysmal type which is attributed to a lesion,
traumatic, infective or vascular, of the
otolithic apparatus. In this condition, there
are no cochlear symptoms and the vertigo
and nystagmus occur with certain critical
positions of the head. However, the patients
are in a younger age group as a rule and
on repetitive positional tests, the nystagmic
response becomes characteristically reduced,
even to the point of abolition,[69] which is

not the case with vertebral artery insufficiency. Abnormalities of the foramen
magnum such as the Arnold-Chiari malformation as well as posterior fossa tumors,
particularly midline cerebellar tumors, may
cause vertigo and nystagmus on retraction
of the head which develop immediately and
continue as long as the position is maintained. These lesions usually can be readily
recognized by the accompanying neurologic
signs but Cawthorne and Hinchcliffe[75] have
reported several cases of metastatic cerebellar tumor in which this type of positional vertigo and nystagmus was the main
finding and it led to investigations that
revealed the correct diagnosis.

It has been suggested[76] that with cervical spondylosis or after injury to the cervical spine, vertigo may occur on neck
movement due to vestibular imbalance
caused by interference with the tonic neck
reflexes. While it might be difficult to
reject this explanation for patients who
manifest vertigo and nystagmus on neck
movement, with pain and other well-marked
evidence of disease of the cervical spine as
well, it is probably an uncommon cause of
the syndrome.

VERTIGO DUE TO DRUGS

A toxic disturbance of the vestibular
mechanism is a well-recognized complication from the administration of certain
drugs. Vertigo sometimes accompanies the
deafness and tinnitus that may occur when
large doses of *quinine* or *salicylates* are
administered. The association of deafness,
tinnitus and vertigo suggests that the site
of the toxic effect is the peripheral cochlear
and labyrinthine structures, with involvement possibly of the eighth nerve also.
The inhalation of *tobacco* smoke by susceptible individuals or *alcoholic* intoxication may cause vertigo which is probably
due to a toxic effect on the central vestibular mechanism. Toxic doses of certain
anticonvulsant drugs, particularly Dilantin,
occasionally cause vertigo although more
commonly the symptoms consist simply of
ataxia, horizontal nystagmus, and dysarthria.

The otic complications of *streptomycin*
therapy have received considerable atten-

tion in recent years. Large doses and long administration are important factors in their occurrence. Symptoms become manifest between 30 and 35 days after beginning treatment[77] and deafness and low-pitched tinnitus sometimes develop with the vertigo. If the drug is promptly discontinued complete recovery is likely to occur. Even if total loss of reactions on vestibular testing remains permanently, the patient usually recovers from any deafness that may have been present. In this event accessory balance mechanisms may compensate for the bilateral labyrinthine loss although some constant unsteadiness of gait and posture may remain.[78] Such patients may complain also of inability to focus objects with the eyes when the head is in motion. Objects seem to dance or oscillate before the patient's eyes when he is walking or riding in a vehicle. These visual phenomena are due to the loss of the vestibulo-ocular reflexes which influence the extra ocular muscles in such a manner as to compensate for movements of the head. In addition to clinical studies, which have shown that streptomycin injures the vestibular nerve peripherally,[79] studies on experimental animals indicate that the localization of lesions after streptomycin is central as well as peripheral. The vestibular ganglion and Deiters' nucleus in the brain stem, together with the nerve, were found to show definite changes.[80]

Psychogenic Dizziness

Many patients who show in their histories and on examination positive evidence of psychoneurosis give "dizziness" or "giddiness" as one of their symptoms. The complaint is often poorly described, and, when pressed, the patient may not be able to do more than reiterate "just a dizzy feeling." Sometimes it is described as "a feeling as if I am going to fall," although the patient never falls and will usually admit that she never even staggers, yet it may keep her confined to the house for long periods. In such cases the sensation would seem to be a symbolic reflection of the inherent sense of insecurity caused by adjustment difficulties relating to the environment. The symptom is continuous, not coming in attacks, and may persist for weeks, months or years. Brain[3] has suggested that it symbolizes the patient's fear of impending collapse—mental, moral and physical.

Dizziness may also be a complaint in some psychotic patients, particularly in schizophrenia and depressive states. Inquiry shows that the word is used to indicate "thick headedness" or an inability to think consecutively resulting from preoccupation or mental blocking.

Although dizziness is common in anxiety states, one must not assume that the dizziness is entirely a product of it. The converse may be true. Patients with paroxysmal vertigo are very prone to develop anxiety states as a result of their fear and apprehension about attacks, and in such cases a careful study of the patient may be necessary to evaluate correctly the symptoms. It should also be emphasized that the symptom of dizziness is not to be considered psychogenic because the patient's description does not indicate true vertigo. The complaint should always be interpreted in the light of the total findings, and other positive evidence must be found before concluding that it is a product of the mental state.

Ocular Vertigo and Motion Sickness

Ocular disorders are not a common cause of vertigo. Vertigo has been described as occurring at the onset of diplopia when an ocular muscle becomes suddenly paralyzed and is attributed to the faulty projection of the visual field of the affected eye. Looking down from heights and watching moving trains from a stationary platform causes vertiginous sensations in certain people due to the discrepancy between the visual perceptions and the proprioceptor impulses from elsewhere in the body.

It was formerly considered that in seasickness and certain other types of motion sickness the ocular factor was prominent in causing the vertigo. However, it is now generally believed that the disturbance is primarily vestibular in all forms of motion sickness, although the nature of the physiologic mechanisms at fault is still a matter of conjecture and theory. The condition has been attributed to excessive stimulation of the peripheral labyrinthine mechanism by the repetitive movement,[81] but the absence of spontaneous nystagmus in the various types of motion sickness has led to the opinion that the cause is excessive stimulation of the macula utriculi rather than the labyrinth. It is of interest that Bard and his associates[82] have cured car sickness in susceptible dogs by isolated removal of the nodulus of the cerebellum, thus apparently localizing a central pathway concerned in the disorder.

SUMMARY

Vertigo is a specific subjective sensation, consisting of a hallucination of movement of the individual or his surroundings. It may result from lesions affecting the vestibular pathways from the labyrinth to the cortex, but in its most developed form it is confined to lesions of the labyrinth or the vestibular structures in the brain stem. Vertigo is encountered most commonly with labyrinthine disturbances which may result from inflammatory, vascular or toxic disorders or from the idiopathic hydrops of the labyrinth that accompanies Ménière's disease. The vertigo arising from disturbed function of the vestibular structures in the brain stem may be due to their direct involvement by vascular lesions or it may result from ischemia caused by impaired circulation in the basilar-vertebral arterial system. Plaques of multiple sclerosis as well as neoplasms, may also involve the vestibular nuclei to produce vertigo. Persistent vertigo following cerebral trauma is the result of damage to the labyrinth or the vestibular nuclei. A particular type of postural vertigo after head injury, where there is paroxysmal vertigo and nystagmus when the head is placed in certain critical positions, is believed due to a traumatic lesion of the otolithic apparatus. Intracranial expanding lesions not directly involving the brain stem may cause vertigo as a result of edema and changes in vascularity in the region of the vestibular nuclei associated with increased intracranial pressure. In subtentorial neoplasms there is likely to be the additional factor of distention of the fourth ventricle which ac-

companies hydrocephalus. Tumors and other lesions involving the eighth nerve may give rise to vertigo as an early symptom but not with anything like the consistency seen with disease of the labyrinth itself. Lesions strictly confined to the cerebellum give rise to a characteristic disturbance of equilibrium but there is no substantial evidence that vertigo results unless the brain stem is involved, directly or indirectly, as well. Destructive lesions of the forebrain rarely cause vertigo. When they do, it is a less severe and less clearly defined variety than that accompanying disorders of the labyrinth and the brain stem. Not infrequently migraine and epilepsy are associated with vertigo. It may occur as the aura of an attack in either condition, and in migraine sometimes it may replace the headache or be present throughout the attack. In rare cases of chronic labyrinthine disease epileptic seizures may develop which appear to be provoked by the excessive spontaneous discharge arising from the vestibular apparatus. (vestibular epilepsy)

The complaints of "dizziness" and "giddiness" lack specific meaning. They are used to include not only vertigo and related sensations but also sensations pertaining to disturbed mental equilibrium and to syncope. Therefore, it is always necessary to obtain an *exact description* from the patient of what he feels in order to evaluate the symptom correctly.

A type of dizziness that may be associated with vertigo or occur alone is particularly important and probably has a basic mechanism similar to vertigo. It consists of sensations of unsteadiness in walking and uncertainty of equilibrium, with often a feeling of some sort of movement within the head, but it lacks the hallucination of movement of the individual or his surroundings that distinguishes vertigo. In cases of cerebral neoplasm, dizziness of this kind is a more common symptom than true vertigo. It is assumed to be due to changes affecting vestibular structures in the brain stem associated with increased intracranial pressure and it is particularly likely to occur with subtentorial tumors where obstruction and distention of the fourth ventricle are present. It occurs also as an aftermath of attacks of true vertigo, is frequently a symptom following head injury and may be present in cerebral vascular disease with or without hypertension. In these various conditions it is commonly brought on by change of posture. The symptoms described as dizziness that occasionally accompany certain cardiovascular diseases likewise may be induced by change of posture or by exertion, but for the most part their nature indicates a relationship to syncope and probably they result from acute cerebral ischemia and anoxia.

It is evident that vertigo and dizziness may be symptoms in a variety of pathologic conditions affecting the peripheral labyrinthine mechanism and the vestibular pathways in the brain. In order to localize the lesion correctly and to arrive at an accurate diagnosis of the cause of these symptoms a carefully taken history and a thorough examination of the patient are always essential.

REFERENCES

1. Jackson, H.: Selected Writings, vol. 1, p. 309, London, Hodder & Stoughton, 1931.
2. McNally, W. J.: The physiology of the vestibular mechanism in relation to vertigo, Ann. Otol., Rhin. & Laryng. 56:514, 1947.
3. Brain, W. R.: Vertigo: its neurological, otological, circulatory and surgical aspects, Brit. M. J. 2:605, 1938.
4. Symonds, C. P.: The clinical significance of vertigo, Lancet 2:959, 1933.
5. Foerster, O.: The motor cortex in man in the light of Hughlings Jackson's doctrines, Brain 59:135, 1936.
6. Lindsay, J. R.: Postural vertigo and positional nystagmus, Ann. Otol. Rhin. & Laryng. 60:1134, 1951.
7. Larsell, O., and Dow, R. S.: Cerebellum; new interpretation, West. J. Surg. 47:256, 1939.
8. Ransom, S. W., and Clark, S.: The Anatomy of the Nervous System, ed. 10, Philadelphia, Saunders, 1959.
9. Kunkle, E. C.: Central causes of vertigo, J. South Carolina M. A. 50:161, 1954.
10. Penfield, W., and Erickson, T. C.: Epilepsy and cerebral localization, Springfield, Ill., Thomas, 1941.
11. Penfield, W.: Vestibular sensation and the cerebral cortex, Ann. Otol. Rhinol. & Laryng. 66:691, 1957.
12. Spiegel, E. A.: Labyrinth and cortex, Arch. Neurol. & Psychiat. 31:469, 1934.
13. Simonton, K. M.: The symptom of dizziness: its significance in general practice, Proc. Staff Meet. Mayo Clinic 16:465, 1941.
14. Burrowes, W. L.: Acute labyrinthitis, Brit. M. J. 2:1182, 1952.
15. Leishman, A. W. O.: Acute labyrinthitis or epidemic vertigo, Lancet 1:228, 1955.
16. Dix, M. R., and Hallpike, C. S.: The pathology, symptomatology and diagnosis of certain common disorders of the vestibular system, Proc. Roy. Soc. Med. 45:341, 1952.
17. Cawthorne, T.: Vertigo, Proc. Roy. Soc. Med. 52:529, 1959.
18. Dedering, D.: Clinical and experimental examinations in patients suffering from MB Menieri including a study of the problem of bone conduction, Acta Otolaryngol. Suppl. x-xi, 1929.
19. Furstenberg, A. C., Lashmet, F. H., and Lathrop, F.: Ménière's symptom complex; medical treatment, Ann. Otol., Rhin. & Laryng. 43:1035, 1934.
20. Shelden, C. H., and Horton, B. T.: Treatment of Ménière's disease with histamine administered intravenously, Proc. Staff Meet. Mayo Clinic 15:17, 1940.
21. Atkinson, M.: The dizzy patient, Eye, Ear, Nose & Throat Monthly 22:53, 1943.
22. Fischer, J. J.: Otologic aspects of vertigo, New England J. Med. 241:142, 1949.
23. Harley, D.: Some observations on the fundamentals of allergy with special reference to its aural manifestations, J. Laryng. & Otol. 62:1, 1948.
24. Balyeat, R. M.: Migraine, Philadelphia, Lippincott, 1933.
25. Lempert, J., et al.: A new theory for the correlation of pathology and symptomatology in Ménière's disease, Ann. Otol. Rhin. & Laryng. 61:717, 1952.
26. Merica, F. W.: Vertigo due to obstruction of the eustachian tubes, J.A.M.A. 118:1282, 1942.
27. Athens, A. G.: Vertigo in hypothyroidism, Minnesota Med. 29:562, 1946.
28. Levy, I., and O'Leary, J. L.: Incidence of vertigo in neurological conditions, Ann. Otol., Rhin. & Laryng. 56:557, 1947.
29. Wright, A. J.: Labyrinthine giddiness, its nature and treatment, Brit. M. J. 1:668, 1938.
30. Fowler, E. P., and Zeckel, A.: Psychosomatic aspects of Ménière's disease, J.A.M.A. 148:1265, 1952.

31. Hallpike, C. S., and Cairns, H.: Observations on the pathology of Ménière's syndrome, J. Laryng. 53:625, 1938.

32. Altman, F.: Dizziness of peripheral vestibular origin, Laryngoscope 55:164, 1945.

33. Lindsay, J. R.:- Labyrinthine dropsy and Ménière's disease, Arch. Otolaryng. 35:853, 1942.

34. Tumarkin, A.: The otolithic catastrophe, Brit. M. J. 2:175, 1936.

35. Williams, H. L., Horton, B. T., and Day, L. A.: Endolymphatic hydrops without vertigo, Arch. Otolaryng. 51:557, 1950.

36. Cawthorne, T. E., Fitzgerald, G., and Hallpike, C. S.: Observations on the clinical features of "Ménière's" disease with especial reference to the results of the caloric tests, Brain 65:161, 1942.

37. Day, K. M.: Hydrops of labyrinth (Ménière's disease) diagnosis—results of labyrinth surgery, Laryngoscope 56:33, 1946.

38. Cawthorne, T.: Ménière's disease, Tr. Am. Otolaryng., Rhin. & Otol. Soc., p. 352, 1946.

39. Hyland, H. H.: The diagnosis of Ménière's syndrome, Bull. Acad. Med., Toronto 19:8, 1945.

40. Furstenberg, A. C.: Symposium on vertigo, Ann. Otol., Rhin. & Laryng. 56:576, 1946.

41. Milliken, C. H., Siekert, R. G., and Whisnant, J. P.: The syndrome of occlusion of the labyrinthine division of the internal auditory artery, Proc. Am. Neurol. Ass. 1959.

42. McNally, W. J., and Stuart, E. A.: Vertigo from the standpoint of the otolaryngologist, Tr. Am. Acad. Ophth. Nov.-Dec., 1941, p. 33.

43. Cushing, H.: Tumors of the Nerve Acusticus, Philadelphia, Saunders, 1917.

44. Edwards, C. H., and Patterson, J. H.: The symptoms and signs of acoustic neurofibromata, Brain 74:144, 1951.

45. Dix, M. R., and Hallpike, C. S.: Discussion on acoustic neuroma, Proc. R. Soc. Med., 51:889, 1958.

46. Dandy, W. E.: Ménière's disease, its diagnosis and a method of treatment, Arch. Surg. 16:1127, 1928.

47. Alexander, L., and Suh, T. H.: Arterial supply of lateral parolivary area of medulla oblongata in man, Arch. Neurol. & Psychiat. 38:1243, 1937.

48. Alpers, B. J.: Vertigo: its neurological features, Tr. Am. Acad. Ophth., Nov.-Dec., 1941, p. 38.

49. Barnett, H. J., and Hyland, H. H.: Tumours involving the brain stem, Quart. J. Med., 83:265, 1952.

50. Cairns, H.: *Quoted by* Symonds (4).

51. Denny-Brown., D. E.: Neurologic aspects of vertigo, New England J. Med. 241:144, 1949.

52. Lindsay, J. R.: The significance of a positional nystagmus in otoneurological diagnosis, Laryngoscope 55:527, 1945.

53. Phillips, D. G.: Vertigo, New Zealand M. J. 45:219, 1946.

54. Fulton, J. F.: The William Withering Memorial Lectures, London, The Clarendon Press, Oxford, 1949.

55. Dow, R. S.: Effects of unilateral and bilateral labyrinthectomy in monkey, baboon and chimpanzee, Am. J. Physiol. 121:392, 1938.

56. Spiegel, E. A., and Alexander, A.: Vertigo in brain tumors with special reference to the results of labyrinth examination, Ann. Otol., Rhin. & Laryng. 45:979, 1936.

57. Abbott, W. D., and Kaump, D. H.: Subdural hematoma, Am. J. Surg. 49:64, 1940.

58. Mollison, W. M., and Cloake, P.: Diagnosis and treatment of vertigo, Tr. M. Soc. London 65:45, 1948.

59. Gowers, W. R.: Borderland of Epilepsy, Philadelphia, Blakiston, 1907.

60. Behrman, S.: Vestibular epilepsy, Brain 78:471, 1955.

61. Linthicum, F. H., and Rand, C. W.: Neuro-otological observations in concussion of the brain, Arch. Otolaryng. 13:785, 1931.

62. Russell, W. R.: Cerebral involvement in head injury, Brain 55:549, 1932.

63. Glaser, M. A.: The cause of dizziness in head injuries, Ann. Otol., Rhin. & Laryng. 46:387, 1937.

64. Friedman, A. P., Brenner, C., and Denny-Brown, D.: Post-traumatic vertigo and dizziness, J. Neurosurg. 2:36, 1945.

65. Phillips, D. G.: Investigation of vestibular function after head injury, J. Neurol., Neurosurg. & Psychiat. 8:79, 1945.

66. Osnato, M., and Gilberti, V.: Post-concussion neurosis — traumatic encephalitis, Arch. Neurol. & Psychiat. 18:181, 1927.

67. Schuster, F. P.: Head injuries with ear symptoms, Southwest Med. 11:116, 1927.

68. Symonds, C. P., and Lewis, A.: Discussion on differential diagnosis and treatment of post-contusional states, Proc. Roy. Med. 35:601, 1942.

69. Harrison, M. S.: Notes on the clinical features and pathology of post-concussional vertigo with special reference to positional nystagmus, Brain 79:475, 1956.

70. McKenzie, K. G.: One aspect of the post-traumatic syndrome in cranio-cerebral injuries, Tr. Am. Neurol. A. 69:103, 1943.

71. Denny-Brown, D.: The sequelae of war head injuries, New England J. Med. 227: 771, 1942.

72. Hutchinson, E. G., and Yates, P. O.: The cervical portion of the vertebral artery, Brain 79:319, 1956.

73. Tissington Tatlow, W. F., and Bammer, H. G.: Syndrome of vertebral artery compression, Neurology 7:331, 1957.

74. Biemond, A.: Thrombosis of the basilar artery and the vascularization of the brain stem, Brain 74:300, 1951.

75. Cawthorne, T., and Hinchcliffe, R.: Positional nystagmus of the cerebral type as evidence of subtentorial metastases, Brain 84:415, 1961.

76. Ryan, G. M. S., and Cope, S.: Cervical vertigo. Lancet, 2:1355, 1955.

77. Snell, F. B.: Some otic complications of streptomycin therapy, Mil. Surgeon 102:202, 1948.

78. Ford, F. R.: Clinical classification of vestibular disorders, Bull. Johns Hopkins Hosp. 87:299, 1950.

79. Glorig, A., and Fowler, E. P.: Tests for labyrinth function following streptomycin therapy, Ann. Otol., Rhin. & Laryngol. 56:379, 1947.

80. Barr, B., Floberg, L. E., Hamberger, A. C., and Koch, H. J.: Otological aspects of streptomycin therapy, Acta Otolaryng. Suppl. 75, 1949, p. 5.

81. Krieg, W. J. S.: Functional Neuroanatomy, Philadelphia, Blakiston, 1942.

82. Bard, P., et al.: Quoted by Fulton (54).

30

Dehydration, Fluid and Electrolyte Imbalances

CYRIL M. MACBRYDE

DEFINITION

Dehydration may be defined as that bodily state resulting from excessive loss of fluid. It is implied that such loss is sufficient to endanger or actually to impair functions for which certain amounts of fluid are necessary. The life of the organism depends upon adequate performance by the body fluids of their essential functions of transportation of nutrient and excretory materials and of temperature and chemical regulation. It is important to remember that dehydration always signifies loss not only of water but of electrolyte, and that, therefore, the term dehydration is incomplete. Likewise it is apparent that dehydration cannot be cor-

rected by replacement of water alone; electrolyte also must be replaced.

The body fluids constitute what Claude Bernard called "the internal environment" of the body.[1] He showed that in mammals the amounts and the constituents of the body fluids varied within relatively fixed limits, variations beyond these limits endangering life. Cannon[2] designated the coordinated physiologic processes that maintain a healthful internal environment as *mechanisms of homeostasis*. When one or more of the regulatory functions breaks down, or when the body is prevented from employing its usual restorative measures, fluid may be lost in excessive amounts. Loss of fluid, which is itself the homeostatic agent of greatest importance, and is the medium in which a number of important regulators exist and are transported, may have serious consequences. In this chapter will be considered the ways in which dehydration may occur and how the body is affected thereby.

DEHYDRATION AS A SYMPTOM

The clinical picture of dehydration is usually easy to recognize. In mild or moderate dehydration, thirst, fatigue, anorexia, nausea and oliguria are observed. With more advanced degrees of dehydration the patient usually complains of extreme thirst, weakness and rapid weight loss. If the fluid loss has been extreme, the patient may be faint, prostrated or in coma, and may suffer from the severe dyspnea (Kussmaul breathing) of acidosis. Physical examination reveals dry mucous membranes; dry, inelastic loose skin; low blood pressure and soft eyeballs; and, often, the expired air smells of acetone. Fever may be present solely as the result of dehydration. Frequently the history reveals one or more influences leading to failure of fluid absorption or to excess fluid loss. Less often, the causes of the dehydration may be obscure, especially when it has been gradual in development. Sudden loss of fluid (as from hemorrhage) does not permit time for the development of dry skin and mucous membranes, but is characterized by weakness, thirst, low blood pressure and clinical evidences of shock.

Clinically three stages or degrees of dehydration may be distinguished: (1) simple dehydration with dry skin and mucous membranes, weight loss, etc.; (2) more advanced fluid loss with dry skin, etc., plus a fall in blood pressure and other evidence of loss of plasma volume —weakness, faintness, fever, weak pulse, shock, coma; (3) the previous manifestations plus signs of renal failure (uremia, acidosis). Severe renal failure may prevent recovery even when water and electrolytes are restored.

CENTRAL NERVOUS SYSTEM EFFECTS

Simple dehydration (pure water loss) results in only mild and inconstant circulatory changes (mild or moderate decrease in cardiac output and prolongation of circulation time, slight fall in blood pressure). However, mental confusion has been noted frequently. The dehydration, blood hypertonicity and hypernatremia may terminate in delirium, coma and respiratory paralysis.

When 12 per cent of the body water has been lost, the victim can no longer swallow; when 15 to 25 per cent has been lost, death usually results. In great heat, death comes much more quickly, from loss of temperature control and an explosive rise in deep body temperature.

CIRCULATORY EFFECTS

In most clinical conditions, there is concomitant loss of water and salt, though often not in the proportions in which they exist in extracellular fluid. When salt loss predominates, the circulatory collapse may be striking, since the differential osmotic pressure of extracellular fluid depends primarily upon sodium and chloride. When Na and Cl concentration in extracellular fluid drops, extracellular water moves into the cells. The Na loss is followed by a loss in circulating plasma proteins with further decrease in plasma volume; there is hemoconcentration and increased viscosity of the blood, fall in cardiac output, drop in blood pressure and prolongation of circulation time.

RENAL EFFECTS

Renal insufficiency with oliguria and azotemia is a common sequel of sodium depletion, since the circulatory collapse may be manifested largely by failure of the renal circulation. Salt limitation plus vigorous diuresis may lower extracellular electrolyte sufficiently to endanger life through renal failure.[55]

WATER BALANCE

The amount of water in the body depends upon the *water balance,* the intake normally equaling the output when the body is in a state of equilibrium. Dehydration occurs when there is a *negative water balance,* resulting from failure of intake to keep pace with a normal output, or from excessive fluid loss in the presence of a normal intake, or from both diminished absorption and accelerated loss.

The normal route of entry for fluid is the gastrointestinal tract, while the routes of exit are the kidneys, the lungs, the sweat glands and the breasts (milk), only a small amount usually being excreted in the stool. Therapeutically, fluid may be introduced into the body through the veins, subcutaneous tissue, peritoneal cavity or bone marrow. As the result of trauma, fluid may be lost from the blood vessels, the lymph vessels and the tissue spaces in wounds, burns, etc. Excessive loss may therefore occur through both normal and abnormal channels.

Clothing and environmental and body temperature cause such fluctuations in the proportion of water intake lost through skin and lungs (totaling from 30 to 50 per cent) that *change in urine volume* when water intake is fixed does not dependably measure changes in water balance. Daily variations in body weight, however, closely reflect changes in total water content of the body. Sudden considerable gain or loss in weight indicates change in water and sodium content primarily.

CAUSES OF DEHYDRATION

Disturbance involving one or more of the routes by which fluid is taken in or lost may lead to dehydration of greater or less degree, depending upon the severity of the disorder and upon the number of routes involved. Often several factors are simultaneously operative in the production of dehydration. Thus, vomiting usually implies not only loss of fluid but failure of intake. Often these two factors leading to dehydration are accompanied by a third, diarrhea. Conditions leading to dehydration include:

1. Failure of fluid intake (unavailable, nausea, psychic disorders, etc.)

2. Failure of absorption (diarrhea, intestinal disorders, etc.)

3. Loss from gastrointestinal tract (vomiting, diarrhea, fistula)

4. Excess renal excretion due to renal factors (failure of tubular reabsorption)

5. Excess renal excretion due to prerenal factors (disturbed body-fluid chemistry)

6. Excessive perspiration or vaporization

7. Loss from wounds, burns, etc. (hemorrhage, transudation of interstitial fluid and serum).

Even the simpler forms of body-fluid disturbance involve a number of physiologic and chemical relationships. When water is not ingested, water deficit develops because of continued loss through lungs, skin and kidneys. When the body is deprived of water the sodium, chloride and water output falls to a minimum as dehydration advances and the concentration in the serum of Na^+ and Cl^- rises with the developing hemoconcentration. Maintenance of the normal total ionic concentration in the extracellular fluid requires renal removal of an equivalent quantity of electrolyte. Should renal function be normal, the kidneys may be able to increase the output of solids while reabsorbing water at a maximal rate, but if there is renal impairment, the urine volume may continue high or even increase (the specific gravity being relatively fixed at a low level) and the dehydration may thus be further exaggerated. For another example, vomiting may result in loss not only of fluid but of considerable amounts of hydrochloric acid in the gastric secretion, while in some cases vomiting results in great loss of the alkaline duodenal content. Such alterations in the acid or base content of the body fluids require adjustments between the various compartments in fluid and electrolyte content and demand compensatory activity by the kidneys. A better understanding of these relationships is possible if we review the anatomy and the physiology of the body fluids.

ANATOMY OF THE BODY FLUIDS

The structure of the body is largely fluid, variously confined within cell walls, the walls of vessels, or in the tissue spaces. The body fluids exist in three forms (Fig. 182): (1) blood plasma; (2) interstitial fluid; and (3) intracellular fluid. Together the blood plasma and the interstitial fluid (including lymph) constitute the *extracellular fluid*. The extracellular fluid constitutes the immediate environment of the organism, in which its cells and tissues exist. The interstitial fluid, which lies between the blood and the lymph vessels and the tissue cells, constitutes the organ of transfer of necessary metabolites between the cells and the vascular system. The blood plasma provides contact with the gastrointestinal tract, the lungs, the kidneys and the skin, so that together the interstitial fluid and the plasma form a fluid structural system for transportation of nutrient and waste substances.

Of the total weight of the body, normally 50 to 70 per cent is in fluid form. Forty to fifty per cent of the body weight is present as intracellular fluid and 15 to 20 per cent as extracellular fluid. Three-quarters of the extracellular fluid is interstitial and one-quarter is intravascular.*

In obese persons, the body weight is nearer to 50 per cent water, in very lean persons nearer 70 per cent water.

Newborn babies have approximately 77 per cent of body weight as fluid and 23 per cent as solid. In the infant, 48 per cent of body weight is accounted for by cellular fluid, 29 percent by extracellular fluid. Thus the newborn baby has nearly twice as much extracellular fluid as the adult in proportion to body weight.[36]

The baby has a much more rapid fluid turnover than the adult, because (1) he is

---

* Studies have indicated that the figures now in common use for the body content of water may be too high. The use of inulin, deuterium (heavy water) and antipyrine have permitted the simultaneous measurement of the extracellular compartment, of total body water, and by difference, the intracellular compartment. Such studies have given figures of 53 per cent (instead of 70 per cent of body weight) for total body fluid, 37 per cent (instead of 50 per cent) for intracellular fluid, and 16 per cent (instead of 20 per cent) for extracellular fluid.[4,5,6,7,32]

From measurements of body water by antipyrine and of body fat by specific gravity in the same persons, one may calculate the water content of lean body mass (fat-free tissue). This figure was found to be quite constant, averaging 71.8 per cent. Thus it is evident that the proportion of water depends upon the amount of fat—the more fat, the lower the percentage of water.

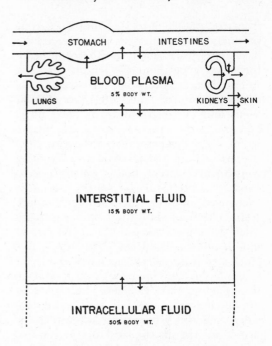

FIG. 182. Composition of extracellular fluid. (Gamble, J. L.: Chemical Anatomy, Physiology and Pathology of Extracellular Fluid, Boston, The Harvard Medical School)

a rapidly growing individual with a high metabolic rate, and (2) because his body surface area (including the intestinal surface area) is two to three times that of an adult in proportion to weight. A baby with no water intake will lose a volume of fluid equal to its extracellular fluid volume in about 5 days, while it will take an adult about 10 days to lose fluid equal to his extracellular fluid volume. Babies and small children are therefore much more vulnerable than adults to water and electrolyte disorders.[36]

The body fluids have several dimensions, including volume, composition, and position. The extracellular fluid is available to us for study; the cellular fluid is not—therefore we focus our attention on the extracellular fluid. It may vary in volume, being excessive or deficient. It may reveal deficits or excesses of various components. In some disease states the position of the extracellular fluid becomes abnormal: for example a disproportionately large percentage of the extracellular fluid may shift from the plasma into the interstitial compartment. Movement of the extracellular fluid takes place chiefly through the heart, the blood vessels and the lymph channels.

The factors governing the structure of the intracellular and the extracellular fluids and the distribution of body water are chiefly concerned with the permeability of the cell membrane to the two chief cations, sodium and potassium. Like other constituents of the body, water is in a dynamic state and is being constantly exchanged between the various compartments. Most of the cation of the intracellular fluid is potassium (for example, in muscle and in blood cells). Sodium is the chief cation of the extracellular fluid (for example, in the interstitial fluid and in the blood serum). Evidence indicates that sodium traverses the cell wall with difficulty, and this accounts to a considerable degree for the specific structure of the two compartments of the body fluids, extracellular and intracellular.[3]*

Potassium, the chief intracellular cation, exists in a state of dynamic equilibrium with the potassium of the extracellular fluids. The mechanism of maintenance of the much higher concentration of potassium within the cells as compared with that in the serum is not yet well understood. It is reasonable to believe that the oxidative energy of the cells has much to do with maintenance of this equilibrium.

It has long been known that the cell membranes are freely permeable to water, oxygen, carbon dioxide, urea and other nutrient and excretory products. Until recently it was believed that they are relatively impermeable to sodium and potassium. Recent studies have led to new concepts and a clearer understanding of water and electrolyte physiology. Use of heavy water and of radioactive isotopes of sodium and potassium have shown that the cells *are permeable* to sodium and potassium,

---

* It has been shown that both sodium and chloride enter cells to a variable degree, depending upon a number of circumstances. Darrow has calculated that normally a quantity of sodium exists within the cells which is equal to about one-ninth of the total extracellular sodium, or to one-half of the "available base."

---

but that this permeability is slow compared with that of water.[4] When heavy water was injected intravenously, equilibrium with total body water was established in 120 minutes. When radioactive sodium was injected, equilibrium with extracellular sodium was attained in 60 minutes, but not with total body sodium until 24 hours. Radioactive potassium requires 15 hours before reaching equilibrium with cellular potassium.

In spite of great fluctuations in the intake of salt and water, in health there is normally great constancy of the serum sodium concentration, the range being 132 to 142 mEq./L. The constancy of the serum sodium concentration is the consequence of the fact that the salts of sodium comprise the major osmotically active solutes in the serum and that a number of physiologic mechanisms operate to maintain in health a total solute concentration in the serum within the narrow limits of 275 to 290 mOsm./L. of water.

The osmotic activity of the serum proteins is of prime importance in the distribution of extracellular fluid between the intravascular and the interstitial compartments but protein normally contributes little to the solute activity of serum. The normal serum protein content of 60 to 70 Gm./L. amounts to only about 1 mOsm./L. because of the large molecular weight of the serum proteins (about 60,000 for serum albumin).

Maintenance of the constancy of the total solute activity of the serum is a function of the interlocking system which may be thought of broadly as the *thirst-neuro-hypophyseal-renal-adrenal axis,* the operations of which will be discussed below in the section on Physiology of the Body Fluids. With the *concentration* of the serum sodium thus regulated, normally the *volume* of the extracellular fluid is dictated by the *quantity* of sodium it contains. For this reason the clinical state of hydration, largely determined by extracellular fluid volume, is in most situations largely a direct function of the extracellular content of sodium.

The important role of sodium in the regulation of *cell* volume has only recently been appreciated. Since with radioactive isotopes it has been shown that cell membranes are permeable to water and to almost all the small solutes of the extracellular fluid, one may ask why the protein content of cells through the osmotic pressure it exerts does not result in a progressive swelling and lysis of all cells. The answer appears to be that the sodium ion through its largely extracellular position sets up a counter osmotic force that just balances the intracellular oncotic pressure and stabilizes the cell volume.

It seems that the extracellular position of sodium is not dependent upon an absolute impermeability of cell membranes to sodium but rather to an active extrusion of the sodium that continuously diffuses into the cells. Through this active transport of sodium ions, in which all body cells are engaged, plus the important but less conspicuous cellular-extracellular exchange of potassium ions, the characteristic difference in ionic composition of cellular and extracellular fluids is maintained and the volume of the cells preserved. It is chiefly the sodium *retained* in the extracellular fluids and the sodium *extruded* from the cells (with the accompanying, usually reciprocal, potassium interchanges) that regulate the respective volumes of the two compartments.[56]

Probably most cells accumulate potassium actively as well as extrude sodium, but whether the extrusion of sodium is coupled in any rigorous, quantitative way to the uptake of potassium remains unsettled. The ability to accumulate K and extrude Na in the presence of large amounts of Na and small amounts of K in the surrounding fluid is a fundamental characteristic of living cells.[57] When death of the cell occurs these ionic gradients are rapidly dissipated. These gradients are maintained by living cells in spite of permeability of cell walls to both ions. Therefore, the relative concentrations of Na^+ and K^+ ions in extracellular and cellular fluids must be the result of steady-state conditions supported by energy derived from cellular metabolism; it is not an equilibrium state resulting from the impermeability of cell membranes to one or more ions, as was thought earlier. The energy inherent in such ionic gradients has been secondarily adapted by certain specialized cells to afford nervous conduction and the excitation phase of muscular contraction.

Our concept of the extracellular fluid has been oversimplified and the inulin space is not the final answer to its measurement. Sodium and chloride diffuse rapidly into collagenous connective tissue, whereas inulin and thiosulfate do not. It has been suggested that the extracellular phase, aside from the plasma in the vascular system, should be partitioned into two subphases: the interstitial fluid which is an ultrafiltrate of plasma, and connective tissue. The inulin space defines only the plasma and the first of these two subphases, while sodium and chloride diffuse rapidly through both subphases before entering more slowly the true intracellular fluid. Not only do sodium and chloride enter the intracellular fluid, but they also cross cell barriers into special fluid pools and other depots. Such pools called *transcellular fluids* include fluids in the gastrointestinal tract, in serous and synovial cavities, in the lower urinary tract, in cerebrospinal fluid and in bile.[4,33] Bone also acts as a sodium and potassium reservoir.[51]

Water balance depends upon control of the amounts of fluid in each of the fluid compartments. Circulation of the blood requires a fairly constant volume in the vascular compartment. The volume of cell fluid to permit proper tissue metabolism must be quite constant. The usual volume of interstitial fluid is apparently ideal, but wide variations may occur without great disturbance of its functions. Water loss by vaporization and perspiration for heat regulation and by urinary excretion of waste products is at the expense of interstitial fluid. Water exchange consists essentially in loss and replacement of extracellular water, chiefly interstitial water. Plasma-volume fluctuations occur, but permissible variations are relatively limited. Cell-volume changes also occur, but these alterations can only be slight.

The chemical structure of the various compartments of the body fluids is illustrated diagrammatically in Figure 183.

By circulation of the blood through *the lungs,* gaseous exchange with the external environment is accomplished. The red blood cells constitute the special vehicle for transportation of oxygen and carbon dioxide between lungs and tissues, this being made possible by the reversible affinity of hemoglobin for these two substances. Water is lost from the lungs through the exhalation of vapor.

Intimate contact of body fluids with the *gastrointestinal tract* provides for the absorption of water and nutrient substances into cells and tissue spaces and thence for transport by the vascular system, and likewise permits excretion into the intestinal tract by the same routes.

Most important of all in maintenance of the constancy of structure of the extracellular fluid are *the kidneys,* which are capable of regulating not only the amount of water that leaves the body by the renal route but the kinds and the amounts of substances in solution in that water. Thus the chemical components of the blood plasma and the interstitial fluid are maintained within homeostatic limits largely by renal regulation.[41,46,47,49,50]

The skin through perspiration and evaporation is concerned with control of water balance and the excretion of certain metabolites. *Insensible perspiration* consists of the water lost invisibly from the skin without loss of salts. *Sweat* contains excretory products (urea, etc.), sodium, and chloride and other salts, and is perceptible or visible. The epidermis or outermost layer of the

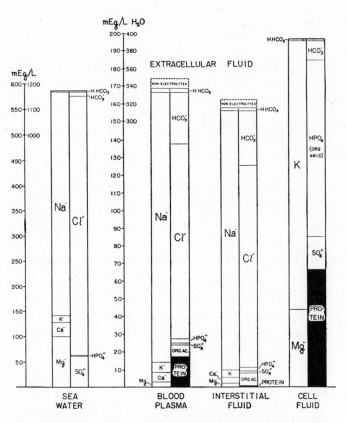

Fig. 183. Chemical anatomy of body fluids in terms of acid-base equivalence. (Gamble, J. L.: Chemical Anatomy, Physiology and Pathology of Extracellular Fluid, Boston, The Harvard Medical School)

skin is continuously active as a factor inhibiting water loss from blood vessels and tissues by the pressure and the covering it affords. The corneal layer of the epidermis, which is of microscopic thickness except in the palms and the soles, is the layer of greatest importance in the inhibition of water loss by diffusion from the underlying tissues. When the protective skin covering is removed by burns or other injury, large quantities of water and electrolytes and of blood proteins may be lost. Thus the "dead," keratinous, ever-desquamating, thin corneum has, nevertheless, an important role in the maintenance of normal water and electrolyte balance.

PHYSIOLOGY OF THE BODY FLUIDS

The functions served by the body fluids are closely interrelated but may be divided as follows:
1. Transportation
   (a) of oxygen and CO_2
   (b) of nutrient materials such as amino acids, glucose, fats, vitamins, minerals, etc.
   (c) of hormones and chemical regulators
   (d) of excretory products such as urea, etc.
2. Temperature regulation
   (a) by shifting the blood to the surface for cooling, or to the interior to prevent heat loss
   (b) by perspiration and evaporation of moisture from the skin surface
3. Osmotic pressure regulation
   (a) plasma-protein effects
   (b) electrolyte effects
4. Acid-base balance regulation
   (a) through respiratory control of carbonic acid
   (b) through renal chemical control.

In addition to the simple function of *transportation,* the aqueous medium in which the tissues and the cells exist provides stable physical and chemical conditions. *Temperature, the hydrogen-ion concentration* and *osmotic pressure* are regulated by the extracellular fluid, and the influences of these factors are exerted in the fluid and through the fluid upon the tissues.

The concentration of sodium in the extracellular fluid is kept quite constant, although there is a slow, continuous interchange of water and of sodium from the extracellular fluid through cell walls.

Water alone will not enter the cells unless there is a decrease in the concentration of extracellular sodium, otherwise the cells would be hypotonic in relation to the extracellular fluid. Water alone likewise cannot leave the cell unless the concentration of extracellular sodium rises. Therefore the state of hydration of the cells depends primarily upon the *concentration of sodium ion in the extracellular fluid.* A major function of the kidney is to regulate the concentration of sodium in the extracellular fluid.

The water and salt intake, the regulatory activity of the kidney and the osmotic pressures acting across semipermeable membranes all operate to maintain a constant internal environment. The degree of hydration and the distribution of body water are usually so well regulated that the osmotic pressure of the fluids is kept quite constant.[4-7]

The *volume,* as well as the osmolality and the pH of body fluids, is maintained within certain limits to permit adequate performance of the various physiologic functions listed. The volume fluctuations in the several fluid compartments which are compatible with health differ considerably: interstitial volumes can vary widely, intravascular volumes moderately, and cell volumes relatively little. There are volume-regulatory mechanisms which are apparently separate and independent of osmoreceptors and of changes in the osmolality of the body fluids. Knowledge of the location of sensitive indicators of volume and their mode of operation is incomplete.[8] "Volume-receptors" have been described within the cranium and in vascular structures within the thorax. After disturbances of osmolality the mechanisms operating to restore normal fluid volumes are better understood. However, when the changes are isosmolar, the processes involved in the correction of aberrations in fluid volume are less clear. Following hemorrhage, for example, even in the absence of the intake of fluid, restoration of intravascular volume soon begins. If water is administered as isotonic glucose, a prompt water diuresis ensues, since glucose is not freely permeable through cell walls, and thus attracts water into the intravascular compartment. However, if water is administered as isotonic NaCl solution, there is no immediate effect upon water excretion. The volume of the body fluids is increased, body weight increases, and there is every evidence of a positive water balance. Over a period of several days there is a delayed response to the expanded fluid volume, diuresis occurs at a moderate rate over a span of days, and during these days there is a negative water balance, so that at the end of the period of adjustment, the previous normal fluid volumes and body weight are restored.

The juxtaglomerular apparatus of the kidney is a volume receptor. A fall in the pressure within the afferent renal arterioles leads to the secretion of renin, the formation of angiotensin II, and promotes the secretion of aldosterone.[68]

TRANSPORTATION

Normally there is wide variation in the amount of fluid taken into the body and excreted daily, but the total intake equals the total output with great constancy. Such equilibrium holds true over a period of a few days, not necessarily for each 24-hour day. This is necessarily so, since otherwise fluid would either accumulate in the body or dehydration would occur. By control of the amounts of fluid absorbed and excreted, stability of the volume of extracellular fluid is established, and thus *constancy of transport* is maintained.

Water Requirement. The water intake is derived from several sources: (1) drinking water; (2) water in food; (3) water formed in combustion of food; (4) water formed in combustion of body substance. The amount of water consumed as such is usually only about one third of the total water intake. The average normal person drinks from 1 to 1.5 liters of liquid daily, except when subjected to active exercise or high temperature, under which conditions the amount drunk may be increased severalfold. Foods furnish water because most of them are high in water

content: meat, about 70 per cent; milk, 87 per cent; and certain vegetables and fruits (cucumbers, watermelon), over 95 per cent. An ordinary diet yields in combustion about 12 ml. of water per 100 calories. The total amount of water required is roughly parallel to the energy metabolism, being approximately 1 ml. per calorie. Thus a sedentary man may need only 1,500 ml. daily, while a physically active man of the same size and weight may require 3,000 ml.

Water Output. Under normal temperate conditions there are certain usual proportions between water intake and its disposal by the various routes, as shown by these average daily figures of the usual ranges for an adult:

Urine	1,000-1,500 ml.
Feces	50- 200
Skin (insensible perspiration) ..	450-1,050
Sweat	100- 500
Lungs	250- 350
Total per 24 hours	1,850-3,600 ml.

Water Deprivation. When the body is deprived of water for any reason, dehydration with a fall in the volume of extracellular fluid occurs, insensible perspiration diminishes and the urine volume greatly and rapidly decreases. The decrease in the urine volume is presumably due to activity of the posterior pituitary antidiuretic hormone. Conservation of water occurs through increased tubular reabsorption until the urine volume becomes minimal and its concentration becomes maximal. Glomerular filtration may fall at this point because of the reduction in blood volume and because of the rise in the colloid osmotic pressure of the plasma. Hemoconcentration occurs. The blood urea rises. As dehydration advances, water is lost out of proportion to salt, which is preferentially absorbed. The concentrations of sodium and chloride in the extracellular fluids rise and draw water from the cells. The cells also yield some potassium, which permits further escape of cellular water. Loss of 10 per cent of body water is disabling to man.[36,42,48]

Sodium Deprivation. One cannot in a short period of days or weeks by using only *dietary restriction* seriously deplete the body sodium, because the urinary output of Na and Cl decreases so promptly. The results of sodium loss through excessive sweating, vomiting, diarrhea, etc., depend upon the amount of water simultaneously lost.[52,54] Loss of both water and salt in hypotonic solution, as in *sweat*, has immediate effects of a primary loss of salt, if water is taken in freely during the sweating. Sweat contains about half the salt per liter (about 75 mEq. of Na) as compared with that present in the plasma, so much salt may be lost during heavy sweating. Sweating greatly accelerates the dehydration of water deprivation, further augmenting the rise of sodium and chloride in the serum. If sufficient water is taken in, of course, the concentration of serum Na and Cl may rapidly fall to normal or subnormal levels as a consequence of salt loss from excessive sweating. If, however, little or no water is taken in, loss of sweat (which is hypotonic—that is, contains more water proportionately than plasma) has primarily the effect of water depletion. Loss of gastrointestinal and digestive secretions, which are isotonic, should presumably deplete sodium and water in equivalent proportions. If water only is ingested, some of the water is absorbed and the remainder is discharged in the vomitus, fistular discharge or stool, carrying salt with it to make it isotonic. These conditions therefore produce salt depletion primarily. In such states the volume of fluid lost usually exceeds the volume ingested, and there is therefore a large deficit of water associated with the salt depletion. Whenever decompression and lavage of the gastrointestinal tract are carried out (as in the treatment of intestinal obstruction), normal saline solution should be employed rather than water, in order to reduce the secretory activity of the digestive glands and of the alimentary canal to a minimum and thus prevent salt loss.

Sodium Excess. Salt taken without sufficient water during dehydration will exaggerate thirst and water loss. Sodium chloride taken in excess of body needs at any time will promote diuresis, providing that the renal mechanisms for excreting salt and water are unimpaired. However, should the ability of the kidney to eliminate salt and water be limited for any reason (circulatory failure, renal damage, hormonal disorder, etc.), overhydration and edema may result.

Whenever the ratio of salt to water is greater in the ingesta than in extracellular fluid, the volume of the latter expands at the expense of intracellular fluid. Diuresis results, and the intensity of the increased water and salt output depends upon the volume and the salt concentration of the ingesta. The same processes are of course operative if the water and the salt are given parenterally. Diuresis results because of the decreased rate of reabsorption of water by the renal tubules, the osmotic effect of the high salt concentration in the glomerular filtrate tending to hold water in the tubules for excretion. The rate of glomerular filtration further increases the degree of diuresis, since it is increased more by hypertonic saline than by an equal amount of water. This is apparently the result of the greater increase in the extracellular fluid volume caused by the higher salt concentration in the blood which draws water from the cells.

Thirst is the desire to ingest liquids. It probably should not be regarded as a simple sensation, due to dryness of the mucous membranes of the mouth and pharynx. Such dryness, which may result from many causes (mouth breathing, inhibition of salivary secretion by atropine, etc.) can, if not associated with body fluid aberration, be corrected by simply keeping the membranes moist, and the so-called thirst disappears.

True thirst is a more widely perceived sensation, more like hunger; it may or may not be associated with dryness of the oropharyngeal membranes. Thirst occurs when (1) cellular dehydration is present, or (2) when extracellular fluid volume is decreased, or (3) when certain hypothalamic centers are stimulated. It seems likely that the cells in the hypothalamic center are sensitive to the relative osmolality of the fluid reaching them, become relatively dehydrated, and relay impulses to higher centers interpreted as thirst. Studies in man suggest that when cell volume of the tissues generally is reduced by 1 or 2 per cent thirst appears.[58,59]

Studies suggesting that there is a "thirst center" in the hypothalamus are based upon observations such as these on animals:[60] (1) injection of a very small amount of hypertonic NaCl into a particular area of the hypothalamus caused intense polydipsia; isotonic NaCl solution produced no such response; (2) electric stimulation of the same area produces water ingestion; destruction of the area by electrocoagulation caused hypodipsia.

Although thirst *usually* indicates true physiological need for water, it is not an accurate indicator of the water *content* of the body. Thus, (1) extracellular fluid volume may be excessive, but if the effective osmolality of the fluid is high (causing cellular dehydration) thirst occurs; also (2) if extracellular fluid volume is low but the osmolality is in normal relation to that of the cells (no cellular dehydration) there will be no thirst.

Inappropriate thirst may be observed in the syndrome of hyponatremia. Here there is reduced vascular volume which results in the stimulus to drink water; such a response does not defend the osmolality of the body fluids. In patients with hepatic cirrhosis, serum proteins may be low and blood volume high; abdominal paracentesis may lead to prompt thirst, and fluid ingestion would further distort extracellular fluid changes in the same direction. Presumably, in these instances, reduction in volume of the extracellular fluid causes cellular dehydration and activates the sensation of thirst.

It is reasonable to suppose that the factors concerned in thirst and the influences upon water balance through the control of the secretion of the antidiuretic hormone of the pituitary are part of the same regulatory mechanism. Wolf's[58,59] calculations of osmometric changes of 1 to 2 per cent cellular dehydration necessary to produce thirst are about the same as those found by Verney as resulting in secretion of ADH.[61] If one compares the effects of giving isosmolal solutions of NaCl (20%) and urea (40%) intravenously, thirst is much greater and water intake is much higher after the NaCl. The cellular membranes are permeable to urea, but relatively impermeable to the Na^+ and Cl^- ions so the *effective* hypertonicity is the most important factor, rather than the total osmolality. Other ions which do not traverse cell membranes freely have similar effects: intake of hypertonic amounts of any such solutes causes thirst. The thirst results in increased water intake, which leads to decrease in the abnormally high solute concentration. Similarly, hypertonicity of extracellular fluids results in increased ADH secretion; renal loss of water is diminished and there is relative fluid retention which favors reduction of the hypertonicity.

Apparently the concentration of solutes in the body fluids, as well as the volume of the body fluids, determines the desire for water.[58-60] It may be that the stimulus to thirst depends upon the water content of the cells (*cellular dehydration*), and that the cells of the mucosa of the tongue, the mouth and the pharynx are often, to the affected person, the most sensitive but not the only indicators. When the body is depleted of sodium chloride, there may be little thirst despite extreme dehydration. On the other hand, increasing the salt content of the body will cause thirst promptly, even when the total body-water content is already adequate or excessive. Severe thirst may occur in such instances apparently as a central sensation, with no dryness of the mucous membranes. The rise in sodium content of the extracellular fluid causes cellular dehydration. The establishment of normal osmotic relationships after aberration in either direction is apt to terminate the sensation of thirst. Thirst occurs normally whenever the extracellular fluid volume is appreciably diminished, by whatever route, whether through water deprivation, perspiration, increased renal or intestinal loss, hemorrhage, massive loss of serum into burns, etc.[45] When extracellular fluid volume falls, some water is given up *from the cellular compartment* and this loss no doubt is the stimulus to the sensation of thirst.

It seems particularly significant that in the experiments of Andersson,[60] in which he demonstrated the presence of a thirst center in the hypothalamus, stimuli which would induce thirst would in many instances also elicit antidiuresis. The nuclei of the anterior hypothalamus which are now known to be the source of antidiuretic hormone[62] must overlap the thirst center. Verney[63] has produced evidence that the osmoreceptors may also be localized in the same nuclei. Thus, thirst center, osmoreceptor and source of antidiuretic hormone are closely integrated anatomically as well as functionally.[56]

Thirst plays a primary role in the operations of the *thirst-neurohypophyseal-renal axis* to maintain constancy of the solute concentration (particularly sodium) of the extracellular fluid. Usually, unless some circumstance prevents it, water intake keeps pace with water loss or promptly makes up for it. Whenever fluid loss is accelerated, intake is increased. In health this response is automatic and is dependent upon the sensation of thirst.

When the sensorium is clouded or the patient is in coma, the physiologic mechanisms to produce thirst may be present, but the sensation cannot be perceived. Obligatory fluid losses may proceed to dangerous or fatal levels of dehydration if the subject is unable to perceive the thirst signal or is unable for any reason to respond to it by appropriate intake of water.

TEMPERATURE REGULATION AND PERSPIRATION

When the temperature of the air is high or when body temperature is elevated by fever, *perspiration* may be greatly increased. However, under normal conditions, exercise is the chief factor leading to increased water loss as sweat. The *evaporation of water* from the body surface constitutes the most important mechanism by which body water influences body temperature. When body or environmental temperature is high, or when work is done and there is no condition to interfere with the ingestion or absorption of water, thirst provides the stimulus and spontaneously the intake is greatly increased, providing adequate fluid for this mode of temperature regulation. Usually less water is excreted in the urine (and feces) under these circumstances, and

more through the lungs, so that water balance figures might be as follows:

Urine	500 ml.
Feces	50
Sweat	4,000
Lungs	500
Total	5,050 ml.

Cardiovascular Factors. To promote elimination of heat and water through the skin, a larger than normal volume of intravascular fluids is diverted to the blood vessels supplying the skin. To serve the purposes of heat elimination a large increase in the minute volume of blood circulating through the skin occurs by reflex. An unacclimatized man forced to work in the heat has a great burden imposed upon his cardiovascular system.

Adrenocortical Factors. Hormones produced by the adrenal cortex regulate in some degree the amounts of sodium, chloride, potassium and water retained by the renal tubules or excreted in the urine. There is an adrenocortical control of the sodium and chloride of sweat also. Normally the concentration of sodium in the sweat is about a third to a half of that of the plasma. The administration of desoxycorticosterone or of adrenocorticotropic hormone reduces the salt content of sweat, as it does that of urine.[9] When the subject was put to work in a hot room and excessive sweating became apparent, there were indications suggestive of increased ACTH and adrenocortical activity: lowered concentration of the NaCl in the sweat, negative nitrogen balance and high urinary uric acid excretion. Under these circumstances with a severe stress calling for salt retention, the administration of desoxycorticosterone (or the restoration of a positive NaCl balance by giving salt) restored nitrogen equilibrium to normal. This is apparently another instance of the pituitary-adrenal system's role in responses to stress and maintenance of homeostasis. Such evidence suggests that acclimatization to heat (and possibly adaptation to strenuous muscular exertion) may consist partly in adrenocortical stimulation via pituitary ACTH, with resultant salt conservation.[37,40,50]

In the acute or early phase of excitation

by pituitary ACTH of adrenocortical activity there is increase in secretion of several steroids of the adrenal cortex, including the most highly potent mineralocorticoid, aldosterone. In the later or persistent phase of adjustment, the salt lost through the sweat glands may be decreased by as much as 95 per cent by aldosterone action, without participation of ACTH or of other hormones of the adrenal cortex.[64]

Neurogenic control of sweating is well recognized, but excessive sweating from this cause is seldom so prolonged as to affect materially total water balance—except when the organism is totally deprived of water.

Sweating associated with exercise, fever, or high environmental temperature may cause extreme dehydration if for any reason the water intake is not correspondingly increased. The usual normal loss of approximately 0.5 Gm. of NaCl through sweat per day may reach 5 to 10 Gm. or more. Extreme exertion in hot environments may cause the loss of 10 or 12 liters of water per day through the skin. Acclimatization may reduce the sweat Na concentration from a normal level of around 75 mEq. to 2 to 5 mEq. per liter.

The movement of air over the skin, as determined by clothing and wind, accelerates water loss. High humidity increases sweating. High air temperature and low humidity increase insensible water loss. As much as 10 liters may be lost through the skin in a few hours on a desert.

Should some factor prevent adequate water intake it is obvious that water balance could not be maintained during heavy perspiration, and dehydration (reduction in extracellular fluid) would soon occur. Even when conservative measures, such as diminution of the urine output (increased tubular reabsorption), are brought into play, excessive perspiration in the presence of normal or decreased water intake would soon result in a serious deficit in body fluid.

Increase in water intake alone will not compensate for excessive fluid loss by perspiration, because not only is water so lost, but electrolyte. Increase of water intake alone results in further loss of both water and NaCl, both by perspiration and through urine. Because of the lowered amounts of total Na and Cl in the cells and the extracellular fluid, the amounts of water in all compartments are reduced to maintain normal physiologic relationships. Adding more water without increasing the Na and Cl intake simply increases the rate of NaCl loss, since the water cannot be retained in the absence of adequate electrolyte, but takes some electrolyte with it when excreted.

Acclimatization. A process of adaptation called "acclimatization to heat" occurs when man is exposed to an environment hotter than that to which he is accustomed. When completed, acclimatization results in a remarkable increase in capacity to live and work in a hot environment without distressing symptoms. The period of time required for adaptation varies from a few days up to about 20 days, being longer for higher temperatures. On the first day of exposure to heat, a normal subject attempting to complete a given work load may collapse with a high rectal temperature and evidence of peripheral vascular failure; the same subject, after exposure to the same amount of heat with a lighter work load over a period of 6 or 7 days, will be able to perform the original task easily, without cardiovascular difficulties and with a much lower rectal temperature.

The acclimatized man develops his ability to work in the hot environment without serious untoward effects through certain physiologic changes. These changes are primarily of two types: (1) alteration in cardiovascular function, and (2) modification of sweat gland activity.

Initially upon exposure to heat or after strenuous exercise or both, there is an acute diversion of blood to the periphery through reflex action, a great increase in the volume of blood circulating through the skin, and thus an acceleration of the rate of heat and water loss. This is a temporary compensatory mechanism operating in all normal persons when the heat or work are not prolonged. However, if work in the heat is continued and adaptation is successfully accomplished, more persistent changes occur: increased plasma and extracellular fluid volumes, increased peripheral circulation, and often an increase in resting cardiac output.

The fully acclimatized man produces a

somewhat larger volume of sweat during performance of a standard work load than does an unacclimatized person. In dry heat this extra water loss through the skin helps eliminate heat from the body by vaporization. In moist heat, however, this advantage is lost, since much of the sweat drips off the body and is of no value in eliminating heat. However, in either case a large sweat volume carries with it a relatively large amount of sodium chloride. The second important mechanism in acclimatization consists in a great reduction in the concentration of sodium chloride in sweat.

Conn[64] studied men performing a standard work load in a "tropical climate room" (temperature 90°F.; relative humidity 80% to 90%). Sweat volume was 5 to 7 liters per day. A typical response during acclimatization was a decrease in the salt concentration of sweat from an initial 3 Gm. per liter to less than 1.0 Gm. per liter by the tenth day, a saving of 10 to 14 Gm. of salt daily.

Men who continued at work in the heat, under the conditions described, had a negative nitrogen balance for the first 10 to 20 days, and showed other evidences of excitation of the pituitary-adrenal axis with liberation of several of the hormones of the adrenal cortex, not mineralocorticoids only. In the first few days of exposure to heat there is intense salt conservation both by the kidneys and by the sweat glands. However, after the first few days under conditions of large sweat volume and average salt intake, the sweat glands continue to be very efficient in salt conservation, but the renal excretion of sodium actually rises (escapes) to attain sodium equilibrium. When the early phase of negative nitrogen balance disappears, low concentrations of sodium in sweat persist as an indicator of continued and intense salt conservation by the sweat glands. Recent studies indicate that increased secretion of the specific adrenocortical mineralocorticoid, aldosterone, accounts for the greatly reduced NaCl content of the sweat. The maintenance of continued augmented aldosterone secretion is independent of pituitary ACTH activity and is not accompanied by a general increase in the secretion of the other adreno-

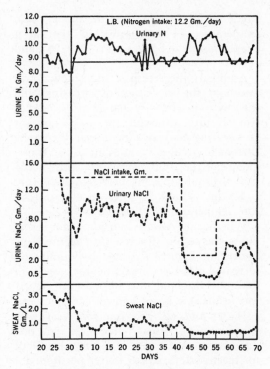

FIG. 184. Metabolic pattern of acclimatization to humid heat and of adjustments that occur upon sudden salt privation. (Mechanism of Acclimatization to Heat, *Advance. Intern. Med.* 3:373-394; Conn[9,64])

cortical hormones. There is thus seen to be an important difference in the physiologic processes of NaCl conservation during exposure to heat between two clearly defined phases: (1) during the early phase (lasting 10 to 20 days under the conditions of Conn's studies) there is acute stress with excitation of the pituitary-adrenal axis; (2) during the persistent phase of acclimatization which follows thereafter, the sweat glands take over the primary role under the influence of independent aldosterone secretion (Fig. 184).

Under normal conditions the renal mechanisms of salt conservation play by far the major role, but with heavy sweating the major salt-saving function of the body is turned over to the sweat glands.

In physically fit persons, work in a hot environment sufficient to elevate body core temperature on each of several successive days leads to adaptation with dramatic reduction of strain. For example, in one study the subject developed on the first day a rectal temperature of 104°F., skin temperature of 99°, pulse of 180; after adaptation these figures were 101°, 96°, and 140.[65]

Acclimatization results in a new lower threshold for the onset of sweating, and thereby induces maintenance of lower skin temperature, although the total amount of sweating may not be much increased. Lessened circulatory burden is a consequence of the ability to maintain the necessary thermal gradient between body core and skin without as great an elevation in core temperature.

Whether the lowered threshold for sweating is the result of a resetting of the regulatory mechanism in the hypothalamus, increased patency of cutaneous vessels, or lowered threshold for response of receptors in the skin is not known.

Water and salt requirements vary with the extent of losses. Some men can produce sweat at the rate of 3 liters per hour for brief periods, up to 1 liter per hour for 8 hours, and as much as 0.5 liter per hour for a 24 hour period. Frequent ingestion of water sufficient to satisfy thirst has demonstrable advantages over restricted or postponed water intake. Before acclimatization, 2 to 4 Gm. of NaCl is required for each liter of sweat. Dietary intake usually provides 10 Gm. or more of NaCl daily—enough to meet ordinary requirements of sweating.

Apparently the normal person receives adequate warning of incipient heat injury through developing faintness, dizziness or fatigue. When workers engaged in very hot industrial jobs are free to rest at intervals as need is felt, heat injury seldom occurs. Persons working in hot environments should be instructed concerning proper increases of NaCl and fluid intake—to prevent dehydration, and not to wait until symptoms are evident.

Persons with impaired circulatory reserve may be unable to respond to the great demand for mobilization of fluid necessary in adjustment to high environmental temperature. Circulatory failure may be precipitated by such a stress.

Persons with adrenocortical insufficiency tend to have abnormally high concentrations of salt in sweat and are less able to adjust to high environmental temperatures. One of the salt-conserving mechanisms available to persons with normal adrenocortical function is reduction of the NaCl in sweat. Salt depletion of the body from any cause results in increased adrenal cortical secretion and reduction in the NaCl concentration in sweat.[9,64,66,67]

It is significant that, during the second phase of acclimatization, reduction of NaCl intake from liberal to very low levels induces a stress response similar to that observed upon first exposure to work in the heat (Fig. 184). Renal conservation of salt again becomes intense and there is a negative nitrogen balance.

Another important aspect of the physiologic processes of adjustment to heat and heavy sweating is concerned with the ability of an acclimatizing man to maneuver himself into a state of positive sodium balance.[64] Upon initial exposure to work in the heat there are very large losses of sodium in sweat. The precipitous fall in sweat sodium plus the drop in urinary sodium which then occur result in a period of active retention of sodium which persists until the total amount restored exceeds that initially lost. The added NaCl plus added water causes expansion of the extracellular fluid volume, which permits long-term cardiovascular adjustment to heat, an essential part of successful acclimatization.

The aldosterone-sweat gland system can reduce salt losses from the skin by as much as 95%; all forms of temperature regulation in hot climates would fail without action of this system in maintaining or even augmenting the volume of the extracellular fluid. Aldosterone plays an essential role in bringing about the cutaneous, renal and cardiovascular adjustments necessary for man's survival in hot climates.

Summary. One may summarize a working hypothesis concerning the sequential processes involved in the physiology of acclimatization as follows: in the initial response to exposure to heat (with a moderate work load and average salt intake) there is heavy sweating with consequent contraction of the extracellular fluid and plasma volumes because of the large amount of NaCl lost in the sweat. There is a reflex diversion of a larger than normal proportion of the intravascular volume to the skin. This diversion results in decreased renal plasma flow; decreased pressure or volume in the afferent renal arterioles stimulates the juxtaglomerular apparatus (this apparatus serving as one site of the vascular volume receptors) and aldosterone secretion is stimulated through the renin-angiotensin system. Because of decreased glomerular filtration rate or increased aldosterone activity upon the renal tubules, or both, urinary sodium may fall virtually to zero. Reduction of the concentration of NaCl in sweat becomes evident about 12 to 24 hours later. Within a few days there is escape from the intense restriction of renal NaCl output; renal salt output rises and tends to fluctuate with NaCl intake. However, the excretion of NaCl in the sweat remains very low, permitting a positive NaCl balance and fluid retention, with gradual expansion of the extracellular fluid volume until a new level of sodium balance and a new fluid equilibrium is established compatible with the acclimatized state.

Untoward Effects of Heat. When the protective mechanisms are able to operate adequately, health may be maintained despite strenuous exertion in a hot environment.

Failure to adjust adequately to heat may occur quickly as in (1) cardiovascular failure or (2) heat stroke; after more prolonged heat stress, as in (3) heat prostration or (4) heat cramps.

Factors which may account for inability to accommodate to heat include: (1) lack of water intake, (2) lack of NaCl intake, (3) adrenocortical deficiency (especially of aldosterone secretion), (4) impaired cardiovascular system, central or peripheral, (5) renal failure, (6) central nervous system disorders (of temperature regulation, of ADH secretion or affecting renal salt conservation).

The state ultimately reached by prolonged perspiration in the absence of adequate replacement of salt and water is called *heat exhaustion* or *heat prostration*. It is characterized by peripheral vascular failure. The patient is dehydrated and may be in shock. The skin is cool, moist,

pale, sometimes cyanotic. Often there are muscular and abdominal cramps. The blood pressure is low, normal or slightly elevated, pulse weak. Restoration to normal is accomplished by treatment of the shock and replacement of NaCl and water.

Heat cramps occur in persons engaged in strenuous activity at high environmental temperature and result from extreme loss of NaCl through sweat while the water intake is kept very high. The shocklike symptoms of heat prostration are less evident, although the two conditions merge. Loss of salt may reach 20 Gm. daily. The hypotonic body fluids cause intracellular overhydration and, through abnormal diffusion conditions in the muscles, severe muscular spasms and pain, particularly in the arms and the legs. The Na and Cl concentrations in the serum are low, and the urinary NaCl output diminishes greatly. In heat prostration the salt and water loss are more proportionate, so that the serum electrolytes are less evidently reduced and the changes tend further to be masked by anhydremia, with hemoconcentration, but the plasma volume falls and the circulation fails.

Cardiovascular failure may be precipitated even in normal persons by exposure to extreme heat; persons with previous cardiovascular impairment, either central or peripheral, are especially susceptible. The acute diversion of blood to the periphery is responsible for the early signs of vascular collapse: rapid pulse, decreased stroke volume, sometimes decreased minute output, severe postural hypotension, fainting or coma, sometimes convulsions. Often there is evidence of vascular engorgement, such as flushing of the face, neck and chest, injection of the sclerae, edema of nasal mucous membranes, edema of hands and feet.

The heart may fail quickly when there is reduced coronary flow from the conditions described above. The heart may fail later due to inability to cope with the increased work demanded by acclimatization, (See discussion above under Acclimatization.)

Heat prostration must be distinguished from *sunstroke* or *heat stroke,* also apt to occur in hot weather. The latter, however, is characterized by loss of temperature control and high fever, reaching as high as 110° F., not necessarily accompanied by dehydration. The pulse is full, blood pressure normal or high, skin hot and flushed. Headache and vertigo are common, and convulsions, coma and death may occur. Ice-water tub baths and the administration of NaCl and water parenterally help to restore temperature control. Apparently both the mechanisms for heat production and heat elimination are involved in the production of heat stroke. Inability to lower the rate of metabolism in response to a sudden rise in environmental temperature seems particularly apt to occur in persons with arteriosclerosis and impaired cardiac reserve. Increased peripheral circulation is suddenly required to facilitate heat loss and a greater burden is thrown upon the heart, so that death may occur either from heart failure or from the hyperpyrexia itself. Diminution or cessation of sweating before the onset of acute symptoms may be observed, and is characteristic, indicating a breakdown in the mechanism of heat elimination. Persons exposed to excessive sunlight or to extremely high temperature may of course suffer from both dehydration and loss of temperature control. Loss of body fluid removes safety factors in temperature control and predisposes to heat prostration or sunstroke.

Considerable amounts of NaCl may be lost in the perspiration. The average NaCl loss by this route is about 5 per cent of the intake, or about 0.5 Gm. daily. Under conditions of very heavy sweating this may be increased to many grams (from 5 to 10 or more). If this salt lack is not made up by adequate NaCl intake, water alone being taken, weakness, vomiting, diarrhea, muscular cramps, convulsions and other signs of salt deficit may occur. This is *water intoxication* due primarily to cellular overhydration, occurring as the result of reduced osmotic pressure of the blood. *Salt hunger* is a definite sensation which usually leads animals and man to correct this lack if NaCl is available. The mechanism of salt hunger is not yet well understood, but apparently it depends upon the salt concentration of the extracellular fluid reaching the taste buds.[6]

OSMOTIC PRESSURE AND ELECTROLYTE REGULATION

Circulation of the extracellular fluid depends partly upon the hydrostatic pressure produced by the heart and partly upon the difference in protein content between blood plasma and interstitial fluid. The work of the heart sustains a higher hydrostatic presure on the arterial side of the capillary bed, and, as a result of this pressure, fluid steadily moves into the interstitial spaces. On the venous side of the capillary bed the plasma proteins provide an osmotic differential which is unopposed and fluid returns to the venous capillaries and the veins.

UNITS OF MEASUREMENT

The desirability of expressing chemical measurements in truly comparable terms has been emphasized by Gamble[3] and the following discussion on units of measurement is quoted from him:

In studying the chemical structure of extracellular fluid, measurements of its components must obviously be stated in terms of chemical equivalence. Only in this way can their relative magnitudes and inter-relationship be correctly displayed. The suitable term is milliequivalents per liter. This value is obtained by dividing milligrams per liter by atomic weight and multiplying by valence.

The form of statement for measurements of the inorganic ions which usage has unfortunately imposed is milligrams per cent. Conversion to milliequivalents per liter for the individual ions is as follows:

	mg. per 100 ml.
Na·	× 10 ÷ 23
K·	× 10 ÷ 39
Ca··	× 10 ÷ 40 × 2
Mg··	× 10 ÷ 24 × 2
Cl′	× 10 ÷ 35
HPO_4'' (mg. P)	× 10 ÷ 31 × 1.8
SO_4'' (mg. S)	× 10 ÷ 32 × 2

The valence of HPO_4 is taken as 1.8 because, at the normal pH of extracellular fluid, 20 per cent of the concentration of this radical carries one equivalent of base,

(BH₂PO₄), and 80 per cent two equivalents, (B₂HPO₄); B representing univalent base. Base equivalence per unit of (HPO₄) is therefore $0.2 + (0.8 \times 2) = 1.8$. The double valency sign is to this small extent inaccurate.

For the concentrations of carbonic acid (H.HCO₃) and of bicarbonate (B.HCO₃) convention prescribes the cumbersome statements: volume per cent CO₂ as carbonic acid and volume per cent CO₂ as bicarbonate. These volume per cent values are converted to milliequivalents per liter by dividing by 2.22.

The base equivalence of protein as milliequivalents per liter is obtained by multiplying grams protein per 100 ml. by the Van Slyke factor, 2.43.

In studying the osmotic features of extracellular fluid, measurements of its components are stated in terms of ionic concentration. In other words valence is disregarded. The suitable term is milliosmols per liter (milligrams per liter divided by atomic weight). The milliosmolar and milliequivalence values for the univalent ions are obviously identical. The chemical equivalence of the divalent ions is twice their milliosmolar value. The term milliosmolar is used instead of millimolar to make clear the additive osmotic effect of individual ions; e.g., the milliosmolar value of a solution of sodium chloride is twice its millimolar value.[3]

Chemical Structure of Body Fluids. Blood plasma and interstitial fluid resemble each other closely, except for the presence in plasma of the considerable amount of protein, whereas in interstitial fluid there is a very small quantity of this nondiffusible component. (See the two middle diagrams, Figure 183.) This difference requires adjustment of the concentrations of the diffusible ions in order to preserve total cation-anion equivalence (Donnan equilibrium) within the interstitial fluid. The diagram of the interstitial fluid reveals that the base equivalence of plasma protein has been replaced by a balanced reduction of cation (note the shorter Na· column), and an increase in diffusible anion (note the longer HCO₃′ and Cl′ columns). This results in a total of equivalents in interstitial fluid which

is less than that in plasma—in other words, the concentration of electrolytes is less. The total of equivalents in plasma stands above that in interstitial fluid by approximately the base equivalence of plasma protein (16 mEq./L.). Owing to its multivalency, the *chemical* equivalence of protein is about 8 times its concentration value.

The difference in *osmotic values* is approximately 2 milliosmols per liter—this being dependent upon the actual difference in ion concentration without regard to valence. The small difference of 2 milliosmols is of great importance in promoting normal extracellular fluid circulation (Fig. 183). If the level of the serum albumin falls below normal levels, fluid may not be returned to the vascular system at a rate sufficient to prevent abnormal extravascular fluid accumulation. If protein is present in extravascular areas in amounts in excess of the very low level normally present in interstitial fluid, such important clinical states as *ascites, edema pericardial effusion*, etc., may result (see Chap. 31). A total value for the nonelectrolytes is placed across the top of the diagrams. The nonelectrolytes include the nutrient substances, such as glucose and amino acids, and the waste products of protein metabolism, such as urea. "The nonelectrolytes demand only expeditious conveyance. The electrolytes constitute a chemical framework on which rests the stability of the physical properties of extracellular fluid. Their transport is in terms of this requirement. This is the meaning of the large prominence of the electrolytes."[3]

In Figure 183 the values may be read on the left of the ordinate. The figures on the right give the total of equivalence (the sum of the values in both columns). The values given are those per liter of water—the space occupied by protein being (for this purpose) disregarded.

Note that Figure 183 shows that the plasma contains more total mEq. per liter of the various ions than interstitial fluid; that is, the plasma is somewhat more concentrated. Likewise, the cell fluid is more concentrated than the plasma. This is due to the presence of protein on one side of a membrane impermeable to it, a higher amount in the cells, a lesser amount in the blood plasma.

Even during good health there are of course numerous minor variations in the electrolyte values. Since water and other substances enter and leave the extracellular fluid irregularly, and since renal adjustments require some time, large deviations may occur in the presence of disease. Recovery is permitted by the elasticity of the electrolyte system.

Cell fluid differs greatly from extracellular fluid (Fig. 183). The two largest ionic constituents of extracellular fluid, sodium ion and chloride ion, do not easily pass the boundaries of the cell wall. In the cell, potassium constitutes the largest base component, while $PO_4^=$ and $SO_4^=$ are the largest anions or acid radicals. Although the two fluids are osmotically balanced and are separated only by a thin sheet of protoplasm, their ionic patterns differ entirely.

As yet data concerning composition of cell fluid are scanty and incomplete. The average composition of muscle cell fluid has been inferred from various indirect measurements to be approximately as follows:

	mEq./L.
Na+	10
K+	150
Mg++	40
HCO3-	10
Cl-	15–20
PO4= and SO4=	150
Protein	40

It seems likely that cells of the various special organs and tissues will be found to have various compositions related to their unique functions.

Bone. The composition of bone is unique as compared to other tissues; only about 20 per cent is water and only about 35 per cent of the solids is protein. The remainder of the solid phase of bone is a latticework of inorganic salts. Of the total body sodium, 30 to 45 per cent is in bone, about 15 per cent in the extracellular phase. The largest part of the sodium present in bone is part of the crystal structure of bone, and 30 to 40 per cent of this is

exchangeable with an isotope of sodium in 24 hours. Potassium is also present in bone and is exchangeable, but in much smaller amounts.

When sodium or potassium deficits occur, they may be shared by bone. Both Na+ and K+ of bone apparently are exchanged with H+ ions in either direction as part of the mechanism opposing distortion of acid-base relationships.

High NaCl intake increases Na storage in bone; hyponatremia leads to mobilization of Na from bone. Since it has been shown that large quantities of sodium may enter or leave bone, it seems evident that exchanges of ions do not necessarily represent extracellular-intracellular shifts, but may result from exchanges between extracellular fluid and bone solids.[51]

Lymph and Lymphatics. Whenever there is an increase in the vascular hydrostatic pressure or in the protein content of the interstitial fluid, tending to cause an increase in the net transfer of fluid from the plasma to the interstitial space, the lymph vessels operate to reduce unphysiologic expansion of the interstitial fluid volume. Normally the volume of lymph reaching the plasma through the lymphatic vessels in an adult is about 1.5 ml. per Kg. body weight per hour, or a total of about 2,400 ml. per day. A considerable amount of protein escapes from the arterial capillaries by transudation from the plasma into the interstitial fluid. The lymphatic capillaries are far more permeable than the blood capillaries and constitute the special channels by which such protein is returned to the plasma. When for any reason the lymphatic capillaries cannot function normally to remove fluid, protein and crystalloids from the interstitial fluid, local accumulations of such fluid may occur, or generalized edema.

The protein content of human leg lymph is normally 0.5 to 0.7 per cent. The lymph flowing from the thoracic duct, since it comes largely from the intestine and liver, varies with the digestive processes and ranges in protein content from 2 to 4.5 per cent.

The Blood Plasma. In Figure 185 are given the normal values for the components of the electrolyte structure of blood plasma. The blood plasma is the most readily accessible portion of the extracellular fluid, and by studying changes in it one can judge the effectiveness of the regulatory mechanisms. The kidneys are the chief regulatory organs, controlling the concentration in the plasma of all its components except two, the carbonic acid and the protein. The carbonic-acid content is under respiratory control. Plasma-protein content depends upon amino-acid supply to the site of plasma-protein manufacture (apparently the liver), normality and adequacy of such manufacture, and upon abnormal protein losses (if any) through kidneys, ascitic fluid, etc.

The total ionic concentration is determined by the sum of the cation values, since the adjustable part of the ionic structure is the anion HCO_3^-. The total ionic concentration is not changed when other anion values are altered, since reciprocal alterations of HCO_3^- occur. Nearly all the base (cation) is sodium, and therefore the efficiency of the renal control of this one electrolyte element is paramount in the maintenance of stability of the osmotic value of the extracellular fluid.

The intake of water and of sodium is variable, and their supply to the body is not regularly related, therefore renal control is constantly in operation. However, the kidney requires time to establish osmotic equality between intracellular and extracellular fluid. Fortunately, a rapid supplementary form of control is available. An immediate prerenal adjustment takes place, depending upon the obligatory extracellular position of sodium, and consisting simply in the transfer of water from one compartment to the other as necessary to produce osmotic equilibrium. For example, if NaCl is taken in excess (beyond isotonic limits in proportion to the water ingested), water moves from intracellular to extracellular fluid. The increased volume of the extracellular fluid is then reduced by the kidney at leisure. Or the contrary takes place: there is a sudden large loss of extracellular electrolyte. Water shifts from the extracellular position into the cells, the excessive intra-

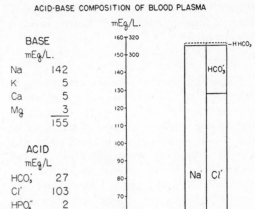

ACID-BASE COMPOSITION OF BLOOD PLASMA

mEq./L.

BASE
mEq./L.

Na	142
K	5
Ca	5
Mg	3
	155

ACID
mEq./L.

HCO$_3^-$	27
Cl'	103
HPO$_4^-$	2
SO$_4^-$	1
ORG AC	6
PROTEIN	16
	155

Fig. 185. A view of the various factors of the acid-base structure of the plasma in true perspective as regards their relative magnitudes. (Gamble, J. L.: Chemical Anatomy, Physiology and Pathology of Extracellular Fluid, Boston, The Harvard Medical School)

cellular-fluid volume being later reduced by excretion through the kidneys. Although either water or salt depletion alone may cause the same degree of contraction in total extracellular volume, the contraction of plasma volume is greater after salt loss. Loss of salt is more deleterious to the circulation than water withdrawal. Salt depletion causes intracellular overhydration, while water depletion causes cellular dehydration. Thus, changes in volume of the two compartments may take place to compensate for alterations in total ion content, thereby permitting maintenance of osmotic equilibrium. The requirements of osmotic balance may be satisfied temporarily by such shifts between the two compartments. It must be recognized, however, that the effects of loss of salt and loss of water, which usually occur together and proportionately, are opposite in character when separate or disproportionate. Salt loss leads to hypotonicity in both compartments and water loss to hypertonicity.

RENAL REGULATION OF BODY FLUIDS

Renal regulation consists essentially in *selective reabsorption* of water and solute substances from the glomerular filtrate by the tubules. Urine formation seems to be the result of simple filtration by the glomeruli, followed by modification of the composition of the glomerular filtrate by tubular absorption and tubular excretion.

The glomerular filtrate contains the same amount of water and the same concentration of contained substances (except for protein) as does the plasma. Some substances are normally practically completely absorbed by the tubules, others partially absorbed. The tubules are capable of adding certain substances to the urine. The distal tubules are the site of ammonia formation and the final adjustment of urinary pH. According to studies of glomerular filtration with inulin, approximately 125 ml per minute of filtrate, amounting to 180 liters in 24 hours, are produced. Urine volume usually does not exceed two liters, therefore almost all the water of the filtrate must be reabsorbed. With this huge amount of water must be reabsorbed all the important constituents of the plasma such as Na and Cl. The renal NaCl excretion (actually lost in the urine) amounts to about 95 per cent of the intake normally, and for the normal adult usually ranges from 6 to 15 Gm. daily. Gamble[3] has calculated that by weight the quantity of Na and Cl together reabsorbed may amount to a kilogram or more per 24 hours. Normally nearly all the water, Na and Cl (99 per cent) and the glucose filtered through the glomeruli are reabsorbed by the tubules, but about 60 per cent of the urea, 18 per cent of the SO_4, 12 per cent of the HPO_4 and 8 per cent of the K is excreted, reabsorption being less active for these substances.

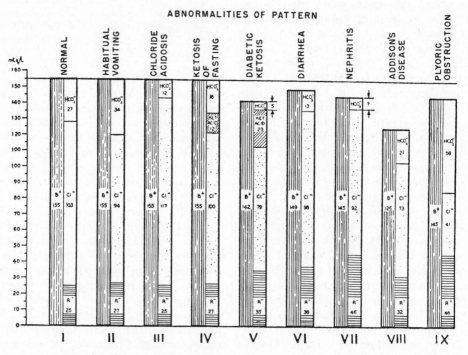

FIG. 186. Eight different types of abnormal patterns in the blood plasma compared with the normal pattern. The numbers within the columns give the concentrations in milliequivalents per liter. (Newburgh, L. H., and Leaf, A.: Significance of the Body Fluids in Clinical Medicine, Springfield, Ill., Thomas, p. 32)

The total daily urinary solute excretion averages normally about 30 to 40 Gm. It varies considerably both as to total amount and as to constituents, depending upon intake of various salts and foods and upon fever, increased destruction of tissue, rate of protein metabolism, etc. Representative average normal figures per liter of urine might be: urea 20 Gm., NaCl 8 Gm., K about 2 Gm., P about 2 Gm., S about 1.5 Gm., uric acid 0.6 Gm., and ammonia 0.6 Gm. The kidney allows excretion of a more dilute urine when the solute load is large; the larger the solute load the nearer the urinary osmolality approaches that of plasma. With heavy solute loads the specific gravity of the urine will approach the isosmolar level of approximately 1.010. Many substances, such as NaCl, Na_2SO_4, urea, sucrose and mannitol will therefore act as osmotic diuretics. Ingestion or parenteral administration of hypertonic salt solutions thus causes diuresis and dehydration.

Normally the greatest variable in daily water loss is sensible perspiration, the output by this route varying from zero to many liters. To preserve water balance two compensatory mechanisms operate: (1) adjustment of water intake as regulated by thirst, and (2) adjustment of water output as regulated by the kidneys. Renal control may vary the concentration through a range varying from four times the concentration of plasma to about one-sixth that of plasma (1400 m. Os./L. to 50 m. Os./L.).

In the absence of renal impairment, the rate of water output by the kidneys depends upon two control systems: (1) defense of the osmolality of the body fluids, and (2) defense of the volume of the body fluids.

The defense of osmolality depends upon the response of the distal renal tubules to the antidiuretic hormone and to the rate of excretion of solutes in the urine.

Volume changes definitely call forth homeostatic protective responses. A drop in extracellular fluid volume causes thirst and results in restriction of renal water loss. The physiologic mechanisms resulting in these defensive responses are not known. It has been suggested that one

mechanism may be the increased *aldosterone* secretion known to result from hemorrhage, dehydration, etc. Previously it had been postulated that the major volume receptors which control salt excretion are probably located in the walls of arteries. A well-documented reflex mechanism with a "volume receptor" leads to aldosterone secretion. The pathway is entirely outside the central nervous system and the connecting links are all humoral. The receptor is in the wall of the afferent arteriole of the glomerulus. It consists of or activates a small group of cells called the juxtaglomerular apparatus; they secrete renin. A *decrease* in stretch of the afferent arteriole activates renin secretion. Renin acts in the blood stream on protein precursors made in the liver which can be split to yield an active polypeptide called angiotensin II. This is the same material previously known to be a potent vasoconstrictor. Small amounts of angiotensin infused into the adrenal artery cause stimulation of secretion of the salt-retaining hormone aldosterone by the cells of the zona glomerulosa of the adrenal cortex. Such stimulation can occur with amounts of angiotensin too small to affect peripheral vascular tone. ACTH can stimulate the adrenal to produce aldosterone, but is much more potent in causing glucocorticoid (cortisone and cortisol) secretion. *Angiotensin is a relatively specific stimulant for aldosterone secretion.*[68]

The various constituents of the glomerular filtrate are acted upon in a number of different ways by the tubule cells. The mechanisms of the differential treatment of all the materials contained in the filtrate are as yet incompletely understood. It seems evident that active work is performed by the tubule cells, because they bring about movements opposite to those exerted through osmotic forces. Through work done by the tubule cells (1) water can be moved from a region of higher concentration to one of lower concentration; (2) solutes can be moved from a region of lower concentration to one of higher concentration.[47,49]

As concerns water, about 85 per cent of the glomerular filtrate is reabsorbed iso-osmotically. Work is involved, however, in conserving the remainder of the water, since it must be absorbed against the osmotic gradient. As the water reaches the lower tubule cells the concentration of the solutes becomes very high, but still the tubules must continue their valiant task of conserving body water and preventing dehydration. It is evident that impairment of renal function may be reflected quickly and most significantly in deranged fluid balance.

Urea is the urinary constituent chiefly responsible for the necessity of work by the renal tubules, since it is present in the urine in the largest amounts and in the highest concentration. If a man excreted one liter of urine it might normally contain about 15 grams of urea, the original glomerular filtrate having contained 30 grams in 180 liters. Hence, in this instance, the urea concentration of the urine is 90 times that of the plasma or the original plasma filtrate.

About 150 grams of glucose enter the upper ends of the tubules in 24 hours, all but 1 or 2 grams being reabsorbed.

The serum sodium and chloride concentrations are kept within rather narrow limits, despite wide fluctuations in the intake of sodium chloride and water, through the work of the renal tubules. If sodium is present in excess, the urine will become higher in sodium concentration than the plasma. However, should water be present in excess, the urine becomes dilute. If sodium conservation is needed, the total volume of the urine may remain the same, but the urine sodium concentration becomes less than that of the plasma.

Water and salts are reabsorbed principally in the proximal portion of the tubules, so that here the approximately 180 liters of water and 1 to 1.5 kilograms of NaCl are restored to the body. In the distal tubules more fluid is absorbed, further concentration of the urine takes place, and the final adjustments of the urinary pH are made, according to whatever the requirements may be at the time in preservation of the body's acid-base balance.

The remarkable exactitude and the deli-cacy of these renal functions are evident when one considers that should the renal tubules be so little impaired as one per cent in their water-retaining ability (through intrinsic renal disease, through hormonal control or otherwise), 1.8 liters in excess of normal might be lost each day in the urine, and dehydration would result.

Hormonal Regulation of Fluid Balance

The renal control of fluid balance is to a large degree under hormonal influence. The hormonal influence is exerted in the activity of the distal renal tubular cells and is concerned with the amount of water reabsorbed by the tubules and with the amounts of certain solutes, particularly sodium and potassium, which are reabsorbed or excreted.

Two types of hormones affect renal tubular control of water and solutes: (1) The neurohypophysial hormone, apparently produced primarily in certain cell groups in the anterior hypothalamus and produced or stored in the posterior lobe (pars nervosa) of the pituitary. It is called *vasopressin,* and for brevity and convenience, ADH. It exerts a major controlling influence on water reabsorption. (2) Certain steroid hormones produced in the cortex of the adrenal gland. There are several of these mineralocorticoids, of which *aldosterone* is by far the most potent in promoting sodium retention and potassium excretion.

In the distal renal tubules there is free permeability of the tubular membrane to water only under the influence of ADH; in the absence of this hormone only very small amounts of water can be absorbed and the tubular fluid passing on to be excreted as urine remains voluminous and dilute. The most striking example of this influence is observed in the disease *diabetes insipidus,* in which the power of the tubules to reabsorb water is greatly impaired and the renal water loss per day, instead of the normal 1.5 or 2 liters may be 10 or 20 liters. Relief of this disorder is possible by administration of antidiuretic hormone. A diuretic influence is apparently exerted by the anterior lobe of the pituitary and the thyroid gland and is normally balanced by the posterior pituitary antidiuretic factor.[10] Urine-concentration tests indicate that patients with diabetes insipidus receiving a limited intake of fluid will continue to secrete urine of low specific gravity, with resultant dehydration and loss of body weight. In any case in which such a response is obtained, the diagnosis of organic damage of the supra-optico-hypophysial tract should be made. The normal antidiuretic effect exerted through the neurohormonal control maintained through the supra-optic nuclei and the posterior lobe of the pituitary gland is lost when the tract is injured bilaterally.

Dehydration or increased osmotic pressure of the blood brings about increased secretion of ADH and increased amounts of ADH have been detected in the body fluids in such states.[11] In the hypothalamus there are "osmoreceptors" which are sensitive to fluctuations of electrolyte concentration of the plasma.[12] Thus release of ADH is controlled by changes in the electrolyte concentration, a rise causing posterior pituitary stimulation (antidiuresis), a fall causing inhibition (relative diuresis).

Evidence indicates that ADH acts directly upon the renal tubules, with stimulation of these cells to absorb more water from the lumen of the tubule. Thus water is retained and urine volume is reduced.

In diabetes insipidus the degree of polyuria varies directly as the nitrogen excretion, which indicates that the kidneys in this disease cannot concentrate urea any better than they can salt. The antidiuretic hormone checks the excretion of water by re-establishing normal absorption in the tubules. The rate of elimination of Na and Cl is not changed by the activity of the hormone. If a normal kidney is already excreting a maximally concentrated urine, the action of additional ADH is not detectable. Thus it is possible with the hormone to inhibit a water diuresis, but not a diuresis induced by salt or urea, because the kidney is concentrating the salt or urea to its maximum ability.

If ADH is administered to a normal subject, the effect depends upon the amount of water available for excretion. If water is withheld, the volume of urine is not altered. If, however, water is given, the usual diuresis is prevented by the ADH, the urine volume is much less than would normally be the case and the specific gravity of the urine remains relatively high. Since ADH does not alter the excretion of salt and other solutes, *water intoxication* may result in normal persons given ADH and allowed large amounts of water.

The specific gravity of urine depends largely upon the concentrations of salts and of urea. In diabetes insipidus the volume of the urine tends to remain very high, its specific gravity very low, as long as fluid intake keeps pace with the water loss. Prolonged water deprivation may limit the output somewhat and raise the specific gravity. Injection of ADH in proper amounts will restore output and specific gravity to normal. If urinary specific gravity is low and volume high because of renal impairment, ADH cannot restore normal conditions.

Hickey and Hare have introduced a test to measure the ability to liberate the antidiuretic principle. Hypertonic chloride solution is given intravenously during water diuresis. If the diuresis is inhibited, the hypothalamico-hypophysial system is presumed to be normal. If there is no inhibition of diuresis, the diagnosis of diabetes insipidus may be made—for hypertonic salt in the body fluids normally calls for water retention through secretion of the antidiuretic hormone.

The simple "concentration test" of renal function depends largely upon the stimulus of water deprivation to promote release of ADH. After 12 hours of nocturnal deprivation of water, at least one of three hourly urine specimens should have a specific gravity of 1.023 or above (Fishberg). If the specific gravity is lower, renal disease is suspected. Progressive diminution of concentrating ability occurs with increasing renal impairment, until the base line is 1.010. This level is reached in the common forms of renal disease (arteriosclerosis, glomerulonephritis) when urea clearance is reduced to about 15 per cent of normal, glomerular filtration rate is only about 20 ml. per minute (compared to the normal 125 ml.), tubular secretory capacity is 20 per cent of normal and the number of nephrons has been reduced by about 40 per cent.

The cells of the distal convoluted tubules do a minimum of osmotic work when the urinary specific gravity is 1.010, for at this point the osmotic concentrations of the fluids at the two cell faces (tubule fluid and interstitial fluid) are approximately equal.[13]

The rate of tubular resorption of sodium, chloride and water is in some degree under the endocrine influence of the *adrenal cortex*. The cortisone group of steroids promote retention of Na, Cl, and water and loss of K. Deoxycorticosterone is some 30 to 50 times as effective in this respect. Aldosterone is effective in even smaller amounts, being some 25 times as potent as deoxycorticosterone in influencing electrolyte and water metabolism.[39,40,75] When the adrenal cortical principles concerned with sodium metabolism are secreted in inadequate amounts, sodium, chloride and water are excreted to a highly abnormal degree and dehydration develops. The clinical picture of the crisis of Addison's disease, with its evidences of prostration, dehydration, low serum Na and Cl, high serum K, and low blood pressure, is due in large part to renal loss of base and water.[37]

We studied adrenal function by measuring urinary 17-OH corticosteroids and 17-ketosteroids in five patients over periods of from one to three months in order to determine the importance of the adrenal in the physiologic conservation of salt (Daughaday and MacBryde[14]). We found no indications of increased pituitary adrenocorticotropic hormone (ACTH) activity or of increased adrenocortical secretion of glucocorticoids or of androgens after salt deprivation.

Nevertheless, sodium was conserved after salt deprivation and it seemed likely that the adrenal cortex played a part in the salt-conservation mechanism. We suggested that: (1) there is an adrenal cortical salt-retaining hormone, the release of which

is independent of ACTH, and that (2) an "idiorenal" mechanism or renal-adrenal influence might affect adrenal steroid activity and be concerned with renal tubular sodium reabsorption.[14]

Conn and his co-workers[9] at about the same time were studying the salt-conserving mechanisms set into operation by heavy sweating; they also concluded that an adrenocortical hormone then not yet identified reduced salt losses partly through the kidneys, but largely through the sweat glands.

Since then the powerful salt-conserving hormone has been found and identified as aldosterone.[39] It exerts a major controlling influence on the amounts of salt excreted in the urine and in sweat.[64,75] Aldosterone is largely or usually secreted independently of ACTH activity. Aldosterone secretion is increased by (1) restricted sodium intake; sodium losses; (2) increased potassium intake; (3) reduction in extracellular fluid; (4) muscular activity; (5) the upright posture; (6) trauma, surgical stress; (7) emotional tension.

When operating physiologically, aldosterone helps to restore effective circulatory volume. In some pathologic states the effective circulatory volume may be decreased by loss of fluid from the circulation into extravascular compartments with resultant production of edema, ascites, etc. The loss of *effective* circulatory volume may cause increased production of aldosterone, although the total body fluid and NaCl content may already be excessive. In a number of pathologic states such secondary *hyperaldosteronism* is known to occur. Among these are (1) congestive heart failure; (2) the nephrotic syndrome; (3) cirrhosis of the liver with ascites; (4) idiopathic hypoproteinemia; (5) renal disease, and (6) idiopathic periodic edema.[75] In many of these conditions there may be sequestration of blood in the venous system and decrease in arterial flow. The volume receptors may not distinguish between decreased volume and decreased pressure; therefore a fall in blood pressure caused by decreased cardiac output or lower peripheral resistance would also lead to salt and water retention.[68]

TYPES OF DEHYDRATION

Dehydration may be classified into three general types:

1. Conditions in which the water deficit exceeds the salt deficit;
2. Conditions in which the salt deficit exceeds the water deficit;
3. Conditions in which the water and salt deficits are present in approximately balanced or isotonic proportions.

PATHOGENESIS OF DEHYDRATION

Water Deficit Predominating

1. Lack of water intake: too ill, too weak, mentally obtunded, nausea, etc. Water loss proceeds through excretion via skin, lungs, etc.
2. Excessive sweating
3. Diabetes insipidus
4. Solute diuresis: this may occur if ill persons are given, either orally or parenterally, excessively concentrated food and fluids. There is inadequate water intake in proportion to the solutes provided; the solutes remove excessive water in the urine.

Salt Deficit Predominating

1. Adrenocortical deficiency
2. Renal salt-wasting diseases
3. Cerebral salt-wasting diseases:
In some cases of cerebrovascular accidents, acute encephalitis, bulbar poliomyelitis, and brain tumors, excretion of large quantities of salt may occur despite hyponatremia. The etiology is not clear. One theory is that there is derangement of neurogenic centers controlling renal tubular salt reabsorption. Some patients with this syndrome seem to have *inappropriate secretion of ADH;* the sequence seems to start with retention of water, then the resulting expansion of body fluids requires excretion of salt.[69] Although these patients have salt loss, if fluid intake has been relatively high, the signs and symptoms may be those of water intoxication. Therapy may require restoration of serum sodium by water restriction as well as by salt administration.
4. Diabetic acidosis (in some cases; in others water loss exceeds salt loss)
5. Low sodium diet plus diuresis.

Isotonic or Balanced Salt and Water Deficit. When there is simple loss of fluid from the gastrointestinal tract, the loss is balanced or isotonic. However, in many clinical conditions the fluid balance status of the patient is also influenced by other factors, especially if the disorder has persisted for some length of time (many hours or days). Thus:

1. Gastrointestinal fluid losses with cessation of intake are accompanied by loss of water from skin, lungs and kidneys: the net effect is of water loss in excess of salt loss.
2. Gastrointestinal losses replaced by water result in net salt loss in excess of water loss.
3. Hemorrhage produces an initial balanced loss; prompt thirst often occurs. If water is provided without salt, and renal losses of salt proceed, there is a net salt deficit.

Multiple Pathogenesis. In the classification given above the primary causes of the various chief types of dehydration have been separately listed: as dehydration occurs clinically, however, there are usually combinations of two or more pathogenetic mechanisms, although often one may predominate. A patient with diabetes mellitus, for example, may develop ketosis and have dehydration with great loss of Na^+ and Cl^-, but may also have vomiting, failure of water intake, and fever with excessive sweating from an infection.

Determination of the Nature of Deficits. In each case in which dehydration is suspected, evaluation of information from the history, the physical examination and laboratory tests will help in the analysis.

THE HISTORY may reveal abnormal factors influencing fluid intake and output, environmental temperature, etc. A knowledge of body weight before the present illness is of great help: sudden loss is usually due to fluid deficit and the amount of weight loss is of help in computing the extent of the deficit. A knowledge of the blood pressure before dehydration is very helpful: an apparently normal blood pressure may actually be hypotensive in a person known previously to have hypertension.

CHART OF FLUID BALANCE

INTAKE   OUTPUT

Day & Time	Body Wt.	Oral	Parenteral	Urine	Vomitus	Diarrhea	Insens. Loss	Sweat	Blood

FIG. 187. Form for clinical record of factors in fluid balance. One should enter volume estimates or actual measurements of causative factors; accurate record should be kept of oral and parenteral fluids used in treatment and of urine and other losses during therapy.

In problems of fluid balance it is of great help to measure whenever possible all fluid accessions and losses, or to estimate them as closely as possible, and to record them on a special balance sheet. As treatment is administered, the character and amount of fluids is entered on the chart (Fig. 187).

THE PHYSICAL EXAMINATION yields important information concerning the effects of water and electrolyte deficits and permits rough estimates of the type and degree of aberrations. One notes the state of consciousness, the color, moisture, texture and turgor of the skin and mucous membranes, the blood pressure, the peripheral arterial pulsations, the temperature and color of the extremities, etc. Deep, rapid respirations suggest acidosis, and in ketosis an acetone odor may be detected on the breath. Alkalosis may be indicated by positive Chvostek and Trousseau signs. Low blood pressure, weak peripheral arterial pulsations, tachycardia and pallor or cyanosis are suggestive of vascular collapse and impaired peripheral blood flow. Such evidences of seriously affected peripheral circulation imply large fluid deficits and extreme dehydration.

LABORATORY DATA. Among the most valuable laboratory aids in the analysis of fluid and electrolyte disorders are:

Hematocrit, Hemoglobin and Total Serum Proteins. These values are helpful in the estimation of the extent of contraction of plasma volume. When proportionately elevated they indicate hemoconcentration due to fluid deficit.

Serum sodium concentration normally ranges from 132 to 142 mEq./L. The serum sodium may be high, low or normal in concentration during dehydration, depending upon the relative amount of water lost from the plasma. When hyponatremia is associated with dehydration, it suggests great deficit in extracellular fluid volume, or hyperglycemia or hyperlipemia.

Hyponatremia with dehydration and significant contraction of fluid volume implies that diuresis has not occurred as it normally does to protect the normal effective osmolality of the body fluids. The absence of such diuresis indicates that fluid volume has been sufficiently reduced to cause secretion of ADH; there must be great contraction of *extracellular fluid volume* to function as an adequate stimulus to promote the secretion of ADH. (One recalls that the *usual* effective stimulus results from an increase in osmolality of the extracellular fluid, with consequent cellular dehydration.)

Hyponatremia With Hyperglycemia. At normal glucose concentrations, the glucose has relatively little effect upon the total osmolality of the extracellular fluid. If, however, hyperglycemia is considerable, glucose increases the osmolality of the extracellular fluid to a significant degree, water is drawn from the cells into the extracellular compartment and the serum sodium concentration is in consequence decreased. The total effective plasma osmolality may be within normal limits when there is hyperglycemia, and hyponatremia and dehydration.

One may calculate the effective tonicity as suggested by Welt.[70] *Method:* Subtract 100 from the patient's blood concentration of glucose in mg. per cent; multiply by 10 to convert to mg. per liter; divide by 180, the molecular weight of glucose. The figure derived indicates the *excess* of glucose in millimols or milliosmols per liter. Divide by 2 since 1 mM of the sodium salts concerned provides 2 mOsm.). Add the figure derived to the serum sodium concentration as determined at the same time. The sum will indicate the effective osmolality or to-nicity of the plasma at the time. If it is between 132 and 142 it may be considered normal; (part of the usual osmolar effect of sodium is, in the presence of excess glucose, significantly exerted by glucose).

Example.
Given:
Serum Na^+ = 115 mEq. or mOsm./L.
Blood glucose = 880 mg. per cent

$$\frac{(886 - 100) \times 10}{180} =$$

43.7 mOsm. glucose /L.

$$\frac{43.7}{2} = 21.8$$

$$115 + 21.8 = 136.8 \text{ mOsm./L.}$$

In this example the tonicity is within normal limits despite the great reduction in the concentration of sodium in the serum.

Hyponatremia with Hyperlipemia. The concentration of serum sodium and other electrolytes is ordinarily expressed per unit volume of serum. It would be more precise to express such concentrations per unit volume of *serum water*. Normally the value for serum water is so large and constant (90 to 93 per cent) that the error is not significant. However, in hyperlipemia the serum lipids occupy a larger volume and the percentage of serum that is water may be drastically reduced to as low as 70 to 80 per cent.[71] An average concentration of sodium of 138 mM./L. in a serum with water content of 93 per cent equals 148.4 mM./L. of serum *water*. If the same concentration were present in the *water* of a lipemic serum containing only 80 per cent water, the concentration per liter of *serum* would be 148.4 × 0.80 = 118.7 mM. Thus a very low serum sodium may be present with no decrease in the effective osmolality of the extracellular fluid.

Serum potassium concentration normally ranges from 3.5 to 5.3 mEq./L. The total quantity of potassium in the extracellular fluids is so small that relatively slight shifts of K into or out of cells cause significant changes in serum K concentration. For example, at a serum K level of 4 mEq., the total K in the extracellular fluids might be 64 mEq. (4mg. × 16 L.). There might occur a 25 per cent loss of extracellular K to 48 mEq., but if this were accompanied by a 25 per cent contraction of extracellular volume to 12 L., the serum K would still be 4 mEq./L. If fluid were taken without K, the extracellular compartment might be re-expanded from 12 to 16 L., still containing only 48 mEq. of K, the concentration now being only 3 mEq./L.

Blood urea nitrogen normally ranges from 8 to 18 mg. per cent. The level of the serum BUN depends upon the rate of formation and the rate of excretion; the rate of excretion depends upon the glomerular filtration rate and the amount that diffuses back through the tubules. When urea is not being formed at an accelerated rate and there is no renal damage affecting excretion or absorption, the serum BUN reflects the adequacy of hydration. In serious dehydration the BUN may be elevated both because of inadequate filtration due to reduced renal blood flow and because of diminished excretion by the tubules into the urine, practically all the water and the urea being reabsorbed.

The urine provides much information concerning the state of hydration and the status of renal function. The volume of urine and its concentration provide significant data. A highly concentrated urine implies adequate kidney function in the presence of a powerful antidiuretic stimulus (or actual severe fluid deficit). A high volume of urine with low specific gravity suggests lack of ADH (diabetes insipidus) or extensive renal disease with great impairment of tubular reabsorption of water. Analysis of the urine for electrolytes may be informative: significant natriuresis in the presence of hyponatremia suggests a salt-wasting disease. Potassium losses in the urine suggest cellular dehydration. Routine urinalysis may reveal albuminuria and other changes suggestive of renal impairment, or glycosuria explaining ketosis and dehydration.

ASSESSMENT OF FLUID AND ELECTROLYTE DEFICITS

Water deficit is suggested by thirst, dry mucous membranes, loss of skin turgor, etc. Biochemical evidences include all the signs of hemoconcentration: elevated hematocrit, hemoglobin and electrolyte values. *Overhydration* occurs if salt-free fluids are given in excess during renal shutdown. The clinical signs are restlessness, apprehension, muscle cramps and sometimes the convulsions of water-intoxication. Low serum Na is the cardinal biochemical finding.

Sodium and Chloride Deficits. Deficits of sodium usually are accompanied by deficits of other extracellular ions, especially chloride, and of extracellular water. History of conditions causing renal sodium loss (chronic glomerulonephritis, low-sodium diet plus excessive diuresis, diabetic acidosis, adrenocortical deficiency) are suggestive. Abnormal loss of gastrointestinal fluids should arouse suspicion. The clinical signs are primarily those of peripheral vascular collapse: cyanosis, cold, clammy skin, rapid thready pulse, hypotension, and severe oliguria. Biochemical signs are those of decreased plasma volume and hemoconcentration plus, in severe cases, evidence of renal failure: elevated blood urea nitrogen and phosphorus, lowered CO_2 combining-power. The serum Na may be low, also the serum Cl, but these determinations may be within normal limits if there is hemoconcentration. They may become low after establishment of normal hydration. *Sodium excess* is accompanied nearly always by excess water retention in the body and edema. The serum sodium is apt to be within normal limits except during periods of water transfer.

Potassium derangements are discussed below under Intracellular Effects of Dehydration. It is essential to remember that intracellular K deficit may be present with normal or elevated serum K.

Bicarbonate and Anion-Cation Balance. The pH of the blood and of the extracellular fluid is determined by the ratio of the bicarbonate and other buffer anions (summed as "buffer base") to the concentration of carbonic acid. Since the latter is regulated by gas exchange in the lungs and the former by metabolic and renal transfers, abnormalities in the anion-cation balance may occur from either primary *respiratory,* or primary *metabolic* disorders. Secondary or compensatory changes may occur

in the other half of the system, however, so that biochemical findings will not always indicate which change is primary; clinical evidence is necessary to permit proper interpretation of the laboratory data.

ACID-BASE BALANCE AND WATER BALANCE

The mechanisms which make possible selective resorption by the tubules are not understood. The average normal diet is predominantly "acid-ash" in character, requiring an excess of excretion of acid over base so that the normal pH of plasma (7.4) may be maintained. This is accomplished by (1) direct saving of base by secretion of acid urine and by (2) substitution of ammonium for plasma base to cover acid radicals as they enter the urine.

The enormous degree of base-conservation constantly taking place is revealed by simply measuring the urinary pH, which is usually between 5 and 7. It must be remembered that urine at pH 6.4 is ten times as acid as blood plasma at 7.4, while urine at pH 5.4 is one hundred times as acid. Thus the acidity of the urine indicates the excretion of large amounts of acid and a corresponding saving of large amounts of base. The most acid urine the kidney can form is pH 4.5. Thus only negligible quantities of strong acids such as sulfuric or hydrochloric can be excreted as free titratable acid. Such strong acids are neutralized by Na^+ or K^+ in the plasma, but through renal tubular activity may be excreted through combination with ammonium ions.

Saving of base by excretion of acid urine (usually about pH 6) is made possible by (1) excretion of certain weak organic acids (such as citric acid) without the base linked to the acid ions in the plasma, by (2) excretion of HPO_4^- as monobasic phosphate rather than as dibasic phosphate as it exists in the plasma, and by (3) conservation of base by failure to excrete bicarbonate in the urine. It is reabsorbed by the tubules, the sodium retained and the CO_2 excreted by the lungs.

Respiratory Regulation. The relatively enormous amount (about 2 lb. daily) of the most abundant end product of metabolism, carbonic acid, is removed by the lungs without expenditure of base. The bicarbonate buffer system is particularly effective in permitting rapid readjustments of pH. Saving of base takes place by the interaction of bicarbonate with the relatively strong acids formed as a result of metabolic activity in the tissues (hydrochloric, sulfuric, phosphoric and lactic acids); the excess of carbonic acid is removed (as carbon dioxide) through the lungs. Carbon dioxide is constantly being formed through oxidative processes in the body and (as carbonic acid) it can quickly combine with excess amounts of alkali to form bicarbonate. Thus, the respiratory protective mechanisms guard against either acidosis or alkalosis and protect the body against loss of electrolytes and water.

"Respiratory acidosis" may occur, with a slight increase in the CO_2 combining power of the plasma when CO_2 is retained in excess (in asphyxia, emphysema, morphine narcosis, etc.). "Respiratory alkalosis" may occur from a decrease in blood carbonic acid due to hyperventilation (in hysteria, encephalitis, at high altitudes, etc.). These primarily respiratory deviations in acid-base balance are not associated with any considerable abnormalities in water balance. Note that the CO_2 content of the plasma is high in respiratory acidosis and low in metabolic or renal acidosis; it is low in respiratory alkalosis and high in metabolic or renal alkalosis.

Renal regulation. The *renal protective mechanisms* are more often deranged and are therefore of the greatest clinical importance. The three chief modes of conserving base are:

1. The three renal mechanisms which permit the excretion of acid urine, permit the return of base (chiefly sodium) to the body, and preserve the stability of plasma pH at approximately 7.4. Through them the base is not normally excreted (a) as B_2HPO_4 or (b) as $BHCO_3$ to any significant extent or (c) with the organic acids. Not only is base conserved but water also, since if these acids took base out with them into the urine, corresponding amounts of water would be excreted.

2. The ammonium-forming ability of the distal renal tubules which permits the saving of Na^+ ions, NH_4^+ ions being substituted for them in combination with acid radicals, the ammonium compounds then being excreted in the urine. Likewise, the renal tubules are able to substitute H^+ ions for base ions.

3. The resorptive powers of the renal tubules are the means through which enormous quantities of sodium (and of water) are returned to the plasma.

These *base-sparing* mechanisms are also *water-sparing,* and the buffer systems are defenses not only against *acidosis* but against *dehydration.*[32,41,42,43,46]

If one assumes that 180 liters of plasma are filtered through the glomeruli per 24 hours and that each liter contains 27 mEq. of bicarbonate, one finds that 4,860 mEq. or nearly one pound (expressed as sodium bicarbonate) is delivered into the tubules daily. Normally only 1 or 2 mEq. escape into the urine each day—the resorption by the renal tubules is practically 100 per cent.

The renal stabilization of body fluid bicarbonate rests upon (1) the renal conservation described above, and upon (2) mechanisms which promote the elimination of acid ions without the base they bind in the blood and permit restoration of that base to the body as bicarbonate.[46,47]

Under certain much less frequent conditions the buffer systems may be brought into play to combat the reverse condition, *alkalosis.* When base is ingested in excessive amounts (for example, sodium bicarbonate in relieving indigestion or treating peptic ulcer), or when chloride is lost (vomiting), an alkaline urine containing considerable amounts of bicarbonate may be excreted. Either acidosis or alkalosis tends to cause diuresis, because the kidney acts promptly to rectify any disturbance in acid-base equilibrium. Therefore, all the buffering and protective systems guarding the acid-base balance also defend body water.

ACIDOSIS AND DEHYDRATION

Acidosis may be defined as reduction in body base. It is usually measured by determining the CO_2 combining-power of the plasma, the normal range being between 55 and 65 volumes per cent (25 to 29 mEq.

per liter). Values below 25 mEq./L. indicate loss of base. Actual measurement of the plasma hydrogen ion concentration may reveal *acidemia,* a true fall in pH resulting from uncompensated loss of base.

A number of conditions leading to acidosis and dehydration may occur. These include:

1. Excess acid ingestion
2. Inadequate base intake
3. Loss of base (vomiting, fistula, diarrhea)
4. Renal failure (acid retention and base loss)
5. Inadequate carbohydrate combustion.

It is apparent that if an excess of acid ions is ingested, base will be required to combine with it and provide for its excretion, and that the base reserve may thus be seriously depleted and considerable amounts of water lost.

If the base supply is curtailed, a deficit may soon develop, for some base is being lost constantly, the average normal sodium excretion in the urine being about 4 Gm. daily.

Gastrointestinal Loss of Base. Very large amounts of base are secreted into the intestine in the alkaline pancreatic secretion, the bile and the duodenal mucosal secretion (Table 30). Normally, practically all the fluid and the base secreted into the intestine are reabsorbed. Any disorder interfering with resorption of this base and water will cause dehydration. The tendency to such dehydration will be increased by the relative chloride excess and resultant increase in chloride and water output through the kidneys. The importance of conserving this fluid and base is emphasized when one observes that the digestive secretions may total 8,200 ml. daily in a person whose blood-plasma volume is 3,500 ml.

The development of severe dehydration and electrolyte depletion from diarrhea caused by various types of dysenteries, food poisoning, and ulcerative colitis is frequent and well-recognized. A similar but less familiar syndrome may occur with certain colonic neoplasms, particularly *villous adenomata* of the rectum and sigmoid.[71A] Symptoms of abdominal distress may be present for months or years before copious passage of mucous occurs. There may be rapid development of severe dehydration with hyponatremia, hypokalemia, azotemia and circulatory collapse. Most of the tumors are benign, but they may become malignant. Often the tumor is within reach of the examining finger or sigmoidoscope, but the tumors may be multiple. Water and electrolyte replacement is life-saving but is of only temporary benefit. Complete excision is necessary to halt the fluid depletion.

Renal failure may lead to base and water loss in several ways. *Glomerular damage* may lead to retention of $PO_4^=$ and $SO_4^=$ and other acid ions that will require base and water for disposal. *Tubular damage* may interfere with resorption of water and base. Inability to secrete a concentrated urine is characteristic of chronic nephritis. For adequate excretion of waste products the urine volume therefore necessarily becomes large and dehydration may occur at any time if for any reason the intake of water is limited. When large amounts of kidney tissue are destroyed (as in polycystic disease, hydronephrosis, etc.), the intake and output of water may be of such proportions as to suggest diabetes insipidus. In chronic nephritis, ammonium production is impaired and base is lost because this usual defense of plasma sodium is not available. This diuretic effect is at least partly responsible for the failure of edema to appear in chronic nephritis until plasma protein is greatly depleted. Thus dehydration may occur in chronic nephritis because of retention of acids, because of loss of base and because of impaired tubular resorption of base, with accelerated water loss.

The normal pH of the body fluids (7.4) is maintained by the kidney, which keeps

TABLE 30. VOLUME OF DIGESTIVE SECRETIONS PER 24 HOURS PRODUCED BY ADULT OF AVERAGE SIZE

Saliva	1,500 ml.
Gastric secretions	2,500
Bile	500
Pancreatic juice	700
Secretion of the intestinal mucosa	3,000
Total digestive secretions	8,200 ml.

the plasma concentration of bicarbonate-bound base at 25 to 29 mEq./L., and by the respiratory system, which stabilizes the plasma carbonic acid level at 1.25 to 1.45 mEq./L. Stability of hydrogen ion concentration does not require fixed values for $H.HCO_3$ and $B.HCO_3$, but depends upon the maintenance of their 1:20 ratio, thus permitting flexibility in control.

The role of the kidneys in maintaining the bicarbonate concentration is a dual one, involving (1) salvage of the filtered bicarbonate and (2) restoration to the body of base utilized in neutralizing acids for renal excretion. In protecting and restoring bicarbonate, normally the renal tubules perform the amazingly efficient task of reabsorbing a pound or more of sodium bicarbonate daily, with loss of less than 0.1 per cent into the urine.

The tubular mechanisms for substituting hydrogen or ammonium ions for sodium ions in the tubular urine are of particular physiologic interest and clinical importance (Fig. 188).[41,46,47,78] Through substitution of these ions, acids may be excreted in free titratable form or in combination with ammonia, without loss of base. Both substitutions are performed in the distal segments of the tubules.[15]

The acidosis and dehydration of renal disease may thus be (1) partly the result of the inability of damaged renal tubules to exchange hydrogen ions and ammonium ions for base at a rate sufficient to compensate for the metabolic load, (2) partly due to failure of the tubules to absorb sodium bicarbonate, and (3) partly from retention of phosphate and sulfate with consequent displacement of bicarbonate.

Sulfonamide drugs block to some extent the renal tubular replacement of sodium ions with hydrogen ions, so that base, normally replaced by hydrogen ions and reabsorbed, is excreted in the urine. Such loss of considerable amounts of base may lead to acidosis and dehydration.

Adrenocortical activity is related to renal response to acidosis.[15,37,40,78] Not only are adrenocortical hormones necessary to adequate absorption by the tubules of sodium and water, but they are necessary for increasing the production of ammonia and

titratable acidity (see Fig. 188). In experimental animals it has been demonstrated that (1) adrenalectomized animals normally cannot conserve sodium during induced acidosis, nor can they adequately increase ammonia and titratable acidity under such conditions; (2) the deficiency in renal re-

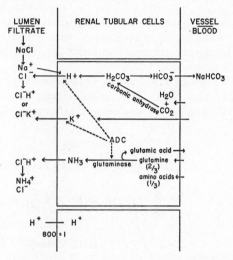

FIG. 188. Sites of action of adrenal cortex hormones (ADC) in renal tubular control of electrolytes. The diagram shows the processes involved in acid-base regulation as they are believed to operate in the distal renal tubular cells. The primary event is the exchange of H^+ ions dissociated from carbonic acid within the tubular cell for base ions in the tubular urine. Base is thus conserved for return to body fluids (Na^+ plus HCO_3^- equals $NaHCO_3$, etc.)

Note that the diffusion of ammonia into the urine is important to neutralize the H^+ ions. Some free H^+ ions may be excreted in the urine, but the capacity of the tubular cells to produce free acid in this way is limited to a concentration gradient of H^+ ions of 800 to 1. NH_4^+ ions, formed by union of H^+ ions with ammonia (two thirds from glutamine, one third from amino acids), reduce the concentration of free H^+ ions, thus reducing the gradient and facilitating flow of H^+ ions into the urine.

The probable sites of action of adrenal cortex hormones (ADC) are shown, indicating their importance in the tubular mechanisms involved in the exchange of hydrogen ions, potassium ions and ammonium ions for sodium ions.[37]

sponse can be corrected with desoxycorticosterone or adrenal cortex extract; and (3)
acidosis causes adrenocortical activation
with decrease in ascorbic acid and cholesterol content of the gland. As yet a complete explanation of the adaptive response of the kidneys to acidosis is lacking,
but an important part is undoubtedly
played by stimulation of the adrenal cortex
in some way by the acidosis, with resultant
stimulation of renal tubular activity by
adrenocortical hormones.

Lack of Carbohydrate Oxidation. Whenever the chief fuel, carbohydrate, is not
available or for any reason cannot be uti-

lized in adequate amounts, acidosis may
develop, with resultant dehydration (Fig.
189). This comes about as the consequence
of (1) destruction of body protoplasm with
release of $PO_4^=$ and $SO_4^=$, which require
base for excretion; of (2) excess Cl^-, from
reduction of the base and the volume of
the extracellular fluid, also requiring base
for excretion; and of (3) ketone-body production due to excess oxidation of fats.
These ketone bodies are excreted partly
as free organic acids and partly combined
with base. All these products require an
increase in the water output. The increase
in the water excretion can only partly be

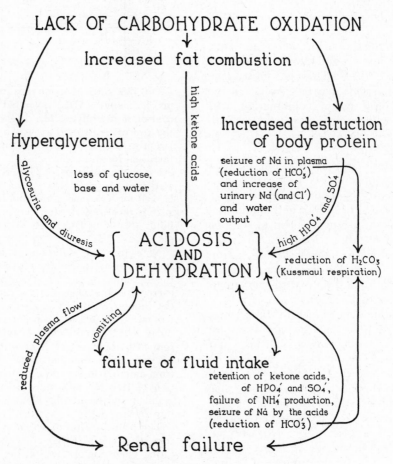

FIG. 189. Diagram illustrating mechanisms involved in the production
of the acidosis and dehydration of diabetic coma.

compensated by increasing the water intake, since in the presence of diuresis a smaller than normal proportion of these substances and of water is reabsorbed by the tubules. Whenever carbohydrate is supplied or its combustion is facilitated these processes are reversed toward normal.

Acidosis and dehydration depending upon failure of normal carbohydrate combustion may occur from:

1. Starvation (failure of intake)
2. Ketogenic (low-carbohydrate) diets
3. Hypoglycemia
4. Loss of carbohydrate from the gastro-intestinal tract (vomiting, diarrhea, fistula)
5. Diabetes mellitus.

Other factors often accompany limitation of carbohydrate combustion and increase the severity of the acidosis and dehydration. Among these factors are limitation of water intake and renal failure. If there is, in addition to loss of available carbohydrate, loss of base and fluid in the intestinal secretions by vomiting, diarrhea or fistula, the acidosis and the dehydration will be much more severe.

Diabetes mellitus constitutes a special and a common cause of acidosis and dehydration (Fig. 189). In the absence of adequate carbohydrate combustion, fat and protein become the main sources of calories. Accelerated combustion of fat causes production of the ketone acids beyond the rate at which they can be metabolized. Accumulation of the organic ketone acids results from the accelerated fat combustion and leads to loss of water and base. Breakdown of body protein and lipids produces an excess of $SO_4^=$ and $PO_4^=$, calling for more base and leading to further water loss. The excessive drain on the reserve of base soon becomes evident, despite a fivefold to tenfold increase in the rate of excretion of titratable acid and of ammonia. Soon the renal compensation fails to keep pace, and the bicarbonate stores are progressively depleted. The blood and other body fluids may be unable to maintain their normal slightly alkaline reaction as reserve base is depleted; acidemia occurs and death may result. The excessively high blood sugar leads to such rapid renal loss of glucose that the tubules cannot reabsorb it all, and severe glycosuria with further water loss results because of the osmotic effect of the hypertonic glucose solution in the tubules. Glucose that escapes resorption in the tubules requires for its excretion the same amount of water required by an osmotically equivalent quantity of salt. Glucose does not replace Na and Cl from the urine but, on the contrary, accelerates their excretion. Glycosuria is therefore especially dehydrating. Vomiting is a common accompaniment of diabetic acidosis, and the dehydration is thus further increased. Chloride is excreted in excess because of the reduction in extracellular-fluid volume made necessary by the reduction in sodium. The carbon dioxide combining-power of the blood plasma (normally about 60 volumes per cent, or 27 mEq./L.) may be reduced to 20 volumes per cent (9 mEq./L.) or less as the patient succumbs to severe diabetic acidosis and lapses into coma. Very deep and rapid "Kussmaul" respiration appears. This is characteristic of severe acidosis and results from stimulation of the respiratory center with consequent effort to expel great amounts of CO_2. The dry, inelastic skin, the dry tongue, the soft eyeballs, the weak pulse and the low blood pressure complete the picture of the shocklike state occurring with extreme dehydration. The severe dehydration causes *renal disability* with further loss of base and retention of $SO_4^=$, $PO_4^=$ and organic acids. The renal failure may be sufficient to result in nitrogen retention and signs of uremia. Reversal of all the pathologic processes is brought about by supplying Na, Cl and water, insulin and carbohydrate in the milder cases and in those without impairment of renal function. If the acidosis is severe or prolonged, if the patient is a small child or an elderly person, if renal function is poor, it may be of considerable benefit to supply base as sodium bicarbonate or sodium lactate as well as that furnished in physiologic NaCl solution. The intracellular ions K^+ and $PO_4^=$ should also be included in the parenteral fluids supplied, if the serum potassium is low.

ALKALOSIS AND DEHYDRATION

If dehydration occurs from vomiting that results primarily in the loss of gastric secretion (HCl), as in pyloric obstruction, alkalosis may accompany it. Signs of tetany may be present. In pernicious vomiting, after prolonged gastric drainage, or following repeated ingestion of large quantities of sodium bicarbonate, the concentration of chloride in the body fluids is reduced and that of bicarbonate is proportionately elevated. Despite the alkalosis, the urine may remain acid and contain essentially no bicarbonate. It appears that as long as the blood chloride is depressed, the kidney preserves bicarbonate, as if, having failed to maintain the normal proportions of the anions Cl^- and HCO_3^-, total concentration at least is maintained. Only when the blood chloride is elevated to normal (and the blood K^+ also, if there has been hypokalemia), is the renal bicarbonate threshold restored to the normal range. Correction of the condition by giving intravenous physiologic NaCl solution is possible, since the body retains the Cl, excreting the excess Na and excreting HCO_3 instead of Cl in the urine until the chloride deficit has been compensated.

When milder degrees of alkalosis are present (or more accurately, states of *alkali excess*), spontaneous adjustment may be very prompt. If as little as 4 Gm. of sodium bicarbonate is ingested, the urine becomes less acid promptly. Through this mechanism either small amounts of base or very large amounts of base may be excreted. This may be accomplished even though the urinary pH may shift from the average normal of 6.0 to reactions only slightly more alkaline than that of the blood plasma. Because of the buffering action exerted by the *high carbonic acid content of alkaline urines,* much larger amounts of base can be eliminated in the urine than one might calculate. The most alkaline urine the kidney can elaborate is about pH 8.0.

Excess intake of the basic salts of sodium may cause a rise in the pH of the extracellular fluids but has little diuretic effect if renal function is normal, since the excess bicarbonate is eliminated by inhibition of its resorption in the tubules. Sodium excess in pathologic states may tend, on the contrary, to produce edema, sodium and water being retained in excess amounts, especially in circulatory or renal failure (see Chap. 31).

Whatever the cause of the alkalosis, the alkali excess must be disposed of, and the usual mode of disposal is diuresis. Alkalosis therefore, in the absence of renal impairment, tends to produce dehydration. Alkalinizing salts such as bicarbonate or citrate promote diuresis but the effects are less pronounced than with acidifying salts, such as ammonium chloride, because distortion of the electrolyte pattern is less severe.

INTRACELLULAR EFFECTS OF DEHYDRATION

Salt loss causes intracellular overhydration, while water depletion causes cellular dehydration. A balanced loss of water and salt results in contraction of both extracellular and intracellular compartments. Excess fluid intake, especially with salt depletion, results in cellular overhydration and may produce the symptoms of water intoxication.

When there is considerable loss of extracellular electrolyte and water, maintenance of osmotic equilibrium may require removal not only of water but of electrolyte from the cells. Dehydration therefore causes some loss of potassium from the cells, accompanying the much larger loss of sodium from extracellular fluid. Thus the interstitial-fluid reservoir does not completely defend the cells, as withdrawal of water and electrolyte does occur. However, since intracellular-fluid volume is two and one-half times that of extracellular fluid, the loss of fluid is proportionately smaller. Measurement of the sodium and the potassium lost, taking into consideration the relative concentrations of these two bases as they exist in the body fluids, will permit calculation of the amounts of fluid lost from each compartment.

POTASSIUM METABOLISM AS RELATED TO ACIDOSIS, ALKALOSIS AND DEHYDRATION

Since potassium is the chief cation of intracellular fluid, derangements of the electrolyte or water metabolism which are severe enough to pass beyond the first-line defenses present in the plasma and in the interstitial fluid may be evident through decrease in the K content of the cells and through alterations of the K concentration of the extracellular fluids. Under normal conditions, 98 per cent of the body potassium is intracellular. Normally, K is present in cell fluid in a concentration of about 150 mEq./L. This is about 35 times its concentration in the blood serum (3.5 to 5.3 mEq./L.). Any considerable deviation from these narrow limits is apt to be associated with *disturbances in the conduction of impulses* through the nerves and in the function of muscle, both skeletal and cardiac. The *conduction system of the heart* is significantly affected by abnormal rise or fall in the serum K.

In the average normal diet, from 2 to 4 grams of K are ingested daily and the renal excretion of K is so regulated that the body remains in K balance. However, when K deficit exists, K is retained, and when there is a K surplus, the excess K is excreted. It should be noted that the renal tubules have not only the ability to absorb K, but they also can actively excrete it. Renal tubular secretion of potassium may occur in severe renal insufficiency and constitutes a mechanism to prevent accumulation of potassium to toxic levels in body fluids.[16] The renal tubules can curtail urinary Na loss almost to zero under certain circumstances, but even in the presence of cellular deficiency of K and low serum K, the urinary excretion of K continues. The rate of K loss in the urine may drop with a low serum K, but there is apparently an obligatory potassium loss in the urine; no such obligatory sodium loss occurs. Approximately 40 mEq. of potassium daily are required daily to avoid a negative K balance from renal loss of K.

Cardiac arrythmias may result from low serum K. A low serum K (and presumably low intracellular K) sensitizes the heart to digitalis and predisposes to digitalis intoxication. In the presence of digitalis intoxication, potassium administration may be indicated.[72] Digitalis should be administered with care to patients depleted of K (after vomiting, diuresis, etc.) Toxic doses of digitalis cause egress of K from myocardial cells and inhibit return of K into the cells. If K is given, hyperkalemia may develop. Elevated serum potassium may have serious myocardial depressant action (see below.)

Muscle metabolism is profoundly disturbed whenever there is severe derangement of intracellular potassium and striking symptoms may be observed involving both (1) *somatic muscles* and (2) *the heart.*

The transfer of glucose from the extracellular fluids into cells requires potassium. Serum K may fall even if K is administered with glucose. Even small *decreases in serum K* may be especially dangerous in two groups of patients: (1) those having severe K depletion, and (2) those receiving digitalis.[73] Such patients should, to prevent the precipitation of dangerous ventricular arrhythmias, be given at least 40 mEq. of K in 5 per cent glucose per hour of treatment.

Toxic doses of digitalis cause release of potassium from the liver and interfere with the uptake of K by the cells of skeletal and cardiac muscle. Therefore, when digitalis intoxication is treated by intravenous infusions of potassium salts, there is ever present the danger of causing *hyperkalemic* cardiac arrhythmias. Apparently such a consequence can be avoided if the oral or intravenous rate of administration is slow, not exceeding 0.5 mEq. of K per minute.[74]

Since it is difficult to judge from the level of the serum K or the amount of urinary K what the state of the intracellular potassium may be, and since certain pathologic states depend primarily upon the serum K concentration, the clinical recognition of abnormalities of K metabolism is more difficult than the diagnosis of Na, Cl and bicarbonate disorders.[44,52,53]

Potassium Deficiency. If intake of potassium is deficient and protracted, the obligatory excretion of K proceeds, with negative K balance resulting from its continued excretion in the urine.

Dehydration and trauma to tissue will accelerate loss of K from cells and thus increase urinary K loss. Abnormal drainages of gastrointestinal fluid cause much loss of potassium (vomiting, gastrointestinal suction, drainage from fistulas, diarrhea, steatorrhea, etc.). Potassium deficiency is especially apt to be found in patients suffering from such disorders who are maintained on the usual potassium-free parenteral fluids.[17]

In diuresis, especially if associated with conditions such as those above (with K loss from cells and little or no K intake), the K loss is accelerated and deficiency is especially apt to occur.

It should be emphasized that when serum Na or Cl is low (abnormal hydration factors being eliminated), there is a body deficit of such ions. In the case of the intracellular electrolyte potassium, however, there is no such relatively simple approach to the assessment of K deficits. Deficiency of K must be suspected primarily from the clinical circumstances, since serum K may be high, normal or low in such states, the blood level reflecting transport levels, and not necessarily tissue or cell content.

ACIDOSIS. In severe degrees of acidosis, hyperkaliemia is likely to occur, but the cells may be relatively depleted of K, and the body K balance may be negative. This may be true, for example, in *diabetic acidosis,* in which there is dehydration, loss of K in the urine (hemoconcentration and loss of K from cells). Before therapy, the serum K is usually normal or elevated, but after treatment is given K excretion decreases, K moves back into the cells, the extracellular fluid volume expands and the serum K may fall precipitously. To prevent serious K deficiency, therapy with fluids containing K may be imperative as soon as the initial *temporary hyperkaliemia* has been abolished. As much as 20 Gm. of potassium may be required in the first 48 hours to make up for the negative K balance, which may have been developing for a number of days.

ALKALOSIS (if renal function is adequate) leads to transfer of sodium from the extracellular to the intracellular fluids, with displacement of K from the cells and its loss in the urine. The K balance may be negative. The serum K may be low (as it often is, if urine volume has been high) or it may be normal or elevated (high K usually occurs if there has been oliguria). Such alkalosis may occur with chloride loss (pyloric obstruction, etc.). Treatment with solutions of NaCl alone will not correct the alkalosis: one must repair the K deficit as well as the Cl deficit before the serum bicarbonate returns to normal. In general, it appears that persons depleted of K tend to develop alkalosis and that alkalosis leads to depletion of K. A renal mechanism is involved, but the details of its operation are as yet incompletely understood.[18] When K is lost from the body either through the kidneys or the gastrointestinal tract much of it is accompanied by Cl taken from the extracellular fluids. This unbalanced loss of extracellular anions is compensated for by a rise in extracellular bicarbonate. This is apparently why acute potassium deficiency is usually associated with alkalosis.[19]

ADRENOCORTICAL HORMONES exert considerable control not only over Na absorption by the renal tubules, but also over the absorption and excretion of K through the renal tubules.[37] Persons with Addison's disease tend to lose Na and retain K. The adrenocortical steroids cause retention of Na and promote the excretion of K. Overdosage with deoxycorticosterone or cortisone may cause abnormally great K loss, with low serum K and serious clinical effects. If potassium intake is deficient while K excretion is kept at a normal or accelerated rate with deoxycorticosterone, foci of necrosis may occur in the heart muscle fibers with death from heart failure. This may occur in the course of treatment of Addison's disease (Goodof and MacBryde[20]). Clinical evidence of deficiency of potassium has been observed in patients treated with ACTH (adrenocorticotrophic pituitary hormone), and with cortisone.[38] In some patients with Cushing's syndrome, hyperactivity of the adrenal cortex is accompanied by evidences of potassium deficiency.

Thus, we have discussed how loss of potassium may occur

1. Through the urine, if intake is inadequate
2. Through tissue destruction
3. Through dehydration, diuresis and polyuria
4. With loss of gastrointestinal fluids

5. With acidosis
6. With alkalosis
7. With adrenocortical hormone effects. All these are mechanisms by which there may occur actual negative potassium balance. There is in these conditions a loss of potassium from the cells and from the body, but at various stages in these various conditions the serum K may be low, normal, or even high. A normal or higher than normal serum K may occur even in the presence of a true K deficit (1) if there is dehydration with hemoconcentration or (2) if the transfer of K from intracellular fluids to the extracellular fluid is rapid.

A *low serum K* may become evident in the potassium deficiency states (1) if diuresis is promoted by the use of parenteral fluids or if dialysis is employed with fluids containing inadequate potassium; (2) if the shift of K from serum to cells is suddenly brought about: (a) by unknown factors, such as those which apparently operate at the onset of an attack of familial periodic paralysis, or (b) by movement of glucose into the cells.[21] It appears that the mechanism by which the serum K is reduced is the formation of a monopotassium salt and its deposition with hexosediphosphate during the process of glycogen formation and storage. In familial periodic paralysis an attack can be produced by the intake of a large quantity of carbohydrate. In the hyperkaliemia of diabetic acidosis or of uremia, glucose and insulin therapy may lower the serum K to normal or subnormal levels; or (c) by adrenocortical steroids; deoxycorticosterone, or large doses of adrenal cortex extract or of cortisone tend to cause K shift from serum into the cells.

A low serum K may occur when there is no true deficiency in the cells or total body tissues. Either (1) dilution of the blood or (2) sudden shift of K into cells may bring about such a temporary lowering of serum K.

Clinical Signs of Potassium Deficiency. A low serum K which indicates cellular deficiency of potassium usually is accompanied by a gradual diminution of strength first. The muscles become flaccid; reflexes cannot be elicited. The patient may complain of weakness only, or of a numb, dead feeling, then partial paralysis, then complete paralysis. The paralyses usually occur mainly in the extremities, ascending from the periphery toward the center. The facial and respiratory muscles often remain unaffected, but frequently respiratory paralysis may endanger life.

In potassium deficiency cardiac arrythmias are apt to occur, especially if the patient has been receiving digitalis.[72,73,74,76] There are *electrocardiographic changes* occurring quite regularly when the serum K is below normal: depressed, broadened T waves, prolonged Q-T interval, and depression of the S-T segment. Now that the flame photometer has greatly facilitated serum K determinations, it is advisable not to depend upon the electrocardiogram alone, but, if it is possible, to determine also the serum K. These two laboratory tests plus a careful analysis of the patient's clinical status usually clarify the pathogenesis of signs and symptoms present and indicate logical therapy.

Potassium Intoxication: Hyperkaliemia. Abnormal elevation of the serum potassium concentration may occur as the result of one or more of the following pathogenic mechanisms:

1. Renal failure from any cause, especially if associated with oliguria or anuria. Hyperkaliemia is rare if the urine volume exceeds 500 ml. per 24 hours. The principal limiting factor in the excretion of potassium is reduction of the glomerular filtration rate.

2. Renal failure with high K intake or Na depletion, particularly when both occur simultaneously. Potassium clearance remains remarkably constant even in severe renal disease. When potassium excretion is limited the urine volume is a significant factor. Thus if there is oliguria and the K intake increases (for example, from the ill-advised administration of orange juice, which contains large amounts of K, or from the breakdown of red blood cells, which occurs with an incompatible transfusion), dangerous hyperkaliemia may suddenly be precipitated.

3. Trauma, tissue destruction, fever, the injection of epinephrine—any stimulus

adequate to cause "the alarm reaction"—may accelerate catabolic processes above the normal rates, and, if K excretion is impaired, hyperkaliemia may result.

4. Dehydration. Increased tonicity of the plasma causes passage of Na into cells and of K into the extracellular fluids. Since dehydration is apt to be associated also with oliguria and with impaired renal function, the tendency toward a high serum K will progress until the dehydration and oliguria are corrected.

5. Infusion of hypertonic fluids: dehydration is increased and the shift of K from cells to plasma is facilitated.

6. Acidosis, especially with the common associated factors of dehydration, oliguria and Na deficit.

7. Alkalosis, when complicated by dehydration and oliguria.

Clinical Signs of High Serum Potassium. The clinical signs of high serum potassium concentration closely simulate those of low potassium concentration: progressive weakness, then flaccid paralyses of the extremities, later, difficulty in phonation and respiration; often cardiac arrhythmias. Because of the clinical similarity of the symptoms occurring with abnormalities of K metabolism in either direction, it is highly desirable, whenever possible, to

follow both the serum potassium and electrocardiographic changes for diagnosis and during and after treatment.[72,73,74,76]

It is important to point out that the electrocardiogram will reveal characteristic alterations, as a rule, before there are serious clinical evidences of hyperkaliemia.[22] These are usually apparent whenever serum K exceeds 7 mEq./L. The changes in the electrocardiogram occurring with the onset and progression of potassium intoxication are usually in this order and are quite constant:[22] (1) development of tall, narrow, pointed T waves; (2) depression of the S-T segment, which tends to become a direct line from the nadir of the S to the apex of the T wave; (3) auriculoventricular block; (4) decreased amplitude and increased duration of P waves; (5) intraventricular block, with lowered R and deeper S waves; (6) prolonged Q-T interval; (7) ventricular arrhythmia; (8) sinus bradycardia; (9) disintegration of the ventricular complexes; and (10) ventricular standstill.

Conclusions Concerning Relationships of Potassium Metabolism to Dehydration. Dehydration may cause loss of potassium in several ways. The serum potassium may be elevated or depressed in dehydration, depending upon a number of factors discussed above. Either acidosis or alkalosis may be present in dehydration, as determined by the pathogenesis of the dehydrated state, but hyperkaliemia is common in acidosis, low or normal serum K in alkalosis (except in severe oliguria). Whenever dehydration is present, disordered potassium metabolism may be expected. Whenever a derangement in potassium metabolism has occurred, abnormalities in fluid distribution have also occurred, usually with loss first of extracellular fluid with later loss of fluid from the cells and withdrawal of potassium from the cells.

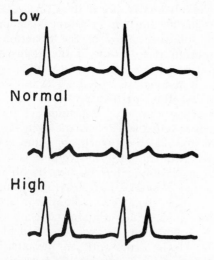

FIG. 190. Changes in the electrocardiogram produced by alterations in serum potassium concentration shown for unchanged heart rate.

DEHYDRATION AND RENAL IMPAIRMENT

Dehydration and renal dysfunction are related in two ways: (1) renal disorder may lead to water loss; (2) dehydration may cause renal failure.

1. The rate of plasma flow through the

kidney, as determined by diodrast-clearance studies, is about 740 ml. per minute. The total volume of blood passing through the kidneys is therefore about 1,300 ml. per minute. This is approximately a quarter of the total cardiac output under basal physiologic conditions. About 125 ml. per minute, or approximately one fifth of the plasma entering the kidney per unit time, are filtered by the glomeruli. Some 99 per cent or more of the glomerular filtrate is reabsorbed by the tubules. From these considerations it is apparent that rapid and efficient movement of extracellular fluid through the kidneys, with rapid renal disposal of waste products but retention of essential materials, is required for maintenance of normal fluid and electrolyte balance.

We have previously considered how derangements of renal function may interfere with water and electrolyte control. When tubular reabsorption is impaired in chronic nephritis, even to a slight degree, fluid loss is excessive and there is a tendency to dehydration. Added to this hazard is the inability of the damaged kidney to manufacture NH^4 with normal rapidity. The relative failure of the ammonium mechanism causes loss of fixed base. Whenever fixed base is lost from the plasma, water must be withdrawn and excreted to preserve the normal total ionic concentration in the plasma. Thus renal disease through impairment of both tubular function and ammonium production may cause dehydration. When, however, there is albuminuria sufficient to lower the plasma albumin, the diminished ability of the plasma to withdraw water from the interstitial fluid may combat the tendency to fluid loss, and if the hypoproteinemia is of sufficient degree, the opposite effect of fluid retention may occur with production of edema.

Not only may renal disease produce dehydration, but serious fluid loss may occur with renal dysfunction resulting from endocrine disorders. Derangement of hormonal control of tubular water absorption produces dehydration in diabetes insipidus, and hormonal disorder causes the sodium, chloride and water loss of Addison's disease.

2. If dehydration is severe, plasma volume may be greatly reduced and the rate of plasma flow through the kidney may fall to such a point that renal function may be seriously impaired. Extreme fluid loss of course affects all tissues and organs, but because of the very large plasma flow necessary to maintain the vital functions of the kidney, evidences of kidney failure quickly become apparent. Retention of waste products soon result in uremia, and the inability of the kidney to manufacture ammonium and to excrete acids causes acidosis. Thus severe dehydration, if it continues for any length of time, is characterized not only by (a) signs of water loss (dry, inelastic skin, dry mucous membranes, soft eyeballs, weight loss) and (b) signs of diminished blood volume (shock, low blood pressure), but by (c) evidence of renal failure (high blood nonprotein nitrogen, high serum potassium, acidosis).

Only in very severe degrees of dehydration does renal impairment appear, however, because of the wide, elastic and adjustable interstitial fluid compartment that protects the plasma volume. A man weighing 70 Kg. has approximately 15 per cent of his body weight as interstitial fluid (10.5 liters) and 5 per cent as plasma (3.5 liters). Many liters of interstitial fluid may be lost before serious reduction occurs in plasma volume. Studies have shown that from one-third to one-half of the extracellular fluid must be removed to produce the clinical picture of dehydration.

DEHYDRATION, SALT DEPLETION AND SHOCK

The adverse effects of extensive loss of body fluid upon the circulation are well recognized. Loss of fluid is an important factor in the production of shock following various types of trauma, including burns. The loss of fluid need not be external, since large amounts of fluid accumulate in the injured region and may be unavailable to the organism, at least temporarily. When shock is associated with such segregation of fluid, intravenous saline solution may produce prompt relief.

The relative importance of (1) *trauma* and its effect upon the nervous system, the circulatory system and the skeletal muscular system, of (2) *salt depletion,* of (3) *water depletion* and of (4) *disturbances of potassium metabolism,* in the production of shock needs clarification. In the absence of trauma, salt depletion may produce a form of peripheral vascular collapse closely resembling traumatic shock.[23] Plasma volume, cardiac output, circulation rate and blood pressure all decline sharply, and plasma protein falls. Water depletion alone, however, fails to produce such striking effects. When water alone is lost to a degree resulting in the same decline in total extracellular-fluid volume as that produced by the salt deficit, there is no peripheral vascular collapse. The cardiac output, plasma volume, mean arterial pressure and circulation rate may slightly decline. Usually little or no protein disappears from the plasma.

It should be noted that in the salt- and water-deprivation studies no close correlation could be established between the degree of drop in the plasma volume and the extent of the decrease in the cardiac output. Therefore the shocklike state produced by sudden salt depletion cannot be explained by diminished plasma volume alone. Withdrawal of NaCl results in a large shift of water from the extracellular to the intracellular phase, with consequent depletion of the former and expansion of the latter. The body fluids become hypotonic and the plasma volume is decreased. The hypotonicity of the body fluids and the lowered plasma-protein content, as well as the lowered plasma volume, deserve attention.[23,42,48] The fate of the protein is not known, but it is probably segregated somewhere within the body. Current concepts picture a continuous exchange between the protein of circulating plasma and that outside the vascular spaces. Salt depletion may displace the normal equilibrium. The greater circulatory collapse produced by salt loss as compared with water loss may be related to the loss of protein from the circulation. Lowering the plasma protein may favor the disproportionate decline in plasma volume, and thus aid in producing the drop in venous return, cardiac output and arterial blood pressure. However, such an explanation must remain for the present hypothetical. It seems quite as logical to consider that the salt depletion injures one or more parts of the cardiovascular system and thus produces shock. As extracellular salt is withdrawn, water moves (in response to osmotic forces) out of the extracellular fluid into the cells. Extracellular dehydration, intracellular overhydration and hypotonicity of both compartments result. Potassium is lost from the cells, and either hyperkaliemia or hypokaliemia may occur, depending upon a number of factors discussed in the section on potassium above. The changes in the sodium and potassium concentration of both intracellular and extracellular fluids alter the conduction of nerve impulses and affect both the physiologic and anatomic integrity of skeletal and cardiac muscle. These changes may directly injure the cells of the heart or blood vessels, producing shock, and indirectly and only incidentally causing loss of circulating protein. That is, the protein loss may be only another evidence of vascular damage and not a contributing factor in producing the shock.

PARENTERAL FLUIDS IN THE TREATMENT OF DEHYDRATION

Although this chapter is concerned with the etiology and the pathologic physiology of dehydration as a symptom, full consideration of the subject requires some mention of attempts to restore body fluids by parenteral injection of solutions or suspensions intravenously, subcutaneously or intraperitoneally. *Three primary aspects of the problem deserve attention:* (1) restoration of total body fluid volume to normal; (2) restoration of solutes (Na, Cl, K, etc.); (3) restoration of acid-base balance. Whether "physiologic" sodium chloride solution or some other form of fluid, such as dilute alkali, glucose solution, whole blood, plasma, etc., is selected, should depend upon the nature and the degree of the fluid loss, with consideration not only of water but of other substances that are constituents of the lost fluids. Chemical examinations of the blood often reveal loss of water, chloride, bicarbonate, plasma protein, hemoglobin, sodium, or potassium. If one is to overcome the dehydration completely, the electrolytes should be restored along with the water. Plasma protein may be needed to re-establish normal circulation and normal interchange of substances between the blood and the intercellular fluid. To accomplish such full restoration of the fluid anatomy to normal, without too much reliance upon aid from renal activity of gastrointestinal absorption, the parenteral fluids given must be similar to normal intercellular fluid, or must at least provide the most essential mineral constituents. Sodium chloride is the most important salt because it is present in body fluids in greatest amount (Fig. 183). The administration of isotonic sodium chloride solution will therefore relieve many of the phenomena of dehydration. However, sodium chloride alone frequently is not capable of providing complete relief of symptoms.[24,32,35,36,70,77]

Isotonic sodium chloride solution is often quite effective if renal function is relatively good, and if the dehydration has not been severe enough to cause considerable withdrawal of potassium from the cells.

When the deficit is primarily of water, one may wish to provide parenteral fluids containing no NaCl (hypernatremia already present).

When base losses exceed those of chloride, one may wish to provide much of the sodium without chloride ion.

With some of these basic considerations in mind we may proceed to review briefly some of the most effective solutions used to replace either intracellular deficits, extracellular deficits or both.

SOLUTIONS FOR INTRACELLULAR FLUID REPLACEMENT

When there has been a significant loss of potassium, use of solutions containing potassium may be urgently indicated.

TABLE 31. COMPOSITION OF DARROW'S SOLUTION

	Gm. per 100 ml.		mEq. per Liter
NaCl	0.40	Na	123
KCl	0.26	K	35
Sodium lactate ...	0.59	Cl	105
		Lactate	53

Potassium chloride in 0.60 per cent solution with 5 per cent glucose is effective and will provide 80 mEq./L. of K. If less NaCl is desired than that in "physiologic" saline solution, but NaCl and K are both needed, a useful solution contains 0.60 per cent KCl and 0.43 per cent NaCl, and provides 80 mEq./L. of K and 73 mEq./L. of Na and of Cl.[26]

Darrow[25] showed that from one third to one half of the extracellular fluid and of the extracellular electrolytes might be lost in severe dehydration with acidosis. He calculated that the following solution provided the most essential electrolytes and would provide an alkaline solution to combat acidosis: 0.40 Gm. NaCl, 0.26 Gm. KCl, 0.59 Gm. of sodium lactate to 100 cc. of water. The amount given was 80 cc. per kilogram of body weight per 24 hours until plasma bicarbonate content and other blood chemical determinations approached normal. It was quite effective in dehydration and acidosis resulting from diarrhea in infants.

A low serum sodium aggravates the untoward effects of a high serum potassium. When the serum K is high, solutions containing K should not be given, but sodium replacement may be important, plus *methods to lower the serum K* (glucose solutions, insulin and perhaps hemodialysis).

When the serum potassium is low and *potassium administration* is indicated, it would seem that the logical accompanying anion would be phosphate. This important intracellular ion is often deficient when K is deficient, and negative potassium balance is apt to be accompanied by a negative phosphate balance. Elkinton and Tarail[26] have suggested the use of one gram of KH_2PO_4 and 4.5 grams of K_2HPO_4 to one liter of solution (glucose, physiologic saline or protein hydrolysate) to yield a solution with pH 7.35 containing 60 mEq. of potassium per liter.

Glucose should probably be given with potassium to facilitate the transfer of K into cells. If the K deficit is severe, 75 to 150 mEq. of K per 24 hours may be administered; if mild, 30 to 50 mEq. may be adequate.

Volume of Fluids. The clinician must judge from the history, the physical findings and the laboratory data and estimate as closely as possible the *total fluid deficit*. It may require several days to make up the total deficiency when it is severe. The daily fluid administered should include (1) maintenance fluids plus (2) fluids to supply deficit.

Maintenance for the nonsweating, nonfebrile resting adult will require about 1,000 ml. (for water of vaporization, "insensible water loss") plus about 1,000 ml. for urinary loss or a total of approximately 2 liters. If there is fever and sweating, one must provide an additional 0.5 to 1.5 liters daily. From 10 to 20 per cent of the body water may be lost during the development of severe dehydration. In infants, between 100 and 300 ml. of fluid per kilogram of body weight may be necessary, given over a period of from 12 to 48 hours. In adults the requirements to cover maintenance plus partial deficit replacement may be 6 liters or more per 24 hours. When feasible, fluids should be given by mouth. When necessary, nasal tube administration is often successful. Subcutaneous or intravenous routes are employed when the need is urgent or there are gastroenteric disturbances. Too rapid or excessive intravenous infusion may precipitate circulatory failure and may be guarded against by frequent measurement of the venous blood pressure, which should be kept within normal limits. Isotonic fluids containing the normal electrolytes and glucose are less likely to embarrass the circulation, but hypertonic solutions and plasma protein attract fluid into the vascular compartment and tend more rapidly to increase blood volume and blood pressure. They may pro-

duce acute circulatory failure with cardiac dilatation and pulmonary edema.

Computation of the fluid deficit will be only approximate, but may be of great importance in directing treatment. Various methods of estimation follow:[33]

1. From body weight.

Example:

Usual wt.	= 70.0 Kg.
Present wt.	= 67.2
Acute wt. loss	= 2.8 Kg.
	= 2.8 liters H_2O

2. From estimated fluid losses.

Example (during 2 days):

Output:

Urine	= 900 ml.
H_2O vaporization	= 3,000
Gastric fluid	= 2,800
Total	6,700 ml.

Intake:

Oral fluids	= 400 ml.
I-V fluids	= 4,000
H_2O oxidation	= 200
Total	4,600 ml.
Balance H_2O	= −2.1 liters

3. From the rise in serum sodium concentration and the estimated total body water, W_1.

$$\text{Deficit } H_2O = W_1 - W_2 = (0.6\ Wt.) - \frac{Na_1 \times (0.6\ wt.)}{Na_2}$$

Example:

Given
$$Wt._1 = 70\ Kg.$$
$$Na_1 = 140\ mEq./L.$$
$$Na_2 = 160\ mEq./L.$$

Then $W_1 = 0.6 \times 70 = 42$ liters

$$W_2 = \frac{140 \times 42}{160} = 37 \text{ liters}$$

Deficit $H_2O = 42 - 37 = 5$ liters

Route and Rate of Fluid Administration. In severe dehydration intravenous infusions are often imperative to restore vital functions. To save life it may be necessary to relieve shock, and to restore as promptly as possible the blood pressure, blood volume, oxygen-carrying power, pH and renal circulation. Initially fluids given intravenously may restore consciousness and the ability to take fluids and nourishment by mouth. Within a few hours oral alimentation may become the route of choice. This is often the case in diabetic coma. Broth and orange juice may provide adequate water, glucose, Na, Cl, and K so that it is not necessary, in many instances, to give glucose or K intravenously.

Caution to prevent hyperkaliemia is imperative in administering K intravenously. Darrow, in treating infants dehydrated by diarrhea, used isotonic sodium chloride solution and dextrose, along with blood or plasma until circulatory and renal function had been restored. Then he gave subcutaneously the solution (now called Darrow's solution) containing NaCl, KCl, and sodium lactate. This solution can also be given orally, with two parts of 5 per cent dextrose in water.

When the serum K is quite low, however, glucose and NaCl solution may further lower it to dangerous levels. The use of KCl in 0.1 to 0.2 per cent solution may be very effective. The rate of K administration intravenously should not exceed a liter (2 Gm. KCl) per hour.[27,28,72,73,74]

SOLUTIONS FOR EXTRACELLULAR REPLACEMENT

1. DEXTROSE 5% IN WATER to provide water without electrolyte. Used in simple dehydration resulting from insensible water loss in patients deprived of fluid.

2. ISOTONIC SODIUM CHLORIDE ("PHYSIOLOGIC" or "NORMAL" SALINE) SOLUTION. This 0.85 per cent NaCl solution contains 145 mEq. per liter of Na and of Cl and is therefore physiologic or isotonic with extracellular fluid only in respect to sodium, while the chloride is relatively high (145:100). Use of this solution if there is no chloride deficit may be dangerous if the kidneys are unable to excrete the chloride excess. When renal regulation is adequate, it is valuable in replacing fluid losses such as those occurring from diabetic ketosis, gastro-intestinal disorders, adrenocortical deficiency, etc.

3. COMBINED SODIUM CHLORIDE AND SODIUM LACTATE SOLUTIONS. An ideal solution to correct hypotonicity when CO_2 is normal can be constructed on the basis of the 140:100 normal proportions of the Na:Cl in the serum. A mixture of 5/7 molar NaCl and 2/7 molar Na lactate will provide the Na and Cl ions in proper proportions. Thus 700 ml. of the solution is prepared easily: combine 500 ml. of molar NaCl with 200 ml. of molar Na lactate.

Other combinations of NaCl and Na lactate[24] can be used to alter the CO_2 combining-power in either direction. A higher proportion of Na lactate may be used if the CO_2 combining-power is decreased.

4. MOLAR SODIUM LACTATE may be used when there is a severe deficit of base.

5. MOLAR SODIUM CHLORIDE is indicated when there is salt depletion with severe deficit of extracellular solute in relation to water as evidenced by hyponatremia and hypochloremia.

6. ONE-SEVENTH MOLAR (ISOTONIC) SODIUM LACTATE is useful in certain acidotic patients whose water requirement is normal but whose extracellular sodium is low in relation to chloride.[24]

7. ONE-SEVENTH MOLAR AMMONIUM CHLORIDE may be used when only chloride is needed, e.g., for the metabolic alkalosis resulting from loss of gastric HCl.

Choice of Fluids. When the cause of the dehydration is known, the type of fluid required is suggested by the nature of the physiologic disturbance. For example, in repeated *vomiting* from pyloric obstruction, dehydration may be accompanied by alkalosis, and the use of a solution containing bicarbonate is contraindicated while chloride is greatly needed. Potassium may be needed also. After *hemorrhage,* dehydration may be extreme, but isotonic saline or lactate-Ringer's solution will be relatively ineffective. Plasma protein may restore the blood volume and relieve the shock, but whole blood, with its red cells and hemoglobin to carry oxygen and relieve anoxia of the tissues, is the only complete replacement therapy. In conditions associated with *starvation* or inability to utilize carbohydrate, glucose solution as well as electrolyte solution is necessary. Thus dehydration with acidosis from diarrhea or loss through a fistula may require not only large amounts of water, salts and base (such as provided in sodium lactate-Ringer's solution) but glucose as well.

In *diabetes,* especially if acidosis or coma occurs and sufficient carbohydrate cannot be ingested, glucose with insulin in large doses to accelerate carbohydrate utilization may be the only direct route to reversal of the processes resulting in the dehydration. The initially high serum K often rapidly falls during treatment of diabetic acidosis until hypokaliemia becomes evident, requiring potassium replacement therapy.[29]

In diabetic acidosis, persons in the younger age groups (with good renal function—and possibly also with good hypothalamic-pituitary-adrenocortical responses to enable them to retain sodium, chloride and water) can usually quite promptly correct even quite severe acidosis if provided with adequate amounts of isotonic NaCl and insulin.

In diabetic acidosis or in any other type of acidosis accompanied by renal inadequacy (infancy, advanced age, chronic nephritis, etc.), the capacity to reabsorb sodium may be diminished, ammonia production may be impaired and the use of alkaline fluids with extra sodium may be beneficial.

When the blood glucose concentration is quite high, there is apparently sufficient available body glucose to allow adequate carbohydrate metabolism for some hours, even with the large doses of insulin usually necessary in the treatment of severe diabetic acidosis. Some authorities believe that dehydration and glycosuria are exaggerated by giving glucose when considerable hyperglycemia is already present and advocate avoidance of the use of glucose solutions, except when necessary to provide sufficient available carbohydrate. Others advocate the prompt use of glucose solutions in all severe diabetic acidosis.

Renal failure, with or without true uremia, often results in severe acidosis, dehydration, loss of chloride and fixed base. The severe acidosis must be relieved without help from the kidneys, too badly impaired to exercise their usual efficient functions of adjusting fluid balance and acid-base balance. The acidosis, the dehydration

and the hypochloridemia may often be relieved by "fortified" lactate-Ringer's solution. Glucose, insulin or dialysis may be indicated to lower the serum K. Intravenous dextrose is valuable and blood may prove important in relieving the anemia so often present.

In *Addison's disease* glucose, salt and water are needed. In *thyroid crisis,* with dehydration accompanying an extremely high metabolic rate, large amounts of glucose, as well as salt and water, are needed. In extensive *burns,* protein, as well as salt and water, is lost, and whole blood or plasma is indicated.

Dextrose solutions alone should seldom be employed in the relief of dehydration, for they may cause further diuresis and increase the dehydration. Likewise, the excessive use of hypotonic solutions is dangerous and may cause water intoxication.

Computation of Electrolyte Deficits. If the blood sodium and CO_2 combining-power are known, deficits in many conditions may be approximated by simple mathematical calculations.[33,34,35] Using 20 per cent of body weight as a rough approximation, one calculates the extracellular fluid volume; this figure is multiplied by the aberration of the serum Na from the normal 140 mEq./L. The product represents the degree of hypotonicity or hypertonicity of the extracellular fluid. If edema is present, the estimated edema volume is added to the estimated normal extracellular fluid volume.

EDEMA WITH HYPONATREMIA.

Example:

> Man normally weighing 70 Kg.
> Very edematous (estimate 10 L.)
> Serum Na = 120 mEq./L.

$$70 \times 0.2 = 14 \text{ L. extracellular fluid}$$
$$10 \text{ L. edema fluid}$$
$$\overline{\hspace{2cm}}$$
$$24 \text{ L. total body fluid}$$

$$24 \times 20 \text{ mEq./L.} = 480 \text{ mEq.}$$

$$\text{Na deficit} = 480 \text{ mEq.}$$

This could be administered by giving 480 ml. of molar NaCl orally or intravenously. Usually one finds that only about half of the administered Na stays in the extracellular fluid, so in 12 to 24 hours the calculations are repeated and more Na is given if indicated.

DEHYDRATION WITH HYPERNATREMIA.
Example:

> 70 Kg. normal weight
> 60 Kg. present weight
> ───────
> 10 Kg. = 10 L. fluid loss

Of this 10 L., approximately 2 L. are extracellular fluid loss.

If serum Na = 160 mEq.L/L., $12 \times 20 = 240$ mEq. of Na must be diluted with water. This could be accomplished with $240/140 = 1.7$ liters of water, which could be given in isotonic form as 5 per cent glucose.

An 8 liter deficit remains to be replaced by a solution close in composition to that of body fluid.

DEHYDRATION WITH HYPONATREMIA. Deficits of sodium may reach 50 per cent of the extracellular sodium (thus totaling as much as 1,000 mEq. in a 70 Kg. adult) before death results from circulatory collapse. Ranges of deficits more commonly encountered, as in diabetic coma or pyloric obstruction, are 300 to 600 mEq. in the average adult.

If the extracellular fluid volume has been reduced and if the serum Na is low, the Na deficit consists of (1) the sodium lost with its proportional share of water, plus (2) the sodium missing from the extracellular fluid left behind (thus resulting in the lowered Na concentration).

1. Acute wt. loss of 1.5 Kg. $\times$ 140 = 210 mEq. of sodium.
2. Normal wt. 70 Kg. $\times$ 0.6 = 42 liters.

> Serum Na = 125 mEq./L.
> Deficit = $15 \times 42 = 630$ mEq.

Total Na deficit = 210 + 630 = 840 mEq.

ACID-BASE IMBALANCE. Deficit of sodium in excess of fixed anion (as in metabolic acidosis in diabetes, renal insufficiency, infant diarrhea, etc).: CO_2 combining-power is low in serum.

Example:
Serum CO_2 = 12 mM./L.; 27 (normal) − 12 = 15 (deficit).
14 (L. extracellular fluid volume) $\times$ 15 = 210 mM. total deficit of base; 210 mM. of base necessary to raise CO_2 to normal.

Theoretically, this would require 210 ml. of molar Na lactate solution. In actual practice 2 or 3 times this amount would probably be required since 50 per cent or more of the Na usually enters the cells.

Chemical measurement of the bicarbonate reserve and the serum sodium, serum potassium, and chloride levels, as well as determination of the blood glucose content and the serum protein and nonprotein nitrogen, is of great help in determining the choice and the amount of fluid replacement to be employed. *Intracellular losses or gains of water or electrolytes cannot be measured directly with the methods now available, therefore estimates must be based upon the history, the physical status and laboratory tests of blood and urine. Whenever possible, frequent follow-up chemical determinations, as well as an initial diagnostic chemical study, are advisable. For example, a blood-protein level, initially apparently normal, may subsequently prove to be subnormal when hydration is restored. Acidosis may be overcorrected if excess amounts of alkaline solutions are employed, and repeated determination of the blood carbon dioxide combining power is an excellent guide to indicate how much of a solution such as lactate-Ringer's should be given, and how often repeated.

Since the concentration of the serum sodium may be an excellent guide for the regulation of replacement of this most important cation of the extracellular fluids, it should be determined before and after therapy, if the means are available, and it will often be found to yield data not deducible from CO_2 and chloride determinations.

The serum potassium concentration is of much greater importance than previously realized, as shown by a number of excellent studies. It may change quickly and should be followed whenever possible, for the clinical signs of hypokaliemia and hyperkaliemia are difficult to distinguish.

The development of the flame photometer, which permits rapid and accurate determinations of serum sodium and potassium, has contributed greatly to the recent rapid advance of knowledge in this field. Rapid determination of the concentration of these cations in the blood permits accurate diagnosis and suggests the type of fluid and electrolyte therapy indicated. It also permits following the results of treatment, and the prompt adjustment of therapy to whatever changing indications may appear.

The electrocardiogram is an important adjunct to chemical measurement of the blood constituents. It is particularly useful in detecting abnormal levels of the serum potassium. The conduction of the cardiac impulse through the auriculoventricular conduction system may be impaired with serum K deviations, and the electrocardiographic tracings generally permit quite accurate deductions as to whether the serum K is high or low, often before clinical signs become evident.

DIURETICS AND DEHYDRATION

The kidneys, through mechanisms described early in this chapter, exert the most important control over the disposition of body fluid. Under certain conditions drugs and other substances may, through increasing the urinary output, cause dehydration. In therapeutics, knowledge of diuretic agents is useful in choosing means to rid the body of excess fluid. Diuretic agents may work in either or both of two ways: (1) by increasing the rate of glomerular filtration; (2) by decreasing the rate of tubular reabsorption.

Substances acting as diuretics may be classified into four major groups,[30] as follows: (1) water and osmotic diuretics; (2) substances increasing colloidal osmotic pressure; (3) acid-forming salts; (4) inhibitors of renal tubular transport. The mechanism of action of the principal members of each group is indicated:

Water. Ingestion of large amounts of water leads to decrease in tubular reabsorption, as the result of decrease in the secretion of the antidiuretic hormone. Water ingestion causes water diuresis.

Osmotic Diuretics. (1) SODIUM CHLORIDE. Isotonic sodium chloride administration increases blood volume and accelerates glomerular filtration.

Hypertonic sodium chloride solution increases the extracellular fluid not only by the volume injected or ingested but by the water withdrawn from the cells, and glomerular filtration is consequently greatly increased. In addition, the rejected sodium chloride limits resorption of water by the tubules. As a result of accelerated output of fluid into the tubules and diminished reabsorption, diuresis occurs.

In clinical edema, it should be noted, water and sodium chloride are not useful diuretics because they may be retained in the interstitial fluid, thus increasing the edema.

The frequently and often tragically demonstrated fact that no fluid intake is preferable to the ingestion of sea water was brought to our attention repeatedly during World War II. Drinking sea water causes dehydration because (1) it may cause vomiting, (2) water is pulled into the intestinal tract by the hypertonic salt solution and excessive quantities of water are excreted in the feces, and because (3) that part of the sodium chloride absorbed requires an increase in the urinary-water output.

"Salt fever," the temperature elevation caused by dehydration, may result from intravenous saline or glucose in excess.

Water intoxication, the condition resulting from excessive water ingestion, with resultant reduction in the osmotic pressure of the blood and cellular overhydration, may be promptly relieved by intravenous administration of hypertonic sodium chloride solution.

(2) POTASSIUM SALTS, in contrast to those of sodium, are effective diuretics in any concentration. Potassium is the main cation of the cells of the body. When present in excess in the extracellular fluid it is filtered through the glomerulus and rejected by the tubules, taking considerable quantities of water with it.

(3) There are certain molecules, such as *urea, glucose* and *sucrose,* which in the

renal tubule require water for excretion because of their limited reabsorption.

Substances altering oncotic pressure are effective diuretics under certain conditions. When edema is present because of low concentration of serum protein (as in nephrosis, malnutrition, chronic diarrhea, etc.), blood or plasma or albumin transfusion may prove extremely successful treatment. Plasma expanders such as dextran mobilize interstitial fluid. Acacia has a similar effect but may produce toxic results.

Acid-forming salts, such as ammonium chloride, ammonium nitrate and calcium chloride, are powerful diuretics. The ammonium salts act by giving up the ammonium to form urea, leaving the anion to demand base from bicarbonate and to require water for excretion. Calcium similarly is freed from chloride by being excreted in the intestine or deposited in bone, and the chloride displaces bicarbonate in the extracellular fluids.

The Xanthines. Caffeine and theophylline and its derivatives (aminophylline), etc., and theobromine apparently act primarily by decreasing tubular resorption. In addition, they seem to increase the rate of glomerular filtration when it is diminished.

The Mercurials. Mercurial diuretics are the most powerful of all diuretics. Their action is exerted through reduction in the ability of the renal tubules to absorb water. The basic mechanism of action of organic mercurials seems to be the inhibition of SH-activated enzyme systems which are essential to provide energy for renal tubular transport. The resorption of Cl^- ion is blocked specifically. H^+ ion transport and bicarbonate resorption are not affected. The loss of fixed cation (chiefly Na) is secondary to the effect on the anion (Cl).

Inhibitor of Carbonic Anhydrase: Acetazolamide (Diamox). This sulfonamide depresses the rate of formation of carbonic acid by the inhibition of carbonic anhydrase, thus greatly reducing the rate of H^+ ion and Na^+ ion exchange in the renal tubule (see Fig. 188). As a result, bicarbonate resorption is incomplete, and titratable acid and ammonia disappear from the urine. The kidney elaborates an increased volume of alkaline urine.

The reabsorption of NaCl depends largely upon the process of ion exchange through which the cells of the renal tubules reabsorb sodium only in proportion to the rate at which they release hydrogen, one H^+ ion being exchanged for one Na^+ ion. The carbonic anhydrase present in the renal tubules catalyzes the formation of $H^+HCO_3^-$, which is strongly ionized, from H_2O and CO_2 (unionized); it thus promotes the liberation of H^+ ions, permitting the excretion of an acid urine and reabsorption of sodium. Acetazolamide, by inhibiting carbonic anhydrase, retards tubular excretion of H^+ ions and reabsorption of Na^+ ions. It also increases excretion of K^+ ions, which compete with H^+ ions for the anions Cl^-, HCO_3^-, etc. The result is accelerated renal loss of HCO_3^-, which carries out Na^+, K^+, and water; there is diuresis and alkalinization of the urine.

Chlorothiazide and Hydrochlorothiazide are potent diuretic agents which promote excretion of sodium and water by inhibiting their reabsorption by the proximal renal tubule. These compounds contain a free sulfanilamide group, but their mode of action differs from that of the carbonic anhydrase inhibitors. The diuresis produced by the thiazide diuretic drugs produces a balanced loss of sodium with its two attendant anions in approximately the proportions in the extracellular fluid; the drug acetazolamide causes a diuresis of sodium and bicarbonate. The thiazides also promote potassium excretion, and potassium depletion must be guarded against.

Aldosterone Inhibitors. An important recent development has been the discovery of agents which block the effect of aldosterone on the renal tubules. These compounds, the spirolactones, are derived from progesterone and are similar to aldosterone structurally. Spironolactone (Aldactone) has been extensively studied. It promotes diuresis by blocking, through competitive inhibition, the sodium-absorbing, water-retaining and potassium-excreting effects of aldosterone on the distal renal tubules (see Fig. 188). The use of spironolactone is particularly indicated when potassium conservation is desired but diuresis is imperative, and when secondary hyperaldosteronism is believed to be a causative factor in edema or ascites (many cases of congestive heart failure, cirrhosis, nephrosis, idiopathic edema, etc).[75]

MISCELLANEOUS DIURETICS

Digitalis is a diuretic only for persons with heart failure, and its effects upon urine flow are exerted through its action on the heart and the circulation. The mobilization of the edema fluid comes first, then the diuresis. Desiccated thyroid may promote the elimination of fluid when fluid retention is caused by low thyroid function.

Choice of a Diuretic. The promotion of diuresis when relative dehydration is desired (that is, the restoration of an overly hydrated to a normally hydrated body state) is often dramatically successful in therapy. The choice of agents is extremely important and depends largely upon the condition of the kidneys. When renal function is impaired, the mercurials, acid-forming salts, potassium salts and urea may be dangerous.

CATHARTICS AND DEHYDRATION

Cathartics are used much too widely and physicians not infrequently see persons who intermittently produce in themselves moderate dehydration by the ingestion of preparations that increase the bulk and the liquid content of the feces. Cathartics act by one of three fundamental mechanisms, any one of which increases the water output through the fecal route. Cathartics are either irritant, bulky or emollient in action. The *irritant preparations,* such as cascara or castor oil, cause rapid propulsion of the intestinal contents, allowing inadequate time for the usual water resorption with resultant elimination of liquid stools. *Bulky laxatives* increase the volume of the intestinal contents and thus are more physiologic in action. They may be inorganic salts that are slowly absorbed from the intestinal tract and thus hold water in the canal due to the osmotic pressure that they exert or they may be hydrophilic colloids or indigestible fiber that resist destruction

in the alimentary canal. Examples of the saline cathartics are magnesium sulfate and sodium phosphate. Agar exerts all three types of laxative action. Agar is rich in indigestible hemicellulose, which provides bulk, is hydrophilic and forms a mucilaginous mass that also acts as an *emollient.* Mineral oil is indigestible and unabsorbable, and acts as a *lubricant* to the fecal contents, preventing their excessive dehydration in the colon.

The saline cathartics may cause dehydration of considerable degree if taken in excessive doses. The mechanism of action of all of them is similar. During the absorption of solutes from the intestinal tract the concentration of the salts tends to become isotonic with that in the blood serum. If the salt happens to be sodium chloride, which is easily absorbed, the salt and, therefore, the water will be removed from the alimentary canal quite rapidly. However, if the solute contains ions that are slowly absorbed—for instance, the cation magnesium or the anions sulfate, phosphate, tartrate and citrate—they are retained in the canal for a comparatively long time and thus draw water through the intestinal wall. The water leaves the extracellular fluid and enters the intestinal tract until the solution of the cathartic salt is rendered isotonic with the body fluids. The bowel becomes distended with liquid and thus the propulsion along the canal is mechanically increased and large amounts of fluid may be lost.

SUMMARY

Loss of water and electrolyte from the body or maldistribution of body water and electrolyte may produce profound disturbances of body physiology. The results of salt loss are more severe than those of water loss alone. Loss of extracelluar electrolyte leads to loss of plasma volume, and is the prototype of the usual clinical conditions grouped under the term *dehydration.*

Water is in a dynamic state, and all body water is being constantly exchanged. Although sodium is the chief cation of the extracellular fluid and potassium the chief cation of the intracellular fluid, these ions are also in a dynamic state, and no part of the body is inaccessible to them. There are variations in the amount of sodium, chloride and potassium in intracellular, as well as extracellular, fluids, and a simple type of osmotic relationship is not sufficient to explain the behavior of body fluids.

The state of hydration of the cells depends primarily upon the concentration of sodium ion in the extracellular compartment. A major function of the kidney is to regulate the concentration of sodium in the extracellular fluid.

When water and salt balance are within normal limits and renal function is adequate, the regulatory processes can usually correct aberrations and preserve a relatively constant internal fluid environment. If, however, serious disturbance occurs in the water and salt balance, or in the renal regulation, it may be difficult to reverse the morbid process and dehydration may result. The symptom *dehydration,* if adequately analyzed and interpreted, may lead to detection of the cause of the water and electrolyte disturbance and its correction.

REFERENCES

1. Bernard, Claude: Leçons sur les propriétés physiologiques et les altérations pathologiques des liquides de l'organisme, Paris, Baillière, 1859.
2. Cannon, W. B.: The Wisdom of the Body, New York, Norton, 1932.
3. Gamble, J. L.: Chemical Anatomy, Physiology and Pathology of Extracellular Fluid, ed. 6, Cambridge, Harvard, 1954.
———: Companionship of Water and Electrolytes in the Organization of Body Fluids, Stanford, Calif., Stanford Univ. Press, 1951.
4. Moore, F. D., *et al.*: Body composition; total body water and electrolytes; intravascular and extravascular phase volumes, Metabolism 5:447-467, 1956.
5. Levitt, M. F., and Gaudino, M.: Measurement of body water compartments, Am. J. Med. 9:208-215, 1950.
6. Wilde, W. S.: Transport through biological membranes, Ann. Rev. Physiol. 17:17-36, 1955.
7. Pinson, E. A.: Water exchange and barriers as studied by the use of hydrogen isotopes, Physiol. Rev. 32:123-134, 1952.
8. Bresler, E. H.: The problem of the volume component of body fluid homeostasis, Am. J. Med. Sci. 232:93-104, 1956.

9. Conn, J. W., and Louis, L. H.: "Salt-active" corticoids reflected in thermal sweat, J. Clin. Endocrinol. 10:12, 1950.
10. Heinbecker, P., and White, H. L.: The role of the pituitary gland in water balance, Ann. Surg. 110:1037, 1939.
11. Gilman, A., and Goodman, L.: The secretory response of the posterior pituitary to the need for water conservation, J. Physiol. 90:113, 1937.
12. Chambers, G. H., Melville, E. V., Hare, R. S., and Hare, K.: Am. J. Physiol. 144:311, 1945.
13. Ray, C. T.: *in* Sodeman, W. A.: Pathologic Physiology, Philadelphia, Saunders, 1961, p. 86-121.
14. Daughaday, W. H., and MacBryde, C. M.: Renal and adrenal mechanisms of salt conservation, J. Clin. Investigation 29:591-601, 1950.
15. Pitts, R. F.: Acid-base regulation by the kidneys, Am. J. Med. 9:356-372, 1950.
16. Leaf, A., Camara, A., and Albertson, A.: Renal tubular secretion of potassium in man, J. Clin. Investigation 28:1526-1533, 1949.
17. Randall, H. T., Habif, D. V., Lockwood, J. S., and Werner, S. C.: Potassium deficiency in surgical patients, Surgery 26:341, 1949.
18. Berliner, R. W.: Renal excretion of water, sodium, potassium, calcium, and magnesium Am. J. Med. 9:541-559, 1950.
19. Darrow, D. C., Schwartz, R., Ianucci, J. F., and Coville, F.: The relation of serum bicarbonate concentration to muscle composition, J. Clin. Investigation 27:198, 1948.
20. Goodof, I. I., and MacBryde, C. M.: Heart failure in Addison's disease with myocardial changes of potassium deficiency, J. Clin. Endocrinol. 4:30-34, 1944.
21. Kolf, W. J.: Serum potassium in uremia, J. Lab. & Clin. Med. 36:719-728, 1950.
22. Merrill, J. P., Levine, H. D., Somerville, W., and Smith, S.: Clinical recognition and treatment of acute potassium intoxication, Ann. Int. Med. 33:797-830, 1950.
23. Elkinton, J. R., Danowski, T. S., and Winkler, A. W.: Hemodynamic changes in salt depletion and in dehydration, J. Clin. Investigation 25:120-129, 1946.
24. Hollander, W., and Williams, T.: Dehydration, Disease-a-Month, Chicago, Year Book Pub., 1958.
25. Darrow, D. C., Pratt, E. L., Flett, J., Jr., Gamble, A. H., and Wiese, H. F.: Disturbances of water and electrolytes in infantile diarrhea, Pediatrics 3:129, 1949.

26. Elkinton, J. R., and Tarail, R.: The present status of potassium therapy, Am. J. Med. 9:200-207, 1950.

27. Hoffman, W. S.: Clinical physiology of potassium, J.A.M.A. 144:1157-1162, 1950.

28. Smith, F. H.: Potassium deficiency in gastrointestinal diseases, Gastroenterology 16: 73-82, 1950.

29. Danowski, T. S., Peters, J. H., Rothbun, J. C., Quashnock, J. M., and Greenman, L.: Studies in diabetic acidosis and coma, J. Clin. Investigation 28:1, 1949.

30. Goodman, L., and Gilman, A.: The Pharmacological Basis of Therapeutics, ed. 2, New York, Macmillan, 1955.

31. Darrow, D. C.: Tissue water and electrolyte, Annual Review of Physiology 6:95-122, 1944.

———: and Pratt, E. L.: Fluid therapy; relation to tissue composition and expenditure of water and electrolyte, J.A.M.A. 143: 365-373, 1950.

32. Weisberg, H. F.: Water, Electrolyte and Acid-Base Balance, ed. 2, Baltimore, Williams & Wilkins, 1962.

33. Elkinton, J. R., and Danowski, T. S.: The Body Fluids; Basic Physiology and Practical Therapeutics, Baltimore, Williams & Wilkins, 1955.

34. Schroeder, H. A., and Perry, H. M.: Disturbances of the internal environment and their correction, Am. J. Clin. Path. 23:1100, 1953.

35. Goldberger, E.: Primer of Water, Electrolyte and Acid-Base Syndromes, Philadelphia, Lea & Febiger, 1962.

36. Snively, W. D.: Body Fluid Disturbances, New York, Grune & Stratton, 1962.

37. MacBryde, C. M.: Adrenal cortex hormones: influence on water balance and electrolyte metabolism, Missouri Med. 51: 740-742, 1954.

38. MacBryde, C. M.: Significance of recent studies with ACTH and cortisone, J. Missouri M. A. 47:905-909, 1950.

39. Reichstein, T.: A new adrenal hormone, Lancet 2:551, 1953.

40. Hills, A. G., et al.: Adrenal cortical regulation of distribution of water and electrolytes in human body, J. Clin. Invest. 32:1236-1247, 1953.

41. Gilman, A., and Brazeau, P.: The role of the kidney in the regulation of acid-base metabolism, Am. J. Med. 15:765-770, 1953.

42. Black, D. A. K.: Body-fluid depletion, Lancet 1:305-311, 1953.

43. Leaf, A., and Newburgh, L. H.: Significance of the Body Fluids in Clinical Medicine, Springfield, Ill., Thomas, 1955.

44. Overman, R. R.: Sodium, potassium and chloride alterations in disease, Physiol. Rev. 31:285-311, 1951.

45. Adolph, E. F., Barker, J. P., and Hoy, P. A.: Multiple factors in thirst, Am. J. Physiol. 178:538-562, 1954.

46. Pitts, R. F.: Modern concepts of acid-base regulation, A. M. A. Arch. Int. Med. 89: 864-876, 1952.

47. Mudge, G. H.: Renal mechanisms of electrolyte transport, in Clarke, H. T. ed.: Ion Transport Across Membranes, New York, Acad. Press, 1954.

48. Robinson, J. R., and McCance, R. A.: Water metabolism, Ann. Rev. Physiol. 14: 115-142, 1952.

49. Smith, H. W.: The Kidney; Structure and Function in Health and Disease, New York, Oxford, 1951.

50. Robinson, S.: Salt conservation by kidneys and sweat glands in men, Fed. Proc. 13: 119-120, 1954.

51. Bergstrom, W. H., and Wallace, W. M.: Bone as a sodium and potassium reservoir, J. Clin. Invest. 33:867-873, 1954.

52. Danowski, T. S.: Fundamental features of metabolism of sodium and potassium, Am. J. Clin. Path. 23:1095-1099, 1953.

53. Blahd, W. H., and Bassett, S. H.: Potassium deficiency in man, Metabolism 2:218-224, 1953.

54. Black, D.: Sodium Metabolism in Health and Disease, Oxford, England, Blackwell, 1952.

55. Schroeder, H. A.: Renal failure associated with low extracellular sodium chloride; low salt syndrome, J.A.M.A. 141:117124, 1949.

56. Leaf, A.: The clinical and physiologic significance of the serum sodium concentration, New England J. Med. 267: 24-30; 77-83, 1962.

57. Leaf, A., and Santos, R. F.: Physiologic mechanisms in potassium deficiency, New England. J. Med. 264:335-341, 1961.

58. Wolf, A. V.: Osmometric analysis of thirst in man and dog, Am. J. Physiol. 161:75, 1950.

59. ———: Thirst, Springfield, Ill., Thomas, 1958.

60. Anderson, B.: Water and electrolyte metabolism in the goat, Acta Physiol. Scand., 288:188, 1953; 33:50, 1955; 35: 312, 1956.

61. Verney, E. B.: Croonian Lecture: The antidiuretic hormone and factors which deter-

mine its release, Proc. Roy. Soc. 135:25, 1947.

62. Bargmann, W., and Scharrer, E.: Site of origin of the hormones of the posterior pituitary, Am. Sci. 39:255-259, 1951.

63. Verney, E. B.: Agents determining and influencing functions of pars nervosa of pituitary, Brit. M. J. 2:119-123, 1948.

64. Conn, J. W.: Aldosteronism in man, J.A.M.A. 183:775-781, 871-878, 1963.

65. Belding, H. S.: Hazards to health: work in hot weather, New England J. Med. 267:1052-1054, 1962.

66. Kuno, Y.: Human Perspiration, Springfield, Ill., Thomas, 1956.

67. Robinson, S., and Robinson, A. H.: Chemical composition of sweat, Physiol. Rev. 34:202, 1954.

68. Laragh, J. H., et al.: Hypotensive agents and pressor substances: effects of epinephrine, norepinephrine, angiotensin II, etc., on the secretory rate of aldosterone in man, J.A.M.A. 174:234-240, 1960.

69. Schwartz, W. B., et al.: A syndrome of renal sodium loss and hyponatremia probably resulting from inappropriate secretion of antidiuretic hormone, Am. J. Med. 23:529, 1957.

70. Welt, L. G.: Clinical Disorders of Hydration and Acid-Base Equilibrium, ed. 2, Boston, Little, Brown, 1959.

71. Albrink, M. J., et al.: The displacement of serum water by the lipids of hyperlipemic serum, J. Clin. Invest. 34:1483, 1955.

71A. Davis, J. E., et al.: Salt and water depletion caused by villous rectosigmoid adenomas, Ann. Surg. 155:806, 1962.

72. Winsor, T.: Potassium and digitalis intoxication, Am. Heart J. 60:151, 1960.

73. Kunin, A. S., et al.: Decrease in serum potassium and cardiac arrythmias, New England J. Med. 266:228, 1962.

74. Lown, B., et al.: Digitalis, electrolytes, and surgical patient, Am. J. Cardiology 6:309, 1960.

75. Bartter, F. C.: The role of aldosterone in normal homeostasis and in certain disease states, Metabolism 5:369-383, 1956.

76. Friedberg C.: Heart, Kidney and Electrolytes, New York, Grune & Stratton, 1962.

77. Maxwell, M. H., and Kleeman, C. R.: Clinical Disorders of Fluid and Electrolyte Metabolism, New York, McGraw-Hill, 1962.

78. Pitts, R. F.: Physiology of the Kidney and Body Fluids, Chicago, Year Book Pub., 1963.

31

Edema

HENRY A. SCHROEDER

DEFINITION

Claude Bernard said:

Animals have really two environments: a *milieu extérieur* in which the organism is situated, and a *milieu intérieur* in which the tissue elements live. The living organism does not really exist in the *milieu extérieur* (the atmosphere if it breathes, salt or fresh water if that is its element) but in the liquid *milieu intérieur* formed by the circulating organic liquid which surrounds and bathes all the tissue elements; this is the lymph or plasma. ... The *milieu intérieur* surrounding the organs, the tissues and their elements never varies; atmospheric changes cannot penetrate beyond it and it is therefore true to say that the physical conditions of environment are unchanging in a higher animal: each one is surrounded by this invariable *milieu* which is, as it were, an atmosphere proper to itself in an ever-changing cosmic environment. Here we have an organism which has enclosed itself in a kind of hot-house. The perpetual changes of external conditions cannot reach it; it is not subject to them, but is free and independent. ... All the vital mechanisms, however varied they may be, have only one object, that of preserving constant the conditions of life in the internal environment.[1]

Edema is merely the result of expansion of the *milieu intérieur,* or the extracellular fluid of the body.

Edema is a sign common to a variety of diseases. It may be defined as any abnormal accumulation of extravascular extracellular (interstitial) fluid. The source of the fluid is the blood plasma. All edema comes from the circulating blood and its composition is similar to that of plasma, containing electrolytes (principally sodium, chloride and bicarbonate), glucose, urea, creatinine, amino acids and various other diffusible crystalloid substances. On the other hand, its protein content depends upon the cause of the edema, varying from the negligible quantities usually encountered in most states of chronic edema to the concentrations approaching those of plasma seen in severe local traumatic conditions.

Edema can be general or localized to a particular area or organ. When it is general, relatively large amounts of water must accumulate in the tissue spaces before swelling can be detected by physical examination. A patient's body weight may increase nearly 10 per cent before "pitting" edema becomes evident. It is obvious that diffusion of such large amounts of water and electrolytes into tissue spaces must be accompanied or preceded by the renal retention of water and electrolytes in order to maintain plasma volume. The normal ratio of plasma to extracellular fluid volume is about 1:3. If the large volume of edema fluid lost from the blood were not replaced, hypovolemia sufficient to induce severe vascular shock would occur. Small localized accumulations of edema fluid may develop without affecting the general circulation; large amounts of necessity must be accompanied by replacement, which usually means retention, and retention requires ingestion or injection.

Knowledge of the pathologic physiology of the formation of edema is incomplete. There appear to be two general groups. The first is composed of those types in which fluid from plasma primarily transudes into tissue spaces, setting in motion a mechanism for its replacement by the renal retention of salt and water and the formation of other elements lost to the circulating blood. The second comprises those types in which the primary derangement is in the renal excretion of salt and water, leading to transudation of fluid from plasma into tissue spaces. In either variety, the composition of the fluid retained may be altered in terms of concentration of electrolytes or acid-base balance. The relative amounts of fluid and electrolytes ingested and the metabolic and the renal losses apparently govern these alterations. Therefore edema is to be considered as a derangement of water and electrolyte balance in one direction; dehydration is its counterpart, although under exceptional circumstances an edematous patient may also be dehydrated (See Table 32, page 754).

PHYSIOLOGIC CONSIDERATIONS

The vascular factors which lead to the formation of edema in general comprise disturbances of one or more of the normal functions governing the exchange of fluid between the intravascular and extravascular fluid compartments. These are: (1) capillary permeability, (2) capillary blood pressure, (3) colloid osmotic pressure of

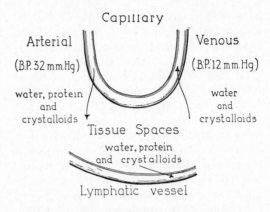

FIG. 191. Principal structures involved in the normal interchange of tissue fluid.

plasma, (4) colloid osmotic pressure of tissue fluid, (5) tissue pressure, and (6) factors influencing the formation and flow of lymph. Figure 191 depicts diagrammatically the principal local vascular structures involved in the normal interchange of tissue fluid.*

The general mechanisms which affect the formation of edema fluid are principally those which concern the regulation of water and electrolyte balance: (1) renal arterial and venous pressure, (2) the renal retention of electrolytes and water as influenced by extrarenal hormonal regulatory mechanisms or by intrinsic renal diseases, (3) the dietary intake of salt and water, (4) the excretion of salt and water by other than renal routes (stool, expired air, sweat and pathologic drainage) and (5) the formation or destruction of plasma proteins.

VASCULAR FACTORS

Capillary Permeability. The area of capillary wall available for fluid interchange

---

* For purposes of simplification in this discussion, the capillary bed is considered as a continuous network of vessels branching from arterioles and then anastomosing into larger channels on their venous ends. This is not actually the case. The capillary system must be considered as being similar to an irrigation system, with arteriovenous anastomoses, side channels, small capillary beds and plexuses which are constantly changing, shutting off blood from some channels and opening others. The capillary bed appears to depart from the general configuration of the arterial and venous systems, each of which resembles a river system with its watershed and tributaries.

is extremely large. It is estimated[2] that in a man who weighs 50 Kg. the area of the capillaries in his skeletal muscles alone is 6,300 m² (over 1.5 acres), that their lengths total 100,000 Km. and that 1 ml. of blood is exposed to a filtering surface of 0.5 to 0.7 m². From animal experiments it has been determined that the capillary wall is so permeable to water and electrolytes that the entire plasma volume of a man would be filtered through his capillaries within ten seconds if there were no forces operating to retain fluid within the blood vascular system.[3] The capillary walls are permeable to all the normal constituents of blood plasma except protein, to which they are only slightly permeable. In general, those substances which are filtered by the glomeruli of the kidney are filtered by the general capillary bed into interstitial fluid spaces. For example, inulin, which is used to measure glomerular filtration rate, also can be used to measure total interstitial fluid volume because its relatively large molecule appears to filter through capillary walls as it is filtered by glomerular capillaries. The ability of any substance to pass through capillary interstices depends probably not only on the size of its molecule but also upon its shape.

Both filtration and diffusion account for the interchange of substances between plasma and cells.[4] Capillaries, however, have diverse structures as seen by the electron microscope. Those of liver, intestine and kidney showed pores of small size, while none were demonstrable in muscle, skin, connective tissue and lung.[5] By infusing of dextran of differing molecular weights, and then measuring the amounts in lymph, it has been shown inferentially that capillaries were completely permeable to molecules of about 20 Å radius, slightly permeable to those of 30 to 40 Å radii, with some residual permeability of much larger molecules. Liver capillaries passed the largest molecules of 200 Å or greater.[6] Diffusion of lipid-soluble substances occurs directly through the capillary wall or perhaps by active transport.[4]

Capillary Blood Pressure. The blood pressure in the capillary provides the force necessary to filter fluid through the permeable capillary walls. The driving force for filtration, therefore, comes from the heart. Blood pressure in the capillaries is controlled principally by the arterioles from which the capillaries arise. Localized arteriolar constriction will reduce blood pressure and flow in capillaries if systemic arterial pressure remains unchanged. Arteriolar dilatation will lead to increased flow and pressure if systemic pressure is unchanged. However, widespread changes in arteriolar diameter are accompanied by changes in systemic blood pressure inasmuch as the arterioles provide much of the peripheral resistance to flow and so govern the level of pressure. From these considerations, it is obvious that the force of filtration which comes from the blood pressure and the amount of fluid filtered from the blood can be altered by changes in arteriolar diameter, changes in systemic blood pressure and changes in the total flow of blood or cardiac output.

As blood passes from arteriole to pre-capillary to capillary there occurs a fall of pressure and a diminution in the amount of fluid within the capillary; further along toward the venular end restoration of fluid in the venule takes place. These changes depend upon pressure gradients. Pressure in the arteriolar limb of the capillary has been shown by direct measurements to be approximately 32 mm. of mercury, whereas the pressure in the venous limb is in the neighborhood of 12 mm.[7] The average pressure in the entire capillary bed is approximately equivalent to the colloid osmotic pressure of the plasma proteins (24 mm.).[7] Owing to the gradient between the arteriolar and the venous ends of the capillary, conditions favor filtration in the arteriolar portion, and reabsorption in the venous portion.

Capillary pressure is extremely variable, depending upon arteriolar vasomotion, total flow, freedom of venous outflow, posture, temperature, neurogenic influences and all other circulatory factors.[8] In a given capillary, at one moment filtration may predominate and at another, reabsorption. Although the volume of fluid entering the tissue spaces varies considerably with circulatory adjustments,[8] the total daily exchange is remarkably constant, neither dehydration nor edema developing normally.

Pressure in capillaries naturally may be altered by venous pressure. A high local or systemic venous pressure may be transmitted retrograde to venules and may alter the normal gradient. Such alterations would result in a tendency for less filtered fluid to be reabsorbed in the venular ends of the capillaries. Although systemic venous pressure measured in brachial or great veins is usually considerably lower (7 mm. Hg) than that obtained in the venular end of the capillary loop (12 mm. Hg), increases in pressure in the upright position (to 35 to 40 mm. Hg) could easily be transmitted to the venules and could influence markedly the reabsorption of fluids in the lower part of the body were it not for the many valves found in medium-sized veins. A high venous pressure, however, may be transmitted through valves if venous distention or congestion is present and thus cause venular stasis.

Therefore, exchange of fluid between blood and tissue spaces is affected by the general level of arterial pressure as related to the state of the arterioles, the general level of venous pressure, the state of the venules and veins, which have vasomotor controls, and by the pressure-flow relationships in any given segment of the circulation. No part of the arterio-venous circulation can be considered as a passive system of tubes. When effective pressure is increased, filtration is also increased; when pressure is decreased, filtration falls.

Colloid Osmotic Pressure of Blood Plasma. Opposing the filtration force of the capillary blood pressure is the colloid osmotic pressure (oncotic pressure) of plasma—minus the colloid osmotic pressure of other tissue fluids. Both plasma and interstitial fluids have considerable oncotic pressure since they both contain approximately the same concentration of electrolytes, urea, sugar and other diffusible materials. The principal difference between them lies in their protein content, which accounts for only about 5 per cent of the total oncotic pressure of plasma.[9] The pressure exerted by plasma protein opposes the filtration of fluids and dissolved substances

and favors the reabsorption of water and of these substances. When capillary pressure is higher than plasma oncotic pressure, filtration will occur; when it is lower reabsorption will take place.

The importance of colloid osmotic pressure in controlling fluid interchange was first demonstrated by Starling in 1896.[10] Having rendered one hind leg of a dog edematous by infiltrating it with hypertonic sodium chloride solution, Starling perfused both hind legs through the femoral arteries with defibrinated blood. The passage of blood through the edematous leg caused the edema to disappear; the returning blood was diluted by the absorbed edema fluid. Blood passing through the control leg remained unchanged. When the experiment was repeated using protein-free salt solution as the perfusing fluid, the edema fluid was not absorbed. Starling thus demonstrated that the absorption of fluid from the edematous limb was dependent upon the presence of protein in the perfusate, and concluded that the protein acted by exerting a difference of osmotic pressure within the vascular system. He later measured the osmotic pressure of the serum colloid directly and found it to be approximately 30 mm. of mercury.

Subsequent measurements of the colloid osmotic pressure of human plasma have shown it to be nearer 25 mm. of mercury than 30.[11] The relatively large protein molecules of the plasma exert their osmotic pull within the capillary because of their inability to pass through most capillary walls. The smaller molecules of electrolytes, urea and sugar, although capable in solution of exerting much greater osmotic pressure, have no effect on fluid exchange as they pass freely through capillary walls. Because of the Donnan equilibrium, some of the crsytalloids of the blood which do not pass freely exert an osmotic effect. The osmotic pressure exerted by plasma albumin is much greater than that exerted by globulin. One gram per cent of albumin (molecular weight about 70,000) exerts a pressure of 5.5 mm. of mercury; one gram per cent of the much larger globulin is responsible for a pressure of only 1.4 mm.[12] The difference is due largely to the smaller molecular weight of albumin, for the pressure is proportional to the number of particles.

Chemical analyses of edema fluid and lymph indicate that the normal capillary endothelium acts as a semipermeable membrane, allowing the free passage of water and crystalloids and at the same time preventing the larger protein molecules of the plasma from escaping into the tissue fluid.[13] The quantitative relationship of the concentrations of protein and salt in blood and edema fluid corresponds closely to that which Donnan proved must exist in an equilibrium established across an inert semipermeable membrane. Since the capillary endothelium normally retains more than 95 per cent of the plasma protein,[8] it may be concluded that the effective colloid osmotic pressure in the body is only slightly less than estimated from measurements made in vitro.

As blood passes along the capillary and filtration of water and dissolved substances occurs, it is obvious that the protein concentration in the blood at the distal end of the capillaries must be increased. An increase in the concentration of plasma protein favors the reabsorption of water; this factor acts on the venular side.

The formation of edema fluids may be profoundly affected by changes in the colloid osmotic pressure of the plasma. Concentration of plasma protein may favor increased reabsorption of tissue fluids and produce dehydration; dilution of plasma protein favors increased filtration and decreased reabsorption of tissue fluids. The balance is probably a very delicate equilibrium, disturbed by small changes.

Colloid Osmotic Pressure of Tissue Fluid. If an appreciable quantity of protein were present in the extravascular fluid, it would tend to counteract the osmotic pressure exerted by the plasma proteins within the capillary. Although regional differences in capillary permeability exist within the body, the amount of protein in the extravascular fluid is normally less than 5 per cent of that present in the blood.[8] Landis and his co-workers have presented indirect evidence that the capillary filtrate from the blood averages only 0.3 per cent protein.[14]

Under normal circumstances, therefore, the colloid osmotic pressure of the tissue fluids is so small that it may be virtually ignored. It becomes significant only under conditions wherein vascular damage causes an increase in the permeability of the capillary endothelium, or when protein removal by lymphatics is disturbed, causing concentration.

Mechanical Pressure in Tissue Spaces. The space available in tissues for the accommodation of extravascular fluid is limited. When the volume of tissue fluid is increased above normal, the tissue elements must be separated and further filtration of fluid is opposed by the pressure required to cause the separation. Accurate measurements of normal tissue pressure are difficult to obtain, and the values reported by different investigators are inconsistent.[8] It is thought that the normal cutaneous tissue pressure amounts to approximately 7 mm. of mercury, whereas subcutaneous tissue pressure is appreciably less, ranging from 2 to 4 mm. of mercury.[15] As the volume of interstitial fluid increases and the tissues are stretched, the tissue pressure rises appreciably.[16]

There is experimental evidence that tissue pressure is an important factor in the prevention of edema. Direct measurements in edematous patients reveal that there is always an elevation in pressure relative to the clinical status of the edema.[16] Warren, Merrill and Stead[17] have observed that when tourniquets are placed about the limbs of a dog for a period of 5 hours, plasma volume can be maintained with much less visible edema if the animal has a relatively tight skin. They conclude that the pressure of interstitial fluid (directly related to tissue tension) is a more important antifiltration factor than the volume of fluid and that the pressure exerts its effect by decreasing filtration at the arteriolar end of the capillary, increasing absorption at the venous end and augmenting the flow of lymph. Finally, it is a common clinical observation that patients who have recently lost weight or who have had previous bouts of extensive edema exhibit a striking tendency to become edematous.[18] Loss of normal tissue elasticity in such cases apparently diminishes the normal mechanical resistance to fluid accumulation. The dependent edema seen sometimes in aged persons may be accounted for by this factor.

The Flow of Lymph. As suggested in Figure 191, the lymphatics play an important role in controlling the interchange of fluids between capillaries and tissue spaces. Fluid within the lymphatic vessels contains appreciable quantities of protein, indicating that the walls of the lymphatics are permeable to the large protein molecules.[19] This finding is not surprising since it is well known that foreign particles, including large bacteria, are rapidly taken up by the lymphatic system when injected into various tissues of the body. That the preservation of normal intercellular fluid volume depends at least in part upon lymph flow is well demonstrated by the compre-

hensive studies of Drinker and his collaborators.[19] For example, such factors as venous congestion and muscular activity (which tend to increase the amount of fluid leaving the capillaries) cause an appreciable increase in the flow of lymph. Similarly, experimental procedures that lower the effective osmotic pressure of the blood, either by injuring the capillary wall or by decreasing the concentration of protein in the plasma, cause an increased amount of fluid to escape from the capillaries into the tissue spaces and thus bring about an increase in the flow of lymph. The importance of the lymphatics is dramatically demonstrated when the normal functioning of lymphatic vessels is impaired.

Extracellular-Intracellular Relationships. The normal compositions of extracellular and intracelluar fluids are shown in Figure

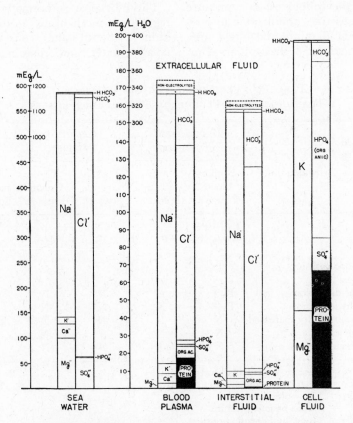

Fig. 192. Chemical anatomy of body fluids in terms of acid-base equivalence. (Gamble, J. L.: Chemical Anatomy, Physiology and Pathology of Extracellular Fluid, Boston, The Harvard Medical School)

192. Cellular membranes are also semipermeable, but of a specialized variety. It is obvious that pronounced changes in extracellular osmotic pressure will influence intracellular fluids as well. The interchange of potassium, magnesium and sodium salts may be affected by changes in concentration of extracellular fluids and may have profound effects upon cellular metabolism. Overhydration or dehydration of cells may occur. These alterations must be borne in mind during any consideration of fluid exchange and regulation.

Summary. The factors favoring filtration of fluid from plasma into tissues are: the blood pressure at the arteriolar end of the capillary minus the colloid osmotic pressure of the plasma minus the mechanical pressure in the tissue spaces plus the colloid osmotic pressure of the tissue fluid itself. The factors favoring reabsorption of fluid from tissues into blood are: the tissue pressure plus the colloid osmotic pressure of plasma minus the colloid osmotic pressure of tissue fluid minus the blood pressure at the venous end of the capillary. During a state of equilibrium the sum of the factors favoring filtration and the sum of those favoring reabsorption are equal. A disturbance or change in either one of these factors will lead either to increased filtration or increased reabsorption until equilibrium is again established (Table 32). This equation can be stated more simply: the colloid osmotic pressure of plasma minus the colloid osmotic pressure of tissue fluid must equal the average intracapillary pressure (half the sum of the pressure at the arteriolar end and the pressure at the venous end) minus the tissue pressure. If edema is formed, one of these four factors is disturbed and transudation of fluid continues until there is an increase in tissue pressure great enough to overcome it or until the disturbed factor itself is restored toward normal.

MECHANISMS CONTROLLING BODY FLUIDS

Fluid balance is normally achieved by regulatory mechanisms mediated by the kidney. The substances concerned are principally water and sodium chloride, al-

TABLE 32. PERIPHERAL FACTORS LEADING TO
TRANSUDATION OF FLUID FROM PLASMA INTO TISSUES

	HYDROSTATIC PRESSURE		OSMOTIC PRESSURE		CHANGE TENDING TO RESTORE EQUILIBRIUM
TYPE OF DISTURBANCE	Capillary Blood Pressure	Tissue Pressure	Plasma Oncotic Pressure	Tissue Oncotic Pressure	
Equilibrium	$\dfrac{P_A + P_V}{2}$ $-$	P_T $=$	OP_P $-$	OP_T	....
Capillary blood pressure increased					
Arteriolar dilatation	$P_A \uparrow$ $-$	N $>$	N $-$	N	$P_V \downarrow$ $P_T \uparrow$
Venous hypertension	$P_V \uparrow$ $-$	N $>$	N $-$	N	$P_T \uparrow$
Capillary permeability increased	N $-$	N $>$	N $-$	$\uparrow$	$P_T \uparrow$
Hypoproteinemia	N $-$	N $>$	$\downarrow$ $-$	N	$P_T \uparrow$
Decreased tissue pressure	N $-$	$\downarrow$ $>$	N $-$	N	$P_T \rightarrow N$

Symbols: P_A = Pressure at arteriolar end of capillary
P_V = Pressure at venular end of capillary
P_T = Tissue pressure
OP_P = Plasma oncotic pressure
OP_T = Tissue fluid oncotic pressure

The dynamic formula from which this simplified one was derived is as follows:

$$\text{Filtration} = P_A - OP_P - P_T + OP_T = P_T - OP_T + OP_P - P_V = \text{Resorption}$$

though other electrolytes and electrolytic substances may play a part. Water is excreted in expired air, in stools, in sweat and insensible perspiration and in urine. Unless pathologic conditions are present, the amount excreted by way of expired air is quite constant, varying with the humidity of the inspired air; about 500 ml. per day are lost through this route. The stools normally contain little water, although in some pathologic conditions they contain so much as seriously to deplete the body and cause shock and death. Insensible perspiration depends upon the environment, as does the amount of sweat. It is not known whether the amount is controlled by other influences than environmental temperature, although sweating has a neurogenic control in part. High environmental temperatures very rapidly may deplete the body of water

and of salt and may cause hemoconcentration and diminish the volume of blood and interstitial fluid (see Chap. 30). The sodium and chloride content of sweat is apparently under hormonal control and is influenced by the activity of the adrenal cortex, the concentrations normally being about one-third that of plasma.

Renal Regulation of Water and Electrolyte Balance. The kidneys perform a marvelously exact function of regulating the water and electrolyte content of the body. To understand this mechanism, one must examine the function of the nephron and consider the several ways in which fluid and electrolyte balance may be affected. The situation in the nephron is basically similar to that in other capillaries and is governed by the same mechanisms: those of filtration and reabsorption. The com-

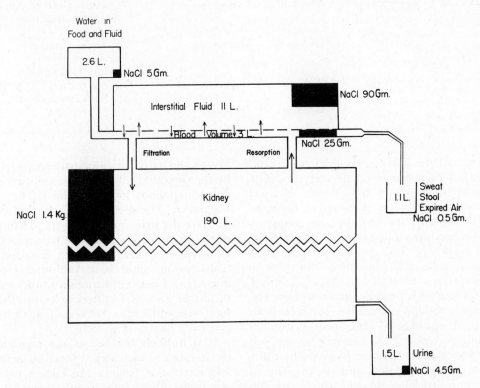

Fig. 193. Diagrammatic representation of the total daily fluid interchange in the kidneys. The volumes are of such magnitude compared with the intake and output that relatively small absolute changes of one function without compensation by another lead to serious imbalance. Sodium chloride exchange is shown by the proportionate black squares. Bicarbonate and other anions have been ignored in the diagram, for simplification, chloride being shown in terms of sodium. There is free interchange of salt and water between blood and tissue fluid.

TABLE 33. PRINCIPAL FACTORS FOUND OR PROPOSED FOR
REGULATING EXTRACELLULAR FLUID VOLUME

SUBSTANCE AFFECTED	FUNCTION OF CIRCULATION	STIMULUS	RECEPTORS	MECHANISMS OR EFFECTS
Retention by Distal Renal Tubules				
Water	Blood volume	Reduced	Left atrium	Vasopressin
	Blood pressure	Reduced	Thyro-carotid	Vasopressin
	Osmolarity	Increased	Midbrain	Vasopressin
Salt	Blood volume	Reduced	Right atrium ⎫	Aldosterone-
	Blood pressure	Reduced	Carotid sinus ⎬	Stimulating Hormone(s) and ACTH
	Osmolarity	Reduced	Unknown ⎭	
Excretion by Distal Renal Tubules				
Water	Blood volume	Increased ⎫		
	Blood pressure	Increased ⎬	Unknown ? passive	(Lack of active hormones ?)
	Osmolarity	Reduced ⎭		
Salt	Blood volume	Increased	Unknown ? passive ⎫	
	Blood pressure	Increased	Unknown ⎬	(Lack of active hormones ?)
	Osmolarity	Increased	Unknown ? passive ⎭	
Intrarenal Retention or Excretion				
Water and Salt	Blood pressure	Reduced	Unknown	Glomerular filtration reduced, tubular reabsorption increased
		Increased	Unknown	Glomerular filtration increased, tubular reabsorption reduced
	Osmolarity	Reduced	Unknown	Proximal tubular reabsorption of NaCl increased
		Increased	Unknown	

plexity of the kidney as a specialized structure for excretion from the body lies principally in the addition to simple capillary filtration and venular reabsorption the structures necessary for reabsorption against osmotic pressure. The tubules perform work, the capillary bed probably does not.* Water, salts, and substances dissolved in plasma are filtered by the glomerular capillaries at a high pressure, about 75 mm. Hg. These substances are then reabsorbed by tubular epithelium back into peritubular capillary blood, some actively by the performance of work, some passively by diffusion or by increased osmotic pressure of efferent arteriolar blood, which contains proteins concentrated by about 20 per cent.

* The mucosa of the gastrointestinal tract and the tubules of sweat and of salivary glands may also perform work against osmotic pressure and be regulated by hormonal influences. Active transport in other capillaries has been suggested.

Water and salts are principally reabsorbed by the proximal tubules, the total during a day being about 190 liters and 1.4 Kg., respectively. The distal tubules further concentrate the urine and adjust its pH to the needs of the body's acid-base balance. Obviously a very small change in filtration or reabsorption could have profound consequences: a 1 per cent variation would result in loss or gain of 1.9 liters of extracellular fluid—the difference between dehydration and early edema (Fig. 193).

It is unlikely that all of the regulatory mechanisms of such a vital function as fluid and electrolyte balance are known. However, several have been found. Powerful intrinsic intrarenal mechanisms exist; in fact, the kidney probably would perform adequately without its extrinsic nervous and hormonal influences, although it could not respond rapidly to small changes. There are direct autonomic nervous effects and at least two hormones, one affecting retention of water and one affecting retention of sodium chloride. The subject is complex, confused, and only partially understood. It is well to examine separately the influences governing osmolarity as affecting: (1) water, (2) sodium chloride, (3) blood volume, and (4) blood pressure (Table 33).

Intrinsic Renal Controls. Glomerular filtration and tubular reabsorption can markedly affect water and electrolyte balances, as will be discussed. In chronic hyponatremia, for example, proximal tubules absorb excessive sodium from glomerular filtrate.[20] There are intrinsic "reflexes" maintaining renal blood flow and oxygen tension in spite of lowered perfusion pressures, the latter, however, occurring at the expense of an acid cortex.[21,22] These mechanisms are highly important and little understood.

Renin, secreted probably from juxtaglomerular cells, appears to cause release of aldosterone (and other adrenal hormones) from the adrenal cortex.[23] The stimulus for release of renin is almost always reduction in renal blood flow. The evidence strongly suggests that the effector substance formed by renin, angiotensin, stimulates the adrenal cortex of dogs[24,25] and, in vitro, of cattle,[26] as well as producing vasoconstriction (See Chapter 12). Thus arterial pressure would be raised and blood volume tend to be restored by the same hormone. The clinical significance of these experiments is unknown.

Hormonal Controls. Active reabsorption of water by the distal tubules is governed by the antidiuretic hormone (ADH), called vasopressin, an octapeptide formed in the paraventricular nuclei and supra-optic area, released from and stored in the posterior pituitary (neurohypophysis). Release, under control from the hypothalamic region, depends largely upon hyperosmolarity.[27] Osmoreceptors, critically sensitive to changes in the concentration of plasma electrolytes, have been indirectly demonstrated in the hypothalamus[28] and perhaps in other areas, governing secretion of vasopressin from moment to moment. Chemical structure is partly species-specific, in that hog

vasopressin differs in one amino acid, lysine, from the primate and other animal ADH hormones, which have arginine. It also constricts smooth muscle of arteries and arterioles, probably through an intermediary mechanism, for it is inactive on the isolated rabbit aortic strip. Excessive amounts can be overcome by opposing influences preventing overhydration; however, no diuretic hormone has been isolated.

Active reabsorption of sodium by the distal tubules is governed mainly by aldosterone, a potent steroid formed by the zona glomerulosa of the adrenal cortex.[30] One manner of release may be through angiotensin.[32] Changes in electrolyte concentrations of adrenal perfusates have failed to show direct effects on adrenal venous contents of this hormone. Adrenocorticotropic hormone (ACTH) apparently affects it only under certain conditions and may not be its principal regulator (although prolonged use in human beings often leads to edema from salt retention). A relatively simple indole substance, structurally related to melanotonin and obtained from the area of the midbrain, "adrenoglomerulotropin," has been found to cause release;[31] its existence has been disputed.[32] While active tubular reabsorption of sodium chloride by aldosterone can be overcome by opposing influences at a new level, preventing cellular dehydration, no natruretic hormone has been isolated or identified. However, a large part of the activity of whole adrenal extracts rests in the amorphous fraction, a fact often forgotten under the enthusiasm of dealing with pure compounds, of which the adrenal contains several.

Nervous Controls. The hormones with target sites in the kidney are apparently somewhat under nervous control. Antidiuretic hormone, released by the neurohypophysis, is affected by volume or stretch receptors in the left atrium and pulmonary veins.[33,34] Impulses are transmitted via the glossopharyngeal and vagus nerves to the medulla and thence to the hypothalamus, the exact central pathways not yet having been discovered. Both stimulatory and inhibitory fibers appear to be present. Similar receptors have been found on the arterial side, at the thyrocarotid junction. Therefore, both arterial and venous pressure may influence the release of vasopressin, making volume, in terms of pressure, and concentration, in terms of osmolarity, mediated by nervous mechanisms in respect to water.

In respect to electrolytes, aldosterone also may be governed in part by nerves. Although the most potent stimulus to aldosterone secretion is a lowering of the intake of sodium chloride, this hormone may also be under control by both volume and pressor receptors, the former apparently situated in the right atrium, while the latter are perhaps in the thyrocarotid junction.[35] Afferent pathways appear to pass via the ninth and tenth cranial nerves to the hypothalamic region. Efferent influences are probably hormonal, through Aldosterone-Stimulating Hormone(s), but also, perhaps, by release of adrenoglomerulotropin.[31] Sympathetic renal nerves also may partly affect sodium retention; when one adrenal is removed from dogs, thereby cutting part of that kidney's nerve supply, sodium and chloride are excreted differentially by the homolateral kidney.[36] The mechanism is unexplained. It must be emphasized that these nervous mechanisms appear to be of secondary physiologic importance, derangements not causing overt disease. Many clinical conditions involving disturbances are not necessarily associated with imbalances of water or electrolytes.

All vital functions are controlled by opposing influences providing readiy adjustable balances under "tension." The perceptive renologist will immediately note that liberation of both antidiuretic hormone (to retain water) and aldosterone (to retain salt) is opposed by lack of release, leaving glomerular filtration rate and tubular reabsorption as the "opposing force" in the net balances of body water and salt. Teleologically speaking, these "forceless" influences leave much to be desired. A near perfect system would include both diuretic and natruretic components. Although suggested, neither has been identified. Furthermore, while there is some explanation of how *blood* volume is regulated, none has been proposed for the regulation of *extracellular fluid* volume, a function obviously under strong homeostatic control.

DISTURBANCES OF REGULATION OF BODY FLUIDS COMMON TO MOST FORMS OF EDEMA

Primary transudation of fluid from blood to tissue spaces in amounts large enough significantly to decrease effective circulating blood volume* is always accompanied either by renal retention of water and electrolytes to repair the deficit or by embarrassment of the circulation. The latter circumstance occurs when the intake of fluids is limited and when available stores are depleted. The initial formation of edema therefore resembles in its circulatory aspects hemorrhage, differing in that red blood cells and usually protein are not lost. The stimulus for salt and water retention probably is common to all conditions involving loss of effective circulating blood volume, affecting the kidneys which govern the retention, and other organs which govern renal regulatory mechanisms. There are several ways by which this can be accomplished.

Changes in Renal Regulatory Mechanisms. Changes in glomerular filtrate of as little as 5 per cent unaccompanied by changes in tubular reabsorption would lead to serious depletion of body fluids or to overhydration. Fortunately reabsorption of both water and electrolytes alters normally when glomerular filtrate changes, maintaining the fluid equilibrium. A change in the amount of salt reabsorbed would lead either to excessive retention or depletion of electrolytes.

Small changes are difficult to measure accurately. Theoretically, they can result from (1) changes in filtration rate, (2) changes in renal blood flow, (3) changes in the rate of reabsorption of water and salt. Combinations are possible. A fall in glomerular filtration rate without change in the rate of reabsorption will lead to retention of fluids. A marked decrease in renal blood flow with less fall in filtration rate will lead to greater retention. Increased reabsorption of salt (with which water is retained) will cause retention. Which of these mechanisms operates is not known definitely; probably all

* The expression "effective circulating blood volume" is used in this review to denote that amount of circulating blood which is adequate to supply the needs of the body.

of them contribute at one stage or another.

Changes in Renal Blood Flow. When insufficient blood is flowing through the kidneys, or blood is shunted away from the kidneys by some external influence, there may be insufficient filtration for excretion of fluids.[37] Under these conditions water and salt may be retained—in themselves they can lead to edema. Some mechanism such as this has been believed to account for the edema of congestive circulatory failure.[38] A similar situation may result when the kidneys are severely diseased, especially in nephrosclerosis and in glomerulonephritis. Insufficient blood may flow through the kidneys to form enough glomerular filtrate to rid the body of excessive water and salt, and edema may accumulate. Diseases affecting the tubules of the kidneys may also interfere with the renal excretion of salt and water by promoting either excessive or insufficient reabsorption.

Elevation of Venous Pressure. If systemic venous pressure is elevated, blood flow through the kidneys may be slowed. Retardation of blood flow may provide a longer amount of time for peritubular capillary blood to remain in contact with renal tubules. Thus, excessive reabsorption of water and salt may occur as a result of renal passive congestion; this has been shown to occur in experimental animals.[39]

Excessive Dietary Intake of Salt and Water. When large amounts of salt are ingested the concentrating ability of the kidneys for this electrolyte may be exceeded. It has been found that man can concentrate salt roughly to 18.0 Gm. per liter of urine. Intakes greater than this result in the retention of salt which is accompanied by retention of water. Edema and increased venous pressure have occurred as a result of excessive dietary salt intake;[40] about 3 to 6 times the normal intake is necessary. As contrasted with man, the dog can excrete large amounts of salt,[41]—about 8 times as much in proportion to body weight. However, excessive intakes of water do not lead to edema unless the kidneys are severely diseased.

Formation of Protein and Red Blood Cells. When an increase in blood volume occurs as a result of the retention of excessive fluids, which is only seen in certain forms of edema, the blood would be diluted by the retained water and salt if hematopoiesis and protein synthesis were not stimulated. Therefore, hypervolemia in which the concentrations of the constituents of the blood are normal is accompanied by an increase in the total amount of plasma proteins and the total number of red blood cells. A return to a normal blood volume must be accompanied by evidence of protein catabolism and red cell destruction, or the blood would become concentrated. The stimuli for these changes are not well understood. Albumin and most globulins are synthesized by the liver. When, through passive congestion, intrinsic disease or dietary deficiency, the rate of synthesis is less than the rate of loss, plasma osmotic pressure will be lowered and the tendency to edema increased.

Stimulus for Renal Retention. Decrease of effective circulating blood volume occurs when interstitial fluid volume is increased by any of the peripheral factors leading to transudation of fluid from plasma to tissues. The common stimulus affects renal regulation of salt and water balances, causing retention of fluids to make up for the loss. The process is halted by the effects of other influences limiting the amount of edema. The total blood volume can be normal, somewhat reduced, or increased, depending upon the primary cause of the edema. This mechanism probably does not act when local accumulations of fluid collect which are too small to affect blood volume seriously. It is possible that all forms of edema except those resulting from primary renal retention of salt and water due to excessive dietary intakes or severe renal disease originate in an affection of this mechanism at some point in its chain of interacting influences.

Alterations in Electrolytes. The concentration and composition of electrolytes may be disturbed seriously in edematous states. In fact, one could consider that pure isotonic edema of itself offers little interference with health, except for the added burden and the presumably delayed interchange of oxygen and metabolites between cell and capillary. Unfortunately, however,

Table 34. Some Stimuli Favoring Sodium and Water Retention
(Partly After Selkurt[42])

Stimulus	Renal Hemodynamics			Retention of Electrolytes		Urine Volume	Effective Blood Volume or Flow
	ERPF	GFR	FF	Na	Cl		
Upright position...............	−	−	+	+	+	−	−
Exercise......................	−	−	+	+	+	−	+
Sleeping......................	0	0	0	+	+	−	−
Sympathetic nervous stimulation..	−	−	+	+	+	±	±
Loss of blood volume...........	−	−	+	+	+	−	−
Lowered cardiac output.........	−	−	+	+	+	−	−
Increased venous pressure........	−	−	±	+	+	−	−
Excessive intake of salt..........	0	0	0	+	+	−	+
Excessive intake of water........	0	0	0	±	±	+	0
DCA.........................	±	+	?	+	+	+	+?
Aldosterone...................	0	0	0	+	+	−	?
Cortisone.....................	0	0	0	±	±	±	?
Norepinephrine................	−	+	+	0	0	±	+?
Vasopressin...................				0	0	−	?
Angiotensin	−	+	+	0	0	−	+?
Increased renal venous pressure...	−	−	±	+	+	−	0
Increased ureteral pressure.......	−	−	±	+	+	−	0
Compression of neck............		0		−	−	±	
Hypoxia......................		+		−	−		

Symbols: ERPF = Effective renal plasma flow.
        GFR = Glomerular filtration rate.
        FF   = Filtration fraction.
        +   = Increased.
        −   = Reduced.

Table 35. Some Stimuli Affecting Urinary Output
(After Gauer et al.[34])

Stimulus	Change in Intrathoracic Circulation	Change in Extrathoracic Circulation	Renal Venous Pressure	Urine Flow
Hemorrhage...................	−	−	−	−
Positive pressure breathing.......	−	+	+	−
Inferior vena caval obstruction above renal veins.............	−	±	+	−
Same below renal veins..........	−	±	−	−
Orthostasis...................	−	±	+	−
Congestion of extremities by cuffs..	−	+	−	−
Same plus 1,500 ml. blood.......	0?	+	0?	0
Blood transfusion...............	+	+	+	+
Negative pressure breathing......	+	−	−	+
Head down tilt.................	+	−	−	+
Immersion of trunk in warm bath.	+	−	+	+
Exposure to cold...............	+	−	+	+

TABLE 36. POSSIBLE COMBINATIONS OF SINGLE COMMON
ELECTROLYTE DISTURBANCES IN REFERENCE TO WHOLE BODY[43]

| | | | EXTRACELLULAR FLUIDS | | |
DESIGNATION	TOTAL BODY WATER	TOTAL BODY SALT	CONCEN- TRATION	TOTAL (BODY WT.)	EXAMPLES
Hypotonic overhydration............	+	N	−	+	Water retention
Hypotonic isohydration.............	N	−	−	N	Salt deprivation
Hypotonic dehydration.............	−	−−	−	−	Adrenal insufficiency
Hypertonic overhydration..........	+	++	+	+	Salt water retention
Hypertonic isohydration...........	N	+	+	N	Salt retention
Hypertonic dehydration............	−	N	+	−	Water deprivation
Isotonic overhydration.............	+	+	N	+	Edema
Isotonic isohydration..............	N	N	N	N	Normal state
Isotonic dehydration...............	−	−	N	−	Simple dehydration

	TOTAL BODY ACID	TOTAL BODY BASE	pH
Absolute acidosis..................	+	N	−
Relative acidosis..................	N	−	−
Absolute alkalosis.................	N	+	+
Relative alkalosis.................	−	N	+
Normal state.....................	N	N	N

NOTE: There are 44 possible combinations of the above and 1 normal state, when one includes the relations of acid to base loss or excess, for each of the above functions can vary independently of another. When metabolic and respiratory acid-base disturbances are included, there are 81 combinations.

when serious water and salt retention is set in motion, the normal checks and balances which keep the *milieu intérieur* at an optimum concentration of salt water and pH may go awry. Not only may renal regulation be altered, but over- or under-production of the renal monitors may occur, leading to marked disorders of concentration and acid-base balance.[43] Since the introduction of the flame photometer in clinical practice, these disorders are being diagnosed much more frequently. In themselves, further disorders may be produced, especially in cellular concentrations of water and electrolytes, which can lead to profound illness and death. Renal insufficiency may be one result.[44]

Table 36 lists the 44 possible combinations of changes in total body water, total body salt, total acid or base and their relations to concentrations of each. A moment

of reflection will show that the subject is not as complicated as it appears on the surface. Obviously if there is an excess of water in the body without adequate salt, extracellular fluid will be hypotonic. If total body water is then decreased in amount, dehydration will result (hypotonic dehydration). There are thus three types of edema or overhydration of the whole body, hypotonic, hypertonic and isotonic, depending upon whether more or less salt or water is present. Only the last does not affect the integrity of the cell by disturbing the Donnan equilibrium. Likewise, acid-base imbalances may be found which can profoundly affect the cells, again from a total of too much or too little, a loss of one or the other. The electrolyte changes in dehydration are discussed in Chapter 30.

Many of these profound disturbances, which probably affect every cell in the body, are the result of eating and drinking excesses or insufficiencies of salt or water during the development of edema, while renal mechanisms are unable to make up for these mistakes. The most frequent alterations are those of hypotonicity and acidosis. Edema (overhydration) resulting from cirrhosis of the liver is especially apt to be hypotonic with respect to cells. In severe anasarca from congestive heart failure hypotonicity is often found. When organic renal disease has caused the edema, both hypotonicity and acidosis may be present. Hypotonic overhydration, like hypertonic dehydration, is especially prone to cause renal insufficiency in respect to the excretion of water, salts and nitrogen, and produce more edema.

Preservation of the *milieu intérieur* is vital to proper cellular function. Hypotonicity of interstitial fluid causes cellular swelling with loss of K and Mg and gain of Na by the cell. Hypertonicity induces shrinkage, but integrity of the cell membrane is disturbed in both conditions in the same direction. Acidity and alkalinity also alter the membrane's function to conserve K and Mg and to repel sodium. Basic enzymatic processes are thus changed and cellular "health" impaired. The ability of the kidneys to restore imbalances may be exceeded, leading to renal failure and death in a manner not well understood. In severe hyponatremia, for example, the kidney fails to excrete water,[44] although it is present in excess.

Of preventable nature are the iatrogenic disturbances resulting from the injection of too much salt or water into patients with limited renal function. The commonest forms of edema in these are hypotonicity and acidosis, due to the prevalent use of intravenous fluids and the mistaken ideas that physiologic saline solution is a diuretic and that water given always will be excreted even when kidneys are damaged.*

* So-called physiologic saline solution is also an acid in effect, containing 145 mEq. of sodium and 145 mEq. of chloride per liter. Extracellular fluid contains approximately 144 and 103 respectively, the balance being composed of bicarbonate and other anions. In order for saline to replace lost body fluids, about 40 mEq. of chloride must be excreted by the kidney as HCl or NH_4Cl.

Intracellular excesses and losses cannot be measured at present; therefore we are forced to consider the measurable extracellular ones. Since limited renal function carries with it limited ability to adjust, we must avoid unnecessary renal work from overloading with electrolytes or water. A diseased kidney cannot make up for our own mistakes and often not for the patient's own errors in ingesting nonphysiologic amounts.

EDEMA CAUSED BY PRIMARY TRANSUDATION OF FLUIDS FROM BLOOD TO TISSUE SPACES

Edema may be caused by multiple disturbances, or it may result primarily from single factors. In the following discussion, the various types of edema will be considered in the light of their most logical explanation. It must be emphasized that all the facts in each instance are not known, and therefore the present classification may be modified when new evidence accumulates. A general class is comprised of those forms of edema resulting from transudation of fluids due to peripheral vascular factors; the sequence of events is: first, transudation, second, loss of effective circulating blood volume and third, restoration of blood volume by stimulation of renal regulatory mechanisms. The accumulation of edema in these conditions usually occurs gradually, small disturbances of equilibrium being followed by corrective measures in a recurring cycle until final equilibrium is attained.

EDEMA DUE TO CHANGES IN CAPILLARY BLOOD PRESSURE

Capillary pressure may be increased either by increased venous pressure or by arteriolar dilatation. The greater flow accompanying the latter may compensate for the increased filtration, many closed capillaries opening and functioning to promote reabsorption; therefore, examples of significant edema due to this are rare. States of peripheral vasodilatation (aortic insufficiency, hyperthyroidism) are not in themselves accompanied by increased interstitial fluids.

Neurologic disease affecting autonomic nervous control of vasoconstriction has been said to cause edema localized to an affected extremity or side, as seen in hemiplegia.[45] Complicating factors are the decreased lymphatic and venous flow associated with muscular inactivity. Perhaps the best example of edema caused by capillary pressure is that seen when an extremity is immersed in hot water; local and general arteriolar dilatation results. The summer edema of the ankles, especially common in women, may be partly a result of arteriolar dilatation, to which is added the increased hydrostatic pressure of the arterial blood column in the erect position (about 110 mm. Hg in the ankles), and of the venous column (about 100 mm. Hg). While surgical sympathectomy of an extremity is not followed by edema, chemical sympathectomy by ganglionic blockade often is associated with minor degrees; both arteriolar and venular tone may be affected.

Edema of the optic disk and the brain resulting from acute and severe arterial hypertension probably represent examples of increased capillary pressure leading to transudation of plasma. Tissue pressure in the eyeball is about 25 mm. Hg; as a result, arteries and arterioles are thin-walled. When extreme vasoconstriction in the whole body occurs, these relatively weaker structures probably cannot constrict to the same degree. The result is that capillaries are forcefully engorged with blood, followed by transudation of fluid (retinal sheen), of local collections of plasma ("cottonwool" exudates) and of blood (hemorrhages).

The walls of the arteries of the brain are also thinner than are those of the rest of the body, being enclosed in a rigid skull where tissue pressure is relatively inflexible. It is possible that cerebral edema (wet brain) resulting from severe hypertension is also caused by insufficiently powerful vasoconstriction relative to the periphery. It must be pointed out that this explanation, while logical from a serious consideration of hemodynamics, is not the commonly accepted one. "Ischemia" is usually said to be the cause. Ischemia, however, directly produces edema in no other tissue.

The most common causative factor of edema is increased venous pressure, causing increased capillary pressure—especially at the venular or reabsorptive end of the capillary network. In 1926 Landis[46] demonstrated that capillary blood pressure may be measured directly by a microcannulation method. Krogh, Landis and Turner[47] studied the relation between venous pressure and the transudation of fluid from capillaries into the tissues of the human arm and showed that fluid accumulates when venous pressure is raised about 15 to 20 cm. of water. When venous pressure in the forearm was elevated above 17 cm. of water, the rate of filtration of fluid into the tissue spaces was found to be directly proportional to the increase in venous pressure. It was concluded that the increase in filtration due to elevation of venous pressure was caused by the resulting rise in capillary pressure. That a rise in venous pressure does cause an elevation of capillary pressure has been repeatedly demonstrated by direct measurements.[7,46] When venous obstruction (partial or complete) causes venous stasis and congestion, there may be added the factor of hypoxia, which leads to increased capillary permeability, and a change in the relative osmotic pressures of plasma and interstitial fluid resulting from filtration of protein into the edema. In this manner edema formation is furthered.

The simplest form of this type is the *edema of posture.* The upright position is associated with a small but definite loss of plasma volume into interstitial spaces, a concentration of protein[48] and a reduction in renal blood flow.[49,50] Therefore, preedema is a normal state. Swelling of the ankles is common in persons whose employment requires long periods of standing with little muscular exertion—elevator operators, for example.* When some degree of

---

* Normal venous return against gravity is accomplished principally by muscular contraction, which "milks" blood upward. This exerts a very active function. The valves in the veins prevent return flow during muscular relaxation. Complete muscular rest of dependent parts therefore favors venous stasis. In the upright position the venous hydrostatic column above the foot is approximately 140 cm. of water (about 100 mm. Hg) higher than right atrial pressure when the veins are full.

venous obstruction and cardiovascular relaxation is added, as is often the case in persons who sleep in the sitting position in busses, trains and aircraft, edema is prone to develop but can hardly be considered pathologic.

Thrombophlebitis, phlebothrombosis (milk leg), constriction of veins by new growths, aneurysms, scarring after trauma, ligature, and other changes which *interfere with venous return* are associated with edema of the area drained by the affected veins. The ability of collateral venous channels to assume total venous flow is enormous, however; simple ligature of a single vein, even a large one, may be followed by little if any edema. Varicose veins are often accompanied by edema; dilatation of their walls renders functionless the valves which normally prevent overdistention and nullify in part the effects of hydrostatic pressure. Probably the long uninterrupted hydrostatic column from heart to foot is the principal factor concerned.

Arteriovenous aneurysms provide direct arterial pressure to the venous circulation and are often accompanied by edema, which may be surprisingly small in view of the great pressure. Arterialization of the venous wall develops; probably collateral circulation not in direct contact with the aneurysm provides most of the venous return. Reversal of the circulation by surgical anastomosis of artery to vein has succeeded in a few instances;[51] experimentally it has been performed on the coronary sinus and femoral vein with only temporary edema developing.

Pulmonary edema represents a special set of circumstances. Pressure in the pulmonary capillaries is only about 9 mm. Hg which provides a large differential between plasma osmotic and filtration or •hydrostatic pressures. In addition, pulmonary lymphatics are widespread and active. Therefore, the lungs have a built-in protection against edema, which breaks down only when high pulmonary venous and capillary pressures exceed net colloid osmotic pressure, and when alveolar edema is formed faster than the lymphatics can remove it. Pulmonary edema results, therefore, from rather extreme disturbances of one or more

factors influencing fluid exchange generally. It can occur from (1) *increased capillary blood volume,* the result of a disproportion of the output of the right and left ventricles, caused by left-sided myocardial failure (as in severe arterial hypertension, aortic insufficiency, or coronary occlusion) or insufficient left ventricular filling or emptying (as in mitral stenosis or insufficiency), leading to increased pressure in pulmonary veins. A simple calculation shows that if the left ventricle pumps continuously as little as 0.01 ml. less blood per beat than the right, over a liter will collect in the lungs in 24 hours. If the disproportion is 1.0 ml., almost 5 liters would collect in one hour, and pulmonary venous pressure would be greatly increased. It has been estimated that pulmonary edema will develop when the lungs contain about 2 to 3 liters extra of blood. Experimental evidence that Starling's hypothesis holds for the lungs has been demonstrated in dogs.[52] Increased blood volume from massive transfusions or infusions, and arteriolar dilatation from drugs may induce it when other factors are operative. (2) *Increased capillary permeability* from the direct action of toxic gases, poisons and respiratory burns, leads to massive serous and bloody edema. (3) *Decreased plasma oncotic pressure* accompanying starvation, hepatic cirrhosis or the nephrotic syndrome carries with it a tendency to pulmonary edema. (4) It is possible that *negative pressure breathing* may cause it when added to another disturbance, for positive pressure breathing favors its control.

Edema of the face may develop during severe respiratory efforts, especially in bronchial asthma and other forms of bronchial or tracheal obstruction; the effort leads to increased venous pressure. The orbital spaces are especially prone to develop fluid because of the very low tissue pressure therein; sometimes edema under the eyes is the first sign of retention of fluids. Edema localized to the upper half of the body is the cardinal sign of obstruction of the superior vena cava.

Increased venous pressure, therefore, provides one of the conditions which leads to edema, and probably constitutes the most

TABLE 37. ESTIMATE OF BLOOD DISTRIBUTION IN THE VASCULAR BED

(After Bazett[53]) *

AREA	VOLUME IN ml.	AREA	VOLUME IN ml.
Heart......................	250	Aorta......................	100
Pulmonary arteries............	400	Systemic arteries..............	450 .
Pulmonary capillaries..........	60	Systemic capillaries............	300
Saccular venules..............	140	Venules......................	200
Pulmonary veins..............	700	Systemic veins................	2,050
Total pulmonary system........	1,300	Total systemic vessels..........	3,100
Heart....................	250	Unaccounted 550. (Probably extra blood in reservoirs of liver and spleen.)	
	1,550		

* This table represents a rough estimate of the situation in a 30-year-old man weighing 63 Kg. and 178 cm. tall, with an assumed blood volume of 5.2 liters. It will be seen that the pulmonary and systemic system account for at least 3 liters and that over 80 per cent of the blood in the peripheral circulation, excluding the capillaries, is in the venous system.

common single factor. Systemic venous pressure can be elevated chronically in three ways: by increase in blood volume, by decrease in venous capacity (by generalized venoconstriction), and probably to a small extent by failure of cardiac filling. However, failure of cardiac filling per se does not contribute to pronounced rises, in view of the relatively small arterial blood volume as compared to the venous volume, unless other factors operate (Table 37). Local venous hypertension can be produced by obstructive or hydrostatic interferences with venous flow. When venous congestion is present to a significant degree, restoration of effective blood volume probably occurs, and total (but not effective) blood volume is increased.

EDEMA DUE TO INCREASED PERMEABILITY OF CAPILLARIES

The capillary endothelium normally holds within the capillaries more than 95 per cent of the protein in the plasma. If the permeability of the capillary wall increases, protein escapes into the extravascular fluid, thereby increasing its effective colloid osmotic pressure and disturbing the reabsorption-filtration equilibrium. This leads to the formation of edema, as has been demonstrated experimentally. Tainter and Hanzlik[54] have shown that the edema produced by paraphenylene diamine is due to injury of the capillary wall, resulting in escape of plasma protein. When edema is produced by acute uranium poisoning, the fluid contains a high concentration of protein, suggesting that the edema is due to capillary damage.[55] The local application of irritants to epithelial surfaces likewise produces edema in the underlying tissues. The common wheal, seen in urticaria and in various skin tests utilized in clinical practice, is in reality a form of local edema. The high protein content of the edema fluid removed from such wheals indicates that the edema formation is due, at least in part, to increased permeability of the capillaries.[56] Both heat and cold, if sufficiently severe, will cause blisters which contain a high concentration of protein.[57] Burns are characteristically followed by serous transudation. Although the edema that accompanies most acute infections is no doubt a relatively complicated phenomenon, the presence of red cells and fluid of high protein content in the tissue spaces indicates that the capillary permeability is much increased. Of particular importance is the observation by Landis[58] that *lack of oxygen*, brought on by such factors as stasis, may cause the wall of a capillary to be permeable to protein. Finally, Fishberg has concluded that the capillaries about the various serous cavities of the body are more permeable than those in subcutaneous tissues, as evidenced by the fact that the protein content of ascitic and pleural transudates is considerably higher than that of subcutaneous fluid.[59] However, it should be pointed out that the relatively high protein content of pleural and ascitic fluid may be due not to increased capillary permeability but rather to a relatively inefficient removal of protein by the lymphatics of the pleura and the peritoneum, as compared with those of the subcutaneous tissues, protein being concentrated as water is reabsorbed. In addition, "tissue" pressure is low in the peritoneal cavity and is negative in the pleural spaces.

Edema is caused primarily by increased capillary permeability in conditions involving anoxia, irritation, sensitivity, trauma, capillary toxins, and certain dietary deficiency states. The edema of acute nephritis may begin in this way. Because proteins are filtered with edema fluid, reabsorption is severely hindered in proportion to the difference in concentrations of plasma and edema. Serous transudates accordingly are absorbed with difficulty and limited in extent by tissue pressure.

Enormous amounts of serous fluid may escape through capillary walls after severe burns and trauma, causing serious circulatory disturbances. Much of the resultant shock is due to mechanical loss of fluid. Renal regulatory mechanisms cannot cope with sudden losses; therefore, replacement is necessary. Saline infusions do little more than increase the amount of edema; readily filtrable, they provide no osmotic difference between plasma and extravascular fluid. Protein is mandatory, therefore, and plasma transfusions are the logical means for replacement. Pressure bandages and plaster casts applied to burned or traumatized extremities before edema has fully developed will often oppose the transudation of fluid by increasing tissue pressure.[60]

The edema from snake bite results from toxic action of venom upon capillaries. Such toxins increase permeability and produce transudation of protein-rich fluid. Allergic edema—whether angioneurotic, from serum sickness, from drugs, or from urticaria—is similar, although localized structures are more commonly involved. The edema of scurvy has been insufficiently studied; increased capillary fragility observed in vitamin C deficiency suggests, however, that the edema may contain protein in increased amounts.

Exudates act in a similar manner. Their high content of protein, which may be greater than that of plasma, provides the conditions for further transudation of water and electrolytes. The effects of capillary damage resulting from cellulitis, infections and other toxic situations are opposed by localized vascular constriction and by tissue pressure. The tense, hard, inflamed area about a local infection (boil) is a familiar example.

When protein is lost from plasma, it is probable that the mechanisms for replacement by the liver are stimulated. The formation of plasma albumin is a relatively slow process.[61] Therefore, the serious consequences of massive serous transudation cannot be nullified by renal attempts at retention of salt and water; artificial or natural replacement of the lost oncotic pressure becomes necessary. Renal retention does not restore blood volume adequately, as has been pointed out. Large amounts of protein may be stored in depots in the body; possibly depletion of these depots occurs after serous transudation.

Massive edema due to increased capillary permeability is the most serious type, for all the factors favoring capillary reabsorption of fluid are affected, with the exception of tissue pressure. Stimulation of all the natural defenses against loss of effective circulating blood volume and loss of plasma osmotic pressure probably takes place, but until some sort of equilibrium can be established, the whole body is seriously affected. In essence, the circulatory status resembles hemorrhagic shock, except for the concentration of red blood cells which occurs.

EDEMA DUE TO DECREASED OSMOTIC PRESSURE OF PLASMA

Rapid lowering of the colloid osmotic pressure of the blood can be accomplished experimentally by bleeding animals at frequent intervals and by injecting after each bleeding only the red cells (plasmapheresis). Utilizing this method in dogs, Leiter[62] showed that chronic hypoproteinemia produced by repeated plasmapheresis caused an accumulation of extravascular fluid when the plasma protein fell to *3 per cent or less*. This observation has been confirmed a number of times.[8]*

The effect of plasma proteins in combating edema formation was demonstrated by Krogh, Landis and Turner.[47] The amount of protein in the circulating blood was found to increase slightly in subjects standing motionless, the upright position causing protein-free fluid to be filtered into dependent tissues. The effect on filtration rate of changes in colloid osmotic pressure of the blood was studied by determining the filtration produced in the forearm by a given venous pressure while the subject stood and while he reclined. A unit rise of colloid osmotic pressure (1 cm. of water) decreased the filtration rate by 0.0027 to 0.0045 ml. per minute per 100 cc. of forearm.

Nutritional or "war" edema is probably caused primarily by disturbances in the synthesis of proteins[63] secondary to starvation, although other undescribed factors may operate. Apparently the body readjusts itself moderately well to chronic starvation; it was not uncommon to find enormous increases in edema when starved war prisoners were provided with their first good meals. Transudation of water and salt through capillaries because of low plasma oncotic pressure can explain most of the clinical findings. Studies of starvation have shown a tendency for the renal mechanisms to retain water and salt. In one case in which hypoproteinemia was apparently associated with ceroid disease of the small intestine and liver, overloading of the circulation with concentrated salt solution revealed no renal deficiency in excretion; retention undoubtedly had been present in view of the edema. This procedure did not deplete, but rather increased, effective circulating blood volume, and the stimulus to retention was probably overcome.[64]

Hypoproteinemic edema is found in certain renal diseases, especially the nephrotic stage of glomerulonephritis. Excessive urinary losses of protein, more than 3.5 Gm. per day, probably exceed the ability of the liver to manufacture albumin. Normally, the glomerulus filters up to 30 or 40 Gm. of protein in 24 hours, almost all of which is reabsorbed by the tubules. Nephrotic glomeruli have increased permeabilities; it is not known whether decreased tubular reabsorption also plays a part, nor whether decreased hepatic synthesis contributes to the lowered plasma albumin. At any rate low plasma colloid osmotic pressure appears to be the fundamental process concerned; blood volume is normal or low, renal retention of salt and water is highly active, and massive isosmotic edema (anasarca) usually results. Losses of essential constituents carried in plasma by albumin (lipids, vitamins, trace metals) may also contribute to the clinical state.

EDEMA DUE TO DECREASED TISSUE PRESSURE

Decreased tissue pressure may be a factor in some forms of edema. When skin and subcutaneous tissues are loose, dependent edema is sometimes noticed; this does not usually represent a pathologic condition. In aged persons and in those who have recently lost considerable weight, evening swelling of the ankles may develop, which disappears over night. Although it is difficult to separate this cause from other factors, such as the increased capillary pressure and slightly diminished oncotic pressure which may be present in such persons, clinical observations that patients recently edematous with stretched tissues gain edema more rapidly than do others with more firm tissues lends support to this conclusion. The ease of fluid formation in the pleural

---

* A simple method for estimating the plasma oncotic pressure is to multiply the concentration of albumin by 5.5 mm. Hg and the concentration of globulin by 1.4 mm. Hg. The total is normally 25 to 30 mm. Hg. Hypoproteinemia is said to be a factor causing edema if the total is less than 20 mm. Methods of measurement of albumin and globulin used in most clinical laboratories are not necessarily accurate, however. Edema may disappear without change in plasma proteins and may not always occur when they are low. The osmotic pressure of proteins changes with the concentration.

and peritoneal cavities, where "tissue" pressure is low or absent, is well known.

EDEMA OF LYMPH STASIS

Lymphatic obstruction can cause edema. After radical operations for carcinoma of the breast with widespread removal of lymph nodes, swelling of the arm on the affected side may develop. After an interval, the swelling may subside partially or completely. Metastatic carcinomatosis of lymph nodes can produce the same result. Lymphangitis may also give rise to edema. Chronic osteomyelitis is often accompanied by edema of the affected part, probably due to obstruction of lymphatic channels. This process can be a contributory factor in other infections associated with cellulitis.

Filariasis in its later stages is accompanied by elephantiasis, often involving one or both legs and the genital organs. The worms become encysted in lymph nodes after hematogenous spread, and the irritation resulting from their presence is believed to interfere with the transport of lymph. Although lymphedema occurs in the initial stages, later ones are characterized by an enormous proliferation of fibrous tissue; the size of the affected extremity is partly due to fibrosis. It is believed that the scar tissue results from infection by organisms of low virulence following trauma to the edematous part. Therefore, elephantiasis may be the result of obstruction to lymph nodes and superimposed lymphangitis.

An uncommon type of lymphedema, the pathogenesis of which is little understood, is primary hereditary trophedema, or Milroy's disease. This condition is characterized by lymphedema in the legs, which is sharply demarcated at the level of a joint and which eventually involves both legs to the groin. The hereditary nature of the disease makes its recognition fairly easy.

As the lymphatics remove the small amount of protein filtered through capillaries, the fluid of lymphedema is rich in protein and its albumin fraction proportionately greater than in plasma. Naturally, tissue oncotic pressure is thus higher and its ratio to plasma greater, interfering with normal capillary reabsorption of fluids. Lymphedema is therefore difficult to remove.

EDEMA CAUSED BY PRIMARY RENAL RETENTION OF SALT AND WATER

Renal retention of salt (and therefore water) can result from (1) ingestion of more salt than normal kidneys can excrete, (2) diminution of the excretory ability for salt by renal parenchymal disease or dysfunction, so that normal intake exceeds output, and (3) stimulation of normal tubular reabsorptive mechanisms by intrinsic disease or by extrarenal hormonal influences.

Ingestion of excessive salt (20 to 30 Gm. per day) by normal subjects is accompanied by a rise in venous pressure and body weight and the appearance of minimal edema; all changes return to normal rapidly when salt is discontinued.[40] Extracellular fluid volume may be increased merely by an excess of salt accompanied by an excess of water in the body.

Certain stages of severe, often terminal, renal disease, especially arteriolar nephrosclerosis and chronic glomerulonephritis with uremia are accompanied by edema. It is probable that this is a result of mechanical retention of salt and water due to the inability of the kidney to excrete them. Pathogenesis is not well understood, and the findings vary widely from excessive retention to excessive excretion. We may postulate that the differences occur because of the variable nature and extent of the lesions in a majority of nephrons; diminished glomerular filtration is always present, and the balance between salt and water retention and excretion depends upon the relative activity of the remaining tubules. If a majority fail to reabsorb, salt will be lost; if a majority reabsorb actively, salt will be retained and edema will appear. The wide disturbance of electrolyte balance seen in uremic states may be to some extent compensatory, for attempts to correct low sodium or chloride levels usually result in edema. Obstructive uropathies lead to edema if water and salt intake exceed output, as do primary renal diseases with diminished renal function.

Steroid substances similar to or identical

with those produced by certain endocrine glands act upon the renal tubules, directly stimulating the reabsorption of salt from glomerular filtrate. Deoxycorticosterone acetate (DCA) has a strong action in this respect; testosterone, progesterone and other allied substances have it to some degree. The daily injection of DCA causes *transient* retention of salt and water, a gain in weight,[65] and in some cases, edema. Patients with adrenal insufficiency may be more prone to develop such edema than those with intact adrenals.[66] Patients treated with large doses of testosterone, estrogen, cortisone, hydrocortisone or progesterone sometimes retain salt and water and may develop mild to severe edema. Aldosterone, 9α-fluorohydrocortisone and its methyl derivative are the most potent salt-retaining substances known.

This phenomenon has provided an analogy to the edema sometimes seen in the premenstrual period. A few days before the menses (concurrent with maturation of the corpus luteum) some women have oliguria, gain weight, and notice ankle edema. As the menses begin, diuresis and weight loss occur coincidentally with the regression in the corpus luteum. The nature of the hormone causing salt retention has not been disclosed.

The edema of Cushing's syndrome may be of similar cause. Considerable endocrine imbalance, especially of the adrenal-pituitary axis, is characteristic of this group of diseases, which can be the result of tumors or hyperplasia of the adrenal cortex, or of pituitary dysfunction. Edema is not always present. The adrenal cortex secretes salt-retaining and possibly salt-losing hormones; retention may depend upon a predominance of the former. Some steroids are initially salt-retaining, then become salt-losing. Patients differ in their reactions to these substances. Stimulation of the adrenal cortex by injection of adrenocorticotropic hormone can result in considerable edema due to retention of salt;[67] the mechanism is probably through the increased reabsorption of salt due to renal stimulation by adrenal cortical hormones other than aldosterone.

The above examples can be considered with some reservations as edema due to primary renal retention of salt. It must be re-emphasized that all edema of any degree is accompanied by renal retention of salt initiated by the low blood volume following transudation. Primary renal edema has its seat in the kidneys alone, or in extrarenal factors stimulating the tubules directly; in other forms the renal element appears to be secondary.

EDEMA DUE TO UNKNOWN CAUSES

A variety of diseases can be accompanied by edema, the cause of which has been insufficiently studied. Speculation as to the factors involved is unrewarding until more facts are known; the mechanisms probably are to be found among those discussed, and not in some new and revolutionary concept.

Edema associated with old age, convalescence and cachexia may be caused by decreased tissue pressure, increased capillary pressure, and/or lowered oncotic pressure. Definitive studies have not been made. The sometimes massive edema of hookworm disease, which may lead to general anasarca, has as its accompaniment anemia, malnutrition, possibly lowered plasma oncotic pressure, and possibly increased capillary permeability. The edema of anemia is unexplained; increased capillary pressure due to vasodilatation, increased capillary permeability due to hypoxia, and retention of salt and water due to renal hypoxia have been considered as explanations. The edema of leukemia may have similar beginnings. The edema of relapsing fever, of malaria and of Raynaud's disease are not understood, although portal hypertension may occur in long-standing chronic malaria. Edema associated with dermatomyositis, disseminated lupus and Raynaud's phenomenon are not explicable at present except when renal disease is an associated factor. Hyperthyroidism is said to give rise to edema, in some instances due to increased capillary permeability, in others possibly secondary to congestive circulatory failure.

The cause of any type of edema can be fairly well understood by (1) examination of the circulatory factors, (2) examination of the renal factors, (3) measurement of the protein content of the fluid and (4) understanding of the known mechanisms of edema formation. These procedures, direct or indirect, are available in most clinical laboratories, and require few special technics.

EDEMA DUE TO MULTIPLE FACTORS
Edema of Portal Venous Obstruction

Portal obstruction is usually the result of intrinsic hepatic disease involving the network of veins in the portal spaces of the lobules of the liver. Scarring of involved hepatic cells, constriction of venous channels and obliteration of some of them occurs as the primary disease progresses. As a result, hepatic venous resistance is increased, leading to portal venous hypertension. The venous drainage of the splanchnic bed is disturbed, therefore, and congestion of the gastrointestinal tract, the spleen and the pancreas causes increased capillary pressure, localized to the peritoneal contents. The situation may be considered analogous to partial venous obstruction in an extremity, except that collateral circulation around the obstructed area is limited. Collateral channels are confined to the hemorrhoidal veins, the retroperitoneal plexus, the lower gastroesophageal veins, and the umbilical network through the obliterated fetal umbilical veins. Although portal hypertension provides the conditions for transudation of fluid into the walls of the intestines, whose capillary vessels are continuously secreting and reabsorbing large quantities of fluid, it is possible that the increased lymphatic drainage induced by the congestion may supply the largest part of the ascitic fluid. Furthermore, the liver itself may "weep" serous exudate as a result of obstruction to lymphatic flow.

Preceding or accompanying the portal hypertension of hepatic disease is the development of abnormalities of the plasma proteins, especially reduction in the albumin content. That this is a consequence of the primary liver disease appears obvious, but the mechanism is not wholly explained. Therefore, decreased plasma oncotic pressure becomes a factor favoring the transudation of fluid into the peritoneal cavity and into tissue spaces.

Another factor leading to venous obstruction of a more general nature is partial *constriction of the inferior vena cava* by enlargement or contraction of the liver. The vena cava passes through a notch between the right and caudate lobes; a ligament (the vena cava ligament) crosses the vein which joins the two lobes and binds it closely to the liver. Partial vena caval obstruction of this nature would lead to little hepatic venous congestion, as the hepatic veins empty into the vena cava above this ligament; however, intrahepatic obstruction in the region of the caudate lobe might produce obstruction of hepatic veins. Therefore, venous obstruction in all subdiaphragmatic areas can result from hepatic cirrhosis; inclusion of the iliac veins leads to dependent edema, and of the renal veins, to disturbances of renal function.

The ascites and dependent edema associated with chronic hepatic disease is the result of increased capillary and decreased oncotic pressure. Other factors providing for the maintenance of ascites are the oncotic pressure of the fluid and the very low "tissue" pressure in the peritoneal cavity. The peritoneal surfaces are well adapted to reabsorption of fluids which may contribute materially to their normal state. However, the oncotic pressure of ascitic fluid is usually much increased, not only in portal hypertension but also in congestive circulatory failure. The electrolyte content is similar to that of plasma, but the protein content can be high, up to 5 Gm. per 100 ml. or more. Obviously the smaller the differential is between plasma and ascitic osmotic pressures, the less readily will fluid reabsorb. So peritoneal capillaries appear either to be more permeable to protein than other capillaries, or protein becomes concentrated because of failure of lymphatic reabsorption.

As emphasized before, the loss of fluid from the circulating blood requires retention of water and electrolytes in order to maintain blood volume. As in other edematous states, the kidneys are stimulated to reabsorb sodium chloride and water. In the urine of patients with cirrhosis has been found antidiuretic substance;[68] whether this comes from the pituitary, liver or other sources has not been determined. The renal disturbance of salt excretion, however, is similar to that found in congestive circulatory failure.[69]

Enormous amounts of protein may be lost from the circulation into ascitic fluid, contributing further to the deficiency of plasma proteins. At levels of 3 Gm. per cent, 300 Gm. would be contained in 10 liters of fluid, or considerably more than that normally present in the whole plasma volume. In actuality, a degree of plasmapheresis occurs when ascites develops, continuing the state.

The several factors which operate to promote the ascites of cirrhosis of the liver have been critically reviewed by Hyatt and Smith,[70] to which the student is referred. From what is known, these authors believe that *portal hypertension* is not the dominant factor in marked ascites, although it is contributory. Likewise, *reduction of plasma proteins* exerts a secondary influence. Retention of sodium (presumably through *aldosterone* and other steroids) and retention of water (presumably through *antidiuretic substances*) are believed to play the major part. The diseased liver conjugates steroids poorly and they may accumulate.

Portal hypertension can result from portal (Laennec's) cirrhosis of the liver, cholangitic or biliary cirrhosis, the invasion of trematodes or flukes into portal venous radicles, schistosomiasis, extensive carcinomatosis, and many other diseases of the liver or portal vein which result in portal venous obstruction. The presence or absence of portal hypertension is probably determined by the extent and number of venules or veins involved. Partial obstruction of the portal vein itself causes pure portal hypertension, which may not be associated with vena caval obstruction, hypoalbuminemia, or ascites.

Edema of Pregnancy

Normal pregnancy is associated with slight ankle edema, frequently during the later stages. Toxemias of pregnancy are characterized by the presence of retention of fluids. The several factors probably operating are: (1) increased capillary pressure, (2) decreased plasma oncotic pressure and (3) renal retention of salt and water.

Increased capillary blood pressure in pregnancy can result from two conditions: direct *pressure upon pelvic veins* by the pregnant uterus and direct transmission of some arterial pressure into veins through the uterine circulation, which contains *arteriovenous anastomoses*. The pregnant uterine circulation has a large blood flow in which the normal artery-to-vein pressure gradient is less than that of most organs. Pregnancy is accompanied by an increase in circulating blood volume. The circulatory state resembles to some extent that pertaining in arteriovenous aneurysm, localized to the lower part of the body. Of equal or greater importance is the partial obstruction of the iliac veins by the large tumor, a situation which causes increased femoral venous pressure and which can lead to phlebothrombosis.

Plasma oncotic pressure is not usually low in normal pregnancy, but in toxemia the albumin concentration may fall to levels contributing to edema. The minor decreases reported,[71] which may amount to 1.0 Gm. per cent of total proteins, contribute, but are not the primary factor.

The importance of positive sodium and chloride balance in the causation of water retention in both normal and toxemic pregnancies is well established.[72,73] It is clear also that an increased excretion of sodium frequently accompanies the commonly observed postpartum diuresis.[74] There is considerable clinical and experimental evidence that the mechanism of salt retention in pregnancy is related to endocrine function. The specific hormones involved and their relative roles, however, are not known. The placenta elaborates estrogen, progesterone, DCA-like substances, and other steroids. Aldosterone in urine is increased. The fetal adrenal cortex is secreting.[75] Maternal blood volume increases, requiring formation of protein and red-blood cells and retention of water and electrolytes. At term, the woman gains about 8 Kg., of which 81 per cent is water requiring 720 mEq. of sodium.[76] Ability to excrete salt is functionally impaired. Taylor and his associates[77] attribute the water retention of pregnancy to the presence of excessive amounts of estrogenic substances and progesterone in the circulation. They report that estrogens and pregnandiol disappear from the urine shortly before the postpartum diuresis. They have also administered doses of estrogens and progesterone during puerperium and have observed that these drugs tend to prevent the usual postpartum loss of sodium.

In conclusion it may be stated that pregnancy edema is due to several factors, the most important of which appear to be: (1) increased intracapillary pressure in the lower extremities resulting from mechanical interference with venous return from the legs, (2) a tendency to hypoproteinemia and (3) electrolyte retention, apparently resulting from the endocrine changes that occur in both normal and toxemic pregnancies.

EDEMA OF BERIBERI

The edema associated with beriberi has been insufficiently studied to delineate the disturbances involved. However, it would appear that the plasma proteins are decreased,[78] that capillary permeability may possibly be increased and that the cardiac disturbances leading to congestive failure may contribute to the retention of water and salt. Under some circumstances it may be difficult to distinguish between beriberi and nutritional edema except by therapeutic tests with vitamins.[79]

Decreased plasma oncotic pressure may explain the presence of the edema which accompanies chronic beriberi without cardiac insufficiency. Although there are "wet" and "dry" forms of beriberi, correlation between plasma proteins and the presence or absence of edema has not been satisfactorily determined. When deficiency of thiamine affects the cardiovascular system a characteristic chain of events is set in motion which is accompanied by tachycardia, *increased cardiac output,* cardiac enlargement and congestive failure. The pathogenesis of this condition is not clear, but a disturbance in the myocardial cells is probably present. Edema in this situation develops as a result of the congestive failure.[80] When plasma oncotic pressure is also lowered by a fall in serum albumin obviously failure will become more marked and the tendency for renal retention of salt and

water will become greater. If increased capillary permeability is also present, which remains to be demonstrated conclusively, transudation will increase.

EDEMA OF CONGESTIVE CIRCULATORY FAILURE

The words congestive circulatory failure are used in this discussion rather than congestive "heart" failure because the same sequence of events leading to edema, increased venous pressure and retention of fluids, may be set in motion by noncardiac or by cardiac factors.[81] In general the primary initiating cause appears to lie in the heart. Obstruction to the inflow of blood into the heart (as in constrictive lesions involving the great veins or tricuspid stenosis) or obstruction to the outflow of blood from the heart (as in constrictive pericarditis) may reproduce peripheral signs of congestive failure exactly similar to those seen when the myocardium itself is damaged. Factors which appear to be important in the pathogenesis of the edema resulting from these causes are shown in Fig. 194.

Decrease in Effective Circulating Blood Volume. In almost all, if not all, cases of congestive circulatory failure the effective circulating blood volume appears to be decreased. As a result of factors arising in the heart itself or decreasing the flow of blood through the heart, the output of the heart is always *decreased* when compared to that of normal subjects, although there is some overlapping.[82] Most measurements have been made at rest; it is probable that the cardiac output in the presence of severe myocardial or valvular disease would increase much less during exertion than necessary to meet the demands of the body for oxygen. Cardiac decompensation, however, may occur in the presence of a *normal* or *high cardiac output* in such conditions as fever, beriberi, thyrotoxicosis, anemia, arteriovenous aneurysm and cor pulmonale. If there is any unitary factor at all in the development of cardiac insufficiency, it must lie in the relation between actual cardiac output and peripheral needs for blood. Therefore, in these conditions the cardiac output should be compared to the level

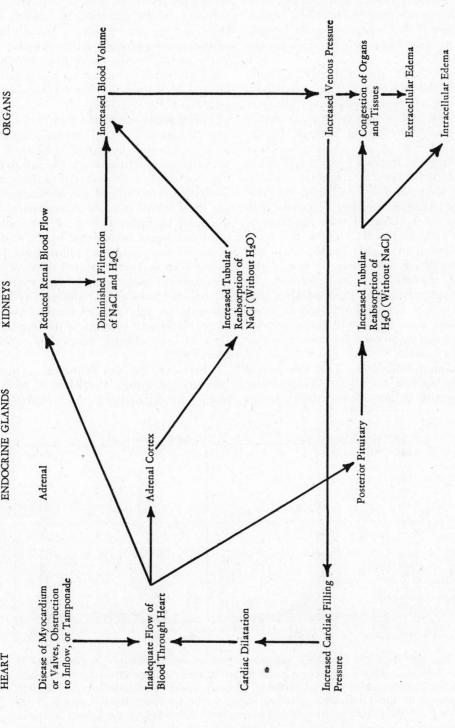

Fig. 194. Diagram of factors operative in producing edema of congestive circulatory failure.

which should be present if failure had not supervened. It has been shown that the output of the failing heart increases very little during exertion.[83] Therefore, congestive failure probably depends upon a deficit of circulating blood in relation to the body's needs.

Alterations in the Kidneys. Changes occur in the function and hemodynamics of the kidneys when congestive failure is present. Renal blood flow is markedly reduced with consequent decrease in the amount filtered by the glomerulus; as a result, filtration fraction is very high.[38] One must postulate efferent arteriolar constriction of severe degree to account for these findings. During exercise, filtration may fall to a level consistent with retention of sodium and chloride.[84] The lowered renal blood flow of itself may predispose to the retention of salt and water because of the lessened amount of filtrate formed. In normal subjects and in those without congestive failure but with a variety of renal conditions, there appears to be no correlation between glomerular filtration rate and sodium excretion.[85]

Extrarenal Influences. This mechanism does not account for all the changes seen in congestive failure, for the ability of the kidney to excrete nitrogen in many cases may be relatively unimpaired. In addition there appears to be present a specific disturbance in the excretion of sodium and chloride by the kidney. When large amounts of hypertonic saline solution are given intravenously to cardiac patients[64] relatively small amounts are excreted; the kidneys of normal subjects excrete the salt rather rapidly (Fig. 195).

This disturbance in the excretion of salt may be caused by renal venous congestion or by extrarenal hormonal influences, especially those derived from the salt-retaining hormone of the adrenal cortex. Evidence of overactivity of the adrenal cortex has been found in chronic congestive failure both by measurements of the sodium concentration of sweat[86] and by the finding of an increase in urinary aldosterone.[87] It is also true that an increased renal venous pressure will lead to diminished excretion of sodium chloride.[88,89] Abnormally small amounts of salt are excreted, however, when the venous pressure is not especially elevated, and dietary restriction controls edema.[90,91]

There may be also disturbances in the excretion of water. Ingestion of water is often unaccompanied by diuresis.[92,93]

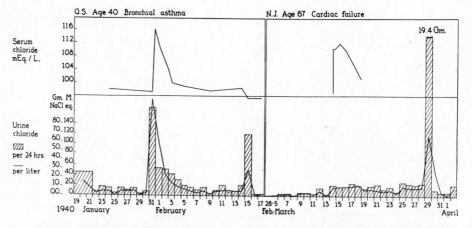

Fig. 195. Inability of cardiac patient to excrete sodium chloride in the urine. In the left-hand chart data from a patient not in heart failure show that the kidney normally will excrete a large excess of chloride when hyperchloremia is artificially induced by the intravenous administration of salt solution. Data depicted in the right-hand chart indicate that in severe congestive heart failure the kidney is unable to respond to such a stimulus. In both instances the administration of salyrgan resulted in an increased excretion of chloride in the urine.[64]

Plasma sodium levels may be somewhat lower than normal, indicating dilution of body fluids. Many cardiac patients appear to have stored excess water, as judged by chloride balance studies during recovery.[91] Antidiuretic substances have been found in the urine.[94] These alterations in water balance probably are principally extrarenal in origin, acting upon the kidneys to promote excessive reabsorption of water by the tubules; diminished excretion by other routes contributes but can hardly explain the findings.[95,96]

Increase in Total Blood Volume. Although the exact sequence of events which leads to the full-blown picture of congestive failure has not been elucidated, the same stimulus operating in other edematous states is functioning, that is, that which arises from an inadequate effective circulating blood volume or flow. The stimulus acts upon the kidneys to retain salt and water in the body in an attempt to re-establish effective blood flow and therefore blood volume. The mechanism most likely concerns the volume receptors. The development of congestive failure is usually a slow process, dependent upon the *gradual accumulation of fluid;* only minor degrees occur immediately following severe myocardial infarction because there is insufficient blood in the circulation to produce edema, other than hepatic or pulmonary. The rarity with which chronic congestive failure follows a first coronary occlusion is difficult to explain. After establishment of failure the following changes have occurred: (1) increase in total blood volume, (2) increase in body weight, (3) renal retention of salt and water, and (4) increase in venous pressure. The increase in total blood volume is usually associated with a normal hematocrit and normal or slightly low plasma proteins. However, the plasma oncotic pressure may be lower than normal, due to relative reduction in the albumin content and in increase in globulin,[97] but is not low enough to cause edema of itself. Since there is usually no great dilution of the blood, hematopoiesis and release from storage or synthesis of plasma proteins must have occurred. Recovery from congestive failure, as might be expected, is associated with concentration and possibly storage of plasma proteins[98] and destruction of blood.[99]

The cause of the elevated venous pressure may be two-fold: first, due to the increased blood volume, most of which is on the venous side of the circulation, and second, venoconstriction, which can exert a profound influence upon total venous volume.[100,101] A third factor is that of inability of the right heart to pump the blood it receives. An examination of Table 37 will show that this must be of minor importance inasmuch as exclusive of the pulmonary system and heart, over 80 per cent of the blood is normally in the veins.

Peripheral Factors. Local factors contributing to the edema of congestive failure arise from two sources: first, increased capillary blood pressure as a result of venous hypertension and second, increased capillary permeability as a result of anoxia. The latter probably does not allow a large amount of protein to escape, since the protein content of edema fluid is usually less than 0.6 Gm. per 100 ml.—although occasionally it has been found as high as 1.0 Gm.[102] There appears to be little or no globulin in the fluid.

Other Factors. The function of the liver may be altered by chronic passive congestion and contribute to a decrease of plasma proteins; hypoxic depression of steroid conjugation may allow salt-retaining hormones to accumulate. Anorexia and malnutrition may occur, leading to further decrease. Absence of lymph flow in the edematous skin has been noted;[103] this may be secondary to the increased venous pressure or to anoxia. In addition tissue pressure may be diminished after repeated attacks of edema.

Summary. The edema of congestive circulatory failure is the result of alterations in almost all the factors leading to edema. The primary disturbance lies in or near the heart and results in diminished effective blood flow. The renal stimulus to retention of salt and water operates. However, the peripheral factors may vary in intensity and in importance from patient to patient, depending upon a number of variable circumstances.

Edema of Renal Disease

All edema involves disturbances of the kidneys and primary renal diseases can cause edema. A working hypothesis divides the edemas secondary to primary renal diseases into two general categories: (1) those in which there is primary failure of excretion of ingested salt and (2) those involving primary failure of retaining plasma protein. The second type leads to hypoproteinemic edema, discussed elsewhere.

Several factors are believed to result in the generalized edema of acute glomerulonephritis secondary to sensitivity to Group A streptococci: (a) Increased capillary permeability, in which the glomeruli take part. (b) Inflammatory edema of the kidney itself, with resultant lowered blood flow. Protein content of edema fluid, however, is characteristic of a transudate. (c) Inflammatory excitation of tubular reabsorption of salt and water. (d) The familiar chain of events involving adrenal steroids, vasopressin and retention of salt and water, induced by lowered blood volume may or may not be operative. (e) Later, hyponatremia or congestive heart failure may contribute.[104] However, these ideas have not been satisfactorily proved.

Edema accompanying late stages of chronic glomerulonephritis, pyelonephritis, arteriolar nephrosclerosis, disseminated lupus, glomerulosclerosis and other destructive renal diseases is probably secondary to "fixation" of intrarenal abilities to conserve or excrete water and salt. Thus, when excesses of either are ingested (or injected), the kidneys cannot respond normally and expansion of extracellular fluid occurs, its tonicity depending upon relative amounts of each retained. When about 200,000 of the 2 million nephrons present in the normal human kidney are left, nitrogen balance may be precariously maintained. As kidneys so damaged are limited in their abilities to synthesize ammonia and excrete acids, complicating factors include acidosis and in end stages, retention of potassium and magnesium, which may promote myocardial insufficiency. Destructive renal diseases rarely damage all nephrons alike; therefore, a wide variety of disturbances may be present, the net result of which determines the effect. Protein-losing disease from damaged *glomeruli* results in nephrotic edema; salt-losing and water-losing disease from damaged *tubules* result in dehydration and polydipsia; while nephrons unable to excrete excesses allow edema to accumulate. All of the other renal factors, however, may contribute and it is difficult to separate them. Circulatory congestion from heart failure, hypoproteinemia from poor intake, lessened synthesis and urinary losses, depletion of body sodium from overzealous treatment may play ancillary roles.

Sometimes the edema and the accompanying nitrogen retention and acidosis can be partly relieved by very careful attention to intakes of salt, water and acids, adjusting them rigidly to the amount excreted. Kidneys are thus relieved of overwork and given a certain degree of "osmotic rest." However, this procedure requires the services of a metabolic ward, a laboratory, and a fine clinical touch; for practical purposes it has been replaced by the use of the artificial kidney.

SUMMARY

Edema is the result of disturbances of one or several factors concerned in the normal interchange of fluid between blood and tissue spaces[105] and in the normal regulatory mechanisms of fluids and salts in the body as a whole. When the normal peripheral factors (capillary blood pressure, capillary permeability, plasma oncotic pressure, tissue pressure) are disturbed in such a way as to lead to transudation of fluid into tissue spaces, the formation of edema is initiated. The resultant loss of effective circulating blood volume affects the regulatory mechanisms of the whole body. Renal retention of salt and water to make up for the loss occurs, probably through the interaction upon the kidney of the renal monitors, aldosterone and vasopressin or similar substances. Edema may also accompany disturbances of these regulatory mechanisms themselves, especially of the kidneys, which can cause edema without loss of effective circulating blood volume. When circulating blood volume or flow are affected primarily, as in the conditions reducing the output of the heart, the regulatory mechanisms are similarly called into play, with a resultant increase in total blood volume which leads to the formation of edema by affecting peripheral factors. Therefore, edema is a sign pointing to local disturbances affecting general bodily functions or to general circulatory disturbances themselves. Analysis of the pathogenesis of each type is important in developing logical methods for therapy.

REFERENCES

1. Smith, H. W.: The Kidney: Structure and Function in Health and Disease, New York, Oxford University Press, 1951, Preface V.
2. Krogh, A.: Anatomy and Physiology of Capillaries, New Haven, Yale, 1922.
3. Landis, E. M.: Micro-injection studies of capillary permeability; relation between capillary pressure and rate at which fluid passes through walls of single capillaries, Am. J. Physiol. 82:217, 1927.
4. Pappenheimer, J. R.: Passage of molecules through capillary walls, Physiol. Rev. 33:387, 1953.
5. Bennett, H. S., Luft, J. H., and Hampton, J. C.: Morphological classifications of vertebrate blood capillaries, Am. J. Physiol. 196:381, 1959.
6. Grotte, G.: Passage of dextran molecules across blood-lymph barrier, Acta chir. scandinav. (Supp. 211) p. 1-84, 1956.
7a. Landis, E. M.: Micro-injection studies of capillary blood pressure in human skin, Heart 15:209, 1930.
7b. ———: Capillary pressure and capillary permeability, Physiol. Rev. 14:404, 1934.
8. Ziverfach, B. W.: Basic mechanisms in peripheral vascular homeostasis, Trans. 3rd Josiah Macy Jr. Conf. on Factors Regulating Blood Pressure, New York, Macy, 1949.
9. Van Slyke, D. D.: Factors Affecting the Distribution of Electrolytes, Water, and Gases in the Animal Body, Philadelphia, Lippincott, 1926.
10. Starling, E. H.: On the absorption of fluids from the connective tissue spaces, J. Physiol. 19:312, 1896.
11. Claussen, F., and Schade, H.: Osmotic plasma pressure and edema, Ztschr. f. klin. Med. 100:363, 1924.
12. Govaerts, P.: Osmotic pressure of serum proteins as factor in edema and arterial hypertension, Compt. rend. Soc. de biol. 91:116, 1924.
13. Loeb, R. F., Atchley, D. W., and Palmer, W. W.: Equilibrium condition between blood serum and serous cavity fluids, J. Gen. Physiol. 4:591, 1922.
14. Landis, E. M., Jonas, L., Angevine, M., and Erb, W.: The passage of fluid and protein through the human capillary wall during venous congestion, J. Clin. Investigation 11:717, 1932.
15. Meyer, F., and Holland, G.: Die Messung des Druckes in Geweben, Arch. f. exper. Path. u. Pharmakol. 168:580, 1932.
16. Burch, G. E., and Sodeman, W. A.: Estimation of subcutaneous tissue pressure by direct method, J. Clin. Investigation 16:845, 1937.
17. Warren, J. V., Merrill, A. J., and Stead, E. A., Jr.: Role of extracellular fluid in maintenance of normal plasma volume, J. Clin. Investigation 22:635, 1943.
18. Harrison, T. R.: Failure of the Circulation, ed. 2, Baltimore, Wood, 1939.
19. Drinker, C. K., and Field, M. E.: Lymphatics, Lymph and Tissue Fluid, Baltimore, Williams & Wilkins, 1933.
20. Goldsmith, C., Rector, F. C., and Seldin, D. W.: Evidence for a direct effect of serum sodium concentration on sodium reabsorption, J. Clin. Invest. 41:850, 1962.
21. Schroeder, H. A., and Steele, J. M.: The behaviour of renal blood flow after partial constriction of the renal artery, J. Exper. Med. 72:707, 1940.
22. Olsen, N. S., and Schroeder, H. A.: Oxygen tension and pH of the renal cortex in acute ischemia and chronic hypertension, Am. J. Physiol. 163:181, 1950.
23. Mulrow, P. J., Ganong, W. F., Cera, G., and Kuljian, A.: The nature of the aldosterone-stimulating factor in dog kidneys, J. Clin. Invest. 41:505, 1962.
24. Ganong, W. F., and Mulrow, P. J.: Evidence of secretion of an aldosterone-stimulating substance by the kidney, Nature 190:1115, (June 17) 1961.
25. Ganong, W. F., Mulrow, P. J., and Boryczka, C. G.: Evidence for a direct effect of angiotensin-II on adrenal cortex of the dog, Proc. Soc. Exper. Biol. & Med. 109:381, (Feb.) 1962.
26. Kaplan, N. M., and Bartter, F. C.: The effect of ACTH, renin, angiotensin-II and various precursors on biosynthesis of aldosterone by adrenal slices, J. Clin. Invest. 41:715, 1962.
27. Chambers, G. H., Melville, E. V., Hare, R. S., and Hare, K.: Regulation of the release of pituitrin by changes in the osmotic pressure of the plasma, Am. J. Physiol. 144:311, 1945.

28. Verney, E. B.: Antidiuretic hormone and the factors which determine its release, Proc. Roy. Soc., London, Series B. 135:25, 1947.

30. Simpson, S. A., Tait, J. F., Wettstein, A., Neher, R., v. Euw, J., Schindler, O., and Reichstein, T.: Konstitution des aldosterons, des neuen mineralocorticoids, Experientia 10:132, 1954.

31. Farrell, G.: Adrenoglomerulotropin, Circulation 21:1009, 1960.

32. Davis, J. O.: A critical evaluation of the role of receptors in the control of aldosterone secretion and sodium excretion, in Friedberg, C. K., ed., Heart, Kidney and Electrolytes, New York, Grune & Stratton, 1962.

33. Gauer, O. H., Henry, J. P., Sieker, H. O., and Wendt, W. E.: The effect of negative pressure breathing on urine flow, J. Clin. Invest. 33:287, 1954.

34. Gauer, O. H., Henry, J. P., and Sieker, H. O.: Cardiac receptors and fluid volume control. in Friedberg, C. K., ed., Heart, Kidney and Electrolytes, New York, Grune & Stratton, 1962.

35. Bartter, F. C., and Gann, D. C.: On the hemodynamic regulation of the secretion of aldosterone, Circulation 21:1016, 1960.

36. Kriss, J. P., Futcher, P. H., and Goldman, M. L.: Unilateral adrenalectomy, unilateral splanchnic nerve resection and homolateral renal function, Am. J. Physiol. 154:220, 1948.

37. Selkurt, E. E., Hall, P. W., and Spencer, M. P.: Influence of graded arterial pressure decrement on renal clearance of creatinine, p-aminohippurate and sodium, Am. J. Physiol. 159:369, 1949.

38. Merrill, A. J.: Edema and decreased renal blood flow in patients with chronic congestive heart failure: evidence of "forward failure" as the primary cause of edema, J. Clin. Investigation 25:389, 1946.

39. Blake, W. D., Wégria, R., Keating, R. P., and Ward, H. P.: Effect of increased renal venous pressure on renal function, Am. J. Physiol. 157:1, 1949.

40. Grant, H., and Reischman, F.: The effects of the ingestion of large amounts of sodium chloride on the arterial and venous pressures of normal subjects, Am. Heart J. 32:704, 1946.

41. Ladd, M., and Raisz, L. G.: Response of the normal dog to dietary sodium chloride, Am. J. Physiol. 159:149, 1949.

42. Selkurt, E. E.: Sodium excretion by the mammalian kidney, Physiol. Rev. 34:287, 1954.

43. Schroeder, H. A., and Perry, H. M., Jr.: Disturbances of the internal environment and their correction, Am. J. Clin. Path. 23:1100, 1953.

44. Schroeder, H. A.: Renal failure associated with low extracellular sodium chloride: The low salt syndrome, J.A.M.A. 141:117, 1949.

45. Weiss, S., and Ellis, L. B.: The circulatory mechanism and unilateral edema in cerebral hemiplegia, J. Clin. Investigation 9:17, 1931.

46. Landis, E. M.: The capillary pressure in frog mesentery as determined by microinjection methods, Am. J. Physiol. 75:548, 1926.

47. Krogh, A., Landis, E. M., and Turner, A. H.: Movement of fluid through human capillary wall in relation to venous pressure and to colloid osmotic pressure of blood, J. Clin. Investigation 11:63, 1932.

48. Thompson, W. O., Thompson, P. K., and Dailey, M. E.: Effect of posture upon composition and volume of blood in man, J. Clin. Investigation 5:573, 1928.

49. Brun, C., Knudsen, E. O. E., and Raaschou, F.: The influence of posture on the kidney function. II. Glomerular dynamics in the passive erect posture, Acta med. Scandinav. 122:332, 1945.

50. White, H. L., and Rolf, D.: Effects of exercise and of some other influences on the renal circulation in man, Am. J. Physiol. 152:505, 1948.

51. Beck, C. S.: Revascularization of the heart, Ann. Surg. 128:854, 1948.

52. Paine, R., Butcher, H. R., Howard, F. A., and Smith, J. R.: Observations on mechanisms of edema formation in the lungs, J. Lab. & Clin. Med. 34:1544, 1949.

53. Bazett, H. C.: Factors Regulating Blood Pressure, Tr. Third Conference, New York, Josiah Macy, Jr. Foundation, 1949, p. 53.

54. Tainter, M. L., and Hanzlik, P. J.: Mechanism of edema production by paraphenylenediamine, J. Pharmacol. & Exper. Therap. 24:179, 1924.

55. Govaerts, P.: Pathogenie de l'œdeme au cours de l'intoxication aiguë par l'urane. Bull. Acad. roy, de méd. de Belgique 8:33, 1928.

56. Lewis, T.: Vascular reactions of skin to injury; reaction to stroking; urticaria factitia, Heart 11:119, 1924.

57. Lewis, T., and Grant, R. T.: Vascular reactions of skin to injury; liberation of a histamine-like substance in injured skin; the underlying cause of factitious urticaria and of wheals produced by burning; and ob-

servations upon nervous control of certain skin reactions, Heart 11:209, 1924.

58. Landis, E. M.: Micro-injection studies of capillary permeability; effect of lack of oxygen on permeability of capillary wall to fluid and to plasma proteins, Am. J. Physiol. 83:528, 1928.

59. Fishberg, A. M.: Hypertension and Nephritis, ed. 4, Philadelphia, Lea & Febiger, 1939.

60. Glenn, W. W., Muus, J., and Drinker, C. K.: Observations on physiology and biochemistry of quantitative burns, J. Clin. Investigation 22:451, 1943.

61. Barnett, C. W., Jones, R. B., and Cohn, R. B.: Maintenance of normal plasma protein concentration in spite of repeated protein loss by bleeding, J. Exper. Med. 55:683, 1932.

62. Leiter, L.: Experimental nephrotic edema, Arch. Int. Med. 48:1, 1931.

63. Kurnick, N. B.: War edema in the civilian population of Saipan, Ann. Int. Med. 28:782, 1948.

64. Futcher, P. H., and Schroeder, H. A.: Studies on congestive heart failure. II. Impaired renal excretion of sodium chloride, Am. J. M. Sc. 204:52, 1942.

65. Perera, G. A.: The adrenal cortex and hypertension, Bull. New York Acad. Med. 26:75, 1950.

66. Soffer, L. J.: Diseases of the Adrenals, Philadelphia, Lea & Febiger, 1946.

67. Forsham, P. H., Thorn, G. W., Prunty, F. T. G., and Hills, A. G.: Clinical studies with pituitary adrenocorticotropin, J. Clin. Endocrinol. 8:15, 1948.

68. Ralli, E. P., Robson, J. S., Clarke, D., and Hoagland, C. L.: Factors influencing ascites in patients with cirrhosis of the liver, J. Clin. Investigation 24:316, 1945.

69. Farnsworth, E. B.: Electrolyte partition in patients with edema of various origins, Am. J. Med. 4:338, 1948.

70. Hyatt, R. E., and Smith, J. R.: The mechanism of ascites, Am. J. Med. 16:434, 1954.

71. Stander, H. J.: Williams' Obstetrics, ed. 8, New York, Appleton, 1941.

72. Freyberg, R. H., Reekie, R. D., and Folsome, C.: Study of water, sodium, and energy exchange during later part of pregnancy, Am. J. Obst. & Gynec. 36:200, 1938.

73. Thompson, H. E., Jr., and Pommerenke, W. T.: Electrolyte and nitrogen metabolism in pregnancy, J. Nutrition 17:383, 1939.

74. Dieckmann, W. J.: Edema in pre-eclampsia and eclampsia, Am. J. Obst. & Gynec. 41:1, 1941.

75. deAlvarez, R. R.: The retention of sodium and water in toxemia of pregnancy, in Moyer, J. H., and Fuchs, M., eds., Edema, Mechanisms and Management, Philadelphia, Saunders, 1960.

76. Seitchik, J.: Fluid and electrolyte metabolism in pregnancy, in Moyer, J. H., and Fuchs, M., eds., Edema, Mechanisms and Management, Philadelphia, Saunders, 1960.

77. Taylor, H. C., Jr., Warner, R. C., and Welsh, C. A.: Relationship of estrogens and progesterone to edema of normal and toxemic pregnancy, Am. J. Obst. & Gynec. 45:547, 1943.

78. Brull, L., Barac, G., Brakier-Zelkowiecz, T., et al.: Les états de carence en Belgique pendant l'occupation allemande de 1940-1944, Liége, Soledi, 1945, p. 286.

79. Youmans, J. B.: Some clinical aspects of dietary deficiencies, South. M. J. 28:843, 1935.

80. Weiss, S., and Wilkins, R. W.: Nature of cardiovascular disturbances in nutritional deficiency states (beriberi), Ann. Int. Med. 11:104, 1937.

81. Dock, W.: Heart failure: the relation of symptoms and signs to its severity and duration, Ann. Int. Med. 29:11, 1948.

82. Altschule, M. D.: Physiology in Diseases of the Heart and Lungs, Cambridge, Harvard, 1949.

83. Hickam, J. B., and Cargill, W. H.: Effect of exercise on cardiac output and pulmonary arterial pressure in normal persons and in patients with cardiovascular disease and pulmonary emphysema, J. Clin. Investigation 27:10, 1948.

84. Merrill, A. J., and Cargill, W. H.: The effect of exercise on the renal plasma flow and filtration rate of normal and cardiac subjects, J. Clin. Investigation 27:272, 1948.

85. Green, D. M., Bridges, W. C., Johnson, A. D., Lehman, J. H., Gray, F., and Field, L.: Relation of glomerular filtration rate and sodium tubular rejection fraction to renal sodium excretion, Am. J. Physiol. 160:306, 1950.

86. Highes, D. J., Turner, H. H., Moseley, A. J., and Merrill, A. J.: Mechanisms of salt and water retention in heart failure, Am. J. Med. 7:249, 1949.

87. Luetscher, J. A., Jr., and Johnson, B. B.: Observations on the sodium-retaining corticoid (aldosterone) in the urine of children and adults in relation to sodium balance and edema, J. Clin. Invest. 33:1441, 1954.

88. Rowntree, L. G., and Fitz, R.: Studies of

renal function in renal, cardiorenal and cardiac diseases, Arch. Int. Med. 11:258, 1913.

89. Burch, G., and Reaser, P.: Rates of turnover of radiosodium in the blood and urine of normal subjects and patients with congestive heart failure, J. Clin. Investigation 26:1176, 1947.

90. Schroeder, H. A.: Studies on congestive heart failure. I. The importance of restriction of salt as compared to water, Am. Heart J., 22:41, 1941.

91. Schroeder, H. A.: Studies on congestive circulatory failure. III. The relation of edema to urinary chlorides, Circulation 1:481, 1950.

92. Fremont-Smith, F., Dailey, M. E., and Thomas, G. W.: Dilution of blood and cerebrospinal fluid in fever, J. Clin. Investigation 6:9, 1928.

93. Fremont-Smith, F.: Mechanism of edema formation, New England J. Med. 206:1286, 1932.

94. Bercu, B., Rokaw, S. N., and Massie, E.: Antidiuretic action of the urine of patients in cardiac failure, Circulation 2:409, 1950.

95. Burch, G. E.: The rates of water and heat loss from the respiratory tract of patients with congestive heart failure who were from a subtropical climate and resting in a comfortable atmosphere, Am. Heart J. 32:88, 1946.

96. Burch, G. E.: The influence of environmental temperature and relative humidity on the rate of water loss through the skin in congestive heart failure in a subtropical climate, Am. J. M. Sc. 211:181, 1946.

97. Luetscher, J. A., Jr.: Electrophoretic analyses of proteins of plasma and serous effusions, J. Clin. Investigation 20:99, 1941.

98. Calvin, D. B., Decherd, G., and Hermann, G.: Plasma protein shift during diuresis, Proc. Soc. Exper. Biol. & Med. 44:578, 1940.

99. Waller, J. V., Blumgart, H. L., and Volk, M. C.: Studies of the blood in congestive heart failure. With particular reference to reticulocytosis, erythrocyte fragility, bilirubinemia, urobilinogen excretion and changes in blood volume, Arch. Int. Med. 66:1230, 1940.

100. Landis, E. M., and Hortenstine, J. C.: Functional significance of venous blood pressure, Physiol. Rev. 30:1, 1950.

101. McDowall, R. J. S.: Nervous control of blood vessels, Physiol. Rev. 15:98, 1935.

102. Bramkamp, R. G.: Protein content of subcutaneous edema fluid in heart disease, J. Clin. Investigation 14:34, 1935.

103. McMaster, P. D.: Lymphatics and lymph flow in edematous skin of human beings with cardiac and renal disease, J. Exper. Med. 65:373, 1937.

104. Daeschner, C. W.: Factors involved in the pathogenesis of renal edema: The role of aldosterone and posterior pituitary antidiuretic hormone, in Moyer, J. H., and Fuchs, M., eds., Edema, Mechanisms and Management, Philadelphia, Saunders, 1960.

105. Pappenheimer, J. R., and Soto-Rivera, A.: Effective osmotic pressure of plasma proteins and other quantities associated with capillary circulation in hindlimbs of cats and dogs, Am. J. Physiol. 152:471, 1948.

The interested reader is referred to the following sources for more detailed data, theories and hypotheses:

Fishman, A. P., ed.: Symposium on salt and water metabolism, Circulation 21:805, 1960.

Friedberg, C. K.: Heart, Kidney and Electrolytes, New York, Grune & Stratton, 1962.

Starr, I.: Our changing viewpoint about congestive failure, Ann. Int. Med. 30:1, 1949.

Tobian, L.: Interrelationship of electrolytes, juxtaglomerular cells and hypertension, Physiol. Rev. 40:280, 1960.

Moyer, J. H., and Fuchs, M., eds.: Edema, Mechanisms and Management, Philadelphia, W. B. Saunders, 1960.

32

Obesity

CYRIL M. MACBRYDE

Obesity is that bodily state in which there is excessive accumulation of fat. Of "all the thousand natural shocks that flesh is heir to" none is more common, or more distressing, or ultimately more serious than its abnormal accumulation. While to the layman corpulence is primarily a cosmetic defect, making its bearer less attractive to his fellows, to the physician it is a symptom that attains the dignity and the importance of a disease.

Obesity may be defined as excess fat deposit in the body causing body weight 15 per cent or more above the optimal weight.

Adiposity may be distinguished from obesity in that the body weight may not exceed normal but the proportion of the body weight composed of fat is excessive.

Obesity is both a physical sign and a symptom. A physical sign is an anatomic abnormality which is evident to the examining physician; on this count obesity easily qualifies, as discussed in the section below on Diagnosis. A symptom is any perceptible change in the body or its functions which indicates an underlying disorder or disease; the disorder indicated by obesity is a prolonged positive energy balance which has resulted in excess storage of fat. Obesity, therefore, whether or not the patient complains of it, deserves attention and serious consideration.

DIAGNOSIS

When adiposity is sufficient, no exact methods are necessary for its determination, inspection alone being adequate. In accurate medical work, however, the diagnosis of obesity is simply the first step; one should also establish the ideal weight and the degree of obesity. One may find the approximate optimal weights according to height, sex and type of body frame by reference to Tables 38–41. More exact determination of the optimal weight for each person can be made by the use of a series of skeletal measurements.[1] The skeletal measurements of wrist circumference, knee circumference, shoulder width and hip width, etc., permit introduction of computations based upon the width and the depth of the body and the heaviness and the size of the skeletal

TABLE 38. DETERMINATION OF THE IDEAL WEIGHT OF BOYS

Height Inches	5 Yrs.	6 Yrs.	7 Yrs.	8 Yrs.	9 Yrs.	10 Yrs.	11 Yrs.	12 Yrs.	13 Yrs.	14 Yrs.	15 Yrs.	16 Yrs.	17 Yrs.	18 Yrs.	19 Yrs.
38	34	34													
39	35	35													
40	36	36													
41	38	38	38												
42	39	39	39	39											
43	41	41	41	41											
44	44	44	44	44											
45	46	46	46	46	46										
46	47	48	48	48	48										
47	49	50	50	50	50	50									
48	..	52	53	53	53	53									
49	..	55	55	55	55	55	55								
50	..	57	58	58	58	58	58	58							
51	..	..	61	61	61	61	61	61							
52	..	..	63	64	64	64	64	64	64						
53	..	..	66	67	67	67	67	68	68						
54	..	..	..	70	70	70	70	71	71	72					
55	..	..	..	72	72	73	73	74	74	74					
56	..	..	..	75	76	77	77	77	78	78	80				
57	..	..	..	..	79	80	81	81	82	83	83				
58	..	..	..	..	83	84	84	85	85	86	87				
59	..	..	..	..	..	87	88	89	89	90	90	90			
60	..	..	..	..	..	91	92	92	93	94	95	96			
61	..	..	..	..	..	..	95	96	97	99	100	103	106		
62	..	..	..	..	..	..	100	101	102	103	104	107	111	116	
63	..	..	..	..	..	..	105	106	107	108	110	113	118	123	127
64	..	..	..	..	..	..	...	109	111	113	115	117	121	126	130
65	..	..	..	..	..	..	...	114	117	118	120	122	127	131	134
66	..	..	..	..	..	..	...	...	119	122	125	128	132	136	139
67	..	..	..	..	..	..	...	...	124	128	130	134	136	139	142
68	..	..	..	..	..	..	...	...	...	134	134	137	141	143	147
69	..	..	..	..	..	..	...	...	...	137	139	143	146	149	152
70	..	..	..	..	..	..	...	...	...	143	144	145	148	151	155
71	..	..	..	..	..	..	...	...	...	148	150	151	152	154	159
72	..	..	..	..	..	..	...	...	...	...	153	155	156	158	163
73	..	..	..	..	..	..	...	...	...	...	157	160	162	164	167
74	..	..	..	..	..	..	...	...	...	...	160	164	168	170	171

Age is taken to the nearest birthday, height to the nearest inch and weight to the nearest pound. These weights are inclusive of ordinary clothing, except shoes, coats, and sweaters. (American Child Health Association, revised by Dr. Thomas D. Wood and Dr. Bird T. Baldwin)

framework. This permits more nearly accurate estimates of individual ideal weights than the tables based only upon height plus the rough estimate of frame caliber as "small," "medium" or "large." Such methods are satisfactory for persons of average muscular development and for those whose proportions of muscle to fat are within average normal limits. However, in two classes of cases one may be misled by using optimal weight tables or by computing ideal weight from skeletal measurements: (1) if muscle bulk is greatly above normal and the proportion of muscle to fat is high; (2) if muscle bulk is below normal and the proportion of fat to muscle exceeds normal

TABLE 39. DETERMINATION OF THE IDEAL WEIGHT OF GIRLS

Height Inches	5 Yrs.	6 Yrs.	7 Yrs.	8 Yrs.	9 Yrs.	10 Yrs.	11 Yrs.	12 Yrs.	13 Yrs.	14 Yrs.	15 Yrs.	16 Yrs.	17 Yrs.	18 Yrs.
38	33	33												
39	34	34												
40	36	36	36											
41	37	37	37											
42	39	39	39											
43	41	41	41	41										
44	42	42	42	42										
45	45	45	45	45	45									
46	47	47	47	48	48									
47	49	50	50	50	50	50								
48	..	52	52	52	52	53	53							
49	..	54	54	55	55	56	56							
50	..	56	56	57	58	59	61	62						
51	..	..	59	60	61	61	63	65						
52	..	..	63	64	64	64	65	67						
53	..	..	66	67	67	68	68	69	71					
54	..	..	..	69	70	70	71	71	73					
55	..	..	..	72	74	74	74	75	77	78				
56	..	..	..	..	76	78	78	79	81	83				
57	..	..	..	..	80	82	82	82	84	88	92			
58	..	..	..	..	..	84	86	86	88	93	96	101		
59	..	..	..	..	..	87	90	90	92	96	100	103	104	
60	..	..	..	..	..	91	95	95	97	101	105	108	109	111
61	..	..	..	..	..	..	99	100	101	105	108	112	113	116
62	..	..	..	..	..	..	104	105	106	109	113	115	117	118
63	..	..	..	..	..	..	...	110	110	112	116	117	119	120
64	..	..	..	..	..	..	...	114	115	117	119	120	122	123
65	..	..	..	..	..	..	...	118	120	121	122	123	125	126
66	..	..	..	..	..	..	...	...	124	124	125	128	129	130
67	..	..	..	..	..	..	...	...	128	130	131	133	133	135
68	..	..	..	..	..	..	...	...	131	133	135	136	138	138
69	..	..	..	..	..	..	...	...	...	135	137	138	140	142
70	..	..	..	..	..	..	...	...	...	136	138	140	142	144
71	..	..	..	..	..	..	...	...	...	138	140	142	144	145

Age is taken to the nearest birthday, height to the nearest inch and weight to the nearest pound. These weights are inclusive of ordinary clothing, except shoes and coats. (American Child Health Association, revised by Dr. Thomas D. Wood and Dr. Bird T. Baldwin)

limits. In such instances, a very muscular man may seem to weigh much more than he should, or contrariwise, a flabby person with atrophic muscles and excessive fat deposits throughout the body may have a total body weight within or even below the optimal range.

Total body weights in excess of the optimal range usually indicate an excessive fat content of the body. A more exact method of measuring the fat storage, as compared to normal, requires the determination of the specific gravity of the whole body by weighing the patient under water.[2] Since human fat has a density of 0.92, whereas the rest of the body has an average density of 1.1, it is possible to calculate the percentage of body fat when the total body density is known. A correction must be made for residual air within the lungs. This is the most accurate method yet devised for calculation of body fat content, but the difficul-

TABLE 40. DESIRABLE WEIGHTS FOR MEN 25 YEARS OF AGE OR OLDER

HEIGHT (with shoes on) 1-inch heels		SMALL FRAME	MEDIUM FRAME	LARGE FRAME
Feet	Inches			
5	2	112–120	118–129	126–141
5	3	115–123	121–133	129–144
5	4	118–126	124–136	132–148
5	5	121–129	127–139	135–152
5	6	124–133	130–143	138–156
5	7	128–137	134–147	142–161
5	8	132–141	138–152	147–166
5	9	136–145	142–156	151–170
5	10	140–150	146–160	155–174
5	11	144–154	150–165	159–179
6	0	148–158	154–170	164–184
6	1	152–162	158–175	168–189
6	2	156–167	162–180	173–194
6	3	160–171	167–185	178–199
6	4	164–175	172–190	182–204

(Metropolitan Life Insurance Company, Statistical Bureau)

TABLE 41. DESIRABLE WEIGHTS FOR WOMEN 25 YEARS OF AGE OR OLDER

HEIGHT (with shoes on) 2-inch heels		SMALL FRAME	MEDIUM FRAME	LARGE FRAME
Feet	Inches			
4	10	92– 98	96–107	104–119
4	11	94–101	98–110	106–122
5	0	96–104	101–113	109–125
5	1	99–107	104–116	112–128
5	2	102–110	107–119	115–131
5	3	105–113	110–122	118–134
5	4	108–116	113–126	121–138
5	5	111–119	116–130	125–142
5	6	114–123	120–135	129–146
5	7	118–127	124–139	133–150
5	8	122–131	128–143	137–154
5	9	126–135	132–147	141–158
5	10	130–140	136–151	145–163
5	11	134–144	140–155	149–168
6	0	138–148	144–159	153–173

(Metropolitan Life Insurance Company, Statistical Bureau)

Derived primarily from data of the Build and Blood Pressure Study, 1959, Society of Actuaries.

ties involved limit its use to research laboratories. However, standards of reference have thus been provided for comparison with the results of simpler procedures.

Formulas have been devised for estimating body fat content from measurements of skin-fold thickness over several specified areas of the body.

The total proportion of body fat has also been estimated by measurement of total body water. The most practical substance so far used in this method (based on the dilution principle) seems to be antipyrine. It is injected intravenously and after time is allowed for diffusion, the concentration of the test substance is measured in samples of the body water afforded by the blood serum. Under normal conditions total water maintains a constant relationship to lean body mass. When total body water is known, lean body mass can be calculated and the fat content of the body determined by subtracting lean body mass from total body weight.

Keys[3] has evaluated and compared the results obtained by the three methods mentioned: (1) densitometry, (2) skin-fold measurements, and (3) body water measurement. When carefully employed there is rough agreement.

Such studies have yielded a considerable amount of useful data. The human body is composed of several major components, which are largely distinct metabolically and which may show a considerable degree of independent variation. In an average young man these components constitute approximately the following percentages of total body weight:

	NORMAL PER CENT
Fat	15
Extracellular water	23
Cells or "active tissue"	58
Bone mineral	4
Body weight	100

In obesity of extreme degree, the percentage of body fat may exceed 50 and even reach 70; in extreme leanness the percentage of body weight made up of fat may be lower than 10 per cent, even as low as 2 per cent.

Normal Fat Storage. Even among persons of normal weight according to the height-age-weight tables, there may be considerable differences in body fat content. This implies, of course, corresponding differences in lean body mass (presumably largely muscle).

"Normal" middle-aged men are much fatter than normal young men if body content of fat is used as the criterion of comparison, rather than height-weight-age tables. This is most clearly shown when men of equal height and weight, but of different ages, are compared.

In the group studied, the mean body fat content of 33 younger (22-29 years) men was 16.5 per cent as compared with 22.6 per cent for 33 older (48-57 years) men matched in height and weight.

The trend for older as compared with younger females was similar, with the difference that females were fatter than males at each age and relative body weight category (Keys[3]).

Women normally have more body fat than men. In the third decade the proportion in normal persons is: females 18 to 24 per cent fat, males 12 to 18 per cent. Adiposity may be considered present if the body fat content of a woman exceeds 30 per cent, of a man 25 per cent.

Problems arise in older age groups in deciding what degree of adiposity may be considered normal with increasing age. The proportion of fat to muscle increases with age in both men and women. The proportion of fat in older men and women tends to be more than 50 per cent higher than in younger persons of the same sex, height and build. They are thus relatively adipose, although they may not be obese.

No rapid clinical method is available to determine accurately the body fat content. Excess adipose tissue is usually evident, however, when physical examination reveals the muscles to be flabby. Such persons take little exercise and fatigue easily.

Persons of any age who have poor muscles are apt to be relatively adipose, although the total body weight may be normal or even subnormal, rather than excessive. More attention should be paid to *adiposity occurring without obesity,* as it may have great clinical significance.

Changing Fat Storage. The importance of actual estimation of body fat is illustrated in two alterations of the nutritional state:

1. In *prolonged undernutrition* there is a progressive loss of both fat and eventually of muscle and other "active tissue," with no change or an increase in extracellular fluid, as calculated in per cent of total body weight.

2. In *developing obesity* the weight gained consists approximately of 80 per cent pure fat and 20 per cent water; the "active tissue" percentage of the total body weight tends to show little or no change.

Fat, Active Tissue, and Basal Metabolism. An additional concept of great importance arises from the study of body content of fat and of "active tissue": computations based on active tissue indicate that most of the classic age and sex differences in basal metabolic rate are merely reflections of the body content of active tissue. The term "active tissue" here employed means all components of the total body weight except fat and water. It thus appears that younger men have higher metabolic rates per square meter of body surface than older men because of a greater proportion of metabolically active tissue and less fat. The higher rates for men as compared with women may be similarly explained.

Hydration and Body Weight. *Variations in hydration* must be taken into account when estimating the degree of corpulence from total body weight. The tables given in this chapter are predicated upon normal hydration. Dehydration may greatly reduce body weight; extracellular fluid may be reduced from the normal of about 23 per cent of body weight to as low as 10 per cent. Calculating for every liter of fluid 2.2 lbs. ("for every pint a pound"), great differences in weight may occur with no change in body content of fat or active tissue. When the body contains excess fluid, it is not always readily detectable. In undernourished persons clinical edema may not be recognizable until the excess fluid constitutes 10 per cent of the total body weight. In extreme cases extracellular fluid may account for not the normal 23 per cent, but as high as 60 per cent of total body weight. When hydrothorax, ascites, edema, etc., are present, calculations may be made, or the abnormal fluid retention must be removed, before body weight measurements may be compared with "ideal" weights in the tables.

It is very helpful when the actual fat content of the body can be computed, but for practical purposes in most cases, weighing the patient, doing a careful physical examination, and comparing the weight with the ideal weight suffice to establish the diagnosis of obesity and its degree.

Tables giving *average* weights at various ages and heights are misleading, for the optimal weight of an adult remains unchanged, but average weights increase in the middle decades. Life insurance companies have found in their statistical studies that even the minor degrees of corpulence (10 to 15 per cent above optimal weight) are accompanied by higher mortality rates. The *optimal* weight figures given in this chapter are derived from such statistical studies, which indicate that such ideal weights are important factors in longevity.

MEDICAL IMPORTANCE OF OBESITY

Incidence. Obesity, of all health defects, is the most common reason for the refusal of standard risk life insurance. In the United States estimates indicate that one fifth of the population over age 30 (about 15 million persons) may be considered overweight (i.e., 10% above "ideal" weight). About 10% of our population is obese (15% over "ideal" weight). About 5.5 million persons in the country, or approximately 3 per cent of the population, are pathologically obese (20% above "ideal" weight).

Penalty of Overweight. Dublin and Lotka[4] found that "the penalty of overweight is one-fourth to three-fourths excess in mortality." Persons who are from 5 to 14 per cent overweight have an excess mortality rate of 22 per cent; those from 15 to 24 per cent overweight, of 44 per cent; those 25 per cent or more overweight, of 74 per cent. The hazard of obesity increases with age, so that persons between 45 and 50 years of age who are 10 pounds overweight have an increase above the average death rate of 8 per cent; when 20 pounds overweight, of 18 per cent; when 30 pounds overweight, of 28 per cent; when 50 pounds overweight, of 56 per cent.

An analysis by Armstrong, Dublin, Wheatley, and Marks[4] of the causes of death among obese persons, as compared with those among persons of normal weight, revealed that deaths from degenerative diseases of the heart, the arteries and the kidneys account for the greatest proportion of the higher mortality. All types of cardiovascular-renal conditions appear to occur more frequently and with greater severity among overweight persons, including in particular heart failure, cerebral hemorrhage and thrombosis, coronary thrombosis and nephritis. More of the obese die from accidents, probably because fat people are less agile. The death rate from diabetes is almost four times as great in obese persons as in normal persons.

Barr[5] calls obesity "a stop signal, a red light of warning" and presents a lucid and stimulating review and discussion of obesity and its consequences. His adaptation and tabulation of data from the very informative insurance studies[4] is given in Table 42. Notice that the death rate from certain diseases of the liver, biliary tract and intestines is higher percentagewise than from the much more common conditions of nephritis, cerebral hemorrhage and coronary artery disease.

In only two of the categories listed is the mortality of the obese less than the standard for normal weight persons. The lower suicide rate is somewhat of a surprise, for although fat persons are supposed to be jolly and placid, many studies indicate a high rate of emotional disorders. A lower death rate from tuberculosis may indicate that abundant nutrition protects against it, but may mean only that few persons who have tuberculosis are overweight when they die.

Many studies have demonstrated[6] that obesity has an adverse influence upon a number of other medical disorders through (1) increasing their incidence (that is, fat people are more apt to develop the condition), (2) increasing the severity of the disease itself, (3) increasing the number and severity of the symptoms caused by the disease or (4) increasing the incidence and severity of complications of the disease. Disorders influenced adversely by obesity in one or more of the four ways mentioned include diabetes, heart disease, hypertension, pulmonary emphysema, acute and chronic nephritis, arteriosclerosis, venous thrombosis and embolism, hepatic cirrhosis, appendicitis, gallbladder disease, degenerative arthritis, varicose veins, cancer and toxemias of pregnancy. Obesity causes increased fetal mortality and greater complications of obstetric delivery. Should these dangers be avoided, the fat person is still more likely than the normal person to be seriously or fatally injured, or to suffer fractures of bones. Should surgery prove necessary, the greater the adiposity the poorer the prognosis. Orthopedic difficulties are commoner among the obese, with flat feet and arthritic changes in the knees and the back occurring as frequent complications, often disabling in severity. Diaphragmatic hernia occurs more frequently in the obese and in some instances has been corrected solely by weight reduction.

Hypertension. Extensive studies have revealed that elevated blood pressure occurs in obese patients in every age group and in both sexes. There is a steady progression, both systolic and diastolic, with each increase in body weight per height of the individual. There is substantial agreement in the reports of Thompson[12] on life insurance company employees; by Master, Dublin and Marks[13] on 74,000 industrial workers, and by Levy, White, Stroud and Hillman[14] on 22,741 Army officers. The latter group found that sustained hypertension among obese persons develops at a rate 2.5 times as high as among persons of normal weight.

Obesity, Atherosclerosis, Blood Lipids, and Diet. In a study of 1,250 consecutive miscellaneous autopsies, Wilens[15] demon-

TABLE 42. RATIO OF ACTUAL TO EXPECTED DEATHS BETWEEN OVERWEIGHT PERSONS AND THOSE CONSIDERED STANDARD RISKS (100 = STANDARD RATE)

CONDITION	MEN	WOMEN
Diabetes	383	372
Cirrhosis of liver	249	147
Appendicitis	223	195
Biliary calculi	206	284
Chronic nephritis	191	212
Liver and gallbladder cancer	168	211
Cerebral hemorrhage	159	162
Coronary disease	142	175
Auto accidents	131	120
Puerperal conditions	—	162
Suicides	78	73
Tuberculosis	21	35

strated a close association between obesity and atherosclerosis, advanced degrees of the arterial change being found twice as often among the obese as among the poorly nourished. Severe generalized atherosclerosis was found in 20.2 per cent of the obese as compared with 10.9 per cent of average weight and with 7 per cent for the underweight in the age group 45 to 54 years. In the age group 55 to 64, the rate was 37 per cent for the obese, 17 per cent for the average-weight. Among cases in age group 65 to 74, the rate was 45 per cent for the obese, 20 per cent for the underweight. Coronary atherosclerosis of advanced degree occurred in a distribution similar to that for generalized atherosclerosis, averaging 40.8 per cent for obese men as compared with 18.7 per cent for average-weight men.

Evidence has long been accumulating, both clinical and experimental, that prolonged hypercholesteremia and atherosclerosis are in some way associated. The characteristic lesion of the atherosclerotic artery is the cholesterol-rich plaque (containing up to 70 per cent cholesterol). The cholesterol in the blood is carried not in simple solution but in lipoprotein complexes, the so-called "giant molecules" of Gofman. The serum cholesterol level is not altered readily by even quite large changes in the cholesterol content of the diet. However, there is a relationship between the total serum cholesterol and the total fat content of the diet. Keys[16] concluded that not the amount of dietary cholesterol, but the *total amount of fat* is the significant factor in controlling blood cholesterol levels. Low-fat diets led to a fall in blood cholesterol. Low cholesterol but high-fat diets gave high cholesterol blood levels.

Walker *et al.*[17] found that weight loss resulted in reduction of the Sf 12 to 100 lipoproteins to which Gofman attributes pathogenic significance in atherosclerosis. Gofman[18] previously had reported higher levels of these bodies in obese persons and reduction in them by low-fat, low-cholesterol diets.

This class of lipoprotein particle is found in higher than normal concentration in the plasma of patients recently recovered from coronary thrombosis; the concentration increases with age and is much higher in males under age 40 than in females, but this sex difference tends to disappear in the older age groups. These observations are in accordance with the incidence of atheromatosis with respect to age and sex.

Short[10] found that 15 per cent of those who were more than 25 per cent overweight for their height had definite electrocardiographic abnormalities. Only 8.5 per cent of persons of average weight and 2 per cent of underweight subjects showed abnormal electrocardiographic changes.

Cholesterol and probably other lipids are implicated in the problems of arterial disease, particularly of the coronary arteries. Obese persons frequently have blood cholesterol levels above normal and they are also particularly subject to coronary occlusion. It is generally agreed that:

1. Arteriosclerosis and atherosclerosis are characterized by deposition of cholesterol in the arterial walls.

2. Patients with coronary artery disease and atheroma have high blood cholesterol for their ages.

3. These conditions are common among people ingesting high fat diets, less frequent in countries where the fat intake is low.

Blood cholesterol can be raised or lowered by increase or decrease in the dietary intake of animal fat.

5. The ingestion of highly unsaturated fat tends to lower blood cholesterol.

The cause of the accumulation of cholesterol (particularly cholesterol esters) in the atheromatous plaques is not clear. Two main theories are proposed: (1) The filtration theory: cholesterol of the blood, present in excess or in an abnormal physicochemical state, is picked up by the arterial wall; (2) The local theory: changes in the arterial wall are primary, resulting in a local uptake of cholesterol from the plasma, or increased synthesis of cholesterol in the arterial wall.

Attempts by many investigators to relate blood lipid levels to coronary atherosclerosis have shown varying degrees of correlation with cholesterol, triglycerides, total β-lipoprotein, β-lipoprotein of Sf 0-12 and 12-400, etc. Some studies suggest that blood cholesterol elevation is as accurate a parameter as an increase in any of the other fractions. In middle age the incidence of coronary thrombosis is 3 to 6 times as high among persons with elevated blood cholesterol as when the level is normal. Correlation with β-lipoprotein cholesterol concentration seems particularly important.

Recent studies indicate that triglyceride levels may be as significant, or more significant than cholesterol levels.[93,94]

Two points deserve emphasis:

1. Atherosclerosis and coronary occlusion occur in many persons who have not been shown to have any blood lipid abnormality.

2. As yet, measurement of none of the blood lipids has served satisfactorily to permit prediction of coronary thrombosis.

Whether significant prevention of atherosclerosis and its consequences will be possible by weight control or specific diet management awaits more conclusive demonstration. The evidence is already highly suggestive that weight reduction in the obese reduces the mortality from cardiovascular disease.[95]

Diets very low in fat but high in carbohydrate may lower blood cholesterol, but elevate blood triglyceride levels, presumably because of increased lipogenesis from carbohydrate.

It has been demonstrated by a number of investigators[96,97,98] that diets low in cholesterol and relatively high in polyunsaturated fats will reduce blood cholesterol and other lipid levels. Not only can the blood lipids be altered in amount and relative composition, but so can the lipids of subcutaneous fat. In a group of men[97] following such an experimental diet for 2 years, there was progressive desaturation of depot fat, the linoleic acid content rising to 24 per cent as compared with 9 per cent in those on conventional diets.

Authoritative medical committees have reviewed the evidence now available and have recommended[99,100] that physicians prescribe diets low in saturated fats, and relatively high in polyunsaturated fats for persons who have suffered atherosclerotic insults, or who are known to be susceptible or predisposed to them. Such suggestions seem justified and commendable, but probably too conservative. If we have dietary measures at hand which can prevent atherosclerosis, should we not recommend them to everyone?

Since our knowledge is limited and the conclusions to be drawn from the information now available are uncertain, should specific diet regulation be recommended for everyone as a preventive public health measure, or be confined to persons known to have atherosclerosis or to be predisposed to it (by heredity, or because of obesity, diabetes, elevated blood lipids, etc.)?

The best answer we can give at present, in view of the high incidence of atherosclerosis in the United States, the relatively high fat (especially saturated fat) diet of a high portion of persons in this country, and the long time it takes to develop atherosclerosis, seems to be this: the optimum diet for everyone should not allow excess calories and should be adequate in protein, vitamins and minerals; the fat content should supply 25 to 35 per cent of the total calories (not 45 per cent or over, as is usual), and the carbohydrate allowance should be moderate. The fats taken should be chiefly polyunsaturated as supplied in fat of fish and in vegetable oils (corn, cottonseed, soya), while foods supplying the saturated fats should be limited (meat-fats, eggs, whole milk, butter, cream, coconut oil, chocolate).

Optimal levels for blood lipids cannot be set with certainty, but these seem desirable: total lipids under 700 mg. per 100 ml., β-lipoprotein under 400 mg., cholesterol under 225 mg.

Heart, Circulation, Respiration. Obesity, dyspnea and limitation of exertion are frequently concomitant and therefore these questions have received much attention: (1) Can obesity alone cause dyspnea? (2) Does obesity per se cause heart disease? (3) Does obesity cause other disorders which may simulate heart disease? (4) Does obesity impair respiration specifically, aside from or in addition to effects it may have upon circulatory organs and function?

These questions are here considered in order:

1. Obesity can cause dyspnea, excessive fatigue and limited capacity for performing muscular work just by *increasing the body load.* In nearly all types of work, mechanical efficiency is impaired by obesity, so that a given task requires greater expenditure of energy, greater oxygen consumption, etc.

2. Obesity alone can be the cause of *pathologic changes in the heart* and of heart failure. In their study of the pathology of adiposity of the heart, Smith and Willius[7] found that the degree of cardiac enlargement in obesity is roughly proportional to the increase in body-surface area and that some of these otherwise normal enlarged hearts may fail. It is axiomatic that dilated and hypertrophied hearts from any cause tend to fail. The eventual weakening of the cardiac musculature results from relative coronary artery insufficiency, even in the absence of occlusive arterial disease.

In many instances there is not only enlargement of the heart but "adiposity of the heart." In this condition there is an increase in the amount of subepicardial fat and of the fat lying between muscle bundles. Such fatty changes differ from the "fatty infiltration" seen in pernicious anemia, carcinoma, etc., in which droplets of fat appear within the cytoplasm of the cardiac muscle cells.

When coronary atherosclerosis occurs in association with obesity as it so frequently does, a secondary cause of heart disease is added to the primary embarrassment of the heart muscle already operative as a consequence of the obesity per se.

Obesity has been shown therefore, to be associated with the development of three types of true heart disease: (1) hypertrophy and dilatation; (2) fatty infiltration of heart muscle; (3) coronary atherosclerosis.

3. Obesity alone may cause dyspnea[8] since reduction in vital capacity results from *mechanical restriction* of respiratory movements by excess fat in the abdominal and thoracic walls.

In obesity, the decreased compliance of the thoracic structures produced by the encircling girdle of adipose tissue has two effects: it mechanically limits respiration, and it increases the mechanical work of breathing several fold.[103]

In obesity, because of the increased work of breathing, the oxygen costs of breathing are greatly increased. Hypoventilation may result partly from the restricted respiration and partly from the greater demand, so that respiration may not only be labored, but it may be inadequate and unable to support proper gaseous interchange in the lungs.[104] The consequences may be serious (see below).

Emphysema may result from prolonged obesity, with permanent reduction of vital capacity even after weight loss.[9,10]

4. Not only may the subcutaneous fat mass interfere with respiration, but there may be *extensive infiltration of the intercostal muscles and diaphragm by adipose tissue.*[91] Poor function of these muscles may account for serious disturbance in gaseous exchange in the lungs even in the absence of circulatory failure. Normal inspiration depends entirely upon contraction of the external intercostal muscles, the levator costarum and the diaphragm. The diaphragm accounts for approximately two-thirds of the inspiratory function.

The *inadequate pulmonary ventilation* results in decrease in arterial oxygen saturation and increase in carbon dioxide retention.[92] In extreme degrees of such derangement, usually with great obesity, there may be somnolence, muscular twitching, cyanosis, secondary polycythemia, and hypertrophy and failure of the right ventricle (pickwickian syndrome).[91,101]

Diabetes. Obesity and diabetes are interrelated in a number of ways, all of which have led to studies which have yielded information about the interlocking pathologic physiology of both conditions. For further discussion of basic concepts see discussion below under Etiology.

Here we are concerned with the medical importance of obesity as related to diabetes. We may list essential points:

1. Mortality: death from diabetes is almost four times as common among the obese.

2. Incidence: the percentage of obese persons who develop diabetes is higher than among persons not overweight, yet among all obese persons this percentage is small.

However, the other way around, the correlation is very high: approximately 40 per cent of diabetics are obese when the diabetes is diagnosed, compared to a 10 per cent incidence of obesity in non-diabetics.

3. Severity: the greater the obesity, the higher the incidence of diabetes. In one series the incidence was 1.5 times normal among those 10 per cent overweight, 3 times normal if 20 per cent overweight, and 8 times normal if 25 per cent overweight.

Weight gain in overweight persons with limited carbohydrate tolerance further reduces glucose tolerance; weight reduction in the obese improves glucose tolerance.

Liver Disease. Obesity has a definite and deleterious effect upon the liver. The most significant relationship seems to be the duration rather than the degree of obesity. Zelman[19] studied liver function in 20 men who were 50 to 100 per cent overweight and not known to be suffering from any other disorder which might affect the liver. Needle biopsy revealed degenerative changes and functional tests revealed deficiencies in practically all of the patients, severe enough to be classed as of moderate degree in approximately one-half of them. Fatty infiltration and higher total metabolism with relative B-complex vitamin deficiency accompanying high carbohydrate diets were considered as probable factors in the liver derangement.

Cancer. The nature of the interrelationship is obscure, but there is widespread agreement that morbidity and mortality from cancer are increased in the presence of obesity. Hertig and Sommers[20] found a

30 per cent greater incidence of endometrial cancer in overweight women. Records of the Metropolitan Life Insurance Company covering a period between 1922 and 1936 reveal that mortality due to certain cancers was higher among overweight persons. Deaths from benign tumors of the uterus were higher among overweight women. Obesity not only is associated with a higher incidence of cancer, but introduces difficulties in its treatment. Hildreth[21] found that the 5-year survival rate in cancer of the cervix treated by irradiation was 37.5 per cent in women weighing over 170 lbs., but 54.6 per cent in those under 170 lbs.

Psychological Consequences of Obesity. Corpulence may lead not only to the physical disorders we have discussed, but to psychologic aberrations. Fat persons may find themselves rejected by others in many life situations; they find that they are handicapped in many normal activities. Recent emphasis has been given to the psychologic factors in the *causation* of obesity; it is important also to realize that serious emotional and psychic *results* of obesity constitute some of its chief dangers.

Summary. In the preceding discussion we have reviewed some of the most significant information indicating that (1) obesity is a serious health hazard and increases the incidence and severity of many of the commonest causes of disability and death; also that (2) obesity is much commoner than it should be.

Since the *degree* and the *duration* of obesity are important factors in causing predisposition to (and establishing irreversibility of) many disorders, *prevention* of excessive weight gain is even more important than its removal.

OBESITY AND GROWTH

It has been amply demonstrated by many studies that undernourished children grow at subnormal rates. The converse of this question arises: do overnourished children grow at supernormal rates? A recent study[106] indicates that this may be true, since greater thickness of body fat was correlated with faster growth rates and earlier maturation in children of both sexes. However, another possibility must be considered: the rapid growth and maturation and the greater fat deposit may both depend upon a growth factor other than calories alone. Nevertheless, the evidence is suggestive and supports the concept that growth and development are to a certain extent functions of nutritional influences.

Various reviews[107] of the interrelationships of nutrition and growth suggest that the well-documented secular growth rate increases (larger recent generations) are at least in part due to better nutrition.

OBESITY AS A SYMPTOM

This brief review of the facts known concerning the consequences of corpulence emphasizes the serious nature of a condition too often neglected, or even viewed as a sign of abundant good health. Often the symptom of obesity may be only a minor complaint as far as the patient is concerned. However, the physician may discover that it deserves major consideration and, possibly, that it lies at the root of many or all of the patient's difficulties. Fortunately, the general public is becoming more conscious of the decreased efficiency accompanying overweight and its ultimate bad effects. Therefore, more frequently now than formerly the chief complaint of patients seeking medical advice is obesity. This state of affairs is desirable for three reasons: first, early recognition and treatment may prevent serious complications; second, when a patient actually complains of being overweight he has already acknowledged that he does not want to be fat, and is more apt to be co-operative in carrying out reduction therapy; third, when the case is studied early, it is easier to discover the cause of the obesity.

THE CAUSE OF OBESITY

Understanding of the reasons for and the mechanism of the deposit of excessive amounts of fat in the body will enable the physician to help his patients prevent obesity and to help get rid of it when it has occurred.

The three chief fuel-producing food-stuff groups are proteins, carbohydrates and fats. All three are to a certain extent stored in the body. However, protein and carbohydrate stores are relatively small and unimportant as energy reservoirs compared to the body stores of fat. Excessive protein storage does not occur. When protein is taken in excess of body needs, part of the excess is simply excreted, but part is converted into fat and stored as such. When too much carbohydrate is taken, all of the body glycogen reservoirs seem first to be filled, then the excess carbohydrate not utilized for fuel or stored as glycogen may be converted into fat. When prolonged fasting occurs, the fat stores may serve as a source of fuel for a long period. The glycogen stores are used up within a short time. The protein, stored chiefly in the muscles, cannot be utilized without an attack upon the very structure of the body. Fortunately, the protein is the last to go. It is evident, then, that excessive intake of fat, or of protein, or of carbohydrate will lead to excessive deposition of fat in the body. In this sense all foods are fattening, although fat itself will, of course, be stored more readily as fat. The ultimate result of a prolonged immoderate intake of food is, therefore, always the same.

A plethora of calories is the only explanation of obesity, all protestations of our corpulent patients to the contrary notwithstanding. The law of the conservation of energy applies to the human body as surely as to any other heat- and energy-producing machine. Energy, or heat as represented by the caloric equivalent of food, can be neither created nor destroyed. When the intake exceeds the output expended in work and heat, the excess will be found stored in the body tissues. In children, when the body is growing, a positive energy balance for tissue building is necessary. However, after growth is complete, the excess calories do not produce useful body tissue but detrimental adiposity. Numerous careful studies by many investigators have demonstrated conclusively that changes in body weight can be predicted accurately when all metabolic influences are known and measured. Newburgh[11] and his collaborators have published analyses of the apparently paradoxical situation in which

weight is maintained temporarily in spite of low caloric intake, revealing that transient water retention is the explanation.

FAT METABOLISM
AND
STORAGE OF FAT

The fat absorbed from the gastrointestinal tract and the fat formed in intermediary metabolism are widely deposited in the fat depots of various tissues. The sites of greatest storage are the subcutaneous tissues, the intramucular tissues, the omentum, the perirenal tissues, the mesentery and the pericardium.

The immediate destination of the absorbed neutral fat is the fat depots of the tissues. Here it remains until needed as a source of fuel.

The average daily fat intake of a normal adult is 70 to 120 Gm., varying greatly with total caloric intake. The fat of food consists mainly of neutral fat (triglycerides) together with small amounts of free fatty acids, lecithin and cholesterol esters. Digestion and absorption of the fats takes place chiefly in the duodenum and proximal jejunum. Formerly it was thought that triglycerides had to be completely hydrolyzed in the intestine to glycerol and three molecules of fatty acid before absorption, but present evidence indicates that such is not the case.

There are three major phases involved in the transfer of fats from the intestinal lumen to the lymphatic system: (1) the intraluminal digestive phase, during which the fat is modified physically and chemically prior to absorption; (2) cellular phase, during which the digested material passes into the intestinal mucosal cells and undergoes many physical and chemical changes, especially in preparation for (3) passage from the intestinal mucosal cells into the lymphatics.

The form in which lipids are absorbed and the rate of absorption depend upon various reactions taking place in the intestinal lumen. For optimal enzymatic activity in digestion and also for absorption, emulsification is necessary. So thorough is emulsification normally that some of the minute fat droplets pass through the intestinal wall without further preparation. Bile salts and lysolecithin are prime factors in emulsification, but protein also helps disperse the lipids. Bile salts also activate intestinal and pancreatic lipolytic enzymes, as well as playing a crucial role in absorption of all the lipids.

Most of the emulsified triglycerides are hydrolyzed to monoglycerides, diglycerides, fatty acids and glycerol. In the mucosal cells the long-chain fatty acids, monoglycerides and diglycerides are incorporated into triglycerides, which enter the intestinal lymphatics. The mucosal cells also utilize long-chain fatty acids for the synthesis of phospholipids and for the partial esterification of the absorbed cholesterol. The greater part of the absorbed lipids is carried by chylomicra (protein-stabilized particles of tri-, di-, and monoglycerides, cholesterol esters, cholesterol and phospholipids) through the lymphatics to the thoracic duct and thus into the general circulation. The distribution of fatty acids in postprandial lymph from the thoracic duct is approximately: glyceride 82 per cent, phospholipids 10 per cent, cholesterol esters 2 per cent and free fatty acids 6 per cent.

Another route is used for a smaller fraction of the products of lipid digestion: after absorption, the unesterified short-chain (12-carbon or less) fatty acids, the glycerol and the steroid hormones (estradiol, cortisol, testosterone, etc.) are transported to the liver by the portal vein.

The anatomical arrangement of the two main routes permits extrahepatic tissue, particularly fat depots, to clear the blood of chylomicra and to utilize absorbed fatty substances directly. In animal studies 60 per cent of the chylomicra may be cleared from the blood in 10 minutes, with 25 per cent of the cleared lipid being in adipose tissue, 23 per cent in muscle and 20 per cent in the liver.

Fate of Fat After Absorption. Fat may be utilized in three chief ways:

1. It is stored as neutral fat (triglycerides) in the adipose tissues.

2. It is built into the structure of all tissues. Structural lipids are as integral a part of the cell architecture as are proteins. In starvation, fat in the depots is drawn upon as a source of energy but the structural lipids are spared (until the situation becomes extreme). Among the structural lipids are:

a. Lecithin (and the related cephalins)

b. Cholesterol esters.

The lipids in these two groups are essential constituents of all cell membranes. Lecithin is a component of the medullary sheath of nerve fibers.

c. Certain specialized lipids such as the sphingomyelins and cerebrosides of the central nervous system.

d. Steroid hormones, such as those of the ovary, testis, and adrenal cortex.

3. It undergoes complete oxidation to yield energy, CO_2 and H_2O.

BLOOD LIPIDS

Normal fasting serum contains highly variable amounts of the various lipids. Cholesterol, phospholipids (fats containing phosphate esters), and triglycerides (esters of glycerol and fatty acids) constitute the principal lipids occurring in blood. The normal ranges in mg. per 100 ml. in fasting serum are:

1. Fatty acids: 250 to 500 mg. (average 300); of these approximately 80 per cent occur in triglycerides and 15 per cent are esterified with cholesterol. The remaining 5 per cent are unesterified free fatty acids presumably bound to albumin.

2. Cholesterol: 150 to 230 mg. (cholesterol esters constitute 65 to 75 per cent of the total).

3. Phospholipids: 150 to 250 mg. Phospholipids contain about 80 per cent fatty acids, 15 to 20 per cent cephalins and 5 per cent sphingomyelins. The synthesis of phospholipids depends largely upon dietary supplies of choline. Lecithin contains choline as part of the molecule and yields choline on hydrolysis.

Total lipids. The normal fasting total serum lipids vary from 470 to 750 mg. per 100 ml. However, determinations of total lipid are not commonly employed; studies are usually confined to estimations of cholesterol (free and esterified), phospholipids, and triglycerides including fatty acids.

Lactescence of plasma or serum is due to macroscopic aggregates of chylomicrons and low-density lipoproteins mostly due to hydrolysis of triglycerides. It is especially observed in blood drawn a few hours after a high fat meal. Lactescence occurring as long as 12 hours after a meal, largely due to chylomicrons, is observed particularly in idiopathic hyperlipemia.

Physiologic hyperlipemia without lactescence is often observed in the blood of normal persons drawn 3 or 4 hours after ingestion of large amounts of fat.

Pathologic hyperlipemia occurs when carbohydrate metabolism is deficient and fats become the main source of calories (low carbohydrate diets, glycogen storage disease, diabetes mellitus, etc.).

Triglycerides and Fatty Acids. Normal fasting triglyceride varies from 0 to 250 mg. per 100 ml. Only negligible amounts of free fatty acids occur in normal fasting plasma. Total fatty acids as determined in the laboratory include triglycerides, cholesterol esters and phospholipids. Determinations of triglycerides are necessary for the differential diagnosis of the idiopathic hyperlipemias. They are usually increased in glycogen storage disease, hypercholesteremia and hyperphospholipidemia.

Phospholipid Elevation. Hyperphospholipidemia may occur in a number of conditions, including uncontrolled diabetes mellitus, nephrosis, hypothyroidism, etc. It is particularly characteristic of xanthomatous biliary cirrhosis, in which the levels may reach 800 to 3,000 mg. per 100 ml.

Cholesterol Elevation. The chief exogenous sources of this lipid are the dietary animal fats, but it is also synthesized in the body. Blood cholesterol content is increased in diabetes mellitus, arteriosclerosis and atherosclerosis, hypothyroidism, nephrosis, xanthomatosis, etc.

The Liver in Fat Metabolism

When fats are to be used, they are withdrawn (by unknown means) from the adipose tissue cells and pass to the liver. In the fasting state, unesterified fatty acids, freed from depot fat by *lipoprotein lipase* are brought to the liver for utilization. Under usual normal conditions the fat content of the liver is essentially unchanged, since the fat is metabolized as fast as it arrives.

Desaturation of fatty acids probably occurs chiefly in the liver, and phospholipids and fats deposited in the liver contain fatty acids that are more unsaturated than are fatty acids in other tissues.

Normally fat is metabolized thus:

1. The triglycerides are hydrolyzed (enzyme: liver lipase), yielding glycerol and fatty acids. The glycerol is utilized via the pathways of carbohydrate metabolism.

2. The fatty acids are oxidized to acetyl-Co-A units containing 2 C each;

3. The acetyl-Co-A units are completely oxidized to CO_2 and H_2O with energy liberation, or

4. The acetyl-Co-A units are recombined to give acetoacetic acid (a 4 C compound). This process is called ketogenesis, since acetoacetic acid is a ketone. This is a normal step in fat metabolism, as ketones are regularly formed by the liver.

5. The liver cannot further metabolize acetoacetic acid; it is distributed to the tissues where it is completely oxidized to yield CO_2, H_2O and energy.

Ketosis occurs if the liver production of acetoacetic acid exceeds the ability of the tissues to utilize it, and ketone bodies accumulate in the blood. The maximum amount which the tissues can use is about 2.5 Gm. of fat per Kg. body weight per day (about 175 Gm. for a 70 Kg. man).

When carbohydrate supply is deficient, increased metabolism of fat may, through all of the steps above, supply energy, prevent further utilization of depleted carbohydrate stores, and thus help to maintain the blood glucose level.

Fatty Liver. Under certain circumstances the liver cells may become abnormally loaded with excess fat. This appears to develop when (1) fat is provided in excess and glucose metabolism is deficient, or (2) the hepatic cells are unable because of functional impairment to normally metabolize and dispose of the fats brought to them. Since a certain minimum amount of glucose is necessary for maintenance of normal function of hepatic cells and also to preserve their anatomic integrity, and since fat metabolism is accelerated whenever glucose metabolism is deficient, (1) and (2) often occur together. However (2) may be primary when toxins, poisons, etc. damage the liver.

Neutral fat and cholesterol esters may accumulate in the liver in many conditions, especially those in which hepatic damage occurs in association with a toxic or infectious disease or prolonged nutritional disorder. Such abnormal fat deposit in the liver occurs in alcoholism, starvation, diabetes mellitus, toxemias of pregnancy, following certain poisons (phosphorus, chloroform, benzol, carbon tetrachloride), with forced fat feeding, low choline intake, etc.

STORAGE OF FAT

The depots of body fat (adipose tissue) constitute the chief fuel reserve of the body and are composed almost exclusively of triglycerides. In contrast to the small carbohydrate reserves of about one pound, fat reserves normally are 10 to 15 per cent of body weight, amounting to 15 to 22 lb. in a 150 lb. person. This is equivalent to an energy reserve of 1000 cal. per Kg. body weight—more than a month's supply of total food energy. In obese persons, the fat reserve may be in great excess of this liberal normal safety factor, and may amount in extreme cases to hundreds of pounds.

It must be emphasized that neutral fat is not deposited in the matrix between cells or fibers. The triglycerides are stored in the cells of adipose tissue. The cytoplasm diminishes in amount as the fat accumulates, until the cell becomes a thin, cytoplasmic nucleated envelope enclosing a large fat droplet. Adipose tissue exists in a state of dynamic equilibrium with the systems regulating energy metabolism: it stores fat when present in excess of immediate metabolic needs, releasing it when required. In some manner not yet well understood, when normal fat depots are taxed to capacity by arriving fat supplies, the tissues are stimulated to grow and new cells are supplied as needed, so new adipose tissue is created to meet the demand.

The triglycerides of adipose tissue are derived from two main sources: (1) from food fat; (2) from carbohydrate.

Normally the triglycerides of the adipose tissue are in a constant state of exchange with the lipids of the plasma. The problem in obesity is to determine why the fat depots remain excessive or keep growing.

When fats are utilized as fuel, the fatty acids are broken down to carbon dioxide and water. Body fat acts as a highly efficient storehouse of energy: the capacity to store protein and carbohydrate is extremely limited, fat storage is almost unlimited. Pure fat yields 9 calories per gram in combustion, pure protein or glucose only 4 calories per gram.

When the body loses fat, however, the metabolic processes also include the loss of water: for each gram of fat stored, there is stored at least 0.25 gram of water.[3] Recent studies showed that the caloric value of labile body tissue in obese subjects was approximately 2.5 calories per gram. Apparently a considerable amount of water is stored and released as part of the caloric response, since pure fat would yield 9 calories per gram.[22]

Fat stores are definitely in the dynamic state, less readily utilizable for calories than glycogen and glucose, but more readily available than protein. When caloric demand is brief, glucose is the chief source; when prolonged, fat becomes the chief source. The deposition and the mobilization of fat is an active metabolic process in adipose tissue.[23] Adipose tissue is supplied by a rich capillary network and is innervated by the autonomic nervous system. In the adipose tissue new fatty acids are synthesized, fatty acids are transformed to other forms of fatty acids, and glycogen also is synthesized. All of these metabolic functions are controlled by a number of hormonal and nervous influences.

Insulin plays an essential part in lipogenesis. New insight into fat metabolism is permitted by the discovery and the elucidation of the role of coenzyme A (CoA).[24,25] It seems well established that carbohydrate is converted into fat primarily by way of pyruvate, which subsequently is decarboxylated to form acetyl CoA. It appears that acetyl CoA is the major precursor of long-chain fatty acids. Thus glycolysis is the first major metabolic process involved in the conversion of carbohydrate to fat, and glycolysis is in turn dependent upon insulin. It seems that any substance which can give rise to acetyl CoA or "active acetate" can be converted to fatty acids. Adipose tissues as well as a number of other tissues have the ability to synthesize fat. When insulin is lacking, fat formation from the 2-carbon precursors, the ubiquitous "active acetate," is inhibited. It may be "too naïve to suppose that excess fat formation tends to exhaust the insulin mechanism; however there is surely a clue herein."[26] Further discussion in the section on Etiology will emphasize the important interrelationships of fat metabolism and obesity to diabetes and hyperinsulinism.

Fats are excreted in relatively large amounts by the intestinal mucosa, to a small degree in the bile, and in minute amounts by the oil glands of the skin. In the feces, fat is normally present in three forms: soap fats (combined fatty acids), free fatty acids and neutral fat. The relative amount of each depends upon the type of fats ingested and upon the efficiency of fat digestion and absorption. In cases of diarrhea, there may be unusually large amounts of fat present in the feces, simply because of the rapid passage of food through the bowel, with poor absorption. When insufficient amounts of pancreatic lipase reach the intestine, the stools are fatty because of incomplete digestion. Absence of bile likewise results in faulty fat digestion with fatty stools.

HUNGER AND APPETITE

The terms *hunger* and *appetite* have been variously defined and are used widely with various connotations. In Chapter 18 the degree of desire for food is discussed particularly in regard to its diminution, called *anorexia*. In this chapter we are concerned with sensations of heightened desire for food, since, if gratified, excessive or too frequent hunger or appetite may lead to obesity.

As used in this chapter, *hunger* has an organic basis in the body's need for food.

The need may be in the tissues, or may simply exist as hunger contractions of an empty stomach, but it can be demonstrated definitely to be due to a chemical need or a physical state. Hunger is a complex sensation and various theories have been proposed to explain it. Hunger is the principal factor controlling food intake, and consequently, body growth and nutrition. Accompanying the sensation of hunger there are frequently strong contractions of the gastric walls ("hunger contractions"). Such contractions may be inhibited and the hunger pangs relieved by filling the stomach with bulky, even inedible, non-nutritive material. Hypoglycemia usually is accompanied by hunger. Tissue need for glucose may exist when hunger is present but the blood sugar level is high or normal. (Patients with diabetes mellitus are characteristically hungry; persons who have been starved for some time may still be hungry and continue to eat after blood glucose exceeds the normal level.) It is likely that hunger due to deficiency of nutrients at the tissue level, as well as at the blood level, exists for other nutrients than glucose. The introduction of nutrients by a route other than the mouth may appease hunger and quiet hunger contractions. Animals often seek and select the specific nutrient for which need exists ("salt hunger," etc.); thus there may be various hungers depending upon the general body state and apparently controlled by one or more central mechanisms. These aspects of the problem are discussed further below under "Role of the hypothalamus and higher brain centers."

Appetite, as contrasted with hunger, is a sensation which may be considered primarily as a psychic phenomenon, rather than basically organic in origin as hunger is. Appetite may be defined as the desire for food whether or not the need exists. Usually appetite accompanies hunger (desire accompanies need), but under certain circumstances this natural association may not occur, and appetite and hunger may be dissociated. Apparently, appetite is largely acquired and is dependent to a great degree upon previous experience, whereas hunger is inborn. A newborn child experiences hunger, not appetite. Conditioned stimuli and responses exert considerable control over appetite. Training and environmental influences are well known to exert profound influences upon national, local or individual desire for certain foods. Thus the psychic element in appetite is illustrated by its highly selective character. Snails or rattlesnake meat to some persons are highly desirable and even their mention may heighten appetite, but to others, even though the food may be nutritious and the person hungry, such foods may destroy appetite.

Hunger usually whets appetites. Foods usually considered unpalatable may be consumed avidly if true hunger is present. Any stimulus that increases hunger is apt also to increase appetite. When alcohol is ingested, or dilute hydrochloric acid, the flow of gastric juices is stimulated, gastric tone is raised and appetite is aroused. Often appetite is increased greatly after a few mouthfuls of food enter the stomach.

A person may be hungry and anorexic, or even nauseated at the same time. If he has an appetite, however, he welcomes food, even though he may not truly be hungry. Attractively prepared foods and pleasant food odors are powerful stimulants to appetite.

ETIOLOGY OF OBESITY

Although the immediate cause of obesity is always a positive energy balance, there are many ways in which it is conceivable that the balance may be tilted toward the positive side. Let us list these, then consider them in order:

POSSIBLE FACTORS IN THE PATHOGENESIS OF OBESITY

1. Digestive factors: is digestion more complete?
2. Absorptive factors: is absorption more efficient?
3. Tissue factors:
   A. Do tissues take up fats more readily?
   B. Do tissues fail to give up fat stores as readily as normal?
   C. Local and general tissue factors: insulin, enzymes.
4. Utilization of energy:
   A. Basal metabolic rate: is it lower?
   B. Specific dynamic action of food: is there less stimulation to increased heat production after intake of food?
   C. "Luxuskonsumption": is obesity the result of a failure to exhibit a rise in total metabolic rate following excess food intake?
   D. Total metabolism: does obesity result from conservation of energy in work, or in carrying out other normal body functions?
   E. Physical activity: does physical inactivity cause obesity?
5. Endocrine factors: role of pituitary disease, adrenal cortex, hypothyroidism, hypogonadism, diabetes mellitus, hypoglycemia.
6. Role of the hypothalamus and higher brain centers.
7. Influence of heredity.
8. Psychologic factors: mental and emotional factors influencing hunger, appetite and food intake.
9. Social factors.

Digestive Factors. Although a lack of some of the essential digestive ferments may lead to a loss from the body of calories as undigested food (for example, protein and fat loss in the feces in pancreatic disease), an excess of digestive enzymes or increased efficiency of digestion has never been demonstrated to occur in obesity. Obesity is, therefore, not explainable on the basis that the food taken into the body is more completely broken down in the gastrointestinal tract of a person who becomes corpulent than in that of a normal person.

Absorptive Factors. It is conceivable that more efficient and more complete absorption of the products of digestion might enable certain persons to gain weight without excessive intake of food. However, Neuenschwander-Lemmer[27] has compared the combustible materials in the feces with those in the food eaten, and in three obese and three normal patients found no essential differences. The utilization of the dietary constituents by the obese was no different in any way from that of the normal subjects in regard to total calories, nitrogen or fat. In this connection it is interesting to compare these figures with those obtained upon a group of nine undernourished persons gaining weight rapidly upon a forced high-caloric intake. Strang, McClugage and Brownlee[28] found practically the same percentage of food ingested to be absorbed in these patients receiving forced feedings as in the obese and the normal patients in the above study. It might have been expected that less efficient absorption would be demonstrated as the result of undue strain upon digestive and absorptive mechanisms, but such was not the case. Supernormal efficiency of digestion or of absorption is, therefore, not present in obesity.

Tissue Factors. If there were a hereditary constitutional tendency of the adipose cells that enabled them to accumulate excessive amounts of fat, obesity would result. This attractive hypothesis was proposed many years ago by von Bergmann.[29] He compared obesity with growth. A child grows, storing the materials necessary for growth, even though his activity consumes great quantities of food. Thus the fat tissues of obese persons might store fat, even though the diet were inadequate to meet other body needs. This is the theory of *lipophilia*.

Hetenyi[30] carried the idea of lipophilia a step farther by postulating that fat deposited in the depots of an obese person is held there, even when needed as fuel. When the fat tissues of a normal person would release it as a source of energy, the obese person's tissues might thus retain the fat.

Neither ingested nor stored fat would be readily or normally available for the energy requirements of an obese person if von Bergmann's and Hetenyi's theories should prove tenable. Increased food intake in the obese would be necessary to fill the requirements for work and heat, while fat was continuously stored. Hetenyi supported this concept by showing that when given an inadequate diet, the level of blood fats in obese persons falls more than in normal subjects. He believed that there was a delay or hindrance in the release of fat by the tissues of the obese patients.

Newburgh interpreted Hetenyi's own data as evidence against this hypothesis. He says that since obese persons have more fat in the blood when food is unrestricted,

they must be either storing less or mobilizing more of it than normal persons. The lowering of the blood-fat level in obese persons by under-feeding might not mean that fat was released less rapidly from adipose tissue, but that fat that was mobilized at a normal rate was oxidized more rapidly.

If it were true that the adipose tissue cells of obese persons resist mobilization of fat in undernutrition, obese persons on restricted diets should exhibit destruction of body protein and a negative nitrogen balance. This would be true because there would be no other source of calories. Glycogen stores are rapidly exhausted in a few days of severe undernutrition. If fat were unavailable, protein would have to be utilized. However, a number of studies have shown that obese persons are *less likely to develop negative nitrogen balance* than normal subjects. Jansen[31] gave 15 medical students a diet of 1,600 calories, including 61 Gm. of protein, daily for several weeks. The average daily nitrogen loss was 2 Gm. Benedict[32] studied 12 normal subjects receiving 1,534 calories and 51 Gm. of protein daily, and noted 3 Gm. daily as the average nitrogen loss. In studying obese persons given a diet yielding 1,375 calories with 90 Gm. of protein daily, Keeton and Dickson[33] found maintenance of nitrogen balance. Even when the caloric intake is extremely low, fat stores can be mobilized sufficiently to spare body protein, as indicated by the fact that Strang, McClugage and Evans[34] found that obese persons did not lose protein when receiving only 440 calories daily and approximately 1 Gm. of protein per kilogram of ideal body weight.

Block,[35] reinvestigating the possible role of lipophilia, found that three obese subjects remained in positive nitrogen balance during a prolonged period of undernutrition. The blood lipids varied in essentially the same manner as in three normal subjects following the same diets. They at first rose, then later fell. The actual weight loss in the obese patients was in very close agreement with that predicted on the assumption that the body fat was utilized for heat production. These results indicate that the theory of lipophilia is untenable as an explanation for the usual type of obesity.

Study of blood fat and fatty acids has not uniformly revealed a greater avidity for these materials in the tissues of obese persons. When Hetenyi fed fat or injected olive oil into obese subjects, he found only a relatively slight rise in blood lipids as compared to that produced in normal persons, which might be interpreted as indicating more rapid fat deposit in the obese. However, other workers have obtained contradictory results. Obese persons commonly have a somewhat higher blood-lipid level than average normal, which certainly might not indicate increased fat storage, and might be the result of increased fat mobilization.

A possible explanation for the conflict in such studies is proposed as a result of recent studies by Schlechter[102] who found, as did Hetenyi, a greater avidity for lipids in the adipose tissue of obese persons. The avidity was most evident in the *static phase* of obesity, less evident in the dynamic phase.

Antoniades and Gundersen[105,110] have recently described an enzyme in adipose tissue which releases insulin from its binding to basic protein in the plasma, thereby permitting the freed insulin to act to promote fat storage. Certain questions arise as the result of such observations: (1) Could differences in the concentrations of such an enzyme in adipose tissues account for generalized adiposity in some persons? (2) Could differences in concentrations of the enzyme explain, by its action on fat synthesis and deposition, the distribution of adipose deposits as they vary between persons and in many clinical states?

The possibility that fat cells in certain persons may react abnormally has been supported by studies of hereditary obesity in yellow mice. Radioactive carbon (C^{14}) is incorporated into their fat depots in an apparently normal manner, but the labeled fat disappeared from the tissues much more slowly than in normal mice.[36] The decrease in fat mobilization thus may be a fat cell disorder, perhaps an enzyme defect, and it can be hereditary. We have then a modern revival of the *lipophilia* theory of von Bergmann.

In the obese diabetic strain of mice, Guggenheim and Mayer[37] found that when C^{14}-labeled acetate was injected into the fasting animal, one-third less C^{14} appeared in the expired air than in normals. The incorporation of fed C^{14} acetate into fatty acids in obese mice was found to be much higher than in nonobese mice. It was concluded that the obese animals do not oxidize acetate as readily as normals and that the acetate which escapes oxidation is incorporated into fat. As a corollary to this theory, lipolysis is decreased due to impaired acetate oxidation.

The disappearance of C^{14}-labeled fat from the depots of obese rats with hypothalamic lesions proved to be just as slow as that found in yellow mice.[38] Therefore the cell defect can be acquired, and could possibly be the result of the obesity rather than its cause. The slow turnover of C^{14} in the obese diabetic mice might be due to some derangements of carbohydrate metabolism or possibly due to the large pool of fat: the abnormal composition of the animal's body. Further such studies on obese mice may yield progressive insight into the mechanisms of human obesity.

Blood lipids are usually elevated when there is a continuously greater demand for fat as fuel as the result of the lack of available carbohydrate. Hyperlipemia occurs in ether narcosis, for example, and in diabetes mellitus. Insulin in these two conditions can reduce or prevent the hyperlipemia, presumably by facilitating the combustion of carbohydrate, by decreasing fat mobilization, and by promoting fat storage. In diabetes mellitus, in malnutrition, in fasting, in certain liver disorders, and in similar conditions in which carbohydrate is lacking or cannot be utilized adequately, the blood lipids are increased and the fatty-tissue reserves are diminished.

Local factors instead of general influences controlling fat storage are known to exist, although their nature is not understood. The author has observed a number of patients who have developed the well-recognized *fat atrophy* that occurs in a relatively small percentage of patients receiving insulin repeatedly at the same subcutaneous site. There must be in certain persons local tissue responses to insulin that differ from the usual response. The author also has observed the more infrequent phenomenon of the development of *lipomata* at the site of insulin injections. Here the local-tissue effect seems to be the exact opposite, although the stimulus, insulin, is the same. In lipomatosis it seems evident that local conditions must be present that facilitate the deposit of fat. Lipomata may resist the mobilization of their contained fat, and remain unchanged during generalized weight loss and reduction in adipose tissue.

Lipodystrophy has been described in a wide variety of forms. It may affect only the face, or one-half of the face, or the legs, or all of the tissues above or below the umbilicus. The type of lipodystrophy that is most common affects women and involves the tissues above the waist. The upper half of the body, the neck and the face may be emaciated, while the girdle region, the buttocks, the hips, the thighs and the legs may be normal or obese. A number of cases of lipodystrophy have been demonstrated to be hereditary, with the exact type and location of the lesion being transmitted (van Leeuwen,[39] Nassauer-Badt[40]).

Consideration of the evident local factors influencing fat storage in such unusual conditions as lipomatosis and lipodystrophy leads to the inviting theory that the tissues in the common type of obesity may possess some such abnormal property that is generally distributed. It is known that blood, liver, pancreas and subcutaneous tissue contain various lipases. These enzymes are capable of causing profound changes locally in tissue fats under certain conditions. Little is known about the physical and the chemical conditions that activate or inhibit these enzyme systems, but they may be important in influencing fat storage. Barr[40a] feels that, since careful study by many able investigators has not revealed the cause of obesity elsewhere, better knowledge of tissue metabolism may yield the answer. He says: "It does not seem improbable that local or general conditions in the body might influence such enzyme systems and that disturbances in fat storage might occur because of their derangement; also that this might occur to a certain extent independent of the supply of fat in the food or the amount of fat or fatty acids in the blood." He feels that if the local deposits of lipomatosis can be explained by local tissue changes, the generalized adiposity in obesity may be due to the ability of the mesenchymal tissues to store and retain large amounts of fat. Such an unusual ability for the mesenchymal tissues might result from heritage, cerebral lesions or endocrine factors.

Utilization of Energy. Basal Metabolic Rate. If it could be demonstrated that when at rest obese persons conserve energy by lowering the rate of metabolic activity, an important influence tipping the scales toward a positive energy balance would be apparent. However, this definitely is not the case. Boothby and Sandiford[41] found that in 81 per cent of 94 obese persons the basal heat production per square meter of body surface was within 10 per cent of the normal. Strouse, Wang and Dye[42] found practically no differences in the basal metabolic rates of normal, overweight and underweight subjects. Grafe[43] studied 180 cases of extreme obesity and found a low basal metabolic rate in only three patients.

Occasionally a very low rate will be found in an obese person, but rates as low are encountered in those who are underweight. Severe hypothyroidism is not regularly accompanied by obesity.

Specific Dynamic Action. Following the intake of food, the heat production is elevated due to a "specific dynamic action" upon metabolism. This is not due to digestion or absorption, since it occurs even after the intravenous injection of glucose or amino acids. Should the metabolism of food be accomplished with less expenditure of energy, obesity might result. On the usual type of diet the total specific dynamic action in 24 hours may amount to 6 per cent of the day's energy output. Plaut's experiments[44] seemed to show a rather uniform tendency toward lowered S.D.A. in obese persons, particularly those identified as hypopituitary in type. Lauter,[45] Strang and McClugage[46] and others have been unable to confirm the demonstration of a lowered S.D.A. in obese persons. Johnston,[47] in a series of studies upon patients with definite destructive pituitary lesions, found the S.D.A. within normal limits. Protein is responsible for the greatest part of the specific dynamic action of food. Dock[48] concluded that at least 80 per cent of the effect is due to the increased heat produced by the hepatic cells during metabolic changes in protein.

While the view generally accepted at present denies that a difference in the specific heat response to food has an important role in the pathogenesis of obesity, it is difficult to reconcile Plaut's positive observations and the confirmatory results of Kestner, Knipping, Liebesny and others with the negative results of later workers. MacBryde[49] reported studies indicating that the *nutritional state* might not be accompanied regularly by an alteration in the S.D.A., but that the *nutritional phase* might be accompanied by alterations in the S.D.A. During periods of weight gain, obese, normal and thin subjects had lower specific dynamic effects from a standard mixed test meal than the same subjects receiving the same meal exhibited in periods of induced weight loss. It is conceivable that heat production dependent upon liver metabolism may vary according to the disposal of amino acids, fatty acids, glucose and other products of digestion reaching the hepatic cells. During periods of storage, heat production might be low, while during periods of active utilization the specific dynamic action might be relatively high. Failure of previous workers to take into account the *phase* of nutrition, while considering the nutritional *state* only, could well account for the divergent results recorded by a number of excellent investigators. From this standpoint it is evident that one could not expect to reveal a mechanism resulting in gain of weight if the studies were done upon obese subjects actively losing weight.

It seems, therefore, that the subject of the specific dynamic action of food is not yet closed. Further studies will be necessary to determine whether other workers can confirm the author's observations that the S.D.A. may be decreased in any subject actively storing, rather than burning, a large proportion of the products of digestion.

"LUXUSKONSUMPTION." When inadequate amounts of food are taken, the basal metabolic rate may be lowered. The body possesses a means by which the combustion of body-tissue stores is retarded during severe undernutrition. Thus, in the cachexia resulting from severe anorexia nervosa, the basal metabolic rate may reach levels of minus 30 per cent, which adds to the difficulty of distinguishing such cases from Simmonds' disease. When feeding is restored toward normal, the basal metabolic rate returns toward normal values. Grafe[50] carried this concept further by postulating that in addition to the metabolic stimuli of activity and the specific dynamic action of food, the total metabolism is determined by the food intake. Excess feeding, according to this theory, could stimulate heat production so that the surplus caloric intake would automatically be dissipated. Obesity would result from a defect in this mechanism, while thinness would develop when the luxus consumption response was too great.

It is difficult to accept these views, since they include the concept that the basal metabolic rate depends primarily upon the previous food intake. Although the basal metabolism may be altered by starvation, it has not been demonstrated that it can be elevated above normal by forced feeding. Normal human beings, as well as all mammals in the basal state, produce heat in proportion to the body-surface area without regard to previously ingested food. Wiley and Newburgh[51] showed that the surface area increases and weight is gained during superalimentation. The basal metabolic rate rises and the total caloric output increases, but the heat production still is in proportion to the surface area. It therefore seems unlikely that a rise in total metabolism prevents obesity in patients who overeat.

TOTAL METABOLISM. Numerous studies have shown that weight changes can be predicted on any diet when all metabolic factors are considered. The total metabolism of obese persons is necessarily greater than that of normal persons of the same height, age and sex. This has been shown in several ways: (1) The surface area of obese persons is greater, but the basal metabolic rate per unit of surface area is the same; therefore, the total basal heat production is greater. (2) A large proportion of the body tissue of corpulent subjects is inactive, fatty, and produces relatively little heat or energy. Therefore, to maintain the same basal metabolic rate per unit of surface area, the *active* tissues of obese persons must have a higher than normal metabolic rate. (3) Obese subjects expend more energy in performing a given amount of work; therefore, the caloric requirement is greater (Lauter[52]). (4) More work to perform a given task is necessary not only by the skeletal muscles but by the heart muscle. Cardiac work at rest may be decreased by as much as 35 per cent by weight reduction in the obese.[53] Part of the fall in total metabolism induced by weight reduction results from decreased cardiac work.

From these facts one can see that obese persons not only cannot get along on less food without losing weight, but they require more food to maintain weight than do thin persons of the same height, age and sex.

However, careful observers have recorded a number of instances in which weight was maintained for considerable lengths of time upon greatly restricted diets. For two weeks, or even longer, Newburgh and his co-workers[11] found that certain obese persons lost no weight or even gained weight upon a very low caloric intake. Diuresis then occurred, so that at the end of approximately three weeks the weight loss was just that calculated from the known caloric balance. The paradox of apparent failure to lose body fat is explained by temporary retention of water.

PHYSICAL ACTIVITY. Obese persons are significantly less active physically when compared to controls matched by age, sex, etc.[108,109] In one such study, obese women walked an average of 2.0 miles per day, nonobese women, 4.9 miles; obese men 3.7 miles, nonobese men 6.0 miles.[108] Obese children engaged in school games and sports only about one-third as much as nonobese children.[109]

In many moderate or early cases of obesity, especially if physical inactivity is an obvious factor, increased exercise may lead to weight loss and better weight control.

From such observations it is tempting to conclude that relative physical inactivity may be a primary factor in the etiology of the majority of cases of obesity.

However, certain considerations cast doubt upon such a sweeping generalization concerning the pathophysiology of most cases of obesity:

1. Obese persons consume more energy for the performance of each item of activity, every breath, every heartbeat, every step. The total metabolism, even with the lessened physical activity, was not significantly lower in 25 obese men.[108] Indeed in 13 of the 25 obese men the calculated total expenditure exceeded that of nonobese controls. Among obese women there was a calculated lower than normal total energy expenditure, as well as lower physical activity.

2. The fact that an obese person expends more energy even when "at rest" may account for his tendency to decrease overt physical exercise: therefore inactivity may result from obesity and may perhaps not be a cause of the obesity.

Nevertheless, the role played by physical inactivity has been unduly minimized in recent years. In our nation children as well as adults are more sedentary than in former generations, ride more, walk less—and are more often obese. It is probable that these facts are inter-related. Sitting requires 60 calories per hour, walking 300, swimming 500, running 900. Obviously a person who is sedentary and eats only average amounts may gain weight. If he is sedentary and eats excessively, he is apt to become obese.

Endocrine Glands. The *distribution* of body fat is largely under the control of the glands of internal secretion. The simplest example of this influence is the difference between typical female adiposity and that occurring in males (Fig. 196). Women tend to deposit the excess fat chiefly in the region of the hips, the thighs and the buttocks, and sometimes in the mammary region, while in men the protuberant abdomen or "bay-window" distribution is characteristic. In Cushing's syndrome, one finds obesity of the face, the neck and the trunk, while the extremities lose subcutaneous fat (Fig. 197). Virilizing tumors of the ovary or adrenal cortex may cause a normal woman to lose the rounded feminine curves of arms, legs, hips, breasts and shoulders, and to assume the angular aspects of the male. Although the distribution of body fat may depend greatly upon the endocrine makeup of the subject, the development of the obesity seldom can be attributed primarily to an endocrine disorder.

PITUITARY DISEASE. Following the report of Fröhlich[54] in 1901, in which he described an obese hypogonadal boy with a pituitary tumor, inadequate hypophysial activity was considered a cause of obesity. Cushing[55] and other workers strengthened this impression when they described obesity following hypophysectomy in animals. Smith,[56] how-

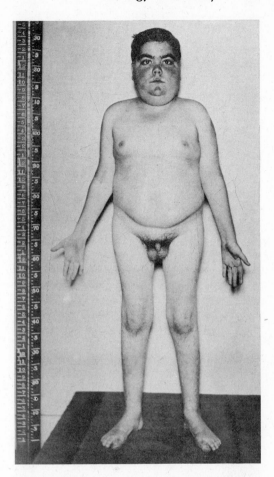

FIG. 197. Cushing's syndrome in a 12-year-old boy. Rubicund, plethoric face; obesity confined to face and trunk.

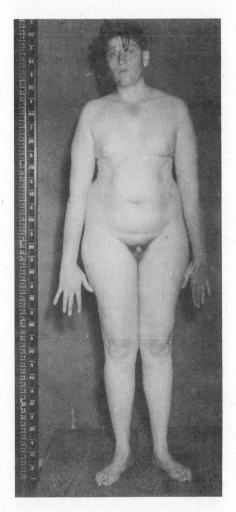

FIG. 196. A 24-year-old eunuchoid male with feminine distribution of fat: over breasts, hips, trochanteric regions and thighs.

ever, demonstrated that obesity occurred only when the *hypothalamus* was injured, and not following destruction or removal of the pituitary alone.

In the earlier clinical observations and also in the experimental work the role of the pituitary was overemphasized; later, when the importance of the hypothalamus was discovered, the part played by the pituitary in the pathogenesis of obesity was too strictly minimized. Both clinical and experimental evidence suggest that (1) damage either to the pituitary or to the hypothalamus separately may cause physiologic aberrations which tend to produce obesity and (2) normally the pituitary and the hypothalamus are integrated functionally through neural and humoral connections—

thus damage to either produces changes in the other, of which obesity is a frequent consequence. As Cushing[55,57] observed, obesity commonly occurs in chromophobe adenomata which are entirely intrasellar, but the obesity is greater if there is pressure on the hypothalamus. Heinbecker *et al.*[58] found that hypothalamic lesions produced greater and quicker adiposity, but that hypophysectomy per se produced less striking weight gain. Reinecke *et al.*[59] found that hypophysectomy led to increased fat content in the rat carcass.

Clinically, as experimentally, destruction of the pituitary alone does not result in obesity, but in pituitary cachexia (Simmonds' disease). Although patients who exhibit signs of hypopituitarism and obesity are frequently encountered, in the great majority of cases it seems that the endocrine disorder is not the cause of the obesity but an associated phenomenon.

The clinical diagnosis of "pituitary obesity," formerly popular, is fortunately disappearing. A preferable term is *neuro-hypophysial obesity,* if there is evidence that the hypothalamus and the pituitary are involved. The term *Fröhlich's syndrome* should be reserved for cases in which there is a known organic lesion of the pituitary-hypothalamic area with hypogonadism and obesity. The report of Fröhlich

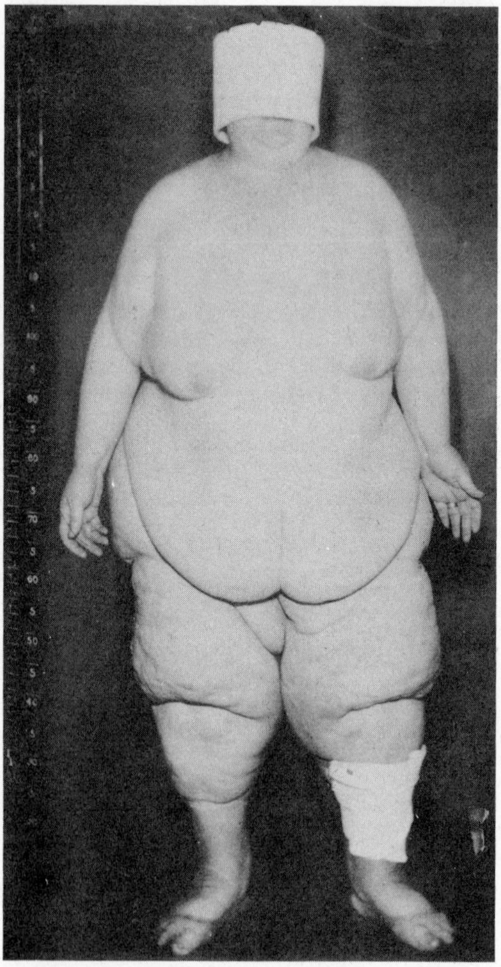

FIG. 198. Generalized, nodular, painful obesity sometimes called adiposis dolorosa or Dercum's disease.

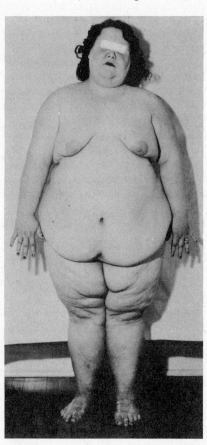

FIG. 199. Adiposogenital dystrophy in a 25-year-old woman. Notice the delicate facial features, the small hands and feet. There was only a small amount of breast tissue present, and menstruation was infrequent and scant.

in 1901 was significant because it first related pathogenically an expanding pituitary tumor with neighborhood pressure symptoms to the obesity and genital hypoplasia exhibited by the 14-year-old male subject. *Adiposogenital dystrophy* is a useful descriptive name without diagnostic implications (Fig. 199). The fact that genital dystrophy accompanies the obesity may indicate that certain pathways influencing the function of the anterior pituitary may be damaged.

HYPERADRENOCORTICISM. Grafting of ACTH-secreting tumors in animals causes obesity.[109]

In hyperadrenocorticism, whether primarily due to adrenocortical hyperplasia or tumor, to pituitary-hypothalamic disorder, or to steroid administration, there is a profound alteration in metabolism of carbohydrate, protein and fat. The tissues lose protein, carbohydrate tolerance decreases, and fat deposits increase. The reason for the location of the excess fat in face, cervical hump and central areas (trunk), while extremities become spare, is unknown. It appears that the obesity of hyperadrenocorticism or Cushing's syndrome is unique, while the tissues are depleted of protein, fat is being deposited in excess.

In Cushing's syndrome there is a peculiar plethoric obesity confined chiefly to the head and the trunk. It is not likely that this syndrome is actually a pituitary disorder due, as originally thought, to a basophil pituitary adenoma. In many cases no such adenoma is present, and the syndrome seems to merge imperceptibly into that associated with adrenocortical hyperplasia or adrenocortical tumors. The cytoplasmic hyalinization and other changes in the pituitary basophil cells described by Crooke have apparently been found in all cases when sought. Three chief hypotheses have been offered to account for the pathogenesis of Cushing's syndrome: (1) Pituitary basophilism, either with Crooke's changes, a basophil tumor, or both, causes excess production of an adrenocorticotrophic hormone; the adrenal cortices then become hyperplastic or neoplastic and an excess production of adrenocortical hormones produces the manifestations of the disease.

Some of the dysfunctions of other endocrine glands may result from the primary pituitary malfunction, some from the adrenocortical hyperfunction. Heinbecker[60] has modified this concept and presents evidence that the primary disturbance is in the hypothalamus. (2) The second hypothesis states that for unknown reasons the primary disturbance arises in the adrenal cortices, with malfunction or hyperfunction expressed anatomically as hyperplasia or neoplasia. The cytologic changes in the pituitary are regarded as retrograde or degenerative in nature. (3) The third hypothesis assumes a dual etiologic process: either the pituitary or the adrenal cortex may be the primary site.

HYPOTHYROIDISM. Evidence against hypothyroidism as the usual cause of obesity has already been cited under consideration of the basal metabolic rate. Obese persons as a rule do not have the dry skin, the slow mental processes, the thin coarse hair, the hoarse voice and other accompaniments of thyroid inactivity. Myxedema is not regularly accompanied by obesity, and overweight in these patients is usually due to abnormal water retention in the body, as demonstrated by Plummer.[61]

DIABETES MELLITUS; HYPERINSULINISM. The clinical and statistical observations that diabetes is not very frequent among obese persons, but that obesity is present in a high percentage (about 40 per cent) of diabetics at the onset of the disease would seem to hold a clue: probably obesity does not "predispose to diabetes" as is so often said, but both conditions may arise from a common cause. It is probably no more accurate to think that obesity leads to diabetes than to believe that diabetes leads to obesity: neither causes the other, but both may be manifestations of the same basic endocrine and metabolic disorders.

Consideration of the interlocking pathologic physiology of the two closely related metabolic disorders, obesity and diabetes, requires a review of certain information:

1. The relative rates of lipolysis and lipogenesis depend upon the rate of glucose utilization. When glucose utilization is deficient, lipolysis exceeds lipogenesis, as in starvation, untreated diabetes, etc. When

there is excess insulin and excess glucose utilization, fat formation in adipose tissue is accelerated and obesity may result.

2. Many obese diabetics have been shown to have normal or hypernormal plasma insulin levels: it would seem that certain tissues (? muscle) are refractory to insulin action, but adipose tissue is not, in such obese persons. Gundersen's observations[110] would support such a concept: protein-bound insulin of serum failed to stimulate glucose uptake by rat diaphragm; adipose tissue, however, contains an enzyme that frees the insulin. Such a situation might explain the concomitant development of diabetes and obesity: obese subjects may have difficulty in freeing insulin for non-adipose tissue and thus may have insufficient insulin action on muscle but increased insulin action in fat depots, promoting fat formation from glucose and facilitating fat storage.

3. Certain observations in many obese persons indicate hyperadrenocorticism in obesity: (a) hirsutism, amenorrhea, hypertension, colored abdominal striae, increased 17-OH and 17-KS steroid excretion (Simkin);[111] (b) decreased glucose tolerance, increased resistance to insulin, increased incidence of diabetes.

4. Insulin may be produced in excess, both because of increased food intake and because of relative insulin refractoriness of certain tissues. The excess insulin may promote accelerated lipogenesis. A number of the same biochemical reactions operate both in the adrenal cortex and in adipose tissues. Insulin produces an increase in lipids and enlargement of each. Insulin, especially in large amounts, increases adrenal glucosteroid production; these steroids in turn play an important role in stimulating increased production of insulin antagonists. A cycle may thus be set up characterized by obesity, functional hyperinsulinism (with or without diabetes) and functional hyperadrenocorticism. If the stresses thus set up are severe enough, or persist long enough, permanent insulin-deficiency diabetes may result from exhaustion of the β cells of the islets of Langerhans.

5. Weight loss, induced by simple restriction of caloric intake, can reverse these processes, at least in the early stages. Obesity may disappear, glucose tolerance return to normal, and excess corticosteroid production subside.[111] The concept is suggested that obesity is not only facilitated by certain endocrine aberrations, but that obesity *causes* certain endocrine disorders. The endocrine disorders may be reversible with abolition of the obesity. It is well recognized that obesity and diabetes are closely related. Joslin[62] among 1,063 diabetic patients found that in 40 per cent obesity preceded the onset of the diabetes. It is also known that patients with tumors of the islets of Langerhans often are driven to excess food intake by hypoglycemia and its associated intense hunger, and may become obese. There is a close relationship between hypoglycemia and the hunger mechanism. It seems possible that a mild degree of hypoglycemia, insufficient to produce symptoms, could be the cause of the desire for excess food. However, sugar-tolerance tests in obese persons do not give consistent results; they often show diabetic-type curves instead of flat or low curves. The work of Ogilvie, described below, may explain these apparent paradoxes. Patients who do show hypoglycemic types of sugar-tolerance curves are sometimes fat, but are usually average or lean, so that functional hyperinsulinism may in some cases, but certainly not in all, be cited as an adequate cause for production of obesity. Obesity has been produced in rats by protamine insulin injections.[63]

Ogilvie[64] observed that, particularly in the earlier stages of adiposity in human beings, the islands of Langerhans showed marked hypertrophy. Ogilvie's studies on glucose tolerance in obese subjects are interesting, and throw light upon the probable interrelationship of these facts connecting the pancreatic islets and obesity. In one-third of his patients sugar tolerance was increased in the early stages of obesity. With advancing age it seemed that the increased or normal tolerance gave way to decreased tolerance, and ultimately this became evident in a considerable proportion of cases as clinical diabetes mellitus. Overeating may therefore be primary, and the repeated ingestion of excessive amounts of carbohydrate may exert progressively greater demands upon the islets. A functional hyperinsulinism may result and obesity develop. In those persons whose islets cannot sustain the prolonged strain there is eventually islet-cell degeneration with production of diabetes mellitus. Subjects with a hereditary or constitutional tendency toward diabetes would thus be more apt to become diabetic as a consequence of obesity, which clinically is true and statistically is quite evident. When the islet cells have high integrity, obesity may develop and persist in consequence of chronic functional hypoglycemia.

McKay, Barnes and Carne[65] have demonstrated that young growing normal rats eat almost twice as many calories and deposit much more body fat when offered only carbohydrate food than they do when offered only protein.

The more recent observations of Schechter[102] and others seem to confirm the classic, older studies of Ogilvie: glucose tolerance was increased in the dynamic phase of obesity, decreased in the static phase.

The obese-hyperglycemic syndrome of mice seems also to represent an endocrine imbalance characterized by excessive secretion of insulin and glucagon by the islets of Langerhans.[109]

It has not yet been demonstrated how the hypothalamic injuries described below produce obesity. There is some evidence that hypothalamic injury causes hyperphagia and that hypothalamic disorders lead to relative hypoglycemia; perhaps three types of functional hypoglycemia may lead to excessive appetite, overeating, and thus to obesity: (1) hereditary or constitutional; (2) acquired through injuries, operations, encephalitis, etc.; (3) acquired through excessive carbohydrate ingestion.

The role of carbohydrate is closely bound with psychic factors in the production of obesity. The interplay between carbohydrate craving, psychic maladjustment and obesity produces a pattern often encountered clinically in various forms.

HYPOGONADISM. It is well known that in man and animals adiposity is apt to occur after removal of the gonads. The disposi-

tion is more placid and there is less tendency to muscular action. More fat is stored and less protein, and the muscles are less well developed. The basal metabolic rate usually falls by about 15 per cent. After the menopause, women exhibit these changes spontaneously, and similar, less evident, changes are found in men past middle life. Clinically, two common types of obesity are (1) that associated with hypogonadism in young women and (2) that which develops at middle age in both men and women. The presence of gonadal secretions in adequate amounts may at least in part account for the maintenance of normal weight in the average young and vigorous man or woman.

Role of the Hypothalamus and Higher Brain Centers. Recent observations[66,67] indicate that certain nuclei in the hypothalamus are essential parts, and perhaps the primary sites of the homeostatic mechanism which normally operates to match food intake to body needs. Stimulation of one of the laterally located pair of nuclei results in increase of food ingestion, whereas bilateral destruction of these nuclei results in rejection of food even to the extreme of starvation and death. A pair of medial nuclei seems to be opposite in function, for their destruction results in hyperphagia. The lateral nuclei seem to be related to hunger and facilitate the eating reflexes. The medial nuclei have been termed "satiety centers" and inhibit feeding reflexes. It is supposed that the feeding reflexes are affected by many neural connections of the hypothalamic centers with cortical, gustatory, olfactory, visual and other areas. The experimental observations have been so consistent in the many animal species that the general concept of lateral "food-drive" nuclei and medial "satiety centers" has been applied to man.

In the prefrontal area of the cerebral cortex a *higher center* has been demonstrated. In man, lesions of this region are not uncommonly associated with abnormal food intake, usually in the direction of *bulimia*. This center is connected through thalamic nuclei with the hypothalamus.

The early observations that patients with pituitary tumors frequently were obese and that operations upon the pituitaries of animals often resulted in adiposity led to the conclusion that pituitary deficiency causes obesity. Erdheim[68] as early as 1904, however, proposed that hypothalamic disorder might cause such obesity, since often at autopsy the pituitary was undamaged in cases of adiposogenital dystrophy, but evidence of extrasellar tumors or compression of the base of the brain was present. Camus, Roussy et al.[69] in a series of studies from 1913 to 1925 found that dogs with an intact hypophysis developed obesity and diabetes insipidus as a result of bilateral lesions of the tuber cinereum extending to a depth of 5 mm. in the direction of the paraventricular nuclei, and concluded that injury to the paraventricular nuclei caused the obesity. Smith's[56] observations on the rat in 1927 further established the importance of the hypothalamus in the pathogenesis of obesity: chromic acid injected into the hypothalamus caused obesity; hypophysectomy did not. Many subsequent workers showed that in this type of obesity, at least, the factors in the pathologic physiology are: a specific type of damage to the hypothalamus; this produces hyperphagia;[70] the hyperphagia results in a greater than normal rate of conversion of carbohydrates to fatty acids. A related observation of Gildea and Man[71] is that in certain patients with clinical evidence of hypothalamic dysfunction there are abnormally high blood levels of fatty acids and cholesterol. Hetherington and Ranson,[72] after a large amount of meticulous work, concluded that hypophysectomy, stalk destruction or destruction of the infundibular region in rats did not cause adiposity. Certain large bilateral symmetrical hypothalamic lesions not involving the hypophysis caused rats to become very obese. The presence of the pituitary or its absence did not influence the development of obesity so produced. Therefore, hypothalamic obesity cannot be explained by considering it to be caused indirectly by pituitary hormonal disturbance.

Heinbecker, White and Rolf[58] in work on dogs, observed that obesity results from bilateral destruction or retrograde degeneration of the paraventricular nuclei, and that hypophysectomy per se also leads to much more slowly developing, lesser degrees of adiposity, presumably due to deficiency of the pituitary tropic hormones. A role in the pathogenesis of obesity has thus been restored to the hypopituitary state by these workers—both in regard to deficiency of the adenohypophysis and of the posterior pituitary lobe (see below). They found that lesions of the posterior hypothalamus, caudal to the paraventricular nuclei, which interrupt fibers whose cell bodies originate in the caudal portions of the paraventricular nuclei (resulting in retrograde degeneration of these structures), resulted in obesity. Similar lesions that did not produce the retrograde degeneration with resultant diminution in the number of cells in the caudal portion of the paraventricular nuclei did not produce obesity. They also found that co-existing loss of cells of the supraoptic nuclei (producing diabetes insipidus) resulted in the development of a greater obesity (75 to 110 per cent gain in 6 months as compared with 50 per cent for the paraventricular nuclear lesion alone). These workers concluded that in the dog the specific lesion resulting in obesity was the paraventricular nuclear degeneration described, and that in the presence of such a lesion a simultaneous decrease in posterior pituitary secretion intensified the resulting obesity.

These observations indicate that (1) hypothalamic disorder is a potent factor in producing obesity, (2) pituitary lesions may play a part, and (3) adrenocortical functional alterations may also be a factor. These investigators postulate that fibers passing caudally from the paraventricular nuclei innervate cells within the brain stem. These cells (according to the hypothesis) secrete a hormone which influences the adrenal cortex or the basophil cells of the adenohypophysis, either or both of which are concerned with the abnormal deposition of fat. These workers and others have observed that production of posterior hypothalamic lesions or transection of the infundibular stalk has resulted in loss of the basophil cells of the adenohypophysis, with concomitant evidence of functional disorders of the adenohypophysis. Low and greatly fluctuating fasting blood glucose values were produced in the dogs operated upon by White, Heinbecker and Rolf,[73] and the unstable levels were considered to be the cause of the hyperphagia occurring after hypothalamic injury.

Brooks, Lambert and Bard[74] produced obesity in 6 out of 12 monkeys following experimentally produced hypothalamic lesions. Weight was more than doubled in mature monkeys in from 8 to 10 months, after which the weight remained relatively constant. In these studies, in contrast to those just cited, the presence of an associated diabetes insipidus had no influence on the obesity, nor did the presence or absence of hypogonadism. The total caloric intake of the obese monkeys was much greater than that of their nonobese controls.

Apparently the obesity caused by hypothalamic lesions is dependent upon the interruption of descending fibers that leave the ventromedial hypothalamic nuclei and normally descend toward the brain stem.

There have been some studies of the metabolism of animals in which obesity was experimentally produced by hypothalamic injuries. Brooks et al.[74] found a greatly increased caloric intake in the monkeys operated upon. Hetherington and Ranson[72] found that (1) all of the animals operated upon became much less active than their controls, and that (2) most of the animals ate a great deal more than their controls. Some of the animals became obese without eating more than their controls, which is probably explainable by the decreased activity.

Long and his associates[75] have made excellent studies of the metabolism in hypothalamic obesity. These may be summarized as follows: (1) Animals began to eat from two to three times as much per day as they did before the production of the lesions. (2) Obesity soon developed. (3) When given only as much food as the controls, only one out of 10 animals operated upon outgained its control. (4) Studies of the basal and the total oxygen consumption and of basal and postprandial respiratory quotients in paired-fed operated (nonobese) and obese operated rats showed no deviations from normal.

The conclusion of Long and his coworkers was that "the development of obesity is apparently a consequence of increased appetite, and is not associated with any fundamental disturbance in metabolism."

It seems clear that dysfunction of nervous elements that originate in or are mediated through certain nuclei of the hypothalamus may produce a great increase in appetite and in food intake so that obesity results. It is not yet clear how the nervous system regulates appetite, but it seems that the hunger mechanism is under control normally, whereas disease or destruction of certain nerve tracts releases hunger from the usual inhibitory regulation.

The nature of the change in blood constituents or tissue metabolism which acts upon the hypothalamic centers is not yet clear. Since the hypothalamus contains temperature-sensitive cells, it has been proposed by Strominger and Brobeck[76] that central action of the specific dynamic action of food might be the effective inhibitor of the feeding center. It is interesting to note that this concept fits well with the observations of MacBryde[49] who found in human beings, whether obese, normal or thin, that there was a decrease in the S.D.A. during the nutritional phase of gaining weight.

Another theory has been proposed by Mayer and Bates[77] in which the glucose available to the central nervous system is the effective mechanism. In experimental animals very small decreases in blood glucose resulted in increased feeding activity. The critical factor is considered to be the rate of glucose utilization by the tissues, thus the hyperphagia of diabetes despite hyperglycemia might result from the inability of the "glucostat" tissue to utilize the glucose in the absence of adequate insulin. It seems possible that inadequate glucose or phosphates or potassium might operate as the trigger mechanism to activate the lateral "feeding nuclei"; perhaps the medial "satiety nuclei" respond to adequate levels and terminate feeding activity.

The problem of the specific stimuli for the hypothalamic centers regulating food intake remains unresolved. However, direct evidence[78] confirms the concept that the feeding centers exhibit special sensitivity to the hunger state. In the rat these centers take up more radioactive glucose, phosphate, or carbonate in the starved than in the fed state. These centers are unique in this regard, since other contiguous hypothalamic areas showed greater uptake during feeding rather than during starvation.

Evidence of hypothalamic disturbance in obese human beings is probably afforded by the cases having diencephalic lesions in which the obesity was previously interpreted as due to pituitary disease. Epidemic encephalitis is frequently followed by the development of obesity. The hypothalamic lesions observed as the result of encephalitis resemble in many respects those known to cause experimental adiposity.

Influence of Heredity. Obesity occurs as a familial characteristic, as demonstrated by Fellows,[79] who found adiposity occurring ten times as often in the families of fat persons as in relatives of normal or lean subjects. When both parents were obese, Gurney[80] found an incidence of adiposity in the offspring of 73 per cent; when one parent was obese, an incidence of 40 per cent; and only 9 per cent when both parents were lean.

Another study[81] disclosed the following frequencies of obesity when both, one, or neither parent was overweight, respectively: 44 per cent, 25 per cent, and 5 per cent. Hypertension, coronary artery disease and diabetes were found to be closely interrelated with obesity, and all showed high familial incidence. The gradations in frequency of this group of disorders were consistent with Mendelian laws but did not correspond with values calculated on the basis of a simple dominant or recessive gene. Since the pathologic physiology of these disorders is known to be interrelated, the etiology is probably complex. Hereditary factors may be influenced by environmental means; this is seen most clearly when one among several siblings, all obese and the offspring of obese parents, learns to control his weight.

It is possible, of course, that family habits of eating instead of a hereditary factor may produce the known high familial incidence of obesity. However, in animals it is easily demonstrable that certain strains resist fattening, while others acquire adipos-ity readily. The observations of Danforth[82] prove that a gene carries the obese characteristic in certain mice. Yellow male mice were mated to females of various colors. Some of the descendants were yellow, while others were not. All litter mates were kept in the same cage and had the same food offered to them. At or subsequent to sexual maturity, the yellow mice gained weight more rapidly than their litter mates. This was especially true of the yellow females. A mendelian dominant gene carries the characters for yellowness and obesity; non-yellow mice of the same litter are not obese. In such obese animals the basal metabolic rate is said to be subnormal and the body temperature low; a hypothalamic hereditary origin of the obesity has been suggested. A hereditary obesity in mice accompanied by hyperglycemia has been described. Such animals spontaneously take a much greater amount of food than non-obese controls. Evidence therefore seems to favor the inheritance of the tendency to develop obesity.

Psychologic Factors. When it is considered that the majority of human beings maintain approximately normal body weight for many years, with relatively little variation, it is evident that food intake is usually well balanced with the caloric demands of the body. It must be supposed that *metabolic requirements regulate hunger and satiety,* so that as a rule people eat what they need and no more. As they get older and activity decreases, moderate degrees of adiposity are common. It seems likely that habits of eating continue beyond the necessity for them. Habit then becomes the regulator of food intake, and appetite becomes the servant of desire, and not of hunger. Appetite may result from the pleasant memories of the joy of eating. Appetite may be dulled or abolished by disturbed mental states, or stimulated by pleasant odors and tastes or by foods that are attractively colored or prepared.

The infrequency with which obesity can be attributed to organic disease, and the common occurrence of emotional disorders resulting in hyperphagia has properly received increasing recognition and emphasis. Reeve[83] found two groups, the first comprising the gaining of distant satisfactions wherein the symbolic value of the symptom, obesity, is paramount. Other students have recognized that the enlarged body may serve the patient as a fortresslike defense against a hostile world, or as a symbol of independence or prowess, or as a means to discourage suitors, to represent a wished-for pregnancy, or to mask emotions. Reeve's second group includes those values and immediate satisfactions gained in the incorporation process, such as the sensory pleasures of food ingestion.

Obese persons in one large study showed immaturity, suspiciousness and rigidity more often than nonobese persons.[113] The immaturity may be expressed in failure to resist impulses, among them the impulse to eat.

When satisfactions of other types are denied, the pleasures of eating may serve in their stead. One of life's genuine delights is open to practically everyone: eating. If social, business or sexual objectives are unattainable, food may serve not only as a defense and a solace but eventually as a substitute. Although obesity is the outcome, it may not be greatly feared, or may even be welcomed. Obesity can be used as an offensive weapon as well as a defensive one. One patient gloried in her corpulence as a means of punishing her wayward husband. Another preferred to remain obese, since she could not find employment because of her great size. A child who is an invalid, or who for any other reason is the object of excessive parental solicitude, is apt to become obese.

Hamburger[84] in an excellent review finds it useful to divide patients into four groups:

1. Overeating as a response to nonspecific emotional tensions.

2. Overeating as a substitute gratification in intolerable life situations.

3. Overeating as a symptom of an underlying emotional illness, especially depression and hysteria.

4. Overeating as an addiction to food.

Brosin[85] gives excellent discussion and reviews of the work in this field. He emphasizes that psychological disorders of appetite may take various forms, resulting in anorexia and weight loss, or hyperphagia and obesity. He wisely cautions against strenuous reducing programs which fail to take into account the basic psychological conflicts in severe cases. He advises doctors to work sensitively and at length with obese patients in middle life or later, pointing out that if one takes away smoking, alcohol and finally food from a person who has few other genuine satisfactions in life, one has the obligation to put something constructive in its place.

However, as Shelton[86] has stated, it is eminently true that all or nearly all obese persons, especially women and children, are unhappy and frustrated, but this may be the psychologic result of the obesity rather than the cause of it. Short boys, excessively tall girls, adolescents with acne, bald persons, hirsute women, disfigured persons, lame persons, etc., suffer from various degrees of inferiority, frustration and unhappiness, but there is no greater incidence of obesity in these groups. On the contrary, most of such unhappy states are apt to result in decreased appetite and weight loss, a common accompaniment of various neuroses, an extreme example being the so-called anorexia nervosa.

Since restriction of carbohydrate alone frequently breaks into the vicious circle of obesity caused by the carbohydrate habit, producing weight loss and improved psychic adjustment, it seems unlikely that the psychologic situation is always primary. Undoubtedly the physiologic abberation is often much more important, or of equal significance, in the etiology.

Habits of eating certain concentrated foods may be present in the absence of any deep-seated psychological abnormality. Habits of physical indolence are apparently more common in persons who become obese. Often re-education concerning diet and the establishment of new habits of diet and of exercise are sufficient to establish and maintain normal weight. Helpful in the development of new habits may be: anorexic drugs; attractive but bulky low-calorie foods (lean meat, fruits, vegetables); antacids; development of interest in sports and physical activities; encouragement and moral support and prolonged follow-up by the physician.

Addiction to food, as to alcohol, is often a symptom of an underlying psychologic maladjustment. Psychiatric study may be needed to disclose the hidden cause of the obesity, or a history taken carefully and sympathetically will yield the necessary clues. Among children, Bruch[87] found very few patients with endocrine factors of importance causing the obesity, but many children ate excessively in response to parental encouragement, or as a means of gaining attention.[112]

The habit of carbohydrate eating, with its resultant recurrent relative hypoglycemia, may be set up in the maladjusted individual who becomes obese, so that the psychic disturbance is thus associated with excessive activity of the islets of Langerhans. Shelton[86] suggested for this common type of corpulence the descriptive term *neuropancreatic obesity*, implying that there may be a functional or organic disorder operating through the hypothalamus associated with functional hyperinsulinism.

Social Factors. According to one study,[113] obesity is seven times as frequent among women of the lowest socioeconomic level as among those of the highest level, and among men the same relationship exists, although to a much lesser degree. The elements in the environment of etiologic significance are not clear: lack of education is believed to be important. When age and socioeconomic variables were held constant, statistically significant differences in 3 out of 9 measures of mental health were observed: obese persons scored more pathologic responses than nonobese controls in measures of immaturity, suspiciousness, and rigidity.

TREATMENT BASED ON ETIOLOGY

Whenever possible, weight reduction is accomplished by specific therapy based on reversing or relieving etiologic factors. This is relatively easy in rare cases only: for example in hypothyroidism, or when an islet tumor can be removed in hyperinsulinism. Since in the common types of obesity relatively obscure physiologic disorder of appetite control is present or there is a neurosis

of which obesity is only a part, treatment is difficult and often unsuccessful. It seems logical to attempt to decrease appetite at the same time a lower calorie diet is supplied. This is not easy, but clinically, high protein diets seem to have this effect.[88] Simple medical psychiatry is usually necessary, so provision of diet lists alone is inadequate. Often expert psychiatric study and treatment are indicated. Other methods of treatment, as well as those mentioned, are summarized in recent articles,[89,90] and include the use of drugs to inhibit appetite, bulky, low-calorie diets and regulated moderate exercise.

SUMMARY

Whatever the remote causes may be, obesity is always the result of food intake in excess of bodily needs. However, certain conditions may exist that may either (1) facilitate storage of fat when the caloric intake remains constant or (2) operate to raise the intake.

Among the etiologic factors considered, certain mechanisms do not seem tenable as possible explanations of the usual type of obesity. Among these are facilitated digestion or absorption, or lipophilia of the tissues. There is no generally accepted demonstration of abnormal utilization of energy. Endocrine abnormalities may cause a decrease in the basal metabolic rate (e.g., hypothyroidism, hypopituitarism or hypogonadism) and may result in decreased muscular activity, thereby causing a tendency to gain weight. Hyperinsulinism may cause an increased food intake. However, such endocrine abnormalities are infrequently encountered, while obesity is extremely common. Functional relative hypoglycemia seems to be seen fairly often and may lead to obesity. It occurs from overeating carbohydrate foods habitually. Hypothalamic disorders clearly may result in obesity. Whether they do so by increasing food intake or decreasing energy output, or both, is not clear. Evidently the increase in food intake is primary as the result of hypothalamic disorders, if the results of animal studies are applicable to human beings. Hypothalamic damage seems to remove the normal inhibitory controls from the hunger mechanism. It may be that there is a connection between relative functional hypoglycemia and hypothalamic disturbance. In some clinical, as well as in some experimental instances, hypoglycemia is a feature of hypothalamic disorder. Decreased basal metabolic rate and decreased muscular activity have been observed in some cases; perhaps these mechanisms also are operative in hypothalamic obesity. Heredity seems to play a definite role and may operate both by decreasing caloric outgo and by increasing the caloric intake. Psychologic factors most often operate to increase food intake, but may cause physical inactivity also. In any case in which obesity becomes pronounced, exercise becomes more and more of a hardship. Therefore, a decrease in energy output as muscular exercise is apt to be a consequence of corpulence, and will likewise contribute to its further development.

More than one factor is usually operative in each case. The brief case history given below is cited not because it is unusual but because similar problems are common; as an instance illustrating the concomitance of multiple etiologic influences it is a typical example.

A young woman, aged 25, came from an obese family. She had always been short, the nose and the mouth were dainty, the chin was small and pointed. The fingers tapered and the breasts were small. The menstrual periods were scanty and irregular. Her basal metabolic rate had always been low. However, her weight remained normal until she married and her husband left shortly thereafter for the Army. His allotment made it unnecessary for her to work. To console herself in his absence she lay around and read love-story magazines and ate huge quantities of ice cream and candy. She became obese rapidly, gaining 25 pounds in 3 months.

Here the groundwork was laid: a hereditary tendency toward obesity, a hypopituitary physique, moderate hypothyroidism. Yet obesity did not develop until (1) food intake increased and (2) energy output as muscular activity was greatly diminished. The precipitating factor was psychologic: her sexual desires and other drives usually expressed in bearing and rearing children, establishing a home, etc., were frustrated; they were sublimated into eating and reading.

Each case of obesity, therefore, deserves careful study. Proper treatment will be evident when the etiologic factors are discovered.

REFERENCES

1. Shelton, E. K.: Optimal weight estimation; the method of Willoughby, Endocrinology 16:492, 1932.
2. Behnke, A. R., Jr., Feen, B. G., and Welham, W. C.: The specific gravity of healthy men; body weight ÷ volume as an index of obesity, J.A.M.A. 118:495-498, 1942.
3. Keys, A.: Obesity measurement and the composition of the body, Proceedings No. 6, Nutrition Symposium Series, National Vitamin Foundation, New York, 1953.
4. Dublin, L. I., and Lotka, A. J.: Length of Life, New York, Ronald, 1936.
   Armstrong, D. B., Dublin, L. I., Wheatley, G. M., and Marks, H. H.: Obesity and its relation to health and disease, J.A.M.A. 147:1007, 1951.
   Dublin, L. I., and Marks, H. H.: Mortality among insurance overweights in recent years, Tr. A. Assoc. Life Insur. M. Dir. America, Oct. 11-12, 1951.
5. Barr, D. P.: Obesity, Red Light of Health, Proceedings No. 6, Nutrition Symposium Series, National Vitamin Foundation, New York, 1953.
6. Rynearson, E. H., and Gastineau, C. F.: Obesity, Springfield, Ill., Thomas, 1949.
7. Smith, H. L., and Willius, F. A.: Adiposity of the heart; a clinical and pathologic study of one hundred and thirty-six obese patients, Arch. Int. Med. 52:911-931, 1933.
   Willius, F. A.: Discussion, J.A.M.A. 101:424, 1933.
8. Prodger, S. H., and Dennig, H.: A study of the circulation in obesity, J. Clin. Investigation 11:789-806, 1932.
9. Kerr, W. J., and Lagen, J. B.: The postural syndrome related to obesity leading to postural emphysema and cardiorespiratory failure, Ann. Int. Med. 10:569-595, 1936.
10. Short, J. J., and Johnson, H. J.: The effect of overweight on vital capacity, Proc. Life Ext. Exam. 1:36-41, 1939.
11. Newburgh, L. H., and Johnston, M. W.: The nature of obesity, J. Clin. Investigation 8:197-213, 1930.
    Wiley, F. H., and Newburgh, L. H.: The doubtful nature of "Luxuskonsumption," J. Clin. Investigation 10:733-744, 1931.
    Newburgh, L. H.: The cause of obesity, J.A.M.A. 97:1659-1661, 1931.

————: Obesity, Arch. Int. Med. 70:1033-1096, 1942.

12. Thompson, K. J.: Some observations on the development and course of hypertensive vascular disease. Proc. 38th Ann. Meeting, Medical Section, American Life Convention, White Sulphur Springs, 1950.

13. Master, A. M., Dublin, L. I., and Marks, H. H.: The normal blood pressure range and its clinical implications, J.A.M.A. 143:1464, 1950.

14. Levy, R. L., White, P. D., Stroud, W. D., and Hillman, C. C.: Overweight. Its prognostic significance in relation to hypertension and cardiovascular-renal disease, J.A.M.A. 131:951, 1946.

15. Wilens, A. L.: Bearing of general nutritional state on atherosclerosis, Arch. Int. Med. 79:129, 1947.

16. Keys, A.: Symposium on Nutrition, Univ. of Buffalo Med. School, Dec. 12, 1953.

17. Walker, W. J., Lawry, E. Y., Love, D. E., Levine, S. A., and Stare, F. J.: Effect of weight reduction and caloric balance on serum lipoprotein and cholesterol levels, Am. J. Med. 14:654-664, 1953.

18. Gofman, J. W., and Jones, H. B.: Obesity, fat metabolism and cardiovascular disease, Circulation 5:504, 1952.

19. Zelman, S.: The liver in obesity, A.M.A. Arch. Int. Med. 90:141-156, 1952.

20. Hertig, A. T., and Sommers, S. C.: Cancer 2:946, 1949.

21. Hildreth, R. C.: J. Michigan Med. Soc. 49:1175, 1950.

22. Dole, V. P., et al.: The caloric value of labile body tissue in obese subjects, J. Clin. Invest. 34:590, 1955.

23. Werthliner, E., and Shapiro, B.: The physiology of adipose tissue, Physiol. Rev. 28:451, 1948.

24. Lipmann, F.: Biosynthetic mechanisms, Harvey Lecture 44:99, 1948-49.

25. Lipmann, F.: Fat metabolism, in Najjar, V. (ed.): A Symposium on the Clinical and Biochemical Aspects of Fat Utilization in Health and Disease, Baltimore, Johns Hopkins Press, 1954.

26. Parson, W., and Crispell, K. R.: Obesity, Disease-a-Month Series, Chicago, Yr. Bk. Pub., February 1956.

27. Neuenschwander-Lemmer, N.: Ueber Ausnutzungsversuche bei fettsüchtigen und normalen Menschen, Ztschr. f. d. ges. exper. Med. 99:395, 1936.

28. Strang, J. M., McClugage, H. B., and Brownlee, M. A.: Arch. Int. Med. 55:958, 1935.

29. Von Bergmann, G.: Oppenheimer's Handbuch der Biochemie 4:212, 1910.

30. Hetenyi, G.: Untersuchungen über die Enstehung der Fettsucht, Deutsches Arch. f. klin. Med. 179:134-141, 1936.

31. Jansen, W. H.: Deutsches Arch. f. klin. Med. 124:1, 1917.

32. Benedict, cited by G. Lusk: Physiol. Rev. 1:523, 1921.

33. Keeton, R. W., and Dickson, D.: Excretion of nitrogen by obese patients on diets low in calories, containing varying amounts of protein, Arch. Int. Med. 51:890-902, 1933.

34. Strang, J. M., McClugage, H. B., and Evans, F. A.: The nitrogen balance during correction of obesity, Am. J. M. Sc. 181:336-349, 1931.

35. Block, M.: Role of lipophilia in the etiology of obesity, Proc. Soc. Exper. Biol. & Med. 49:496-499, 1942.

36. Salcedo, J., and Stetten, D.: Turnover of Fatty Acids in Congenitally Obese Mouse, J. Biol. Chem. 151:413, 1943.

37. Guggenheim, K., and Mayer, J.: Studies of pyruvate and acetate metabolism in the hereditary obese-diabetes syndrome of mice, J. Biol. Chem. 198:259, 1952.

38. Mankin, H., Stevenson, J., Brobeck, J., Long, C., and Stetten, D.: The turnover of body fat in obesity resulting from hypothalamus injury studied with aid of deuterium, Endocrinology 47:443, 1950.

39. van Leeuwen, H. C.: Ztschr. f. klin. Med. 123:534, 1933.

40. Nassauer-Badt, A.: Ueber partiellen symmetrischen infantilen Fettschwund und sein familiaren Vorkommen, Inaugural dissertation, Frankfurt, 1929.

40a. Barr, D. P.: The pathogenesis of obesity and lipodystrophy, New Internat. Clin. 3:135, 1941.

41. Boothby, W. M., and Sandiford, I.: Summary of the basal metabolism data on 8,614 subjects with especial reference to the normal standards for the estimation of the basal metabolic rate, J. Biol. Chem. 54:783-803, 1922.

42. Strouse, S., Wang, C. C., and Dye, M.: Studies on the metabolism of obesity. II. Basal metabolism, Arch. Int. Med. 34:275-281, 1924.

43. Grafe, E.: Metabolic Diseases and Their Treatment (translated by M. G. Boise), Philadelphia, Lea, 1933.

44. Plaut, R.: Deutsches Arch. f. klin. Med. 142:266, 1923.

45. Lauter, S.: Zur Genese der Fettsucht, Deutsches Arch. f. klin. Med. 150:315-365, 1926.

46. Strang, J. M., and McClugage, H. B.: Am. J. M. Sc. 182:49, 1931.

47. Johnston, M. W.: J. Clin. Investigation 11:437, 1932.

48. Dock, W.: Am. J. Physiol. 97:117, 1931.

49. MacBryde, C. M.: The specific dynamic action of a mixed meal and its relation to obesity, J.A.M.A. 108:589, 1937.

50. Grafe, E., and Graham, D.: Ueber die Anpassungsfähigkeit des tierischen organismus an überreichliche Nahrungszufuhr, Ztschr. f. physiol. Chem. 73:1-67, 1911.

——— and Koch, R.: Deutsches Arch. f. klin. Med. 106:564, 1912.

51. Wiley, F. H., and Newburgh, L. H.: The doubtful nature of "Luxuskonsumption," J. Clin. Investigation 10:733-744, 1931.

52. Lauter, S.: Klin. Wchnschr. 5:1695, 1926.

53. Master, A. M., Stricker, J., Grishman, A., and Dack, S.: Effect of undernutrition on cardiac output and cardiac work in overweight subjects, Arch. Int. Med. 69:1010-1018, 1942.

54. Fröhlich, A.: Ein Fall von Tumor der Hypophysis Cerebri ohne Akromegalie, Wien. klin. Rundschau 15:883-886; 906-908, 1901.

55. Cushing, H.: The Pituitary Body and Its Disorders, Philadelphia, Lippincott, 1912.

56. Smith, P. E.: Harvey Lectures, 1929-30, Baltimore, Williams & Wilkins.

57. Cushing. H.: Neurohypophysial mechanisms from the clinical standpoint (Lister Memorial Lecture), Lancet 2:119, 175, 1930.

———: Papers Relating to the Pituitary Body, Hypothalamus and Parasympathetic Nervous System, Springfield, Ill., Thomas, 1932.

58. Heinbecker, P., White, H. L., and Rolf, D.: Experimental obesity in the dog, Am. J. Physiol. 141:549-565, 1944.

59. Reinecke, R. M., Samuels, L. T., and Bauman, K. L.: Growth and metabolism of young hypophysectomized rats fed by stomach tube, Endocrinology 33:87-95, 1943.

60. Heinbecker, P.: The pathogenesis of Cushing's syndrome, Medicine 23:225-247, 1944.

61. Plummer, W. A.: Body weights in spontaneous myxedema, Tr. Am. A. Study Goiter, p. 88-98, 1940.

62. Joslin, E. P.: J.A.M.A. 76:79, 1921.

63. MacKay, E. M., and Callaway, J. W.: Proc. Soc. Exper. Biol. & Med. 36:406, 1937.

64. Ogilvie, R. F.: Sugar tolerance in obese subjects: a review of sixty-five cases, Quart. J. Med. 4:345-358, 1935.

65. MacKay, E. M., Barnes, R., and Carne, H. O.: Influence of diet with high protein content upon appetite and deposition of fat, Am. J. Physiol. 135:187-192, 1941.

66. Anand, B. K., and Brobeck, J. R.: Hypothalamic control of food intake in rats and cats, Yale J. Biol. & Med. 24:123, 1951.

67. Anand, B. K., Dua, S., and Schoenberg, K.: Hypothalamic control of food intake in cats and monkeys, J. Physiol. 127:143, 1955.

68. Erdheim, J.: Ueber Hypophysengangsgeschwülste und Hirncholesteatome, Sitzungsb. d. k. Akad. d. Wissensch. Math.-naturw. Wien 113:537, 1904.

69. Camus, J., and Roussy, G.: Pituitary syndromes, Rev. Neurol. 38:622-639, 1922.

70. Brobeck, J. R., Tepperman, J., and Long, C. N. H.: Experimental hypothalamic hyperphagia in the albino rat, Yale J. Biol. & Med. 15:831-853, 1943.

71. Gildea, E. F., and Man, E. B.: The hypothalamus and fat metabolism, A. Research Nerv. and Ment. Dis., Proc. (1939) 20:436-448, 1940.

72. Hetherington, A. W., and Ranson, S. W.: J. Comp. Neurol. 76:475, 1942; Endocrinology 31:30, 1942.

73. White, H. L., Heinbecker, P., and Rolf, D.: Effects of removal of anterior lobe of hypophysis on some renal functions, Am. J. Physiol. 136:584-591, 1942.

74. Brooks, C., Lambert, E. F., and Bard, P.: Fed. Proc. 1, Part 2, p. 11, 1942.

75. Long, C. N. H., Brobeck, J. R., and Tepperman, J.: Endocrinology 30:1035, 1942.

76. Brobeck, J. R.: Physiology of appetite, Proceedings No. 6, Nutrition Symposium Series, National Vitamin Foundation, New York, 1953.

77. Mayer, J., and Bates, M. W.: Blood glucose and food intake in normal and hypophysectomized, alloxan-treated rats, Am. J. Physiol. 168:812, 1952.

78. Larsson, S.: On the hypothalamic organisation of the nervous mechanism regulating food intake, Acta physiol. scandinav. 32: Supp. 115, 1954.

79. Fellows, H. H.: Studies of relatively normal obese individuals during and after dietary restrictions, Am. J. M. Sc. 181:301-312, 1931.

80. Gurney, R.: Arch. Int. Med. 57:557, 1936.

81. Thomas, C. B., and Cohen, B. H.: Familial occurrence of hypertension, coronary artery disease, obesity and diabetes, A.M.A. Ann. Int. Med. 42:90-127, 1955.

82. Danforth, C. H.: Hereditary adiposity in mice, J. Heredity 18:153-162, 1927.

83. Reeve, G. H.: Psychological factors in obes-

ity, Am. J. Orthopsychiat. 12:674-679, 1942.

84. Hamburger, W. W.: Emotional aspects of obesity, Med. Clin. North America 35:483-499, 1951.

85. Brosin, H. W.: The psychology of overeating, Proceedings No. 6, Nutrition Symposium Series, National Vitamin Foundation, New York, 1953.
————: Psychiatric aspects of obesity, J.A.M.A. 155:1238, 1954.

86. Shelton, E. K.: The role of carbohydrate in the production of obesity (presidential address, Association for the Study of Internal Secretions, 1944).

87. Bruch, H.: Psychiatric aspects of obesity in children, Am. J. Psychiat. 99:752-757, 1943.

88. Fryer, J. H., et al.: A study of the interrelationship of the energy-yielding nutrients, blood glucose levels and subjective appetite in man, J. Lab. and Clin. Med. 45:684, 1955.

89. MacBryde, C. M.: Treatment of Obesity, in Conn, H. F., ed.: Current Therapy, Philadelphia, Saunders, 1962.

90. MacBryde, C. M.: Obesity, in Cecil & Loeb, eds.: Textbook of Medicine, ed. 10, Philadelphia, Saunders, 1959.

91. Fadell, E. J., et al.: Fatty infiltration of respiratory muscles in the pickwickian syndrome, New England J. Med. 266:861-863 (April 26) 1962.

92. Said, S. I.: Abnormalities of pulmonary gas exchange in obesity, Ann. Int. Med. 53:1121, 1960.

93. Albrink, M. J.: Lipoprotein pattern as a function of total triglyceride of serum, J. Clin. Invest. 40:536, 1961.

94. Seller, R. H., et al.: Use of I^{131} in study of lipid in coronary artery disease, Am. J. Med. 27:231, 1959.

95. Dublin, L., and Marks, H.: Reduction in predicted mortality following weight reduction in obese persons, Proceedings No. 6, Nutrition Symposium Series, National Vitamin Foundation, p. 106-116, New York, 1953.

96. Kinsell, L.: Diets low in cholesterol and high in polyunsaturated fats, in L. Kinsell, ed.: Adipose Tissue as an Organ, New York, Grune & Stratton, 1962.

97. Dayton, S., et al.: A controlled clinical trial of a diet high in unsaturated fat, New England J. Med. 266:1017-1023 (May 17) 1962.

98. Goldsmith, G. A.: Serum lipids and atherosclerosis, J.A.M.A. 176:783-790, 1961.

99. Central Committee for Medical and Community Program (American Heart Association): Circulation 23:133-136, 1961.

100. Council on Foods and Nutrition: The regulation of dietary fat, J.A.M.A. 181:411-429, 1962.

101. Ward, W., and Kelsey, W.: The Pickwickian syndrome. A review of the literature and report of a case, J. Pediat. 61:745-750, 1962.

102. Schechter, P.: Some metabolic characteristics of essential obesity, Am. J. Clin. Nutr. 10:433-442, 1962.

103. Naimark, A., and Cherniack, R. M.: Compliance of the respiratory system and its components in health and obesity, J. Appl. Physiol. 15:377, 1960.

104. Kaufman, B. J., Ferguson, M. H., and Cherniack, R. M.: Hypoventilation in obesity, J. Clin. Invest. 38:500, 1959.

105. Antoniades, H. N., and Gundersen, K.: Studies on the state of insulin in blood: dissociation of purified human blood insulin complexes by incubation with adipose tissue extracts in vitro, Endocrinology 68:36, 1961.

106. Garn, S. M., and Haskell, J. A.: Fat thickness and developmental status in childhood and adolescence, Am. J. Dis. Children, 99:746-751, 1960.

107. Nutrition Reviews 14:172, 229, 1956; 15:193, 1957; 19:36, 1961.

108. Chirico, A., and Stunkard, A. J.: Physical activity and human obesity, New England J. Med. 263:935-940, 1960.

109. Mayer, J.: Obesity: physiologic considerations, Am. J. Clin. Nutr. 9:530-537, 1961.

110. Gundersen, K., and Antoniades, H. N.: Biological activity of insulin complexes examined by rat diaphragm tissue assay, Proc. Soc. Exp. Biol. & Med. 104:411, 1960.

111. Simkin, B., and Arce, R.: Steroid excretion in obese patients with colored abdominal striae, New England J. Med. 266:1031-1035 (May 17) 1962.

112. Bruch, H.: The Importance of Overweight, New York, Norton, 1957.

113. Moore, M. E., Stunkard, A., and Srole, L.: Obesity, social class, and mental illness, J.A.M.A. 181:962-966, 1962.

33

Weight Loss and Undernutrition

CYRIL M. MACBRYDE

DEFINITIONS

Weight loss and undernutrition are physical conditions resulting from a negative nutritive balance; they occur when the output or consumption of one or more essential nutrients exceeds the supply.

Weight loss does not necessarily imply *malnutrition,* since if the nutritive defect is of calories only, other dietary essentials being supplied in adequate amounts, stored fats only may be lost, and that may even be desirable (as in obesity). Likewise, weight loss may indicate an improvement in the physical condition when excessive amounts of fluid are eliminated (as in edema).

Undernutrition may or may not be associated with *thinness* (subnormal body weight) and is therefore not to be considered simply the opposite of obesity. When thinness without any other nutritional defect is present, the problem is primarily caloric, due to inadequate intake of or interference with the absorption or storage of energy-supplying and fat-forming foods.

There are differences in the concepts of various authorities and in their definitions of thinness and undernutrition. Some have suggested that undernutrition is indicated by body weight ten per cent or more below the optimal; others[30] have considered true undernutrition to begin at the point when the small reserves of body protein are gone and body tissue protein is called upon to furnish calories.

Undernutrition. A broader definition is necessary for a proper concept of the problem and for good clinical practice. Let us define undernutrition as any deviation below good nutrition. Good nutrition is essential for normal growth; for normal development, maintenance and function of all body organs and tissues; for reproduction; for optimal working efficiency; for maximal resistance to infection, and for the ability to repair injury. Undernutrition exists whenever it can be demonstrated that a nutritive deficiency is responsible for subnormal response in any of these categories.

Usually undernutrition is not simple but complex, in the sense that there is not a deficiency of a single nutrient, but several deficiencies, and these are apt to be interrelated. The terms undernutrition or malnutrition imply that the negative nutritive balance has been of sufficient degree to endanger or impair body structure or function.

One or more specific types of undernutrition may occur in the presence of normal or excessive body fat. Obesity and various types of undernutrition may therefore coexist. Obesity itself is a type of *mal* (abnormal)-nutrition.

MEDICAL IMPORTANCE OF WEIGHT LOSS AND UNDERNUTRITION

When the body weight originally is near the optimum and neither excess fat nor excess fluid is present, weight loss that is progressive and not easily corrected is of great importance and its study may reveal serious disease.

In Chapters 2 and 32 tables of optimal or ideal weights for various heights and ages and for both sexes are given. Usually serious degrees of thinness are apparent upon inspection only, but the tables are useful in estimating the number of pounds variation from desirable levels. It must be kept in mind that the presence of excess fluid or fat may give apparently normal or high weights in some persons with malnutrition.

When the physician is confronted with a patient who gives a definite history of progressive weight loss or shows physical evidence of it, he must search for the cause of the negative caloric balance and also for other possible associated evidences of nutritional failure. Although statistically, people of normal or somewhat subnormal body weight live longer than obese persons, patients of optimal weight seem to live longest and to enjoy the best health. The physician must not encourage his patients to keep thin, for stored calories provide a safety factor in times of stress or disease. When fashion dictates a suboptimal weight for his patients, he should combat it and instruct in the methods of establishing the optimal weight and nutrition for each person.

States of undernourishment *without weight loss* may exhibit various evidences of *specific nature*. Such specific evidence of physical changes or functional derangement is often distinctive enough to indicate the etiology of the nutritive disorder. However, many persons consider themselves

relatively well, but suffer from various *ill-defined symptoms* many of which can be traced to malnutrition. A study of 610 male industrial workers[2] revealed that 158 (approximately 25 per cent) gave evidence of suboptimal nutrition, particularly with respect to thiamine, riboflavin, ascorbic acid, calcium and phosphorus. No cases of florid or acute deficiency diseases were seen, but suboptimal nutrition and obesity were widespread among all age, income, work and ethnic groups. Dietary faults frequently observed included inadequate consumption of milk and vitamin-C-rich fruits and vegetables, and excess intake of unenriched bread and pastries, sweetened beverages and candy.

Often thorough investigation reveals that the undernutrition is the primary condition, but frequently the nutritive defect may be the presenting abnormality that leads to the discovery of other disease conditions which caused the malnutrition.

The medical significance of the discovery of a nutritive defect has three aspects:

1. The cause of a primary nutritional disorder may be detected and often may be eliminated or corrected.

2. If the disturbed nutrition is found to be secondary to some other disorder, the latter may be diagnosed and properly treated.

3. Recognition of a nutritive defect *and* another disease condition usually directs proper attention to each and improves the prognosis of both, whether or not they are causally related. Restoration of nutrition to normal exerts a favorable influence on practically all disease conditions.

WEIGHT LOSS AND UNDERNUTRITION AS SYMPTOMS

The symptom of weight loss may not be emphasized by the patient, but unless there is an obvious explanation, it always should receive serious consideration by the physician. With or without weight loss, lack of energy, weakness and easy fatigue are usually associated symptoms of an inadequate supply of calories. When not only the energy principle (calories) but certain other essential nutrients are lacking, there may be a wide variety of symptoms, according to the specific food elements involved.

In the absence of weight loss or subnormal body weight, the evidences of undernutrition may be easily overlooked in the history or physical examination unless they happen to be striking. One of the primary purposes of this chapter is to describe the chief symptoms of malnutrition (of which weight loss is only one) and to discuss the mechanisms of their development. The protean symptomatic manifestations of nutritional deficiencies require constant alertness to permit their detection in early or mild stages. It is, of course, in these early stages that diagnosis is of the greatest importance, for by the time florid signs have appeared, correction may be difficult or irreparable damage may have been done. For example, after a compression fracture of an osteoporotic vertebra has occurred, the diagnosis of chronic protein deficiency plus prolonged calcium lack is important, but earlier diagnosis to prevent fractures is much preferable.

GROWTH: NUTRITIVE ASPECTS

During the early part of life, growth is the most striking characteristic of the organism—all the essential nutrients must be supplied in generous amounts for normal growth and development to take place. As maturity is reached, the necessity for a great positive balance of tissue-building elements ceases, and maintenance of tissues (with intake and expenditure equalized) is sufficient. Even structures usually considered as relatively static, such as the bones, actually have an active metabolism, losing and replacing constituents steadily. Therefore, the necessity for good nutrition does not end with the growth period. Optimum health and vigor require during the mature years not only calories for energy, but structural materials and chemical regulators of the metabolic machinery.

HORMONAL-NUTRITIONAL INTERRELATIONSHIPS
HORMONES → NUTRITION

These reciprocal relationships are important and complex. *Pituitary growth hormone* is anabolic, promoting nitrogen, phosphorus, potassium, sulfur and water storage in the proportions to form cells and protoplasm. *Androgens* have a similar effect, facilitating the incorporation of amino acids into protein. *Estrogens* have protein anabolic effect, but it is considerably less marked than that of androgens. Androgens promote calcium and phosphorus retention indirectly, their primary effect being upon the protein matrix of bone, thus laying the groundwork for calcification. The estrogens are thought to have a specific stimulating effect upon osteoblasts, and to have a greater effect upon Ca and P storage than androgens. Giving both of the two gonadal hormones has a greater effect upon bone formation than either alone.

The administration of *insulin* promotes protein and fat synthesis. In insulin lack, protein breakdown is increased and gluconeogenesis is required, both as a preliminary step in the oxidation of amino acids and as a way of forming oxaloacetate to facilitate the complete oxidation of fatty acids.

The effect of *thyroid hormone* is to increase the breakdown of protein. Patients with hyperthyroidism tend to be in negative balance for all the constituents of protoplasm.

The effect of the *adrenal cortical steroids* is to stimulate protein breakdown and gluconeogenesis; a diabetic state may result. Sodium retention by the renal tubules is facilitated, and urinary potassium loss is increased. The adrenocortical types of steroids now are employed so widely in therapeutics that it is imperative to be familiar with signs of overdosage (moon-face, edema, hypertension, glycosuria, etc.).

NUTRITION → ENDOCRINE GLANDS

In the preceding section, we have mentioned some of the chief effects of hormones on nutrition. There are also important effects of nutrition upon the endocrine glands. The synthesis of *pituitary hormones* is impaired in malnutrition, especially protein deficiency.[9] Microscopic examination of the anterior pituitary in malnourished persons has shown atrophy, and in some cases, degenerative lesions.[31] The *adrenal glands* in malnourished persons are small and exhibit lipid depletion. *Thyroid* hypo-activity results from lack of pituitary thyro-tropin. Decrease in *gonadal function* is among the earliest signs of malnutrition and is secondary to lack of pituitary gona-dotropin. Even when careful metabolic and endocrine laboratory studies are util-ized, it may be difficult to distinguish pri-mary pituitary failure from hypopituitar-ism secondary to malnutrition.[21a]

AGING AND MALNUTRITION

The processes of aging have important reciprocal interrelationships with nutrition: aging is apt to cause nutritive disorders; nutritive defects accelerate the degenerative changes usually associated with physiologic aging. Elderly persons suffer from mal-nourishment often because of the frequency with which economic, psychological and organic problems beset them. One must be on guard not to accept degenerative changes as the inevitable erosion of the years.[16,27] The nutritional status of aging persons is not dependent alone upon food, impaired digestion or absorption, etc., but also upon factors such as *stress*. In elderly persons cold, heat, emotional strain, etc., may be followed by nitrogen and other losses which may be cumulative and more difficult to replace than in younger people.[32]

Good nutrition slows and poor nutrition speeds the processes of physiologic aging. Various observations support this concept: in starvation (anorexia nervosa, etc.) the senile appearance of the subject is strik-ing; frequently nutritive failure in old age is mistaken for evidence of senescence it-self, but often great improvement in nutri-tion causes an apparent rejuvenation; catabolic processes (e.g., the osteoporosis of the spine in Cushing's syndrome) may closely simulate the changes associated with aging (senile osteoporosis), etc.

Loss of anabolic influences may cause body changes characteristic of advanced years even in the very young (e.g., progeria in certain dwarfs with pituitary failure). Loss of the anabolic influence of the sex hormones (estrogen, testosterone) may pro-duce fatigue, muscle atrophy, osteoporosis, fine wrinkling of the skin, loss of hair, etc.,

and other changes usually associated with aging. Proper use of sex hormones may greatly relieve signs of premature aging in hypogonadal persons.

CAUSE OF WEIGHT LOSS AND THINNESS

No matter how puzzling the picture may seem, there is (when hydration is normal) only a single cause of weight loss or sub-normal body weight: insufficient calories are being supplied to meet the metabolic needs. It may be true either that the actual number of *calories assimilated* by the body is inadequate or that the *caloric expendi-ture* is excessive, or both factors may be operative, but always there is a negative caloric balance or (in the case of failure to gain) an insufficiently positive balance.

It often seems that certain persons eat more than enough to gain weight but re-main thin, even when no metabolic dis-turbance is present and when absorption and assimilation are normal. Frequently there is a familial tendency to leanness, just as in some families obesity is common. The eating habits of families are, of course, important, and one may be able to demon-strate that certain families as a whole are "small eaters" or that the bulk of their diet is apparently great, but foods low in caloric value are consistently chosen instead of those high in caloric value.

Certain strains of animals tend to be thin, while others get fat, even when both receive the same diet, so that a hereditary predisposition to leanness seems evident. In human beings the evidence is less clear, but it also seems to favor inheritance in some cases.

Local tissue factors are of some impor-tance, probably not in the usual kinds of thinness, but undoubtedly in rare and pe-culiar instances of failure to deposit fat locally in certain areas. Such conditions are known as *lipodystrophy,* and the region in which little or no fat is deposited may be the upper half of the body, the legs only, or the face; or even only one side of the face, etc. The variety most frequently seen occurs in women, the upper half of the body being lean and emaciated, while from the hips down fat is deposited in normal or excessive amounts. The disorder seems to be hereditary, even the type and the location of the lesion being transmitted.

Fat atrophy occurs locally in some persons following repeated subcutaneous injections, especially of insulin.

Psychologic factors are of great importance in regulating food intake. *Appetite* is to a large degree dependent upon habit, training and emotional status. The appearance, the color, the taste, the smell and even the memory of food exert strong influences. When in emotional turmoil, most persons are apt to develop moderate or severe anorexia. When the emotional disorder is extreme, the psychoneurosis known as *anorexia nervosa* may be present, and true emaciation may result. Prolonged nervous tension with lack of appetite may be at least partially the result of overactivity of the sympathico-adrenal system, with inhibition of the parasympathetic motor system to the gastrointestinal tract, and perhaps similar inhibition of secretion of the digestive juices.

Appetite and Hunger. Appetite is the desire for food, a psychologic state which may accompany hunger, but may be present without it. Hunger is a sensation, a physiologic state related in human beings to perception of general weakness, certain sensory impulses from the alimentary tract, and perhaps to decrease in the circulating blood glucose.[3,4]

Hypothalamus and Higher Nerve Center Regulation of Food Intake. Hyperphagia is induced experimentally in animals by bilateral medial lesions in the neighborhood of the ventromedial nuclei. Aphagia (complete failure of eating) occurs if lesions are produced in certain lateral hypothalamic areas. Animals becoming obese after medial lesions abruptly stop eating when lateral lesions are created.

The neural complex for the regulation of feeding seems to be analogous to the mechanisms which regulate circulation, respiration, body temperature and many other variables. That is, the control is eventually effective through the facilitation or inhibition of feeding reflexes. When feeding alone is concerned, regulation at the hypothalamic level occurs, but when other variables are introduced, such as sensation, emotion, volition, choices between foods, etc., the cerebral cortex probably contributes to the regulation.

The pathologic physiology of hunger, appetite, satiety, weight gain and weight loss, anorexia, etc., are discussed also in Chapters 18 and 32 and in recent excellent reviews.[3,4]

Nutritional factors are the common pathways through which the various influ-

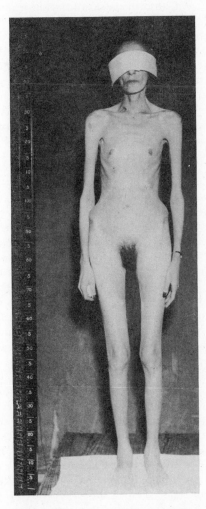

Fig. 200. Appearance resembling pituitary cachexia (Simmonds' disease) from severe anorexia nervosa. Woman, 33 years old, with senile aspect, emaciation, loss of hair and breast tissue and amenorrhea.

ences on body weight and nutritive status must be exerted. Thus, the thin person who because of a neurosis cannot take enough calories differs from the thin person unable to eat because of abdominal distress caused by a peptic ulcer. In one case, the cause may be purely psychologic and in the other purely physical; or, as often happens, the psychologic and the physical elements may become closely intertwined and be present in both instances. Nevertheless, the cause of the weight loss and other symptoms of undernutrition is *inadequate food intake,* if absorption, assimilation and metabolism are normal.

Similarly, weight loss from chronic diarrhea occurs from *failure to assimilate calorigenic nutrients,* whether from a psychogenic ulcerative colitis or from tuberculous enteritis. Likewise, weight loss from prolonged fever or excessive muscular activity results from excessive *caloric expenditure,* just as it does in hyperthyroidism.

CAUSES OF SPECIFIC NUTRITIVE DEFICIENCIES

Failure to maintain adequate stores of energy-producing material such as fat may be thought of as a *general* nutritive defect, depending upon proper caloric balance. Carbohydrate, the chief usual source of calories in the average normal diet, is usually implicated, but fat also often plays an important role. Subnormal carbohydrate or fat intake causes thinness or weight loss; loss of carbohydrate as glucose in the urine (diabetes), or of fat in the stool (steatorrhea) has a similar result, etc.

Other nutritive defects may be considered more *specific:* for example, although calorie intake may be adequate, proper growth and maintenance of muscle and other tissue proteins depend upon protein intake and balance. The calorie foods cannot take the place of the tissue foods nor of other nutrients needed for many different and special functions.

Calcium, iron, iodine and the other mineral essentials; sodium, potassium, magnesium and the other electrolytes; and each of the essential vitamins must be available in certain specific amounts to maintain normal structure and function. Each of the essential nutrients may be thought of as having its own metabolism. The positive and negative phases of the metabolic cycle for each nutrient must be in such balance that adequate amounts may be utilized without production of deficits, otherwise evidences of nutritional failure will appear. Insufficient intake, excess destruction or elimination may affect one or more of the important elements in nutrition, either separately or, more often, in various characteristic combinations, depending upon their function in the body.

As with calories, so with other nutrient essentials such as water, minerals and vitamins. Undernutrition with respect to any one of these elements results when a negative balance for that specific nutrient occurs, or when the balance is insufficiently positive to satisfy metabolic requirements.

The various types of undernutrition occur because of inadequate intake, defective absorption, impaired utilization, excessive destruction or elimination of one or more of the necessary food substances. The materials required for optimal growth and development, health and efficiency are water, certain minerals and vitamins, carbohydrate, fat and protein.

INADEQUATE INTAKE

Anorexia and Starvation. Loss of appetite and failure to ingest adequate quantities of one or more necessary foods will eventually result in malnutrition. The loss of appetite may result from any of a great number of *organic* conditions; for example, gastritis, gastric cancer, heart failure, nephritis, febrile diseases, any condition associated with severe pain, many neoplastic diseases, etc. However, anorexia often is *psychic* in origin and may be a feature of alcoholism and various neuroses or psychoses. If disinterest in food and failure to ingest an adequate diet persist, partial or complete starvation occurs. The starvation may be *general* or *specific:* in anorexia nervosa all foods are shunned, but in some simple "distastes" only one food is avoided. For example, some persons have an aversion to milk and develop calcium deficiency; others may be vegetarians and develop anemia because of lack of protein, iron, etc.

Occult Dietary Deficiencies. Often the diet may be apparently normal, but concealed defects are present. Those who fail to ingest sufficient amounts of the proper types of foods often have easy access to them; others receive improper diets because of circumstances beyond their control.

The average undistorted diet is apt to be adequate as regards many of the food essentials without much effort as to choice of foods, but certain important nutrients may be taken in inadequate amounts. The majority of intelligent people make some attempt to utilize the modern knowledge of food values in selecting their diets. However, it has been shown that a considerable proportion of the apparently healthy normal population shows some evidences of undernutrition because many persons fail to ingest a variety of foods balanced to contain all the essential nutrients in adequate amounts. It is evident that although there are powerful physiologic demands directing our unconscious choices of foods that reinforce and assist our conscious selections, these mechanisms often fail. Man and the animals do not always instinctively select a good diet.

POVERTY is frequently the cause of inadequate intake, since the protein- and the fat-containing foods are more expensive to produce and cost more than carbohydrate, which furnishes calories but is poor in "protective" qualities.

IGNORANCE is often to be blamed, for the dissemination of knowledge is far behind the advances in the available information. There is some excuse for the lay person who has had little or no opportunity to learn about proper diet. Physicians, dietitians and educators in the fields of medicine, hygiene and public health must bear the responsibility of acquiring and disseminating authentic knowledge concerning proper food selection and preparation. The physician particularly and his co-worker, the medical dietitian, must be careful that they do not, through ignorance or inattention, prescribe therapeutic diets that may be of value in correcting one condition but

may precipitate nutritional failure because of inadequacies. The physician responsible for the care of a patient must realize that even in apparently purely mechanical conditions nutritional considerations may be of great importance. For example, immobilization of a fractured bone causes calcium and phosphorus loss and calls for attention to the intake of these elements and of vitamin D.

Efforts should be made to educate physicians, educators, dietitians, nutritionists, public-health officers and the public concerning the nutritive values of foods and their proper preservation and cooking. Even if the food originally is high in vitamins and minerals, large amounts of these essential nutrients may be destroyed in *food preparation*. The salts may be washed out by soaking, or may be lost if cooking juices are thrown away. The refining of cereals such as wheat, with removal of the germ and the bran layer, causes great reduction of the vitamin-B content. Water-soluble vitamins may be thrown away with the cooking water. Vitamins of the B-complex and ascorbic acid are rendered inert by alkalis. Heating of foods containing ascorbic acid may result in complete inactivation of the vitamin if air is present and oxidation takes place. The losses of vitamin B_1 (thiamine) in foods under conditions comparable with those in baking may be as high as 50 per cent.

In the United States many diets are deficient in thiamine (vitamin B_1), nicotinic acid, ascorbic acid and calcium, and recognizable clinical deficiency states often result in spite of adequate caloric intake and the maintenance of normal body weight. Refined cereals, white bread and sugar are often taken in excess to the neglect of fruits, vegetables, milk, meat and whole-wheat products.

CLIMATE AND SUNLIGHT. There is one essential nutrient not derived primarily from food. It is vitamin D. Few foods other than eggs, fish liver or fish-liver oils contain appreciable amounts of it. Most of the requirement is supplied through the chemical changes produced in cholesterol through irradiation of the skin by *sunlight*. During a large part of the year in cold or in temperate climates, sunlight and outdoor activity are so limited that vitamin-D deficits are common. This is especially the case in children, in whom, because of rapid skeletal growth, the requirement is high.

TRADITION AND HABIT. A third factor in malnutrition among the apparently normal part of the population is traditional adherence to certain types of food. Deficient diets are often followed consistently because of individual, familial, racial, regional or religious habits.

FADS. Food faddism, such as vegetarianism, etc., is not uncommon and may cause many different types of deficiencies.

ALCOHOLISM. Chronic alcoholism is apt to cause nutritional disorders because (1) alcohol supplies calories without all the other necessary nutrients; (2) alcohol often precipitates nausea, vomiting, diarrhea and its use frequently causes anorexia; (3) it often results in liver damage, peptic ulcers, etc., which are then the further causes of nutritive defects; (4) it often is associated with psychiatric disturbances, neglect of proper diet, food faddism, etc.

ORGANIC DISEASE. The factors leading so-called normal people to poor food selection have been mentioned. Failure of intake of the necessary foods may also result from organic disease of many types. Affections of the mouth, the tongue and the pharynx such as dental disorders, gingivitis, glossitis, tonsillitis and ulcerations of various sorts, often cause restriction of the diet to liquids over a considerable period. Inflammatory, ulcerative, neoplastic or obstructive disease, or surgical changes involving the gastrointestinal tract may interfere with normal food intake or be accompanied by vomiting, nausea or anorexia. Loss of appetite, sometimes with nausea or vomiting, is frequent in many organic disorders, such as cardiac conditions, nephritis and intracranial disease.

PSYCHIC DISORDERS. Fatigue, nervous tension, emotional states, psychoneuroses and psychoses often affect the functions of the alimentary canal or cause loss of interest in food.

DRUG THERAPY. Many commonly used drugs may cause anorexia, nausea or vomiting (e.g., morphine, codeine, salicylates,

digitalis), or diarrhea (mercurials, antibiotics, etc.) and thus interfere with nutrition.

Not only may drugs interfere with intake, but absorption and utilization may suffer (see section following).

THERAPEUTIC DIETS. In the treatment of disease therapeutic diets are often employed, and inadvertently there may be prescribed a diet so deficient in one factor or more that a nutritive disorder results. In *peptic-ulcer* therapy, tomato juice and citrus fruits may be forbidden and vitamin-C deficit may occur. In the treatment of *diabetes,* care must be taken not to give a diet too low in the B-complex vitamins when bread and other cereals are restricted. In *allergic* conditions, milk or other foods may be eliminated from the diet and calcium deficiency or other types of malnutrition may be produced. Therapeutic diets for weight reduction in *obesity* are apt to be deficient not only in calories but in other nutrients, and to prevent malnutrition the physician must in many instances ensure the intake of certain essentials while total calories are restricted. Thus a generous allowance of skimmed milk will provide adequate calcium and phosphorus intake, eggs and meat will provide protein and iron, and it may be advisable to supply supplements of vitamins A and D (because of restricted fats), B complex (because of restricted wheat and cereals) and C (because of limited citrus fruits).

NUTRITIONAL DISORDERS often interfere with food intake and thus may set up a vicious circle which tends to perpetuate and intensify the malnutrition, frequently making what was a simple, perhaps single nutrient deficit into a complex, multiple deficit. Thiamine deficiency and nicotinic acid deficiency are particularly known to cause anorexia and nausea. Anorexia is characteristic of pernicious anemia and other B_{12}-deficiency states.

INADEQUATE ABSORPTION OR UTILIZATION

Even though a proper amount of all the necessary nutrients is ingested, they may not be absorbed or utilized because of mechanical, chemical or bacterial dysfunction in the alimentary canal. Chronic diarrhea, from whatever cause, by reason of the excessively rapid passage through the body, may fail to permit time for proper digestion and absorption of water, salts and vitamins, as well as of some of the carbohydrate, the protein and the fat. When certain enzymes (such as pancreatic lipase) are lacking, food elements are lost (in this case fats, with steatorrhea). When bile is excluded from the intestine, fats and fat-soluble vitamins (A, D, E and K) are poorly digested and absorbed, and fats and insoluble calcium soaps are excreted. Such calcium loss, if prolonged, may lead to osteomalacia and result in pathologic fractures. Proteins may be inadequately digested and absorbed when gastric hydrochloric acid and pepsin are lacking. Other examples are the poor absorption of iron in the absence of adequate hydrochloric acid and poor calcium absorption with deficient vitamin D.

Vitamin B_{12} is inadequately absorbed in the absence of the intrinsic gastric factor; also B_{12} deficiency with macrocytic anemia may result from interference with its assimilation caused by other gastrointestinal disorders (see discussion further on in this chapter under vitamin B_{12}).

The malabsorption syndrome is the term now used to designate a group of related conditions described in the past as tropical sprue, nontropical sprue, celiac disease and idiopathic steatorrhea. In all of these diseases there is a severe chronic diarrhea with bulky stools containing excess lipid. In children (celiac disease) there is growth failure. Affected patients lose weight, have flat glucose tolerance curves; depleted reserves of iron, folic acid and B_{12} (with microcytic or macrocytic anemia); vitamin K deficiency (with hypoprothrombinemia and hemorrhages); hypoproteinemia with edema; hypocalcemia with tetany, rickets or osteomalacia; and frequent electrolyte disturbances. The etiology is obscure—it is not clear whether the abnormalities found in the small intestine are primary. Biopsies of jejunal mucosa have shown short, blunted villi and the microvilli are sparse, blunted and fused; these changes reflect a major loss of the bowel absorptive area.

The anemia when macrocytic in type responds to B_{12} or folic acid therapy, but the anemia is often mixed in type and may be concomitantly or primarily due to iron deficiency. Vitamin B_{12} and folic acid in acquired deficiencies cause improvement in the intestinal mucosa but in congenital celiac disease have not reversed mucosal changes. Gluten-free diets have induced remissions in celiac disease and non-tropical sprue and alterations of villi toward the normal pattern have been observed following prolonged periods of such therapy.[37]

It is not clear whether the malabsorption syndrome is due primarily to a mucosal defect, a toxic or antibody immune response (to gluten, and possibly to other nutrients) or some other mechanism. However, it is evident, that during the florid phase many important nutrients are lost in the stools and that during remission (with cessation of diarrhea) rapid repair of deficits begins promptly.

Drug therapy with antibiotics or sulfa drugs can destroy bacteria constituting the normal flora of the intestinal tract which are engaged in synthesizing vitamin K and various members of the B complex group. Most of such synthesis occurs in the colon and it seems that a small part at least of such vitamins thus are supplied to human beings. Even a small supplement from this source may be important to persons consuming diets containing minimal amounts of the vitamin or its precursors.[26]

An excess of phosphorus in the diet will decrease calcium absorption. An excess of calcium diminishes iron absorption. Antacids decrease iron absorption and may perpetuate anemia in peptic ulcer therapy, etc. Aluminum hydroxide greatly decreases phosphorus absorption.

In spite of adequate intake and absorption, assimilation and utilization may be interfered with. Thus in chronic alcoholism there may develop *hepatic cirrhosis* with inability to form serum albumin from the protein materials that reach the liver in adequate amounts through the circulation. Likewise, *hepatic parenchymal damage* may prevent adequate conversion of glucose to glycogen and its storage in the liver; or may hinder utilization of vitamin K and formation of prothrombin. *Bone-marrow damage* may prevent adequate utilization of protein and iron and other materials to form hemoglobin and red blood cells and other elements of the blood, such as white blood cells and platelets.

In *diabetes mellitus* glucose is adequately absorbed and present in the blood in excessive amounts, but it cannot be adequately utilized in the absence of sufficient insulin. Large amounts of glucose, as well as of sodium chloride and of water, escape from the body through the kidneys in the characteristic polyuria.

EXCESSIVE ELIMINATION OR ABNORMAL LOSS

Serious nutritional disturbance may result from excessive elimination of substances important to the body through normal channels or from losses through abnormal routes. Examples of excessive excretion through normal routes include diarrhea, the polyuria of diabetes just mentioned, diuresis, excessive sweating, the albuminuria of nephritis, the calciuria of hyperparathyrodism, the blood loss of menorrhagia, etc. Examples of losses through abnormal routes are blood loss from wounds; blood protein, salt and water loss from burns, vomiting, fistulae, etc.

Nutritional disorders frequently cause diarrhea, thus setting up a vicious circle. Nutritive deficiencies especially apt to result in diarrhea include those of nicotinic acid (pellagra), and of protein (kwashiorkor).

INCREASED METABOLISM

In certain conditions, the total metabolism may be accelerated so as to require a much greater supply than normal of all nutrient materials. Whenever the demand is augmented but is not satisfied, or sufficient nutrients cannot be ingested or otherwise administered, undernutrition will occur.

Examples of *pathologic conditions*, in which attention must be paid to the very high nutrient requirements as the result of a generalized increased metabolism, are hyperthyroidism and fevers. Chronic low-grade infections such as tuberculosis, brucellosis, tonsillitis and arthritis may keep a patient underweight by accelerating the metabolism even without the production of fever. In such instances, the acceleration

of metabolism apparently results from the action of toxins. Neoplastic diseases (cancer, sarcoma, leukemia, Hodgkin's disease, etc.) may cause tissue destruction locally and general toxic effects with increase in the metabolic rate and resultant weight loss.

Trauma, either accidental or surgical, may cause profound metabolic reactions accompanied by large losses of proteins, vitamins and other nutrients.[22] Such losses have in the past been considered as inescapable and obligatory but recent studies indicate that vigorous nutritive efforts may prevent the negative nitrogen balance, etc., and promote quicker recovery.[20]

Physiologic conditions in which metabolic demands are unusually high are pregnancy, lactation, periods of prolonged strenuous muscular activity, and the periods of great activity and rapid growth of childhood.

PATHOLOGIC PHYSIOLOGY

When any of the above etiologic factors becomes of sufficient magnitude or persists for a sufficient period of time, the metabolic balance for one or more essential nutrients becomes negative. The nutrient is withdrawn from the body tissues normally containing it; therefore, tissues and organs depending upon the nutrient for performance of certain functions may receive it in inadequate amounts. At this stage assay of the blood (or tissues) may reveal low levels of the nutrient (for example, low ascorbic acid levels, low serum potassium concentration, etc.). Such low biochemical levels may continue for prolonged periods, but if the level drops farther, or demand for the nutrient suddenly increases, functions dependent upon the nutrient falter and anatomic manifestations may appear. For example, in *ascorbic acid* deficiency there occurs failure in the formation and maintenance of intercellular materials, increased capillary fragility and bleeding into the gums; in *potassium* deficiency there is diminution in neuromuscular irritability, paralyses of skeletal muscle, failure of heart muscle action and finally definite anatomic changes in the muscles.

The usual order of change in the pathologic physiology of nutritional disease is:

1. Negative balance of the nutrient factor
2. Tissue depletion
3. Biochemical change
4. Functional alterations
5. Anatomic defects

Further discussion of these stages of nutritive failure will be found later in this chapter in the section, Effects of Malnutrition.

EFFECTS OF DISEASE ON NUTRITION

As indicated in the previous section on etiology and pathologic physiology, various types of illness, of either organic or functional nature, may affect the intake, the absorption and the utilization or the excretion of the various necessary food elements, or may increase certain metabolic demands. For example, during fevers, or after surgery, intake of calories, protein and vitamins usually are diminished and losses may be accelerated at the very time when metabolism is increased and demands are heightened. These adverse influences upon nutrition are here recalled for the purpose of emphasizing that not only does disease affect nutrition, but as discussed below, nutrition exerts important effects upon disease.

EFFECTS OF NUTRITION ON DISEASE

When illness develops, the state of nutrition is important in determining the course of the disease. For example, the prognosis for a very poorly nourished person who develops tuberculosis is apt to be bad, and a patient with scurvy who requires surgical therapy for an obstructed intestine is in a precarious condition.

The physician must recognize the presence, the type and the degree of the malnutrition and treat it. At the same time he must treat any incidental or accompanying or causative specific disease. Often the outcome will depend more upon correction of the malnutrition than upon any therapy directed toward the other malady.

CLUES IN THE HISTORY

Since patients with many nutritive disorders do not exhibit characteristic physical findings until the undernourished state is far advanced, the diagnosis of undernutrition often depends upon obtaining clues in the history. One usually will not think of making any special tests for nutritional failure unless the history suggests the lack of some necessary foods in the diet or some derangement that may have prevented proper intake, absorption or utilization or may have caused excessive losses or increased metabolic requirements. If the physician asks the proper questions, the presence or the absence of the etiologic factors may be discovered. The fact that the patient is underweight or is losing weight is particularly suggestive. An adult who for some time has not included in his *daily diet* the following foods may in many instances have an undernourished state of some type, depending upon the essential foods missing: one pint of milk, one egg, 4 slices of whole-wheat bread or their equivalent, one serving of meat, two servings of vegetables, two servings of fruit (one citrus), 3 teaspoonfuls of butter, or its equivalent in cream or fortified margarine. Inquiry in regard to the frequency with which these "protective" foods (that is, high in content of vitamins, minerals and protein) are taken will give the physician a fairly good indication of the probable existence of nutritional deficiency. Most persons who are not underweight or losing weight will be found to ingest sufficient carbohydrate, fat and minerals, with the possible exceptions of calcium and iron. The most commonly deficient elements are proteins, calories and vitamins. Thinness alone suggests simply lack of sufficient calories. Obesity does not preclude undernutrition with respect to minerals, vitamins or protein, but indicates only an excess of calories.

ESSENTIAL FOODS

Foods as we eat them, such as milk, eggs, meat, wheat and other cereals, fruits, vegetables, butter and oils, starches, etc., must be broken down into basic units before

TABLE 43. THE SIX NUTRITIONAL GROUPS
AND THEIR BASIC UNITS

GROUP	UNITS
1. Water	Water
2. Electrolytes and minerals	Various electrolytes such as sodium chloride, etc., and various minerals such as calcium, iron, copper salts, etc.
3. Carbohydrate	Glucose (dextrose)
4. Fat	Fatty acids and esters
5. Protein	Amino acids (and small peptids)
6. Vitamins	Thiamine, riboflavin, etc.

they can be absorbed and utilized. The six groups of nutrients with the basic units derived from them are listed in Table 43. A complete diet includes adequate amounts of all the essential nutrients in each of the six groups. Some of the required substances in this biochemical classification of the basic units that actually enter the blood for utilization are simple and some are complex. The various groups are highly interdependent in their nutritional and metabolic activity. The nutrients must be supplied not only in certain amounts but in certain proportions.

FUNCTIONS OF FOODS

The functions of the various nutrients must be adequately performed to maintain the anatomic integrity and the physiologic efficiency of the body. Therefore, not only must the nutrients be supplied and absorbed in proper quantity, but certain proportions must be maintained between them to ensure an optimum state of the cells and the tissues. For example, an increase in the salt intake requires a proportionately greater supply of water to keep the electrolyte composition of the extracellular fluid within normal limits. Likewise, an increase in the carbohydrate combustion demands an increase in the available thiamine.

The nutrient elements may be classified according to three general functions: (1) as *structural* or supportive material (for bone, cartilage, skin, connective tissue, stroma of individual organs and cells; and for the blood plasma, the interstitial fluid and the lymph that together constitute the organ of transport, the extracellular fluid); (2) as *fuel* (for body heat, muscular activity and work, as well as for the energy for numerous complex intermediate metabolic processes), and (3) as *catalytic* substances or chemical regulators.

Each nutrient element performs more than a single function and every essential nutrient falls into more than one of the three categories. For example, by far the chief function of carbohydrate is to supply fuel, but some is used in the construction of special conjugated proteins in cartilage and some is needed in the formation of certain enzymes. Fats are used primarily for fuel, but adipose tissue furnishes some structural support: fats serve largely as fuel-storage materials. The fatty substances known as phospholipids and cerebrosides are important constituents of tissues and organs. Fats supply the essential fatty acids (linoleic and arachidonic); they carry the fat-soluble vitamins A, D, E and K and facilitate the absorption of calcium and phosphorus.

Energy is supplied by the combustion of food: from fat, 9 calories per Gm.; from protein, 4 calories per Gm.; from carbohydrate, 4 calories per Gm. The basal metabolism (minimum heat production at rest, 12 to 14 hours after the last meal) varies with surface area, age and sex. The total metabolism includes caloric requirements for basal metabolism plus specific dynamic action of food, plus physical activity. Allowance of about 5 per cent must be made for the specific dynamic action of food: that is, an average of approximately 5 per cent of the total caloric value of the food is expended in preparing the food for use by the body and is not available for energy purposes.

Numerous careful studies have determined the energy requirements for various activities. Mental work is of little consequence in raising caloric needs—probably only a 3 to 4 per cent increment above basal levels being necessary. Physical activity raises metabolism greatly: for sitting or standing, about 10 per cent of the basal calories; for walking on the level at 3 miles per hour, about 1 calorie per hour per pound of body moved. This for a 70 Kg. (154 lbs.) man of 1.8 square meters surface area at 40 calories per sq. m. per hour = 72 basal calories per hour plus 154 calories per hour for walking, or an increment of over 200 per cent. Heavy labor or strenuous sports may increase the energy expenditure by as much as 800 per cent to 1,500 per cent.

A sedentary clerk's daily requirement will be about 2,400 calories; a moderately active salesman, 3,000; a painter or carpenter, 3,500; a mason or sawyer, 4,500 to 6,000.

Economy of energy metabolism is observed under certain conditions, nutritive balance being maintained with a very low caloric intake. The basal metabolic rate may decrease during undernutrition to minus 30 per cent or lower (Lusk[14]). Following severe illness this conservation mechanism may be of great importance. As nutrition and energy metabolism are restored to normal, the basal metabolic rate again rises to a normal level.

Carbohydrate and fat together supply about 90 per cent of the calories in the average normal diet. In the poorer types of diets, used especially in the lower economic groups, carbohydrate supplies from about 60 to 70 per cent; fat, from 20 to 25 per cent; and protein, about 5 per cent. In better diets, about 50 per cent of the total calories is derived from carbohydrate, from 35 to 40 per cent from fat, and 10 per cent or more from protein. Fats are expensive to produce, and during times of famine or of war, fat is apt to be the nutrient most seriously curtailed. In Madrid in 1941, fat furnished only about 10 per cent of the calories of the average diet and in 1942, Belgium and Finland were restricted to only about a fifth of their prewar fat consumption. In 1944, there was widespread mass starvation in Holland, with severe malnutrition, the result of prolonged consumption of only about 1,000 calories of food daily. About 20 per cent of one group studied had hunger edema, indicating protein starvation and hypopro-

teinemia, with consumption of body protein for caloric needs, the usual energy foods, carbohydrate and fat, being lacking.[5]

FATS

The term *lipid* includes true fats and other fatlike substances. Three types of lipids are important in nutrition.

1. Neutral fats are combinations of fatty acids and glycerol. Most of the food fats belong to this group, and most of the adipose tissue of the body is in this form.

2. Phospholipids contain phosphoric acid and a nitrogenous base in addition to the fatty acid and glycerol molecule. The phospholipids such as lecithin and cephalin are important constituents of cell protoplasm.

3. Sterols are combinations of fatty acids and sterols of high molecular weight. Cholesterol is the only sterol occurring as such in the body. It is found in practically every living tissue but especially in the brain, blood, skin and adrenal cortex. Irradiation of cholesterol or of its derivatives in the skin is believed to be the body's mode of making vitamin D. Cholesterol is apparently the "mother-substance" from which are manufactured the sex hormones and the adrenocortical hormones, which are of steroid structure.

CARBOHYDRATE

Glucose, derived from the sugars and starches of the food, is the form of carbohydrate circulating in the blood. It provides a quick source of energy. Glucose is stored as glycogen in the liver, whence it may be released as required to maintain a circulating blood glucose level of about 100 mg. per 100 ml., and to provide for energy demands. Carbohydrate taken in excess of the body's immediate needs is converted into fat and stored in fatty tissues, where it serves as a source of fuel for future needs. As much as 200 to 300 Gm. of glycogen may be stored in the liver, and considerable amounts are also present in the muscles and in the skin. The intake of carbohydrate food among normal persons varies widely, ranging around 300 Gm. daily in the average normal adult of 70 Kg.

body weight (154 lb.) whose total caloric requirement is approximately 2,500 calories daily, but ranging much higher when caloric demands are greater.

PROTEIN

Proteins are very complex organic compounds, containing carbon, hydrogen, oxygen, nitrogen and usually sulfur. The presence of nitrogen distinguishes protein, the average protein containing 16 per cent N. Some specialized proteins also contain iron, phosphorus, iodine, copper and other inorganic elements.

Proteins are composed of simpler substances called *amino acids.* Analysis of protein hydrolysates has revealed 20 different amino acids widely distributed in proteins. The human body can manufacture many amino acids, but it cannot produce certain others in amounts adequate to meet body needs. Nitrogen balance and rate of growth have been used to determine whether the various amino acids are essential in the diet (i.e., cannot be made in the body in adequate amounts). Evidence indicates that for growth of rats (and probably of humans) there are 10 *essential* amino acids. However, only eight of these are needed to maintain nitrogen equilibrium in the human adult, histidine and arginine not being required (Table 44).

It should be emphasized that the "nonessential" amino acids are just as important in human nutrition as the essential ones. The terms are confusing, but traditional.

TABLE 44. CLASSIFICATION OF THE AMINO ACIDS

ESSENTIAL	NONESSENTIAL
Arginine	Alanine
Histidine	Aspartic acid
Isoleucine	Cystine; cysteine
Leucine	Glutamic acid
Lysine	Glycine
Methionine	Hydroxyproline
Phenylalanine	Proline
Threonine	Serine
Tryptophane	Tyrosine
Valine	

The nonessential ones can be formed in the body from other sources; the essential ones must be furnished as such in proteins in the diet. Radioactive carbon (C^{14}) has been used to demonstrate the biogenesis of the nonessential amino acids. The C^{14} is found in tissues in the amino acids which are nonessential, while the essential amino acids contained none of the tracer fed in labeled precursors (sugar, acetic acid, CO_2).[1]

Proteins are classified as complete, partially complete or totally incomplete or of high or low "biologic value," according to the adequacy with which they supply all the amino acids necessary for construction of body tissues. For example, the protein of milk (casein), though poor in cystine, is *complete,* because it alone can provide fully for life, growth and vigor. Gelatin, by contrast, is *incomplete,* of low biologic value (no tryptophan or valine; inadequate tyrosine and cystine) and will not support growth or maintain nitrogen equilibrium. The proteins of meat and eggs are of high biologic value.

For efficient protein synthesis, both the essential and the nonessential amino acids must be available simultaneously and in sufficient quantities. The production of proteins in the body is limited not only by the supply of essential amino acids but also by the speed and efficiency with which the so-called nonessentials are made available. The availability of the nonessential acids depends upon the proper function of the conversion mechanisms and it seems probable that some of the disturbances of protein formation, for instance in liver disease, may be the consequence of a failure in the formation of the nonessential amino acids.[11]

Proteins compose the major portion of the solid matter of muscles and glandular tissues. All cells and all body fluids (except bile and urine) contain protein. Serum proteins are of great value in the regulation of osmotic pressure and of fluid interchange. Proteins are amphoteric (may behave as either acid or alkali) and are of great importance in the regulation of acid-base balance. The hormones of the pituitary, pancreas (insulin) and thyroid (thyroxine) are proteins of specific structure and function. Enzymes (trypsin, pepsin, amylase, etc.) are protein in nature. Resistance to disease is in large part determined by protein substances called *antibodies.*

Protein constitutes about 75 per cent of the dry weight of the tissues of the body. Proteins are most important as structural material, and in the plasma and the red cells contribute to the essential properties of blood. Proteins are also necessary for the formation of enzymes and hormones and thus also furnish catalytic substances and chemical regulators. Protein materials, therefore, with the minerals (calcium and phosphorus for bone, iron for hemoglobin, etc.) constitute the metabolic machinery of the body. Of all the food essentials, protein is probably closest to the vital processes; its very meaning is derived from the Greek root meaning primary or first.

When protein nutrients are supplied in excess of the requirements for replacement of structural needs, they are converted into fat and stored. When caloric intake is inadequate, fat stores are used. This is also true of carbohydrate stores, which, however, being relatively scant, are quickly exhausted. Under such circumstances body protein will be used for fuel. Under conditions of complete starvation Lusk has estimated that 87 per cent of the calories will come from adipose tissue and 13 per cent from protein tissue; after fat stores are exhausted, body protein may become the chief source of calories. To maintain normal function, protein intake per day should be a minimum of one gram per kilogram of body weight, and 1.5 Gm. is probably nearer the optimum level. This means 105 Gm. for a 70 Kg. (154-lb.) man.

NITROGEN BALANCE may be maintained only if all the essential amino acids are supplied and absorbed in adequate amounts. If the daily protein intake is only 40 or 50 Gm. per day for a 70 Kg. person, it is especially important that the dietary protein be of high biologic value; with higher intakes the safety factor is much greater. Nitrogen balance can be preserved and the destruction of body protein for fuel can be avoided if adequate calories from carbohydrate and fat are available. The "protein-sparing" effect of carbohydrate is greater, for it directly supplies essential glucose; fat supplies calories, but cannot alone supply adequate glucose to avoid gluconeogenesis from protein.

WATER

Water (1) furnishes the vehicle for absorption of nutrients into the body; (2) constitutes the chief ingredient of the extracellular fluid, and thus provides the means of transport; (3) provides for excretion and secretion, and (4) is responsible, by evaporation from lungs and skin, for about 25 per cent of body heat loss, and so contributes to temperature regulation. When water intake is undisturbed, little attention to the intake is usually necessary. Excesses of water are easily disposed of unless some factor interferes with excretion (circulatory failure, nephritis, hypoproteinemia, etc.). Water enters the body as water and also as a constituent of other foods, both liquid and solid (the latter are in some cases actually from 70 to 80 per cent water) and as water of oxidation. The water requirements vary greatly with the temperature of the environment, with bodily exertion and heat production and with salt intake; under extreme conditions they may be as high as 10 liters per day. The minimum requirements of an average normal man in a temperate environment are usually from 1.5 to 3 liters per day. For a discussion of water and electrolyte requirements under various conditions see Chapter 30.

VITAMINS

A number of potent organic compounds occurring in minute quantities in natural foodstuffs have been designated as *vitamins;* they perform specific and vital functions in the cells and tissues of the body.

The vitamins differ widely in chemical structure, natural distribution and physiologic function.

Vitamin deficiency is often not detected

until after deprivation has been prolonged, since stores of vitamins may have been present and are only gradually exhausted.

Vitamins act primarily as part of enzyme systems in important metabolic reactions. *Nicotinic acid,* for example, becomes a component in two important coenzymes (I and II), both concerned in glycolysis and tissue respiration.

Vitamins in many instances, perhaps in all, exert their specific activity when serving as the prosthetic group of an enzyme. *Riboflavin* enters into several enzyme systems, its broad activity thus probably accounting for the variety of symptoms resulting from its deficiency. *Thiamine* serves as a part of the enzyme cocarboxylase. *Biotin* and coenzyme R are identical.

Vitamins were at first named for their curative properties or were given a convenient letter designation more or less in the order of their discovery: vitamin A, the antiophthalmic factor, vitamin B_1, the antiberiberi factor, etc. Many of the vitamins have now been chemically identified, and the chemical names are usually to be preferred: ascorbic acid instead of vitamin C; thiamine instead of vitamin B_1, etc. However, in some instances descriptive names may be retained instead of the more awkward longer chemical names: e.g.: folic acid instead of pteroylglutamic acid.

Some of the vitamins are groups of related character, e.g., the B complex vitamins, of which some 15 have been described. They are grouped together chiefly because all are water-soluble and all can be obtained from the same sources, notably liver and yeast.

The vitamins can usefully be separated into two types: (1) water-soluble vitamins (ascorbic acid, B complex) and (2) fat-soluble vitamins (carotene, vitamins A, D, E and K).

The two types of vitamins differ in absorption, storage and excretion. Since the water-soluble vitamins are diffusible, impaired absorption is seldom encountered (except for B_{12} in pernicious anemia). However, the fat-soluble vitamins, normally absorbed with the lipids in foods, may be inadequately absorbed when fat digestion or absorption is impaired (biliary obstruction, steatorrhea, etc.).

The water-soluble factors are excreted in the urine. Even with high dosage, toxic accumulation is unlikely. Likewise, storage supplies may last only a few months. The fat-soluble factors are not excreted in the urine and storage capacity for them is much greater; overdosage and toxic accumulation is possible within a short period of time; therapeutic amounts may be supplied at long intervals because of slow destruction and excretion, the effects persisting often for many months or a year or more.

At present, the following vitamins are recognized as necessary for man: carotene and vitamin A, vitamin D, vitamin K, thiamine, riboflavin, niacin, pyridoxine, folic acid, vitamin B_{12} and ascorbic acid.

Human requirements are not established or defined for the following: biotin, inositol, pantothenic acid, vitamin E (the tocopherols) and the flavanoids (vitamin P).

MINERALS

Minerals make up a total of about 4 per cent of the body weight; of this about one-half (2 per cent of the total) is calcium; one-fourth (1 per cent of the total) is phosphorus; and the remaining 1 per cent is composed of potassium, sulfur, sodium, chlorine, magnesium and iron. These 8 elements are vital to the body economy.

At least 5 of the so-called "trace minerals" (found in very small amounts in the body) are also necessary: iodine, copper, manganese, cobalt and zinc.

The minerals serve four chief purposes in the body:

1. They compose a large part of the skeletal framework and the teeth. The bony structures are the main depots for calcium, phosphorus, magnesium, sodium, and the trace minerals.

2. They take part in the formation of many organic compounds, such as nucleoproteins and phospholipins, thus forming an integral part of all cells. Muscles hold large amounts of magnesium, potassium, phosphate and sodium.

3. They circulate in the body fluids as

inorganic salts, as dissociated ions and in more or less loosely-bound combinations, playing a vital part in the control of acid-base equilibrium and water balance (Na, Cl, K, especially); neuromuscular irritability (Ca, Mg, K, Na); blood-clotting (Ca); membrane permeability (Ca); muscle contraction; and the transfer of energy (P), etc.

4. They make up essential parts of compounds of paramount importance: iron in hemoglobin, iodine in the thyroid hormone, as essential parts of enzyme systems, etc.

REQUIREMENTS OF SPECIFIC NUTRIENTS IN HEALTH AND DISEASE

IN HEALTH

The nutritional requirements for healthy normal persons under average conditions and under conditions of physiologic stress (such as increased muscular activity, pregnancy, etc.) have been fairly well defined, in terms both of the basic units and the actual natural foods as they are consumed. In terms of the basic units they are approximately as given in Table 45 when the energy expenditure is about 2,500 calories daily.

The normal requirements for an average adult are present in an average normal diet that includes carbohydrate and fat sufficient to supply the necessary calories plus the following protective foods: one pint of milk, one egg, one serving (3 to 4 ounces) of meat, 3 teaspoonfuls (15 Gm.) of butter, 4 servings of whole-grain bread or cereal, 2 vegetables other than potato (one green) and 2 fruits, one of which is raw and one preferably citrus or tomato. Wholesome natural foods such as those mentioned should be selected, since these provide not only calories but necessary protein, vitamins and minerals.

Alcoholic drinks supply calories but fail to furnish other important nutritive materials. Alcohol supplies 7 calories per ml. (a 12 ounce bottle of beer furnishes 170 calories; 1 ounce of whisky, 105 calories). Use of alcoholic beverages in excess may decrease the desire for and intake of more

TABLE 45. APPROXIMATE NORMAL DAILY REQUIREMENTS

1. Water	3,000 ml.
2. Electrolytes (salts of Na, K, Mg, etc.)	10 Gm.
and minerals (calcium, 0.8 Gm; Fe, 12 mg., etc.)	1 Gm.
3. Carbohydrate	300 Gm.
4. Fat	120 Gm.
5. Protein	70 Gm.
6. Vitamins (vitamin A, 5,000 units; thiamine, 2 mg.; riboflavin, 3 mg.; nicotinic acid, 20 mg.; ascorbic acid, 75 mg.; vitamin D, 500 units)	100 mg.

wholesome, complete foods and may cause nutritive disorders.

High carbohydrate diets, even when supplemented with vitamin concentrates, often fail to provide the essential nutrients necessary to good health because of omission of protective foods. The common tendency to supply carbohydrate and fat (the fuel foods) to the partial exclusion of protein, salts, minerals and vitamins (the foods necessary for construction and operation of the metabolic machinery) leads to certain relatively frequent deficiencies. These are related chiefly to inadequacies of the following: calcium, iron, vitamins A and D, vitamin B complex, ascorbic acid, and proteins that contain the essential amino acids and are therefore of high biologic value. The fact that many persons prefer white bread to darker breads may lead to B-complex deficiencies. The use of "enriched bread" containing added thiamine, nicotinic acid and iron is a logical step in the prevention of such deficiencies when inadequate amounts of the whole cereal foods are ingested.

Optimal intake of the necessary foods in normal persons depends upon various factors affecting metabolic demands, such as age, sex, size, muscular activity, pregnancy, lactation and growth. Table 46 gives the *recommended daily allowances* for specific nutrients of the Committee on Foods and Nutrition of the National Research Council. In this table the figures given allow for the various influences affecting normal persons and also allow in most instances a margin of safety of about 30 per cent. That is, these are not minimal daily requirements, but those that are considered *safe allowances,* since it is known that some persons because of individual characteristics require more than minimal or average amounts of certain nutrients, and since in many instances the approximate requirements are known, but exact limits are not.

In Table 46 we note the proportionally very high requirements of infants and young children which are necessary for their great activity and rapid growth. At age 6 months, the caloric requirement is about 120 cal. per Kg., at one year about 100 cal., at age 6 years, about 80 cal., at age 12 years about 60 cal., as compared to a requirement of about 30 cal. per Kg. for a relatively sedentary adult. Protein and other requirements show a similar range. The child at 3 years needs about 3 Gm. of protein per Kg. of body weight, the child of 12 years about 2 Gm., and the adult about 1 Gm. The rapid appearance of clinical manifestations and the more serious results of nutritive disorders in the young are explained by their high requirements.

In Disease

The nutrient requirements during abnormal conditions such as in (1) primary undernutrition, (2) undernutrition secondary to disease, and (3) in malnourished states in which nutritional disturbance is an incidental accompaniment of or has caused (4) organic disease are, of course, varied and complex. Single deficiencies are uncommon. Lack of several or many food elements is detectable in most instances. When a single deficit is present, a characteristic picture of a single-deficiency disease may appear, such as scurvy due to lack of ascorbic acid, or hypochromic anemia due to lack of iron. However, usually the syndromes are partial and mixed. Under Causes of Specific Nutritive Deficiencies many of the organic, functional and psychic disturbances have been mentioned, with explanations of the ways in which such conditions interfere with nutrition. In each instance the requirements of the

various nutrients either (1) to prevent malnutrition or (2) to correct it would depend upon the character, the severity and the duration of the malady.

The occurrence of disease highlights the necessity for *optimal* nutrition, not just minimal nutrition during health. Optimal nutrition implies provision of the materials essential not only for structure, fuel and chemical regulation, but for storage of reserves against unusual demands. Thus a previously thin person who because of illness becomes unable to take adequate calories may soon show signs of serious malnutrition. Likewise, a patient with poorly controlled diabetes may quickly exhaust his low supply of liver glycogen after a short period of vomiting, and also may soon become dehydrated because of the previously existing polyuria. A child with a bare minimum of vitamin-D stores may develop rickets when confined indoors because of a series of respiratory infections.

Increased Nutritional Requirements During Disease

A great increase in the demand for certain nutrients occurs in certain pathologic conditions. Some of the most important disorders will be considered as they affect the various necessary food elements:

Water and Salts. Water and electrolyte needs are considered together because they are intimately connected metabolically.

Normal requirements for water vary tremendously, especially with the temperature of the environment and the water lost by insensible evaporation and perspiration. Averages for adults range from about 1 to 3 liters per day. An approximate standard for diverse persons is 1 ml. per calorie of food. Much of the water is contained in prepared foods, the balance is ingested in liquids.

Sodium chloride requirements vary with many conditions, especially with water intake and output. An adequate intake of NaCl is about 5 Gm. daily, while average adult intakes usually range higher than necessary (8 to 15 Gm. daily).

The demands for salt and water will be increased in any disease in which there is

TABLE 46. FOOD AND NUTRITION BOARD, NATIONAL RESEARCH COUNCIL RECOMMENDED DAILY DIETARY ALLOWANCES,[1] REVISED 1958*

	AGE YEARS	WEIGHT KG. (LB.)	HEIGHT CM. (IN.)	CALORIES	PROTEIN GM.	CALCIUM GM.	IRON MG.	VITAMIN A I.U.	THIAMINE MG.	RIBO-FLAVIN MG.	NIACIN MG.	ASCORBIC ACID MG.	VITAMIN D I.U.
Men......	25	65 (143)	170 (67)	3200[2]	65	0.8	12	5000	1.6	1.6	16	75	
	45	65 (143)	170 (67)	2900	65	0.8	12	5000	1.5	1.6	15	75	
	65	65 (143)	170 (67)	2600	65	0.8	12	5000	1.3	1.6	13	75	
Women....	25	55 (121)	157 (62)	2300[2]	55	0.8	12	5000	1.2	1.4	12	70	
	45	55 (121)	157 (62)	2100	55	0.8	12	5000	1.1	1.4	11	70	
	65	55 (121)	157 (62)	1800	55	0.8	12	5000	1.0	1.4	10	70	
	Pregnant (3rd trimester)			Add 400	80	1.5	15	6000	1.5	2.0	15	100	400
	Lactating (850 ml. daily)			Add 1000	100	2.0	15	8000	1.5	2.5	15	150	400
Infants[3]....	0–1/12[4]												
	1/12–3/12	6 (13)	60 (24)	kg.x120	kg.x3.5[3]	0.6	6	1500	0.3	0.4	3	30	400
	4/12–9/12	9 (20)	70 (28)	kg.x110	kg.x3.5[3]	0.8	6	1500	0.4	0.7	4	30	400
	10/12–1	10 (22)	75 (30)	kg.x100	kg.x3.5[3]	1.0	6	1500	0.5	0.9	5	30	400
Children...	1–3	12 (27)	87 (34)	1200	40	1.0	7	2000	0.6	1.0	6	35	400
	4–6	18 (40)	109 (43)	1600	50	1.0	8	2500	0.8	1.2	8	50	400
	7–9	27 (59)	129 (51)	2000	60	1.0	10	3500	1.0	1.5	10	60	400
Boys.......	10–12	35 (78)	144 (57)	2500	70	1.2	12	4500	1.3	1.8	13	75	400
	13–15	49 (108)	163 (64)	3200	85	1.4	15	5000	1.6	2.1	16	90	400
	16–20	63 (139)	175 (69)	3800	100	1.4	15	5000	1.9	2.5	19	100	400
Girls......	10–12	36 (79)	144 (57)	2300	70	1.2	12	4500	1.2	1.8	12	75	400
	13–15	49 (108)	160 (63)	2500	80	1.3	15	5000	1.3	2.0	13	80	400
	16–20	54 (120)	162 (64)	2400	75	1.3	15	5000	1.2	1.9	12	80	400

* Designed for maintenance of good nutrition of healthy persons in the U.S.A. (Allowances are considered to apply to persons normally vigorous and living in temperate climate.)

1. In planning practical dietaries, the recommended allowances can be attained with a variety of common foods which will also provide other nutrient requirements less well known; the allowance levels are considered to cover individual variations among normal persons as they live in the United States subject to ordinary environmental stresses.

2. These calorie recommendations apply to the degree of activity for the average active man and woman. For the urban "white-collar" worker they are probably excessive. In any case, the calorie allowance must be adjusted to the actual needs of the individual as required to achieve and maintain his desirable weight.

3. The recommendations for infants pertain to nutrients derived primarily from cow's milk. If the milk from which the protein is derived is human milk or has been treated to render it more digestible, the allowance may be in the range of 2–3 Gm. per Kg. There should be no question that human milk is a desirable source of nutrients for infants even though it may not provide the levels recommended for certain nutrients. (See discussion in text.)

4. During the first month of life, desirable allowances for many nutrients are dependent upon maturation of excretory and endocrine functions. Therefore no specific recommendations are given.

an excessive loss or inadequate intake. The most common conditions are fairly well known and involve the *loss of gastrointestinal secretions* by vomiting, diarrhea or intestinal fistulae. Another common cause of water and electrolyte loss is *excessive sweating* under conditions of increased environmental temperature or fever. In *diabetes mellitus,* water and salt loss may be chronic and mild with moderate dehydration, or acute and severe with extreme dehydration, as in diabetic acidosis or coma.

The amount of water and electrolyte that may be lost in a few hours or in a day under these conditions may reach the equivalent of several liters of isotonic saline solution. In other words, there may be, for example, a loss of 4 liters of water or more containing 36 Gm. or more of sodium chloride. The physician should be able to recognize, from the history alone, the existence, if not the degree, of such losses and should promptly be impressed, therefore, by the need for replacement. Patients will seldom know exactly how much fluid they have lost by vomiting or diarrhea, but the mere presence of these symptoms should immediately suggest the need for meeting such losses. Not only *replacement* but *correction of the cause* of gastrointestinal upset, or in diabetes the correction of the metabolic status, with abolition of the glycosuria and ketosis or acidosis, etc., is necessary to relieve permanently the salt and water deficit.

The term *dehydration* is often applied to the result of such loss of water and electrolyte, and this term is an accurate one, provided its variations are understood. Dehydration really means loss of water. The variations concern the substances that accompany this loss of water. In the type just described, the fluid depletion includes loss of salt in approximately isotonic concentration, that is, for every liter of water 9 grams of salt are lost. In other types of dehydration—as, for example, in that which follows extensive burns, pneumonia, peritonitis or intestinal obstruction—the water lost contains not only electrolyte but also protein. Because the protein concentration in the fluid approaches that of plasma, this type of dehydration may be called plasma dehydration, and it will be discussed later under protein requirements.

Dehydration may involve loss of water primarily, with very little loss of electrolyte. This occurs when there is *no water intake,* but no vomiting, diarrhea, etc. Because water is necessary for the vital processes, it will be obtained from body stores as long as life lasts. Under these conditions the various body tissues become progressively depleted of fluid: first extracellular water is lost, then cellular water, until finally death occurs. There is a significant difference between this type of dehydration and that which follows vomiting, diarrhea, etc., because only small amounts of salts are lost. Indeed, the percentage of body solids increases, both extracellular and intracellular fluid compartments become hypertonic, and death is said to occur because of the accumulation of these substances in the body. This is the reason that water alone in *starvation plus dehydration* may greatly prolong life. From the practical point of view, it is obvious that the fluids administered in this type of dehydration must contain relatively little electrolyte in order to avoid increasing further the osmotic pressure in the fluids of the body. Instead of administering normal saline solution to such patients, water in the form of glucose solution should be given, containing perhaps only 2 Gm. per liter of sodium chloride rather than 9 Gm. per liter. The small amount of electrolyte is added only because in water deprivation there is some actual loss of salt at the onset and complete replacement requires that it be included. Although deprivation of water is a basic cause for this simplest variety of dehydration, insensible loss through the skin under conditions of high environmental temperature will accelerate the progress of fluid depletion of this type.

For a detailed discussion of the requirements of water, sodium, chloride, potassium, etc., under various disease conditions causing depletion, see Chapter 30.

Energy Needs. True *increased requirements* for calories (not due to inadequate absorption or excessive excretion of nutrients) in disease occur in hyperthyroid states, in fever, in cancer and in other neoplastic diseases. A patient at rest in bed ordinarily requires no more than from 10 to 15 calories per pound (approximately 25 to 30 calories per Kg.) of body weight, or about 2,000 calories for an average-sized person.

The need for calories in *fever* increases at a rate of about 7 per cent per degree Fahrenheit. Fever is often, in addition, accompanied by destructive processes that break down body tissue and cause excessive elimination of structural elements in the urine (e.g., calcium and phosphorus in osteomyelitis, nitrogen in cancer).

In *hyperthyroidism* the increase in caloric requirements results from (1) a basal metabolism that is accelerated, plus (2) an increment resulting from the purposeless hyperkinesia so common in the disease, plus (3) an inefficiency of motor activity that requires greater than normal energy expenditure for normal purposeful motion. Thus, a patient suffering from thyrotoxicosis and having a basal metabolic rate of plus 50 per cent requires more than an increase of 50 per cent in his caloric intake to maintain a normal energy balance and to prevent weight loss. His true total energy requirements while resting (in bed or chair 16 hours daily, sleeping 8 hours) may be calculated (approximately) as follows:

Patient is a man, age 35; height, 67 inches, weight, 154 pounds.

Basal caloric requirement (if normal) for 24 hours would be 1.8 sq. meters (surface area) × 39.5 cal. for 24 hours = ...	1,706 calories
Add 50 per cent due to thyrotoxicosis	853
Add 20 cal. × 16 hours for hyperkinesia	320
Add 10 cal. × 16 hours for inefficiency (though resting)	160
	3,039
Add 10 per cent for specific dynamic action of food.........	304
Total	3,343 calories

Since patients with hyperthyroidism usually have lost weight, the exact needs

should be exceeded and 4,000 or 5,000 calories should be given to permit storage of protein, fat, carbohydrate, calcium and other essential nutrients of which these patients have been depleted.

Physiologic conditions increasing the total caloric need as well as raising specific protein, mineral and vitamin demands are *pregnancy, lactation* and prolonged and repeated *strenuous exertion.* Abnormally high environmental temperatures imposed by climate or industry may raise the requirement for all nutrients.

Psychologic conditions, if maniacal in type and accompanied by delirium and by hyperactivity, may raise all requirements.

Protein Needs. Although the normal person requires per day about 0.5 Gm. of protein per pound of body weight to maintain nitrogen balance (1 Gm. per Kg.), the needs are increased tremendously in certain types of disease. All protein foods vary in composition; body requirements demand that the protein be of good biologic value. Increased protein needs may be divided into two groups according to whether the loss is actual or metabolic. The *actual* increases are those which result from direct loss of protein from the body in one or more ways. These may be listed as follows:[15]

1. Loss of hemoglobin and plasma protein in hemorrhage.

2. Loss of plasma protein as such from the surface of burns and wounds.

3. Loss of plasma protein into the tissue cavities, i.e., peritonitis, empyema.

4. Loss of plasma protein into tissue, e.g., burns, pneumonia, intestinal obstruction, tissue trauma.

Metabolic loss of protein occurs by excessive destruction of tissue protein which is often called toxic destruction. This occurs in the following conditions:

1. After operation or injury, as a part of the so-called alarm reaction.

2. Infections of various kinds.

3. So-called toxic states that may follow infections long after fever and other evidence of infection have subsided.

4. The progressive cachexia associated with malignant neoplasms.

5. Immobilization or bed rest, with consequent muscle atrophy, etc.

The amount of protein lost in excess of the normal requirements may be tremendous. In terms of actual loss, as much as 50 Gm. a day has been observed to escape from the surface of burns and other wounds. In a single hemorrhage of 1 liter, 150 Gm. of hemoglobin and 50 Gm. of plasma protein are lost. When the losses are metabolic the amount may reach larger proportions. In a case of pneumonia, for example, the daily loss of nitrogen may be 40 Gm. per day, which (×6.25) means the destruction of 250 Gm. of dry tissue protein. This really means the loss of over two pounds of intact tissue protein, such as muscle.[15]

These figures explain the rapidity with which tremendous loss of weight may occur following a variety of diseases in which the loss of protein becomes excessive.

Vitamin Needs. Relatively little information is available in regard to the increased needs for various vitamins in disease. This undoubtedly will be forthcoming as further study reveals the metabolism of the various conditions. A few of the known facts may be discussed.

The requirements for *thiamine* are known to be dependent upon the metabolism of glucose. By analogy, any condition in which more calories as carbohydrate are required probably also will require more thiamine. The modern industrial processing of foods often separates the vitamin B complex from its natural union with carbohydrate in whole grains and plants, so that nature's effort to ensure automatic proportional ingestion of these two nutrient elements is frequently thwarted. In the orient, the use of polished rice led to the recognition of beriberi as a deficiency disease and to the discovery of the B vitamins. As might be expected, the intake of thiamine can with safety be greatly reduced if the diet is rich in fat but low in carbohydrate. This is explained by the fact that co-carboxylase, a thiamine complex, is needed for carbohydrate but not for fat metabolism.

In the sudden drastic alteration in metabolism occurring with rapid regulation of severe diabetes, signs of thiamine deficiency may appear (such as leg pains, reflex changes, and peculiar mental symptoms). Such symptoms are a reflection of the sudden shift from fat to carbohydrate as the chief source of energy, the need for thiamine suddenly becoming very great and exceeding the supply, and the whole process being accelerated by the frequent use of large doses of insulin.

In fevers and in hyperthyroidism there is a general increase in metabolic demands, largely supplied as a rule by increasing the carbohydrate intake. Signs of thiamine deficiency may appear if the intake of that vitamin is not also increased.

The amounts of thiamine required in the various diseases are difficult to estimate exactly, but from the practical point of view the precise need is perhaps not so important, since it is easy to meet even tremendously increased requirements by the simple expedient of giving large repeated doses. Between 0.5 and 1 mg. daily per 1,000 calories is needed for prophylaxis, while about ten times such doses given orally or parenterally are advisable if deficiency signs are apparent.

In some experimental work, vitamin-C requirements during infection (tuberculosis, rheumatic fever, etc.) have been shown to be considerably greater than normal. King and Menten found that resistance of guinea pigs to diphtheria toxin was decidedly increased when supplies of ascorbic acid were adequate. Guinea pigs adapt to cold environments much better when they have adequate intakes of ascorbic acid.

The requirements for *vitamin C* may be increased tremendously in certain surgical conditions. There is definite evidence that large amounts of ascorbic acid are utilized or destroyed in extensive inflammation and in postoperative conditions and burns. This evidence is based upon the fact that the vitamin frequently disappears from the plasma following injury, even though the tissues were saturated with it beforehand. Moreover, it has been observed that tremendous doses of ascorbic acid, i.e., one gram or more per day, may be required if the normal plasma level is to be maintained in such cases. High concentrations of ascorbic acid have been found to occur in the tissue fluids at operative sites. This may explain the low plasma ascorbic-acid levels after injury or operation. The vitamin may be mobilized when needed at the site of any area of inflammation or injury. Vitamin C is known to have an important beneficial influence upon wound healing. These observations may be related and may provide another example of protective activities of the body.

EFFECTS OF MALNUTRITION

The effects of malnutrition may long be concealed, with little or no physical evidence, and with symptoms so ill-defined that the subject may not seek advice, or may simply be considered a psychoneurotic even after advice is sought and some medical investigation has been undertaken. The detection of undernourished states should, of course, be early, before florid signs of nutritional failure appear.

FIVE STAGES OF NUTRITIVE FAILURE

Five successive stages of nutritional failure may be distinguished:

1. **Negative Balance.** In this early stage demand is so great that supply cannot keep pace, or supply is deficient, or both factors are operative in regard to one or more nutrient factors.

2. **Tissue Depletion.** In this stage, first the stores are used up, then the normal supplies of the nutrient in the cells and the tissues and the fluids are drawn upon. The fact that the body carries as a rule certain protective reserves allows tissue depletion to proceed for considerable periods before other more evident effects become manifest. Tissue depletion may be advanced before symptoms develop.

3. **Biochemical Disturbances.** When abnormalities in the tissues and the fluids reach a certain point, there may be measurable chemical changes in the blood and the tissues. For example, after the tissue protein has been greatly depleted, the amounts and the types of serum proteins begin to change, the usual alteration consisting of a considerable fall in total serum protein, affecting chiefly the albumin fraction, with a smaller relative decrease in the serum globulin.

Measurements of the body water content may be accomplished by various dilution methods, using antipyrine, deuterium oxide, etc. In undernutrition there is (in the absence of dehydration) an increase in the percentage of body weight as extracellular fluid. There seems to be replacement of fat and cellular structures with water.

Electrolytes (Na, K, Cl, bicarbonate) in the blood may be determined, but possible alterations in the blood volume must be kept in mind, since dilution or concentration will alter serum or plasma levels. In Chapter 30 is given a detailed discussion of dehydration and electrolyte disorders; in Chapter 31 excess body fluid and edema is discussed.

Vitamin A and its provitamin carotene are found in the blood, and levels vary with intake and liver stores. The vitamin circulates in the fasting state chiefly (80 per cent) as the alcohol form. The elevation after oral intake is due largely to an increase in the ester form, which disappears in about 24 hours.

In some instances a low level of ascorbic acid in the blood is discovered before signs of vitamin-C deficiency have occurred. A deficiency of prothrombin, as indicated by a lengthened prothrombin time, may indicate lack of vitamin K. When the blood pyruvic-acid level is elevated, thiamine may be depleted.

Determination of the amounts of calcium, phosphorus and alkaline phosphatase is useful in detecting disturbances of nutrition affecting the bones. Thus, the calcium or phosphorus levels may be low in rickets and the phosphatase level is elevated. In tetany associated with rickets, the calcium level is low, the phosphatase high; but in idiopathic or hypoparathyroid tetany, the serum calcium is low, phosphate high and phosphatase normal, because the bones are not affected. Thus endocrine disorders may sometimes be distinguished from vitamin-D or calcium malnutrition.

Measurement of the serum iron and the hemoglobin content of blood may reveal iron deficiency. Determination of the serum protein-bound iodine content reflects the status of iodine and thyroid-gland metabolism.

These are some of the chemical tests which have proved helpful in revealing early stages of malnutrition. Present chemical technics are as a rule inadequate to detect nutritional deficiency before functional or anatomic evidence of malnutrition has occurred. However, progress in this direction has been rapid, and certain newer tests seem promising.

4. Functional Changes. When the operation of the body's functions becomes impeded, the patient is apt to become aware of the disturbance, but neither the subject nor the physician may at first recognize the cause. The first two stages, tissue depletion and biochemical disturbances, may have been operating over a considerable period of time. The first symptoms may be characteristic—such as paresthesiae or leg pains in thiamine deficiency, or sore gums in scurvy—but they may be obscure and confusing: for example, dyspnea and edema may at first suggest heart failure rather than its occasional cause, anemia; or a badly disturbed mental state may suggest an organic brain disease rather than pellagra. Aching legs in children have often been called growing pains when they were really the sign of rickets.

Fatigue, lack of energy, faintness, dizziness, a tendency to collapse on prolonged standing, backache, legache, chilliness and numbness were prominent symptoms of functional nature observed among the starved population of Holland during the recent war. Pulse rates often fell to 40 per minute and systolic blood pressures to 80 mm. of mercury. Body temperatures of 95° F. indicated the low vitality.

5. Anatomic Lesions. It is as a rule difficult to separate functional from anatomic changes, and, of course, they are not separate, but really part of the same process. However, functional disturbances may be present for a long time before actual physical manifestations of malnutrition appear. The commonest physical evidence is weight loss. This may at first be slight and slow, but if the cause is not removed and the nutrition corrected, it may progress to emaciation. The fat padding is lost first and later the muscles waste. Pallor may appear; there may be hemorrhages into the skin, edema of the legs, dermatitis, collapse of vertebrae, etc. Certain special types of anatomic examination may help to identify the disorder as nutritional: for example, x-rays of bones for osteoporosis and rickets and study of the number and the type of the red blood cells in anemia. The chief clinical syndromes and the chief anatomic evidences occurring in various deficiency states are given in Table 47.

Occasionally one sees a more or less pure single-deficiency state, but more often the deficiency is multiple and the clinical picture presented is a complex of several deficiency states: e.g., weight loss, occurring with scurvy and rickets, or fatigue and thinness plus anemia, dermatitis, polyneuritis, cheilosis, etc.

Extreme undernutrition may result in death. Less severe degrees of nutritional failure may cause extreme emaciation, loss of practically all body fat, muscle atrophy and extreme weakness that may continue for years. The skin becomes dry and rough, inelastic and wrinkled; the hair becomes dry, brittle and gray, and breaks and falls out; teeth may become carious and may loosen and fall out. The gums may soften, bleed and atrophy. There are signs of pituitary, thyroid and gonadal failure in many extreme cases, so that the final physical appearance is very similar to that seen as the result of complete pituitary failure (Simmonds' disease).

CLINICAL MANIFESTATIONS OF MALNUTRITION

When undernutrition occurs it is apt to be concealed or barely evident in the beginning and even after long periods, if mild in degree. The mild or early states of nutritive failure do not produce any weight loss in many instances, and since weight loss is mistakenly apt to be (to both patient and physician) a sine qua non of undernutrition, the condition is often allowed to go unrecognized. Malnutrition should always be suspected and looked for even in the absence of presenting symptoms or physical signs, whenever the history indicates a negative nutritive balance.

TABLE 47. EFFECTS OF MALNUTRITION

FACTOR LACKING	FOODS LACKING	RESULTS
Calories	Carbohydrates, fats	Thinness, lack of energy, failure to grow
Protein	Eggs, meat, milk, wheat, corn, rice, peas, beans	Muscle wasting, hypoproteinemia, anemia, edema, osteoporosis, fractures of bone
Calcium	Milk	Defective bones and teeth, rickets; osteomalacia and tetany in pregnancy
Vitamin A	Green vegetables, carrots, tomatoes, milk, eggs, butter, fish-liver oils, sweet potatoes	Xerosis of conjunctiva and cornea, nightblindness, follicular hyperkeratosis
Vitamin B_1 (thiamine)	Whole cereals, milk, meat (especially liver and pork)	Beriberi, polyneuritis, anorexia, constipation
Vitamin B_2 (riboflavin)	Milk, eggs, liver, green vegetables	Cheilosis, glossitis, ocular disorders
Nicotinic acid (niacin)	Milk, lean meat, liver	Pellagra, stomatitis, glossitis, dermatitis, mental symptoms
Vitamin B_{12} (cyanocobalamin)	Muscle meats, eggs, wheat germ, liver	Hyperchromic macrocytic anemia
Folic acid	Leafy vegetables, liver	Macrocytic anemia, glossitis, diarrhea
Vitamin C (ascorbic acid)	Oranges, lemons, grapefruit, tomatoes	Scurvy, capillary fragility, hemorrhages, anemia
Vitamin D (calciferol)	Fish, fish-liver oils, milk, eggs, liver (sunlight)	Rickets, osteomalacia
Vitamin K	Green leaves: spinach, cabbage, kale, cauliflower; also egg yolk, liver *plus* exclusion of bile from intestinal tract or intestinal lesions or liver disease	Prothrombin deficiency; hemorrhages resulting from prolonged bleeding and clotting time
Iodine	Fish, iodized salt	Goiter; functional thyroid disorders; cretinism in offspring
Iron	Meat, liver, eggs, beans, prunes, peas, wheat, oatmeal, spinach	Hypochromic anemia, especially during growth, menstruation, pregnancy, blood loss

The term *subclinical* is often applied to the early and mild stages of undernutrition, corresponding to the periods of tissue depletion and biochemical change. Vague ill-health may be the first symptom of which the patient complains, with general malaise and an inability clearly to define the feeling of deviation from good health. Later it may be noted that lack of energy and easy fatigability are present.

As functional changes become more evident, anatomic changes are apt to appear and the physician can often, by physical examination and biochemical tests, identify the several types or single type of malnutrition present. The physician's effort should always, of course, be directed toward early discovery of the nutritive defect, so that irreversible damage may be prevented.

Clinically, probably the commonest nutritional defect is thinness with failure to gain or negative caloric balance with weight loss. Perhaps the disturbance next most frequent is dehydration, with negative salt and water balance, seen often after diarrhea, vomiting, etc., and in diabetes. Probably the most common of all chronic deficiencies is that of iron, producing iron-deficiency anemia. The various vitamin deficiencies are probably next in frequency, and are usually multiple and complex. Hypoproteinemia, the most striking result of a protein deficit, is a late stage; when edema appears, muscle wasting and protein loss have usually been going on for some time.

Each of the effects of malnutrition (see Table 47) is a symptom or pathologic state requiring some analysis and interpretation.

Loss of Weight. Does weight loss always indicate malnutrition? Obviously not, for the weight lost may represent unwanted excess salt and water and may indicate improved health—for example, after digitalization for heart failure. Likewise, weight gain in a thin person is not necessarily a good sign, for if malnutrition and hypoproteinemia were present, the gain may consist of edema fluid.

Weight loss may represent loss of excessive fat and may improve physiologic performance. Obesity may be viewed mistakenly as a sign of good health, but it may mask protein, mineral or vitamin deficiencies. Whenever muscle and other protein structures of the body begin to waste, weight loss is a serious symptom.

Failure to Grow. Children may fail to grow properly when deprived of essential nutrients, the most important of which for growth seem to be protein, calcium, phosphorus, iron, and vitamin D. They also need the calorie-producing foods and other vitamins for optimal growth. However, failure to grow may occur from various other causes, and possible causes that must be especially considered are hypothyroidism and lack of the pituitary growth hormone, as well as chronic infections.

Lack of Energy, Easy Fatigue, Muscular Weakness. Fatigue and weakness are typical signs of malnutrition and, in early or mild cases, often the only signs.

A diet inadequate in calories may bring about an impairment of physical efficiency within a matter of days.[12]

In prolonged semistarvation, muscle strength is diminished greatly and muscle endurance is still more strikingly decreased.[8,29] In severely malnourished persons, energy expenditure above the rate of 300 calories per hour results in collapse from muscular and circulatory-respiratory failure.[21b]

Headache, sweating, vasomotor instability, dizziness, "light-headedness" or faintness may occur.

Many different types of malnutrition first become apparent through these symptoms: lack of calories for energy, protein deficiency, thiamine deficiency, iron lack, anemia, etc.

Fatigue on an organic basis must be distinguished from fatigue on a nervous basis. Fatigue and lethargy are in a high percentage of cases due to *psychic disorders* ranging from the mildest to the most severe. Dissatisfaction with life is apt to result in withdrawal from activities, loss of interest in the routine duties of the day, depression and mental and physical inactivity. If such symptoms progress they may develop into the complete withdrawal of the schizophrenic or of the severe depressive psychoses. More complete treatment of this subject is given in Chapter 25 on Nervousness and Fatigue.

Often the lack of energy is the result of *organic disease* which can in many ways already discussed adversely affect energy metabolism.

When a *nutritive defect* is primarily at fault a history suggestive of factors favoring malnutrition may be obtainable, or a history of weight loss and muscle atrophy or physical evidences of undernutrition may be present.

Nervous Irritability. In addition to the depressive types of psychic disorders mentioned in the preceding paragraph, other psychological effects of malnutrition may occur such as irritable types of nervous tension, gum-chewing or cigarette-smoking of excessive and compulsive degree, emotional instability, etc.

Physicians who prescribe dietary reducing regimens are apt to encounter resentment and hostility among patients as well as "irritability, depression, decrease in self-initiated activity, loss of sexual drive, social introversion," etc., called the "semistarvation neurosis" as seen in a study of 36 young male volunteers.[24]

Delay in Convalescence. The duration of disability following trauma or disease is shortened significantly by adequate nutrition. Negative nitrogen balance and other manifestations of "the catabolic phase" are not considered inevitable now.[20,22]

Poor Wound Healing. An important role in the healing of wounds is played by the state of nutrition. Proteins, ascorbic acid, riboflavin and vitamin A are the nutrients principally involved in the healing of wounds.[22]

Dehydration. Ordinarily dehydration may be detected early; it causes symptoms even when it has been present only a short time. In this respect it differs from carbohydrate, fat, protein, vitamin and mineral malnutrition, in which the symptoms as a rule appear comparatively late. Exhaustion, mental obtundity, dry inelastic loose skin, dry tongue and mouth, soft eyeballs, vascular hypotension, often acidosis and shock, are the usual evidences of extreme dehydration. Profound prostration will soon follow any extensive loss of water and salt that cannot quickly be repaired. For a fuller discussion of these points, see Chapter 30.

Anorexia. The common idea that an undernourished or partially starving person is apt to be ravenous for food is largely erroneous. Usually those persons who exhibit the largest appetites are husky manual workers with great caloric requirements and obese persons who do not need the calories but enjoy eating. A malnourished person as a rule has a *poor appetite* that can often be *improved* by proper nutrition. Persons who have been partially starved find it very difficult to ingest a diet anywhere near normal in the early stages of treatment, and a prolonged period of training is often necessary.

The above considerations are important when the anorexia is the result of malnutrition alone. When the anorexia is caused by an organic or psychic disorder, and the effect of the malnutrition in depressing appetite is an additive factor, it can be seen that correction of anorexia and restoration of normal food intake may be a task of some proportions and ramifications. It is essential that the cause of the anorexia be discovered. It is only when the symptom of anorexia itself is understood in the particular case that the physician can expect to plan a therapeutic program to correct it, and thus to correct the malnutrition. (See Chap. 18.)

Impaired hepatic function has been shown to follow malnutrition. Fatty infiltration of the liver (often with hepatomegaly), develops in starvation, in pellagra, in kwashiorkor, and in many diseases of inanition, such as ulcerative colitis, tuberculosis and alcoholism. In many instances the fatty liver precedes the development of hepatic cirrhosis. Lack of glucose supply with inadequate glycogen storage renders the liver more susceptible to toxins and interferes with liver-cell metabolism. Lack of *choline* when the intake is high in fat and low in protein is known to produce liver damage. *Inositol* acts synergistically with choline in reducing the fat content of fatty livers in experimental animals. Recent experimental evidence indicates that hepatic injury (cirrhosis) results from insufficient protein intake in association with lack of some as yet unidentified vitamin-B factor. A decrease in the protein content of the liver with impairment of liver function has been shown to follow the induction of hypo-albuminemia in dogs by dietary means.

Protein Deficiency. Severe degrees of loss of body protein may occur with no decrease in the circulating blood proteins. Protein deficiency is not synonymous with hypoproteinemia. By the time a definite fall in the serum albumin has occurred there has been extreme depletion of tissue protein. At present there is no way of measuring the various milder and intermediate stages of protein deficiency. It is evident that the integrity of the body-tissue proteins is actually much more important than the serum-protein level. Weight loss and depletion of the body's fat stores is usually apparent before protein loss. In estimating the degree of protein deficit present one must depend upon the indirect evidence obtained by studying the fate of protein ingested or injected into the body. Such studies have yielded data indicating that a tremendous decrease in tissue protein is always present before the protein deficit is reflected in a fall in the circulating protein in the blood. A fall of about 30 Gm. in tissue proteins must take place before serum proteins decrease 1 Gm.

One must consider not only the total quantity of protein but its quality. Protein deficiency may occur even in the presence of the usually adequate intake of one gram or more per kilogram of body weight, if the protein is poor in certain essential amino acids. Protein to be adequate in all respects for body needs must furnish all the essential amino acids. To ensure this, it is recommended that proteins derived from *animal sources* constitute at least 65 per cent of the total protein intake. When cereal proteins furnish a large part of the protein intake, protein synthesis may be inadequate, since certain amino acids (lysine, etc.) may be lacking. When sufficient calories are supplied to provide for energy needs, the usually recommended daily allowance of one gram per kilogram of body weight allows a safety margin of almost 100 per cent, if the proteins are of good quality.

Consideration of protein deficiencies as they may produce or affect clinical conditions is important in various normal or physiologic states and in certain pathologic or disease conditions (Table 48).

The causes of protein deficiency, as far as the mechanism is concerned, are the same as for the other nutrients: inadequate intake (either qualitatively or quantitatively); inadequate digestion, absorption or utilization, increased metabolism and excessive excretion or loss. However, it is of considerable importance to remember certain special features of protein metabolism:

TABLE 48. CONDITIONS AFFECTING AND
AFFECTED BY PROTEIN METABOLISM

Physiologic
  Growth
    Muscle and tissue formation
    Bone formation
    Blood formation
  Pregnancy
  Lactation
  Appetite and hunger
  Absorption of other nutrients
  Immunity and resistance
Pathologic
  Fatigue
  Convalescence
  Wound healing
  Edema
  Obesity
  Impaired gastrointestinal absorption
  Wasting diseases
  Liver disease
  Kidney disease

liver disease may lead to inadequate synthesis of plasma protein; *kidney disease* may result in severe protein loss (albuminuria), while protein losses after wounds and burns and from hemorrhage, peritonitis or ascites may be great.

Protein deficiency is apt to result in disorders of *fluid transport* through development of hypoalbuminemia, with resultant *edema,* and sometimes *ascites.*

It must not be forgotten that *hemoglobin* requires protein as well as iron for its manufacture, and that either iron or protein deficiency or both may cause anemia.

A good protein matrix is necessary to build and maintain *bone.* Adequate bone growth in children requires not only calcium, phosphorus and vitamin D, but proper protein. In the aged, osteoporosis may occur with deformity and fractures resulting from protein loss from the bone matrix. In Cushing's syndrome, or after prolonged administration of corticosteroids, protein is lost as well as calcium, and the bones become fragile.

The widespread misconception that protein foods are *always* harmful in kidney disease must be combated, for often recovery is possible only after restoration of a positive protein balance.

Proteins are of great importance in *defense against infection* and bacterial invasion. Recent investigations in acquired immunity suggest that antibody production is a phase of protein metabolism and that protein deficiency may impair the production of *antibodies,* with resultant loss of acquired immunity and increase in the susceptibility to infection. Protein deficiency impairs *phagocyte* formation also. It appears that protein is likewise necessary for the production of toxins, antitoxins and antigens. Hypoproteinemia may develop rapidly in overwhelming infections and in shock, but the mechanism of its development is not understood.

KWASHIORKOR is the name applied to a syndrome occurring primarily in tropical and subtropical areas, chiefly in children of the postweaning period (ages 1 to 3 years), in underprivileged populations, and caused by protein deficiency. Often it occurs as the child is deprived of maternal milk and is given almost a pure carbohydrate diet, which may be quite adequate in calories. The nutritive defect appears to be primarily a deficiency of protein foods, imbalance of amino acids, and lack of accessory food factors associated with protein metabolism. Classically one finds growth failure, mental changes (apathy and irritability), weakness and atrophy of skeletal muscles, edema, dermatoses, hair loss and depigmentation, gastrointestinal symptoms (anorexia, vomiting and diarrhea), anemia and hypoalbuminemia. Adult residues include hepatic cirrhosis and a high incidence of primary hepatoma.[38]

When an extreme stage of protein deficiency is reached as the result of any process causing a negative protein balance, and hypoproteinemia, anemia and edema are present, the need for prompt analysis of the symptoms, discovery of the cause and reversal of the pathologic processes is obvious. Less obvious and more recently discovered indications for establishment of a highly positive protein balance include acute as well as chronic *liver disease*. The tendency to hypoalbuminemia in cirrhosis of the liver has long been recognized, but only recently has attention been called to the fact that high amounts of protein as well as of carbohydrate are of value in protecting liver cells against noxious agents. Such measures have proved helpful in hepatitis of various sorts, including infectious hepatitis, toxic hepatitis and subacute yellow atrophy. The sulfur-containing amino acids *methionine* and *cystine* appear to be the protein components of greatest importance in protecting the liver from toxic hepatitis.

Choline, inositol, and certain other fractions of the vitamin B complex, as well as protein, have been shown to be important in the preservation of normal liver structure and function.

IN SURGICAL CONDITIONS, attention to the protein supply is imperative because injuries and wounds cause negative balance and intake is usually greatly limited. Wound healing is adversely affected by protein deficiency.

HYPOPROTEINEMIA may be masked or concealed under two specific circumstances especially: (1) in *dehydration,* the initial serum protein determination may be normal, but the level may fall as dilution occurs when normal hydration is established, and (2) in certain conditions the rise in *serum globulin* may be sufficient to mask the fall in serum albumin, if total protein alone is measured. The term *hypoalbuminemia* is preferable to hypoproteinemia, since it is the albumin fraction that is decreased.

Because of its small molecular size, albumin is responsible for the major part of the osmotic tension of the serum proteins under ordinary conditions. The osmotic tension exerted normally by serum albumin is about five times that of serum globulin. Often the rise in serum globulin may equal or exceed the fall in serum albumin, so total protein values may be misleading. In the study of edema as related to nutritional disorders, the serum albumin level is the important factor.

Mineral Deficiencies. Mineral deficits occur as the result of a variety of abnormal conditions which may be grouped in three general classes:

1. SEVERE UNDERNUTRITION, e.g., loss of K, Mg, Fe, P and Ca from tissues, of Na, Cl and water from the extracellular fluids; deficient intake, or excessive losses, as in sweating, polyuria, vomiting, diarrhea, etc.

2. RENAL DISEASE. In certain types of renal disease the kidneys lose much of their ability to conserve the chief base of the blood plasma and interstitial fluids, sodium; chloride and potassium losses may also occur.

3. HORMONAL DISORDERS, e.g., Ca and P loss in hyperparathyroidism; Na and Cl loss in adrenocortical deficiency; Na, Cl, K losses in diabetes mellitus.

SODIUM, CHLORIDE AND POTASSIUM. For discussion of water, sodium, chloride and potassium metabolism and manifestations of their derangements, see Chapters 30 (Dehydration) and 31 (Edema).

The diet is more likely to be deficient in calcium than in any other mineral element. Mineral deficiencies most frequently seen clinically are those of calcium, phosphorus, iodine or iron. These minerals deserve special discussion because of the frequency and importance of the clinical manifestations associated with their lack or loss.

CALCIUM AND PHOSPHORUS deficit in adults may exist for years with gradually developing demineralization of the bones that finally may reach attention only after a vertebra has collapsed or some other bone has been fractured.

When the fault lies in deficient intake of calcium, phosphorus or vitamin D in growing children, rickets results; weakening of adult bones on the same pathologic basis results in the condition of poor calcification known as *osteomalacia*. If the calcium intake of the pregnant woman is inadequate, calcium for the fetal skeleton is withdrawn from her bones and osteomalacia may result. Calcium and vitamin D deprivation is a common cause of hypocalcemic tetany during infancy, pregnancy and lactation. *Osteoporosis* is the term used to describe the poor calcification and diminished strength of bony structures resulting from a defect in the formation of the bone matrix. When protein derangement occurs (disuse, malnutrition, old age, Cushing's syndrome, etc.) and the bone matrix is not normally formed or is depleted, calcification of bone may not proceed normally, or calcium and phosphorus may actually be lost from the bones and from the body, even when the intake of calcium, phosphorus and vitamin D is normal. When both mineral and protein deficiencies are present, *osteomalacia* plus *osteoporosis* may be present (e.g., senile bone changes with pathologic fractures are commonest in persons who have chronic deficits in Ca and P and vitamin D). X-ray evidence usually shows that the anatomic process was far advanced before symptoms occurred. Occasionally aching pain in the bones may be present without fracture or malformation of the bones. A history of dislike for milk (usually with overindulgence in coffee) should suggest possible calcium deficiency. Large amounts of calcium and phosphorus are necessary for construction of the growing skeleton of children. In childhood, calcium and phos-

phorus deficit may be manifested in poor growth as well as in the deformities of rickets and in poor teeth.

The calcium or phosphorus depletion (usually both) may be caused by inadequate intake of these minerals and of vitamin D, or by losses due to pregnancy, lactation, immobilization (as in casts), hyperthyroidism or hyperparathyroidism, impaired bile secretion, chronic diarrhea (sprue and similar diseases). Hypocalcemia and osteomalacia may result from steatorrhea. Rarely is hypocalcemia due to a true nutritional calcium deficiency in adults, although low calcium intake and vitamin-D lack cause hypocalcemia and tetany in children. The level of serum calcium is primarily under the control of the parathyroid hormone. Serum calcium tends to remain normal even when intake of calcium is low and bones are much depleted of calcium.

The manifestations of calcium deficiency are evident in aberrations from normal in its control over blood clotting, the rate and the rhythm of the heart beat, the state of neuromuscular transmission of impulses and the permeability of membranes, as well as in structural abnormalities in bones and in teeth. For example, hypocalcemia may so alter membrane permeability that the volume and the pressure of the cerebrospinal fluid rise and papilledema and epileptiform convulsions occur.

IRON deficiency in men is uncommon, while it is relatively frequent in women and in children. This is because iron is essentially a "one-way substance" that after absorption is retained and avidly conserved; upon release from cells it is stored or utilized again and again for formation of hemoglobin.[10]

If iron for hemoglobin formation is not available in adequate quantities, the maturation of red blood cells is retarded, the number released from the bone marrow is subnormal, and each red cell has a subnormal hemoglobin content. The characteristic manifestation of iron deficiency is hypochromic, microcytic anemia, primarily a lack of hemoglobin, although the red blood cells are often reduced in number. Accompanying the anemia there may be glossitis; cheilosis; esophagitis and indigestion with the Plummer-Vinson syndrome; brittle, flat or spoon-shaped fingernails (koilonychia); and, with very low hemoglobin, such symptoms as pallor, weakness, fatigue, dyspnea and edema.

The normal adult human absorbs an average of 5 to 10 per cent of iron from foods; with a dietary intake of 12 to 15 mg. absorption amounts to approximately 0.6 to 1.5 mg. daily. The amount of iron utilized for hemoglobin synthesis per day is about 20 to 25 mg. The normal adult catabolizes enough hemoglobin per day to release 20 to 25 mg. of iron. Only about 5 per cent is excreted in feces, urine, sweat, cells desquamated from the skin, etc., so that iron lost from the body totals about 1 mg. daily on the average and daily absorption tends to replace daily loss: the body tends to remain in iron balance. When iron deficiency is present there is normally greater absorption (up to 20 per cent or more) of the dietary intake, and a positive iron balance may persist until body stores are replenished.

The body of a normal adult contains approximately 2.5 to 5.5 Gm. of iron, depending largely upon the body weight and the circulating mass of hemoglobin. About 50 to 60 per cent of this total is found in hemoglobin, about 10 to 20 per cent in myoglobin; the important cellular enzyme portion is relatively small; the remainder is stored chiefly in organs rich in reticuloendothelial cells (liver, spleen, bone marrow).[34]

At birth the child receives from the mother a somatic inheritance of about 375 mg. Children may not take in enough iron during the period of growth while the needs for iron are increasing, and thus anemia may develop. Women, because of blood loss at menstruation and increased demands and loss with pregnancy and childbirth, may have at times or chronically a *negative iron balance* with resultant anemia. The annual loss through menstruation averages about 300 mg. Iron ingested is absorbed or eliminated in the stools; it is not excreted in the usual sense. Very small amounts are eliminated in the urine. These facts make it evident that iron deficiency in adult males means blood loss, whereas in women or children the intake may not be sufficient to balance the usual or increased demands.[5b]

In chronic infections, hypoferremia precedes the anemia, which is caused by impaired hemoglobin formation.[13]

IODINE intake is the principal factor determining the iodine content of the thyroid gland, the principal storehouse for iodine. The requirement for iodine is small, about 0.002 mg. daily per Kg. body weight or a total of 0.1 mg. to 0.3 mg. daily for the adult. Iodized salt is needed in many areas to insure such supply. Requirements for iodine are increased in adolescence and pregnancy.

Goiter (enlargement of the thyroid gland) results from thyroid hyperplasia due to iodine deficiency. The most urgent reason for stressing iodine as a preventive measure is not the goiter which may occur in the affected woman but the profound thyroid deficit which may result in her offspring. Cretinism occurs in the infant when the pregnant woman is so depleted of iodine that none is available for development of the thyroid of the fetus.

A normal adult thyroid gland weighs about 25 Gm. and contains 8 to 10 mg. of iodine. Normally the thyroid gland maintains an iodine concentration of about 40 mg. per 100 grams. When this concentration falls below 10 mg. per 100 grams, hyperplasia ensues and goiter may develop, with or without various types of functional thyroid disturbance (hyperthyroidism or hypothyroidism). Iodine is an important and necessary constituent of the thyroid hormone, and is thus of fundamental importance in body growth and function, exercising constant control over the rate of metabolism in all tissues.

Vitamin Deficiencies. VITAMIN A is of great nutritional importance as a growth factor. It acts as an important nutritive element in the metabolism of epithelial tissues. The normal epithelium atrophies in vitamin-A deficiency and is replaced by proliferating basal cells that become keratinized. Vitamin A is necessary in the regeneration of visual purple in the retina.

Clinical manifestations of vitamin-A deficiency are chiefly, therefore, failure to grow, xerophthalmia, dermatosis and night blindness. The precursors of vitamin A are all the carotenoid pigments commonly called carotene. The greatest source of vitamin A is food containing carotene. The skin conditions known as keratosis pilaris, ichthyosis, follicularis, etc., are probably the same or closely related, and are due to vitamin-A lack. The presence of such hyperkeratosis, usually with small pustules, especially on the extensor surfaces of the arms and legs, is especially suggestive.

THE VITAMINS OF THE B COMPLEX have such varied and important functions and the specific indications of their lack have been so fully treated elsewhere that only the chief clinical manifestations that will lead to the suspicion of nutritive failure will be recited here.

Vitamin B₁ (thiamine) exerts an important influence in carbohydrate metabolism because it is essential for the oxidation of the intermediate metabolite, pyruvic acid. Since the brain and the nerves subsist primarily upon carbohydrate, profound disturbance of cerebral and peripheral nervous-tissue function is caused by thiamine lack. Severe deficiency results in beriberi, neuritis and cardiovascular dysfunction. Anorexia is a very early and suggestive sign, also ill-defined fatigue, mental depression, irritability, and peculiar aches and paresthesiae in the legs. Thiamine requirement increases greatly with acceleration of metabolism, especially of carbohydrate.

Vitamin B₂ (riboflavin) is an important constituent of living animal cells. It enters into the formation of the prosthetic groups of several flavoprotein enzymes. Mammalian tissues have a number of different flavoprotein enzyme systems each containing a specific protein (apoenzyme) and a riboflavin-containing prosthetic group (coenzyme). These enzymes are essential in oxidative systems in living cells; thus it is axiomatic that cellular growth cannot evolve in the absence of riboflavin. Manifestations suggestive of riboflavin deficiency are cheilosis (maceration in each

angle of the mouth, reddening of the lips along the line of closure, and thin, shiny, denuded mucosa); scaly, greasy desquamation in the nasolabial folds; corneal vascularization, conjunctivitis and glossitis. The requirement is 2 to 3 mg. daily.

Nicotinic acid deficiency is manifested by the lesions characteristic of pellagra: dermatitis, glossitis and stomatitis, and gastrointestinal disorders with diarrhea. The mental symptoms of pellagra may be due partly to nicotinic-acid deficiency and partly to thiamine deficiency. The human requirement for nicotinic acid is difficult to determine because part of the daily needs can be met by metabolic conversion in the tissues from the amino acid tryptophan. Deficiencies of thiamine, of riboflavin, or of pyridoxine may lead to impaired formation of nicotinic acid. The requirement is 10 to 20 mg. daily.

Vitamin B₆ (pyridoxine) is active in the body in the form of phosphorylated pyridoxal or pyridoxamine. As such, the vitamin serves as a prosthetic group in enzyme systems which are of fundamental importance in the metabolism of amino acids. In man seborrhealike skin lesions about the eyes, the nose and the mouth accompanied by glossitis and stomatitis can be produced within a few weeks by feeding a diet poor in B-complex plus daily doses of the vitamin-antagonist desoxypyridoxine.[19] Between 1951 and 1953 a number of infants in the United States developed hyperirritability and convulsions from taking a commercially distributed feeding formula which proved to be deficient in pyridoxine.[6,18] The vitamin is widely available in natural foods, and the requirement is about 1 to 2 mg. daily.

VITAMIN C (ascorbic acid) is necessary for the normal development and maintenance of intercellular cement substance, ground substance and collagen in connective-tissue supporting structures, in bone matrix, tendons and cartilage, and in the smaller blood vessels. It is important in the formation of teeth and bones. It occupies an important position in cellular respiration. Vitamin-C lack retards wound healing. The needs for ascorbic acid are greatly increased in febrile diseases, hyperthyroidism and other states of accelerated metabolism. Abundant vitamin C seems to be necessary at the normoblast stage of erythrocyte development. Scurvy is now relatively rare, but less severe subclinical forms of ascorbic-acid deficiency with easy bruising, capillary fragility, appearance of petechiae, etc., are not uncommon.

Ascorbic acid facilitates the absorption of iron from the intestinal tract. The conversion of folic acid to the metabolically active form, folinic acid, requires ascorbic acid. From observations made in studies on premature and young infants, vitamin C also appears to be related to the metabolism of the two amino acids tyrosine and phenylalanine.

During infections such as tuberculosis, pneumonia, rheumatic fever, etc., additions above a normal intake are required to maintain desirable tissue levels. It seems clear that ascorbic acid is important in providing resistance to infections. An intake of 10 to 20 mg. of ascorbic acid is sufficient to protect an adult from developing overt evidence of scurvy, but higher intake is advisable to maintain desirable tissue and plasma ascorbic acid levels. The daily intakes recommended by the National Research Council (see Table 46) are 30 to 60 mg. for infants and children, 75 to 100 mg. for adolescents, 75 mg. for adults, and 100 to 150 mg. during pregnancy and lactation. These standards are based on observations that such requirements are necessary to maintain tissue stores near saturation and to hold plasma fasting levels near 1.0 mg. per ml.[41,42]

VITAMIN D is essential in promoting calcium and phosphorus absorption and normal bone development, and in preventing osteomalacia and rickets. When administered in adequate amounts with sufficient ingested calcium, it is effective in treating hypocalcemia, will elevate serum calcium and prevent tetany. Aching limbs, poor growth and the typical deformities of rickets are the characteristic signs of vitamin-D deficit in childhood which should be prevented or detected earlier. When lack of vitamin D plus calcium deficiency is severe and prolonged in adults, bone deformities

and pathologic fractures characteristic of osteomalacia may result. Dental growth and maintenance of sound teeth depend, among other factors, upon adequate supplies of D.

In pregnancy and lactation the vitamin-D requirements are increased, and in these states special attention to the supply of this vitamin and of adequate calcium and phosphorus is necessary.

VITAMIN K deficiency is manifested as a tendency to hemorrhage in consequence of a lowered prothrombin content of the blood. Vitamin K is essential for the maintenance of prothrombin in the blood plasma. Prothrombin, a part of the plasma-protein complex, is one of the components of the blood which is necessary for proper coagulation. It is apparently produced in the liver. If the liver is removed or is severely damaged, the concentration of prothrombin in the blood decreases.

In the absence of vitamin K, the prothrombin level falls even if the liver is intact. Under normal conditions there are two sources of vitamin K. Vitamin K_1 is ingested with the food: since it is very widely distributed and only minimal amounts are required, dietary deficiency is rare. A second source is that supplied by the bacterial flora in the intestinal tract. Many bacteria, including members of the normal intestinal flora, produce vitamin K_2. These naturally occurring compounds are fat-soluble. In order for vitamin K to be properly absorbed (as with other fat-soluble vitamins such as A and D), it is necessary that the amount of bile in the intestine be adequate, that the intestinal absorptive surface be sufficient, and that the intestinal contents do not pass too rapidly.[40,41,42]

Any condition which seriously interferes with intestinal absorption may be a cause of vitamin K deficiency. However, since the requirement of the vitamin is so small, and since prothrombin activity usually must be reduced to less than one-third of normal before a bleeding tendency becomes manifest, impaired absorption alone seldom causes bleeding unless bile salts are absent from the bowel.

If there is faulty absorption plus impaired liver function, the effect in lowering prothrombin activity is additive. Some degree of liver deficiency is common in biliary tract disease. Often surgery is necessary in such conditions. Preoperative determination of prothrombin activity is important to prevent postoperative bleeding. Treatment with vitamin K may be indicated.

When bleeding results from low plasma prothrombin activity, the hemorrhage usually occurs at a site of local trauma due to accidental injury, surgery, or pre-existing disease. Ecchymoses into the skin are apt to occur first, rather than the petechiae that occur as initial signs of vitamin C deficiency. Vitamin K is essential in facilitating prothrombin formation by the liver, but the vitamin does not make up part of the prothrombin molecule. Bile salts are not absolutely essential to vitamin-K absorption, but greatly aid it. Only small amounts of the vitamin are stored, and deficiency may be apparent in one week after its intake or absorption ceases. It is believed that the normal human adult need not take this vitamin in his diet since it is synthesized by bacteria in the intestine. The facts that clinical evidence of avitaminosis K are found in the newborn (before the bacterial flora becomes established) and in adults when there is destruction of intestinal organisms by antibiotic or sulfonamides are in consonance with this view.

Prothrombin deficiency occurs in many conditions with impaired liver function, with biliary fistulas, biliary obstruction (obstructive jaundice), sprue, steatorrhea, ulcerative colitis, during severe infections, as a toxic effect of certain drugs (sulfonamides, salicylates).

Hemorrhagic disease of the newborn and the bleeding occurring with obstructive jaundice (inadequate absorption of the fat-soluble vitamin K) may be relieved or prevented with vitamin K.

When vitamin K is given in the fat-soluble form (menadione), in the presence of obstructive jaundice or a biliary fistula, bile salts should also be given to facilitate its absorption. Water-soluble quinones with vitamin K activity are available to use if fat absorption is impaired.

The vitamin may be given prophylactically to the mother before delivery or to babies during the first week of life to prevent prothrombin deficiency in the newborn.

When liver parenchymal involvement prevents utilization of vitamin K in the formation of prothrombin, the hypoprothrombinemia may be irreversible if the liver damage cannot be repaired.

OTHER B-COMPLEX NUTRITIONAL FACTORS

Vitamin B$_{12}$ (Cyanocobalamin). This red, crystalline compound containing cobalt, phosphorus and nitrogen is the "EMF" (erythrocyte maturation factor) or the "extrinsic factor." Classic addisonian pernicious anemia is a *conditioned deficiency disease* caused by lack of a specific substance secreted by the normal gastric mucosa known as the "intrinsic factor" of Castle. Since the extrinsic and the intrinsic factors are ineffective when either is given alone in pernicious anemia, Castle originally postulated that the two interacted in some way to produce the antianemia factor which is present in liver. This view is untenable now that cyanocobalamin is known to be both the extrinsic factor and the liver principle.[35]

Absorption of B$_{12}$ is facilitated by intrinsic factor, but is limited even in normal persons. The preferred route for administration of cyanocobalamin is intramuscular since huge doses (over 100 times as much) are required orally unless it is combined with a source of intrinsic factor. Absorption is mainly from the ileum. Ability to absorb B$_{12}$ is decreased by extensive gastro-intestinal resections, bowel anastomoses, idiopathic steatorrhea, etc., and in the elderly. The vitamin occurs almost exclusively in foods of animal origin (especially kidney, liver, muscle meats and milk) in the form of a protein complex. Proteolytic enzymes release it in the upper gastrointestinal tract. It is synthesized by many bacteria, among which *Streptomyces griseus*, *Streptomyces aureofaciens* and *Bacillus subtilis* are commercial sources. Herbivorous animals obtain B$_{12}$ from micro-organisms in the rumen and it is probable that these organisms are the main sources of the vitamin in animal tissues. Omnivorous animals like man ingest vitamin B_{12} in foods of animal origin (meat, milk, eggs, cheese).

Vitamin B_{12} is highly effective in the treatment of pernicious anemia, producing satisfactory clinical and hematologic response and preventing the progress of neurologic lesions. It is thus obviously a nutritive factor of importance, but its place in normal nutrition is uncertain.

In addisonian pernicious anemia, the gastric mucosal atrophy is probably due to an hereditary genetic defect. *Total gastrectomy, gastritis, gastric cancer,* etc., operate through a similar mechanism in producing macrocytic anemia in some instances of these conditions. Occasionally in *pregnancy*, gastric acidity and intrinsic factor secretion are progressively inhibited until after delivery. The presence of the broad fish tapeworm in the upper intestine in some way interferes with the action of intrinsic factor sufficiently, in persons with apparently minimal amounts of this enzyme, to produce macrocytic anemia.

Extreme and prolonged B_{12} deficiency produces the clinical picture of pernicious anemia, the manifestations usually appearing in this order.[28] (1) Inflammation, followed by atrophy of tongue, oral mucosa and mucous membranes of the gastrointestinal tract. (2) Macrocytic anemia with megaloblastic bone marrow. The red cells are large and have only about half the normal life (60 days instead of 120). Therefore serum bilirubin is elevated somewhat. White cells and platelets are formed at slow rates. (3) Degeneration of the peripheral nerves, the posterior and the lateral columns of the spinal cord, the cerebrum and the cerebellum.

Nutritional Macrocytic Anemia. Diets extremely low in animal protein may directly fail to provide sufficient vitamin B_{12}. Patients with nutritional macrocytic anemia do not respond to B_{12} unless the bone marrow is megaloblastic. In the United States inadequate intake is rare as a cause of macrocytic anemia; faulty absorption and assimilation may occur with intestinal dysfunctions. The deficit in nutritional macrocytic anemia is more often *folic acid de-*

ficiency than B_{12} deficiency and often there is associated lack of *ascorbic acid.*

Pernicious and related macrocytic anemias exhibit low levels of serum vitamin B_{12} and respond to the administration of B_{12} itself or to B_{12} in the form of highly refined liver extract.[6] Combined system disease of the spinal cord is virtually confined to patients with achylia gastrica. Lingual and gastrointestinal disturbances are common to all of the macrocytic anemias, but vary in severity in different clinical syndromes. The blood and the bone marrow pictures overlap completely. When the anemia results from inadequate intake or intestinal dysfunction, various other evidences of associated or secondary nutritional disorders are apt to be present. In pernicious anemia, the diet is not ordinarily strikingly defective until the anemia is severe; the nutritive derangement is then the result of the illness, not its cause.

Folic Acid. The terms *pteroylglutamates* and *folic acid* are currently applied to a group of compounds included among the B-complex factors. Knowledge of the pteroylglutamate content of foods is very incomplete, but it is known that fresh green leafy vegetables, cauliflower, kidney and liver are rich sources.

Ascorbic acid facilitates the conversion of folic acid to folinic acid, its metabolically active form. Studies of the growth requirements of bacteria and of the histochemical changes in man and animals resulting from deficiencies of vitamin B_{12} or of folic acid reveal that profound and widespread derangements of nucleic acid metabolism are involved. The rapidly dividing cells of the body are among the first affected: the production of red cells and leucocytes in the bone marrow; the reproduction of the cells of the intestinal mucosa. Both folic acid and B_{12} are concerned with early stages of the synthesis of purines and pyrimidines, which together with ribose sugars and phosphoric acid, form the master molecules of both nuclear deoxyribonucleic acid (DNA) and cytoplasmic ribonucleic acid (RNA).[35]

Folic acid deficiency can be both a cause and a result of intestinal malabsorption. When the condition is an acquired deficiency disease, as in tropical sprue, therapy with folic acid may reverse the atrophic changes in the small intestine. When the defect is primary in the intestine, as seems to be the case in celiac disease, folic acid fails to correct the intestinal disorder, but a gluten-free diet may be successful. See the discussion earlier in this chapter on the malabsorption syndrome. Intestinal resections, strictures and blind loops cause loss of absorptive surface and there may also be detrimental effects exerted by bacterial growth through competing for folic acid or by causing injury to the absorptive surface of the intestine. Vitamin B_{12}, fats, calcium, iron, etc. may also be poorly absorbed. Folic acid, unlike B_{12}, is readily absorbed under normal conditions, from the upper part of the small intestine.

Maternal and infantile deficiencies of folic acid probably result from increased demand when intake is inadequate. In liver cirrhosis the metabolic conversion of folic to folinic acid may be disturbed.

Folic acid appears to be necessary for the transformation of megaloblasts into red blood cells; it is not, however, the maturation factor present in liver extract, nor is it the extrinsic factor. Folic acid usually causes remission in pernicious anemia, but response may be incomplete and relapse may occur during treatment; furthermore, neurologic lesions may progress during therapy. On the other hand, folic acid produces a satisfactory remission in sprue, tropical macrocytic anemia, "refractory megaloblastic anemia," the macrocytic anemia occurring in some cases of hepatic cirrhosis, the macrocytic anemia of pregnancy, and the megaloblastic anemia of infancy.

Some work indicates that B_{12} may be necessary to make available the naturally occurring pteroylglutamates. The role of folic acid in human nutrition needs much further clarification.

Choline, a constituent of lecithin, occurs in many foods, both animal and vegetable: liver, heart, kidney, sweetbreads, brain, egg yolk, nuts, roots and green leafy vegetables.

Choline is an essential component of acetylcholine and of the phospholipids.

With methionine, cystine and creatine, it performs an important function in the general metabolic process of transmethylation. It promotes growth, facilitates fat transport, aids protein metabolism, and indirectly is important in promoting normal carbohydrate metabolism. Lack of choline produces in certain experimental animals liver changes similar to Laennec's cirrhosis in man. Choline has been used with favorable results in treating human hepatic cirrhosis, presumably by mobilization of fatty acids from the excess fat deposits in the liver. Its exact position in human nutrition has not yet been determined.

Inositol. A number of studies indicate that inositol acts synergistically with choline in reducing abnormal hepatic fat deposits in experimental animals. In view of its lipotropic activity, it is probably significant that inositol is a constituent of certain phospholipids. Little is known of the nutritional value of inositol in man.

In diabetes mellitus inositol excretion in the urine is high. Apparently it competes with glucose for resorption by the renal tubular cells. In diabetes mellitus and in healthy persons during glycosuria from intravenous infusions of glucose, the reabsorption mechanism is inhibited and large amounts of inositol appear in the urine.[7b] Whether this is harmful is not known. These facts and its high content in heart muscle suggest that it may play a role in human nutrition.

Vitamins: Relationship of Adequate vs. Supernormal Intake to Health and Vigor. There is no evidence to support the view that a *higher than adequate normal* intake of any or all vitamins will improve health or energy production or will facilitate growth or resistance to infection. However, when one or more vitamin deficiencies exist the effect of supplying the factors lacking is strikingly beneficial.

Hypervitaminosis. Not only is excessive vitamin intake valueless in enhancing health, but it may cause serious deleterious effects. Such results from vitamin overdosage have been reported in human beings taking massive amounts of vitamins A or D.

Hypervitaminosis A has caused hard,

tender lumps in the extremities and cortical thickening of underlying bones. Additional findings in some patients include fissures of the lips, loss of hair, dry skin, jaundice and hepatomegaly.

Hypervitaminosis D causes bone resorption and metastatic calcification occurs. There is hypercalcemia, hyperphosphatemia, and hypercalciuria. Calcium is deposited in the kidneys especially, as nephrocalcinosis or renal lithiasis; renal failure with uremia may result.

MALNUTRITION AS CAUSE OF DEATH

Death from malnutrition may be manifest, or obscure. That is, when the patient has obviously been suffering from a severe nutritive deficit (perhaps not susceptible of correction, such as anorexia or vomiting from carcinoma of the stomach), it is sometimes impossible to avoid death from starvation, and its cause is clearly apparent. However, the starvation may not be apparent when the cause is not so obvious: for example, in protein deficiency due to chronic nephritis, or in cerebral and peripheral nerve disturbance due to thiamine deficiency. When attention is directed primarily to only one aspect of a problem—for example, the surgical removal of a toxic goiter—death may occur because of failure to recognize and provide for the associated nutritional disturbances. The physician's responsibility consists in recognizing the nutritional aspects of all types of disease and in perceiving the abnormal practices and situations that may lead to malnutrition, so that these factors may be corrected before nutritive defects occur.

SUMMARY

The early detection of the processes leading to weight loss and undernutrition is a task of paramount importance to the physician, the nutritionist and the public-health officer. In analyzing and interpreting the symptoms indicative of malnutrition, the physician has a complex problem, since the symptoms often suggest other etiologies and frequently are vague and, as a rule, multiple in origin, due to the lack of several nutrients. An understanding of the influ-

ences leading to nutritive failure, plus knowledge of the essential nutrients and of the indications of their lack, as discussed in this chapter, will prepare the physician to appreciate the significance of symptoms due to malnutrition.

REFERENCES

1. Albanese, A.: Protein and amino acid requirements of man, *in* Albanese, A., *ed.:* Protein and Amino Acid Requirements of Mammals, New York, Acad. Press, 1950.
2. Babcock, M., et al.: Nutritional status of industrial workers, Milbank Mem. Fund Quart. 32:323, 1954.
3. Brobeck, J. R.: Physiology of hunger, appetite and satiety, *in* Wohl, M. G., and Goodhart, R. S., *eds.:* Modern Nutrition in Health and Disease, Philadelphia, Lea & Febiger, 1960.
4. Brosin, H. W.: The psychology of appetite, *in* Wohl, M. G., and Goodhart, R. S., *eds.:* Modern Nutrition in Health and Disease, Philadelphia, Lea & Febiger, 1960.
5a. Burger, G. C. E., Sandstead, H. R., and Drummond, J.: Starvation in western Holland: 1945, Lancet 2:282, 1945.
5b. Cartwright, G., et al.: Symposium on Nutritional Aspects of Blood Formation, New York, National Vitamin Foundation, 1955.
6. Coursin, D. B.: Convulsive seizures in infants with pyridoxine-deficient diets, J.A.M.A. 154:406, 1954.
7. Daughaday, W., and Larner, J.: The renal excretion of inositol in normal and diabetic human beings, J. Clin. Invest. 33:326, 1954.
8. Davidson, C. S., et al.: A nutritional survey of starvation in a group of young men, J. Lab. & Clin. Med. 31:721, 1946.
9. Ershoff, B. H.: Nutrition and the anterior pituitary, Vitamins & Hormones 10:79, 1952.
10. Finch, C. A., et al.: Iron metabolism: The pathophysiology of iron storage, Blood 5:983, 1950.
11. Geiger, E.: Digestion, absorption and metabolism of protein, *in* Wohl, M. G., and Goodhart, R. S., *eds.:* Modern Nutrition in Health and Disease, Philadelphia, Lea & Febiger, 1960.
12. Keys, A., Brozek, J., et al.: The Biology of Human Starvation, Minneapolis, Univ. of Minn., 1950.
13. Krammer, A., Cartwright, G. E., and Wintrobe, M. M.: The anemia of infection, Blood 9:183-188, 1954.
14. Lusk, G.: Physiological effects of undernutrition, Physiol. Rev. 1:523, 1921.

15. MacBryde, C. M., and Elman, R.: Nutritional Requirements in Acute and Chronic Disease, Advances in Internal Medicine, New York, Interscience, 1946.

16. MacBryde, C. M.: Aging, malnutrition and hormones, J. Clin. Nutrition 1:469, 1953.

17. McLester, J. S., and Darby, W. J.: Nutrition and Diet in Health and Disease, Philadelphia, Saunders, 1952.

18. Molony, C. J., and Parmelee, A. H.: Convulsions in young infants from B_6 deficiency, J.A.M.A. 154:405, 1954.

19. Mueller, J. F., and Vilter, R. W.: Pyridoxine deficiency in human beings, J. Clin. Invest. 29:193-201, 1950.

20. Pareira, M., Conrad, E., Hicks, W., and Elman, R.: Therapeutic nutrition with tube feeding, J.A.M.A. 156:810-816, 1954.

21a. Perloff, W., et al.: The starvation state and functional hypopituitarism, J.A.M.A. 155:1307-1313, 1954.

21b. Pollack, H., et al.: Calories expended in military activities, Bull. U. S. Army Med. Dept. 74:110, 1944.

22. Pollack, H., and Halpern, S. H.: Therapeutic Nutrition, Washington, D. C., National Academy of Sciences and National Research Council, 1952.

23. Rose, W. C.: Amino acid requirement of man, Fed. Proc. Am. Soc. Exper. Biol. 8:546, 1949.

24. Schiele, B., and Brozek, J.: Experimental neurosis resulting from semi-starvation in man, Psychosom. Med. 10:31, 1948.

25. Sebrell, W. H., and Harris, R. S., eds.: The Vitamins, New York, Acad. Press, 1954.

26. Smith, D. T.: Disturbance of normal bacterial ecology by the administration of antibiotics, with the development of new clinical syndromes, Ann. Int. Med. 37:1135, 1952.

27. Stieglitz, E. J.: Nutrition problems of geriatric medicine, A.M.A. Handbook of Nutrition, New York, Blakiston, 1951.

28. Vilter, R. W.: Vitamin B_{12}, in Wohl, M. G., and Goodhart, R. S., eds.: Modern Nutrition in Health and Disease, Philadelphia, Lea & Febiger, 1960.

29. Wilson, M. W., et al.: Influence of various levels of thiamine intake on physiologic response, J. Am. Dietet. Ass. 25:221, 1949.

30. Youmans, J. B.: Undernutrition, in Cecil, R. L., and Loeb, R. F., eds.: Textbook of Medicine, ed. 10, Philadelphia, Saunders, 1959.

31. Zubiran, S., and Gomez-Mont, F.: Vitamins and Hormones 11:97, 1953; Ann. Int. Med. 42:1259, 1955.

32. Watkin, D. M., and Stieglitz, E. J.: Nutrition in the Aged, Chapter 36 in Wohl and Goodhart.[33]

33. Wohl, M., and Goodhart, R.: Modern Nutrition in Health and Disease, ed. 2, Philadelphia, Lea & Febiger, 1960.

34. Moore, C. V.: Iron, Chapter 10 in Wohl and Goodhart.[33]

35. Castle, W. B.: Disorders of the Blood, in Sodeman, W., ed.: Pathologic Physiology, Philadelphia, Saunders, 1961.

36. Best, C. H., and Lucas, C. C.: Choline Malnutrition, chapter 7 in Jolliffe, N., ed.: Clinical Nutrition, New York, Hoeber-Harper, 1962.

37. Gardner, F. H., and Strauss, E. W.: Disorders related to disturbed absorption of the small bowel, Advances in Internal Medicine 10:137, 1960; Sprue and other malabsorption syndromes, in Harrison, T., et al., eds.: Principles of Internal Medicine, ed. 4., New York, McGraw-Hill, 1962.

38. Brock, J., and Hansen, J.: Protein Deficiency, Chapter 3 in Jolliffe.[39]

39. Jolliffe, N.: Clinical Nutrition, ed. 2, pp. 1-87, New York, Hoeber-Harper, 1962.

40. Follis, R. H., Jr.: Deficiency Disease, Springfield, Ill., Thomas, 1958.

41. Proudfit, F., and Robinson, C.: Normal and Therapeutic Nutrition, ed. 12, New York, Macmillan, 1961.

42. Control of Malnutrition in Man, American Public Health Assn., New York, 1960.

43. Brock, J.: Recent Advances in Human Nutrition, Boston, Little, Brown, 1961.

34

Pigmentation of the Skin

Harold Jeghers and Herbert Mescon

FACTORS INVOLVED IN NORMAL SKIN PIGMENTATION

The living human skin normally contains pigments responsible for skin color. Abnormal skin pigmentation can be appreciated only when the range and the many modifying factors of normal skin coloration are thoroughly understood. Consequently, a considerable portion of our presentation of skin pigmentation will be devoted to the normal skin color.

Methods of Analysis of Skin Color

At the very beginning of his examination, the doctor discovers much of importance merely by noting the color of his patient's skin. In optical terms, we say that the eye has been stimulated by light reflected from the skin. When properly interpreted, the message carried by this reflected light can prove helpful in appraising the clinical status of the patient.

Observation of skin color of patients admitted to a hospital at night should be re-

The authors acknowledge the contribution of Edward A. Edwards, co-author of this chapter in previous editions.

peated later in bright daylight. Many hospital rooms and wards are too dark, even during the day. If this is true, the bed should be moved temporarily to a sun porch or to the bright side of a ward to permit proper inspection of the body surface.

Light impinging on the skin is not simply reflected from the very surface. The human skin is translucent. Light penetrates the various layers of the epidermis, the dermis and even the more superficial strata of the subcutaneous tissue (Fig. 201). We may think of these layers as a series of colored screens, since normally each contains some pigment. The term *pigment* is used here to denote any colored material present in the skin, whether deposited in the tissue proper or present in the blood passing through the skin—and not merely melanin, too often thought of as the only important skin pigment. This broad concept of skin pigment is necessary to understand properly normal and abnormal skin color. As the light strikes each layer of the skin, a portion is absorbed, some is transmitted, and some is reflected. Of each portion transmitted some will be reflected from a deeper layer. Thus, each reflected

855

portion returns to the surface modified by the pigment of the complex skin structure. The reflected light carries two varieties of information. In its aggregate, it can be appreciated as skin color. Secondly, by analysis of this reflected light, one can determine the contributions of the various pigments to the color.

The human eye is an admirable instrument for the first type of information, that is, color per se. Even this function is at times poorly performed, due to the prevalence of poor color sensitivity, as well as the rarer forms of color blindness. Moreover, it is impossible to record or to tell others the color of a skin area in any fashion qualitatively reproducible. This difficulty is resolved to a certain extent by the use of color comparators, such as color charts or color tops.

An entirely objective measurement and recording of color is possible through the use of the spectrophotometer, a technic first used in 1926 by Sheard, Brown and Brunsting for the analysis of the skin color.[1,2,3,4] The highly accurate Hardy recording spectrophotometer, introduced in 1935, was used by Edwards and Duntley and their associates[5,6,7,8] and by Buckley and Grum[64,65] for additional and expanded studies not previously possible. As a result of such investigations, analysis of skin color has been placed on a rational basis and is now explainable in both quantitative and qualitative terms. The use of this instrument must still be looked upon as a re-

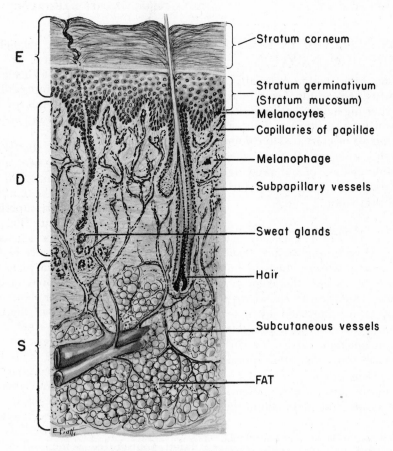

FIG. 201. Composite picture of the histologic appearance of the skin (semidiagrammatic). (E) The extent of the epidermis. (D) The dermis (corium). (S) The subcutaneous tissue. (E. A. Edwards)

PLATE 4

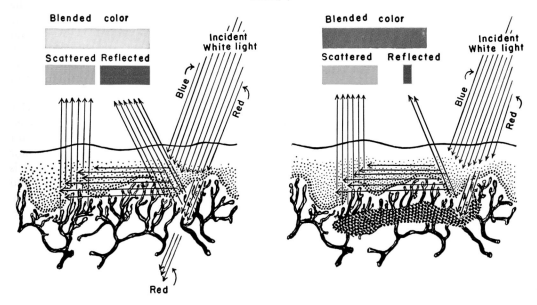

(*Left*) Incident white light (composed of spectral rays—violet, indigo, blue, green, yellow, orange and red) strikes the skin with differential absorption, transmission and reflectance at each layer. Note the reflection of some red rays from the hemoglobin in papillary capillaries and the transmission of other red rays through living tissue to give the red color of transillumination. The turbidity of the lower layers of the epidermis scatters the blue rays back to the surface. The composite of reflected red and scattered blue light blended gives to normal skin its "flesh-color" appearance.

(*Right*) The large mass of pigment present in the dermis (corium) absorbs most of the red spectral light rays, permitting reflection or transmission of only a small portion of them. Blue spectral light rays are scattered not only from deeper layers of the epidermis (as is true normally) but also from the pigment mass, resulting in a marked increase in the amount of blue light returned to the skin surface. The composite of the increased scattered blue light and minimal reflected red light gives the skin over the pigment mass a blue color. The mass in the dermis represents any of the types of pigment described in the text under Scattering Phenomenon, Blue Coloration. (Courtesy of Edward A. Edwards)

search procedure and not directly utilizable for clinical practice, but much which is applicable to medicine has been learned through its use. The objective measurement of color is expressed in terms synonymous with those used by the physicists. Thus, the physicist expresses color in terms of *dominant wave length, relative brightness* and *excitation purity* to correspond with *hue, brightness* and *saturation.*

Lerner and his co-workers[76,77] have developed a relatively simple quantitative method for measuring skin color by photography and reflectance measurements, which is a useful additional method of study.

The eye is inaccurate and may fail entirely in appreciating the second variety of information contained in the skin reflectance: the identity and relative quantity of the pigments contributing to the color. It is particularly for this kind of information that spectrophotometry has been so useful.

A material is a pigment by virtue of absorbing some particular wave lengths in the visible spectrum. A pure white substance has absorption entirely outside the visible

spectrum. A substance is pure black in color because of complete absorption of all light rays within the visible spectral range. Gray color of a substance is due to partial but uniform absorption of all visible spectral rays; light gray representing less absorption than a dark gray. Any color is produced by absorption of some and reflection of other light rays from the visible spectrum. The total light reflected from the skin contains the absorption bands of each pigment in the skin, identifiable by spectrophotometry. In the accompanying reproduction of curves obtained by the use of the Hardy instrument (Figs. 204, 207, 208, 209, 211, 212, 213, 214), the reflectance values of the skin, or transmission values of solutions of pigments, are shown for all wave lengths from the violet limit of visibility at 400 millimicrons, to the red limit at 700 millimicrons. Each pigment has a zone or zones characteristic of it which are known as its *absorption bands.* The finding of such bands in the curve indicates the presence of the corresponding pigments. Moreover, since the extent of light absorption is pro-

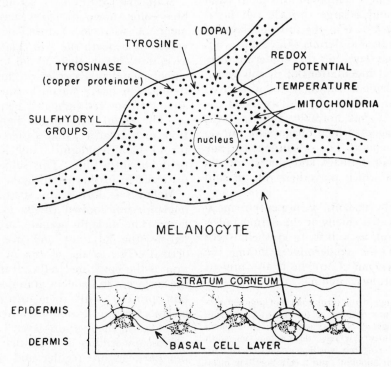

FIG. 202. "Biochemical factors controlling melanin formation." (Fitzpatrick and Lerner: A.M.A. Arch. Dermat. & Syph. 69:133)

portional to the amount of pigment present, one can give an estimate of the quantity of the pigment.[5,6]

Analysis of human skin color by means of spectrophotometry is indicative of the importance of the science of physics to medical research.[9] However, in actual practice physicians judge skin color by total visual impression. With a proper understanding of basic science concepts, this provides considerable useful information for routine clinical diagnosis.

THE SOURCES OF SKIN COLOR

Figure 201 gives in semischematic form the characteristic histologic appearance of a section of the skin with emphasis on the components important in skin color. On the surface of the skin is the keratinized layer (stratum corneum). Beneath this is a small clear layer which represents the stratum lucidum (present only in the palms and soles) and the stratum granulosum. Above the dermis and beneath the clear layer is the stratum germinativum (stratum mucosum). Collectively these various layers are called the *epidermis*. The stratum germinativum is composed of a small basal cell layer and a larger prickle cell layer. Melanocytes* exist at the junction layer of the epidermis and dermis (Fig. 202).

The basal layer of the epidermis contains conical indentations of dermis which contain terminal capillary loops derived from the superficial subpapillary blood vessels. The dermis normally contains cells (melanophages*) which phagocytize but do not form melanin. The subcutaneous tissue contains hair follicles and shafts and fat cells, all of which play their role in skin color.

Ordinarily, melanin is present in melanocytes, located chiefly at the dermoepidermal junction, as well as in epithelial cells throughout the epidermis including the stratum corneum. Carotene is also present in the stratum corneum.

---

* The change in the terminology of pigment-producing cells was decided at the Third Conference on the Biology of Normal and Atypical Pigment Cell.[50,51] Under this new terminology an adult melanin-producing cell is called a "melanocyte" instead of a "melanoblast" and a cell engulfing melanin a "melanophage" instead of a chromatophore.

Four pigments and the additional optical effect called *scattering* have been found responsible for normal skin color.[5] Whether the sweat glands contribute to color, however, is not clear. The main pigments of the dermis are oxyhemoglobin and reduced hemoglobin present in the papillary capillary projections and superficial subpapillary vascular plexuses. The pigments of the subcutaneous layer include carotene in the fat and oxyhemoglobin and reduced hemoglobin present in the deeper vascular plexuses.

Scattering consists of a rearrangement of light as it passes through a turbid medium, whereby the reflected light shows a preponderance of the lower wave lengths (blue colors).[5] In other words, the light is rendered "more blue" or "less red." All the skin pigments are yellow or red in hue. Spectrophotometrically, brown is a yellow of low purity. The skin is turbid, particularly in the basal layers of the epidermis. The resultant scattering offsets to some extent the otherwise extreme redness of the pigments (Plate 4) and gives a composite color which we appreciate as "flesh color."

Scattering additionally accounts for the blue color shown by heavy masses of pigment of whatever nature, lying deeply within or beneath the skin (Plate 4). Rare exceptions occur, such as the red color of cinnabar and green color of chromate tattooing. The heavy mass of pigment absorbs almost all the red light rays penetrating to it. The major part of the light reflected from such an area is that scattered from the turbid basal epidermis, and is therefore predominantly blue. This subject will be discussed in further detail later.

Melanin is formed by specialized cells (melanocytes) located chiefly in the basal layer. The melanin granules are transmitted to the adjacent and overlying epidermal cells. In the process of keratinization as the epidermal cells advance toward the surface, the pigment granules they contain proceed with them. An occasional melanocyte can also be visualized proceeding toward the keratin layer.[71] Electronmicroscopy studies indicate that the melanin particles are regular and constant in form and configuration.[57] A congenital inability to form melanin is seen in albino individuals. The formation of melanin is a vital process. As the basal cells are pushed superficially in the growth of the epidermis, the cells become progressively lifeless and the granules of melanin disintegrate. In a fair-skinned person, melanin granules are not only fewer in number but smaller in size and occupy one or two lower layers of epithelium. In persons of darker complexion melanin granules are larger in size and more numerous, occupying somewhat more rows of cells. Edwards and Duntley[5] noted that the disintegration of

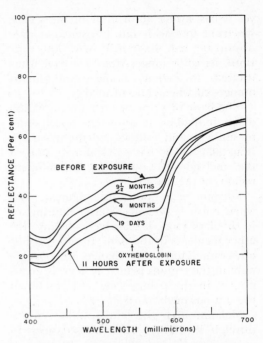

FIG. 204. Spectrophotometric curves of the skin after a single exposure to sunlight. Hyperemia (oxyhemoglobin bands at arrows) is maximum at 11 hours, melanin at 19 days and melanoid at 4 months. Blood stagnation, as registered by evidence of reduced hemoglobin (blunting of oxyhemoglobin bands and depression of peak between them) persists from the early disappearance of the hyperemia for the entire duration of the experiment. (Edwards and Duntley: Science 20:235)

DISTRIBUTION OF MELANIN

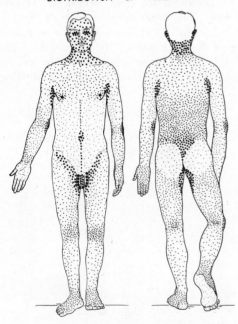

FIG. 203. The bodily distribution of melanin. Note primary areas of accentuation in the eyelids, the axillae, the nipples, the areolae, the nape of the neck, the umbilicus, the linea nigra and the genitoanal region. Accentuation on the face due to sunlight exposure and at the elbows and knees due to friction. Note the small amount of melanin on the palms and soles.

With the exception of the eyelids, the ears, the axillae, the perineum and the penis, the data were derived from spectrophotometry. The scalp was omitted from consideration. (Edwards and Duntley: Am. J. Anat. 65:1)

melanin gives rise to a diffuse derived pigment which they term *melanoid* whose exact chemical composition or significance is still to be determined. It appears to have an absorption band in the visible violet at 400 mμ and to give the skin a yellowish sallow appearance if present in excess. Others[78] feel that melanin in fine particulate form occurring in the stratum corneum, in conjunction with strong hemoglobin absorption bands in the 400 to 420 mμ range, could account for the changes noted in the skin reflectance curve in this range.

Although present in the skin in particulate form, melanin behaves spectrophotometrically as though in solution. It shows its greatest absorption in the ultraviolet, yet it has strong absorption in the visible spectrum too, with fair transmission only toward the red. Examined in various dilutions, its color ranges from a brown when diluted, to yellow, orange, and finally orange-red when concentrated.

The basic or primary melanin formation of an individual is unrelated to exposure to sunlight and follows a definite pattern (Fig. 203). Szabo has painstakingly studied the melanocyte population in different regions of the body.[70]

Melanin is a powerful pigment, and when much is present, as after tanning, or in the dark races, it effectively obscures the other pigments in the skin. In such people, observations on color change are possible only in the regions primarily poor in melanin, as in the palms, soles and certain of the mucous membranes.[78]

Melanin may give rise to blue effects, through scattering, when massed deep in the epidermis. Normally this may obtain in the eyelids and axillae, where the material is present in dermal melanophages (chromatophores) or in a hairy area which has been shaved, as in the male cheek, where melanin is present in the deep-lying hair bulbs.

Melanin appears to be the main pigment of the hair, though some additional pigments have recently been discovered. Pheomelanin, a yellow granular alkaline soluble pigment, found in red hair may be derived from tryptophan as well as tyrosine.[66] Variations in hair color correspond to the difference noted in varying dilutions of the melanin.

Oxyhemoglobin and Reduced Hemoglobin. The constant perfusion of the cutaneous and subcutaneous tissues by blood forces one to consider the pigments of the blood as cutaneous pigments. The vessels penetrated by light and thus contributing

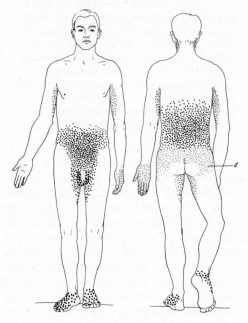

DISTRIBUTION OF VENOUS BLOOD

Fig. 205. The bodily distribution of predominantly venous blood. Areas not included here or in Figure 206 show no special predominance, except that investigation was not made of the regions noted under Figure 203. (Edwards and Duntley: Am. J. Anat. 65:1)

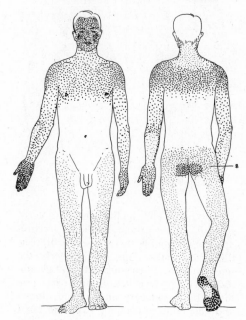

DISTRIBUTION OF ARTERIAL BLOOD

Fig. 206. The bodily distribution of predominantly arterial blood. Areas not included here or in Figure 205 show no special predominance, except that investigation was not made of the regions noted under Figure 203. (Edwards and Duntley: Am. J. Anat. 65:1)

to skin color, are arranged in three beds: (1) vessels of the dermal papillae, mainly capillaries; (2) the subpapillary plexus, made up predominantly of veins; and (3) the subcutaneous vessels, in which only the large veins are prominent visually. The subpapillary venous plexus presents the largest surface area of the three vascular beds. The subcutaneous veins show up mainly as blue, owing to the phenomenon of scattering. It is apparent, then, that the blood pigments exert their effect on skin color mainly according to their presence in the papillary and subpapillary networks.

What are the pigments involved? Those of the blood plasma, yellow in color, but usually quite pale, are without much effect on normal skin color. Hemoglobin constitutes the important pigment material. Hemoglobin exists in the red cells in both the reduced and the oxidized form. Each has a distinct absorption spectrum and color. Oxyhemoglobin, the more brilliantly red of the two, is especially characterized in the spectrum by absorption bands at 542 and 576 millimicrons. Reduced hemoglobin is darker and less red, or (one might say) more blue. Its curve shows a single band at 556, replacing the twin bands of oxyhemoglobin. The proportion of hemoglobin which is oxidized varies with the class of vessel under scrutiny. Thus, in arteries, the quantity of oxidized hemoglobin is from 90 to 95 per cent; in the veins it is about 50 per cent; while in the capillaries the value lies between the arterial and venous levels. The subpapillary venous plexus has a larger surface area than the papillary capillary network. This is the main reason why the oxyhemoglobin bands in most areas of the skin are considerably replaced by those of reduced hemoglobin. In some areas, the fine veins are unusually prominent, while the capillaries are poorly developed. Such areas of venous preponderance are to be found in the lower trunk and on the dorsa of the feet (Fig. 205). In certain areas, on the contrary, the arterial flow and capillary perfusion are comparatively great, with a corresponding prominence of oxyhemoglobin. This is especially true in the head and neck, the palms, the soles and in the skin over the ischial tuber-

osities. To the eye, these areas are considerably redder than the surrounding skin (Fig. 206).

The over-all contribution of hemoglobin to skin color will vary with the total quantity of that material, as in anemia or polycythemia. *Rapid changes in skin color are due entirely to changes in vessel caliber, in blood flow and the degree of hemoglobin oxidation* (Fig. 207). Arterial dilatation results in an increased capillary perfusion, with reddening of the skin, due to the

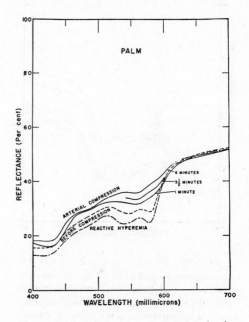

FIG. 207. The effects of ischemia in changing the appearance of the palm. A manometer cuff on the arm was quickly inflated above systolic pressure. In 1 minute, the curve has lost its evidence of oxyhemoglobin, and the general shape of the curve shows this to be due mainly to an increase in the reduced form.

As ischemia continues, the 3½- and 6-minute curves show less and less absorption by reduced hemoglobin, indicating a progressive diminution of blood in the skin. Vasoconstriction of cutaneous vessels may be responsible. In these relatively bloodless curves, the absorption band of carotene at 482 mμ previously obscured now becomes evident. On deflation of the cuff, reactive hyperemia is evidenced by the greatly increased absorption with strong evidence of oxyhemoglobin. (Edwards)

presence of more hemoglobin, while arterial constriction or obstruction induces the opposite effect—a pale skin, due to a reduction in the quantity of hemoglobin viewed, and a diminution in the degree of its oxidation. The capillaries are probably not capable of change in caliber independ-

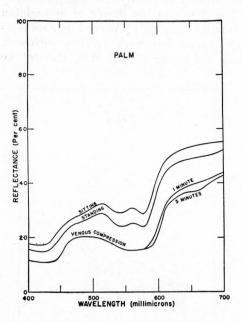

FIG. 208. Venous distention in the skin in response to posture and to venous compression. The palm becomes darker with the subject standing and the hand dependent. The increased absorption is caused by the presence of more hemoglobin, but the slight blunting of the twin bands of oxyhemoglobin and the general shape of the curve show this to be due mainly to an increase in the reduced form.

Compression of the arm by a manometer cuff inflated below diastolic pressure gives a further increase in the amount of reduced hemoglobin present. With continued compression, the amount of reduced hemoglobin increases for about 5 minutes, at which time the veins seem to have reached their limit of distensibility. The portion of the curve shown reveals further reduction of the hemoglobin present, but no increase in total amount. Fatigue of the veins with further distensibility would undoubtedly occur with greatly prolonged compression. The absorption band at 660 mμ in the 5-minute curve is unexplained. (Edwards)

ent of such changes in the arteries or veins. Interference with venous outflow depends upon posture, venous constriction or obstruction. Under these circumstances, both the quantity and ratio of reduced hemoglobin are increased (Fig. 208). A comparison of visual analysis of vascular change with spectrophotometric examination demonstrates that the eye appreciates quite well the increase in quantity and ratio of reduced hemoglobin under these circumstances.

An obstruction to venous outflow may exist simultaneously with either arterial constriction or dilatation, adding the bluer hue of reduced hemoglobin to the paleness of the arterial constriction or to the ruddiness of arterial dilatation.

Cyanosis is appreciated when reduced hemoglobin is present in concentrations of 5 Gm. or more per 100 ml. of blood. Cyanosis may be general (because of insufficient aeration) or local (because of obstruction to the venous flow).

An intensely red skin does not necessarily mean arterial dilatation and increased capillary flow. The hands and feet may occasionally be cold, but still bright red, with evidence of highly oxygenated hemoglobin. Such findings suggest the lack of utilization of oxygen by the tissues. This is seen when the part is subjected to extreme cold, for very little oxygen exchange takes place at low temperature levels. It may be that lowered tissue utilization of oxygen when it exists in other conditions, such as lowered metabolism, may influence skin color. In other instances, such a change would appear to depend upon the opening of the normal arteriovenous communications of the hands or feet. Of course, it may be seen also in the presence of abnormal arteriovenous fistulae as well, especially when the fistulae are multiple and small.

Carotene is the yellow pigment of the subcutaneous fat. The term is used here to include a group of related carotenoids. It is found likewise in the cornified superficial layer of the epidermis and in the sebaceous glands, and also in the blood plasma[5] in a slight and variable amount.

Carotene shows absorption bands at 455

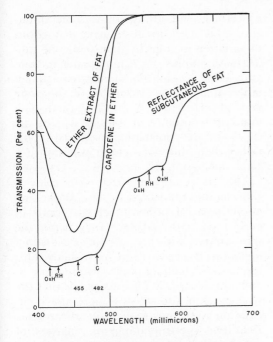

The reflectance of the removed subcutaneous fat from a cadaver, compared with the transmission of its ether extract and with a known solution of carotene in ether. The absorption of carotene at 455 and 482 mμ are evident in all three curves. Only the band at 482 mμ is pronounced in the curves of living skin. Absorption bands of hemoglobin are noted in the fat specimen. Some of the pigment has been oxidized by exposure to the air. (Edwards and Duntley: Am. J. Anat. 65:1)

and 482 millimicrons (Fig. 209). Its color in concentrated form is a golden yellow. Spectrophotometric analysis of skin color has shown that carotene is an important normal skin color component. It shows regional variations in quantity closely resembling the pattern of arterial preponderance (Fig. 210). Carotene, being lipid soluble, is present maximally in lipid-rich subcutaneous areas (buttock and breast) and in those areas where surface lipid is high either from sebum secretion (face) or from lipids released in areas of most active keratinization, i.e., palms and soles.

The human subject obtains carotene mainly through the ingestion of fruits and vegetables. Intestinal absorption of caro-

tene requires the presence of dietary fat and bile acids. In the liver enzymatic conversion to vitamin A takes place. Excess carotene is either destroyed metabolically or excreted in sebum and possibly, to some minor degree, in the urine.

More than 30 pigments constitute the lipochrome or carotenoid group of pigments widespread in nature in plants and some animal substances. The majority have a yellow color, others are yellow to red in hue. Only four of these (alpha-carotene, beta-carotene, gamma-carotene and cryptoxanthine) have provitamin A activity and these collectively or separately are the ones commonly known as carotene, and are the carotenoid pigments most important in skin color in man.

Normal Sweat and Sebum. These have not been found to affect skin color appreciably. When allowed to accumulate excessively, the secretion may obscure the skin's surface. However, sebum contains a little

DISTRIBUTION OF CAROTENE

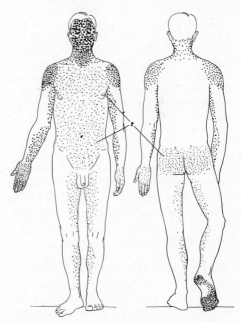

Fig. 210. The bodily distribution of carotene. With the exception of the regions listed under Fig. 203, which were not examined, the unshaded areas were particularly poor in carotene. (Edwards and Duntley: Am. J. Anat. 65:1)

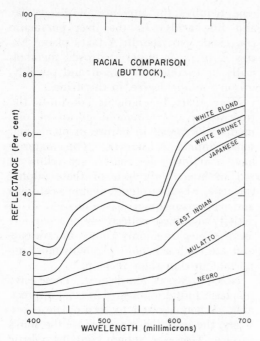

FIG. 211. Comparison of readings from the buttocks of males of different racial groups. This area was chosen as one whose pigment content would be minimally disturbed by exposure to sunlight. The curves vary only in their melanin content. Note how readily the oxyhemoglobin and carotene absorption bands can be seen in the spectral reflection curve in the white blond and their obliteration by the increased melanin in the skin of those more heavily pigmented. (Edwards and Duntley: Am. J. Anat. 65:1)

carotene, and when intake of this substance is unusually high, areas of much sebaceous secretion may appear yellow. This accounts, in part, for the characteristic localization of the yellow color to the greasy portion of the face in carotenemia.

PATTERNS OF NORMAL SKIN COLOR

BASIC PATTERN AND INDIVIDUAL VARIATION

Classifications of patterns of skin pigmentation are to be mentioned in reference to race, sex and age. It is important to emphasize, however, that the skin color of any two individuals falling into the same category, as far as these factors are concerned, will always show some difference. It is often unsafe to make deductions of variation in color by comparing one subject with another. It is much safer to compare differences in color of one area with another in the same person, or of the same area at different times. The spectrophotometric reflectance of normal skin of the cheek and the explanation for its red-yellow rather than blue-violet visual appearance is given in Figure 212.

Age. It is apparent that skin color is considerably influenced by age. Darkening of the areas of primary melanin occurs in both sexes with puberty. In general, the skin darkens with age. At times a distinct melanosis is seen in senile individuals. This seems to be due to a progressive increase in melanin deposit. Evidence suggests that the younger skin also shows a more active circulation and a greater quantity of carotene. Definitive spectrophotometric analyses of age changes in skin color are not available.

The regional distribution of the pigments has been individually portrayed (Figs. 203, 205, 206, 210). It is apparent that different regions of the body vary in skin color because of their particular content of the pigments. Differences in thickness of the skin are also of undoubted importance, for a heavy epidermis will cause more scattering. Thickening of the cornified epidermis may add greater quantity of carotene and possibly melanin. Areas where the stratum corneum is thinnest, as mucous membrane surfaces, accentuate the hemoglobin pigments.

Rapid variations in color, due to changes in blood vessel caliber and flow, are particularly marked in the hands, the feet and the face. One should attempt to approximate basal conditions before giving much weight to changes in color in these regions.

RACIAL VARIATIONS

Spectrophotometry has confirmed histologic evidence that variations in the content of melanin are alone responsible for the differences in color of the various races.[15,78]

Gates and Zimmerman[52] have correlated racial coloration with melanin in the epidermis, but not with the sparse amounts of the pigment in the melanophages of the dermis. Shizume and Lerner[53] have found approximately the same level of pituitary melanocyte-stimulating hormone in Negroes as in whites.

The colors of the skins of the races can be arranged in a series conforming to the graduations of color in solutions of melanin of varying strength[5] (Fig. 211). No evidence has been found to support the theory which is occasionally stated that the pigmentation of the dark races is due to pigment not normally found in the white, or to an increase of the ordinary pigments other than melanin.

The heavy melanin deposit of the dark races, especially of the Negro, considerably obscures the other pigments.[78] Nevertheless, regions of the body with the least melanin deposit, such as the palms and soles, may still furnish valuable information regarding skin color.

Sex Differences and the Effects of the Sex Hormones

Spectrophotometry indicates that the ruddier appearance of the male is caused by the presence in the skin of more blood (hemoglobin) and melanin than in the female. Contrariwise, the female possesses more carotene than does the male.

The regional patterns of pigment distribution vary somewhat in the two sexes. Females show stronger areas of primary melanization in the nape of the neck, the linea nigra and axilla than do males. The contrast in amount of melanin deposit, between areas richly supplied and those poorly supplied, is more marked in the female than in the male. The buttocks of the female shows a slight arterial preponderance, rather than a venous one as in the male. Finally, females show good evidence of carotene in the breast, abdomen and buttocks, regions which are poor in carotene in the male.

Study of castrated men and ovariectomized women gives evidence that much of the sex difference in color is genetic and not subject to complete disappearance, or reversal, on removal of the gonads. This is not to gainsay that the gonads affect skin color considerably through their in-

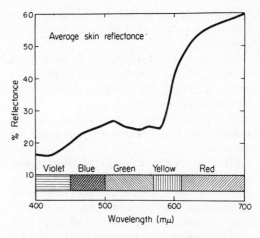

Fig. 212. Reflectance curve; average skin left cheek. Note the dips at approximately 415, 542 and 575 mμ. These are due to oxyhemoglobin. They are blunted when there is more reduced hemoglobin which has a band at 555 mμ. The absorption slope from 465 to 510 mμ. is due to carotenoids which has a maximal absorption band at 480 mμ. In general, more red and yellow are reflected and less green blue and violet. This explains the visual appearance of normal skin. (Buckley, W. R., and Grum, F.: Reflection Spectrophotometry; use in evaluation of skin pigmentary disturbances. Arch. Dermat. 83: 249-261)

ternal secretions. It is noteworthy that reactions to these sex hormones take place in the entire skin of the human, rather than in specialized zones as in other animals. A possible exception is the areolar hyperpigmentation resulting from direct application of estrogen cream.

Effects of Castration in the Male. From visual observations, it was believed that the pale sallow skin of the male castrate was due to a deficiency in melanin, but spectrophotometry indicates that melanin production in the castrate or eunuchoid individual is only slightly diminished.

The factor mainly responsible for the abnormal color of the castrate is a pronounced reduction in cutaneous blood flow, the hemoglobin being reduced in quantity and in the degree of oxidation. Areas characterized by a large venous bed showed evidence of venous dilatation and stagnation, with a real increase in reduced hemoglobin.

Carotene is substantially increased in the skin of the castrate, and could be a factor in giving the sallow appearance to these individuals.

All of the changes enumerated can be reversed by the administration of male sex hormone.

The Hormonal Control of Skin Color in the Female. The effects of the sex hormones are well shown in the female by the changes after ovariectomy, as well as those incident to the menstrual cycle.

As in the male, removal of the gonads causes a diminution in superficial cutaneous blood flow, with a lowered amount of hemoglobin and a relative increase in its reduced form (Fig. 213). Administration of estrogen is followed by an increased blood flow and an increase in oxyhemoglobin. Progestin increases the degree of

oxidation of hemoglobin, but does not consistently increase the total hemoglobin present. The simultaneous administration of both products gives the paradoxical result of a diminution of the quantity of hemoglobin, with a predominance of the reduced form. The spectrophotometric evidence available fails to show any changes in melanin attributable to variations in estrogen or progestin levels. However, there have been reports of chloasma resulting from progestational oral contraceptives.[87]

It will be recalled that, contrary to the situation in the male, the output of the sex hormones in the female fluctuates widely in different times of the menstrual cycle. Early, before ovulation, neither estrogen nor progestin is present in appreciable quantity. At this time the woman's skin resembles that of the ovariectomized subject. After midcycle there is greatly increased superficial blood

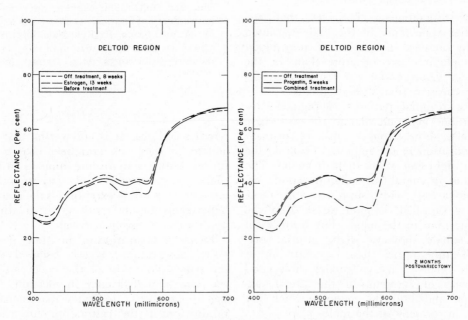

FIG. 213. Spectrophotometric curves of the deltoid region of an ovariectomized subject. On the left, the pretreatment curve is low in hemoglobin content, and with dominance of the reduced form. After treatment with estrogen, the curve shows a real increase in oxyhemoglobin. With cessation of treatment, the curve reverts to its pretreatment character.

On the right the administration of progestin produces a marked increase in oxyhemoglobin. The combined use of progestin and estrogen diminishes the hemoglobin content, causing the curve to revert to its off-treatment level. (Edwards and Duntley: Am. J. Obst. & Gynec. 57:501)

flow, with a maximum in the premenstrual period. This is consistent with the high estrogen production of the ovulation and postovulation period. Progestin is produced more tardily, in the premenstrual period, and the combined effect of the two hormones finally lowers the cutaneous circulation to the level observed at the beginning of the cycle (Fig. 214).

SKIN COLOR CHANGES AFTER EXPOSURE TO SUNLIGHT

These depend as much on blood vessel effect as on melanin and melanoid formation. Edwards and Duntley[7] followed these changes after a single heavy exposure (Fig. 204). The initial hyperemia and redness increased to a maximum 11 hours after exposure. An increase in

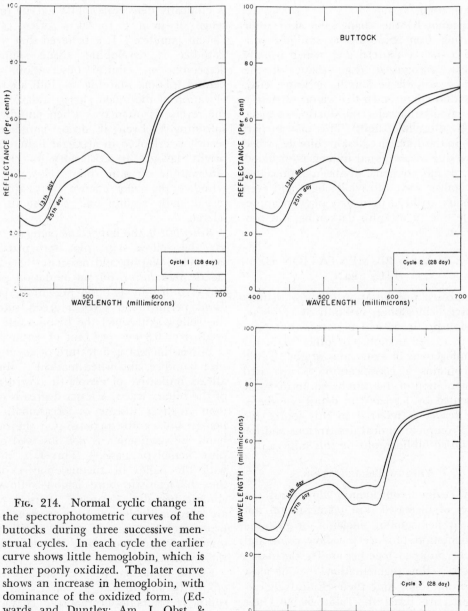

FIG. 214. Normal cyclic change in the spectrophotometric curves of the buttocks during three successive menstrual cycles. In each cycle the earlier curve shows little hemoglobin, which is rather poorly oxidized. The later curve shows an increase in hemoglobin, with dominance of the oxidized form. (Edwards and Duntley: Am. J. Obst. & Gynec. 57:501)

melanin was apparent in two days and reached its maximum on the nineteenth day. The early hyperemia was followed by a venous enlargement and stasis, which contributed considerably to the darkness of the tanned skin.

Since all persons are customarily exposed to sunlight, with much variation in the potency of actinic rays as well as in the area of skin exposed, the effect of sunlight exposure always must be considered by physicians in their evaluation of skin color.

Fortunately, the changes in skin color resulting from exposure to sunlight produce a surface pattern area which usually can be recognized (e.g., shape of the bathing suit, sleeve length, neckline, etc.).

Findlay[80] has shown that vasoconstriction and vasodilation affect production of melanin by ultraviolet light. This may in part explain the difference in skin color described above due to hormonal influence on blood flow. It has not generally been appreciated that longer wave ultraviolet light and even ordinary artificial light may play an appreciable role in melanin darkening and production.[81,82]

INCREASED PIGMENTATION OF THE SKIN

Increased pigmentation of the skin may involve hemoglobin, melanin or carotene, physiologically normal pigments (but present in excess amounts) or other pigments of endogenous or exogenous origin. Table 49 contains a classification of increased pigmentation of the skin based on material presented by Jeghers[10] in detail elsewhere. The reader is referred to this source for more complete clinical descriptions and for a detailed bibliography on this subject.

Yellow Pigmentation

By curious coincidence, almost all the causes of increased skin pigmentation not due to hemoglobin, melanin or metallic pigmentation produce a yellow color and can be grouped together under the designation "yellow pigmentation."[10] The most important ones and their clinical characteristics are listed in Table 50.[10] These possibilities should be investigated in any patient presenting a predominantly yellow color of the skin.

Jaundice is the commonest cause of a yellow skin color. A small amount of bilirubin, as indicated by an icterus index of 4 to 6 or a quantitative van den Bergh of 0.1 to 0.5 mg. per cent, is normally present in the blood. However, this small amount is not detectable even spectrophotometrically in normal skin color. The icterus index must reach 20 to 25 before jaundice is clinically detectable. The icterus index range of from 6 to 20 is often called "latent jaundice." It is believed that when jaundice is developing, tissue staining, detectable on clinical observation, lags behind plasma staining as indicated by elevation of the blood icterus index, while the reverse is often true when jaundice is subsiding.[10] Even if deep, jaundice is readily overlooked in artificial light. Only bright daylight is satisfactory for clinical observation of skin color. However, in jaundice the color change is usually detected most readily and earliest in the sclerae.

Bilirubin is the important pigment causing the yellow skin color recognized as jaundice. Watson and associates[11,12] show clearly that *biliverdin,* an oxidation product of bilirubin, is often present in jaundiced persons and gives a green tint to the yellow skin when the blood value exceeds over 0.3 mg. per cent of serum.

Biliverdinemia is a feature of regurgitation jaundice, and when marked is almost always indicative of neoplastic obstruction of the biliary tract. A lesser degree is common in liver disease or occasionally in benign biliary obstructions. On the other hand, biliverdinemia is not observed on a pure hemolytic basis.[12] This fact, along with the pallor of anemia, may explain the characteristic pure lemon yellow of chronic hemolytic jaundice. Persons who are chronically jaundiced may develop a bronze color suggestive of the addition of some degree of melanosis, in addition to their yellowish-green skin color.

Elastic tissue has been called *bilirubinophilic* because of its great affinity for bilirubin. It is believed that the character-

TABLE 49. CLASSIFICATION OF PIGMENTATION OF THE SKIN

NORMAL PIGMENTATION OF THE SKIN	INCREASED PIGMENTATION OF THE SKIN	DECREASED PIGMENTATION OF THE SKIN

Skin color in health is produced by a composite of the four following pigments in normal amounts
  CAROTENE
  MELANIN
  OXYHEMOGLOBIN
  REDUCED HEMOGLOBIN
plus the optical effect of
  SCATTERING PHENOMENON
due to turbidity of normal epidermis
	YELLOW PIGMENTATIONS (see Table 50)
	HEMOGLOBIN PIGMENTATIONS (see Table 51)
	MELANIN PIGMENTATIONS (see Table 52)
	METALLIC PIGMENTATIONS (see Table 53)
	EXAGGERATED SCATTERING PHENOMENON produced by excess of normal or presence of abnormal pigments in the corium (Table 54)
	MISCELLANEOUS PIGMENTATIONS
		DIMINISHED AMOUNT OF HEMOGLOBIN (ANEMIA)
		DECREASED OR ABSENT MELANIN
		EDEMA OF THE SKIN
		DIMINISHED BLOOD FLOW TO THE SKIN
		SCAR TISSUE
		MACERATED OR DESQUAMATING SKIN

TABLE 50. DIFFERENTIAL CHARACTERISTICS

CLINICAL CONDITION	PIGMENT RESPONSIBLE	SKIN COLOR	CHARACTERISTIC LOCALIZATION
Carotenemia.........	Carotene	Canary yellow Lemon yellow Orange yellow	Palms, soles, alae nasi; occasionally diffuse. Absent in sclerae and mucous membrane
Jaundice (hemolytic)..	Bilirubin	Lemon yellow with pallor	Sclerae, mucous membrane and diffuse skin
Jaundice (hepatic and obstructive)	Bilirubin and biliverdin	Light yellow, dark yellow, orange, saffron or yellowish-green	Sclerae, mucous membrane and diffuse skin
Myxedema..........	Carotene	Sallow yellow, old ivory tint	Palms, soles and face
Ingestion quinacrine hydrochloride	Quinacrine hydrochloride	Yellow to greenish-yellow	Diffuse skin—accentuated exposed portion and body folds. Minimal or absent sclerae and mucous membranes
Chronic uremia......	Urine chromogens Carotene (?) Diminished hemoglobin	Yellowish—pallor Yellowish—tan Buckwheat tint	Accentuated on skin exposed to light. Absent sclerae and mucous membrane
Industrial staining....	Various yellow chemicals	Yellows of various hues	On exposed skin (face, hands, ankles and hair). Absent in sclerae or mucous membrane
Picric acid ingestion (simulated jaundice)	Picric acid and breakdown derivatives	Yellow	Sclerae, mucous membrane and diffuse skin
Generalized xanthomatoses of skin	Cholesterol and cholesterol esters	Golden yellow Chamois yellow	Patchy on skin even when diffuse. None on sclerae or mucous membrane
Local discolorations of old ecchymosis, Cullen's sign, Grey-Turner's sign, etc.	Bilirubin and derivatives	Initially blue due to scattering phenomenon; later greenish-yellow to yellow	At site of trauma; Cullen's sign at umbilicus or in abdominal scars; Grey-Turner's sign on left flank
Lycopenemia........	Lycopene	Orange yellow	Skin diffusely involved; most marked on palms and dorsa of hands, forearms, face and soles.

Comparative Range of Intensity of Skin Color *	Mechanism of Production	Specific Aids to Diagnosis	Comment
X to XX	Excess ingestion of carotenoid foods. Low B.M.R.(?) Diminished liver function(?)	Three-layer test of serum	Carotenemia is often a factor in skin color in Simmonds' disease and in the male castrate.
X to XXX	Hemolysis of blood with bilirubin retention	Icterus index; quant. test for bilirubin; lack of bile in urine	Modified by pallor of anemia
X to XXXX	Regurgitation of bile pigments into blood	Icterus index; quant. tests for bilirubin and biliverdin; bile in urine	Melanosis may develop when jaundice is chronic
X	Diminished metabolism impairs utilization of carotene.	Low B.M.R.; normal icterus index	Skin color modified by myxedematous condition of skin and anemia
X to XXX	Direct staining of epidermis of skin	History; specific urine tests for the medication	Blue spots due to scattering phenomenon, due to pigment deposited in corium or in cartilage noted rarely
X	Retention of urinary chromogen with deposition in tissues; oxidized to yellow color on exposed surfaces	Blood chemistries and urinalysis	Melanosis stimulated in some instances
X to XXXX	External staining of exposed skin and hair	Occupational history	Some yellow chemicals produce liver damage and true jaundice as well as staining skin directly.
X to XX	Picric acid and derivatives deposited in skin and mucous membrane	Urine orange to red in color; specific tests of urine for picrates; history	May also occur with use of picric acid ointments
X to XX	Deposition of lipoids in skin	Biopsy of skin shows local lipoids	Characteristic color seen best in the common xanthomata palpebrarum
X to XXX	Breakdown of blood or hemorrhagic fluid in tissues	Clinical observation only	Depends on local formations of bilirubin, biliverdin and derived pigments
X to XX	Excess ingestion of tomatoes	History; increased serum carotenoids with spectrophotometric confirmation of lycopene	Specific histologic and histochemical changes in liver

* X indicates skin color is barely detectable clinically. XX, XXX and XXXX indicate increasingly marked change in skin color.

istic distribution of jaundice, with its accentuation in the sclerae, mucous membranes and certain portions of the skin in the upper part of the body, reflects the greater amount of elastic tissue which these areas contain. Meakins[13] has shown clearly that jaundice cannot be detected in an edematous skin.

Clinically, carotenemia results when an excess of carotene (carotenoid pigments) stains the serum and skin. The term *carotenoderma* is sometimes used to indicate excess tissue staining with carotene.[10,14] The color of carotenemia is best detected where the skin has a heavy layer of stratum corneum (palms and soles) and areas of the face (forehead, nose and cheeks) which are rich in sebaceous gland activity. It is absent in the sclerae and mucous membranes of the mouth.[79] A reliable bedside test for its detection is by comparison of the physician's palm, if normal in color, with the palm of a person suspected of being carotenemic.

Carotenemia results from prolonged excess ingestion of foods rich in carotene, its use as medication, lowered body metabolism (e.g., myxedema, Simmonds' disease, etc.), which hinders conversion of carotene to vitamin A in the liver, diminution of androgenic hormonal activity (e.g., the male castrate), and possibly to some minor degree with renal failure. A mild degree is physiologic in the normal skin color of women as compared with men.[5] Carotenemia was at one time common in diabetic patients, probably because of the high lipochromic diet formerly used, although it was claimed by some to be due to diminished conversion of carotene to vitamin A in the liver. Theoretically liver disease can cause carotenemia by preventing the conversion of carotene to vitamin A, which takes place in this organ, but if severe, the yellow color of carotenemia would be masked if there was jaundice. Carotenemia per se is harmless and gradually disappears when excess intake or underlying metabolic cause is corrected. The various circumstances under which carotenemia is of clinical interest are given in Table 50. The exact role of the xantho-

phylls, as a group, in contributing to normal or abnormal yellow color of the skin is not clear.[64] Elevated levels have been noted in hypothyroidism, nephrotic syndrome and hyperlipemic xanthomatoses. The spectral absorption curve for xanthophyll is somewhat similar to B-carotene. *Lycopene,* the familiar orange-red pigment of tomatoes, is a carotenoid pigment, which, when ingested in excess, may produce a pigmentary syndrome known as lycopenemia.[67] It differs from carotenemia in the source of the carotenoid pigment, the presence of elevated lycopene levels in the serum, a deeper orange skin color and specific histologic changes in the liver.

Medication. Quinacrine hydrochloride, a drug utilized at times in the therapy of amebiasis, tapeworm infestation and malaria, is an example of medication which may produce a striking yellow skin pigmentation after a week or so of continuous use. It produces a diffuse yellow skin color as a result of direct staining of tissues usually easily distinguished from jaundice by absence or minimal staining of the sclerae.[10] Rarely, pigmentation changes in the deeper layers of the skin or mucous membrane may produce a blue color due to the scattering phenomenon.[15,83]

Recently, yellow pigmentation of the teeth induced by tetracycline has been reported in a high percentage of young children who received this antibiotic for control of pulmonary infections associated with cystic fibrosis.[85] The offspring of a woman who received tetracycline therapy for cystic acne during pregnancy also showed yellow-brown pigmentation of the teeth.[86]

Patients with chronic uremia often manifest a skin color which has a distinct pale yellow or yellowish-tan hue.[10] The pallor can be readily explained by the severe anemia so common in this condition. The yellowish skin discoloration has been attributed to retention in the skin of chromogens ordinarily excreted in the urine and responsible for its normal amber or yellow color. Excretion of a pale urine is characteristic of long-standing renal failure. The oxidative influence of light on the skin tends to accentuate the yellowish color

TABLE 51. CLASSIFICATION OF HEMOGLOBIN PIGMENTATIONS

TYPE	SKIN COLOR PRODUCED	CLINICAL SIGNIFICANCE
Predominance of reduced hemoglobin	Varies from purplish-blue to heliotrope	Clinically recognized as cyanosis
Predominance of oxyhemoglobin.	Red	Color characteristic of blush, flush, erythema, inflammation, arteriolar dilatation, etc.
Increased amount of hemoglobin.	Reddish-blue	Caused by polycythemia vera; blood contains normal amount of oxygenated hemoglobin as well as increased amounts of reduced hemoglobin
Methemoglobinemia.	Chocolate blue	Various causes. See Reference #19
Sulfhemoglobinemia.	Lead or mauve-blue	Various causes. See Reference #19
Carboxyhemoglobinemia.	Cherry red	Carbon monoxide poisoning
Cyanhemoglobinemia.	Bright red	Seen as bright red spots in persons dead from hydrocyanic poison
Nitricoxidehemoglobinemia.	Bright red	Seen on exposure to nitrate explosion in closed space

on the exposed portions of the skin. Retention of carotenoid pigments has also been postulated as a cause for a yellowish skin color in uremia but is not generally accepted. At times chronic uremia appears to lead to an increase in melanin pigmentation. Malnutrition and trauma from scratching may be important causes of this melanosis.

A large number of yellow chemicals used in industry can stain externally the exposed portions of the skin and even the hair a distinct yellow color. This characteristic color distribution, absence of staining of the mucous membrane and sclerae and the occupational history make the diagnosis easy. Such persons are often referred to as "industrial canaries." The yellow color in certain instances is accentuated on exposure to light.[10]

The importance of knowing about this condition lies in the fact that exposure to some of these industrial chemicals may also damage the liver with resultant true jaundice and thus confuse the clinical problem.

Ingestion of picric acid or its absorption from ointments applied to open wounds can closely simulate jaundice by the ability of this yellow chemical to stain both the skin and mucous membranes.[10] Simulation of jaundice in this fashion was apparently a common means of malingering by soldiers in some armies during World War I. This substance is toxic and occasionally produces liver disease with true jaundice. In a similar manner, the metabolic stimulant dinitrophenol, formerly used extensively for weight reduction, can stain tissues yellow. Because its toxic effects are now well known one rarely sees it used at present.

Xanthomas are yellow and usually localized. Occasionally, xanthomatosis produces diffuse skin infiltration with a resultant yellowish-orange type of skin discoloration.

There are a number of dermatologic disorders characterized by a yellow color of a local lesion.[16,17] They are not likely to be confused with the type of skin discoloration discussed in this section.

Blood diffused through the subcutaneous tissues in the nature of an ecchymosis, hematoma, suffusion, etc., causes at first a purplish-blue or blue discoloration from the exaggerated "scattering" effect. As the blood pigments break down, bilirubin, biliverdin and other similar pigments are formed. Therefore, diffuse blood in tissues can produce localized areas of yellow discoloration (bilirubin) or yellowish-green discoloration (bilirubin and biliverdin). Cullen's sign consists of this type of discoloration about the umbilicus or scars in the abdominal wall and is diagnostic of ruptured tubular pregnancy or of hemorrhagic pancreatitis.[10] Grey-Turner's sign is a similar discoloration in the left flank and is diagnostic of hemorrhagic pancreatitis[10] or retroperitoneal hematoma as from ruptured aneurysm.

The lesions of urticaria pigmentosa may give a yellow color.[16] At times, freckles look yellowish-tan. The skin at times in the male castrate and in subsiding suntan may manifest a sallow, yellow appearance.[5,7] However, ordinarily melanin does not produce a striking yellow skin color. Its closest approximation is to give a yellowish-brown or tan.

Hemoglobin Pigmentation

As explained previously, reduced hemoglobin and oxyhemoglobin in the small blood vessels of the superficial and to a greater degree the deeper subpapillary plexuses play an important role in normal skin color. Many deviations from this normal pattern are seen in clinical practice as a result of changes in the nature of hemoglobin from normal. These conditions are tabulated in Table 51.[10]

All the hemoglobin pigmentations have in common the feature that the color change is most readily detected on clinical observation in the portions of the body where the keratinized layer of the epidermis is thinnest or absent and stratum mucosum most superficial. These are the lips, the palpebral conjunctivae, the fingernails and the mucous membranes of the mouth. Abnormal hemoglobin colors are accentuated in the areas shown in Figure 206 where oxyhemoglobin is normally predominant. Abnormal hemoglobin colors are also conditioned by the physiologic factors governing circulation in the superficial capillaries. Patients with carcinoid syndrome may have a periodic bright red to reddish-purple flush which may be in the "blush areas" or generalized. It is probably the result of vasodilatation or vasodilatation with stasis.

Melanin pigment in skin, if sufficient in amount, may effectively screen out the specific absorption pattern of any hemoglobin color change and prevent its clinical recognition. A representative example is the difficulty of detecting erythema and cyanosis in the skin of a Negro.

The palms and the soles, the fingernails, the lips and the palpebral conjunctivae should be inspected for hemoglobin color change in the darker racial groups because of the minimal or absent melanization in these areas.

Cyanosis results when the reduced hemoglobin in blood reaches 5 Gm. per cent. Apparently this is an average value, since Comroe and Botelho[18] have shown by the use of an oximeter for standardization that even trained observers (anesthetists, cardiologists, etc.) vary greatly in the ease with which they detect its presence by clinical observation in experimental subjects exposed to progressively increased degrees of anoxia. The blue color of cyanosis varies in tone and hue from deep purplish-blue to heliotrope and is influenced by numerous clinical factors. The purplish-blue hue is likely to be seen when carbon dioxide retention (which dilates vessels) accompanies anoxia. Cyanosis due to suffocation is a representative example. A false impression of cyanosis occasionally may be gained by inspection of the lips. The vermilion border may be quite blue due to dermal melanin in dark skinned people, particularly of Mediterranean origin. For a detailed discussion of the mechanism of cyanosis see Chapter 17.

Predominance of oxyhemoglobin explains almost all clinical situations characterized by a red skin color. In most instances the explanation is simply an increase in number or dilatation of the superficial skin vessels or an increase in rapidity of superficial skin blood flow so that the red color of oxyhemoglobin dominates the total skin color to a greater degree than normal. Representative examples of this are the red-flushed skin of fever, emotion, alcoholism and the various erythemas. At times, increases in the size and number of superficial capillaries are responsible (e.g., inflammation). Also at times, the skin is bright red because oxygen absorption by tissues is impaired because of low temperature. The tongue looks beefy red in a deficiency glossitis because of desquamation of the superficial, opaque, whitish, avascular filiform papillae (analogous to the stratum corneum of the epidermis) with resultant more superficial position of the lingual mucosa and papillary capillary projections.

Patients with true polycythemia appear to have a flushed, slightly cyanotic appearance which is called *erythremia*. It represents the full effect of the red oxyhemoglobin tinted with the blue of an increased amount of reduced hemoglobin because of the incapacity in this condition for oxygenating the hemoglobin increment. Peripheral capillary stasis further exaggerates these color changes.

Persons exposed to *carbon monoxide* fumes develop carboxyhemoglobinemia with a peculiar cherry-red color quite unlike the red of oxyhemoglobin. It disappears within half an hour after cessation of the exposure. In cases with fatal issue, the color persists. The bright red skin spots occasionally seen with cyanhemoglobinemia due to hydrocyanic poison also persist after death. The normal pink skin color of oxyhemoglobin disappears after death and instead one notes the bluish blotches and mottling of unoxygenated hemoglobin in dependent areas, to which the blood moves because of influence of gravity.

Whereas a clinically recognizable cyanosis requires the presence in the blood of 5 Gm. of reduced hemoglobin per 100 ml. of blood, a comparable skin color results from 1.5 Gm. of methemoglobin and less than 0.5 Gm. of sulfhemoglobin.[19] Methemoglobinemia produces a chocolate-blue skin color and sulfhemoglobinemia a mauve-blue one. Because of the small amount of these abnormal hemoglobin pigments necessary to produce cyanosis, individuals so affected are often quite comfortable and without symptoms, in contrast with the distress frequently noted when true cyanosis is present. This is especially true where the underlying condition is benign, as in idiopathic methemoglobinemia.

Although cyanosis is ordinarily related to hemoglobin changes in red cells, it may also occur after hemolysis, in which methemoglobin and metalbumin are present in the plasma.[19]

MELANIN PIGMENTATIONS (MELANOSIS)

Melanosis is a term commonly used to denote increased melanin pigmentation of the skin. Inasmuch as this pigment is an important component of skin color normally, it becomes clinically significant only when increased or markedly decreased in amount. Any increase in the degree of melanization is relative, since the degree of melanization normal for a person of one complexion or racial group may be abnormal for another.

Melanin pigmentation in any individual can be best judged by contrasting it with its previous intensity (sometimes readily done from old photographs), by comparing one area of the body to another, and by comparison with other members of the same family of like basic complexion. Frequently the relatives have noticed and commented on a change in the person's complexion.

Fitzpatrick, Seiji, and McGugan[68] have proposed a clinically useful classification of disturbances in human melanin pigmentation due both to decreased as well as increased amounts. Table 52 contains this classification. Inasmuch as all normal persons have melanocytes in their skins, everyone has the potential for developing melanosis if affected with any of the systemic diseases listed in this classification. Only the albino with his generalized defect of melanin formation in the skin remains immune.

Metabolism of melanin. Melanin is a normal endogenous body pigment. Over the years many of the older controversial aspects of the mechanism of its formation and its biochemistry have become clarified. The reader is referred to the important papers by Lerner and Fitzpatrick,[21] Fitzpatrick and Lerner,[54] Lorincz[62] and Lerner,[63] for a more detailed discussion of the metabolism of melanin and for a complete bibliography.

Melanin is formed by specialized cells

TABLE 52. DISTURBANCES OF HUMAN MELANIN PIGMENTATION.*

TYPE	DECREASED PIGMENTATION White (or Lighter than Normal)	INCREASED PIGMENTATION	
		Brown or Black	Gray, Slate or Blue †
GENETIC OR NEVOID	Albinism, oculocutaneous ‡ Albinism, localized cutaneous Vitiligo (may be diffuse) Phenylketonuria (hair & iris) Infantile Fanconi's syndrome (hair)	Neurofibromatosis (*café au lait*) Polyostotic fibrous dysplasia (Albright's syndrome) Ephelides (freckling) Xeroderma pigmentosum Acanthosis nigricans (juvenile type) Gaucher's disease ‡ Niemann-Pick disease ‡	Oculodermal melano-cytosis (nevus of Ota) Dermal melanocytosis (Mongolian spot)
METABOLIC		Hemochromatosis ‡ Hepatolenticular disease ‡ (Wilson's disease) Porphyria ‡ (congenital & cutanea tarda)	Hemochromatosis ‡
NUTRITIONAL	Kwashiorkor (hair)	Kwashiorkor Pellagra (may be diffuse) Sprue (may be diffuse)	Chronic nutritional insufficiency
ENDOCRINE	Hypopituitarism ‡ Addison's disease (vitiligoid)	ACTH & MSH producing pituitary tumors ‡ ACTH therapy ‡ Pregnancy (may be diffuse) Addison's disease ‡ Estrogen therapy (nipple)	
CHEMICAL	Arsenical intoxication Hydroquinone, mono-benzyl ether Chloroquin & hydroxy-chloroquin (hair) Guanonitrofurazone Chemical burns (with loss of melanocytes)	Arsenical intoxication ‡ Busulfan ‡ Photochemical (drugs, tar)	Fixed drug eruption Quinacrine toxicity

called melanocytes, located at the epidermo-dermal junction and derived embryologi-cally from the neural crest region.[20,21,54,68] (Figures 202 and 216). Melanin is also formed in the hair bulb, mucous mem-brane, uveal tract, retina and the lepto-meninges.

Under certain stimuli, to be discussed later, melanocytes normally in clear-cell form, enlarge, become dendritic and form melanin, which accumulates as micro-scopic granules in palisade cells of the basal layer of the epidermis, and is present in decreasing amounts in each outward layer of the rest of the epidermis. The number of melanin granules plays a greater role in

the degree of intensity of the skin color than does the size of the individual granule. Relatively little reaches the melanophages of the corium except in the region of the eyelids and axillae of some persons. Mela-nin is absent in the epidermis of albinos, present in the least amount in blonds, somewhat more in brunets and still more in the darker racial groups.[10]

Melanin in humans is formed from the amino acid tyrosine, which acts as the physiologic substrate in a complex enzy-matic action. Lerner and Fitzpatrick[21] reviewed the evidence for the present be-lief that the enzyme tyrosinase (a copper-protein complex) is a single enzyme with

TABLE 52. DISTURBANCES OF HUMAN MELANIN PIGMENTATION (*Continued*)

TYPE	DECREASED PIGMENTATION WHITE (OR LIGHTER THAN NORMAL)	INCREASED PIGMENTATION BROWN OR BLACK	GRAY, SLATE OR BLUE†
PHYSICAL	Thermal burns (with loss of melanocytes) Trauma (with loss of melanocytes)	Ultraviolet light Heat Alpha, beta & gamma radiation Trauma (for example, chronic pruritus)	
INFECTIONS & INFLAMMATIONS	Pinta Leprosy§ Fungous infections§ Postinflammatory§ (atopic dermatitis, drug eruptions & so forth) Vogt-Koyanagi syndrome	Postinflammatory (dermatitis, exanthems, drug eruptions)	Pinta (exposed areas)
NEOPLASMS	Leukoderma acquisitum centrifugum (halo nevus) In sites of melanoma after disappearance (therapeutic or spontaneous) of tumor	Urticaria pigmentosa Adenocarcinoma with acanthosis nigricans	MALIGNANT MELANOMA,‡ advanced (generalized dermal pigmentation syndrome, with melanuria)
MISCELLANEOUS	Scleroderma§ (circumscribed & systemic types) Canities (hair) Alopecia areata (hair)	SCLERODERMA, SYSTEMIC‡ CHRONIC HEPATIC INSUFFICIENCY‡ WHIPPLE'S SYNDROME‡ Melasma (chloasma)	

* This classification includes disorders of interest to physicians in general; many pigmentary disorders not listed are of special interest to the dermatologist.

† Gray, slate or blue color results from the presence of *dermal* melanocytes, or phagocytized melanin in dermis.

‡ Small cap type indicates that pigmentary change is diffuse, not spotty, and there are no identifiable borders.

§ Usually *partial* loss of pigmentation; viewed with the Wood's light, the lesions are not chalk white, as in vitiligo.

Fitzpatrick, T. B., Seiji, M. and McGugan, A. D.: Medical Progress: Melanin pigmentation, New England J. Med. 265:328.

two activities: catalyzation of the oxidation of the amino-acid tyrosine to DOPA and the oxidation of DOPA in turn to melanin. It is important to emphasize that a complex series of chemical reactions constitute the intermediate stages of this reaction and thus the formation of melanin is subject to a variety of controlling factors other than the basic enzymatic reaction itself. These reactions as schematized by Fitzpatrick et al.[68] are shown in Figures 215 and 216.

The metabolic requirements for tyrosine are largely satisfied by conversion of phenylalanine to tyrosine by enzymatic action in the liver. Dietary tyrosine ordinarily plays a minor role (Fig. 219).

The paths of excretion of melanin include (1) from the skin by desquamation and (2) by drainage through the lymphatics, to the blood stream and excretion through the kidney. The amount in the urine is at times grossly visible (melanuria), a condition most likely to result from extensive metastases from melanotic tumors.

Lerner and Fitzpatrick[21] list the many biochemical factors regulating the formation of melanin. Some substances (e.g., DOPA) catalyze the tyrosine-tyrosinase reaction. Other substances (e.g., sulfhydryl compounds) inhibit tyrosinase by virtue of their ability to bind the copper necessary for this enzymatic action. If the sulfhydryl groups are oxidized the inactivated copper is released with increased tyrosinase reaction. A pH higher than the optimal range prolongs the induction period of tyrosine oxidation, while at lower values of pH tyrosinase activity is reduced. The tyrosine-tyrosinase reaction increases with limited rise in temperature. The redox (oxidation-reduction) potential, if high, is associated with a long tyrosine induction period. The amount of the physiologic substrate tyrosine is naturally important. Lastly oxidation is important; melanin being light-colored in reduced form and darker (black) in oxidized form. Fitzpatrick and his associates[54,68] have pre-

sented these facts in diagrams (Figs. 202, 215 and 216).

External (Physical) Causes. In many instances of melanosis the factor responsible is the external application of a physical agent to the skin.[22]

Because of the ubiquity of exposure to sunlight, melanosis due to ordinary exposure is accepted as a component of normal skin color and called *tan*. Only when the exposure is excessive is the increase of melanization likely to be noticed. Even here it has no clinical significance unless confused with melanosis due to internal causes. Exposure to some artificial source of ultraviolet radiation acts the same as

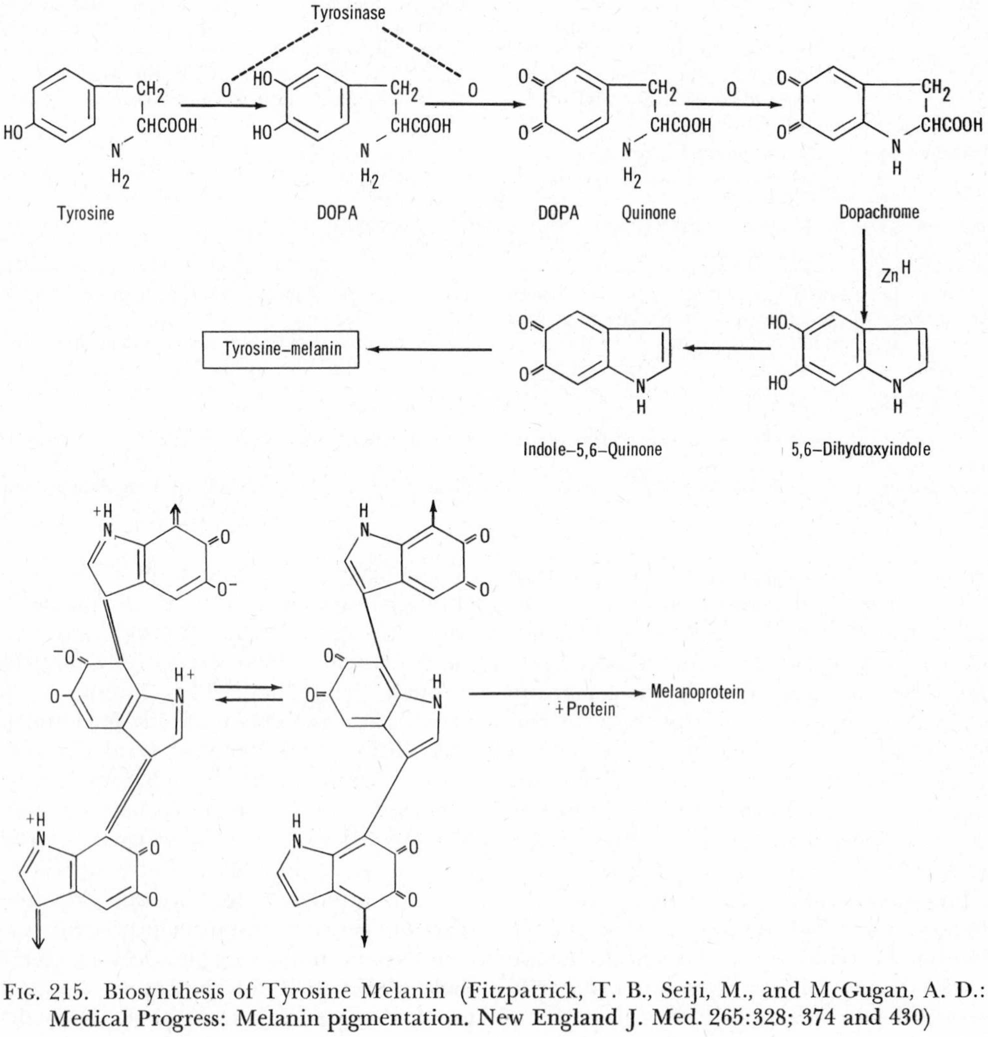

Fig. 215. Biosynthesis of Tyrosine Melanin (Fitzpatrick, T. B., Seiji, M., and McGugan, A. D.: Medical Progress: Melanin pigmentation. New England J. Med. 265:328; 374 and 430)

exposure to natural sunlight. Those with light complexions (blond) tan less readily and to a lesser degree than those of dark complexion (brunet).

Melanin resulting from ultraviolet exposure is deposited only in the epidermis and never in the dermis, and therefore is of a brownish hue.[22] The mechanism by which ultraviolet irradiation stimulates melanosis is complex and is believed to include:[21,23] (1) catalyzing the oxidation of tyrosine to DOPA so that the DOPA so formed can catalyze tyrosine-tyrosinase enzyme reaction (Fig. 215), (2) oxidation of melanin already present in the skin, (3) diminishing the concentration of sulfhydryl groups in the epidermis which normally are the natural inhibitors of tyrosinase, (4) decreasing the redox potential of the skin and (5) elevating the temperature of the skin either directly or by producing an erythema.[21,23]

The skin of albinos and the vitiliginous area of otherwise normal skin manifest erythema and serious burning on exposure to ultraviolet radiation because of failure of melanization in skin with these defects.

The skin may be photosensitized to actinic rays by the application of certain substances externally and possibly by their presence internally. At times a marked melanosis may develop with only a very limited exposure to sunlight. The deposition of melanin pigment in this condition occurs in the upper dermis as well as the epidermis, with a resultant grayish-brown color.[22] This type of pigmentation may persist much longer than the ordinary melanosis due to actinic rays. Dihydroxyacetone has become increasingly popular as a topical agent to produce a bronze appearance of the skin to simulate suntan. It apparently combines with material in the outer keratin layer, and is removed as the

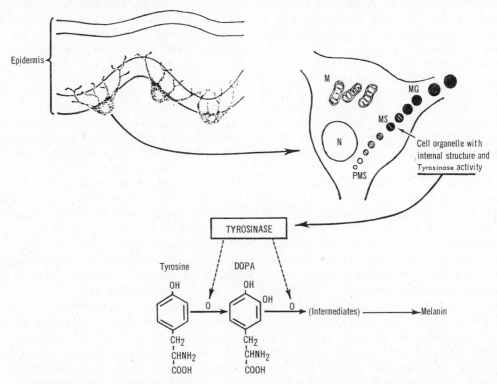

Fig. 216. Melanogenesis in human skin as seen in the light microscope and the electron microscope and at the molecular level. (M) Mitochondria; (N) Nucleus; (PMS) Promelanosomes; (MS) Melanosomes; (MG) Melanin granules. (Fitzpatrick, T. B., Seiji, M., and McGugan, A. D.: Medical progress: melanin pigmentation, New England J. Med. 265: 328; 374 and 430)

keratin is normally shed in a few days. The pigmented compound has not been chemically characterized, but it is definitely not melanin. It does not have the protective activity against sunburning that melanin possesses.

The alpha rays of thorium-x and to a lesser degree beta and gamma roentgen and radium rays stimulate melanization. In dark brunets this may occur without a preceding erythema, although usually it follows an erythema.[22]

The application of *heat* to the skin in any form sufficient to produce prolonged or repeated erythema leads to melanosis of the areas so exposed. The classic clinical example is the reticular pattern of melanin pigmentation which follows *erythema caloricum* due to repeated application of hot water bottles to the abdomen for pain. Melanosis from heat is attributed to an increase in the rate of sulfhydryl oxidation which releases bound copper and to an increase in the tyrosinase reaction as well as direct acceleration of the enzymatic oxidation of tyrosine.[21]

Application of any of these physical agents to a degree sufficient to destroy skin (second and third degree burns) destroys the melanocytes so that the resultant scar tissue has less pigment (both melanin and hemoglobin) than normal and by contrast appears whiter or less pigmented than normal skin.

Irritation of the skin by application of caustic chemicals may produce melanin through the production of severe erythema.

Mechanical irritation of the skin, if long continued, may produce local erythema and eventually melanosis. Classic examples clinically are the melanized areas in the groin from wearing of a truss for hernia and in the axillae from the use of crutches.

An interesting example of melanosis predominantly of external origin commonly seen in every hospital receiving the indigent and neglected type of patient is the so-called *vagabonds' disease* or *beggars' melanosis.*[10] The pigmentation characteristically is more marked on the covered than the exposed portions of the body and especially noticeable over areas where the

clothes chafe. Lack of bathing or removal of dirty clothes and presence of body pediculi with resulting irritation, increase in heat in body folds and scratching are the main factors. However, such individuals are usually malnourished so that internal factors may contribute to the melanization.

Severe pruritus is common in chronic uremia, chronic obstructive jaundice and Hodgkin's disease. It is likely that continual scratching by patients with these diseases acts as a form of constant mechanical irritation and contributes to the melanosis occasionally seen in these conditions.

It is characteristic of all forms of melanosis due to external physical agents that the degree of melanization gradually diminishes when the exciting factor is removed.

Internal (Systemic) Causes. The types of melanosis of chief importance in clinical practice are those which result from internal causes. No attempt will be made here to discuss all the dermatologic disorders with melanosis although some may be of systemic origin. Beerman and Colburn[73] have concisely reviewed them and Cowan[72] has reviewed the ocular pigmentary disturbances. This chapter is concerned primarily with the mechanism of melanosis in the conditions which can be considered of prime interest to the field of internal medicine (Table 52). The following several paragraphs will attempt to group and explain them according to the basic physiologic disturbance responsible,[21] rather than to discuss them purely from the viewpoint of their presence in a wide variety of apparently unrelated diseases. In most instances the origin of melanosis is in nutritional, endocrine, nervous, or dermal causes or in some combination of these.

MELANOSIS OF NUTRITIONAL ORIGIN. There seems but little doubt that many instances of melanosis can be explained on the basis of metabolic disturbance of nutritional origin. At the end of World War II[21,25,26] it was noted that pigmentation was common in persons held for long periods in prison or concentration camps under starvation regimens. The mechanism of the melanosis here is difficult to evaluate, since the nutritional deficiency in humans is invariably of complex origin. An interesting speculation has centered about the possibility that the predominantly vegetable diets of these starved people contained proportionally less sulfhydryl amino acids (cystine and methionine), which normally inhibit melanin formation, than the amino-acid melanin precursors phenylalanine and tyrosine.[21]

In addition, there is a strong possibility that the malnutrition may have been associated with deficiency of certain factors in the diet or that an inadequacy of total caloric content may have secondarily produced abnormalities of endocrine function.

Melanosis is common in pellagra (niacin deficiency) and occurs both with the low-grade chronic variety and following the subsidence of an acute pellagrous dermatitis. The mechanism for this melanosis[21] is considered to be similar to that which follows the various types of erythematous reactions due to physical agents, as described previously. This is probably true for the type following the acute phase of pellagrous erythema. In low-grade chronic pellagra hyperkeratosis and pigmentation of pressure areas without much erythema is at times a prominent feature. Release of sulfhydryl inhibition of melanin formation may be a factor.

Pigmentation is at times a prominent feature in scurvy (vitamin-C deficiency). Both melanosis and hemosiderosis (due to purpura in the skin) must be considered to explain changes in skin color in this disorder.[21] General malnutrition might also play an important role in some instances.

Although extremely rare in the United States,[10] melanin pigmentation has been noted in the skin of patients with vitamin-A deficiency. It exhibits a peculiar localization to the site of the hyperkeratotic follicular lesion so characteristic of this disease.

Lerner and Fitzpatrick[21] attribute the pigmentation in all three of these vitamin deficiencies to the release in the epidermis of normal sulfhydryl inhibition of tyrosinase, with the reason for the production of the decrease in sulfhydryl group different in each of them. In pellagra the mechanism is that characteristic for any postinflammatory variety; in vitamin-A deficiency, diversion of sulfhydryl for increased keratin formation; and in scurvy, from deposition of iron and copper in the skin as a result of the hemorrhagic tendency.

MELANOSIS OF HORMONAL ORIGIN. The generally accepted clinical impression that the endocrine system plays a major role in the control of melanin metabolism finds increasing experimental and scientific support in the medical literature.[69,74,75] The pituitary gland seems to play the dominant role followed in importance by the adrenals, leaving estrogen and progesterone and other endocrine substances a lesser but not well-established significance.

The often confirmed observations of the darkly pigmented appearance of the acromegalic and the characteristic pallor of hypopituitarism (Simmonds' disease) give firm clinical support to the idea that the pituitary gland in humans is concerned in some way with melanin metabolism. The concept of a separate melanophore hormone, produced in the pars intermedia of the pituitary gland, has been accepted for lower forms of animal life.[10]

The presence of melanocyte-stimulating hormone (M.S.H.) in man is now well documented.[69] This concept received renewed interest with reports of melanosis developing in a white male receiving ACTH (pituitary adrenocorticotropin), which substance on analysis was found to contain a significant amount of melanophore hormone (intermedin).[21,30] This could explain pigmentation reported to be due to use of pituitary preparations.[21] Previous evidence suggested that melanocyte-stimulating hormone (M.S.H.) present as a contaminant was responsible in earlier reports of increased melanin pigmentation with ACTH preparations. Lerner and McGuire[77] recently showed that chemically pure ACTH has skin-darkening properties in very large doses.

Lerner and associates[63,69] in excellent reviews discuss the polypeptide nature and separate identity of α- and β-melanocyte-stimulating hormones (M.S.H.) secreted by the intermediate lobe of the pituitary. The reader is referred to these papers for a detailed background of this subject. This secretion has been described for many years as intermedin, melanophore-dilating principle, melanophore hormone, etc., and generally accepted as significant in the pigmentation of fish and amphibia. Recent studies have now determined the presence of M.S.H. in human blood and urine. The highly active biologic effect of M.S.H. in humans is indicated by the ability of a few micrograms to influence melanocytes in humans with a prompt detectable increase in skin pigmentation with diminution to previous skin color a few weeks after cessation of its use.[61]

The pattern of secretion and activity of M.S.H. resembles that of other pituitary hormones, as Calkins[31] had postulated previously. Thus, the level of its urinary excretion is raised when adrenal cortical activity is low, as in Addison's disease or after adrenalectomy. Of interest was the observation of a greatly increased M.S.H. production during pregnancy,[53,61] a period when melanization of the eyelids, the nipples and the areolae of the breast is increased and the linea nigra of the abdomen appears. The level of M.S.H. production is low in panhypopituitarism, which correlates with the pale skin color associated with this disorder.

Several products of the adrenal are antagonistic to the action of M.S.H. Epinephrine and norepinephrine have an inhibiting action and appear to block its action on the melanocyte. This is in accord with clinical observation that in instances of Addison's disease in which the adrenal medulla is destroyed along with the cortex, the cutaneous pigmentation is greater than with the presence of only cortical insufficiency. Cortisone and hydrocortisone diminish melanin production[61] possibly through inhibition of M.S.H. production.

Hall, McCracken and Thorn[49] have studied skin pigmentation, in relation to adrenal cortical function, by means of the Hardy spectrophotometer. They found that a great diminution in cutaneous blood flow accompanied the melanization of Addison's disease or surgical adrenalectomy.

Cortisone caused a lowering of melanin skin content in patients with intact adrenals. Darkening of the skin with use of ACTH apparently depends on an increase in cutaneous blood flow as well as melanin formation. They suggested that the latter effect may be due to some other product of the pituitary accompanying the ACTH as a contaminant.[49]

The almost invariable presence of melanosis in Addison's disease has served to center considerable attention on the relation of the adrenal glands to melanin metabolism. A voluminous literature[10,21] attests to the various theories and extensive research concerning this problem.

It is generally believed that the adrenal hormones inhibit melanization under certain circumstances, as evidenced by the striking hyperpigmentation which occurs in animals following adrenalectomy, or in humans following surgical removal of adrenal cortex or the destruction or atrophy of the adrenal gland from disease.[21]

The various theories[10,21,32,33] to explain melanosis in Addison's disease include: (1) loss of sympathetic nervous inhibition of melanization occasioned by failure of the adrenal stimulation; (2) failure of the diseased adrenal gland to utilize the precursor of epinephrine, which results in its conversion to melanin; (3) diminished storage in the adrenals of vitamin C, which normally has an inhibiting effect on melanin formation; (4) depression of blood level of sodium from adrenal cortical failure, with resultant increased oxidation of ascorbic acid and diminution of its concentration, leading, in turn, to loss of its inhibitory influence on melanin formation; (5) through the possible influence of the adrenal gland in regulating the metabolism of sulfhydryl compounds, with resultant decrease in their concentration in the skin and loss of their inhibiting effect on melanin[21] formation; and (6) loss of control of melanogenesis by a pituitary-adrenal axis in which normally the adrenal hormones inhibit release of M.S.H. or its peripheral action on melanocytes.[21,31,53,61]

This latter idea best explains the known facts and was discussed in more detail previously. Figure 217 from the paper by Lerner, Shizume and Bunding[61] clearly presents this concept in a diagrammatic fashion.

Both clinical observations and laboratory studies have established clearly that primary adrenal cortical insufficiency causes melanosis, whereas adrenal cortical insufficiency secondary to hypopituitarism does so only rarely.[10,21,34,61]

The frequent observation of vitiligo in Addison's disease, with deep melanosis and marked patchy depigmentation irregularly distributed, is striking.

We have mentioned already the influence of the gonads in determining the color of the skin in the normal male and female, the deviations from normal changes which occur in castrated men and ovariectomized women and the reversibility of each of these with the appropriate sex hormone therapy. The gonads normally control skin color not only through their influence on melanization but also the skin

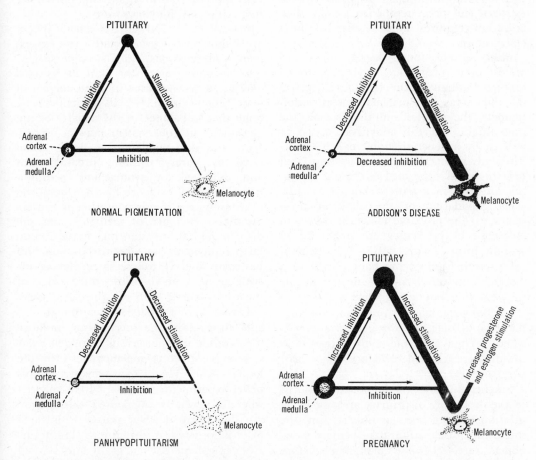

Fig. 217. (*Upper left*) Normal pigmentation. "Hydrocortisone inhibits the output of MSH by the pituitary gland. Noradrenaline and adrenaline inhibit the action of MSH on the pigment-forming cells." (*Upper right*) Addison's disease. "MSH output is increased because hydrocortisone inhibition of the pituitary is decreased. If the adrenal medulla is destroyed, the inhibition of MSH by adrenaline and noradrenaline is removed." (*Lower left*) Panhypopituitarism. "MSH output is decreased because of decrease in pituitary function." (*Lower right*) Pregnancy. "MSH output, progesterone and estrogens are increased. Progesterone may have a direct MSH-like action." (Lerner, Shizume and Bunding: J. Clin. Endocrinol. & Metab. 14:1463)

content of hemoglobin, carotene and melanoid.[5,6,8]

Oral administration of estrogen in women prior to the menopause has been reported as increasing the degree of melanization in the nipples, areolae and linea nigra.[27] Similar hyperpigmentation is said not to develop when estrogens are used after the menopause, perhaps because of diminished functional activity of the pituitary gland at this time of life. Application of estrogen-containing ointment to the skin has been reported as producing areas of increased melanization. The influence of estrogen and progesterone on human melanization requires more study for final clarification.

Melanosis of some degree occurs in almost every pregnancy. It is manifested as pigmentation of the face, accentuation of the areas of primary melanization (namely, the nipples and the areolae, the linea nigra and the anovulvar areas) as well as by a generalized increase.[10,27] Occasionally the facial pigment is accentuated over the cheeks, the bridge of the nose and the forehead in a pattern known as chloasma gravidarum or the mask of pregnancy.[10] The probable factors involved in melanosis of pregnancy are presented in graphic form in Figure 217. As a general rule, termination of pregnancy leads to a marked diminution in the degree of the pigmentation but leaves some sequelae in the form of permanent residue in the nipples, the areolae, the linea nigra and elsewhere. These are commonly accepted as presumptive clinical evidence of a past pregnancy.[10]

Further influence of the gonads is noted in the darkening of primary areas of melanization in both sexes at puberty and the interesting observation that benign melanomas rarely become malignant before puberty.[28]

Numerous examples of in-vitro and in-vivo experiments in animals are on record which demonstrate the influence of the sex hormones on melanin metabolism.[10,21,29] Arrhenoblastoma, the masculinizing tumor of the ovary, has been reported as producing darkening of the skin. Apparently both estrogens and androgens increase melanin skin pigmentation. However, the biochemical nature of this action is still obscure.

There is also the possibility that the thyroid gland is concerned with melanin metabolism, as suggested by the common occurrence of melanosis in hyperthyroidism—especially when chronic.[10] Lerner[63] recently has surveyed the present status of this endocrine gland in relation to melanin pigmentation.

It is of considerable interest that the precursor of melanin, tyrosine, is chemically quite similar to the thyroid hormones, thyroxine and di-iodotyrosine.

MELANOSIS OF NERVOUS ORIGIN. There are a number of clinical and a few experimental observations which strongly suggest that melanization of the skin in humans may be subject (at least in some degree) to neurogenic control.[10,21] It is believed by some that imbalance in the activity of the autonomic nervous system may be important, with skin pigmentation being stimulated by parasympathetic predominance and inhibited by sympathetic predominance. Further evidence for the role of the nervous system in pigmentation is the occasional occurrence of vitiligo along the distribution of a cutaneous nerve. Similarly, repigmentation of a vitiliginous limb has been observed following accidental severing of that nerve, while the vitiligo of the controlateral limb remained the same.

Lerner and Fitzpatrick,[21] although unable to explain the mechanism, indicate the possible role of certain neurogenic factors in controlling melanogenesis in the human skin. They cite in support of this belief experiments reported by Haxthausen wherein normally pigmented skin gradually depigmented when grafted to an area of vitiligo, whereas vitiliginous skin gradually repigmented when grafted to normal skin. They also comment on the fact that the pigmentation of acanthosis nigricans, which in adults may be due to an abdominal visceral carcinoma (especially of the stomach), often develops when the lesion involves the celiac plexus or chromaffin system.

Melanosis is common in neurofibromatosis.[10] The congenital neurocutaneous syndrome of melanosis of the skin and central nervous system and the tendency for a skin pigment spot to localize over a spina bifida occulta are examples of the curious association of nervous lesions with melanosis.[10] Other types have been described.[10,21,63]

MELANOSIS WITH SKIN DISEASE. A variety of skin diseases are known to produce melanosis.[20] Any dermatologic disorder which produces an inflammatory response may be followed by melanosis, for reasons previously discussed.

It is likely that certain systemic diseases with end-organ response in the skin may produce melanosis by changes in skin metabolism of a localized nature. *Arsenic* apparently produces melanosis by its deposition in the skin with resultant binding of epidermal sulfhydryl substances which results in removal of the inhibition of the tyrosinase enzyme.[21] Arsenic may also act to produce skin inflammation. The melanosis seen with scleroderma and dermatomyositis probably results from the local changes of the skin which occur in these conditions.

The reader is referred elsewhere for further information on this group.[20,24,73] There remains little doubt that certain systemic diseases produce melanosis through an influence exerted locally on the skin as an end organ.

Clinical Picture. Melanin normally present in the skin is not of uniform intensity over the entire body but is accentuated in certain areas called primary zones (Fig. 203). These include the eyelids, the axillae, the nipples, the areolae, the umbilicus, the linea nigra, the genital region, the nape of the neck and the anal region. In women the nape of the neck, the linea nigra and the axillae are more heavily melanized than these areas in the male. Szabo[70] has shown marked variations in the number of melanocytes in the epidermis in different regions of the body.

Likewise, the pattern of melanosis is not one of uniform increase in intensity over the entire skin but is subject to accentuation in certain areas which vary with the disease responsible or with exposure to external factors influencing melanin metabolism.

Although derived from the Greek meaning *black,* melanin in the epidermis ordinarily produces a yellowish-tan, tan or brown color but may occasionally appear black. When melanin is present in melanophages in the upper dermis without much in the epidermis it produces a slate-gray color; when present deep in the dermis a blue color occurs due to the scattering phenomenon.[5,10,20]

In most instances the abnormal melanosis shows accentuation in the groin, the axillae, under the breasts, between the buttocks, in skin folds, etc.—all areas of higher than average skin temperature. It is well known that increased temperature accentuates melanin formation. Friction from belts, trusses, buttons, waist bands, garters, areas of chafing, etc., may likewise predispose to local areas of accentuation. Still another pattern is for the accentuation to occur in the normally accentuated primary zones of melanization, such as the nipples, the areolae, the linea nigra, the genital areas and anal areas. Another common pattern is preponderant melanosis of portions of the skin exposed to sunlight. Pigmentation of the face may be uniform or accentuated in areas as in the "mask of pregnancy." At times the eyelids become heavily melanized. The hair may rarely participate by darkening but cases of Addison's disease have been observed with prematurely white hair. Not uncommon is the development of melanization of the mucous membranes of the oral cavity and, at times, of the eye and of the vagina. Even the nail bed may show melanosis.

With a few exceptions (e.g., acanthosis nigricans, arsenic poisoning, etc.) the melanoses of internal origin generally have a similar histologic picture, consisting of an increase in the number and density of melanin particles (melanosomes). For the most part, therefore, a skin biopsy in melanosis tells only that the pigment is melanin, as was usually surmised from the history and clinical inspection.

A few diseases produce a melanotic skin picture which, on clinical inspection, is characteristic of or at least suggestive of the basic systemic disease responsible. These include the "rain drop" appearance and hyperkeratosis of arsenic poisoning; the wrinkled, velvety and often papillomatous pigmentation of the neck, axillae and groin seen in acanthosis nigricans; the ocular pingueculae and melanosis of Gaucher's disease; the blue cartilaginous areas of the ears and nose, the sclerae and ear drums, of ochronosis; the facial mask and nipple-areolae accentuation of pregnancy, chloasma uterinum and estrogen therapy of young women; the perifollicular skin and ocular localization of vitamin-A deficiency, etc.

As a general rule, however, the pattern of melanosis without an increase in the number of melanocytes is not distinctive of the underlying disease. The degree and pattern of melanosis from the same disease may vary greatly from one person to the next, including, at times, the ordinarily distinctive ones mentioned above. The melanosis of certain localized hyperpigmented lesions is often distinctive enough to be readily recognized on clinical inspection (i.e., neurofibromatosis, Albright's syndrome, xeroderma pigmentosum, Peutz-Jeghers syndrome, etc.).

Freckles (ephelides) are the commonest of this variety of melanosis. The pigmentation is in the form of clearly demarcated yellowish-brown to tan areas, varying in size and shape but predominantly small and most prevalent on the exposed parts of the body. They are absent in infancy, appear in childhood, never occur on the palms, soles or inside the mouth, are more prominent in summer and tend to fade in late adult life. The tendency to develop freckles is an inherited dominant characteristic. Except for occasional confusion with melanosis due to disease their main significance is cosmetic.

Except possibly albinos, all persons have the potential of developing a melanotic neoplasm. Aside from the color of the local lesion and its metastases, persons with this condition in an advanced stage often have melanuria and may rarely develop a generalized darkening of the skin due to release from the tumor of precursors of melanin which are oxidized to this pigment in the epidermis.[55] This is one of the few instances where melanin not produced locally by melanocytes can darken the skin;[21] it likewise occurs in ochronosis, in which an intermediate product of the catabolism of tyrosine, namely homogentisic acid, accumulates in the extracellular fluid and is deposited and darkens in cartilage, an area where melanocytes do not occur.[10,21,54]

Mongolian spots (aggregates of dermal melanocytes) are blue in color and most commonly are located over the sacral areas but may occasionally occur elsewhere. They are most common in certain of the darker races but are seen infrequently in white babies. Such spots persist for a variable number of years after birth and eventually disappear.[10,35]

The common pigmented nevus varies from flesh color to brown to blue-black depending upon the amount and depth of pigment-laden nevus cells.

The tendency for the skin pigmentation in Albright's syndrome to occur in unilateral, irregularly marginated patchy areas in roughly the same body location as the bone lesion is a distinctive clinical pattern. Also easily recognized are the smoothly marginated *café-au-lait* spots so commonly associated with neurofibromatosis.

The pigmentation pattern characteristically associated with the generalized form of intestinal polyposis (Peutz-Jeghers syndrome) occurs as small melanin spots distributed in an acral fashion inside and about the mouth, on the face, more prominent on the lower than the upper lip and occasionally on the fingers and toes.[48] This pigmentation has thus far not been associated with polyposis limited to the stomach, the large bowel or the rectum.

The others falling into this group are too rare to warrant discussion here.

Melanin Pigmentation of Mucous Membranes. Histologic observations have shown that melanin-producing cells (melanocytes) are present in the oral mucosa of most white persons. Grossly visible melanin areas in the mouth (melanoplakia) are normally unusual in white persons of light complexion, are occasionally noted in those of dark complexion and are very frequently observed in Negroes. Therefore, melanoplakia has the most diagnostic significance if seen in a person of light complexion or if it develops in a person in whom the mouth is known to have been clear of melanin spots by previous examination. In the darker racial groups, melanosis of the tongue rather than of the buccal mucosa proper may be suggestive of disease. The melanocytes in the mouth are subject to the same internal stimuli as those in the skin, so that melanoplakia occurs frequently in diseases which produce marked melanosis of the skin (Table 52). It is possible that the melanocytes in the oral mucosa may react to local physical factors in the mouth very much as do those of skin. Heat, chemical irritation and friction may be important in this regard.[10,36,37]

It is of interest that melanocytes have also been demonstrated in the conjunctiva. At times, diseases which produce skin melanosis also result in an external ocular melanosis. However, this is less frequent than melanoplakia.

Melanocytes are also present in the nail bed, as indicated by the occasional occurrence of melanization here in Negroes[38] and its rare occurrence in white persons who have certain of the systemic diseases which produce severe melanosis.

Metallic Pigmentation

Under certain conditions abnormal skin color results from the deposition in skin of a group of pigments (not normally present) which have in common the fact that all are metallic. The various skin pigmentations resulting can be classified as metallic pigmentation and are presented in tabular form in Table 53.[10]

Most metallic pigments responsible for skin pigmentation are exogenous in origin. The important exception is hemosiderin, an iron-containing pigment which results from local or general destruction of blood or from some defect in endogenous iron metabolism. The term *hemosiderosis* has been used in a general sense to depict deposition of this substance in body tissue.[10] In the skin it localizes in the superficial corium and if present leads to pigmentation, not only directly but also by stimulating melanin formation.

Hemochromatosis. Basically this condition is characterized by a defect in endogenous metabolism of iron with deposition of hemosiderin in certain visceral and endocrine organs as well as the skin. The mechanism for skin pigmentation is not entirely clear but appears to involve deposition of hemosiderin in the corium and of melanin in the deep epidermis. The former pigment causes a bluish-black, slate or lead color while melanin is responsible for a brownish hue. The classic *bronze color* occasionally seen in this disease appears to depend on the combination of these two skin pigments. Copper is also deposited in the skin. The presence of iron and copper in the skin could bind the sulfhydryl substances and increase the degree of melanization by releasing inhibition of tyrosinase.[21] Likewise, deposition of hemosiderin in endocrine organs with resultant functional changes is characteristic of hemochromatosis, as witness the almost constant pancreatic involvement causing diabetes mellitus. The gonads, pituitary and adrenals are commonly involved, which could account, in part, for some of the melanosis. Cirrhosis could also be a factor.

Exogenous Hemosiderosis. Here the disease results from injection of an excess of blood in the form of repeated transfusions.[39] The excess hemosiderin resulting from the breakdown of this blood is deposited in the skin and organs and produces skin pigmentation in a manner similar to hemochromatosis.

To some degree, repeated hemolysis of internal origin leads to hemosiderin deposition but probably only rarely is it sufficiently marked to account for skin pigmentation. These cases are difficult to evaluate since many also receive transfusions of blood.

Hemosiderosis of the Lower Legs. Extravasation of blood in the skin of the lower legs, particularly if repeated or of chronic duration, leads to deposition of hemosiderin in the corium and stimulation of melanin formation with production of a tan, brown, copper or sepia skin color.[10] This type of pigmentation is limited to the area below the knees and above the upper level at which the shoe exerts a protective pressure and is more marked anteriorly

TABLE 53. CLASSIFICATION OF THE METALLIC PIGMENTATIONS

Type	Pigment Responsible	Where Deposited	Skin Color	Circumstances for Its Causation	Clinical Significance
Hemochromatosis	Melanin and hemosiderin	Generalized in epidermis and corium	Tan; slate gray; bronze	Endogenous defect in iron metabolism. Melanin stimulated by local action of hemosiderin in skin	Skin pigmentation characteristic of this disease and rarely absent. Usually both melanin and hemosiderin are present
Hemosiderosis of skin from chronic hemolysis	Hemosiderin; melanin secondary	Generalized in corium	Tan; slate gray; bronze	As a result of repeated blood transfusion, especially if excess hemolysis occurs	Quite rare. Suspect with use of many blood transfusions
Hemosiderosis of the lower legs	Hemosiderin; melanin secondary	Deeper epidermis and corium of legs	Brownish, copper hue, sepia	Limited to legs below knee and above shoe line. Due to hydrostatic pressure increase in legs plus local capillary or blood hemolytic factor	Seen most commonly in venous stasis of leg veins, leg trauma, sickle-cell disease, chronic purpuric eruptions, congenital hemolytic jaundice, Mediterranean anemia, Gaucher's disease, Cushing's syndrome and some rare dermatologic disorders. See reference 10
Argyria	Silver	Generalized in corium	Gray to blue	Deposited in skin regardless of route of entry to body. Color exaggerated by exposure to the sun	Chiefly of cosmetic importance; closely simulates cyanosis
Bismuthia	Bismuth	Generalized in corium	Gray to blue	Deposition in skin over diffuse area	A rare cause of generalized skin pigmentation
Bismuth line	Bismuth sulfide	Gums near teeth	Black	Deposited in gums of persons receiving bismuth, especially if tartar deposits on teeth are present	Diagnostic of bismuth treatment. Location limited to the mouth
Chrysiasis	Gold	Upper corium predominantly	Gray, grayish-blue to bluish-green	May follow prolonged use of gold therapy. Concentrated in areas exposed to the sun	Cosmetic; gold more toxic than silver
Hydrargyria	Mercury	Epidermis and corium of local areas	Brown or slate gray (Red-cinnabar)	Of local origin. Produced by rubbing mercury creams on skin, expecially the face and neck	Chiefly cosmetic. Simulates systemic causes of facial pigmentation. Rare sensitization.
Lead line	Lead sulfide	Gums near teeth	Black	Deposition in gums of lead sulfide. Local mechanism is similar to bismuth line	Lead does not pigment the skin. Lead line in gums is diagnostic of lead poisoning (Rule out lead exposure)
Iron pigmentation	Basic ferric acetate	Corium	Brown	Produced by tattoo of corium. When iron salts are used on skin lesion lacking epidermal covering	Local areas only. Of cosmetic importance
Chromium	Chromium oxide	Corium	Green	Tattoos	Local areas only. Of cosmetic importance. Rare sensitization.

than posteriorly. The pigmentation may be diffuse or localized to small areas, particularly about ulcers or areas of trauma. The most characteristic example seen clinically is the pigmentation noted in association with varicose veins, especially if ulceration occurs. Hemorrhagic diathesis, venous stasis in the leg veins, increased capillary fragility and changes in tissue pressure are all predisposing factors.[10] Some of the more common diseases responsible are listed in Table 53. Because of the many local causes of hemosiderosis in the legs, this area should never be used for biopsy study for hemochromatosis.

Metal Ions in the Skin. Any silver compound which enters the body, regardless of the route of administration, results in deposition of silver in the corium of the skin and when a sufficient threshold is reached becomes clinically visible and is known as argyria. Exposure to sunlight greatly accentuates its recognition. While some degree of melanization may result, the main color is from the silver itself, which, because of its location in the corium, produces a slate-gray, lead or bluish-gray skin color. Clinically argyria is of importance because of the disagreeable skin discoloration and the ease with which it is confused with cyanosis.

Chrysiasis (from gold) and bismuthia (from bismuth) occur rarely and simulate argyria in the mode of production and the clinical appearance. As a general rule, bismuth produces a dark line on the gum similar to that produced by lead.

Mercury preparations, if rubbed into the skin, produce a local area of discoloration. Metallic iron can tattoo the skin if it reaches the corium through a defect in the epidermis but cannot act systemically to influence skin color. The red and green colors of tattoos are due to mercury (cinnabar) and chromium, respectively.

EXAGGERATED SCATTERING PHENOMENON: BLUE COLORATION

As previously explained, normal "flesh" color of the skin is dependent on the fact that "scattering" adds a blue component to offset the predominant red color reflected

from the hemoglobin (Plate 4). It has been mentioned also that the same phenomenon explains the blue color seen over a heavy mass of pigment of whatever nature.

Scattering accounts for the blue color of a surprisingly wide variety of conditions encountered in medical practice.[10] The blue color of a large superficial subcutaneous vein is perhaps the best-known example. The mass of blood within the lumen of the vein, although dark red in color by reflected light if seen outside of the body (Plate 4), acts as a deep pigment substance to absorb the light reaching it. The light reflected from the tissues overlying the blood mass is scattered in the turbid vein wall and the deep part of the epidermis, to emerge as a blue color (p. 858).

The tattoo artist produces a blue color in the skin by the use of black ink, the degree of blue produced being proportional to the amount of black ink and depth in the dermis at which the needle deposits the particles. The blue color of the skin which results from road accidents in which dark-colored dirt is scraped into the skin and that which results from powder marks from explosion are other examples. A curious type of blue atrophic skin spots is seen in drug addicts who flame the hypodermic needle for sterilization purposes and produce blue tattoo marks by depositing carbon soot particles in the dermis or subcutaneous tissues. At times hypodermic injections of medication do the same thing. Similar spots have been noted from the bites of pubic pediculi.

The blue sclerae associated with fragilitas ossium is explained by the greater transparency of the sclerae in this condition which allows white light to penetrate to the pigmented coat of the eye with resultant absorption there, and greater preponderance in the reflected light of rays scattered in the sclera itself. Greater transparency of the sclerae at birth may account for the tendency to blueness of its color in the newborn. Rarely, individuals are born with their melanocytes located in the deep dermis instead of the lower epidermis over part or even most of their skin. Such persons exhibit a striking blue skin color in

TABLE 54. CLASSIFICATION OF DERMAL PIGMENTATION
(Apparent Blueness: Due to Scattering Phenomenon)

Genetic.....................	Blue nevus
	Mongolian spot (abnormally placed melanocytes in the dermis)
	Nevus of Ota
	Racial (in the eyelids, axillae and nails of certain normal individuals)
	Incontinentia pigmenti
Chemical...................	Mercury (contained in face creams)
	Heavy metal intoxication (silver, bismuth, gold, lead)
	Carbon particles (tattoo, accidental pencil implant, drug addicts)
	Fixed drug eruption
Nutritional.................	Chronic malnutrition (splotchy, slate-gray pigmentation noted in prisoners of war, and experimental human starvation)
Metabolic..................	Hemochromatosis (due to hemosiderin particles in the dermis)
	Ochronosis (polymerized homogentisic acid in the dermis)
Neoplastic.................	Primary melanoma arising from blue nevus and nevus of Ota
	Metastatic malignant melanoma nodule in the dermis
	Malignant melanoma with melanuria and dermal pigmentation
	Pigmented basal-cell carcinoma
	Glomus tumor
	Hemangioma and hemangiosarcoma
	Neurofibromatosis*
Infectious and inflammatory....	Pinta
	Chronic inflammatory dermatoses
	Pediculosis pubis (maculae ceruleae)
Circulatory................	Purpura and hemosiderosis
	Cyanosis
	Methemoglobinemia
	Sulfhemoglobinemia

Classification from Fitzpatrick, Montgomery and Lerner: J. Invest. Dermat. 22:163.
*Presently considered as genetic in origin (see table 52)

such areas. This unusual condition is only of cosmetic importance, since the skin is otherwise normal. A more common variety is the so-called *Mongolian spot,* localized commonly but not exclusively over the sacral area at birth. It is due to a collection of functioning dermal melanocytes in this area which tend to lose their activity as the child develops, with gradual return of normal skin color. The blue phase of pinta has been demonstrated as due to deposition of melanin in the dermis. The blue color of the ears and nose or even the skin in ochronosis is due to pigment deposited in the cartilage of the ear or nose or at times deep in the skin.[9,10] During World War II, use of quinacrine hydrochloride for malaria rarely was noted to produce areas of blue color over the nose, fingernails, palate, etc., apparently the result of deposition of this substance or stimulation of some other pigment deep in the dermis.[15] A syndrome

mimicking ochronosis has been described after prolonged local use of a preparation containing resorcin[84] in treatment of a chronic leg ulcer. The patient had dark urine containing black resorcin polymers.

The blue or purplish color of a deep ecchymosis due to a collection of pigment mass (free blood) in the subcutaneous tissue is another representative example.

The blue color of hematomas and the blue appearance of the umbilicus or of thin abdominal scars when the peritoneal cavity contains free blood are still other examples.

Fitzpatrick, Montgomery and Lerner[55] discuss other disorders which produce a dermal pigmentation capable of producing a blue skin color as a result of the scattering phenomenon. The excellent classification proposed by these authors is given in Table 54.

The bluish discoloration occasionally noted about the eyelids and in the axillae may be due to the fact that these areas in some normal people contain melanin in the dermis as well as the epidermis. The blue sheen of the shaven cheek or axillae of a person with dark hair results from "scattering" because of the darkly pigmented hair shafts in the deep dermis.[5,10] The reader is referred elsewhere[10] for references to the literature on this subject and for a key to available published colored plates. Those not familiar with this form of skin color will profit greatly by a study of such colored illustrations.

MISCELLANEOUS PIGMENTATIONS

There are a few conditions capable of producing abnormal pigments not readily classified in one of the afore-mentioned groups. Most of these are of academic interest and only rarely affect skin color to a degree to be of clinical importance. A few which come to mind are hematin in malaria, methemalbumin, porphyrins, etc. In the group would fall also the skin discolorations produced by the injection or ingestion of colored medicinal or testing substances. These are all self-evident and will not be discussed.

DECREASED SKIN PIGMENTATION

Most commonly, abnormal skin color reflects an increase of normal pigments or the presence of abnormal pigments. However, abnormal skin color at times may result from the diminution of the amount of one or more of the normal pigments or modification of their appearance, by some anatomic or physiologic factor. Such changes may be just as indicative of disease as increase in skin pigmentation and fit usually into one of the following categories.

ANEMIA

The degree of pallor produced by anemia is ordinarily proportional to the loss of hemoglobin. Like any color change produced by hemoglobin, the pallor of anemia is most readily detected in nonmelanized areas (i.e., the lips, the palpebral conjunctivae and the transparent fingernails). Skin color in anemia patients varies for reasons other than diminution of hemoglobin alone. *Hemolytic anemia* may produce a combination of pallor and jaundice as exemplified by the lemon-yellow pallor of severe pernicious anemia. Certain anemias may be associated with the skin deposition of hemosiderin. Vitiligo is not uncommon in anemia. Modern descriptions of hypochromic anemia in adolescent girls no longer include a greenish-yellow pallor. Melanin skin pigmentation occurs in refractory normochromic anemias, some cases of idiopathic microcytic hypochromic anemia and pernicious anemia, as well as certain erythroblastic types of anemia. It may hide skin pallor and be associated at times with a spotty type of melanin pigmentation of the oral mucosa. The yellow pallor of certain hemolytic anemias may be modified by the presence of hemoglobinemia and methemoglobinemia.

DECREASE IN MELANIN PIGMENTATION

The great attention ordinarily paid in clinical practice to increased melanin pigmentation of the skin has overshadowed to a considerable degree the appreciation that there are many biochemical factors which inhibit melanin formation rather than increase it, leading to a decrease in skin pigmentation. Lerner and Fitzpatrick[21] have reviewed the many inhibitors of melanin formation. Most of these are of importance in vitro or in vivo in animals. Some, however, have been shown to be significant as melanin inhibitors in humans, and others appear theoretically possible. The implications of this phase of melanin metabolism have received little attention in regard to its relation to skin color in disease.

Albinism results not as formerly believed from the inherited absence of melanocytes in the skin and the eyes, but rather the inability of the melanocytes to convert tyrosine to melanin, the defect being genetically controlled.[54] Melanocytes are said to be present in albino skin in numbers comparable to normal white skin.[56] There is no lack of the substrate tyrosine. The defect is therefore an inherited enzymatic abnormality. This has been pictorially presented by Fitzpatrick *et al.* (Fig. 218).[68] Albinism can occur in any racial group. The entire skin, eyes and hair of such individuals are completely lacking in melanin. The skin appears pale or a whitish-pink, the hair white and the irides pink in color.

Partial albinism also occurs. It is controlled by a dominant gene, with lack of pigment being limited to part of the skin or hair but with the eyes (as a rule) being normally pigmented.[40] This type can be confused easily with vitiligo. History will usually reveal that in albinism the lesion has been present since birth.

Vitiligo (leukoderma) represents an acquired loss of melanin pigmentation in one or more areas of the skin. It is readily recognized by its patchy distribution and, although extensive at times, almost never covers the entire body. It is more noticeable in persons normally heavily melanized (e.g., Negroes) and at times is readily overlooked in light blonds. Paradoxically, patches of vitiligo not uncommonly coexist in the very skin which shows areas of hyperpigmentation due to systemic disease.

Vitiligo may result from (1) a variety of skin diseases which anatomically involve the melanocytes, (2) systemic disturbances which inhibit melanin formation biochemically and (3) possibly from nervous influence.

A common form of vitiligo occurs in persons otherwise healthy; it appears to be functional in nature, simulating in many ways the pattern of alopecia areata. This type may disappear as readily as it develops or may persist indefinitely; it may change in location with recurrence or recur in identical areas.

Vitiligo occurs not infrequently in *Addison's disease,* depigmentation and pigmentation being intermingled in irregular patches.

Vitiligo is common in *hyperthyroidism* and may be due to increased sympathetic activity in this disease,[10] or to increased conversion of the melanin precursor tyrosine to thyroxine.[21] Areas of vitiligo have been noted in a Negro patient who was being treated with thiouracil.[41] This drug is known to act as an inhibitor of melanin in vitro by combining with the copper of the copper-tyrosinase complex. Thiouracil taken orally resulted in normal urine color in a patient with marked melanuria associated with metastatic melanoma.[42] The reader is referred to the recent review by Lerner[63] for a discussion of mechanisms responsible for vitiligo.

Oliver, Schwartz and Warren[43] have de-

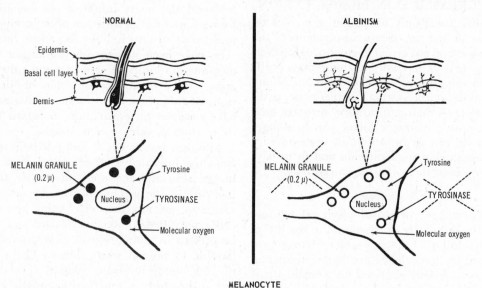

FIG. 218. The Biochemical Lesion in Albinism. Note presence of "amelanated melanin granules" probably due to inability of tyrosinase mechanism. (Fitzpatrick, T. B., Seiji, M., and McGugan, A. D.: Medical Progress: melanin pigmentation, New England J. Med. 265:328; 374 and 430)

scribed an occupational vitiligo in which depigmentation occurred in the areas in contact with rubber-wear containing *p*-benzylhydroquinone. Apparently this substance acts as a melanin inhibitor not only in vitro but also locally by penetration when applied to human skin. The vitiliginous areas usually remelanized slowly with cessation of application of this chemical to the skin. Hydroquinone added to diets of certain experimental animals has produced depigmentation of the hair, with return of hair pigmentation on a normal diet.[44]

Recent studies by Lerner and Fitzpatrick[58] indicate that monobenzyl ether of hydroquinone ointment can be used locally to lighten hyperpigmented skin areas such as freckles, lentigo lesions, melasma of pregnancy, etc. Occasionally, marked contact type dermatitis from this substance has

been reported. This substance can diminish the pigmentation of the normal skin of Negroes as well as hyperpigmentation of skin in whites but does not affect normal white skin color nor the color of the eyes and hair. Applied locally to the skin of a pregnant Negress to produce depigmentation, it caused no change in skin color of her fetus in utero, a point verified at the time of delivery. This substance apparently acts through the ability of hydroquinone to interfere with enzyme reactions. Regeneration of skin color may require two or more months after cessation of its use. Some interesting studies of therapeutic interest with regard to vitiligo have centered on the observation that 8-methoxy-psoralen used locally on vitiliginous skin areas followed by exposure to solar or artificial ultraviolet radiation may occasionally initiate remelanization.[59,60] In practice,

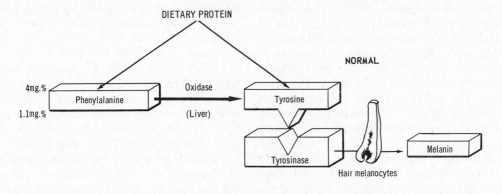

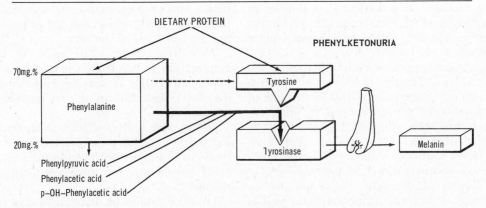

FIG. 219. Pathogenesis of Decreased Melanin Pigmentation in Phenylketonuria. Inhibition of tyrosine-tyrosinase mechanism by phenylalanine and other aromatic metabolites. (Fitzpatrick, T. B., Seiji, M., and McGugan, A. D.: Medical progress: melanin pigmentation, New England J. Med. 265:328; 374 and 430)

local use of the psoralens has been largely discontinued because of the occurrence of marked contact dermatitis, and systemic administration has replaced it.

It is apparent that the function of melanocytes in areas of the normal skin can be inhibited metabolically by one mechanism with the formation of vitiligo while simultaneously those in other areas are stimulated with resultant melanosis.

Generalized Diminution of Melanin Pigment of the Skin. A number of systemic disorders produce a generalized decrease in melanization of the skin which may become clinically recognizable as pallor.

Paleness of the skin is characteristic of the male castrate. This is only in part due to diminished melanization.

Lack or diminution of melanin skin pigmentation has been noted commonly in Simmonds' disease,[34] a disorder attributable to a destructive process of the anterior lobe of the pituitary gland. This clinical finding is of great differential value in distinguishing between true Addison's disease and its simulation by secondary adrenal failure due to hypopituitarism.[10,21,34] Hypothyroidism is characterized by pallor, even in the absence of edema or anemia. There is poor circulation to the skin and decrease in melanization.

Comment has been made that children with the rare disease phenylketonuria have pale or light-colored skin which fails to tan on exposure to sunlight. It is due to an inborn error of metabolism in which the essential amino acid phenylalanine cannot be converted into tyrosine. In vitro, phenylalanine exerts an inhibitory effect on tyrosinase. Dietary restriction of phenylalanine in these cases results in increase of pigmentation toward normal.[68] This concept has been admirably schematized by Fitzpatrick and his associates (Fig. 219). Dietary source of tyrosine alone may not be an adequate source of melanin.[21,54]

Edema of the skin diminishes the intensity of melanin pigmentation as well as the color of hemoglobin.[10]

Negro babies have a rather light skin color at birth and show a progressive degree of melanogenesis until a peak is reached in the sixth to eighth postnatal week.[47]

Depigmentation of many test animals, including cattle, results from the use of copper-deficient diets.[21] The counterpart of this in humans has not been reported but is theoretically possible. As previously mentioned, copper is necessary for the tyrosine-tyrosinase enzyme reaction.[21]

Diets deficient in the filtrate factors of the vitamin-B complex readily produce depigmentation of the hair in many test animals.[21] Gray hair and skin depigmentation have been reported in children on vitamin deficient diets, with return to normal pigmentation after adequate treatment.[45]

A number of studies indicate that the pigmentation of Addison's disease has been markedly diminished in intensity by the administration of ascorbic acid in large doses.[10] Ascorbic acid inhibits melanin formation and may also act to reduce melanin already present in the skin.[21,54]

EDEMA OF THE SKIN

Edema of the skin is associated with pallor. The structural elements of the integument are rendered more distant from each other, separated, as they are, by the fluid. Light penetrating the skin, in its limited path of travel into and out of this structure, thus meets a diminished quantity of pigment. To this effect may be added the changes in the transmissibility of the tissues and perhaps significant reactions of the blood vessels, which may aid in producing the whiteness of the skin.

The characteristic white pallor of edematous skin is best shown in a child with nephrosis. Pallor is striking even though the red blood cell count may be almost normal.

Edema also hides melanin, as shown by the partial loss of pigmentation noted at times in a subject with Addison's disease made edematous by deoxycorticosterone therapy.[10]

Jaundice cannot be detected in skin edematous prior to its onset. Unilateral body edema may occur as a trophic phenomenon in certain types of cerebrovascular disease. If jaundice then occurs in such a person, it may be limited unilaterally to the non-edematous side.[46] This explains the mechanism of unilateral jaundice.

The characteristic white color of an intracutaneous skin wheal is another representative example of the ability of fluid in the skin to give this appearance.

It is evident that edema of the skin may strikingly influence its color. Therefore, one must use caution in evaluating skin color in edematous areas.

DIMINISHED BLOOD FLOW TO THE SKIN

One notes a striking pallor of the skin, if for any reason blood flow to the papillary capillary projections and the superficial subpapillary plexuses is temporarily diminished. This serves to minimize the hemoglobin component of normal skin color. This is seen during syncope, early in Stokes-Adams syndrome, early in arterial emboli or other types of arterial obstruction, in peripheral circulatory collapse, etc.

Some persons (even though their hemoglobin content is normal) appear pale because of the inadequacy of the papillary and subpapillary vascular network or the flow of blood through these areas. That the pallor of the skin of a castrate results in part from such inadequate blood flow has already been discussed.

Inadequate blood flow in the tissues, if persistent, leads to stasis cyanosis, often mottled, so that one notes blotchy blue areas against a pale background. The characteristic ashen-gray color of peripheral circulatory collapse can be attributed to the combination of the pallor of poor capillary circulation of the skin combined with some degree of cyanosis of peripheral stasis origin.

SCAR TISSUE

Scar tissue when new is vascular and pink, when completely formed and healed is avascular and white. The white color is indicative in part of the minimal amount of melanin and hemoglobin pigment which it contains. Its optical characteristics resemble edematous tissue, and it even more strikingly reflects white light—with little differential absorption or reflection of the light rays within the visible spectrum.

MACERATED OR DESQUAMATING SKIN

Areas of the skin with these changes, similar to scar tissue, appear to have less than the normal amount of pigmentation and are white in color.

The coated tongue looks white because the filiform papillae, which have thickened and become opaque, along with debris collected between them, hide the deeper pigments and reflect white light without differential light ray absorption. With desquamation of the white filiform papillae, the mucosa with its prominent capillary projections is exposed and one then sees the red color of a smooth atrophic tongue.

VALUE OF COLORED ILLUSTRATIONS IN MEDICAL EDUCATION

The old proverb that "one picture tells more than a thousand words" is even more true when changed to read "one colored picture, etc." Word descriptions of color of the skin have distinct limitations. Most helpful in teaching students the color appearance of the skin in disease is actual observation of patients. Unfortunately patients suitable for depicting a particular condition may be available only at odd intervals in any given institution. Next most useful would be the use of movies, lantern slides and photographs in color. The great expense entailed in preparing these has limited the number of colored photographs or illustrations published in monographs and medical journals, and those available are widely scattered. There is considerable educational value in systematically studying those available in the literature. For this purpose the reader is referred elsewhere[10] for a guide to many of the colored plates available in the journal literature depicting abnormalities in the color of the skin in disease. Others can be found by perusal of standard texts and systems of medicine.

SUMMARY

Careful inspection of the color of the skin and mucous membranes (plus the use of the spectrophotometer when possible) yields significant information in a large number of disorders.

The normal skin color depends upon various factors, chief among which are: the proportion of the light which is reflected and that which penetrates, and the depth of penetration; the amounts and proportions of the various pigments (melanin, oxyhemoglobin and reduced hemoglobin, carotene); and the phenomenon of scattering.

In health, skin coloration varies greatly between races and greatly among persons of the same race; with age and sex, with tanning from sunlight, with relative vascularity of the skin and vasomotor phenomena (flushing, vasoconstriction, etc.) and in different regions of the body. An understanding of the factors influencing normal skin coloration is necessary to permit interpretation of possible deviations from normal.

Abnormally increased pigmentation can be classified as due to (1) increased yellow components, (2) increased hemoglobin pigment of various types, (3) increased melanin or (4) increased content of metal deposits. Recognition of the specific cause of the abnormal increase may be of great diagnostic value and observation of alterations in the degree of pigmentation may allow deductions concerning the results of tnerapy, the prognosis, etc., in many conditions.

Decreased skin pigmentation occurs in partial or complete albinism, in vitiligo, in anemia, in certain endocrine states, in edema and in skin with diminished blood supply. Proper interpretation of the pathologic physiology resulting in such losses of skin coloration is of great medical importance.

This chapter summarizes present knowledge concerning normal and abnormal skin pigments, methods of recognizing and measuring them, and the mechanisms and significance of abnormalities and alterations in skin coloration.

REFERENCES

1. Sheard, D., and Brown, G. E.: The spectrophotometric analysis of the color of the skin, Arch Int. Med. 38:816, 1926.

2. Sheard, C., and Brunsting, L. A.: Color of skin as analyzed by spectrophotometric methods; I. Apparatus and procedures, J. Clin. Investigaton 7:559-574, 1929.

3. Brunsting, L. A., and Sheard, C.: Color of skin as analyzed by spectrophotometric methods; II. Role of pigmentation, J. Clin. Investigation 7:575-592, 1929.

4. ———: Color of skin as analyzed by spectrophotometric methods; III. Role of superficial blood, J. Clin. Investigation 7:793-813, 1929.

5. Edwards, E. A., and Duntley, S. Q.: Pigments and color of living human skin, Am. J. Anat. 65:1-33, 1939.

6. Edwards, E. A., Hamilton, J. B., Duntley, S. Q., and Hubert, G.: Cutaneous vascular and pigmentary changes in castrate and eunuchoid men, Endocrinology, 28:119-128, 1941.

7. Edwards, E. A., and Duntley, S. Q.: Analysis of skin pigment changes after exposure to sunlight, Science 90:235-237, 1939.

8. ———: Cutaneous vascular changes in women in reference to the menstrual cycle and ovariectomy, Am. J. Obst. & Gynec. 57: 501-509, 1949.

9. Jeghers, H.: Skin color in health and disease, M. Physics 2:984-988, 1950.

10. ———: Pigmentation of the skin, New England J. Med. 231-88-100, 122-136 and 181-189, 1944.

11. Watson, C. J.: Bile pigments, New England J. Med. 227:665 and 705, 1942.

12. Larson, E. A., Evans, G. T., and Watson, C. J.: A study of the serum biliverdin concentration in various types of jaundice, J. Lab. & Clin. Med. 32:481-488, 1947.

13. Meakins, J. C.: Distribution of jaundice in circulatory failure, J. Clin. Investigation 4: 135-148, 1927.

14. Jeghers, H.: Skin changes of nutritional origin, New England J. Med. 228:678 and 714, 1943.

15. Lutterloh, C. H., and Shallenberger, P. L.: Unusual pigmentation developing after prolonged suppressive therapy with quinacrine hydrochloride, Arch. Dermat. & Syph. 53:349, 1946 (see colored plate).

16. Weidman, F. D.: Pathology of yellowing dermatoses; 1. Non-xanthomatous (jaundice, carotinemia, blood pigmentation, melanin, colloid degeneration and elastic degeneration), Arch. Dermat. & Syph. 24: 954, 1931.

17. Montgomery, H.: Cutaneous manifestations of diseases of lipoid metabolism, M. Clin. North America 24:1249, 1940.

18. Comroe, J. H., Jr., and Botelho, S.: Unreliability of cyanosis in recognition of arterial anoxemia, Am. J. M. Sc. 214:1, 1947.

19. Finch, C. A.: Methemoglobinemia and sulfhemoglobinemia, New England J. Med. 239:470, 1948.

20. Becker, S. W., and Obermayer, M. E.: Modern Dermatology and Syphilology, ed. 2, Philadelphia, Lippincott, 1940.

21. Lerner, A. B., and Fitzpatrick, T. B.: Biochemistry of melanin formation, Physiol. Rev. 30:91, 1950.

22. Becker, S. W.: Skin; Melanin pigmentation produced by physical agents, M. Physics 1: 1430-1433, 1944.

23. Fitzpatrick, T. B., Lerner, A. B., Calkins, E., and Summerson, W. H.: Mammalian tryosinase; melanin formation by ultraviolet irradiation, Arch. Dermat. & Syph. 59: 620, 1949.

24. Becker, S. W.: Pigmentary diseases of the skin, Clinics 3:886, 1944.

25. Keys, A.: Caloric undernutrition and starvation, with notes on protein deficiency, J.A.M.A. 138:500, 1948.

26. Burger, G., Sandstead, H., and Drummond, J.: Starvation in western Holland, Lancet 2:282, 1945.

27. Davis, M., Boynton, J., Ferguson, J., and Rothman, S.: Studies on pigmentation of endocrine origin, J. Clin. Endocrinol. 5: 138, 1945.

28. Pack, G. T., and LeFevre, R.: Age and sex distributions and incidence of neoplastic diseases at Memorial Hospital, New York City, with comments on "cancer ages," J. Cancer Res. 14:167, 1930.

29. Hamilton, J. B.: Influence of the endocrine status upon pigmentation in man and in mammals, in The Biology of Melanomas, New York Academy of Sciences, 1948, vol. 4, p. 341.

30. Sprague, R. G., Power, M. H., Mason, H. L., Albert, A., Mathieson, D. R., Hench, P. S., Kendall, E. C., Slocumb, D. H., and Polley, H.: Observations on the physiologic effects of cortisone and ACTH in man, Arch. Int. Med. 85:199, 1950.

31. Calkins, quoted by Lerner and Fitzpatrick, Reference 21.

32. Lea, A. J.: Influence of sodium chloride on the formation of melanin, Nature 155:428, 1945.

33. Sodeman, W. A.: Addison's disease, Am. J. M. Sc. 198:118, 1939.

34. Sheehan, H. L., and Summers, V. K.: The syndrome of hypopituitarism, Quart. J. Med. 18:319, 1949.

35. MacFarlane, E.: The sacral spot in Bengal, Science 95:431, 1942.

36. Monash, S.: Normal pigmentation of oral mucosa, Arch. Dermat. & Syph. 26:139, 1932.

37. Laidlow, G. F., and Cahn, L. R.: Melanoblasts in gum, J. Dent. Research 12:534, 1932.

38. Monash, S.: Normal pigmentation in nails of Negro, Arch. Dermat. & Syph. 25:876, 1932.

39. Schwartz, S. O., and Blumenthal, S. A.: Exogenous hemochromatosis resulting from blood transfusions, Blood 3:617, 1948.

40. Macklin, M. T.: Genetic aspects of pigment cell growth in man, in The Biology of Melanomas, New York Academy of Sciences, 1948, vol. 4, p. 144.

41. Hellerstein, H. K., quoted by Lerner and Fitzpatrick, Reference 21.

42. White, A. G.: Effect of tyrosine, tryptophane and thiouracil on melanuria, J. Lab. & Clin. Med. 32 (pt. 2) :1254, 1947.

43. Oliver, E. A., Schwartz, L., and Warren, L. H.: Occupational leukoderma, Arch. Dermat. & Syph. 42:993, 1940.

44. Martin, G. J., and Ansbacker, S.: Confirmatory evidence of the chromotrichial activity of p-aminobenzoic acid, J. Biol. Chem. 138: 441, 1941.

45. Gillman, T., and Gillman, J.: Powdered stomach in the treatment of fatty liver and other manifestations of infantile pellagra, Arch. Int. Med. 76:63, 1945.

46. Page, I. H.: Ipsolateral edema and contralateral jaundice associated with hemiplegia and cardiac decompensation, Am. J. M. Sc. 177:273, 1929.

47. Zimmerman, A. A., and Cornbleet, T.: The development of epidermal pigmentation in the Negro fetus, J. Invest. Derm. 11:383, 1948.

48. Jeghers, H., McKusick, V. A., and Katz, K. H.: Generalized intestinal polyposis and melanin spots of the oral mucosa, lips and digits, New England J. Med. 241:993 and 1031, 1949.

49. Hall, T. C., McCracken, B. H., and Thorn, G. W.: Skin pigmentation in relation to adrenal cortical function, J. Clin. Endocrinol. 13:243, 1953.

50. Gordon, M.: Pigment Cell Growth: Proceedings of the Third Conference on the Biology of Normal and Atypical Pigment Cell Growth, New York, Acad. Press, 1953.

51. Fitzpatrick, T. B., and Lerner, A. B.: Terminology of pigment cells, Science 117:640, 1953.

52. Gates, R. R., and Zimmerman, A. A.: Comparison of skin color with melanin content, J. Invest. Dermat. 21:339, 1953.

53. Shizume, K., and Lerner, A. B.: Determination of melanocyte stimulating hormone in urine and blood, J. Clin. Endocrinol. 14: 1491, 1954.

54. Fitzpatrick, T. B., and Lerner, A. B.: Biochemical basis of human melanin pigmentation, A.M.A. Arch. Dermat. & Syph. 69: 133, 1954.

55. Fitzpatrick, T. B., Montgomery, H., and Lerner, A. B.: Pathogenesis of generalized dermal pigmentation secondary to malignant melanoma and melanuria, J. Invest. Dermat. 22:163, 1954.

56. Becker, S. W., Jr., Fitzpatrick, T. B., and Montgomery, H.: Human melanogenesis: Cytology of human pigment cells, A.M.A. Arch. Dermat. & Syph. 65:511, 1952.

57. Kenney, J. A., Jr.: Skin pigmentation: A review of recent advances in knowledge and therapy, J. Nat. M. A. 45:106, 1953.

58. Lerner, A. B., and Fitzpatrick, T. B.: Treatment of melanin hyperpigmentation, J.A.M.A. 152:577, 1953.

59. Lerner, A. B., Denton, C. R., and Fitzpatrick, T. B.: Clinical and experimental studies with 8-methoxypsoralen in vitiligo, J. Invest. Dermat. 20:299, 1953.

60. Kanof, N. B.: Melanin formation in vitiliginous skin under the influence of external applications of 8-methoxypsoralen, J. Invest. Dermat. 24:5, 1955.

61. Lerner, A. B., Shizume, K., and Bunding, I.: The mechanism of endocrine control of melanin pigmentation, J. Clin. Endocrinol. 14:1463, 1954.

62. Lorincz, A. L.: Pigmentation, Chapter 22, pages 515-563, in Rothman, S.: Physiology and Biochemistry of the Skin, Chicago, Univ. Chicago Press, 1954.

63. Lerner, A. B.: Melanin pigmentation, Am. J. Med. 19:902, 1955.

64. Buckley, W. R. and Grum, F.: Reflection spectrophotometry: Use in evaluation of skin pigmentary disturbances, Arch. Dermat. 83:249, 1961.

65. ———: Reflection spectrophotometry: II Effect of quinacrine on skin color, Arch. Dermat. 83:249-261, 1961.

66. Fitzpatrick, T. B., Brunet, P., and Kukita, A.: The nature of hair pigment in The Biology of Hair Growth, New York Academic Press, 1958.

67. Reich, P., Schwachman, H. and Craig, J. M.: Lycopenemia: A variant of caro-tenemia, New England J. Med. 262:263, 1960.

68. Fitzpatrick, T. B., Seiji, M. and McGugan, A. D.: Medical progress: Melanin pigmentation, New England J. Med. 265:328, 374 and 430, 1961.

69. Lerner, A. B. and McGuire, J. S.: Effect of alpha- and beta-melanocyte stimulating hormones on the skin color of man, Nature 189:176, 1961.

70. Szabo, G.: Quantitative histological investigation on melanocyte system of human epidermis, pp. 44-125, in Gordon, M., ed. Pigment Cell Biology, New York, Academic Press, 1959.

71. Birbeck, M. S. C., Breathnach, A. S., and Everall, J. D.: An electronmicroscope study of basal melanocytes and high level clear cells (Langerhans cells) in vitiligo, J. Invest. Dermat. 37:51, 1961.

72. Cowan, A.: Ocular pigment and pigmentation; 18th annual de Shweinitz lecture, A.M.A. Arch. Ophth. 55:161-173, 1956.

73. Beerman, H., and Colburn, H. L.: Some aspects of pigmentation of the skin, Am. J. Med. Sci. 231:451-475, April 1956.

74. Deutsch, S., and Mescon, H.: Melanin pigmentation and its endocrine control. New England J. M. 257:222-226, Aug. 1957; 268-272, Aug. 1957.

75. Lerner, A. B.: Hormonal control of pigmentation, Ann. Rev. Med. 11:187-194, 1960.

76. Lerner, A. B., and McGuire, J. S.: Effect of alpha- and beta-melanocyte stimulating hormones on the skin color of man, Nature 189:176-179, 1961.

77. ———: Melanocyte-stimulating hormone and adrenocorticotrophic hormone: their relationship to pigmentation, New Eng. J. Med. 270:539-546, 1964.

78. Buckley, W. R., and Grum, F.: Reflection spectrophotometry. III. Absorptioñ characteristics and color of human skin, Arch. Derm. 89:110-116, 1964.

79. Abrahamson, I. A., and Abrahamson, I. A.: Hypercarotenemia, Arch. Derm. 68:4-7, 1962.

80. Findlay, G. H.: Cutaneous vasoconstrictors, primary pigmentation and the grey-blue reaction, Brit. J. Derm. 73:238-243, 1961.

81. Pathak, M. A., Riley, F. C., and Fitzpatrick, T. B.: Melanogenesis in human skin following exposure to long-wave ultraviolet and visible light, J. Invest. Derm. 39:435-443, 1962.

82. Monash, S.: Immediate pigmentation in sunlight and artificial light, Arch. Derm. 87:686-690, 1963.

83. Tuffanelli, D., Abraham, R. K., and Dubois, E.: Pigmentation from antimalarial ther-

apy: its possible relationship to the ocular lesions, A.M.A. Arch. Derm. 88:419-426, 1963.

84. Thomas, A. E., and Gisburn, A.: Exogenous ochronosis and myxedema from resorcinal, Brit. J. Derm. 73:378-381, 1961.

85. Sternberg, T. H. and Bierman, S. M.: Unique syndromes involving the skin in-

duced by drugs, food additives and environmental contaminants, Arch. Derm. 88:779-788, 1963.

86. Madison, J. F.: Tetracycline pigmentation of teeth, Arch. Derm. 88:58-59, 1963.

87. Esoda, E. C. J.: Chloasma from progestational oral contraceptives, Arch. Derm. 87:486, 1963.

35

Itching (Pruritus)

Stephen Rothman and Arthur L. Shapiro

MECHANISM OF ITCHING

Two hundred years ago, itching (pruritus) was defined as "an unpleasant cutaneous sensation which provokes the desire to scratch," and this simple definition is still the best. The sensation arises in free nerve endings of richly ramifying axons in the epidermis or in the corresponding epithelial layer of the transitional mucous membranes. Itching cannot be elicited from skin areas denuded of their epidermis. The whole tegument is able to receive impulses that lead to the perception of itching. There is an increased responsiveness in the mucocutaneous junctions of the anus, the external auditory canals and the nostrils.

Stimulation of the nerve endings is brought about by chemical, mechanical, thermic and electric stimuli acting from the outside as well as from the inside. If the stimulus, in addition to its effect on the nerve endings, simultaneously also acts irritatingly on epidermal cells or capillary vessel walls, an inflammatory lesion develops. At the site of this lesion, after subsidence of the itching, an increased itching

excitability persists for many hours or even days, regardless of whether or not the anatomic lesion has subsided. In this state of increased excitability, the threshold for adequate stimuli is lowered and the responses are exaggerated. Furthermore, inadequate stimuli, such as light touch, light strokes, pressure, release of pressure, and temperature stimuli elicit intense itching sensations. For example, the spot of a long-forgotten insect bite starts to itch again when it is lightly rubbed or pressed upon or exposed to sudden temperature changes. This state of itching hyperexcitability was interpreted recently by Graham et al. as being caused by a barrage of noxious impulses from the site of injury producing a segmental excitatory state in the cord.

If this re-awakening of the itching sensation recurs several times in the same spot and is responded to by vigorous scratching, the itching excitability rapidly increases, and soon a vicious cycle develops consisting of increasingly violent scratching and increasingly intense itching. This development is greatly facilitated and seriously aggravated by a proliferative reaction

900

of the epidermis in response to repeated mechanical stimulation. The classical form of this reactive epidermal thickening is called "lichenification" (Fig. 220), and is dealt with in the paragraph on sequelae to scratching. In pathologic conditions, the itching-scratching cycle becomes a tormenting affair. It may last many hours, and the scratch paroxysm may cease only because of total somatic and psychic exhaustion of the patient.

In understanding the mechanism of itching certain fairly well-established conceptions are useful. The nerve endings mediating the pruritic sensation are made more sensitive by *increased capillary dilatation*. Heat thus increases the symptom, while cold and vasoconstriction diminish it. Epinephrine and ephedrine tend to diminish pruritus through their vasoconstrictive action. In many inflammatory skin lesions the sensibility of the itching nerve endings is heightened mainly because of hyperemia, and if such lesions are stimulated either chemically by pathologic metabolic products or mechanically, itching and the itching-scratching cycle arise with particular ease. On the other hand, any measure which decreases arterial hyperemia and the other signs of acute inflammation is likely to decrease the sensation of pruritus which has originated with the inflammatory process. Thus, corticotropin and adrenal corticoids, the latter in systemic as well as local application, often have a dramatic antipruritic effect, merely by virtue of their anti-inflammatory action. *Tissue anoxia* due to venous stasis results in itching and is relieved when the blood flow becomes adequate (tight clothing, venous varicosities). Ultraviolet irradiation, x-rays or local anesthetics by their direct action on the nerve endings may temporarily decrease their sensitivity sufficiently long to interrupt the itching-scratching cycle and stop the excessive peripheral stimulation.

Itching hyperexcitability may be elicited, not only by peripheral mechanisms, but also centrally. The perception of itching has an *integrating center* in the hypothalamus and the excitability of this center can be influenced pharmacologically. The

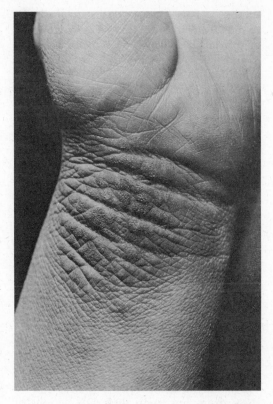

Fig. 220. Lichenification in neurodermatitis.

subcortical center is under a higher control in the cortex. In animal experiments, scratch movements become greatly enhanced after bilateral ablation of the frontal cortex. Psychogenic pruritus occurs in man and will be discussed later.

The foregoing considerations indicate that two factors determine whether or not in a given pathologic process itching is produced: the intensity and the quality of the itching stimulus and the itching excitability which under pathologic conditions may be greatly enhanced by either peripheral or central influences.

Thomas Lewis and his associates advanced the theory that itching is always brought about by the release of histamine or a histamine-like substance, whatever the primary—physical or chemical—stimulus may be. According to this theory, itching and urticarial reaction ("triple response") are co-ordinated phenomena both produced by mediation of released "H-substance." This theory seems to be well founded when it is applied to itching in anaphylactic and allergic skin reactions. It cannot be accepted, however, as an explanation for pruritus without visible gross or microscopic changes as in pregnancy, diabetes, diseases of the liver and lymphoblastomas, for in concentrations that evoke itching, histamine also causes visible changes.

The heuristic theory of Lewis has been quite spectacularly confirmed by the advent of *antihistaminic drugs*. These drugs exert a hitherto unparalleled symptomatic effect on urticarial itching eruptions. However, in conformity with what has been said in the previous paragraph, low dosages of antihistaminics first relieve pruritus, while urticaria still remains. Also, the symptomatic effect of these drugs is constant and reliable only when itching is based upon liberation of histamine. The antipruritic effect of antihistaminics which occasionally occurs in other conditions (i.e., neurodermatitis, pruritus ani, etc.) is not based upon the antihistaminic potentialities of these drugs but upon their side actions of general sedation or local analgesia.

Shelley and Arthur have reported that certain proteolytic enzymes, the endopeptidases, are uniquely effective chemical stimuli for the production of pruritus in man. They have postulated that release or activation of proteases in the epidermis plays a significant role in the pathomechanism of itching. They maintain that the action of proteolytic enzymes is independent of histamine release.

ANALYSIS OF ITCHING AS A SYMPTOM

Diagnostic Evaluation of Itching

Whether or not a cutaneous disorder elicits itching depends more on the nature of the etiologic agent than on the nature of the morphologic elements. For this reason the value of the itching symptom in determination of etiology is considerable, particularly in the differential diagnosis of morphologically similar eruptions. For example, there is a vast variety of cutaneous manifestations of syphilis, cutaneous tuberculosis and leprosy, but none evokes itching. The fact that syphilids do not cause any subjective symptom is particularly of great diagnostic value, because syphilis, the "great imitator," produces in its secondary period not only the roseola, which closely resembles toxic drug eruptions, but also lichenoid, psoriasiform, varioliform, etc., eruptions and in its tertiary period chronic granulomatous lesions that are similar to itching lymphoblastomas. In addition to chronic infectious granulomas, the large groups of nevi and benign and malignant neoplasms of the skin also can be ruled out when itching is present.

Of course, for diagnostic evaluation, the presence or the absence of the itching sensation must be established beyond doubt. This is easy when scratch marks are present. But such marks are sometimes hard to differentiate from spontaneous lesions, and they are by no means always present in itching conditions. Thus, one must largely depend on the patient's statements, which are not necessarily reliable. A patient sometimes will complain of itching, although the lesion is asymptomatic, because when a lesion is elevated or has an uneven rough surface the patient often palpates that lesion, strokes it, or scratches it, and such mechanical irritation elicits a "minimal pruritus" in the nonitching lesion as well as in normal skin. Some patients will deliberately deny the itching, mainly because they feel that they have been "guilty" in scratching. Most commonly, however, the complaint of itching is exaggerated rather than understated.

To have a clear picture, it is never sufficient simply to ask the patient whether he itches or not. One also must ask the following questions: (1) Are you disturbed in your sleep by itching at night and do you wake up finding yourself scratching? (2) Can you forget about your itching in the daytime when your attention is distracted? (3) Can you stop scratching easily when you make up your mind to do so? (4) Does itching arise only in certain situations, such as warm environment, cold weather, undressing, rubbing of a piece of clothing at that spot, etc.?

We may classify the disorder as an obligate itching condition only if it definitely disturbs the patient's sleep. Otherwise the itching is a more or less accidental symptom of minor diagnostic value, because most of the inflammatory cutaneous lesions may itch occasionally as a result of increased hyperexcitability of the nerve endings. When this is the case, the patient will answer our Question 1 with "No"; Questions 2 to 4 with "Yes."

It often has been claimed that more pronounced itching at night is characteristic of one or the other skin disease, particularly of scabies. However, this is not so. The intensifying of itching at night is a common feature of all conditions with obligate itching. This is partly due to the warming of the skin in bed, partly to the absence of the distractive perceptions of daytime activities. In addition, there seems to be a daily periodicity in the tonus of cutaneous capillaries, possibly in association with the daily periodicity of body temperature changes. A maximum of capillary dilatation seems to occur in the early evening hours when the body temperature is highest. This is assumed because the daily exacerbation of itching frequently starts a few hours before the patient goes to bed, and because increased blood flow to the skin intensifies itching excitability.

In any case, for diagnostic purposes it is essential to know whether or not pruritus awakens the patient at night, in order to separate obligate and facultative itching conditions.

On this basis the following classification can be made:*

Obligate itching disorders:

1. Pediculosis, scabies and related mite infestations, insect bites and other external injuries resulting in urticarial wheals
2. Contact dermatitis (both primarily toxic and allergic), caused by exposure to chemical or physical agents
3. Urticaria and toxic eruptions
4. Neurodermatitis, prurigo, strophulus (miliaria)
5. Pruritus due to pregnancy, liver dis-

---

* Rare cutaneous disorders such as prurigo nodularis, urticaria pigmentosa, etc., are not included.

eases, lymphoblastoma, malignant internal neoplasms, kidney insufficiency
6. Dermatitis herpetiformis
7. Lichen planus

Facultative itching disorders (with great variety in intensity, largely depending upon the degree of inflammation):

1. Asteatosis (xerosis, dry skin)
2. Pruritus due to diabetes
3. Psoriasis
4. Seborrheic dermatitis
5. Pityriasis rosea
6. Skin infections due to pyogenic organisms and fungi
7. Local anoxia due to varicose veins, tight clothing, etc.
8. Mechanical irritation

Nonitching disorders:

1. Developmental anomalies
2. Atrophies, degenerations and hyperplasias
3. Benign neoplasms
4. Malignant neoplasms
5. Dermotropic virus infections
6. Chronic infections granulomas (tuberculosis, syphilis, etc.)
7. Lupus erythematodes
8. Pigmentary anomalies
9. Trophic and deficiency diseases
10. Diseases of sweat glands, sebaceous glands, hair follicles and nails

DIAGNOSTIC VALUE OF SCRATCH MARKS AND THEIR SEQUELAE

Proper analysis of the complaint of itching often involves observation of the presence or the absence of scratch marks and skin changes secondary to scratching. The motor response to itching in man is carried out in different ways, namely, by scratching with the free ends of the fingernails, by rubbing with the fingertips or with the nail plates of the fingers, by rubbing one extremity with the other, by kneading movements, by pinching and sometimes by simple pressure.

Excoriations, either punctiform or linear bloody crusts, result only from scratching with the sharp edges of the nail, and it is a notorious fact that in a great number of itching conditions such marks are not found. They are not present, or only ex-

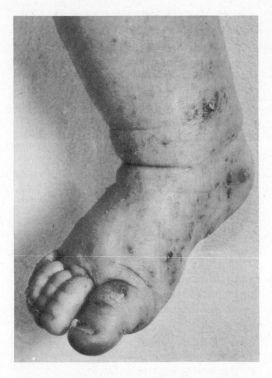

Fig. 221. Scabies. Torn-off burrows on medial aspect of heel.

ceptionally, in urticarial eruptions, whether of external or internal origin, nor are they found in lichen planus, and sometimes they are conspicuously absent in lichenified lesions of neurodermatitis. The nails of the neurodermatitis patient are often shiny, smooth and polished as though they had been cared for by careful manicuring, and this indirect sign bears witness that the patient is suffering from one of the most tormenting itching skin diseases. The patient does not "scratch"; he merely "rubs" and polishes his nails on his own skin. The eyebrows are often rubbed off, so that only a few sparse hairs remain.

In lichen planus the disproportion between severe complaints of itching and almost complete absence of scratch marks is rather characteristic. This is mentioned in order to demonstrate that the scratching technic is obviously different in different diseases.

A special technic is exerted in "prurigo of Hebra" and related conditions. The small elevated itching papules are torn off in their entirety as soon as they are formed, and only a flat bloody crust is

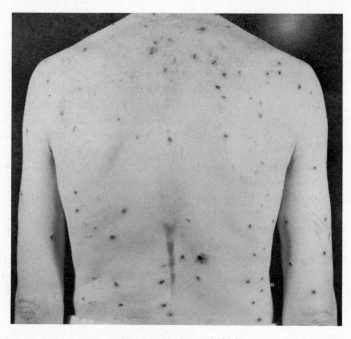

Fig. 222. Neurotic excoriations.

FIG. 223. Eczema due to pollen. It is difficult to decide whether the punctiform lesions are dried crusts of broken vesicles or scratch marks.

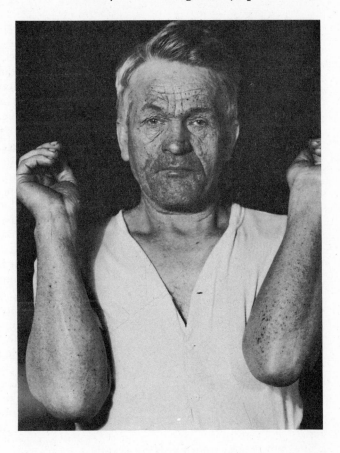

FIG. 223. Eczema due to pollen. It is difficult to decide whether the punctiform lesions are dried crusts of broken vesicles or scratch marks.

left. In scabies, too, entire lesions are torn off—vesicles, papules and burrows, together with the sarcoptes and the ova in them (Fig. 221).

In neurotic excoriations the flat (normal) skin surface is torn off by digging or picking movements, again leaving a bloody crust (Fig. 222). Depending upon the depth of injury a pitting scar may or may not result. Usually, after the crust

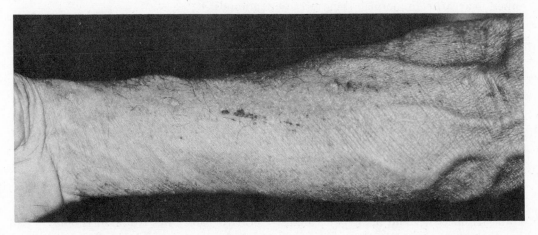

FIG. 224. Linear scratch marks and epidermal thickening in chronic dermatitis.

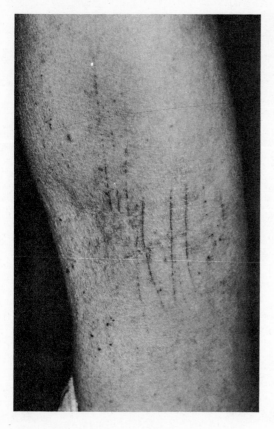

Fig. 225. Linear scratch marks in flexural neurodermatitis.

secondary to the scratch excoriations, often occur in the form of pustules, impetigo, furuncles, lymphangitis, cellulitis, erysipelas and acute suppurative lymphadenitis. Staphylococcic infections of the hair follicles are particularly common in pruritus due to diabetes and in exfoliative dermatitis due to arsenical poisoning.

Correct recognition of scratch marks has diagnostic significance, not only because they are objective signs of itching and scratching, but also because of their characteristic localization they may lead to a final diagnosis, For instance, linear scratch marks on the nape of the neck and on the upper back often lead to the discovery of head-lice infestation that otherwise would remain undetected. Scabies sometimes can be diagnosed only by the localization of scratch marks in cases where most burrows are torn off or removed by scrubbing in the bath tub.

A common sequela of scratching in chronic itching conditions is the gradual enlargement of subcutaneous lymph nodes. Such "buboes," histologically displaying only chronic inflammatory changes, may develop insidiously, mainly in the groin and in the axillae without any clinically manifest acute pyogenic infection. The enlarged glands are hard and indolent. The lymph node enlargement is often a source of diagnostic errors, when one endeavors to differentiate Hodgkin's disease or other lymphoblastomas from chronic dry neurodermatitis or prurigo on purely clinical grounds.

Another common consequence of chronic scratching is lichenification which is represented by deepening of the normal skin lines with formation of infiltrated, slightly elevated, shiny rhomboidal fields in between the lines (Fig. 220). In its classical form lichenification occurs only in dry diffuse neurodermatitis, and in circumscribed neurodermatitis, also called lichen simplex chronicus of Vidal. But similar changes, also due to epidermal thickening, are seen in chronic allergic eczema, particularly in industrial cases, in prurigo and in lymphoblastomas. Although there is no doubt that lichenifica-

has fallen off, a hyperpigmented spot remains for several weeks.

Punctiform scratch marks, with the tiny crusts at about equal distance from each other, may arise in normal skin, because scratching first causes a pilomotor reaction (prepapular phase of Jacquet) and continued scratching leads to the excoriation of the slightly elevated follicular surfaces.

It is often difficult to differentiate punctiform scratch marks from dried tiny hemorrhagic vessicles (Fig. 223).

Long linear scratch marks (Figs. 224 and 225) often parallel because of simultaneous use of several nails, indicating uninhibited scratching, are mainly seen in pediculosis, scabies, pruritus due to pregnancy, lymphoblastomas, liver diseases, kidney insufficiency and malignant tumors. In all these conditions pyogenic infections,

tion arises from mechanical irritation, it cannot be produced experimentally, at will, by scratching. Its development requires a certain predisposition. The great readiness to develop lichenification in response to mechanical irritation is one of the most outstanding features of neurodermatitis.

Scratching or stroking, not severe enough to damage the skin, evokes a localized vascular response. Linear mechanical stimuli of low intensity produce a white line (dermographia alba) due to constriction of the superficial cutaneous capillary vessels. Stronger stimuli elicit vasodilatation manifested by a red line (dermographia rubra). In individuals who are hypersensitive to mechanical stimuli wheal formation may follow scratching; this is known as *factitial urticaria*. In such individuals one can "write" protruding letters on the skin and therefore the condition is also called *dermographia elevata* (Fig. 226). Whereas white and red dermographism are physiologic vascular reactions, factitial urticaria is a pathologic state. It has an allergic mechanism proved by the fact that the urticarial sensitivity to mechanical stimuli can be transferred passively with the patient's serum to normal persons. Antihistaminic drugs influence favorably both the itching and whealing in this condition.

GENERALIZED PRURITUS

Pruritus Due to Tissue Anoxia

This type of pruritus has not yet been explored experimentally, and the knowledge about it is based purely on clinical observations.

Venous stasis may lead to itching in the stasic area when the superficial cutaneous veins are involved and the blood flow to the skin is slowed. The classical example is pruritus as a prominent part of the symptom complex associated with venous varicosities. It is true that the pruritus does not parallel the severity of the varicose condition. Still, there can be little doubt that the itching is of circulatory origin, because it is relieved after successful treatment of the varicosities. We have often observed prompt and complete disappearance of itching after application of a well-fitting zinc-gelatin boot. Also, it is obvious that such itching originates directly from stasis and not by interposition of inflammatory processes (stasic dermatitis), because itching is felt in areas that do not display signs of inflammation either grossly or microscopically.

Itching due to stasis usually does not reach exasperating intensities. It is felt most intensely when the stockings are removed or, to a lesser degree, when they are put on. In daytime it may be completely forgotten, and usually it does not disturb the patient at night. In contrast with this relatively mild degree of itching, scratching is wild and often done with the nails, so that excoriations result. If the condition persists for several months, diffuse thickening of the epidermis develops in consequence of chronic scratching.

For symptomatic relief of itching in stasis, local applications of ichthyol pastes and ointments are used in mild cases; tar preparations are usually effective in more severe cases. These work by relieving the inflammation and diminishing the sensitivity of the nerve endings. The most effective therapy, of course, is the correction of the stasis.

It seems that even physiologically the

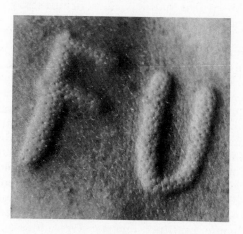

Fig. 226. Factitial urticaria or dermographia elevata. The letters were produced by mild stroking of the skin.

relatively slow circulation in the lower extremities, particularly in the region of the shin bone, increases the itching susceptibility. In nonitching or moderately itching eruptions, such as psoriasis or lichen planus, lesions of the legs always itch more intensely and are scratched more than anywhere else. It is the habit of many people whose skin is perfectly normal to scratch their shins when they undress or go to bed. One of the writers, in a study on senile skin changes, once examined the inmates of an old-age asylum, all over 70, asking them as to whether or not they scratch their skin, and, if so, where. Of the 80, 45 volunteered the answer that "it feels good to scratch the shins in the evening."

This observation leads to the difficult problem of the existence of "senile pruritus." Obviously, senile degeneration and atrophy of the skin is not prurigenic, because pruritus is completely absent in cases of far-progressed senile cutaneous changes, and many cases of exasperating pruritus that are labeled as senile pruritus do not display such changes. Nevertheless, some authors claim that the administration of male sex hormone preparations is valuable in so-called *senile pruritus*. It is possible that peripheral arteriosclerosis of the cutaneous vessels with consequent local anoxemia increases itching hyperexcitability and thus drives the patient into a vicious itching-scratching cycle, but such a mechanism has never been proved. One must think of such a possibility when there are definite signs of peripheral arteriosclerosis and when the pruritus has developed gradually. However, in most cases that are diagnosed as "senile pruritus," the pruritus has nothing to do with senility. An old man or woman may itch from the same causes as do younger patients, but these causes are less thoroughly investigated in the case of old people because of the belief that there exists an idiopathic senile pruritus. One of the writers has seen examples of so-called "senile pruritus" due to: (1) kidney insufficiency with high nonprotein nitrogen values; (2) carcinoma of the stomach, and (3) drugs. One should be particularly skeptical about accepting the diagnosis of senile pruritus when there has been a sudden onset of intense generalized itching.

PRURITUS DUE TO ASTEATOSIS

There is a harmony in the sensory status of the normal skin (the so-called "eudermie" of Jacquet), in which the weak physiologic impulses arising from sensory stimuli of everyday life, such as slight rubbing, slight changes in temperature and pressure, scarcely enter the consciousness and do not cause any discomfort. For the maintenance of this harmonious condition in man, a greasy cover is required on the skin surface. This cover is supplied by the sebaceous glands on most parts of the body and by lipids of scales on the palms and the soles. *Decrease in sebaceous gland activity* leads to a disturbance of the sensory status with decreased itching thresholds, i.e., by increased itching susceptibility. Physiologically, the amount of oily secretion is a function of the atmospheric temperature. It decreases with decreasing temperature, and at from 10° to 15° C. is only one-half as much as it is at 25° C. This effect of cold is the cause of *pruritus hiemalis,* popularly known as "winter itch." Of course, "dryness" of the skin—or in scientific terms "asteatosis" or "xerosis," meaning lack of grease on the surface — does not occur only in cold weather. Many people in moderate climates have dry skin throughout the year. The efficiency of sebaceous-gland function depends upon a great number of internal and external factors. The main internal factor is the inherited constitution of the integument, and a great influence on the sebaceous gland function is exerted by the *glands of internal secretion.* Hypogonadism is often accompanied by skin dryness, as is hypopituitarism. Some authors believe that hypothyroidism is a cause of asteatosis although itching is not characteristic of myxedema. External factors, in addition to atmospheric temperature, are moisture of the air and the use of *water and soap* with great variations of the latter's influence according to the temperature of the water, duration of the contact with water, quality of soap, technic of washing (rubbing, scrubbing, tub bath, shower bath), etc.

The asteatotic skin feels "dry" and rough on palpation and displays fine adherent scales on the surface. The characteristic sign is a superficial cracking of the horny layer in the form of a network of fine pink lines usually in a square or a rhomboidal pattern. It is more pronounced on the extensor surfaces of the extremities, particularly on the legs, than elsewhere. Secondary to the dryness, a mild inflammatory reaction may develop in the form of nonsharply limited erythematous isolated patches. The itching caused by asteatosis is usually moderate, appears in spells, particularly upon undressing and when the skin is exposed to abrupt changes of the external temperature. It usually does not awaken the patient, but often makes it difficult for him to fall asleep.

The nondermatologist practitioner, unfortunately, is not at all familiar with the extremely common picture of asteatosis. He may recognize the condition if there is real "chappiness" with deep rhagades, but this form, mainly occurring on the hands, is not the one that elicits pruritus.

In practice, asteatosis sometimes is mistaken for ichthyosis (which does not itch), or in other cases a desperate search is made for systemic causes of pruritus, and when no cause can be found, the case is often labeled as "senile pruritus" if the patient is over 40. It is highly desirable that asteatosis become better known in general practice because the correct diagnosis implies prompt and often dramatic relief by simple therapeutic procedures: restrictions in the use of water and soap, and massage of an indifferent lubricant into the skin. In our experience, ointment bases containing cholesterol or its derivatives, such as anhydrous lanolin or Aqua-

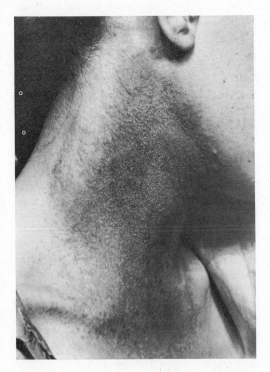

FIG. 227. Eczematous type of allergic reaction with intra-epidermal vesicle formation. The allergen in this case was resorcinol.

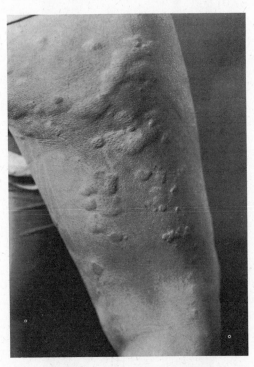

FIG. 228. Urticarial type of allergic reaction. This reaction is most commonly seen in hypersensitivity to drugs and foods.

phor, are greatly superior to any other lubricant in substituting for the natural greasy cover of the skin.

ITCHING AS AN ALLERGIC MANIFESTATION

There are two types of hypersensitivity reactions of the skin, both associated with considerable itching. One is the eczematous type in which the reaction between allergen and the (hypothetical) antibody takes place in the *epidermis cells;* its typical clinical lesion is the intraepidermal vesicle (Fig. 227). The other is the urticarial type in which the hypersensitivity reaction occurs in the *vessel walls of the dermis,* probably in the endothelial cells; its typical clinical lesion is the urticarial wheal (Fig. 228) or, in the case of lower intensities, the erythematous macule (Fig. 229). Roughly, it is correct that allergens acting from the outside are more likely to lead to eczematous reactions ("contact dermatitis") and allergens reaching the skin via the blood stream provoke erythematous-urticarial eruptions ("toxic erythema," "toxic eruption"). However, this is not a rule without exceptions. Drugs, such as quinine and organic arsenicals, administered internally may lead to eczematiform reactions if allergy develops, and insect bites or sunshine cause urticarial wheals by acting from the outside.

In this connection it should be pointed out that in cutaneous allergic reactions it is not the visible lesion that "causes" itching; this is obvious from the fact that both eczematous vesicles and urticarial wheals often are preceded by itching and both last longer than the itching does. What happens is that by the allergic tissue reaction irritating substances are formed which cause two independent phenomena: (1) the anatomic (inflammatory) lesion provoked by cell injury and (2) the itching, provoked by stimulation of sensory nerve endings. In allergic reactions based on histamine liberation, both phenomena are present, although the eruptions may be preceded by itching for several hours. This is the case, for instance, in serum sickness and in urticarial eruptions due to food or drug allergy. In the eczematous type of hypersensitivity, however, it may occur that in low concentrations the irritating substance stimulates the itching nerve endings without causing cellular damage that would lead to visible changes.

Itching and itching eruptions due to allergens acting from the outside (leaves

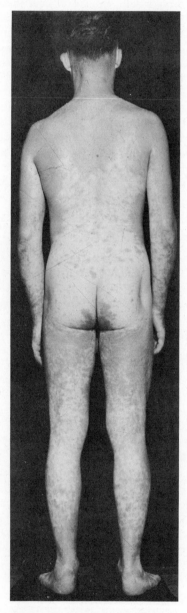

FIG. 229. Macular erythematous eruption caused by hypersensitivity to dilantin.

and flowers of plants, animal hair, an immense number of chemicals and physical agents, such as heat, cold and light, etc.) are most intense on the uncovered parts of the body, and such regional distribution always arouses suspicion of a contact dermatitis (Fig. 223). If the allergen acts from the inside, the pruritus and pruritic eruption are either generalized or at least widely disseminated and, in most cases, symmetrically distributed.

Pruritus of Psychogenic Origin

There is an itching of purely psychic origin. Merely imagining the presence of biting insects may provoke itching and scratching in centrally hyperceptive individuals. The intensity of peripherally induced itching always depends upon the central excitability. Thus it often happens that itch stimuli, for instance, a rough woolen garment, do not cause discomfort to some and cause intolerable itching to others. On the other hand, pruritus simply due to morbid imagination must be a rare condition, as it is not encountered in true psychoses such as schizophrenia, manic-depressive insanity or in compulsion hysteria.

Parasitophobia, a condition in which the patient tries to convince the physician that parasites are crawling on his skin, showing him small scales and dust particles, is always a sign of a severe psychosis, but it does not represent an itching disorder. The patient's complaint is not at all focused on itching; he does not claim to be compelled to scratch; his imagination is completely centered on the presence of crawling parasites.

Similarly, in **neurotic excoriations**, a common syndrome in psychoneurotic individuals, the patients hardly complain of itching. They claim that lesions like acne papules or pustules erupt on their skin; they readily admit that they feel a compulsion to "pick" on these lesions, and that it is not intolerable itching that compels them to do so (Fig. 222).

The psychogenic factor, however, plays a tremendous role in the development of an itching-scratching cycle. Patients suffering from neurodermatitis, most of them psychically unstable individuals, become most easily victims of such a cycle. But the development of the cycle also depends upon the degree of the increased itching susceptibility in the periphery, and if that is high, as it is for instance in Hodgkin's disease, persons with absolutely normal psyche will not be able to avoid the cycle.

In generalized pruritus which lasts more than a few days, one must be extremely cautious when diagnosing "nervous itching." Many cases of severe internal diseases, of scabies and pediculosis and of asteatosis remain undetected because the physician, dealing with a "nervous person," thinks too readily that he has found the answer to itching in this "nervousness." Paradoxically enough, in localized itching, pruritus ani and pruritus vulvae, the psychogenic origin is more common or the psychogenic factor more important than in generalized pruritus.

Emotional urticaria, also called cholinergic urticaria, is the only itching disease the psychosomatic mechanism of which is relatively well understood. Patients suffering from this disease are, overwhelmingly, young females who break out with generalized urticaria when they get excited. They respond with urticaria to external application of heat as well as to emotional stimuli because they are *allergic to acetylcholine* which is released in the skin in response to either emotional or heat stimuli. To local application of acetylcholine these patients display a local triple response, as though from histamine, and they break out with generalized urticaria on systemic administration of acetylcholine. When heat is applied locally, the released acetylcholine reaches the central nervous system via the blood stream and elicits there a widespread nervous impulse leading again to release of acetylcholine at the nerve endings, causing generalized urticaria. This disease represents one of the rare cases of allergy to a physiologic metabolic product.

Pruritus Due to Pregnancy

Frequently pregnant women suffer from intense generalized pruritus during the last month of pregnancy. This pruritus is often misdiagnosed as scabies and is made considerably worse by antiscabetic treatment. In the appearance of the skin there is some superficial similarity to scabies and pediculosis because of the numerous linear and punctiform scratch marks. The frequently present diffuse but uneven pigmentation (in addition to the usual pigmentation of pregnancy) and superficial pyogenic lesions constitute a picture resembling "vagabonds' disease." This diagnostic error, however, is by no means unavoidable, because the diagnosis of scabies should, whenever possible, be based on the demonstration of clinically typical burrows in typical locations and preferably upon microscopic demonstration of the animal organisms.

The pruritus due to pregnancy is characterized by rather sudden onset and early generalization, by exasperating intense itching sensation day and night and by sudden disappearance of the itching within the first few days after delivery. Characteristically, it is a disease of the last month of pregnancy, but occasionally it may start at any time during the last trimester. It is a pruritus appearing without accompanying cutaneous changes of the skin. The visible changes are secondary and are due to scratching, rubbing and consecutive secondary infection. It is seen in entirely normal pregnancies in which no other signs of "toxemia" are found and in which the fetus is entirely normal. That this pruritus is caused by the pregnancy itself, probably by *metabolic products of the fetus* that are foreign to the maternal organism is evidenced by its sudden disappearance after the baby is born and by its stereotype repetition in following pregnancies. As a matter of fact, if once a mother has been afflicted by pruritus due to pregnancy, it is highly probable that the same condition will occur in all following pregnancies.

For symptomatic relief of pruritus in pregnancy, generalized ultraviolet irradiations with suberythematous doses are the method of choice. Their effect is often dramatic. The patient who spent a number of sleepless nights and is completely exhausted somatically and psychically will have a satisfactory night's sleep after the first irradiation. This immediate effect can almost be regarded as having diagnostic value because no other condition responds so promptly. The usual external applications for symptomatic relief of itching, such as calamine lotion, calamine liniment, mentholated alcohol (0.25 per cent), etc., have only limited value.

In addition to the pure form of pruritus gravidarum, toxic eruptions, mainly of the erythematous and urticarial type, may appear in the last month of pregnancy and cause considerable itching. These eruptions also end abruptly after delivery, and there is little doubt that they have the same pathomechanism as has simple pruritus, in originating from metabolic products of the fetus. In urticarial eruptions, the symptomatic effect of ultraviolet light is considerably less than in simple pruritus.

A less common form of itching in pregnancy is that associated with the eruption called *herpes gestationis*. The clinical picture of this eruption is identical with that of dermatitis herpetiformis or Duhring's disease, but it is different by being clearly connected with the state of pregnancy. It appears at any time during the second half of pregnancy, disappears within a few weeks postpartum, recurs in subsequent pregnancies, but never recurs outside of the periods of gestation. The eruption is often preceded by pruritus without visible changes and only after several days do the first signs, erythematous patches, urticarial lesions and finally the characteristic grouped vesicles and bullae appear. A characteristic sign is eosinophilia in the blood and in the blisters. The itching becomes as intolerable as it is in pruritus gravidarum. The disease is generally considered "toxic." However, this toxic state obviously must be different and more serious than that in pruritus gravidarum, because miscarriages or early death of the infant often have been reported. However, the prognosis for the mother is good. Herpes gestationis is not associated with eclampsia and never changes into pemphigus. It is not to be confused with impetigo herpetiformis, a rare lethal disease of pregnancy, the eruption of which does not itch.

DIABETIC PRURITUS

There is no simple relationship between the degree of diabetes and the symptom of itching. On the contrary, it is conspicuous that patients with mild diabetes, and particularly in the incipient phase, suffer more commonly from pruritus than those with severe forms of diabetes. Pruritus may be the very first subjective symptom of the disease, and this initial pruritus will often subside in spite of the fact that the diabetes remains uncontrolled or even turns worse. Two patients under observation may have the same level of blood sugar, identical tolerance curves, identical sugar excretion in the urine, and still one patient will suffer from intolerable pruritus, while the other will not itch at all. Different degrees of acidosis do not explain this situation, because diabetic acidosis does not cause itching. The concentration of glucose in the skin (or in the epidermis) also is irrelevant; glucose when injected into the skin in high concentrations does not cause itching. Yet, there is no doubt that there is a "diabetic pruritus" in which diabetes is the causative agent, for this pruritus disappears promptly when adequate treatment is initiated, and reappears following dietary indiscretions or if the treatment becomes inadequate.

The relationship of pruritus and diabetes is complicated because diabetes provokes itching by causing dryness of the skin, and the tendency to develop this dryness shows great individual constitutional (possibly familial) variations. It also depends on the bathing habits of the patients and other external factors. It has been demonstrated that both water evaporation from the skin surface and sebaceous secretion are decreased in diabetes. Decrease of sebaceous gland secretion greatly increases itching susceptibility. As a matter of fact, diabetic pruritus can often be well controlled by treatment of the asteatosis only, with lubricants and by restriction of the use of water and soap, without controlling the diabetes.

How diabetes causes asteatosis is not understood, and no data are available as to the variations of asteatosis with varying degrees of the metabolic disturbance. However, clinical experience shows that poorly controlled diabetes causes dehydration and that the skin may become quite dry and seems to be much less oily than normal.

It is remarkable that in juvenile diabetes, itching is uncommon, an observation which can be associated with the fact that asteatosis is rarely seen in the age group of from 8 to 24 years.

Clinically, a patient who seeks the physician's advice for generalized pruritus will be particularly suspect of the presence of diabetes when his skin displays clinical signs of asteatosis, when the intensity of itching shows seemingly unexplained variations (probably dependent on atmospheric temperature and use of soap and water), and when scratching leads to pyogenic infections, particularly of the follicles, with a readiness that is far above the average. Otherwise the scratch marks in diabetes are not conspicuous. There might be none or a few punctiform hemorrhagic crusts. Linear scratch marks are infrequently seen. There is no particular predilectional localization of the itching, except that pruritus vulvae is apparently much more common in diabetic than in nondiabetic women.

Textbooks often enumerate diabetes among the causes of pruritus ani. The authors have not yet seen or heard of a case in which localized pruritus ani was proved to be due to diabetes. In cases of pruritus vulvae in diabetic women, the external genitalia and the vagina should be examined for monilia infection. This infection may cause pruritus vulvae.

The extended cutaneous monilia infection of intertriginous areas, involving axillae, submammary folds, umbilical fold, groin and intergluteal folds in fat women is almost pathognomonic for diabetes. Clinically the lesions are characterized by sharply limited, bright-red moist surfaces with overhanging scales on the edges and with irregularly arranged satellite pustules in the neighborhood. This infection causes intense itching. Diagnosis is made by microscopic and cultural demonstration of monilia.

Pruritus, Liver Disease and Jaundice

Itching is present in about 20 to 25 per cent of jaundiced patients. That disturbance in liver function is one of the causes of generalized pruritus is satisfactorily evidenced by the sudden disappearance of exasperating itching after cholecystectomy or operations for malignancy, after subsidence of hepatitis, etc., and by recurrence of itching with relapse of the morbid process.

A review of the literature and of 64 consecutive cases of jaundice observed in Albert Merritt Billings Hospital of the University of Chicago reveals that the presence or the absence of itching cannot be predicted from any of the standard laboratory examinations (icterus index, van den Bergh, blood serum cholesterol level, galactose tolerance). Likewise, analyzing our material, we found no correlation between pruritus and the mechanism by which the jaundice arose. Table 55 shows that pruritus occurs in jaundice of any sort, independent of whether it is due to malignancy, common duct stone or stricture, drugs or infection. However,

Table 55. Jaundice and Pruritus

Etiology	Cases	Pruritus Present	Per Cent
Neoplasm	9	3	33
Common duct obstruction other than neoplasm (stone, stricture, congenital malformation)	9	3	33
Infectious hepatitis	29	4	14
Drug poisoning (arsenic, T.N.T., cincophen)	9	4	44
Syphilis (hepatic)	1	0	0
Cirrhosis (hepatic)	1	0	0
Causes unknown	6	3	50
Total	64	17	26.5

the table also shows, as far as one can draw conclusions from the relatively small number of cases, that pruritus is more frequent in icterus secondary to neoplasm, common duct stone and stricture (33 per cent) and to toxic liver damage due to drugs (44 per cent) than in infectious hepatitis (14 per cent). This is true even though detailed analyses reveal that the icterus index may be considerably higher in some of the nonitching patients with hepatitis than in some of the severely itching patients with, for instance, a stricture of the common duct.

Pruritus is obviously not dependent upon the depth of the discoloration, i.e., on the concentration of bile pigment in the skin. A patient with severe icterus may have no itching, whereas a patient with a mild degree of icterus, even though due to the same etiologic factor, may have severe itching. It is true that in the individual case the pruritus disappears as the jaundice decreases and, contrariwise, the itching may become more severe as the icterus deepens. However, itching also may come and go while the jaundice persists, and itching often precedes and disappears earlier than the clinical jaundice. Finally, itching also occurs in liver diseases unaccompanied by icterus. Thus it is obvious that accumulation of bile pigment in the skin is not the cause of pruritus in liver disease.

When jaundice and pruritus coexist there are evidently chemical changes that either stimulate the nerve endings directly or alter the sensitivity of the nerve endings to external stimuli. It is not known what effect, if any, the altered blood chemistry has upon the itching center in the hypothalamus. Increase in bile acids has been advanced as the chemical change in the blood causing pruritus. This assumption has been substantiated by the studies of R. L. Varco who found that the pruritus due to chronic hepatic disease disappeared rapidly if external biliary drainage was established, but that itching recurred following oral administration of small quantities of bile salts.

Recently, a number of investigators have

demonstrated that pruritus associated with primary biliary cirrhosis or incomplete biliary obstruction is relieved by oral administration of a basic anion exchange resin. This bile acid-sequestering resin causes increased fecal excretion of the bile acids and results in lowered serum bile acid concentration.[3,6]

Hepatogenic pruritus is in most cases generalized. In spite of extreme intensities of itching visible scratch marks and eczematization are rarely seen. Associated with itching in jaundice one occasionally sees erythematous spots and urticaria. Elevated dermographism (factitial urticaria) is common and the elevated stripes are noticeably darker than the surrounding skin in the icteric patient. It was reported that arsphenamine icterus itches only exceptionally. In our series 1 out of 3 cases of

arsphenamine icterus was accompanied by itching.

Symptomatic relief of pruritus associated with jaundice is obtained by ultraviolet irradiations with suberythematous doses or, even more dramatically, by soft x-ray irradiations with small doses (30 to 80 roentgens). Such therapy apparently operates to produce a relative anesthesia of the nerve endings. Biliary drainage as suggested by Varco may be a justifiable surgical procedure in severe, chronic cases.

Pruritus Due to Lymphoblastoma

This group includes myeloid and lymphatic leukemia, lymphosarcoma, mycosis fungoides and Hodgkin's disease.

In all these conditions the first subjective symptom of the disease frequently is generalized pruritus, which reason alone

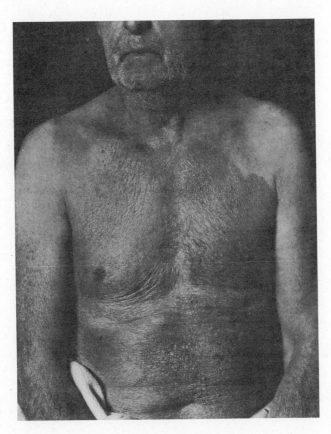

Fig. 230. Mycosis fungoides. Intensely pruritic arciform erythematous premycotic lesion.

prompts the patient to seek medical aid. This initial pruritus without visible lesions is extremely rare in myeloid leukemia, not uncommon in lymphosarcoma and in lymphatic leukemia, and extremely frequent in mycosis fungoides and in Hodgkin's disease (approximately 25 per cent of cases).

Common in all these conditions is the frequent development of exfoliative dermatitis (generalized "erythroderma") with exasperating itching. The clinical picture is characterized by diffuse generalized erythema and lamellous scaling. Histologically, one may find all transitions between the common signs of inflammation and highly specific cellular infiltrates. Similar transitions between "toxic" and "specific" tissue changes are also seen in those non-generalized, disseminated, circumscribed, inflammatory lesions that usually precede the tumor formation, more often in mycosis fungoides and in Hodgkin's disease than in leukemia. These lesions may be simply erythematous patches (Fig. 230), or urticarial, vesicular, bullous or purpuric in nature. Sometimes there may be oozing and crusting lesions, or they may simulate other dermatoses such as prurigo (Fig. 231), lichen planus, psoriasis and parapsoriasis. All these eruptions are primarily "toxic" without characteristic cellular elements, but they may later develop specific infiltrates.

Mycosis fungoides presents particularly polymorphous eruptions in the so-called premycotic stage. The single lesions are always sharply limited, and bizarre configurations, such as circinate, arciform or arabesquelike forms are frequently seen. As long as the cutaneous infiltration of these lesions is slight, the clinical diagnosis is difficult. It is usually the exasperating itching (remaining completely uninfluenced by the usual procedures for symptomatic relief) that first awakens the suspicion that the eruption, which may simulate psoriasis or some other common dermatosis, is mycosis fungoides or one of the other lymphoblastomas. In this early phase the diagnosis must be made by microscopic examination of a skin biopsy specimen. Later on, however, when the cutaneous infiltration is easily palpable, the clinical picture becomes more characteristic. It is a rule that plaques with definite dermal

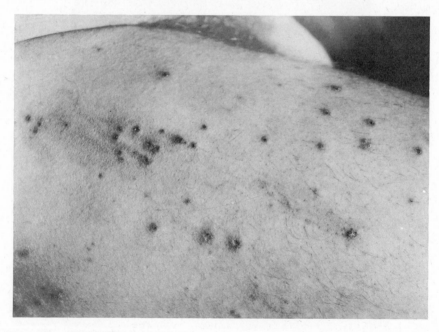

Fig. 231. Prurigolike eruption in lymphosarcoma. In contrast with prurigo neurotic excoriations, the edges of the lesions are infiltrated.

infiltration which itch intensely are manifestations of some kind of lymphoblastoma. In this situation, the symptom of itching is of paramount significance in the differentiation of lymphoblastoma from other cutaneous infiltrates, such as occur in syphilis, tuberculosis, leprosy and deep mycotic infections, which do not itch.

In sharp contrast with premycotic lesions, the fully developed tumors of mycosis fungoides (tomatolike reddish-brown growth with rapidly developing crateriform ulcerations on the top (Fig. 232) are not pruritic at all; neither are the cutaneous tumors in lymphatic leukemia. In Hodgkin's disease, however, all cutaneous manifestations, the diffuse infiltrative plaques as well as the nodular lesions, are equally accompanied by tormenting itching.

Cutaneous manifestations of myelogenous leukemia are rarely seen. However, in a few cases, violently itching nodular cutaneous infiltrates have been reported as due to this blood dyscrasia.

Symptomatic relief of itching in cutaneous manifestations of lympoblastomata can be achieved by x-ray therapy, nitrogen mustard, corticotropin and adrenal steroids. All these measures act indirectly by reducing the infiltrate of the primary process.

PRURITUS DUE TO INTERNAL MALIGNANT TUMORS

Little attention has been paid to the generalized pruritus that is caused by the presence of internal malignant tumors. In the American literature this syndrome was first discussed by Becker, Kahn and Rothman in 1942. The etiologic role of the tumor in pruritus was manifested in several cases by the disappearance of the itching after removal of the tumor and its recurrence with the reappearance of the tumor. The following unpublished case is reported as an illustration.

A 70-year old machinist was admitted to the Dermatology Clinic of Albert Merritt Billings Hospital on February 23, with the complaint of severe generalized itching of 6 months' duration. Physical examinaton revealed dry, scaling skin with senile atrophic changes, diffuse hyperpigmentation and numerous scratch marks. The patient was obviously in great distress because of the itching, and his family reported that for several months he spent his nights scratching and was unable to sleep. Attempts to relieve the pruritus by symptomatic treatment with routine external applications and sedatives failed completely.

Laboratory examinations revealed normocytic anemia, and 4-plus benzidin reaction in the

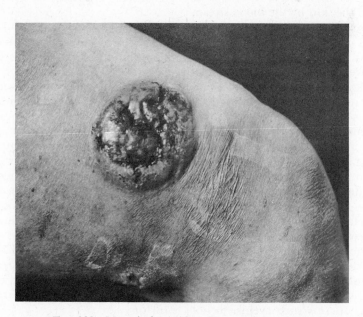

FIG. 232. Mycosis fungoides. Nonpruritic tumor.

stool. X-ray examination of the stomach showed a carcinoma of the lesser curvature near the antrum.

Subtotal gastrectomy was performed on April 9. On the second day after operation, the patient gratefully volunteered that his itching had completely disappeared. His postoperative course was uneventful. He remained under observation until September.

In malignancy, as in lymphoblastomas, the simple generalized pruritus often represents only the introductory phase to the outbreak of itching eruptions which may be prurigolike or toxic in nature. The latter eruptions may simulate erythema multiforme, dermatitis herpetiformis, acute lupus erythematodes and may develop into exfoliative dermatitis. In most of these eruptions, as well as in simple pruritus, a great tendency to early intense diffuse hyperpigmentation is noted. This is more marked in internal malignancy than in Hodgkin's disease.

Pruritus and inflammatory eruptions have been interpreted as being due to toxic substances formed by the tumor cells, or by their decomposition products circulating in the blood stream. However, some of the itching eruptions were interpreted as being not of toxic but of metastatic origin. It was assumed that single tumor cells transported to the skin by the blood stream are decomposed in the skin with accompanying local inflammation. Evidence of such a process was seen in cases in which metastases developed from primarily itching papular lesions. Thus the analogy to pruritus and to itching eruptions in lymphoblastoma is close, in so far as no sharp line can be drawn between "toxic" and "metastatic" manifestations. True final neoplastic metastases of malignant tumors of the skin do not itch, even as no itching accompanies the indolent "tumors" of mycosis fungoides and of lymphatic leukemia. One may conclude that in these conditions, as long as there is vigorous defense in the skin against the elements of foreign growth, the cellular decomposition is sufficiently massive to result in the production of toxic substances causing itching and inflammatory reactions, whereas such events do not occur when the growth becomes uninhib-

ited. Hodgkin's disease is a remarkable exception in so far as its cutaneous tumors, as well as its toxic manifestations, itch.

Pruritus due to internal malignant tumors seems to be rare. Over a period of seventeen years only 10 cases were reported. But there is no doubt that the number of cases would greatly and suddenly increase if more attention were paid to the syndrome by general practitioners and surgeons. Pruritus apparently may occur as a consequence of any kind of malignant tumor of any localization, mostly as a late manifestation and usually after considerable necrosis of the tumor cells has occurred. It was often reported as a terminal symptom. However, the case quoted above, among others, demonstrates that pruritus may be an early symptom and as such may have diagnostic significance. Simple pruritus with hyperpigmentation occurs more frequently with carcinomas of the gastrointestinal tract than with growths in other locations. Itching eruptions were described also in cancers of the breast, of the bronchi, of the pancreas, the uterus, the tongue and also in cases of sarcoma of the thyroid gland. In many of these cases evidence was presented for the causal connection between tumor and itching eruption.

PRURITUS IN KIDNEY INSUFFICIENCY

Pruritus in kidney insufficiency is due to the retention of nitrogenous substances in the blood. This conclusion is drawn from the fact that itching is observed only in those cases of kidney damage in which the nonprotein nitrogen of the blood is elevated. Itching is never observed in nephritis or nephrosis unaccompanied by retention of waste products. It is not known which of the retained nitrogenous compounds is responsible for the itching. It is claimed that urea does not irritate the cutaneous sensory nerve endings of the skin if injected intradermally. A priori, one would assume that uric acid is more likely to be the itch-provoking agent. Reliable investigations, however, have not been made to clarify the mechanism of uremic pruritus.

Itching in uremia is generalized and is

usually associated with a dirty yellowish-brown discoloration of the skin. Scratch marks are seen in abundance in the more severe degrees of itching. The intensity of the pruritus, however, is not proportionate to the severity of the uremia.

LOCALIZED PRURITUS

Pruritus Ani

In the discussion of pruritus ani, textbooks list a considerable number of causative factors: proctitis and colitis, high alkaline pH in the rectum and the colon, intestinal parasites, hemorrhoids, allergy to or primary irritative effect of food, antibiotics and other drugs taken orally, allergy to fecal material, fungus infection or allergic "-id" reactions to distant foci, diabetes, intestinal neoplasm and so forth. In practice, however, while such causes are occasionally found, in the majority of cases of chronic pruritus ani, which is mainly a disease of adults, none of these factors can be demonstrated.

In about 50 per cent of the cases of pruritus ani there is an association with neurodermatitis ("atopic eczema"). Patients with a neurodermatitis constitution have a great tendency to lichenification of the skin in response to scratching or to other forms of mechanical irritation. Neurodermatitis is often associated with eosinophilia, and a familial or individual association with asthma or hay fever ("atopy") may be present, but the cutaneous manifestation never has been proved to be due to an allergic mechanism. Since these patients are high strung and emotionally unstable, sedative therapy is important.

In addition to patients with neurodermatitis, "idiopathic" pruritus ani may arise also in individuals of an emotionally well-balanced personality with no functional disorders. In such cases the pruritus may start with an accidental mechanical irritation of the anus during the wiping action following a bowel movement or with irritation by hard stool particles. This irritation may be maintained by the rubbing of the anus with toilet paper during cleansing and finally may drive the patient into a vicious cycle of itching and scratching.

An auxiliary factor is venous stasis in the external hemorrhoidal ring of veins, but hemorrhoids otherwise play no part in the causation of itching. Disordered intestinal function, either constipation or diarrhea, and spasm of the anal sphincter are further auxiliary factors. Therefore, great emphasis has to be put on the regulation of bowel movements in the management of pruritus ani.

Physiologically, the anus and the perineum display a great readiness to itching as the itching nerve endings are particularly numerous in this region (Fig. 233). An area of increased itching sensitivity may, therefore, easily be set up here in response to scratching.

Discussion of the alleged relation of pruritus ani to suppressed emotions, particularly to psychogenic disturbances in the sexual sphere, as it has been interpreted by psychoanalysts, is beyond the scope of this paper. In some instances manipulation of the genital, the perineal and the rectal areas might be an indication of unsatisfied sexual desire. In these cases psychiatric study may prove advisable. However, it should be emphasized that in pruritus ani highly satisfactory therapeutic results can usually be obtained with only mild sedatives and local measures directed toward elimination of external irritation.

The authors are unable to confirm the numerous statements in the literature that pruritus ani is often the manifestation of a systemic organic disease. Pruritus, when due to a systemic disease, is practically always generalized.

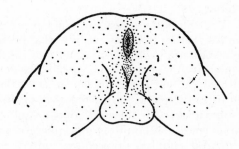

Fig. 233. Relative density of itching points in the male anogenital region. (Longo: Arch. de fisiol. 36:197)

PRURITUS VULVAE

Pruritus vulvae is most commonly functional in origin and is then frequently found in patients with neurodermatitis or in patients who display a similar syndrome of nervous exhaustion and emotional instability. Treatment in these cases is symptomatic and emphasis is laid upon sedation.

However, local irritation as the cause of pruritus vulvae also must be investigated. Such irritating factors are: vaginal discharge of any kind; glycosuria in diabetes (by the easy fermentation of urine droplets retained on the genitals); trichomonas vaginalis infection, etc. Monilial infection of the external genitalia is common with or without diabetes and may cause intolerable itching.

Lichen sclerosus et atrophicus, a patchy degenerative and atrophizing process, when occurring on the vulva, may cause marked pruritus, particularly in children. In the latter, pinworm infestations or gonorrheic vulvovaginitis also may cause vulvar pruritus.

When vulvar pruritus occurs during or after the menopause, it is frequently assumed that the itching is due to estrogen deficiency. As a matter of fact, replacement therapy with natural or synthetic estrogenic substances sometimes causes rapid disappearance of itching. However, the direct relationship of pruritus to the menopause never has been proved experimentally, and strict criticism must be used in evaluating the results of estrogenic replacement therapy, because pruritus vulvae is frequently purely functional, very commonly so in the menopause, and the psychic suggestion connected with the treatment cannot be excluded.

The clinical appearance of pruritus vulvae varies from no visible change to eczematization with excoriations and thickening of the epithelium up to classical lichenification. Kraurosis vulvae is similar in its initial phase. Neglected cases of pruritus vulvae with lichenification are often misdiagnosed as kraurosis and unnecessarily extended surgical procedures are performed. One should keep in mind that in its initial phase kraurosis vulvae can only be diagnosed by histologic examination. It becomes clinically recognizable only in its atrophic phase. Also, one should remember that pruritus vulvae with lichenification is an extremely common ailment, whereas kraurosis vulvae is a rare disorder. Early microscopic diagnosis is the clue to rational therapy.

Psoriasis of the genital and anal area is highly pruritic and is manifested by sharply circumscribed, red, shiny plaques without scaling. Its diagnosis is difficult unless typical psoriatic lesions are found elsewhere.

Despite the close proximity of the vulva and the anus, itching of both areas is not usually concomitant. Both pruritus vulvae and ani have the tendency to spread to the perineum, but not further. When pruritus ani and vulvae coexist, the clinical response to treatment is usually different. Pruritus ani tends to disappear sooner, and relapse of vulvar pruritus is more common.

OTHER FORMS OF LOCALIZED PRURITUS

Localized pruritus of the external auditory canal and of the eyelids is almost exclusively a partial symptom of neurodermatitis. Occasionally itching of the ear canals is caused by fungous infection or by the irritation from a chronic discharge due to otitis media.

Localized pruritus of the nostrils is common in children suffering from intestinal parasites. The same localization of pruritus has been reported as a symptom of tumor of the brain with increased intracranial pressure. This is a remarkable localization in view of the results of animal experiments in which the nostrils were found to be sites of predilection for itching of central origin.

SUMMARY

A detailed history is needed for evaluation of the severity of itching and of its diagnostic significance. It is helpful to differentiate obligate and facultative itching conditions. Punctiform and linear scratch marks and other sequelae of scratching, such as pyogenic infections, thickening of the epithelium, lichenification and chronic lymph node enlargement, are present in some itching disorders, but may be completely absent in others.

The nature of the immediate stimulus to the nerve endings is unknown in pruritus due to pregnancy, diabetes, lymphoblastomas, internal malignancies and kidney insufficiency. In all these conditions the degree of the pruritus does not parallel the severity of the disease. In diabetes, asteatosis of the skin is an important auxiliary factor. According to recent data, accumulation of bile acids is responsible for the pruritus in liver diseases and in obstructive disorders of the biliary tract, often associated with jaundice.

In the itching cutaneous lesions of lymphoblastomas and internal malignancies no sharp line can be drawn between "toxic" and "metastatic" manifestations. Apparently the products of tumor cells, either blood-borne or locally released in the skin, may cause pruritus. "Tumors" of leukemia, mycosis fungoides and the malignant metastases do not itch, whereas the nodular lesions of Hodgkin's disease are intensely pruritic.

Psychogenic factors are important in many forms of pruritus, especially in pruritus ani and pruritus vulvae and in so-called neurodermatitis.

REFERENCES

1. Becker, S. W., and Obermayer, M. E.: Modern Dermatology and Syphilology, ed. 2, Philadelphia, Lippincott, 1947.

2. Becker, S. W., Kahn, D., and Rothman, S.: Cutaneous manifestations of internal malignant tumors, Arch. Dermat. & Syph. 45: 1069-1080, 1942.

3. Carey, J. B., and Williams, G.: Therapy for pruritus of jaundice, J.A.M.A. 176:432-435, 1961.

4. Dunbar, H. F.: Emotions and Bodily Changes, New York, Columbia, 1946.

5. Graham, D. T., Goodell, H., and Wolff, H. G.: Neural mechanisms involved in itch, "itchy skin" and tickle sensations, J. Clin. Invest. 30:37-49, 1951.

6. Hashim, S. A., and Van Itallie, T. B.: Use of bile acid sequestrant in treatment of pruritus associated with biliary cirrhosis, J. Invest. Dermat. 35:253-254, 1960.

7. Jacquet, L.: Troubles de la sensibilite, *in* Besnier, Brocq and Jacquet's La Pratique Dermatologique, vol. 4, p. 330, Paris, Masson, 1904.

8. Lewis, T.: Clinical Science, Illustrated by Personal Experiences, London, Shaw, 1934.

9. Rothman, S.: Physiology and Biochemistry of the Skin, pp. 120-152, Chicago, Univ. Chicago, 1954.

10. Shapiro, A. L., and Rothman, S.: Pruritus ani, a clinical study, Gastroenterology 5: 155-168, 1945.

11. Shelley, W. B. and Arthur, R. P.: Neurohistology and neurophysiology of itch sensation in man, Arch. Dermat. 76:296-323, 1957.

12. ————: The peripheral mechanism of itch in man, Ciba Foundation Study Group, Pain and Itch, Boston, Little, Brown, 1959.

13. Varco, R. L.: Intermittent external biliary drainage for relief of pruritus in certain chronic disorders of the liver, Surgery 21: 43-45, 1947.

Index